a LANGE medical book

CURRENT
Diagnosis & Treatment
Nephrology & Hypertension

Edited by

Edgar V. Lerma, MD
Clinical Associate Professor of Medicine
Section of Nephrology
Department of Internal Medicine
University of Illinois at Chicago College
of Medicine/Associates in Nephrology, SC
Chicago, Illinois

Jeffrey S. Berns, MD
Professor of Medicine and Pediatrics
University of Pennsylvania School of Medicine
Renal-Electrolyte and Hypertension Division
Philadelphia, Pennsylvania

Allen R. Nissenson, MD
Emeritus Professor of Medicine
David Geffen School of Medicine at UCLA
Los Angeles, California
Chief Medical Officer
DaVita Inc.
El Segundo, California

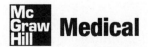

New York   Chicago   San Francisco   Lisbon   London   Madrid   Mexico City
Milan   New Delhi   San Juan   Seoul   Singapore   Sydney   Toronto

Current Diagnosis & Treatment: Nephrology & Hypertension

2 3 4 5 6 7 8 9 0 WFR/WFR 14 13 12 11 10

ISBN 978-0-07-144787-4
MHID 0-07-144787-3
ISSN 1943-832X

Notice

Medicine is an ever-changing science. As new research and clinical experience broaden our knowledge, changes in treatment and drug therapy are required. The authors and the publisher of this work have checked with sources believed to be reliable in their efforts to provide information that is complete and generally in accord with the standards accepted at the time of publication. However, in view of the possibility of human error or changes in medical sciences, neither the authors nor the publisher nor any other party who has been involved in the preparation or publication of this work warrants that the information contained herein is in every respect accurate or complete, and they disclaim all responsibility for any errors or omissions or for the results obtained from use of the information contained in this work. Readers are encouraged to confirm the information contained herein with other sources. For example and in particular, readers are advised to check the product information sheet included in the package of each drug they plan to administer to be certain that the information contained in this work is accurate and that changes have not been made in the recommended dose or in the contraindications for administration. This recommendation is of particular importance in connection with new or infrequently used drugs.

This book was set in Minion by Aptara®, Inc.
The editors were James Shanahan and Harriet Lebowitz.
The production supervisor was Catherine Saggese.
Project management was provided by Satvinder Kaur, Aptara, Inc.
The cover designer was Mary McKeon.
The book designer was Alan Barnett Design.
Worldcolor/Fairfield was printer and binder.

Cover photos: Background: Polycystic disease. Credit: Chris Bjornberg/Photo Researchers, Inc. Right: Kidney, scan. Credit: James Cavallini/Photo Researchers, Inc. Top left: Pulmonary hypertension, angiography. Credit: James Cavallini/Photo Researchers, Inc. Bottom: Credit: Samuel Ashfield/Photo Researchers, Inc.

This book is printed on acid-free paper.

International Edition: ISBN 978-0-07-128742-5; MHID 0-07-128742-6
Copyright © 2009. Exclusive rights by The McGraw-Hill Companies, Inc., for manufacture and export. This book cannot be re-exported from the country to which it is consigned by McGraw-Hill. The International Edition is not available in North America.

Contents

Authors   vii
Preface   xiii

1. Approach to the Patient with Renal Disease   1

Edgar V. Lerma, MD

I. Fluid & Electrolyte Disorders

2. Disorders of Extracellular Volume: Hypovolemia & Hypervolemia   7

David H. Ellison, MD

3. Disorders of Water Balance: Hyponatremia & Hypernatremia   22

Clancy Howard, MD, & Tomas Berl, MD

4. Disorders of Potassium Balance: Hypokalemia & Hyperkalemia   32

Michael Emmett, MD, & Michael R. Wiederkehr, MD

5. Acid–Base Disorders   42

John H. Galla, MD, Ira Kurtz, MD, Jeffrey A. Kraut, MD, Gregg Y. Lipschik, MD, & Jeanne P. Macrae, MD

Metabolic Alkalosis   42
John H. Galla, MD

Metabolic Acidosis   45
Ira Kurtz, MD, & Jeffrey A. Kraut, MD,

Respiratory Acid–Base Disorders   54
Gregg Y. Lipschik, MD, & Jeanne P. Macrae, MD

6. Disorders of Calcium Balance: Hypercalcemia & Hypocalcemia   60

Stanley Goldfarb, MD

7. Disorders of Phosphate Balance: Hypophosphatemia & Hyperphosphatemia   69

Keith A. Hruska, MD

8. Disorders of Magnesium Balance: Hypomagnesemia & Hypermagnesemia   79

Meryl Waldman, MD, & Sidney Kobrin, MD

II. Acute Renal Failure

9. Acute Kidney Injury   89

Muhammad Sohail Yaqub, MD, & Bruce Molitoris, MD

10. Hepatorenal Syndrome   99

Florence Wong, MD, FRACP, FRCP(C)

11. Rhabdomyolysis   109

James P. Knochel, MD

12. Contrast-Induced Nephropathy   113

Steven Brunelli, MD, & Michael R. Rudnick, MD

13. Tumor Lysis Syndrome   117

Brian Stephany, MD, & Martin Schreiber, Jr, MD

14. Acute Renal Failure from Therapeutic Agents   124

Ali J. Olyaei, PharmD, & William M. Bennett, MD

15. NSAIDs & the Kidney: Acute Renal Failure   138

Mark A. Perazella, MD

16. Obstructive Uropathy   146

Beckie Michael, DO

III. Chronic Renal Failure

17. Chronic Renal Failure & the Uremic Syndrome   149

Gregorio T. Obrador, MD, MPH

18. Anemia & Chronic Kidney Disease   155

Robert Provenzano, MD

19. Cardiovascular Disease in Chronic Kidney Disease   160

Nadia Zalunardo, MD, FRCP(C), & Adeera Levin, MD, FRCP(C)

20. Renal Osteodystrophy   170

William G. Goodman, MD

21. Chronic Renal Failure & the Uremic Syndrome: Nutritional Issues   181

Kamyar Kalantar-Zadeh, MD, PhD, MPH, & Joel D. Kopple, MD

22. Slowing the Progression of Chronic Kidney Disease   201

Maarten W. Taal, MBChB, MD

IV. Glomerular Disorders

23. Nephrotic Syndrome versus Nephritic Syndrome   211

Isaac Teitelbaum, MD, & Laura Kooienga, MD

24. Minimal Change Disease   217

Elaine S. Kamil, MD

25. Focal Segmental Glomerulosclerosis   222

Debbie S. Gipson, MD, MS, & Howard Trachtman, MD

26. Membranous Nephropathy   229

Fernando C. Fervenza, MD, PhD, & Daniel C. Cattran, MD, FRCP(C)

27. Immunoglobulin A Nephropathy & Henoch–Schönlein Purpura   242

Meryl Waldman, MD, & Gerald B. Appel, MD

28. Membranoproliferative Glomerulonephritis   249

Howard Trachtman, MD

29. Goodpasture's Syndrome/Anti-Glomerular Basement Membrane Disease   255

Sian Finlay, MD, & Andrew J. Rees, MD

30. Postinfectious Glomerulonephritis   259

Bernardo Rodriguez-Iturbe, MD, & Sergio Mezzano, MD

31. Vasculitides   265

Patrick H. Nachman, MD, & Cynthia J. Denu-Ciocca, MD

32. Lupus Nephritis   276

James E. Balow, MD

33. Plasma Cell Dyscrasias   281

Richard J. Glassock, MD, & Arthur H. Cohen, MD

34. Thrombotic Microangiopathies   288

Cynthia C. Nast, MD, & Sharon G. Adler, MD

35. Glomerular Disorders due to Infections 296

Jeremy S. Leventhal, MD, Michael J. Ross, MD, Kar Neng Lai, MBBS, MD, Sydney C. W. Tang, MD, PhD

HIV-Associated Nephropathy
Jeremy S. Leventhal, MD, & Michael J. Ross, MD

Hepatitis-Associated Glomerulonephritis
Kar Neng Lai, MBBS, MD, & Sydney C. W. Tang, MD, PhD

V. Tubulointerstitial Diseases

36. Acute Tubulointerstitial Nephritis   313

Edgar V. Lerma, MD

37. Chronic Tubulointerstitial Nephritis   320

Edgar V. Lerma, MD

38. Urinary Tract Infection   329

Kamaljit Singh, MD, Sampath Kumar, MD, Ronald Villareal, MD, & Edgar V. Lerma, MD

39. Reflux Nephropathy   337

Hiep T. Nguyen, MD, & Emil A. Tanagho, MD

40. Nephrolithiasis 345

Elaine M. Worcester, MD, & Fredric L. Coe, MD

VI. Hypertension

41. Primary (Essential) Hypertension 353

Peter D. Hart, MD, & George L. Bakris, MD

42. Secondary Hypertension 359

William J. Elliott, MD, PhD, Priya Kalahasti, MD,
Sey M. Lau, MD, Joseph V. Nally, Jr., MD, &
Celso E. Gomez-Sanchez, MD

General Approaches
William J. Elliott, MD, PhD

Renovascular Hypertension
Priya Kalahasti, MD, Sey M. Lau, MD, &
Joseph V. Nally, Jr., MD

Endocrine Hypertension
Celso E. Gomez-Sanchez, MD

Coarctation of the Aorta
William J. Elliott, MD, PhD

Sleep Apnea
William J. Elliott, MD, PhD

43. Hypertension in High-Risk Populations 374

David Martins, MD, Keith Norris, MD, Tiina Podymow,
MD, & Phyllis August, MD, MPH

Hypertension in African-Americans
David Martins, MD, & Keith Norris, MD

Hypertension in the Elderly

Hypertension in Pregnancy
Tiina Podymow, MD, & Phyllis August, MD, MPH

44. Refractory Hypertension 394

Luis M. Ruilope, MD, & Julian Segura, MD

45. Hypertensive Emergencies & Urgencies 401

William J. Elliott, MD, PhD

VII. Cystic & Genetic Diseases of the Kidney

46. Cystic Diseases of the Kidney 405

Qi Qian, MD, & Vicente E. Torres, MD, PhD

**47. Familial Hematurias: Alport Syndrome &
Thin Basement Membrane Nephropathy** 422

Clifford E. Kashtan, MD

48. Fabry Disease 426

Robert J. Desnick, PhD, MD

49. Sickle Cell Nephropathy 430

Jon I. Scheinman, MD

VIII. Renal Replacement Therapy

50. Hemodialysis 437

Michael V. Rocco, MD, MSCE, & Shahriar Moossavi,
MD, PhD

51. Peritoneal Dialysis 444

Brenda B. Hoffman, MD

52. Continuous Renal Replacement Therapy 453

Frank Liu, MD, & Ravindra Mehta, MD

53. Renal Transplantation 463

Phuong-Thu Pham, MD, Julie Yabu, MD, Phuong-Chi
T. Pham, MD, & Alan H. Wilkinson, MD, FRCP

IX. Kidney Disease in Special Populations

54. Diabetic Nephropathy 483

Yalemzewd Woredekal, MD, & Eli A. Friedman, MD

55. Pregnancy & Renal Disease 492

Priya Anantharaman, MD, Rebecca J. Schmidt, DO,
& Jean L. Holley, MD

56. Aging & Renal Disease   **507**

Nada B. Dimkovic, MD, & Dimitrios G. Oreopoulos, MD

X. Special Topics in Nephrology

57. Interventional Nephrology: Endovascular Procedures   **517**

Theodore F. Saad, MD

58. Interventional Nephrology: Peritoneal Dialysis Catheter Procedures   **529**

Stephen R. Ash, MD, FACP

59. Poisonings & Intoxications   **540**

James F. Winchester, MD, & Donald A. Feinfeld, MD

Index   547

Authors

Sharon G. Adler, MD
Professor and Chief, Division of Nephrology and
   Hypertension, David Geffen School of Medicine at UCLA
   and Cedars-Sinai Medical Center, Los Angeles, California
Thrombotic Microangiopathies

Priya Anantharaman, MD
Assistant Professor of Medicine, Robert Byrd Health
   Sciences Center - West Virginia University,
   Morgantown, West Virginia
Pregnancy & Renal Disease

Gerald B. Appel, MD
Professor of Clinical Medicine, Nephrology Division,
   Department of Medicine, Columbia University College
   of Physicians and Surgeons, New York, New York
Immunoglobulin A Nephropathy & Henoch–Schönlein Purpura

Stephen R. Ash, MD
Director of Research, Ash Access Technology, Inc.,
   Lafayette, Indiana
*Interventional Nephrology: Peritoneal Dialysis Catheter
   Procedures*

Phyllis August, MD, MPH
Professor of Research in Medicine, Weill Cornell Medical
   College, New York, New York
*Hypertension in High-Risk Populations: Hypertension
   in Pregnancy*

George L. Bakris, MD
Professor of Medicine, Pritzker School of Medicine,
   University of Chicago, Chicago, Illinois
Primary (Essential) Hypertension

James E. Balow, MD
Professor of Medicine, Uniformed Services University
   of the Health Sciences, Bethesda, Maryland
Lupus Nephritis

William M. Bennett, MD
Professor of Medicine (retired), Oregon Health & Sciences
   University, Portland, Oregon
Acute Renal Failure from Therapeutic Agents

Tomas Berl, MD
Professor of Medicine, University of Colorado,
   Denver, Colorado
Disorders of Water Balance: Hyponatremia & Hypernatremia

Steven Brunelli, MD
Assistant Professor of Medicine, Harvard Medical School,
   Boston, Massachusetts
Contrast-Induced Nephropathy

Daniel C. Cattran, MD, FRCP(C)
Professor of Medicine, University of Toronto,
   Toronto, Ontario
Membranous Nephropathy

Fredric L. Coe, MD
Professor of Medicine, Nephrology Section, University
   of Chicago, Chicago, Illinois
Nephrolithiasis

Arthur H. Cohen, MD
Professor of Pathology and Professor of Medicine, UCLA
   School of Medicine, Los Angeles, California
Plasma Cell Dyscrasias

Cynthia J. Denu-Ciocca, MD
Assistant Professor of Medicine, Department of Medicine,
   University of North Carolina, Chapel Hill, North Carolina
Vasculitides

Robert J. Desnick, PhD, MD
Professor and Chairman, Department of Genetics and
   Genomic Sciences, Mount Sinai School of Medicine,
   New York, New York
Fabry Disease

Nada B. Dimkovic, MD
Professor, Toronto Western Hospital, Toronto, Canada
Aging & Renal Disease

William J. Elliott, MD, PhD
Professor of Preventive Medicine, Internal Medicine and
   Pharmacology, Rush Medical College of Rush
   University at Rush University Medical Center, Chicago,
   Illinois
*Secondary Hypertension: General Approaches, Coarctation
   of the Aorta, Sleep Apnea Hypertensive Emergencies &
   Urgencies*

David H. Ellison, MD
Professor of Medicine, Division of Nephrology and
   Hypertension, Oregon Health and Science University,
   Portland, Oregon
*Disorders of Extracellular Volume: Hypovolemia &
   Hypervolemia*

Michael Emmett, MD
Clinical Professor of Medicine, Department of Internal
Medicine, Baylor University Medical Center, Dallas, Texas
*Disorders of Potassium Balance: Hypokalemia &
Hyperkalemia*

Donald A. Feinfeld, MD
Professor of Medicine, Division of Nephrology and
Hypertension, Beth Israel Medical Center - Albert
Einstein College of Medicine, New York, New York
Poisonings & Intoxications

Fernando C. Fervenza, MD, PhD
Associate Professor of Medicine, Division of Nephrology
and Hypertension, Mayo Clinic College of Medicine,
Rochester, Minnesota
Membranous Nephropathy

Sian Finlay, MD
Consultant in Acute Medicine, Acute Medicine,
Dumfries and Galloway Royal Infirmary, Lockerbie,
Scotland
*Goodpasture's Syndrome/Anti-Glomerular Basement
Membrane Disease*

Eli A. Friedman, MD
Distinguished Teaching Professor, Department of
Medicine - Renal Division, State University of New York
(SUNY)-Downstate
Medical Center, Brooklyn, New York
Diabetic Nephropathy

John H. Galla, MD
Professor Emeritus of Medicine, University of Cincinnati,
Cincinnati, Ohio
Acid–Base Disorders: Metabolic Alkalosis

Debbie S. Gipson, MD, MS
Associate Professor, UNC Kidney Center,
University of North Carolina, Chapel Hill,
North Carolina
Focal Segmental Glomerulosclerosis

Richard J. Glassock, MD
Emeritus Professor of Medicine, David Geffen School
of Medicine at UCLA, Los Angeles, California
Plasma Cell Dyscrasias

Stanley Goldfarb, MD
Professor of Medicine, Renal Electrolyte and Hypertension
Division, University of Pennsylvania School of Medicine,
Philadelphia, Pennsylvania
Disorders of Calcium Balance: Hypercalcemia & Hypocalcemia

Celso E. Gomez-Sanchez, MD
Professor of Medicine, Division of Endocrinology,
University of Mississippi Medical Center, Jackson,
Mississippi
Secondary Hypertension: Endocrine Hypertension

William G. Goodman, MD
Renal Osteodystrophy

Peter D. Hart, MD
Associate Professor of Medicine, Rush University Medical
Center, Chicago, Illinois
Primary (Essential) Hypertension

Brenda B. Hoffman, MD
Associate Professor of Clinical Medicine, Department
of Medicine, University of Pennsylvania School of
Medicine, Philadelphia, Pennsylvania
Peritoneal Dialysis

Jean L. Holley, MD
Clinical Professor of Medicine, University of Illinois,
Urbana-Champaign, Urbana, Illinois
Pregnancy & Renal Disease

Clancy Howard, MD
Disorders of Water Balance: Hyponatremia & Hypernatremia

Keith A. Hruska, MD
Professor of Pediatrics, Internal Medicine, Cell Biology and
Physiology, Division of Biology and Biomedical Sciences,
Washington University in St. Louis School of Medicine,
St. Louis, Missouri
*Disorders of Phosphate Balance: Hypophosphatemia &
Hyperphosphatemia*

Priya Kalahasti, MD
Clinical Associate, Department of Nephrology and
Hypertension, Cleveland Clinic Foundation,
Cleveland, Ohio
Secondary Hypertension: Renovascular Hypertension

Kamyar Kalantar-Zadeh, MD, PhD, MPH
Associate Professor of Medicine, Pediatrics and
Epidemiology, UCLA Schools of Medicine & Public
Health, Torrance, California
*Chronic Renal Failure & the Uremic Syndrome: Nutritional
Issues*

Elaine S. Kamil, MD
Professor of Pediatrics, David Geffen School of Medicine
at UCLA, Los Angeles, California
Minimal Change Disease

Clifford E. Kashtan, MD
Professor of Pediatrics, University of Minnesota Medical
School, Minneapolis, Minnesota
*Familial Hematurias: Alport Syndrome & Thin Basement
Membrane Nephropathy*

James P. Knochel, MD
Clinical Professor, Internal Medicine, University of Texas
Health Science Center at Dallas, Dallas, Texas
Rhabdomyolysis

Sidney Kobrin, MD
Professor, Renal Division, Hospital of the University of
Pennsylvania, Philadelphia, Pennsylvania
*Disorders of Magnesium Balance: Hypomagnesemia &
Hypermagnesemia*

Laura Kooienga, MD
Renal Fellow, University of Colorado School of Medicine,
Denver, Colorado
Nephrotic Syndrome versus Nephritic Syndrome

Joel D. Kopple, MD
Professor of Medicine and Public Health, Division of
Nephrology and Hypertension, David Geffen School of
Medicine at UCLA, Torrance, California
Chronic Renal Failure & the Uremic Syndrome: Nutritional Issues

Jeffrey A. Kraut, MD
Professor of Medicine, David Geffen School of Medicine
at UCLA, Los Angeles, California
Acid–Base Disorders: Metabolic Acidosis

Sampath Kumar, MD
Clinical Instructor, Rush University Medical Center,
Chicago, Illinois
Urinary Tract Infection

Ira Kurtz, MD
Professor of Medicine, Division of Nephrology, David Geffen
School of Medicine at UCLA, Los Angeles, California
Acid–Base Disorders: Metabolic Acidosis

Kar Neng Lai, MBBS, MD
Chair of Medicine, Department of Medicine, University of
Hong Kong, Hong Kong, China
*Glomerular Disorders due to Infections: Hepatitis-Associated
Glomerulonephritis*

Sey M. Lau, MD
Special Fellow in Nephrology, Department of Nephrology
and Hypertension, Cleveland Clinic Foundation,
Cleveland, Ohio
Secondary Hypertension: Renovascular Hypertension.

Edgar V. Lerma, MD
Clinical Associate Professor of Medicine, Section of
Nephrology, Department of Medicine, University of
Illinois at Chicago College of Medicine/Associates in
Nephrology, S.C., Chicago, Illinois
*Approach to the Patient with Renal Disease
Acute Tubulointerstitial Nephritis
Chronic Tubulointerstitial Nephritis
Urinary Tract Infection*

Jeremy S. Leventhal, MD
Fellow in Nephrology, Division of Nephrology, Mount
Sinai School of Medicine, New York, New York
*Glomerular Disorders due to Infections: HIV-Associated
Nephropathy*

Adeera Levin, MD, FRCPC
Professor of Medicine, University of British Columbia,
Vancouver, British Columbia
Cardiovascular Disease in Chronic Kidney Disease

Gregg Y. Lipschik, MD
Clinical Associate Professor, Department of Medicine,
University of Pennsylvania School of Medicine,
Philadelphia, Pennsylvania
Acid–Base Disorders: Respiratory Acid–Base Disorders

Frank Liu, MD
Assistant Professor of Medicine, Division of Nephrology
and Hypertension, Weill Cornell Medical College,
New York, New York
Continuous Renal Replacement Therapy

Jeanne P. Macrae, MD
Associate Professor of Clinical Medicine, Department of
Internal Medicine, State University of New York (SUNY)
Downstate College of Medicine, Brooklyn, New York
Acid–Base Disorders: Respiratory Acid–Base Disorders

David Martins, MD
Assistant Professor of Medicine, Charles Drew University,
Los Angeles, California
*Hypertension in High-Risk Populations: Hypertension in
African-Americans*

Ravindra Mehta, MD
Professor of Clinical Medicine, Division of Nephrology,
University of California, San Diego Medical Center,
San Diego, California
Continuous Renal Replacement Therapy

Sergio Mezzano, MD
Professor of Medicine, Division of Nephrology, Universidad
Austral Valdivia, Valdivia, Chile
Postinfectious Glomerulonephritis

Beckie Michael, DO
Clinical Associate Professor of Medicine, Department
of Medicine/Nephrology, Jefferson Medical College,
Philadelphia, Pennsylvania
Obstructive Uropathy

Bruce Molitoris, MD
Professor of Medicine, Department of Medicine, Division
of Nephrology, Indiana University School of Medicine,
Indianapolis, Indiana
Acute Kidney Injury

Shahriar Moossavi, MD, PhD
Assistant Professor Internal Medicine/Nephrology, Division
of Nephrology, Wake Forest University Health Sciences,
Winston-Salem, North Carolina
Hemodialysis

Patrick H. Nachman, MD
Associate Professor of Medicine, Division of Nephrology
and Hypertension, School of Medicine, University of
North Carolina Kidney Center, Chapel Hill,
North Carolina
Vasculitides

Joseph V. Nally, Jr., MD
Professor of Medicine, Department of Nephrology and
Hypertension, Glickman Urological and Kidney Institute
at the Cleveland Clinic, Cleveland, Ohio
Secondary Hypertension, Renovascular Hypertension

Cynthia C. Nast, MD
Professor of Pathology, Department of Pathology, David
Geffen School of Medicine at UCLA and Cedars-Sinai
Medical Center, Los Angeles, California
Thrombotic Microangiopathies

Hiep T. Nguyen, MD
Assistant Professor, Harvard Medical School, Boston,
Massachusetts
Reflux Nephropathy

Keith C. Norris, MD
Professor of Medicine, Charles Drew University,
Los Angeles, California
*Hypertension in High-Risk Populations: Hypertension in
African-Americans*

Gregorio T. Obrador, MD, MPH
Dean, Universidad Panamericana School of Medicine,
Mexico City, Mexico
Chronic Renal Failure & the Uremic Syndrome

Ali J. Olyaei, PharmD
Associate Professor of Medicine, Oregon Health & Sciences
University, Portland, Oregon
Acute Renal Failure from Therapeutic Agents

Dimitrios G. Oreopoulos, MD
Professor of Medicine, Toronto Western Hospital,
Toronto, Canada
Aging & Renal Disease

Mark A. Perazella, MD
Associate Professor of Medicine, Yale University School of
Medicine, New Haven, Connecticut
NSAIDs & the Kidney: Acute Renal Failure

Phuong-Chi T. Pham, MD
Associate Clinical Professor of Medicine, David Geffen
School of Medicine at UCLA, Los Angeles, California
Renal Transplantation

Phuong-Thu T. Pham, MD
Associate Professor of Medicine, David Geffen School of
Medicine at UCLA, Los Angeles, California
Renal Transplantation

Tiina Podymow, MD
Associate Professor, Nephrology, McGill University,
Montreal, Quebec
*Hypertension in High-Risk Populations: Hypertension
in Pregnancy*

Robert Provenzano, MD
Associate Clinical Professor of Medicine, Wayne State
University School of Medicine, Detroit, Michigan
Anemia & Chronic Kidney Disease

Qi Qian, MD
Assistant Professor, Mayo Clinic School of Medicine,
Rochester, Minnesota
Cystic Diseases of the Kidney

Andrew J. Rees, MD
Marie Curie Professor, Institute of Clinical Pathology,
Medical University of Vienna, Vienna, Austria
Goodpasture's Syndrome/Anti-Glomerular Basement

Michael V. Rocco, MD, MSCE
Vardaman M. Buckalew Jr. Professor, Department of
Medicine, Section on Nephrology, Wake Forest University
School of Medicine, Winston-Salem, North Carolina
Hemodialysis

Bernardo Rodriguez-Iturbe, MD
Professor of Medicine, Hospital Universitario, Universidad del Zulia, Maracaibo, Zulia, Venezuela
Postinfectious Glomerulonephritis

Michael J. Ross, MD
Assistant Professor of Medicine, Division of Nephrology, Mount Sinai School of Medicine, New York, New York
Glomerular Disorders due to Infections: HIV-Associated Nephropathy

Michael R. Rudnick, MD
Associate Professor of Medicine, University of Pennsylvania School of Medicine, Philadelphia, Pennsylvania
Contrast-Induced Nephropathy

Luis M. Ruilope, MD
Professor of Medicine, Complutense University, Madrid, Spain
Refractory Hypertension

Theodore F. Saad, MD
Professor, Nephrology, Christiana Care Health Systems, Newark, Delaware
Interventional Nephrology: Endovascular Procedures

Jon I. Scheinman, MD
Professor of Pediatrics, Division of Pediatric Nephrology, University of Kansas, Kansas City, Kansas
Sickle Cell Nephropathy

Rebecca J. Schmidt, DO
Professor, Department of Medicine, Section of Nephrology, West Virginia University School of Medicine, Morgantown, West Virginia
Pregnancy & Renal Disease

Martin J. Schreiber, Jr., MD
Chairman, Nephrology and Hypertension, Glickman Urological and Kidney Institute at the Cleveland Clinic, Cleveland, Ohio
Tumor Lysis Syndrome

Julian Segura, MD
Refractory Hypertension

Kamaljit Singh, MD
Assistant Professor of Medicine, Rush University Medical Center, Chicago, Illinois
Urinary Tract Infection

Brian Stephany, MD
Associate Staff, Department of Nephrology and Hypertension, Cleveland Clinic Foundation, Cleveland, Ohio
Tumor Lysis Syndrome

Maarten W. Taal, MBChB, MD
Special Lecturer, University of Nottingham Medical School at Derby, Derby, England
Slowing the Progression of Chronic Kidney Disease

Emil A. Tanagho, MD
Chairman, Emeritus and Professor, Department of Urology, University of California at San Francisco, San Francisco, California
Reflux Nephropathy

Sydney C.W. Tang, MD, PhD
Associate Professor of Medicine, Department of Medicine, The University of Hong Kong, Hong Kong, China
Glomerular Disorders due to Infections: Hepatitis-Associated Glomerulonephritis

Isaac Teitelbaum, MD
Professor of Medicine, University of Colorado, Aurora, Colorado
Nephrotic Syndrome versus Nephritic Syndrome

Vicente E. Torres, MD, PhD
Professor of Medicine, Department of Nephrology and Hypertension, Mayo Clinic School of Medicine, Rochester, Minnesota
Cystic Diseases of the Kidney

Howard Trachtman, MD
Professor of Pediatrics, Albert Einstein College of Medicine, New Hyde Park, New York
Focal Segmental Glomerulosclerosis
Membranoproliferative Glomerulonephritis

Ronald Villareal, MD
Nephrology Fellow, University of Illinois at Chicago, Chicago, Illinois
Urinary Tract Infection

Meryl Waldman, MD
Nephrologist, Kidney Disease Section, National Institutes of Health (NIH), National Institute of Diabetes and Digestive and Kidney Diseases (NIDDK), Bethesda, Maryland
Disorders of Magnesium Balance: Hypomagnesemia & Hypermagnesemia
Immunoglobulin A Nephropathy & Henoch–Schönlein Purpura

Michael R. Wiederkehr, MD
Professor, Department of Nephrology, Baylor University
   Medical Center, Dallas, Texas
Disorders of Potassium Balance: Hypokalemia & Hyperkalemia

Alan H. Wilkinson, MD
Professor of Medicine, David Geffen School of Medicine at
   UCLA, Los Angeles, California
Renal Transplantation

James F. Winchester, MD
Professor of Clinical Medicine, Albert Einstein College
   of Medicine, New York, New York
Poisonings & Intoxications

Florence Wong, MD, FRACP, FRCP(C)
Associate Professor, University of Toronto, Toronto,
   Ontario
Hepatorenal Syndrome

Elaine M. Worcester, MD
Professor of Medicine, University of Chicago,
   Chicago, Illinois
Nephrolithiasis

Yalemzewd Woredekal, MD
Assistant Professor of Medicine, Department of Medicine
   - Renal Division, State University of New York (SUNY)-
   Downstate Medical Center, Brooklyn, New York
Diabetic Nephropathy

Julie Yabu, MD
Assistant Clinical Professor, University of California at San
   Francisco, San Francisco, California
Renal Transplantation

Muhammad Sohail Yaqub, MD
Associate Professor of Clinical Medicine, Indiana University
   School of Medicine, Indianapolis, Indiana
Acute Kidney Injury

Nadia Zalunardo, MD, FRCP(C)
Clinical Assistant Professor, Division of Nephrology,
   University of British Columbia, Vancouver, British
   Columbia
Cardiovascular Disease in Chronic Kidney Disease

Preface

The first edition of *Current Diagnosis & Treatment: Nephrology & Hypertension* features practical, up-to-date, referenced information on the care of patients with diseases involving the kidneys and hypertension. It also covers dialysis and transplantation, as well as new areas of specialization, such as critical care nephrology and interventional nephrology. This book emphasizes the clinical aspects of renal care while also presenting important underlying principles. *Current Diagnosis & Treatment: Nephrology & Hypertension* provides a practical guide to diagnosis, understanding, and treatment of the medical problems of all adult patients in an easy-to-use and readable format.

INTENDED AUDIENCE

In the tradition of all Lange medical books, this new Current in Nephrology and Hypertension is a concise yet comprehensive source of up-to-date information. For medical students, it can serve as an authoritative introduction to the specialty of nephrology and an excellent resource for reference and review. Residents in internal medicine (and other specialties) and most especially, nephrology fellows in training, will appreciate the detailed descriptions of diseases and diagnostic and therapeutic procedures. General internists, family practitioners, hospitalists, nurses and nurse practitioners, physician assistants, and other allied health-care providers who work with patients with kidney diseases will find this a very useful reference on management aspects of renal medicine. Moreover, patients and their family members who seek information about the nature of specific diseases and their diagnosis and treatment may also find this book to be a valuable resource.

COVERAGE

Fifty-nine chapters cover a wide range of topics, including fluid, electrolyte, and acid-base disorders, acute and chronic kidney failure, glomerular and tubulointerstitial diseases, hypertension, systemic diseases with renal manifestations, renal replacement therapies, renal transplantation, geriatric nephrology, and interventional nephrology.

These and many other diseases are covered in a crisp and concise manner. Striking just the right balance between comprehensiveness and convenience, *Current Diagnosis & Treatment: Nephrology & Hypertension* emphasizes the practical features of clinical diagnosis and patient management while providing a comprehensive discussion of pathophysiology and relevant basic and clinical science. With its consistent formatting chapter by chapter, this text makes it simple to locate the practical information you need on diagnosis, testing, disease processes, and up-to-date treatment and management strategies.

The book has been designed to meet the clinician's need for an immediate refresher in the clinic as well as to serve as an accessible text for thorough review of the specialty for the boards. The concise presentation is ideally suited for rapid acquisition of information by the busy practitioner.

ACKNOWLEDGMENTS

We wish to thank our contributing authors for devoting their precious time and offering their wealth of knowledge in the process of completing this important book. These authors have contributed countless hours of work in regularly reading and reviewing the literature in this specialty, and we have all benefited from their clinical wisdom and commitment.

We are especially grateful to two authors who have helped in reviewing and editing selected sections of the book: Dr. Sharon Adler, for her valuable contributions to the chapters on Glomerular Diseases, and Dr. George Bakris, for recommending excellent contributors for the chapters on Hypertension.

We would like to thank Harriet Lebowitz for her expert assistance in managing the flow of manuscripts and materials among the chapter authors, editors, and publisher. Her attention to detail was enormously helpful. This book would not have been completed without the help of Arline Keithe, Mary Saggese, Satvinder Kaur, and of course, the unwavering support of James Shanahan.

Edgar V. Lerma, MD
Jeffrey S. Berns, MD
Allen R. Nissenson, MD
December, 2008

Approach to the Patient with Renal Disease

Edgar V. Lerma, MD

▶ General Considerations

A patient with renal disease can present either as an initial outpatient or inpatient consultation. Some patients may be referred because of abnormal urinary findings, such as hematuria or proteinuria, which may have been incidentally discovered during routine clinical evaluation or as part of initial employment requirements. Depending on the stage of renal disease, they can present with mild edema or generalized pruritus, as well as more advanced signs and symptoms of uremia, such as decreased appetite, weight loss, and even alterations in mental status. In general, the symptoms and signs of patients with renal disease tend to be nonspecific (Table 1–1). Still others would present only with elevation in serum creatinine.

To narrow the differential diagnosis, it is necessary to first determine whether the disease is acute, subacute, or chronic on presentation. However, there is usually an overlap in these stages, and at times, it is not exactly clear. Certainly, a patient who presents with an elevated serum creatinine that was documented to be normal a few days previously has an acute presentation, whereas a patient who presents with a previously elevated serum creatinine that has been rising steadily over the past several months to years has a chronic disease. Oftentimes, acute exacerbations of chronic renal disease are common presentations.

The next question concerns which segment or component of the renal anatomy is involved. This is subdivided into prerenal, postrenal, or renal (Table 1–2).

Prerenal disease refers to any process that decreases renal perfusion, such as intravascular volume depletion, hypotension, massive blood loss, or third spacing of fluids. It can also be due to congestive heart failure, whereby decreased effective circulating volume decreases blood flow toward the kidneys (see Chapter 9).

Postrenal disease refers to any obstruction that impedes urinary flow through the urinary tract. Examples include benign prostatic hypertrophy or cervical malignancy (see Chapter 16).

Renal involvement is further subdivided into vascular, glomerular (see Chapters 23–35), or tubulointerstitial disease (see Chapters 36 and 37), depending on which segment is involved.

▶ Assessment of Glomerular Filtration Rate (GFR)

The most common method of assessing renal function is by estimation of the glomerular filtration rate (GFR). The GFR gives an approximation of the degree of renal function. Daily GFR in normal subjects is in the range of 150–250 L/24 hours or 100–120 mL/minute/1.73 m^2 of body surface area. GFR is decreased in those with renal dysfunction, and is used to monitor renal function in those with chronic kidney disease. It is also used to determine the appropriate timing for initiation of renal replacement therapy.

To date, there are several methods by which GFR is measured, namely serum creatinine concentration, 24-hour creatinine clearance, as well as estimation equations such as the Cockroft–Gault formula and the Modification of Diet in Renal Disease (MDRD) Study formula (Table 1–3).

Using the serum creatinine alone to estimate renal functioning is inaccurate for several reasons. First, a small amount of creatinine is normally secreted by the tubules, and this amount tends to increase as progressive renal decline occurs, thereby overestimating the true GFR value. Similarly, there are factors that increase serum creatinine without truly affecting renal function, such as dietary meat (protein) intake, volume of muscle mass, and medications that interfere with tubular secretion of creatinine such as cimetidine, trimethoprim, and probenecid. Elderly patients, those with cachexia, amputees, as well as patients with spinal cord injury or disease tend to have less muscle mass, hence, lower serum creatinine values (Table 1–4).

Table 1–1. Symptoms and signs at presentation of patients with renal disease.

Easy fatigability
Decreased appetite
Nausea and vomiting
Generalized pruritus
Shortness of breath
Sleep disturbances
Urinary hesitancy, urgency, or frequency
Microscopic or gross hematuria
Proteinuria
Frothy appearance of urine
Flank pain, mostly unilateral (may be bilateral)
Mental status changes, eg, confusion
Pallor
Weight loss or gain
Lower extremity "pitting" edema
Ascites
Pulmonary edema or congestion
Pleural or pericardial effusion
Pericarditis
Uncontrolled hypertension

Table 1–2. Causes of acute renal failure.

Prerenal
Intravascular volume depletion
  Blood loss
  Gastrointestinal losses, eg, vomiting, diarrhea
  Third spacing or redistribution of fluids, eg, burns, pancreatitis
Hypotension
  Myocardial infarction
  Sepsis
Decreased renal perfusion
  Congestive heart failure
  Renal artery stenosis
  Medications, eg, nonsteroidal anti-inflammatory drugs, ACE inhibitors, angiotensin receptor blockers and diuretics in the setting of volume depletion

Renal
Glomerular
  Rapidly progressive glomerulonephritis, thrombotic thrombocytopenic purpura
Tubular
  Acute tubular necrosis
    Ischemic
    Nephrotoxic
    Endogenous: Rhabdomyolysis
    Exogenous: Radiocontrast nephropathy, aminoglycosides, cisplatin
Interstitial
  Acute tubulointerstitial nephritis, eg, drugs (antibiotics), infections
Vascular
  Vasculitides, eg, ANCA-mediated diseases, renal artery/vein thromboses

Postrenal
Obstructive uropathy
  Intrinsic: Nephrolithiasis, papilary necrosis, prostate/bladder diseases
  Extrinsic: Retroperitoneal fibrosis, cervical carcinoma

ACE, angiotensin-converting enzyme; ANCA, antineutrophilic cytoplasmic antibody.

The 24-hour urine collection is used to determine creatinine clearance. Obviously, its main limitation is that it is cumbersome, and particularly in elderly individuals or those with either fecal or urinary incontinence, either an incomplete or prolonged (over 24 hours) urine specimen collection tends to provide erroneous information.

To determine if a 24-hour urine collection is complete, the following reference is used:

$$\text{For males, Urine creatinine} \times \text{Urine volume} = 20\text{–}25 \text{ mg/kg/24 hours}$$

$$\text{For females, Urine creatinine} \times \text{Urine volume} = 15\text{–}20 \text{ mg/kg/24 hours}$$

A common method of assessing GFR is by the use of estimation equations:
Cockroft–Gault formula:

$$\text{Creatinine clearance} = \frac{(140 - \text{Age in years}) \times \text{Weight (kg)}}{\text{Plasma creatinine} \times 72}$$

Due to less muscle mass in females, a factor of 0.85 is multiplied by the creatinine clearance to arrive at the estimated GFR.

This formula also has limitations, eg, it tends to overestimate GFR in patients who are morbidly obese and/or have significant edema.
MDRD formula:

$$\text{GFR} = 175 \times \text{Serum creatinine}^{-1.154} \times \text{Age}^{-0.203} \times [0.742 \text{ if female}] \times [1.21 \text{ if black}]$$

This is the formula recommended for use when staging chronic kidney disease (CKD). According to recent published reports, the MDRD formula is reasonably accurate in patients with stable CKD. Similar to the Cockroft–Gault formula, it appears to be inaccurate in morbidly obese individuals, in normal subjects, and in populations of different ethnicities from outside the United States. In the latter, the MDRD formula tends to overestimate GFR due to differences in body mass and dietary habits.

Table 1–3. Methods to estimate renal function.

Serum creatinine
Inaccurate with early or advanced stages of kidney disease
Affected by age, gender, muscle mass, and some medications

24-hour urine creatinine clearance
Cumbersome
Can overestimate the true GFR

Estimation equations
Cockroft-Gault formula
  Highly dependent on serum creatinine (see above) MDRD Study
    formula
  Not tested in different populations, eg, the elderly and obese, or
    ethnicities

Radioisotopic clearance
Best measure of GFR
Invasive
Uses radioisotopes
Available only in certain academic institutions

GFR, glomerular filtration rate; MDRD, Modification of Diet in Renal
Disease.

▶ Clinical Findings

A. Symptoms and Signs

The majority of patients with renal disease are asymptomatic, and on routine examination are only incidentally discovered to have abnormal laboratory findings, eg, elevated serum creatinine and/or abnormal findings on urinalysis.

For those with symptomatic renal disease, most of the symptoms are nonspecific (see Table 1–1) and can be referred to almost any body organ. Examples include constitutional

Table 1–4. Factors that can affect levels of BUN and creatinine, independent of renal function.[1]

Increase BUN
High protein intake, eg, high meat diet, hyperalimentation
Gastrointestinal bleeding
Corticosteroids
Tetracycline
High catabolic state

Increase creatinine
High protein intake, eg, creatine supplements
Trimethoprim
Cimetidine (blocks tubular secretion of creatinine)
Ketones (interfere with the Jaffe reaction, used in some laboratories
  to measure creatinine)

[1]Low BUN and creatinine is usually observed in those with decreased muscle mass, eg, muscle wasting diseases and amputees.
BUN, blood urea nitrogen

symptoms such as generalized weakness, lack of energy, decreased appetite, shortness of breath, and difficulty sleeping. Some patients can present with symptoms referable to the urinary tract such as gross hematuria or flank discomfort. Although abnormalities in urination such as increased urgency or frequency may commonly indicate underlying urologic pathology, they are also seen in infections or inflammatory diseases involving the urinary tract.

B. Laboratory Findings

1. Urinalysis—The most important diagnostic test used in the patient with renal disease is the urinalysis. The urine specimen is obtained by doing a midstream catch for males, while in females, the labia majora should be cleaned and then separated to avoid contamination. Once collected, the urine specimen should be examined within 60 minutes of voiding.

Initially, a dipstick examination is performed, and this includes assessment of the urine specific gravity, pH, protein, blood, glucose, ketones, bilirubin, nitrite, and leukocyte esterase (Table 1–5).

Table 1–5. Interpretation of urinalysis findings.

Dipstick testing
Specific gravity
  Reflects the ability to concentrate urine in states of volume depletion
pH
  Normal range: 4.5–8
  <5.3: Renal tubular acidosis
  >7.0: Infection with urease-producing organisms, such as *Proteus*
Blood
  1–2 red blood cells per high power field
  Seen in glomerulonephritides, nephrolithiasis
Glucose
  Seen in poorly controlled diabetes, Fanconi syndrome
    (type 2 proximal renal tubular acidosis)
  Not reliable for the diagnosis of diabetes
Protein
  Detects only albumin, hence insensitive in detecting
  microalbuminuria
Nitrite
  Indicates the presence of microorganisms that convert urinary nitrate
  to nitrite
Leukocyte exterase
  Pyuria

Microscopy
Casts
  Hyaline
    Nonspecific
  Granular
    Nonspecific
    Acute tubular necrosis: Pathognomonic "muddy-brown" granular casts

(continued)

Table 1–5. *Continued*

Waxy and broad
    Nonspecific
    Advanced renal disease
Fatty
    Nephrotic syndrome: Oval fat bodies that appear as "Maltese crosses" on polarized micoscopy
Red blood cells
    Sine qua non of glomerulonephritis
White blood cells
    Urinary tract infections, eg, pyelonephritis, cystitis
    Tubulointerstitial nephritis
    Renal tuberculosis
Crystals
    Uric acid
        Requires an acidic urine pH
    Calcium phosphate and calcium oxalate
        Require an alkaline urine pH
    Magnesium ammonium phosphate (struvite)
        Seen in urinary tract infections caused by urease-producing organisms, eg, *Proteus* and *Klebsiella*
    Cystine
        Diagnostic of autosomal recessive cystinuria
Epithelial cells
    If >15–20, may be indicative of poorly catched urine specimen
Myoglobin
    Rhabdomyolysis

Microscopic examination of the urine sediment corroborates the findings on the initial dipstick analysis. The presence of various crystals, cells, casts, bacteria, and fungal elements is then reported (see Table 1–5).

Certain patterns of findings on urinalysis are indicative of certain specific diagnoses. For instance, in the patient presenting with acute renal failure, the finding of muddy brown, granular casts points to acute tubular necrosis, whereas the presence of red blood cell casts and dysmorphic red blood cells is indicative of glomerulonephritis. High grade proteinuria may be suggestive of glomerular disorders.

2. Urinary indices—Measurement of urine sodium (urine Na) in a random urine specimen is helpful in the differential diagnosis of acute renal failure. Urine Na <20 mEq/L points to prerenal causes of acute renal failure, eg, intravascular volume depletion due to fluid losses or sequestration, hypotension, sepsis, etc. On the other hand, urine Na >40 mEq/L suggests acute tubular necrosis (ATN). To adjust for the influence of urine output, the following equation is recommended:

$$\text{Fractional excretion of Na } (F_{E_{Na}}\%)$$
$$= \frac{\text{Urine Na} \times \text{Plasma creatinine} \times 100}{\text{Plasma Na} \times \text{Urine creatinine}}$$

An $F_{E_{Na}}$ <1% points to prerenal disease, while an $F_{E_{Na}}$ >2% suggests ATN. Limitations to the use of urinary indices include prior infusion with normal saline or administration of diuretics. This is discussed in Chapter 9.

C. Imaging Studies

In the evaluation of the patient with renal disease, various radiographic studies are available. Usually, they are performed either alone or in combination, to diagnose the different pathologies affecting the genitourinary tract (Table 1–6).

By far, the most common imaging modality used is that of renal ultrasonography, because it is safe, easy to do, and avoids the use of radiation or contrast media that can be nephrotoxic. Important detailed information that can be obtained through ultrasonography includes the size and shape of the kidneys, the presence of calculi, and differentiation between the presence of a mass or cyst. Asymmetry of the kidneys usually indicate a unilateral disease process. The presence of hydronephrosis is an indication of obstruction along the ipsilateral ureter (if unilateral) or at the level of the bladder or lower (if bilateral).

Increased echogenicity is a common finding that signifies chronic medical renal disease.

The plain film of the abdomen gives information about the kidney size and shape, as well as radiopaque (calcium containing) calcifications. Common limitations include its inability to detect radiolucent stones (uric acid).

Computed tomography (CT) scanning provides more detailed information about the structure of the kidneys, as it

Table 1–6. Imaging studies and various renal indications.

Renal ultrasonography
Renal failure
Microscopic and/or gross hematuria
Proteinuria/nephritic syndrome
Obstructive uropathy/hydronephrosis
Nonobstructing stones in the renal collecting system or proximal ureter
Renal allograft rejection
Percutaneous renal biopsy

CT scan with contrast enhancement
Renal vein thrombosis
Renal infarction

CT scan without contrast
Renal parenchyma infection, eg, abscess, pyelonephritis
Nephrocalcinosis
Renal artery stenosis
Retroperitoneal fibrosis
Percutaneous renal biopsy

Intravenous pyelography
Obstructive uropathy/hydronephrosis, eg, stones, papillary necrosis

CT, computed tomography

can also differentiate simple from complex cysts. Noncontrast-enhanced spiral CT scan is the imaging modality of choice for the diagnosis of nephrolithiasis. CT angiography is used in staging of renal cell carcinoma, as well as in demonstrating renal vein thrombosis. Its main disadvantages are the use of large volumes of contrast media as well as radiation.

Magnetic resonance imaging (MRI) also provides detailed structural information about the kidneys. In the past, magnetic resonance angiography (MRA) with gadolinium contrast has been used extensively in the evaluation of the renal vasculature, eg, renovascular diseases. However, recently, with several published reports on nephrogenic systemic fibrosis linked to the use of gadolinium, there has been a significant decline in its use. In fact, some experts recommend not using gadolinium as contrast agent in those with an estimated GFR of less than or equal to 30 mL/minute, including those who are dependent on renal replacement therapy or dialysis.

Renal angiography is commonly used in the diagnosis of renal artery stenosis. Because iodinated contrast media is used, caution is advised, especially in patients with baseline renal insufficiency due to increased risk of contrast-induced nephropathy.

The main indications for radionuclide studies [radioisotope scanning with ^{99m}Tc dimercaptosuccinic acid (DMSA)] include early detection of urinary obstruction and urine leak, as well as vesicoureteric reflux (voiding cystourethrogram).

Retrograde and antegrade pyelography are used primarily during placement of ureteral stents or nephrostomy tubes. Because they utilize radiation and potentially nephrotoxic contrast media, other noninvasive imaging modalities such as ultrasonography and CT scanning have been used more commonly in the diagnosis of urinary tract obstruction, including identification of the site of obstruction.

D. Special Tests

Renal biopsy—Percutaneous renal biopsy is used in situations in which evaluation of the patient's history, physical examination, as well as noninvasive testing (including serum and urine tests and imaging studies) has failed to reveal a diagnosis.

The major indications for doing a renal biopsy include (1) unexplained persistent hematuria or proteinuria, especially if associated with progression of renal dysfunction, i.e., rise in serum creatinine, (2) nephrotic syndrome, (3) acute nephritis, and (4) unexplained acute or rapidly progressive renal decline.

The most common complication arising from a percutaneous renal biopsy is bleeding. The patient's ability to coagulate normally should be ascertained by closely monitoring the coagulation profile (partial thromboplastin time, prothrombin time, international normalized ratio, platelet count, and bleeding time). Patients should also be advised to hold off on acetylsalicylic acid and/or nonsteroidal anti-inflammatory drugs at least 1 week prior to the planned renal biopsy.

Patients requiring maintenance chronic anticoagulation should be placed on heparin, which can be discontinued on the day prior to the biopsy.

Postbiopsy, most patients develop transient microscopic hematuria, while transient gross hematuria has been described in 3–10% of cases. Rare case reports of arteriovenous fistulas arising as complications of renal biopsies as demonstrated by color Doppler studies have been described in the literature.

The major contraindications to percutaneous renal biopsy can be divided into (1) those involving the kidneys and (2) those involving the patient. Examples of contraindications affecting the kidneys are the presence of multiple cysts either unilaterally or bilaterally, the presence of a renal mass, a solitary functioning kidney, the presence of active renal or perirenal infection, and unilateral or bilateral hydronephrosis. Patient-related contraindications include an uncooperative patient, uncontrolled severe hypertension, intractable bleeding disorder, and morbid obesity. It must be noted, however, that with the exception of intractable bleeding disorder, most of the contraindications are relative rather than absolute. Therefore, the actual clinical situation often dictates whether a contraindication can be overridden. Recently, it has been shown that percutaneous renal biopsy may be performed in those with solitary kidneys. Several published reports have demonstrated that even for those with solitary functioning kidneys, the risk of general anesthesia (during open renal biopsy) far outweighs the risk of requiring surgery and subsequent nephrectomy. Therefore, in selected cases, percutaneous renal biopsy may be performed in the presence of a solitary functioning kidney.

▶ Complications

A. Hematuria

Hematuria can be either gross or microscopic. Gross hematuria is the presence of red or brown urine. In the initial evaluation of a patient with gross hematuria, it must be determined whether the urine discoloration is truly secondary to pathologic bleeding within the urinary tract. Patients who are menstruating or postpartum should not be evaluated for hematuria. In the absence of actual bleeding the urine may appear grossly red following the intake of certain medications, such as rifampin, phenothiazine, or phenazopyridine (analgesic), or the intake of beets in certain predisposed individuals. It is also important to differentiate hematuria from other causes of red urine such as hemoglobinuria and myoglobinuria. The latter is usually seen in those with acute rhabdomyolysis.

Microscopic hematuria is defined as the presence of more than two red blood cells (RBCs)/hpf. It is usually detected incidentally by urine dipstick examination.

Careful history taking is of paramount importance in the evaluation of patients with hematuria. Important historical information usually provides diagnostic clues. For instance, the occurrence of concomitant flank pain with radiation to the ipsilateral testicle or labia suggests underlying nephrolithiasis, burning on urination or dysuria may point to possible urinary tract infection, and a recent upper respiratory tract infection may suggest either postinfectious glomerulonephritis or even IgA nephropathy. A family history of hematuria is also vital, as certain diseases tend to run in families, such as polycystic kidney disease or even sickle cell nephropathy. Likewise, thin basement membrane disease and benign familial hematuria tend to occur in families, and notably have a rather benign course despite the presentation. Exercise-induced hematuria is seen in adolescents who exercise vigorously.

In elderly individuals, or those above 50 years of age, the finding of gross or microscopic (even transient) hematuria should trigger an extensive evaluation to rule out malignancy involving the genitourinary tract. The incidence of bladder cancer and other malignancies involving the kidneys and the ureters is significantly elevated, particularly in those with a prolonged history of chronic smoking and analgesic use. The occurrence of symptoms of increased urgency and frequency with hematuria in this population should suggest urinary tract obstruction secondary to either benign prostatic hypertrophy (BPH) or prostatic malignancy.

Using urine microscopy, the presence of dysmorphic RBCs or RBC casts should suggest glomerular disorders as the primary etiology of hematuria. This is one of the indications for performing a percutaneous renal biopsy.

B. Proteinuria

Normal urine protein excretion is 150 mg/day. Anything above this value is considered overt proteinuria. Proteinuria usually implies that there is a defect in glomerular permeability. In general, proteinuria can be classified into three types: (1) Glomerular, (2) tubular, or (3) overflow.

Glomerular proteinuria includes diabetic nephropathy and other common glomerular disorders (see Chapters 36–40). It is usually caused by increased filtration of albumin across the glomerular capillary wall. There are also causes of glomerular proteinuria that have a rather benign course, such as orthostatic and exercise-induced proteinuria. These latter causes are characterized by significantly lower degrees of proteinuria, <2 g/day.

Tubular proteinuria is usually seen in those with underlying tubulointerstitial diseases. They often have defective reabsorptive capacities in the proximal tubules, such that the proteins, instead of being normally reabsorbed, are excreted in the urine. In contrast to glomerular proteinuria, whereby macromolecules such as albumin are leaked out, in tubular proteinuria, it is mostly low-molecular-weight proteins, such as immunoglobulin light chains.

Lastly, overflow proteinuria is exemplified by multiple myeloma, where there is an overabundance of immunoglobulin light chains secondary to overproduction. Simply put, proteinuria occurs because the amount of protein produced basically exceeds the maximum threshold for reabsorption in the tubules.

Whereas both glomerular and tubular proteinuria are secondary to abnormalities involving the glomerular capillary and tubular walls, respectively, in overflow proteinuria, the problem is the overproduction of certain proteins.

When performing a urinalysis, the dipstick examination can detect only albumin, and not the low-molecular-weight proteins. In fact, it can detect it only when proteinuria is >300–500 mg/day. Hence, one of its most important limitations is its inability to detect microalbuminuria, which corresponds to the earliest phase of diabetic nephropathy. However, the sulfosalicylic acid test (SSA) can detect all types of proteins in the urine, including low-molecular-weight proteins.

Quantification of the degree of proteinuria is accomplished by performing a 24-hour urine collection, which can be cumbersome, especially in elderly individuals or those with concomitant fecal or urinary incontinence.

The urine protein-to-creatinine (using a random urine specimen) ratio has been shown to have a good correlation with 24-hour urine protein determination.

Orthostatic or postural proteinuria, by definition, is characterized by increased urine protein excretion in the upright position and normal urine protein excretion in the supine position. It is a benign condition, seen mostly among adolescents, the mechanism of which is not clearly understood. The diagnosis is established by performing a split urine collection, the protocol for which is as follows: (1) The first morning void is discarded, (2) a 16-hour upright collection is obtained between 7 AM and 11 PM, with the patient performing normal activities and finishing the collection by voiding just before 11 PM (the times can be adjusted according to the normal times at which the patient awakens and goes to sleep), (3) the patient should assume a recumbent position 2 hours before the upright collection is finished to avoid contamination of the supine collection with urine formed when in the upright position, and (4) a separate overnight 8-hour collection is obtained between 11 PM and 7 AM.

Patients with orthostatic proteinuria do not progress to end-stage renal disease; in fact, proteinuria resolves spontaneously in the majority of affected patients.

Disorders of Extracellular Volume: Hypovolemia & Hypervolemia

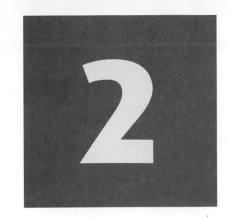

David H. Ellison, MD

EVALUATION OF THE EXTRACELLULAR FLUID VOLUME

▶ General Considerations

Disorders of extracellular fluid volume are disorders of sodium balance and total body sodium content. The terms volume contraction and volume expansion are frequently employed as shorthand to indicate extracellular fluid (ECF) volume contraction and expansion, respectively. Because ECF volume control systems are largely distinct from systems that regulate plasma osmolality, disorders of ECF volume are commonly distinguished from disorders of water balance. The term dehydration is commonly used to indicate ECF volume depletion; strictly, its use should be reserved for depletion of water (as in diabetes insipidus) rather than ECF volume.

Disorders of ECF volume have long presented a challenge in the understanding of body fluid volume regulation. In the normal subject, if ECF is expanded, the kidney will excrete the excessive amount of sodium and water, thus returning ECF volume to normal. What has not been understood, however, is why the kidneys continue to retain sodium and water in edematous patients. Neither total ECF nor its interstitial component, both of which are expanded in the patient with generalized edema, is the modulator of renal sodium and water excretion. Rather, some body fluid compartment other than total ECF or interstitial fluid volume must be the regulator of renal sodium and water excretion.

The term effective blood volume was coined to describe this undefined body fluid compartment that signals the kidney, through unknown pathways, to retain sodium and water in spite of expansion of the total ECF volume. It was first suggested that the kidney is responding to a decline in cardiac output, providing an explanation for sodium and water retention in low-output cardiac failure. This idea, however, did not provide a universal explanation for generalized edema, because many patients with decompensated cirrhosis who avidly retain sodium and water have normal or elevated cardiac output. The venous component of the plasma in the circulation was also proposed as the modulator of renal sodium and water excretion because a rise in the left atrial pressure is known to cause a water diuresis and natriuresis, mediated in part by a suppression of vasopressin and an increase in secretion of atrial and B-type natriuretic peptides. These factors also cannot fully explain ECF volume homeostasis, because renal sodium and water retention are hallmarks of congestive heart failure—a situation in which pressures in the atria and venous component of the circulation are increased.

The arterial portion of body fluids is the remaining component that may be pivotal in the regulation of renal sodium and water excretion. The relation between cardiac output and peripheral arterial resistance [termed the effective arterial blood volume (EABV)] has been proposed as a regulator of renal sodium and water reabsorption. In this context, either a decrease in cardiac output or vasodilation of the arterial tree may cause arterial underfilling and thereby initiate and sustain a sodium and water-retaining state.

Two major compensatory processes respond to arterial underfilling. One is very rapid, consisting of a neurohumoral and systemic hemodynamic response. The other is slower and involves renal sodium and water retention. In the edematous patient, these compensatory responses have usually occurred to varying degrees when the patient is seen. Whether a primary fall in cardiac output or peripheral arterial vasodilation is the initiator of arterial underfilling, the compensatory responses are quite similar and involve the stimulation of the sympathetic nervous system, the renin/angiotensin system, and vasopressin. With a decrease in ECF volume, as occurs with acute gastrointestinal losses, sufficient sodium and water retention can occur to restore cardiac output to normal and terminate renal sodium and water retention before edema forms. Such may not be the case with low-output cardiac failure because even these compensatory responses may not restore cardiac output to normal. Because of the compensatory processes described above, mean arterial pressure is an insensitive indicator of arterial fullness.

HYPOVOLEMIA

ESSENTIALS OF DIAGNOSIS

▶ History of blood loss, gastrointestinal losses, or excessive sweating.

▶ History of diuretic use.

▶ Tachycardia and postural hypotension.

▶ The jugular venous pulse is not visible.

General Considerations

Hypovolemia reflects a decrease in ECF volume (normal body fluid volumes are given in Table 2–1). The ECF volume declines when losses (NaCl losses or losses of ECF) exceed input. Simply reducing dietary NaCl intake leads to a modest decline in ECF volume, with a reduction in total body Na content approximating the reduction in daily Na intake in millimoles. Typical western diets include 4–6 g of Na (43 mmol/g of Na). Although reduced NaCl intake can lead to mild ECF volume depletion, the effects are usually not clinically significant because normal kidneys can reduce urinary NaCl excretion to very low levels.

ECF losses frequently occur via one of four routes: gastrointestinal, renal, integumentary, or into a "third space." A history of vomiting or diarrhea frequently precipitates ECF volume depletion, especially because gastrointestinal disorders are frequently associated with reduced intake. Excessive renal losses typically occur secondary to intrinsic salt-wasting disorders of the kidney, to the administration of salt-wasting diuretic drugs, or to osmotic losses via the urine, such as occur during poorly controlled diabetes.

Clinical Findings

A. Symptoms and Signs

A history of previous renal disease, familial salt wasting, or diuretic use points to salt wasting (see Table 2–2). Symptoms of polyuria, polydipsia, and polyphagia suggest diabetes. Generic symptoms of ECF volume depletion include thirst and salt craving. Patients with Addison's disease frequently manifest symptoms of lassitude. Individuals with inherited salt wasting frequently describe the desire to drink pickle juice or ingest large amounts of salty foods. When ECF volume depletion is more severe, the symptoms result from reduced plasma volume; these include weakness and eventually loss of consciousness.

1. Skin and mucous membranes—If the skin on the thigh, calf, or forearm is pinched in normal subjects, it will immediately return to its normally flat state when the pinch is released. The speed at which the skin returns to its normal

Table 2–1. Body fluid distribution.

Compartment volume in 70-kg person	Amount	Volume (L)
Total body fluid	60% of body weight	42
Intracellular fluid (ICF)	40% of body weight	28
Extracellular fluid (ECF)	20% of body weight	14
Interstitial fluid	Two-thirds of ECF	9.4
Plasma fluid	One-third of ECF	4.6
Venous fluid	85% of plasma fluid	3.9
Arterial fluid	15% of plasma fluid	0.7

flat state after being pinched is often called "skin turgor." A diminished turgor has frequently been suggested to indicate depletion of the ECF volume, but a systematic review found this sign to have no diagnostic value in adult patients. In contrast, dry axillae may suggest ECF volume depletion, whereas moist axillae argue against it. Dryness of the mucous membranes of the mouth and nose and longitudinal furrows on the tongue have also been shown to indicate ECF volume depletion.

Table 2–2. Salt-wasting disorders.

I. Renal
  A. Chronic kidney disease
  B. Postacute renal failure
  C. Postobstructive
  D. Renal tubular acidosis
II. Extrarenal
  A. Mineralocorticoid deficiency
    1. Addison's disease
    2. Isolated hypoaldosteronism
  B. Natriuretic peptide-mediated
    1. Cerebral salt wasting
    2. SIADH
III. Drug-induced
  A. Solute diuresis
    1. Mannitol
    2. Urea
    3. Glucose
    4. Bicarbonate
  B. Diuretics
    1. Proximal
    2. Loop
    3. DCT
    4. CCT

SIADH, syndrome of inappropriate secretion of antidiuretic hormone; DCT, distal convoluted tubule; CCT, cortical collecting tubule.

2. Pulse and arterial blood pressure—Changes in pulse rate and arterial pressure may indicate ECF volume depletion. When the ECF volume depletion is mild, only postural changes may be evident. Clinicians measuring postural changes should wait at least 2 minutes before measuring the supine vital signs and 1 minute after standing before measuring the upright vital signs. Counting the pulse for 30 seconds and doubling the result is more accurate than 15 seconds of observation. In normovolemic individuals, a postural pulse increment of more than 30 beats/minute is uncommon, affecting only about 2–4% of individuals.

The most helpful physical findings in the setting of blood loss are severe postural dizziness (preventing measurement of upright vital signs) or a postural pulse increment of 30 beats/minute or more. Postural changes on sitting are much less reliable. After excluding those unable to stand, postural hypotension has no incremental diagnostic value.

3. Jugular venous pressure—The reduction in the vascular volume observed with hypovolemia occurs primarily in the venous circulation (which normally contains 70% of the blood volume), thereby leading to a decrease in venous pressure. As a result, estimation of the jugular venous pressure is useful to confirm the diagnosis of hypovolemia and to assess the adequacy of volume replacement. Details concerning examination of the jugular venous pressure are presented below (ECF volume expansion). It is important to remember that a low jugular pressure (wherein the jugular pulse cannot be observed) may be normal and is consistent with, but never diagnostic of, hypovolemia.

B. Laboratory Findings

Most information concerning the state of ECF volume is obtained from the history and physical examination. Laboratory tests provide additional information, in some situations. It is worth reemphasizing that abnormalities of serum sodium concentration do not indicate the ECF volume. A hyponatremic patient may be hypovolemic, euvolemic, or hypervolemic, depending on clinical circumstances. Nevertheless, abnormal values for serum Na concentration suggest consideration of volume disorders. Further, abnormalities of serum K, Cl, or HCO_3 also suggest disorders of ECF volume. Hypokalemic metabolic alkalosis is most commonly associated with ECF depletion. Yet hypokalemic alkalosis may also be associated with hypervolemia; thus constellations of electrolyte abnormalities are not generally used to diagnose disorders of ECF volume.

Some laboratory findings do provide useful indications of ECF volume depletion. The ratio of blood urea nitrogen to creatinine, when expressed in mg/dL, frequently exceeds 20:1, when azotemia results from depletion of the ECF volume. Hemoconcentration and increases in serum uric acid concentration may also be observed. In the setting of acute renal failure, a fractional sodium excretion less than 1% suggests prerenal azotemia, which may be the result of ECF volume depletion. Yet prerenal azotemia also occurs in the setting of congestive heart failure, where the ECF volume is expanded. Thus, urine chemistry may help to determine the state of the "effective" arterial volume, but is less useful for determining ECF volume itself. As described above, hypokalemic metabolic alkalosis may be associated with an ECF volume depleted or expanded state. A urine Cl concentration of less than 10–15 mM is taken as evidence that the alkalosis is related to ECF volume depletion and should be chloride responsive.

C. Imaging Studies

Depletion or expansion of the ECF volume may be estimated by ultrasound or echocardiography. This approach is often restricted to patients in the intensive care unit but appears to be reliable. The diameter of the inferior vena or its collapse during inspiration indicates ECF volume depletion.

D. Special Tests

A measured central venous pressure provides definitive evidence of the filling pressure of the venous circulation. Placement of a pulmonary artery catheter can provide information about the left-sided filling pressure, but this technique has become less commonly employed because controlled studies suggest that it does not improve outcome.

▶ Differential Diagnosis

Many times, the differential diagnosis of ECF volume depletion is clear. On some occasions, however, the etiology is less obvious. Individuals may ingest diuretics surreptitiously, leading to hypokalemic alkalosis with volume depletion. In this situation, the urine Na and Cl concentration may be increased despite ECF volume depletion, making the diagnosis difficult. In contrast, bulimia will cause ECF volume depletion and metabolic alkalosis, in association with a very low urinary Cl concentration.

Several rare inherited or acquired diseases of kidney ion transport present with renal salt wasting. Depending on their severity and the clinical setting, salt-wasting disorders may present as unrelenting polyuria with extreme depletion of the ECF volume leading rapidly to death or as mild but troubling syndromes in which depletion of the ECF volume is nearly undetectable. Several clinical features, however, are typical of most salt-wasting disorders. These features include malaise, lassitude, fatigability, and salt craving. When mild, these symptoms can be subtle enough to lead to diagnostic difficulty. A classification of salt-wasting disorders is shown in Table 2–2.

▶ Complications

Progressive and severe hypovolemia causes organ dysfunction, including prerenal azotemia. The kidney is especially sensitive to depletion of the ECF volume or the EABV and responds by increasing retention of NaCl and water. These effects tend to restore ECF volume, but prerenal azotemia can also lead to uremia and acute tubular necrosis, if the ECF volume depletion remains untreated.

When even more severe, hypovolemia can lead to a state of shock in which the perfusion of vital organs is inadequate to meet physiological needs. In this setting, frank hypotension is present, the patient is cool and often dusky, and the mentation is impaired.

Treatment

The essential factors in treating hypovolemic conditions are to remove ongoing precipitants and correct the ECF volume depletion. Clearly, the physician should address ongoing blood, gastrointestinal, or sweat losses appropriately. When excessive diuretic use has contributed to ECF volume depletion, diuretics should be discontinued.

The choice of repletion method depends on the severity of symptoms, the nature of the losses, and the presence of superimposed disorders of osmolality (see Table 2–3). Mild ECF volume depletion frequently responds to provision of dietary NaCl and water. One of the most common causes of ECF volume depletion worldwide is infectious diarrhea, especially in children. Oral rehydration solutions (ORS) have become the standard by which all but the most serious cases are treated (see Table 2–4). These have had a dramatic impact on mortality.

When the ECF volume depletion is more severe, resuscitation with intravenous fluids is indicated. Intravenous saline or Ringer's lactate have been shown to restore ECF volume and hemodynamic stability effectively. Using albumin or starch-containing solutions does not appear to improve effectiveness. Ringer's lactate has the advantage of avoiding hyperchloremic acidosis, except in patients who have ongoing lactic acidosis, in whom the administered lactate will not be metabolized.

The rate of crystalloid administration cannot be derived from empirical formulas. In general, crystalloid may be administered at a rate 50–100 mL/hour greater than ongoing losses, unless the patient is profoundly depleted. For patients who are profoundly hypotensive or in septic shock, a goal-directed approach that combines early central venous pressure (CVP) monitoring with crystalloid administration to maintain the CVP at 8–12 mm Hg has been shown to improve outcomes. Repeated 500-mL boluses of crystalloid can be given every 30 minutes to achieve a CVP of 8–12 mm Hg. One exception to this rule is for patients who are bleeding. In this situation, blood products rather than crystalloids are recommended, with the goal of increasing the hematocrit up to a maximum of 35%. Values above this are associated with potential complications.

When ECF volume depletion is persistent, owing to ongoing renal losses, maneuvers to reduce those losses or to supplement intake are useful. Ingestion of a high salt diet or the use of the synthetic mineralocorticoid, fludrocortisone, may be useful to treat patients with inherited or acquired salt-wasting disorders.

Prognosis

The prognosis of hypovolemia is usually excellent, as long as corrective maneuvers are instituted promptly. Most authorities attribute substantial reductions in childhood mortality to the use of oral rehydration solutions to treat infectious diarrhea in developing countries.

Rivers E et al: Early goal-directed therapy in the treatment of severe sepsis and septic shock. N Engl J Med 2001;345:1368. [PMID: 11794169]

Wills BA et al: Comparison of three fluid solutions for resuscitation in dengue shock syndrome. N Engl J Med 2005;353:877. [PMID: 16135832]

Table 2–3. Treatment of ECF volume depletion in children.

	No Signs of Dehydration	Some Dehydration	Severe Dehydration
Mental state	Well, alert	Restless, irritable	Lethargic
Appearance of eyes	Normal	Sunken	Sunken
Thirst	Not thirsty	Thirsty, drinks eagerly	Drinks poorly
Skin pinch	Normal	Returns slowly	Returns very slowly
Estimated degree of dehydration	<5% or <50 mL/kg	5–10% or 50–100 mL/kg	>10% or >100 mL/kg

Suggested treatment	Treat at home
	  Give more fluids than normal
	  Give zinc supplements
	  Continue to feed child
	  Reassess if worsening
		Rehydration at health center; give ORS-based on weight; assess response; give zinc, food on discharge	Intravenous rehydration in hospital where possible; if not available, nasogastric ORS is suggested

ECF, extracellular fluids; ORS, oral rehydration solutions.
(Reproduced with permission from Cheng AC: *J Clin Gastroenterol* 2005;39:757.)

Table 2–4. Composition of oral rehydration solutions (ORS).

	Recommended rehydration therapy			Not recommended	
	"Standard" ORS (WHO, 1975)	Reduced-osmolarity ORS (WHO, 2002)	Rice-based ORS (eg, Ceralyte)	Gatorade	Coke
Glucose (g/L)	111	75	—	—	—
Carbohydrate (g/L)	—	—	40	60	110
Sodium (mEq/L)	90	75	50–90	20	6
Potassium (mEq/L)	20	20	20	3	
Chloride (mEq/L)	80	65	40	14	26
Citrate (mEq/L)	10	10	30	3	
Osmolarity (mOsm/L)	311	245	225–275	350	650

(Reproduced with permission from Cheng AC: *J Clin Gastroenterol* 2005; 39:757.)

EXTRACELLULAR FLUID VOLUME EXPANSION (EDEMATOUS DISORDERS)

► General Considerations

Starling's law states that the rate of fluid movement across a capillary wall is proportional to the hydraulic permeability of the capillary, the transcapillary hydrostatic pressure difference, and the transcapillary oncotic pressure difference. Normally, fluid leaves the capillary at the arterial end because the transcapillary hydrostatic pressure difference favoring transudation exceeds the oncotic pressure difference. In contrast, fluid returns to the capillary at the venous end because the oncotic pressure difference exceeds the hydrostatic pressure difference. Because serum albumin is the major determinant of capillary oncotic pressure, which acts to maintain fluid in the capillary, hypoalbuminemia can lead to excess transudation of fluid from the vascular to interstitial compartment. Although hypoalbuminemia might be expected to lead commonly to edema, several factors act to buffer the effects of hypoalbuminemia on fluid transudation. First, an increase in transudation tends to dilute interstitial fluid, reducing the interstitial protein concentration. Second, increases in interstitial fluid volume increase interstitial hydrostatic pressure. Third, the lymphatic flow into the jugular veins, which returns transuded fluid to the circulation, increases. In fact, in cirrhosis where hepatic fibrosis causes high capillary hydrostatic pressures in association with hypoalbuminemia, the lymphatic flow can increase 20-fold to 20 L/day, attenuating the tendency to accumulate interstitial fluid. When these safety factors are overwhelmed, interstitial fluid accumulation can lead to edema. Another factor that must be borne in mind as a cause of edema is an increase in fluid permeability of the capillary wall (an increase in hydraulic conductivity). This is the cause of edema in association with hypersensitivity reactions and angioneurotic edema and may be a factor in edema associated with diabetes mellitus and idiopathic cyclic edema.

Although these comments refer to generalized edema (ie, an increase in total body interstitial fluid), it should be noted that generalized edema may have a predilection for specific areas of the body. The formation of ascites because of portal hypertension has already been mentioned. With the normal hours of upright posture, accumulation of the edema fluid in the dependent parts of the body should be expected, whereas excessive hours at bed rest in the supine position will predispose to edema accumulation in the sacral and periorbital areas of the body.

In discussing causes of ECF volume expansion below, emphasis will be placed on diagnosis and treatment of the ECF volume expansion itself. Other chapters (for nephrotic syndrome) or other volumes in this series (for congestive heart failure and cirrhotic ascites) should be consulted for additional details about specific diagnostic and treatment approaches.

CONGESTIVE HEART FAILURE

 ESSENTIALS OF DIAGNOSIS

► History of dyspnea on exertion, orthopnea, and edema.

► Rales, an S3, and edema.

► The jugular pressure exceeds 3 cm above the sternal angle.

► Pulmonary vascular congestion is present on chest x-ray.

► Determination of B-type natriuretic peptide concentration is useful, when the cause of dyspnea is in doubt.

▶ Clinical Findings

A. Symptoms and Signs

Early clinical symptoms of cardiac failure occur before overt physical findings of pedal edema and pulmonary congestion. These symptoms relate to the compensatory renal sodium and water retention that accompanies arterial underfilling. The patient may present with a history of weight gain, weakness, dyspnea on exertion, decreased exercise tolerance, paroxysmal nocturnal dyspnea, and orthopnea. Nocturia may occur since cardiac output and therefore renal perfusion may be enhanced by the supine position. This is also why patients with congestive heart failure may lose considerable weight during the first few days of hospitalization without the administration of diuretics. Although overt edema is not detectable early in the course of congestive heart failure, the patient may complain of swollen eyes on awakening and tight rings and shoes, particularly at the end of the day. As much as 3–4 L of fluid can be retained before overt edema occurs.

1. Jugular venous pressure—As discussed above, the jugular venous pressure provides evidence of the state of the venous circulation on the right side of the heart and is very useful in evaluating patients with dyspnea. Many clinicians recommend estimating the CVP by assessing the internal jugular vein, but most formal analyses indicate that estimates of venous pressure can also be made from the external jugular vein, which runs across the sternocleidomastoid muscle. The patient should initially be recumbent, with the trunk elevated at 15–45° and the head turned slightly away from the side to be examined. The right-sided veins are preferred for assessment of venous pressure.

The external jugular vein is identified by placing the forefinger above the clavicle and pressing lightly. This will occlude the vein, which will then distend as blood continues to enter from the cerebral circulation. The external jugular vein can usually be seen more easily by shining a beam of light obliquely across the neck. At this point, the occlusion should be released and the vein occluded superiorly to prevent distention by continued blood flow. The venous pressure can now be measured, since it will be approximately equal to the vertical distance between the upper level of the fluid column within the vein and the level of the right atrium (estimated as being 5–6 cm below the sternal angle). The normal venous pressure is 1–8 cm H_2O or 1–6 mm Hg (1.36 cm H_2O is equal to 1.0 mm Hg).

Occasionally, the external jugular vein is kinked at the base of the neck. In this setting, there is an increase in the external jugular venous pressure that does not reflect a similar change in right atrial pressure. This possibility should be suspected if an elevated venous pressure is found in a patient with no evidence or history of cardiac or pulmonary disease.

Alternatively, the internal jugular vein can be examined. In this case, the venous pulsations are best distinguished from arterial pulsations by their diffuse, multiphasic negative deflections (representing three troughs, the x, x_1, and y descents, respectively). In most situations, moreover, the venous pressure declines during inspiration, whereas the arterial pressure does not.

Although precise estimates of jugular venous pressure may be attempted, these techniques have had limited accuracy in controlled studies. Comparisons of measured and estimated jugular venous pressures suggest that clinicians tend to underestimate the venous pressure. Based on reviews of empirical trials, it has been suggested that the clinicians should attempt to determine only whether the jugular pressure is more than 3 cm H_2O above the sternal angle. If so, the venous pressure is elevated. More precise estimates of the jugular venous pressure do not generally add diagnostic information.

Measurement of the CVP is useful because it is often related directly to the left ventricular end diastolic pressure (LVEDP). There are clinical settings, however, in which the CVP does not provide a reliable estimate of the LVEDP. First, some patients with pure left-sided heart failure exhibit normal CVP when the LVEDP is elevated. Conversely, the central venous pressure overestimates the LVEDP in patients with pure right-sided heart failure or cor pulmonale. These patients may have high central venous pressures even in the presence of inadequate left-sided filling pressures; as a result, the CVP cannot be used as a guide to therapy.

2. Cardiac and pulmonary examinations—A laterally displaced point of maximal impact suggests heart failure. Third heart sounds also carry both diagnostic and prognostic value in this situation. The presence of rales is also suggestive of a state of expanded ECF volume.

3. Extremities—Two-thirds of body fluid resides inside cells (ie, intracellular fluid, see Table 2–1) and one-third resides outside cells (ECF). The patient with generalized edema has an excess of ECF. The ECF resides in the vascular compartment (plasma fluid) and between the cells (interstitial fluid). In the vascular compartment, approximately 85% of the fluid resides on the venous side of the circulation and 15% on the arterial side. An excess of interstitial fluid constitutes edema. With digital pressure the interstitial fluid can generally be moved from the area of pressure and thus has been described as "pitting." If digital pressure does not cause pitting, either interstitial fluid cannot move freely or edema is absent. Pitting is more frequently demonstrated by using gentle pressure for longer periods of time rather than stronger pressure for shorter periods. Nonpitting edema can occur with lymphatic obstruction (ie, lymphedema) or regional fibrosis of subcutaneous tissue, which may occur with chronic venous stasis.

B. Laboratory Findings

For dyspneic patients, the serum concentration of B-type natriuretic peptide may provide useful information above that provided by the history and physical examination. Although the test has only marginal value for classifying patients whose dyspnea is easily determined to be either cardiac or pulmonary, based on clinical parameters, it is very useful when the diagnosis is less than clear. Thus, determination of B-type natriuretic peptide concentration should be reserved for dyspneic patients in whom a diagnosis is in doubt. Occult hypothyroidism or hyperthyroidism may present as congestive heart failure and are treatable; these conditions may be diagnosed with appropriate laboratory testing.

C. Imaging Studies

1. Chest x-ray—For dyspneic patients in whom ECF volume expansion is suspected, a PA and lateral chest radiograph is important, since the presence of pulmonary venous congestion, interstitial edema, or Kerley-B lines is helpful in confirming the presence of volume overload and heart failure.

2. Echocardiogram—The echocardiogram provides invaluable information concerning the state of left ventricular contractility. Categorization of heart failure into "systolic" dysfunction versus "diastolic" dysfunction provides both prognostic and therapeutic information. Some evidence about LVEDP can also be obtained.

► Differential Diagnosis

Patients with heart failure typically present with either edema or dyspnea. Edema may also result from nephrotic syndrome, cirrhosis of the liver, or local factors. Nephrotic-range proteinuria (>3.5 g/day) in the setting of hypoproteinemia suggests an important component of nephrosis. Typical stigmata of hepatic cirrhosis, and laboratory abnormalities suggesting the same, are often diagnostic of liver disease. Perhaps the most common diagnostic difficulty, however, is to determine whether dyspnea is the result of pulmonary or cardiac disease. As discussed above, the constellation of typical historical and physical findings of heart failure may point strongly to it as etiology, precluding the need for additional tests. When doubt is present, determination of the B-type natriuretic peptide level and, occasionally echocardiography, may prove invaluable.

► Treatment

Treatment of systolic dysfunction involves the use of angiotensin-converting enzyme (ACE) inhibitors, β-adrenergic blocking drugs, digitalis glycosides, and aldosterone blocking drugs. Details of specific treatments can be found in the companion volume, *Current Diagnosis and Treatment in Cardiology.* The current discussion will focus on treatment of ECF volume overload itself.

A. Dietary Salt Restriction

The daily sodium intake in this country is typically 4–6 g (1 g of sodium contains 43 mEq; 1 g of sodium chloride contains 17 mEq of sodium). By not using added salt at meals, the daily sodium intake can be reduced to 4 g (172 mEq), whereas a typical "low-salt" diet contains 2 g (86 mEq). Diets that are lower in sodium chloride content can be prescribed, but many individuals find them unpalatable. If salt substitutes are used, it is important to remember that these contain potassium chloride; therefore potassium-sparing diuretics (ie, spironolactone, eplerenone, triamterene, amiloride) should not be used with salt substitutes. Other drugs that increase serum potassium concentration must also be used with caution in the presence of salt substitute intake [eg, converting enzyme inhibitors, β-blockers, and nonsteroidal anti-inflammatory drugs (NSAIDs)]. When prescribing dietary therapy for an edematous patient, it is important to emphasize that sodium chloride restriction is required, even if diuretic drugs are employed. The therapeutic potency of diuretic drugs varies inversely with the dietary salt intake.

B. Diuretic Drugs

All commonly used diuretic drugs act by increasing urinary sodium excretion. They can be divided into five classes, based on their predominant site of action along the nephron (Table 2–5). Osmotic diuretics (eg, mannitol) and proximal diuretics (eg, acetazolamide) are not employed as primary agents to treat edematous disorders. Loop diuretics (eg, furosemide), distal convoluted tubule diuretics (eg, hydrochlorothiazide), and collecting duct diuretics (eg, spironolactone), however, all play important, but distinct, roles in treating edematous patients. The goal of diuretic treatment of heart failure is to reduce ECF volume and to maintain the ECF volume at the reduced level. This requires an initial natriuresis, but at steady-state urinary sodium chloride excretion returns close to baseline despite continued diuretic administration.

Importantly, an increase in sodium and water excretion does not prove therapeutic efficacy if ECF volume does not decline. Conversely, a return to "basal" levels of urinary sodium chloride excretion does not indicate diuretic resistance. The continued efficacy of a diuretic is documented by a rapid return to ECF volume expansion that occurs if the diuretic is discontinued.

When starting a loop diuretic as treatment for edema, it is important to establish a therapeutic goal, usually a target weight. If a low dose does not lead to natriuresis, it can be doubled repeatedly until the maximum recommended dose is reached (Table 2–6). When a diuretic drug is administered by mouth, the magnitude of the natriuretic response is determined by the intrinsic potency of the drug, the dose, the bioavailability, the amount delivered to the kidney, the amount that enters the tubule fluid (most diuretics that act from the luminal side), and the physiologic state of the individual. Except for proximal diuretics, the maximal natriuretic potency of a diuretic can be predicted from its site of action. Table 2–5 shows that loop diuretics can increase fractional Na excretion to 30%, distal convoluted tubule (DCT) diuretics

Table 2–5. Physiological classification of diuretic drugs.

Osmotic diuretics
Proximal diuretics
   Carbonic anhydrase inhibitors
      Acetazolamide
Loop diuretics (maximal $FE_{Na} = 30\%$)
   Na-K-2Cl inhibitors
      Furosemide
      Bumetanide
      Torsemide
      Ethacrynic acid
DCT diuretics (maximal $FE_{Na} = 9\%$)
   Na-Cl inhibitors
      Chlorothiazide
      Hydrochlorothiazide
      Metolazone
      Chlorthalidone
      Indapamide[1]
      Many others
Collecting duct diuretics (maximal $FE_{Na} = 3\%$)
   Na channel blockers
      Amiloride
      Triamterene
   Aldosterone antagonists
      Spironolactone
      Eplerenone

DCT, distal convoluted tubule; CD, collecting duct.
[1]Indapamide may have other actions as well.

can increase it to 9%, and Na channel blockers can increase it to 3% of the filtered load. The intrinsic diuretic potency of a diuretic is defined by its dose–response curve, which is generally sigmoid. The steep sigmoid relation is the reason that loop diuretic drugs are often described as "threshold drugs." When starting loop diuretic treatment, it is important to ensure that the dose reaches the steep part of the dose–response curve before adjusting the dose frequency. Because loop diuretics act rapidly, many patients will note an increase in urine output within several hours of taking the drug; this can be helpful in establishing that an adequate dose has been reached. Because loop diuretics are short-acting, any increase in urine output more than 6 hours after a dose is unrelated to drug effects. This is the reason that most loop diuretic drugs should be administered at least twice daily, when given by mouth.

The bioavailability of diuretic drugs varies widely, between classes of drugs, between different drugs of the same class, and even within drugs. The bioavailability of loop diuretics ranges from 10 to 100% (mean of 50% for furosemide, 80–100% for bumetanide and torsemide). Limited bioavailability can usually be overcome by appropriate dosing, but some drugs, such as furosemide, are variably absorbed by the same patient on different days making precise titration difficult. It is customary to double the furosemide dose when changing from intravenous to oral therapy, but the relation between intravenous and oral dose may vary. For example, the amount of sodium excreted during 24 hours is similar when furosemide is administered to a normal individual by mouth or by vein despite its 50% bioavailability. This paradox results from the fact that oral furosemide absorption is slower than its clearance, leading to "absorption-limited" kinetics. Thus, effective serum furosemide concentrations persist longer when the drug is given by mouth because a reservoir in

Table 2–6. Ceiling doses of loop diuretics.[1]

	Furosemide (mg)		Bumetanide (mg)		Torsemide (mg)	
	IV	PO	IV	PO	IV	PO
Renal Insufficiency						
GFR 20–50 mL/minute	80	80–160	2–3	2–3	50	50
GFR <20 mL/minute	200	240	8–10	8–10	100	100
Severe acute renal failure	500	NA	12	NA		
Nephrotic syndrome	120	240	3	3	50	50
Cirrhosis	40–80	80–160				1
	1–2	10–20				10–20
Congestive heart failure	40–80	160–240	2–3	2–3	20–50	50

[1]Ceiling dose indicates the dose that produces the maximal increase in fractional sodium excretion. Larger doses may increase net daily natriuresis by increasing the duration of natriuresis without increasing the maximal rate. GFR, glomerular filtration rate.
(Reproduced with permission from Brady HR, Wilcox CS, eds: *Therapy in Nephrology & Hypertension*, WB Saunders, 1999.)

Table 2–7. Complications of diuretics.

Contraction of the vascular volume

Orthostatic hypotension (from volume depletion)

Hypokalemia (from loop and DCT diuretics)

Hyperkalemia (from spironolactone, eplerenone, triamterene, and amiloride)

Gynecomastia (spironolactone)

Hyperuricemia

Hypercalcemia (thiazides)

Hypercholesterolemia

Hyponatremia (especially with DCT diuretics)

Metabolic alkalosis

Gastrointestinal upset

Hyperglycemia

Pancreatitis (DCT diuretics)

Allergic interstitial nephritis

DCT, distal convoluted tubule.

the gastrointestinal tract continues to supply furosemide to the body. This relation holds for a normal individual. Thus, it is difficult to predict the precise relation between oral and intravenous doses.

Complications of diuretic therapy are shown in Table 2–7. Although hyponatremia may be a complication of diuretic treatment, furosemide can help to ameliorate hyponatremia in some patients with congestive heart failure when combined with ACE inhibitors, probably by improving cardiac output. Hypokalemia and hypomagnesemia are frequent complications of diuretic treatment in patients with heart failure because of secondary hyperaldosteronism. This increases sodium delivery to the distal sites at which aldosterone stimulates potassium secretion. Severe renal magnesium wasting may also occur in the setting of secondary hyperaldosteronism and loop diuretic administration. Since both magnesium and potassium depletion cause similar deleterious effects on the heart, and potassium repletion is very difficult in the presence of magnesium depletion, supplemental replacement of both of these cations is frequently necessary in patients with cardiac failure. These complications have become less common with the advent of antimineralocorticoid receptor antagonist treatment.

One concern about aldosterone blockade is hyperkalemia. It is currently recommended that serum potassium be monitored 1 week after initiating therapy with an aldosterone blocker, after 1 month, and every 3 months thereafter. An increase in serum potassium of 5.5 mEq/L should prompt an evaluation for medication such as potassium supplements or NSAIDs that might be contributing to the hyperkalemia. If such factors are not detected, the dose of aldosterone blocker should be reduced 25 mg every other day. It is prudent to avoid use of aldosterone blockers in patients with a creatinine clearance less than 30 mL/minute and to be cautious in those with a creatinine clearance between 30 and 50 mL/minute. Those patients should be followed up even more closely than recommended above.

Ely EW, Haponik EF: Using the chest radiograph to determine intravascular volume status: the role of vascular pedicle width. Chest 2002;121:942. [PMID: 11888980]

Sandham JD et al: A randomized, controlled trial of the use of pulmonary-artery catheters in high-risk surgical patients. N Engl J Med 2003;348:5. [PMID: 12510037]

Wang CS et al: Does this dyspneic patient in the emergency department have congestive heart failure? JAMA 2005;294:1944. [PMID: 16234501]

DIURETIC RESISTANCE

 ESSENTIALS OF DIAGNOSIS

▶ Inadequate diuresis despite maximal doses of loop diuretics.

▶ Exclude occult nephrotic syndrome.

▶ Exclude complicating drug use, such as NSAIDs.

▶ Exclude excessive dietary NaCl intake (24-hour Na excretion measurement).

▶ General Considerations

Patients are considered to be diuretic resistant when an inadequate reduction in ECF volume is observed despite near maximal doses of loop diuretics.

▶ Clinical Findings

A. Symptoms and Signs

The major symptoms and signs of diuretic resistance are those that indicate ECF volume expansion, as described above. The most troublesome cause of diuretic resistance is progression of the underlying disease, because this situation may be difficult to address. Yet, it is always important to seek evidence of reversible or unexpected causes, so that appropriate and effective treatment can be designed (see Figure 2–1). Perhaps the most common cause of diuretic resistance is impaired diuretic delivery to the active site. Most diuretics, including the loop diuretics, DCT diuretics, and amiloride, act from the luminal surface. Although diuretics are small molecules, most circulate tightly bound to protein and reach the tubule fluid primarily by secretion, and diuretic resistance occurs when drugs do not reach the tubule fluid at sufficient levels. Uremic anions, NSAIDs, probenecid, and penicillins all inhibit loop and DCT diuretic secretion into the tubule fluid. Thus, a

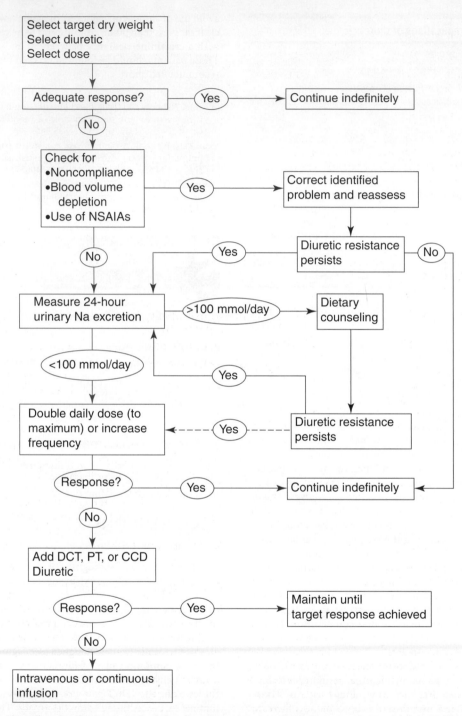

▲ **Figure 2–1.** Algorithm for the treatment of the diuretic-resistant patient. NSAIA, nonsteroidal anti-inflammatory agent; DCT, distal convoluted tubule; PT, promixal tubule; CCD, cortical collecting duct. (Reproduced with permission from Brady HR, Wilcox CS, eds: *Therapy in Nephrology & Hypertension,* WB Saunders, 1999.)

history of renal failure or use of one of the above-mentioned drugs should always be sought. Chronic kidney disease shifts the loop diuretic dose–response curve to the right, requiring a higher dose to achieve maximal effect. Patients with chronic kidney disease are often given doses below those that are required to achieve therapeutic efficacy.

B. Laboratory Findings

One common cause of apparent diuretic resistance is excessive dietary sodium chloride intake. When sodium chloride intake is high, renal sodium chloride retention can occur between natriuretic periods, maintaining the ECF volume expansion. A careful history of dietary salt intake is always essential, but measuring the sodium excreted during 24 hours can be useful in diagnosing excessive intake. If the patient is at steady state (the weight is stable), then the urinary sodium excreted during 24 hours is equal to the dietary sodium chloride intake. If sodium excretion exceeds 100–120 mmol/day (approximately 2–3 g sodium/day), then dietary sodium chloride consumption is too high and dietary counseling should be undertaken. If the sodium excretion exceeds 100–120 mmol/day this also indicates that the patient is not diuretic resistant; this rate of sodium excretion should be sufficient to induce negative salt balance.

As noted above, diuretic resistance is common in chronic kidney disease. Further, diuretic treatment itself, especially in the setting of ACE inhibitors, may predispose to acute renal failure. Both acute and chronic renal failure lead to diuretic resistance, and measurement of blood urea nitrogen and serum creatinine is always important.

▶ Treatment

Several strategies are available to achieve effective control of ECF volume in patients who do not respond to full doses of effective loop diuretics.

A. Combination Diuretic Therapy

A diuretic of another class may be added to a regimen that includes a loop diuretic (see Table 2–8). This strategy produces true synergy; the combination of agents is more effective than the sum of the responses to each agent alone. DCT diuretics are the class of drug most commonly combined with loop diuretics. They inhibit adaptive changes in the distal nephron that increase the reabsorptive capacity of the tubule and limit the potency of loop diuretics. Further, DCT diuretics have longer half-lives than loop diuretics. These drugs therefore prevent or attenuate NaCl retention during the periods between doses of loop diuretics, thereby increasing their net effect. When two diuretics are combined, the DCT diuretic is generally administered some time before the loop diuretic (1 hour is reasonable) in order to ensure that NaCl transport in the distal nephron is blocked when it is flooded with solute. When intravenous therapy is indicated, chlorothiazide

Table 2–8. Combination diuretic therapy (to add to a ceiling dose of a loop diuretic).

Distal convoluted tubule diuretics
Metolazone 2.5-10 mg PO daily[1]
Hydrochlorothiazide (or equivalent) 25-100 mg orally daily
Chlorothiazide 500-1000 mg intravenously
Proximal tubule diuretics
Acetazolamide 250-375 mg daily or up to 500 mg intravenously
Collecting duct diuretics
Spironolactone 100-200 mg daily
Amiloride 5-10 mg daily

[1]Metolazone is generally best given for a limited period of time (3–5 days) or should be reduced in frequency to three times per week once extracellular fluid volume has declined to the target level. Only in patients who remain volume expanded should full doses be continued indefinitely, based on the target weight. (Reproduced with permission from Brady HR, Wilcox CS, eds: *Therapy in Nephrology & Hypertension*, WB Saunders, 1999.)

(500–1000 mg) may be employed. Metolazone is the DCT diuretic most frequently combined with loop diuretics because its half-life is relatively long (as formulated in Zaroxylin®) and because it has been reported to be effective even when renal failure is present. Other thiazide and thiazide-like diuretics, however, appear to be equally effective, even in severe renal failure. The dramatic effectiveness of combination diuretic therapy is accompanied by complications in a significant number of patients. Massive fluid and electrolyte losses have led to circulatory collapse during combination therapy and patients must be followed carefully. The lowest effective dose of DCT diuretic should be added to the loop diuretic regimen; patients can frequently be treated with combination therapy for only a few days and then placed back on a single drug regimen; when continuous combination therapy is needed low doses of DCT diuretic (2.5 mg metolazone or 25 mg hydrochlorothiazide) administered only two or three times per week may be sufficient.

B. Continuous Diuretic Infusion

For hospitalized patients who are resistant to diuretic therapy, a different approach is to infuse loop diuretics continuously (see Table 2–9). Continuous diuretic infusions have several advantages over bolus diuretic administration. First, because they avoid peaks and troughs of diuretic concentration, continuous infusions prevent periods of positive NaCl balance (postdiuretic NaCl retention) from occurring. Second, continuous infusions are more efficient than bolus therapy (the amount of NaCl excreted per mg of drug administered is greater). Third, some patients who are resistant to large doses of diuretics given by bolus have responded to continuous infusion. Fourth, diuretic response can be titrated; in the intensive care unit where obligate fluid administration must

Table 2–9. Continuous infusion of loop diuretics.

Diuretic	Starting bolus (mg)	Infusion rate (mg/hour)		
		GFR < 25 mL/minute	GFR 25–75 mL/minute	GFR > 75 mL/minute
Furosemide	40	20 then 40	10 then 20	10
Bumetanide	1	1 then 2	0.5 then 1	05
Torsemide	20	10 then 20	5 then 10	5

GFR, glomerular filtration rate.

be balanced by fluid excretion, excellent control of NaCl and water excretion can be obtained. Finally, complications associated with high doses of loop diuretics, such as ototoxicity, appear to be less common when large doses are administered as continuous infusion. Total daily furosemide doses exceeding 1 g have been tolerated well when administered over 24 hours. One approach is to administer a loading dose of 20 mg furosemide followed by a continuous infusion at 4–60 mg/hour. In patients with preserved renal function, therapy at the lower dosage range should be sufficient. When renal failure is present, higher doses may be used, but patients should be monitored carefully for side effects such as ECF volume depletion and ototoxicity.

C. Ultrafiltration

When therapy with diuretic drugs fails, ultrafiltration using hemodialysis equipment or a specialized ultrafiltration apparatus has been used. Although this approach is not recommended for routine use, the response to volume removal via ultrafiltration may be more sustained than after an equivalent volume removal via diuretics.

Salvador DR et al: Continuous infusion versus bolus injection of loop diuretics in congestive heart failure. Cochrane Database Syst Rev:CD003178, 2005. [PMID: 16034890]

HEPATIC CIRRHOSIS

 ESSENTIALS OF DIAGNOSIS

▶ History of alcoholism or viral hepatitis.
▶ Stigmata of chronic liver disease including jaundice and spider angiomata.
▶ Signs of portal hypertension including ascites.
▶ Laboratory abnormalities include elevated bilirubin and reduced albumin.

General Considerations

The pathogenesis of the renal sodium and water retention is similar in all varieties of cirrhosis, including alcoholic, viral, and biliary cirrhosis. Studies in both humans and animals indicate that renal sodium and water retention precedes the formation of ascites in cirrhosis. Thus, the classic underfill theory, which attributed renal sodium and water retention of cirrhosis to ascites formation with resultant hypovolemia, seems untenable as a primary mechanism. Since plasma volume expansion secondary to renal sodium and water excretion occurs prior to ascites formation, the overflow theory of ascites formation was proposed. This postulated that an undefined process, triggered by the diseased liver (eg, increased intrahepatic pressure), causes renal sodium and water retention that then overflows into the abdomen because of portal hypertension. This overflow theory, however, predicts that renal salt retention and ascites formation would be associated with decreased levels of vasopressin, renin, aldosterone, and norepinephrine. Because these hormones rise progressively as cirrhosis advances from the states of compensation (no ascites) to decompensation (ascites) to hepatorenal syndrome, the overflow hypothesis also does not seem to explain the renal sodium and water retention associated with advanced cirrhosis. The peripheral arterial vasodilation theory is compatible with most of the known observations in patients during the various stages of cirrhosis. According to this theory, cirrhosis causes arterial vasodilation and a decline in blood pressure; hypotension stimulates renal NaCl retention. The cause of the primary arterial vasodilation in cirrhosis is not clear, but is known to occur early in the course of the disease before ascites formation. The opening of existing splanchnic arteriovenous shunts may account for some early arterial vasodilation. Later, anatomically new portosystemic and arteriovenous shunting secondary to the portal hypertension may also occur.

Treatment

Options for treating cirrhotic ascites and edema include dietary NaCl restriction, diuretic drugs, large volume paracentesis, peritoneovenous shunting, portosystemic shunting (usually transjugular portosystemic shunting or TIPS), and liver transplantation (see Figure 2–2). Each of these approaches has a role in the treatment of cirrhotic ascites, but most patients can be treated successfully with dietary restriction, diuretics, and, when necessary, large volume paracentesis.

A. Diuretics

The initial therapy of cirrhotic ascites is supportive, including dietary sodium restriction and cessation of alcohol. When these maneuvers prove inadequate, diuretic treatment should begin with spironolactone. Spironolactone has several advantages over loop diuretics in this situation. First,

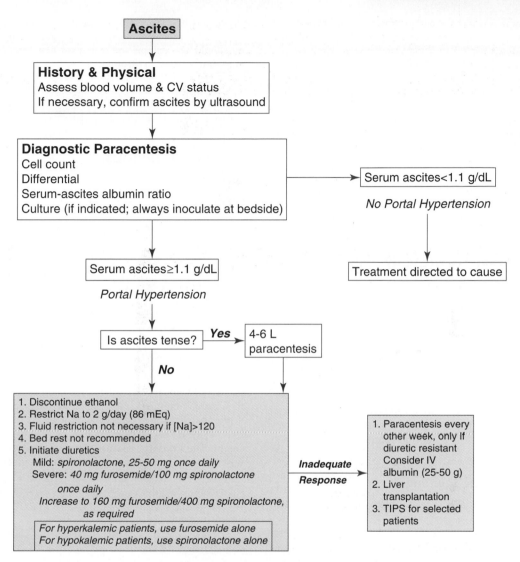

▲ **Figure 2–2.** Algorithm for treatment of ascites. TIPS, transjugular intrahepatic portosystemic shunting. (Reproduced with permission from Brady HR, Wilcox CS, eds: *Therapy in Nephrology & Hypertension,* 2nd edition, WB Saunders, 2003.)

spironolactone is more effective than furosemide as a single agent in reducing cirrhotic ascites. Second, spironolactone is a long-acting diuretic that can be given once per day in doses ranging from 25 to 400 mg/day. Third, unlike most other diuretics, hypokalemia does not occur when spironolactone is administered. Hypokalemia increases renal ammoniagenesis and can precipitate encephalopathy.

The most common side effects of spironolactone are painful gynecomastia and hyperkalemia. Gynecomastia is less common with the more selective antagonist, eplerenone, which may be substituted, but less information concerning its effectiveness in treating cirrhotic ascites is available.

Amiloride, another K-sparing diuretic, can be used as an alternate, although spironolactone tends to be more effective. For patients who do not respond to a low dose of spironolactone, spironolactone can be combined with furosemide, starting at 100 mg spironolactone/40 mg furosemide (to a maximum of 400 mg spironolactone/160 mg furosemide). This regimen has the advantages of once per day dosing and minimal hypokalemia.

The appropriate rate of diuresis depends on the presence or absence of peripheral edema. Because mobilizing ascitic fluid into the vascular compartment is slow (approximately 500 mL/day), the rate of daily diuresis should be limited to

0.5 kg/day if peripheral edema is absent. In the presence of edema, most patients can tolerate up to 1.0 kg/day of fluid removal. Since ascites in the decompensated cirrhotic patient is associated with substantial complications including (1) spontaneous bacterial peritonitis (50–80% mortality), which does not occur in the absence of ascites; (2) impaired ambulation, decreased appetite, and back and abdominal pain; (3) elevated diaphragm with decreased ventilation predisposing to hypoventilation, atelectasis, and pulmonary infections; and (4) negative cosmetic and psychological effects, the treatment of the ascites with diuretics and sodium restriction is appropriate. The approach outlined above is successful in approximately 90% of patients and complications are rare. In earlier studies in which there were complications of diuretic therapy, more aggressive diuretic regimens were often used.

B. Large Volume Paracentesis

Total paracentesis in increments over 3 days or, more commonly, at one setting has been shown to have few complications; in some studies paracentesis appears to have a lower incidence of complications than does diuretic treatment. When peripheral edema is absent, albumin (6 g for each liter of ascitic fluid removed) may be infused to reduce hemodynamic compromise. The use of albumin remains controversial in patients with concomitant edema. Patients often favor paracentesis over diuretic treatment because symptoms improve more rapidly, but diuretics and salt restriction continue to be primary approaches and are required between paracentesis, even in those patients who cannot be maintained on diuretics alone.

C. Portosystemic Shunting

Portosystemic shunting is now usually performed via TIPS. Uncontrolled trials suggested that TIPS increases urine output, reduces ascites, and reduces diuretic usage. In a meta-analysis TIPS was found to be effective in reducing ascites, but was also shown to carry a substantial complication rate, including inducing encephalopathy. Therefore it remains reserved for truly refractory patients who will not receive a liver transplant. Similar considerations apply to peritoneovenous (LeVeen) shunting. In controlled trials, peritoneovenous shunting was shown to reduce ascites more effectively than paracentesis or diuretics, but this was associated with a high rate of complications, and there was no survival advantage of the shunt.

D. Liver Transplantation

The development of ascites in a previously compensated cirrhotic patient is an indication for liver transplantation. In view of the morbidity and mortality associated with decompensated cirrhosis, liver transplantation is an important treatment for the ECF volume expansion that accompanies

cirrhotic ascites. Worsening of ascites in a previously stable individual is most often caused by progressive liver disease but should also compel the search for hepatocellular carcinoma and portal vein thrombosis.

Albillos A et al: A meta-analysis of transjugular intrahepatic portosystemic shunt versus paracentesis for refractory ascites. J Hepatol 2005;43:990. [PMID: 16139922]

NEPHROTIC SYNDROME

ESSENTIALS OF DIAGNOSIS

▶ Signs of ECF volume expansion, including edema.
▶ Proteinuria greater than 3.5 g/day.
▶ Hypoalbuminemia.
▶ Hyperlipidemia may or may not be present.
▶ Kidney function may be normal or impaired.

▶ General Considerations

Another major cause of edema is the nephrotic syndrome, the clinical hallmarks of which include proteinuria (>3.5 g/day), hypoalbuminemia, hypercholesterolemia, and edema. Nephrotic edema may be mistaken for congestive heart failure, if evidence for proteinuria or hypoalbuminemia is not sought. The lower the plasma albumin concentration, the more likely the occurrence of anasarca; the degree of sodium intake is, however, also a determinant of the degree of edema. The nephrotic syndrome has many causes (see Chapter 23). This discussion will focus on treatment of ECF volume expansion in nephrosis.

▶ Pathogenesis

The pathogenesis of ECF volume expansion in nephrotic syndrome is more variable than the pathogenesis in congestive heart failure or cirrhotic ascites. Traditionally, ECF volume expansion in nephrotic syndrome was believed to depend on underfilling of the arterial circulation. Several observations have raised questions about this hypothesis and a role for primary renal sodium chloride retention in the pathogenesis of nephrotic edema has been suggested. While "primary" renal NaCl retention may contribute to nephrotic edema in many patients, it is not often the only mechanism, and it appears therefore that nephrotic syndrome reflects a combination of primary renal sodium chloride retention and relative underfilling. The major consequence of the presence of a component of primary renal sodium retention is that nephrotic patients often tolerated relatively aggressive diuretic regimens without undue consequences.

▶ Treatment

The initial focus of therapy must be aimed at treatable systemic causes of nephrotic syndrome such as systemic lupus erythematosus or drugs (eg, phenytoin, NSAIDs) (see chapters on specific disease processes for additional details).

A. Diuretics

The treatment of the edema in nephrotic patients involves dietary sodium restriction and diuretics, as in other volume expansion disorders. Because nephrotic patients may not be as underfilled as patients with cirrhosis or congestive heart failure, diuretics are often tolerated well. Loop diuretics are always used as initial therapy. For several reasons, however, nephrotic patients are often quite resistant to these drugs. Although low serum albumin concentrations may increase the volume of diuretic distribution and albumin in the tubule lumen may bind to diuretics, these factors are not considered to be predominant causes of resistance. Rather, diuretic resistance likely reflects a combination of reduced glomerular filtration rate (from the ongoing glomerular disease) and intense renal sodium chloride retention (reflecting both primary renal sodium retention and a redistribution of fluid from the vascular compartment to the interstitium).

B. Albumin

Administration of albumin to patients with the nephrotic syndrome can be costly and cause pulmonary edema. Mixing albumin with a loop diuretic (6.25 g albumin per 40 mg furosemide) may induce a diuresis in severely hypoalbuminemic patients. Coadministration of furosemide and albumin may be more effective than either albumin or furosemide alone, but only marginally so. In general, albumin should be reserved for the most refractory patients who are severely hypoalbuminemic.

Wilcox CS: New insights into diuretic use in patients with chronic renal disease. J Am Soc Nephrol 2002;13:798. [PMID: 11856788]

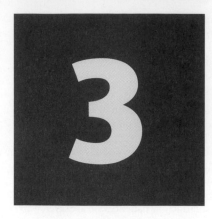

Disorders of Water Balance: Hyponatremia & Hypernatremia

Clancy Howard, MD, & Tomas Berl, MD

HYPONATREMIA

ESSENTIALS OF DIAGNOSIS

▶ Hyponatremia develops due to an excess of total body water in relation to total body sodium.

▶ Determination of extracellular volume status and urinary indices aids in the classification of hyponatremia.

▶ General Considerations

Hyponatremia is present when the serum sodium concentration falls below 135 mEq/L. In healthy subjects, the sodium concentration is closely regulated to remain between 138 and 142 mEq/L despite wide variations in water intake (Figure 3–1). When excess water is ingested, the normal kidney dilutes the urine, excretes excess water, and prevents the development of hyponatremia. Hyponatremia develops when the intake of water exceeds the ability to excrete it leading to dilution of total body sodium.

▶ Pathogenesis

Sodium concentration is the major determinant of plasma osmolality, therefore hyponatremia usually indicates a low plasma osmolality. Plasma osmolality can be estimated by the following equation:

$$\text{Plasma Osm} = (2 \times [\text{Na}]) + ([\text{BUN mg/dL}]/2.8) + ([\text{Glucose mg/dL}]/18)$$

Low plasma osmolality rather than hyponatremia, per se, is the primary cause of the symptoms of hyponatremia. Hyponatremia not accompanied by hypoosmolality does not cause signs or symptoms and does not require specific treatment.

The limitation in the kidney's ability to excrete water in hyponatremic states is, in most cases, due to the persistent action of antidiuretic hormone (ADH, vasopressin). ADH acts at the distal nephron to decrease the renal excretion of water. The action of ADH is, therefore, to concentrate the urine and, as a result, dilute the serum. Under normal circumstances, ADH release is stimulated primarily by hyperosmolality. However, under conditions of severe intravascular volume depletion or hypotension, ADH may be released even in the presence of serum hypoosmolality. Disease states characterized by a low cardiac output or systemic vasodilation result in "effective" intravascular volume depletion and may also stimulate ADH release.

Importantly, ADH alone is not sufficient to cause hyponatremia. Only when the intake of water exceeds its excretory capacity can hyponatremia result. In some cases, massive water ingestion or a defective urinary concentrating mechanism can cause hyponatremia despite the complete absence of circulating ADH.

▶ Clinical Findings

A. Symptoms and Signs

The symptoms and signs of hyponatremia most likely result from cellular and cerebral edema. Headache, lethargy, confusion, weakness, psychosis, ataxia, seizures, and coma can all occur. Although no consistent correlation between the degree of hyponatremia and neurologic manifestations exists, patients with seizures and altered sensorium generally have serum sodium concentrations less than 120 mEq/L.

Understanding the physiology of water movement is essential to understand the symptomatology and proper treatment of the disorders of water balance. In hyponatremia, the fall in plasma osmolality causes osmotic movement of water from the hypotonic extracellular compartment into relatively hypertonic cells. When the movement of water into cells occurs rapidly and exceeds the ability of the cells

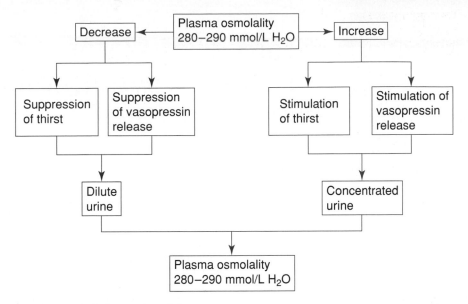

▲ Figure 3–1. Normal control of plasma osmolality.

to compensate, cellular edema occurs and the symptoms of hyponatremia can result. Over a period of days the cells of the brain are able to adapt to a decreased extracellular tonicity by losing osmolytes, thereby decreasing intracellular tonicity. Once cells have adapted, rapid correction of hyponatremia can leave the extracellular space relatively hypertonic. This causes water to move out of cells into the hypertonic extracellular space causing cellular dehydration. In the brain, this can lead to central pontine myelinolysis (CPM).

Consequently, acute hyponatremia developing over less than 48 hours is more likely present with typical symptoms due to the lack of complete cerebral adaptation. In contrast, hyponatremia developing over more than 48 hours, even when severe, may be entirely asymptomatic due to the adaptive capacity of the brain.

B. Laboratory Findings

Typical clinical findings of hypovolemia include diminished skin turgor, flattened neck veins, dry mucous membranes and axillae, orthostatic hypotension, and tachycardia. In mild cases, hypovolemia may not be clinically apparent but usually results in renal sodium avidity and a urinary sodium concentration of less than 10 mEq/L. Vomiting is sometimes accompanied by metabolic alkalosis that obligates urinary bicarbonate and sodium losses, increasing the urinary sodium concentration to greater than 20 mEq/L. In this situation, hypovolemia can be confirmed by measuring the urinary chloride concentration, which is typically less than 10 mEq/L in this setting. Renal volume losses generally occur due to the administration of diuretics and result in a urinary sodium concentration greater than 10 mEq/L.

An increased extracellular volume may be evidenced by distended neck veins, pulmonary edema, ascites, or lower extremity edema. Hypervolemic hyponatremia is generally due to volume-retaining states such as congestive heart failure, cirrhosis, nephrotic syndrome, or advanced renal failure. In the absence of diuretic administration, hypervolemic hyponatremia is usually accompanied by "effective" hypovolemia and, consequently, a urinary sodium concentration less than 10 mEq/L.

Clinical determination of euvolemia is confirmed by the absence of signs of hypovolemia or hypervolemia. The urinary sodium concentration is greater than 20 mEq/L.

▶ Differential Diagnosis

Hyponatremia should be approached systematically using an algorithm. The first step involves determining whether the observed hyponatremia is associated with a decreased, normal, or even elevated plasma osmolality (Figure 3–2).

A. Hyponatremia with a Normal or High Plasma Osmolality

Hyponatremia can be present in the absence of hypoosmolality when one of two situations is present. In the most common situation, osmotically active substances unable to enter the cell, such as glucose (in the absence of insulin), mannitol, or glycine (employed in hysteroscopy, laparoscopy, and transurethral resection of the prostate), cause water to move from the intracellular to the extracellular space. This water movement dilutes the extracellular sodium resulting in hyponatremia but, importantly, not hypoosmolality. Since serum tonicity does not change, symptoms of hyponatremia do not

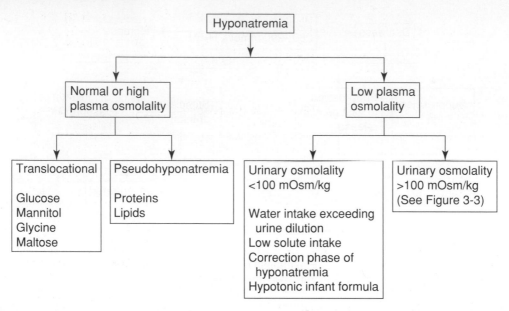

▲ **Figure 3–2.** Initial approach to hyponatremia.

develop. When hyperglycemia is present, the underlying sodium concentration can be estimated by adding 1.6–2.4 mEq/L to the reported sodium concentration for every 100 mg/dL increase in the plasma glucose.

When present, severe hyperlipidemia or hyperproteinemia alter the usual ratio of serum water to solute. Since most clinical laboratories assume a constant ratio and perform a dilution of the serum prior to measuring sodium concentration, the serum water content is overestimated resulting in the reporting of incorrect or "pseudohyponatremia." This error can be avoided by measuring the sodium concentration in undiluted serum using a sodium-selective electrode.

B. Hyponatremia with Low Plasma Osmolality and Low Urine Osmolality

Most often, hyponatremia is associated with a low plasma osmolality. In these cases, determination of the urinary osmolality allows differentiation between hyponatremia resulting from a functioning urinary diluting system that is overwhelmed by hypotonic fluid administration (urine osmolarity <100 mOsm/kg) and hyponatremia resulting from an inability to appropriately dilute the urine (urine osmolarity >100 mOsm/kg)(Figure 3–2).

Hyponatremia that develops despite normal urinary dilution is caused by excessive fluid ingestion or inadequate solute intake, or develops during the correction phase of hyponatremia.

Primary polydipsia is a common problem in psychiatric patients, particularly in those with schizophrenia. In contrast to the syndrome of inappropriate antidiuretic hormone (SIADH), primary polydipsia develops despite maximally suppressed ADH secretion and a maximally dilute urine. Though psychogenic stress may cause defects in urinary dilution, the primary cause of the hyponatremia is the ingestion of massive quantities of water that overwhelm the renal excretory capacity. Urine output in these patients is typically very high.

Subjects that ingest very little dietary solute may develop an ADH independent impairment in renal water excretion. Modest increases in water intake may lead to hyponatremia despite maximal urinary dilution. Poorly nourished, chronic beer drinkers classically develop this condition but other malnourished patients may be similarly affected.

C. Hyponatremia with a Low Plasma Osmolality and Elevated Urine Osmolality

When hyponatremia is associated with low plasma and elevated urinary osmolality it is useful to classify patients based on extracellular volume status (Figure 3–3). Since total body sodium content is the primary determinant of extracellular volume, patients with low, normal, or high extracellular volumes have low, normal, or high total body sodium contents, respectively. Hyponatremia occurs due to an increase in total body water relative to total body sodium.

D. Hyponatremia with Extracellular Volume Depletion

In hypovolemic hyponatremia nonosmotic release of ADH occurs in response to hypovolemia. Despite serum hypoosmolality, circulating ADH causes urinary concentration, water retention, and hyponatremia.

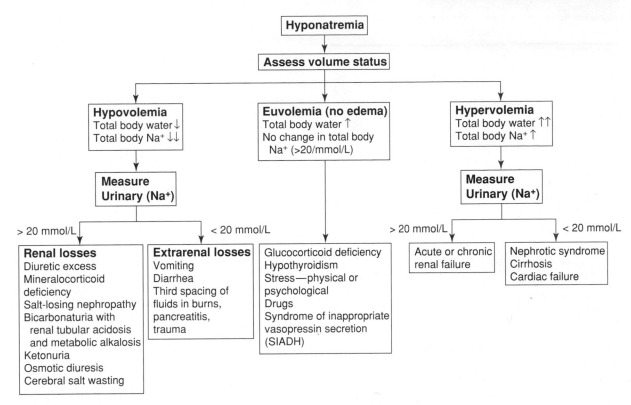

▲ **Figure 3–3.** Approach to hyponatremia with elevated urinary osmolality. (Adapted with permission from Johnson RJ, Freehaly J (editors): *Comprehensive Clinical Nephrology*, 2nd ed. Mosby, 2003.)

A patient with hypovolemia has a deficit of total body sodium resulting from either extrarenal or renal sodium losses. Extrarenal sodium loss can occur from the gastrointestinal tract in the form of vomiting or diarrhea, skin, or through third-space fluid sequestration. Common causes of renal sodium loss occur following diuretic administration or osmotic diuresis. Rarer causes of renal sodium loss occur due to cerebral salt wasting, salt-losing nephropathy, or mineralocorticoid deficiency.

E. Hyponatremia with Normal Extracellular Volume

Euvolemic hyponatremia is the most common form of hyponatremia in hospitalized patients. Normally, euvolemic hyponatremia develops due to inadequate urinary dilution evidenced by an inappropriately elevated urine osmolality (urine osmolality > 100 mOsm/kg H_2O).

1. Syndrome of inappropriate antidiuretic hormone release—SIADH is the commonest cause of euvolemic hyponatremia but remains a diagnosis of exclusion (Table 3–1).

Under normal circumstances, in the setting of hypoosmolality and euvolemia, ADH is maximally suppressed

and urine is maximally dilute. In SIADH, however, ADH is inappropriately released and the urine, consequently, is concentrated. Despite abnormal water handling, sodium regulatory mechanisms remain intact and patients do not become hypervolemic. Hypouricemia is commonly seen in SIADH due to both dilution and increased uric acid elimination.

SIADH is most commonly associated with medication administration (Table 3–2). With widespread use, selective serotonin reuptake inhibitor (SSRI) antidepressants deserve

Table 3–1. Essential diagnostic criteria for the syndrome of inappropriate vasopressin release (SIADH).

Decreased extracellular fluid effective osmolality (<270 mOsm/kg H_2O)
Inappropriate urinary concentration (>100 mOsm/kg H_2O) Clinical euvolemia
Elevated urinary Na^+ concentration (>20 mEq/L) under conditions of a normal salt and water intake
Absence of adrenal, thyroid, pituitary, or renal insufficiency or diuretic use

Adapted with permission from Johnson RJ, Freehally J (editors): *Comprehensive Clinical Nephrology*, 2nd ed. Mosby, 2003.

Table 3–2. Drugs associated with hyponatremia.

Vasopressin analogs
Desmopressin (DDAVP)
Oxytocin

Drugs that potentiate renal vasopressin
Chlorpropamide
Cyclophosphamide
Nonsteroidal anti-inflammatory agents
Acetaminophen

Drugs that enhance vasopressin release
Chlorpropamide
Clofibrate
Carbamazepine-oxycarbazepine
Vincristine
Nicotine
Narcotics
Antipsychotics/antidepressants
Ifosfamide

Drugs that cause hyponatremia by unknown mechanisms
Haloperidol
Fluphenazine
Amitriptyline
Thioradazine
Fluoxetine
Metamphetamine (MDMA or Ecstacy)
Selective serotonin reuptake inhibitors

Adapted with permission from Johnson RJ, Freehally J (editors): *Comprehensive Clinical Nephrology*, 2nd ed. Mosby, 2003.

mention as frequent causative agents, particularly among the elderly. Malignancy, pulmonary or central nervous system (CNS) disease, infection, and trauma are responsible for the remainder of cases. SIADH is also been frequently described in association with human immunodeficiency virus (HIV) infection.

In SIADH, inappropriate urinary concentration may be due to either exogenous ADH secretion or potentiation of the effect of ADH on the nephron. Rarely, ADH is appropriately suppressed by hypoosmolality, but at an unusually low level. This "reset osmostat" has been described in the elderly, in pregnant women, and in paraplegics.

2. Glucocorticoid deficiency—In both primary and secondary adrenal insufficiency, a deficiency of glucocorticoid is associated with elevated ADH levels and impaired water excretion. A standard cortisol stimulation test can be used to exclude glucocorticoid deficiency. If present, administration of replacement doses of glucocorticoid correct the hyponatremia.

3. Hypothyroidism—Hyponatremia occurs in some patients with severe hypothyroidism. Though not clearly defined, ADH-dependent and ADH-independent mechanisms have been implicated. The hyponatremia associated with hypothyroidism is readily reversed by administration of levothyroxine.

4. Postoperative hyponatremia—Postoperative hyponatremia occurs mainly in the setting of excess infusion of hypotonic fluids following invasive procedures. Hyponatremia in the postoperative setting may also occur following the administration of isotonic fluids if serum ADH is elevated. Since sodium handling mechanisms are typically intact, excess infused sodium is excreted, water is retained, and hyponatremia results. Hyponatremia in the postoperative setting has been associated with the development of cerebral edema and catastrophic neurologic events. Premenopausal women appear to be at particular risk of developing complications.

F. Hyponatremia with Excess Extracellular Volume

In hypervolemic hyponatremia, both total body sodium and total body water are increased, but total body water is increased to a greater amount. Edematous disorders such as congestive heart failure, cirrhosis, and nephrotic syndrome trigger renal sodium retention and consequent hypervolemia. These disease states all have a low effective circulating arterial volume that results in excessive thirst and ADH release. The degree of hyponatremia often correlates with the severity of the disorder and is an important prognostic factor. In the absence of diuretic administration, the urinary sodium concentration is less than 10 mEq/L. Advanced acute or chronic renal failure may also be associated with hyponatremia if the intake of water exceeds the ability to excrete it.

▶ Treatment

A. Euvolemic Hyponatremia

Most commonly, euvolemic hyponatremia develops slowly and is often relatively asymptomatic. The principal risk in adapted patients is not hyponatremia, per se. Rather it is overzealous correction that either decreases the serum sodium further or increases it too quickly. Accordingly, therapy for asymptomatic patients is conservative, consisting initially of water restriction and, if possible, removal of the inciting etiology.

In most cases, restricting fluid intake to less than 1 L/24 hours will be sufficient to allow the sodium to rise slowly. Unless hypovolemia is suspected clinically, 0.9% saline should not be given empirically as it will in most cases of euvolemic hyponatremia cause the serum sodium to fall further and may precipitate neurologic symptoms.

In some patients with severely impaired urinary dilutional capacity, clinically achievable water restriction is not sufficient to correct the hyponatremia. In these patients, treatment with demeclocycline may decrease urinary concentration and allow greater ingestion of water. Vasopressin (V_2-receptor) antagonists (Tolvaptan) have recently been described to promote excretion of electrolyte-free water or 'aquaresis' thereby making them attractive treatment options for treatment of euvolemic hyponatremia. Such was described in the SALT-1 and 2 (Study of Ascending Levels of Tolvaptan in Hyponatremia) trials, performed in an outpatient setting. A combined V_1/V_2-receptor antagonist (Vaprisol) is currently approved for parenteral use in the US.

Rapid correction is indicated in patients with acute (<48 hours), symptomatic hyponatremia. Though safe, full correction is not necessary. Rapid correction can be achieved by the administration of hypertonic saline and concomitant furosemide.

When symptomatic, the treatment of chronic euvolemic hyponatremia is made dually challenging by the urgent need for correction and attendant risk of overrapid correction and CPM. Therapy must therefore be undertaken with caution in the intensive care unit.

Patients presenting with euvolemic hyponatremia accompanied by seizures require emergent treatment with hypertonic 3% saline at an initial rate of 1–2 mL/kg/hour. Once the serum sodium rises 10% or neurologic symptoms resolve, conservative therapy should be adopted.

Patients who are obtunded but not seizing do not require treatment with hypertonic saline. The goal in the treatment of moderately symptomatic, euvolemic hyponatremia is to force the excretion of excess total body water at a rate that will result in a safe rate of rise of the serum sodium concentration. The goal rate of rise of sodium should not exceed 1 mEq/L/hour or 12 mEq/day to minimize the risk of developing CPM. Excess total body water is estimated by the following equation:

$$\text{Body water excess (L)} = 0.6 \times \text{Wgt (kg)} \times [1 - ([Na]/[\text{Desired } [Na]])]$$

The estimated time of correction can be calculated by dividing the desired change in sodium concentration by the goal rate of rise. Since there is no need to acutely correct the sodium concentration to a normal value, an increase in sodium concentration of 10% should be the initial goal. Division of the total body water excess by the estimated time of correction will result in the goal rate of water excretion.

Low doses of loop diuretic are used to initiate diuresis. Initially, the urinary volume, sodium, and potassium concentration should be measured hourly. Urinary, sodium, potassium, and water losses exceeding the goal rate should be corrected intravenously. The serum sodium must be monitored closely to ensure an appropriate rate of rise. If the sodium concentration increases rapidly, intravenous 5% dextrose should be given to decrease it to the desired level.

During treatment of euvolemic hyponatremia, as the underlying cause is corrected, a brisk water diuresis may result. Untreated, this rapid loss of hypotonic urine will correct the serum sodium too quickly and put the patient at increased risk of developing CPM. Water diuresis should be treated by replacing approximately 75% of the urine output with 5% dextrose (D_5W) with close monitoring of the serum sodium.

If the urine output is very high, water repletion alone may be impractical. In this case, the urine output can be slowed by the administration of exogenous desmopressin.

B. Hypovolemic Hyponatremia

The treatment of hypovolemic hyponatremia involves removing the stimulus for ADH release by correction of the volume deficit and allowing renal excretion of excess water. In acute hyponatremia (<48 hours), developing over less than 48 hours, the brain has not had sufficient time to compensate for the extracellular hypoosmolality. Thus, acutely, cellular swelling and cerebral edema constitute the major risk. Asymptomatic patients should be treated with volume restoration with isotonic 0.9% saline. Once extracellular volume is restored, the stimulus for ADH release will be removed allowing renal excretion of water and a return to a normal sodium concentration.

The treatment of chronic hypovolemic hyponatremia is complicated by presumed cerebral adaptation to hypoosmolality and, therefore, the risk of overrapid correction of the serum sodium. When hypovolemic hyponatremia has been present for more than 48 hours or is unknown, the volume deficit should, in the absence of hemodynamic instability, be corrected slowly with 0.9% or 0.45% saline. As in euvolemic hyponatremia, the serum sodium concentration should be monitored closely and should not be allowed to rise at a rate greater than 1 mEq/L/hour or 12 mEq/L in 24 hours.

As extracellular volume is restored ADH release will be suppressed and a brisk water diuresis may result. This diuresis may result in an unsafe rise in the plasma sodium concentration and should be treated in a manner similar to the water diuresis occurring during correction of euvolemic hyponatremia.

C. Hypervolemic Hyponatremia

Hypervolemic hyponatremia is generally chronic and relatively mild. Treatment involves sodium and water restriction, the use of loop diuretics, and management of the underlying disorder. V_2-receptor antagonists (Tolvaptan) have been shown to promote excretion of electrolyte-free water thereby making them another option for treatment of hypervolemic hyponatremia. Furthermore, the EVEREST (Efficacy of Vasopressin antagonism in Heart Failure Outcome Study with Tolvaptan) and ACTIV (Acute and Chronic Therapeutic Impact of a Vasopressin Antagonist in Congestive Heart Failure) trial, demonstrated a significant improvement in hospitalized patients treated for acutely decompensated heart failure, in terms of clinical signs and symptoms. As expected, the most common side effects are dry mouth and increased thirst. It must be noted however, that the EVEREST trial did not show long term benefit in terms of cardiovascular events or mortality in the CHF population.

Decaux G: Treatment of symptomatic hyponatremia. Am J Med Sci 2003;326:25. [PMID: 1286112]

HYPERNATREMIA

ESSENTIALS OF DIAGNOSIS

▶ Hypernatremia develops as a result of a relative deficiency of total body water to total body sodium.

▶ Urinary osmolality is useful in distinguishing renal and extrarenal water loss.

▶ General Considerations

Hypernatremia is present when the serum sodium concentration exceeds 145 mEq/L. The renal concentrating mechanism represents the first defense against hypernatremia, but thirst becomes the operant mechanism preventing hypernatremia when the renal concentrating mechanism is impaired or overwhelmed (Figure 3–1). Thirst is such an effective defense that hypernatremia typically does not develop, even in the setting of severe diabetes insipidus, unless the thirst mechanism is impaired or access to water is restricted.

As in hyponatremia, the approach to hypernatremia involves categorizing patients into low, normal, or elevated total body volumes.

▶ Clinical Findings

Symptoms and Signs

Hypernatremia is always reflective of a hyperosmolar state. In response to hyperosmolality, water shifts from the relatively hypotonic intracellular space to the extracellular compartment resulting in decreased cellular volume. In the CNS, depending on the acuity and severity, changes in cellular volume are associated with a spectrum of neurologic symptoms. Irritability, lethargy, muscle spasticity, seizures, coma, and death may all occur. If hypernatremia develops over more than 24 hours, the brain adapts by accumulating intracellular osmolytes that act to restore cellular tonicity and volume. Chronic hypernatremia may, therefore, be less symptomatic at the same degree of hypernatremia than if it had occurred acutely. Due to the accumulation of osmolytes, chronic hypernatremia carries the attendant risk of cerebral edema if rapidly corrected.

▶ Differential Diagnosis

Hypernatremia is also best approached systematically using an algorithm (Figure 3–4).

A. Hypernatremia with Low Extracellular Volume

Hypernatremia with low total body volume occurs when patients sustain losses of both sodium and water. Relatively greater losses of water than sodium result in hypernatremia.

Due to decreased total body sodium, patients typically exhibit clinical signs of hypovolemia. The underlying causes of hypovolemia are similar to those seen in patients with hypovolemic hyponatremia and may occur due to either renal or extrarenal losses. The fundamental divergence that leads to hypernatremia, as opposed to hyponatremia, in this situation is the lack of sufficient water replacement.

Extrarenal loss of hypotonic fluid may occur via the skin or the gastrointestinal tract. Burned patients are particularly susceptible to loss through the skin. Gastrointestinal losses by way of protracted vomiting or diarrhea commonly lead to hypovolemic hypernatremia. Renal loss of hypotonic fluid frequently occurs due to the effect of loop diuretics but may be associated with osmotic diuresis due to glucose with severe hyperglycemia or urea associated with high protein tube feedings. Massive urinary losses are seen in some patients following the relief of a prolonged urinary tract obstruction or during the polyuric recovery phase of acute tubular necrosis.

As in hypovolemic hyponatremia, urinary electrolytes are helpful in clarifying the source of fluid loss if it is not clinically apparent.

B. Hypernatremia with a Normal Extracellular Volume

Hypernatremia with normal body volume occurs as the result of loss of water without loss of sodium. Without sodium loss, the signs of systemic hypovolemia are characteristically absent. Extrarenal loss of water can occur through the skin through sweating or through the respiratory tract. High environmental temperature, fever, and mechanical ventilation are common causes of euvolemic hypernatremia. Rarely, water deficits may occur due to a primary defect in thirst.

As in hypovolemic hypernatremia, euvolemic hypernatremia can occur only if water losses exceed water replacement. Extrarenal water losses are evidenced by a normally functioning renal concentrating mechanism and are, therefore, manifested by oliguria and a maximally concentrated urine (urine osmolality >700 mOsm/kg H_2O).

Primary renal loss of water occurs due to diabetes insipidus, which results from either the failure to synthesize or secrete ADH (neurogenic diabetes insipidus) or the failure of urinary concentration despite adequate circulating levels of ADH (nephrogenic diabetes insipidus). Both disorders are manifested by the inability to concentrate the urine, polyuria, and secondary polydipsia.

Diabetes insipidus may occur as either a complete or partial syndrome. In complete diabetes insipidus, either circulating ADH, or the renal response to it, is absent, resulting in production of large volumes of dilute urine (urine osmolality <100 mOsm/kg H_2O). Partial diabetes insipidus manifests as a less severe defect in urinary concentration. Despite massive urinary losses, in patients with an intact thirst mechanism and access to water, fluid intake is typically adequate to replace urinary losses and hypernatremia is often absent.

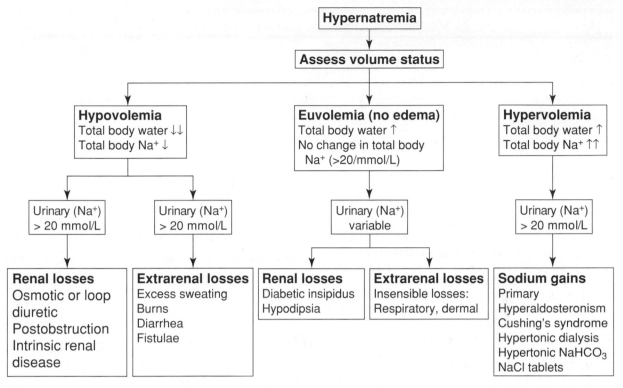

▲ **Figure 3-4.** Approach to hypernatremia. (Adapted with permission from Johnson RJ, Freehaly J (editors): *Comprehensive Clinical Nephrology*, 2nd ed. Mosby, 2003.)

1. Diagnosis of diabetes insipidus—Diabetes insipidus must be considered in the differential diagnosis of any patient with polyuria and polydipsia. Polyuria due to osmotic diuresis from glucose, mannitol, urea, or diuretics can be excluded by demonstrating a urinary concentration greater than 150 mOsm/kg H_2O.

Neurogenic diabetes insipidus, nephrogenic diabetes insipidus, and compulsive water drinking all present similarly with polyuria and a maximally dilute urine (urine osmolality <100 mOsm/kg H_2O). A measured plasma osmolality below 270 mOsm/kg H_2O strongly suggests a positive water balance and supports the diagnosis of compulsive water drinking. Conversely, a serum sodium concentration greater than 143 mEq/L or plasma osmolality >295 mOsm/kg H_2O suggests diabetes insipidus and effectively excludes compulsive water drinking. Water deprivation testing is useful in differentiating difficult cases.

During the water deprivation test, patients fast to ensure that no fluid is consumed during the testing period. Urine osmolality is measured hourly, and serum osmolality is measured every 6 hours. Vital signs and body weight must be monitored closely as patients with diabetes insipidus may rapidly become volume depleted. Fluid deprivation is continued until the body weight has declined 3%, the plasma osmolality is ≥295 mOsm/kg H_2O, or the urine osmolality is unchanged over three consecutive measurements. At this point the plasma vasopressin level is measured and, subsequently, 5 units of aqueous vasopressin is administered subcutaneously. Urinary osmolality is again measured after 60 minutes.

In patients with complete diabetes insipidus, the urine remains dilute despite water deprivation. Vasopressin levels and response to exogenous vasopressin differentiate neurogenic from nephrogenic diabetes insipidus (Table 3–3).

2. Neurogenic diabetes insipidus—Since vasopressin is produced in the hypothalamus and released from the posterior pituitary gland, any disease process involving the hypothalamic–pituitary axis may lead to vasopressin deficiency and neurogenic diabetes insipidus. Common causes include head trauma, pituitary surgery, infection, primary or metastatic malignancy, thrombosis, and granulomatous disease (Table 3–4). Congenital forms have been described but are rare. Computed tomography or magnetic resonance imaging of the hypothalamic – pituitary region may reveal the etiology of neurogenic diabetes insipidus. Normally the posterior pituitary produces a bright spot on T1-weighted images that may be characteristically absent in neurogenic diabetes insipidus.

Table 3–3. Interpretation of the water deprivation test.

	Urinary osmolality after dehydration (mOsm/L H$_2$O)	Plasma arginine vasopressin after dehydration (pg/mL)	Increase in urinary osmolality with exogenous vasopressin
Normal	>800	>2	Increase < 10%
Complete Neurogenic Diabetes Insipidus	<300	Undetectable	Increase > 50%
Partial neurogenic diabetes insipidus	300−800	<1.5	Increase 10−50%
Nephrogenic diabetes insipidus	<300−500	>5	Increase < 50%
Compulsive water drinking	>500	<5	Increase < 10%

Adapted with permission from Johnson RJ, Freehaly J (editors): *Comprehensive Clinical Nephrology*, 2nd ed. Mosby, 2003.

3. Nephrogenic diabetes insipidus—Nephrogenic diabetes insipidus also may be acquired or congenital. Though hundreds of mutations involving the vasopressin (V2) receptor or aquaporin-2 water channel have been discovered, the acquired form is much more common. Any advanced form of chronic renal failure may result in an impairment of urinary concentrating ability, though frank polyuria is uncommon. Some forms of renal disease, listed in Table 3–5, can result in clinically significant defects in urinary concentration despite relatively preserved renal function. Various pharmacologic agents, particularly lithium and demeclocycline, are also associated with the development of nephrogenic diabetes insipidus. Electrolyte disorders and obstructive uropathy comprise most of the remaining cases.

4. Gestational diabetes insipidus—An unusual form of diabetes insipidus resistant to vasopressin has been described in pregnancy. Rather than renal insensitivity to the hormone, placentally derived circulating vasopressinase neutralizes circulating vasopressin. Desmopressin (DDAVP) is not affected by vasopressinase and is effective in treating the disease.

C. Hypernatremia with an Increased Extracellular Volume

Hypernatremia with an increased total body volume is the least common form of hypernatremia and is most often associated with administration of hypertonic sodium chloride or hypertonic sodium bicarbonate during resuscitative efforts. Salt water drowning, hypertonic hyperalimentation solutions,

Table 3–4. Causes of Neurogenic Diabetes Insipidus.

Hereditary
  Autosomal dominant
  Autosomal recessive (Wolfram syndrome)

Acquired
  Head trauma
  Pituitary surgery
  Neoplasia
    Primary (craniopharyngioma, pituitary, suprasellar tumors)
    Metastatic (lymphoma, leukemia, breast or lung carcinoma)
  Vascular
    Aneurysm
    Cerebrovascular accident
    Postpartum necrosis (Sheehan's syndrome)
    Pregnancy (transient)
  Infection
    Meningitis
    Encephalitis
    Tuberculosis
    Syphilis
  Granulomatous
    Sarcoid
    Histiocytosis
    Eosinophilic granuloma
  Autoimmune

Table 3–5. Causes of Nephrogenic Diabetes Insipidus.

Hereditary
  X-linked
  Autosomal dominant
  Autosomal recessive

Acquired
  Chronic renal disease
    Polycystic kidney disease
    Obstructive uropathy
    Sickle cell anemia
    Any other
  Drug induced
    Lithium
    Demeclocycline
    Amphotericin
    Foscarnet
  Electrolyte disorders
    Hypokalemia
    Hypercalcemia

and dialysis against a high sodium content dialysate may also result in hypervolemic hypernatremia. Excess mineralocorticoid states such as occur in Cushing's syndrome and primary hyperaldosteronism can manifest with a slightly elevated total body volume and clinically insignificant hypernatremia.

▶ Treatment

In the clinical setting, hypernatremia is preventable. Clinicians must be aware of the obligate water losses of their patients and either provide access to water or intravenous repletion. Very young, very old, restrained, and water-restricted patients are at particular risk. The importance of prevention of hypernatremia is underscored by the associated increase in mortality in patients who develop hypernatremia in the hospital setting.

Once present, appropriate therapy for hypernatremia depends on the volume status, the time course over which the hypernatremia developed, and the degree of symptomatology demonstrated by the patient. Therapy should always be guided to reverse the underlying etiology once patients are clinically stable. Acute hypernatremia occurring over less than 24 hours may be rapidly corrected as little cerebral adaptation is likely to have occurred. Chronic hypernatremia must be attended to quickly, but the serum sodium concentration should be decreased by no more that 1–2 mEq/L/hour to minimize the risk of cerebral edema.

A. Hypovolemic Hypernatremia

Initial therapy of severe hypernatremia and hypovolemia involves the restoration of the volume deficit with isotonic (0.9%) saline. Since the osmolality of isotonic saline is typically lower than the serum osmolality of the patient, with administration the serum sodium concentration will fall. Once signs of circulatory compromise are resolved, the remainder of the sodium and water deficit should be carefully replaced with 0.45% saline.

B. Euvolemic Hypernatremia

Correction of euvolemic hypernatremia requires the estimation and replacement of the water deficit. Ongoing insensible, gastrointestinal, and renal losses must also be accounted for and corrected. The water deficit is estimated from the following equation:

$$\text{Water deficit (L)} = 0.6 \times [\text{body weight (kg)}] \times [([\text{Na}^+]/140) - 1]$$

Symptomatic acute hypernatremia should be treated by rapid replacement of the water deficit. Once neurologic symptoms have resolved, the remainder of the deficit may be replaced over 24–48 hours.

Symptomatic chronic hypernatremia requires urgent therapy, however, the serum sodium concentration should not be allowed to decrease at a rate faster than 1 mEq/L/hour.

To estimate the hourly water replacement rate the following equation may be utilized:

$$\text{Hourly water replacement rate (mL/hour)} = [\text{Water deficit (mL)}/([\text{Na}^+] - 140)] + \text{ongoing water losses (mL)}$$

The water deficit may be replaced either enterally as water or intravenously as 5% dextrose in water. During treatment the serum sodium concentration and neurologic status should be monitored closely. A rapid decline in the sodium concentration or deterioration (after improvement) in neurologic status suggests the development of cerebral edema and requires temporary discontinuation of water replacement.

Patients with neurogenic diabetes insipidus and an intact thirst mechanism do not develop hypernatremia if water is available. Treatment is aimed at relieving the inconvenience of persistent polyuria and polydipsia. In the acute setting after trauma or hypophysectomy, aqueous vasopressin is preferred because of its short duration of action. Chronically, desmopressin acetate (DDAVP) is more commonly utilized due to its longer duration of action and minimal vasopressor activity. DDAVP is generally administered intranasally every 8–24 hours. but may also be administered intravenously or subcutaneously if required.

Patients with nephrogenic diabetes insipidus do not respond to exogenous vasopressin. They are consequently reliant on an intact thirst mechanism. If identifiable, correction of the underlying etiology of acquired nephrogenic diabetes insipidus may ameliorate the symptoms over time. In resistant cases, the combination of a low-salt diet and therapy with thiazide diuretics has met with some success in producing mild volume contraction and decreased urinary flow. Nonsteroidal anti-inflammatory drugs are helpful as adjunctive therapy for some patients. Amiloride may be useful in lithium-induced nephrogenic diabetes insipidus to block lithium ion uptake by the collecting duct.

C. Hypervolemic Hypernatremia

Hypervolemic hypernatremia requires the removal of excess sodium, which can be achieved by the administration of diuretics. Water replacement is also necessary in some cases. For those with significantly impaired renal function, dialysis can be employed.

Adrogue HJ: Hypernatremia. N Engl J Med 2000;342:1493. [PMID: 10816188]

Gheorghiade M et al: Short-term clinical effects of tolvaptan, an oral vasopressin antagonist in patients hospitalized for heart failure: Results of the EVEREST Clinical Studies. JAMA 2007; 297: (12) 1332–1343.

Sanghi p et al: Vasopressin antagonism: a future treatment option in heart failure. Eur Heart J 2005; 26: 538–543.

Schrier RW et al: Tolvaptan, a selective oral vasopressin V2-receptor antagonist, for hyponatremia. N Engl J Med 2006; 355: 2099–2148.

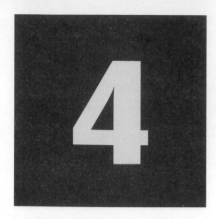

4

Disorders of Potassium Balance: Hypokalemia & Hyperkalemia

Michael Emmett, MD, & Michael R. Wiederkehr, MD

DISORDERS OF POTASSIUM BALANCE

▶ General Considerations

Potassium is the principal cation of the intracellular fluid (ICF) where its concentration is between 120 and 150 mEq/L. The extracellular fluid (ECF) and plasma potassium concentration [K] is much lower—in the 3.5–5.0 mEq/L range. The very large transcellular gradient is maintained by active K transport via the Na-K-ATPase pumps present in all cell membranes and the ionic permeability characteristics of these membranes. The resulting greater than 40-fold transmembrane [K] gradient is the principal determinant of the transcellular resting potential gradient, about −90 mV with the cell interior negative (Figure 4–1). Normal cell function requires maintenance of the ECF [K] within a relatively narrow range. This is particularly important for excitable cells such as myocytes and neurons. The pathophysiologic effects of dyskalemia on these cells result in most of the clinical manifestations.

Individual potassium intakes vary widely—a typical Western diet provides between 50 and 100 mEq K per day. Under steady-state conditions, an equal amount is excreted, mainly in urine (about 90%), and to a lesser extent in stool (5–10%) and sweat (1–10%). Normally, homeostatic mechanisms maintain plasma [K] precisely between 3.5 and 5.0 mEq/L. Rapid regulation of potassium concentration is needed to prevent potentially fatal hyperkalemia after every meal and is largely due to transcellular K shifts. The normal postprandial rise in insulin concentration moves both K and glucose into the intracellular compartment, where 98% of total body K (~3000 mEq) is located. Postprandial insulin release is primarily related to increased plasma glucose concentrations but hyperkalemia also directly stimulates pancreatic β-cells to release insulin. Insulin deficiency and/or resistance increase plasma [K]. Epinephrine and norepinephrine also rapidly regulate transcellular K balance and become especially important during and following vigorous exercise.

Hyperadrenergic states such as alcohol withdrawal and hyperthyroidism, β-sympathomimetics such as the tocolytic terbutaline, and theophylline poisoning often generate hypokalemia due to translocation of K from the ECF into cells.

Metabolic alkalosis stimulates cellular K uptake whereas some forms of hyperchloremic and other inorganic (mineral) acidoses enhance movement of K out of cells. However, the common organic metabolic acidoses (lactic and ketoacidosis) do not directly cause any K shift. Respiratory acid–base abnormalities generally have small effects. Although it had been assumed that the alkalemia produced by respiratory alkalosis would move K into cells, the opposite has been found, ie, a small *increase* in plasma [K] due to associated α-adrenergic stimulation. Respiratory acidosis increases plasma [K] slightly. Hyperosmotic conditions that shift fluid out of cells are an important cause of K translocation to the ECF. Finally, hypokalemia per se moves K from the intracellular to the extracellular space.

▶ Potassium Metabolism

Potassium absorption in the small intestine is not specifically controlled. Although colonic epithelial cells can increase K secretion in response to chronic hyperkalemia (patients with chronic kidney disease), the net effect on K balance is minor. Although the [K] in stool water may be high, the quantity of water in formed stool is small—thus absent diarrhea, total stool K excretion is low and most ingested K is absorbed.

Potassium excretion is principally into the urine and the main regulator of body K balance is the kidney. Potassium is freely filtered (600–800 mEq/day) and then largely reabsorbed in the proximal tubule and thick ascending loop of Henle. The K load delivered to the cortical collecting duct (CCD) is about 10–15% of filtered K and the intraluminal [K] of fluid entering this segment is low. It is here that major regulation of K excretion occurs. Sodium (Na) reabsorption and K and H secretion in the CCD is dependent on the amount of Na delivered to this segment, the "absorbability"

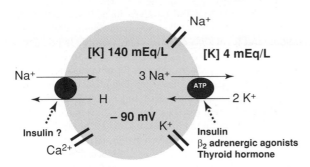

▲ **Figure 4–1.** Transcellular ion movement. Most cells contain these pumps, antiporters, and channels. The effects of insulin, catecholamines, and thyroid hormones on K transport are shown.

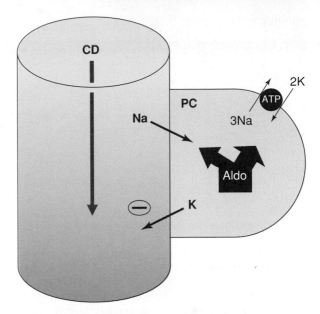

▲ **Figure 4–2.** K handling by the cortical collecting duct. Aldosterone has multiple effects on electrolyte transport in the cortical collecting duct (CCD). Sodium (Na) absorption increases through stimulation of basolateral Na-K-ATPase activity and the increased number and "open state" of the luminal Na channel (ENaC). The influx of Na causes a negative charge to develop within the lumen. This stimulates K (and H) secretion into the lumen down electrical and chemical gradients. Volume-contracted states result in little Na delivery to the CCD (due to avid more proximal absorption) so that K (and H) secretion is slight despite high aldosterone levels. Volume- expanded states enhance delivery of Na to the CCD and cause physiologically adequate levels of K (and H) secretion due to suppressed aldosterone levels.

of the anion, and the activity of the mineralocorticoid aldosterone. In the CCD, Na is absorbed through epithelial Na channels (ENaC) present on the luminal surface of the predominant (principal) cells in this segment. The absorption of large amounts of Na, especially when delivered with an anion not easily absorbed (Cl, HCO₃, and others), generates a negative charge within the lumen and enhances the secretion of K and H (Figure 4–2). Aldosterone regulates the rate of Na absorption through these channels at multiple levels. It affects the rate of energy (ATP) generation, the activity of Na-K-ATPase pumps, and the number and "open state" of the ENaC channels themselves.

In normal individuals, an inverse relationship exists between aldosterone activity and CCD Na delivery. A high salt intake will expand ECF volume, inhibit renin and aldosterone levels, and increase distal delivery and excretion of Na. High distal Na delivery counterbalances low aldosterone activity and the net effect is normal CCD K and H secretion and excretion. Conversely, a low salt intake contracts the ECF, stimulates renin and aldosterone levels, and markedly reduces distal CCD Na delivery and excretion. In this case, low CCD Na delivery is linked to high aldosterone activity and again normal K and H secretion and excretion is maintained. This reciprocal interplay between aldosterone activity and distal Na delivery is physiologic and acts to simultaneously maintain both volume and electrolyte homeostasis.

Pathophysiologic conditions exist when high CCD Na delivery combines with high aldosterone activity or low CCD Na delivery coexists with low aldosterone activity. In the first circumstance, the magnitude of CCD Na absorption increases markedly and results in excessive K and H secretion, thereby generating hypokalemia and metabolic alkalosis. Conversely, the second scenario causes a major reduction in CCD Na reabsorption and very low rates of K and H secretion leading to hyperkalemia and metabolic acidosis. Increased CCD Na delivery together with high aldosterone levels occurs in patients with primary hyperaldosteronism and as a result of thiazide and/or loop diuretics. Reduced CCD Na delivery together with low aldosterone activity occurs in some forms of hyporeninemic hypoaldosteronism and when aldosterone antagonists are given to patients with disorders with reduced "effective" intra-arterial volume such as hepatic cirrhosis or congestive heart failure.

► Clinical Findings

Nerve, cardiac conduction, and muscle cells are especially sensitive to changes in transcellular voltage and therefore are most affected by hypokalemia or hyperkalemia. Figure 4–3 shows how either condition can cause muscle weakness.

Hypokalemia increases the resting potential across the myocyte membrane, ie, the cell becomes more negative and less sensitive to excitation. Severe hypokalemia thus leads to a *hyper*polarization block and flaccid paralysis. It may also

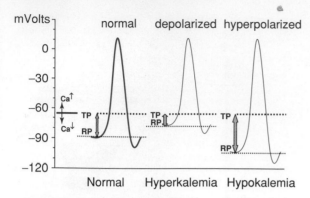

▲ Figure 4-3. Cell depolarization and hyperpolarization depend on extracellular potassium. An action potential is generated when the cell depolarizes from its resting potential (RP) to the threshold potential (TP). Hyperkalemia moves the RP closer to the TP and results in depolarization muscle paralysis. Hypokalemia hyperpolarizes the cell and thereby impairs depolarization. The flaccid paralysis caused by hypokalemia or hyperkalemia is clinically similar. Calcium raises the TP, ameliorating the effects of hyperkalemia, while hypocalcemia has the opposite effect.

cause rhabdomyolysis and paralytic ileus. Renal manifestations include metabolic alkalosis, nephrogenic diabetes insipidus, and formation of renal cysts. Chronic hypokalemia has been implicated in the development of hypertension.

Hyperkalemia reduces the resting potential, ie, the cell becomes less negative. Following depolarization, the cell is unable to adequately repolarize and becomes unexcitable. Severe hyperkalemia causes a *de*polarization block and flaccid paralysis. Clinical manifestations include fatigue, myalgia, and muscle weakness (especially lower extremity), hyporeflexia, paresthesias, muscle cramps, electrocardiogram (ECG) changes, and cardiac arrhythmia (Figure 4–4). Muscle weakness may progress to ascending paralysis, hypoventilation, and respiratory failure.

The clinical manifestations of an abnormal plasma [K] vary greatly and depend on (1) its magnitude, (2) acuity of onset, (3) the relative contributions of K shift versus change in total body K, and (4) coexisting abnormalities that either potentiate or blunt the [K] effects, including underlying heart disease, drugs (digoxin, antiarrhythmic agents), hypocalcemia or hypercalcemia, cardiac pacing devices, and others.

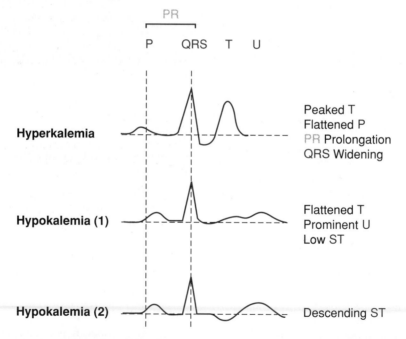

▲ Figure 4-4. Electrocardiographic tracings with hypokalemia and hyperkalemia. Hyperkalemia initially causes peaking ("tenting") of T waves and then progresses to widening of the QRS and PR intervals, sinus bradycardia and arrest, atrioventricular (AV) block, fusion of QRS with T (sine wave appearance), idioventricular rhythm, and finally ventricular tachycardia and fibrillation, and asystole. Hypokalemia causes ST depression, flattening of the T waves, and prominent U waves. This progresses to fusion of the T and U waves into a single wave and the ST segment becomes negative and descending. The QT interval lengthens, especially if hypocalcemia or hypomagnesemia is present. Atrial and ventricular arrhythmias may develop.

The resting membrane potential is determined by the ratio of intracellular and extracellular [K] (K_i/K_e). An acute K shift into or from the intracellular space alters intracellular [K] only minimally since it is quantitatively so large; about 3000 mEq or 98% of total body K is within cells. However, the effect on the extracellular concentration can be dramatic because the total quantity of K outside of cells is only about 60 mEq. Therefore, acute K shifts will markedly affect the K_i/K_e ratio and can cause profound cellular hyperpolarization or depolarization with muscular, neurologic, and cardiac symptoms (Figure 4–5). In contrast, states of chronic K depletion reduce both intracellular and extracellular K levels and have a much smaller effect on K_i/K_e with fewer and less severe clinical manifestations. Furthermore, K shifts produce much more rapid changes in plasma [K] and thus the effects are often more dramatic than with states of total body K depletion or excess. This has important clinical implications: A dialysis patient with a chronically elevated [K] who presents with a [K] of 6.5 mEq/L and minimal ECG effects may not require urgent intervention. However, a diabetic patient with chronic kidney disease who develops acute hyperglycemia and a rapid [K] rise to 6.5 mEq/L may manifest major ECG changes, which mandate quick action.

Comorbid illness such as coronary heart disease will amplify the clinical importance of dyskalemia by increasing the risk of serious arrhythmia. Hyperkalemic effects on cardiac conduction are well documented and are the principal reason it constitutes a medical emergency (Figure 4–4). The cardiac risks of hypokalemia are less well established. Although increased risk of ectopy is established for patients with acute myocardial infarction and those treated with digoxin and other antiarrhythmic agents, its importance for most other patients remains unclear.

Calcium has important effects on myocyte depolarization. Hypocalcemia reduces the depolarization threshold potential and renders the cardiac myocyte more excitable. Conversely, hypercalcemia reduces membrane excitability by increasing the depolarization threshold (Figure 4–3). This calcium-related shift of the depolarization threshold reverses the cardiac toxicity of hyperkalemia. Coexisting hyperkalemia and hypocalcemia is a particularly pernicious combination and is common in patients with severe kidney failure.

Gennari FJ: Disorders of potassium homeostasis. Hypokalemia and hyperkalemia. Crit Care Clin 2002;18:273. [PMID: 12053834]

Macdonald JE, Struthers AD: What is the optimal serum potassium level in cardiovascular patients? J Am Coll Cardiol 2004;43:155. [PMID: 14736430]

HYPOKALEMIA

 ESSENTIALS OF DIAGNOSIS

► Serum [K] below 3.5 mEq/L.
► Most commonly caused by use of thiazide or loop diuretics, vomiting/nasogastric suction, and diarrhea (or laxatives).
► Reduction of total body K stores.
► Excretion less than 20–30 mEq K per day.
► Osmotic diuresis.

► Diagnosis & Complications

A serum [K] below 3.5 mEq/L defines hypokalemia, and Table 4–1 lists some of the causes and clinical conditions associated with this disorder. The most common causes of hypokalemia are the use of thiazide or loop diuretics, vomiting/nasogastric suction, and diarrhea (or laxatives). These etiologies are usually readily apparent unless the patient is

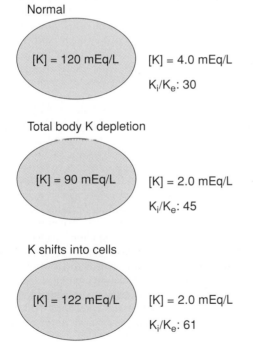

Normal

[K] = 120 mEq/L   [K] = 4.0 mEq/L

K_i/K_e: 30

Total body K depletion

[K] = 90 mEq/L   [K] = 2.0 mEq/L

K_i/K_e: 45

K shifts into cells

[K] = 122 mEq/L   [K] = 2.0 mEq/L

K_i/K_e: 61

▲ **Figure 4–5.** K distribution with intracellular K shift versus K depletion. The resting membrane potential is determined by the ratio of intracellular and extracellular potassium (K_i/K_e). Total body K depletion reduces both intracellular and extracellular [K]. The K_i/K_e ratio increases and the cell becomes hyperpolarized. A transcellular shift of K into cells slightly increases intracellular [K] and markedly reduces extracellular [K]. Therefore, the K_i/K_e ratio increases markedly and cellular hyperpolarization is severe and often produces clinical symptoms.

Table 4–1. Hypokalemia.

Renal losses
  Diuretics
  Vomiting, nasogastric suction
  Osmotic diuresis (uncontrolled diabetes and others)
  Drugs
    Excretion of nonreabsorbable anions
    Fludrocortisone and others
    Licorice (see text)
    Tubular toxicity (aminoglycosides, cisplatinum, and others)
  Primary hyperaldosteronism
  Liddle syndrome
  Cushing's disease
  Renal tubular acidosis type I and type II
    (when treated with NaHCO₃)
  Bartter and Gitelman syndrome
  Magnesium deficiency
Extrarenal losses
  Diarrhea, laxatives
  Ileostomy/short bowel
  Ureteral diversion into colon
Transcellular shift
  Insulin
  β₂-Adrenergic agonists
  Thyrotoxicosis
  Periodic paralysis
  Theophylline
    Barium
Rapid expansion of cell mass
  Anabolic states

covertly using drugs or vomiting. A more elaborate evaluation is necessary when these frequent causes are excluded. It is then important to determine whether hypokalemia is primarily due to an intracellular shift of K or to excessive K renal or gastrointestinal losses (sometimes combined with reduced intake).

Hypokalemia due to transcellular K shifts may generate impressive clinical presentations. Examples include several forms of hypokalemic periodic paralysis, the administration of β₂-agonists to treat obstructive lung disease or premature labor, theophylline poisoning, and conditions that enhance β-agonist activity such as hyperthyroidism and hypothermia. Insulin also drives K into cells and promotes hypokalemia. Barium poisoning and chloroquine overdose block K exit from cells and cause K accumulation within the ICF and profound hypokalemia. Another cause of K accumulation within cells is a rapid expansion of cell mass that occurs during refeeding after prolonged starvation, with rapidly growing tumors, and when patients with severe pernicious anemia are treated with vitamin B₁₂.

Patients with hypokalemic periodic paralysis often have a dramatic clinical presentation. At least two distinct subtypes of this syndrome have been characterized: A rare familial form (usually due to an autosomal dominant mutation

affecting a calcium channel) and a more common hyperthyroid-associated form. Hyperthyroid periodic paralysis is especially prevalent among young men of Asian (or less often Hispanic) ancestry. They typically present with profound acute muscle paralysis affecting mainly proximal limb muscle groups with sparing of ocular and respiratory muscles. Deep tendon reflexes are generally absent. Paralysis often develops after a period of exercise (which increases β-agonist activity) or following ingestion of carbohydrates (which increases insulin). Clinical signs and symptoms of thyrotoxicosis may be subtle. A prior history of recurrent episodes of weaknesses is common. Plasma [K] is usually below 2 mEq/L, and both hypophosphatemia and mild hypomagnesemia may be seen. Acute treatment with exogenous K salts is appropriate, but rebound hyperkalemia often develops since total body K is normal. Treatment with β-blockers such as propranolol is helpful and correction of the hyperthyroid state is usually curative. The pathophysiology of this disorder is thought to include the effect of thyroid hormone on the Na-K-ATPase, an exaggerated insulin response, the hypera drenergic state of hyperthyroidism, genetic and racial predisposition, and probably inherited mutations of muscle ion transport that remain subclinical until magnified by the hyperthyroid state.

A reduction of total body K stores may be due to gastrointestinal loss, renal loss, or both. The 24-hour urine potassium excretion helps define the etiology. A patient with hypokalemia should excrete less than 20–30 mEq K per day. If this is found, renal losses are generally excluded and either gastrointestinal losses or a transcellular shift should be considered. Higher excretion rates indicate renal K wasting. However, one caveat is that some renal K losses occur intermittently, with intervening periods of appropriate K conservation. For example, diuretics cause excess renal K losses but urine K excretion falls to an appropriately low range when the diuretic effect wears off. Similarly, vomiting or nasogastric suction causes excess renal K loss during the active phase, but K excretion becomes very low in the "equilibrium phase."

If a 24-hour urine collection cannot be accomplished, an alternative useful measurement is the transtubular [K] gradient, or TTKG. This calculation attempts to correct the urinary [K] for the increase generated by distal water reabsorption after the tubular fluid has exited the CCD. In theory, the TTKG approximates the [K] gradient in the cortical collecting tubule, and is calculated as

$$TTKG = \frac{U[K] \times P[Osm]}{P[K] \times U[Osm]}$$

A TTKG below 2–3 indicates appropriate renal K conservation in a patient with hypokalemia. However, the TTKG becomes uninterpretable if urine osmolality is less than plasma osmolality or if distal nephron sodium delivery is very low, ie, urine sodium below 20 mEq/L.

Assessment of a patient's volume status and blood pressure provides additional diagnostic clues. Patients with hypokalemia, volume expansion, and hypertension may have primary or exogenous hypermineralocorticoidism. An increased plasma aldosterone level (normal 5–20 ng/dL) *and* a simultaneous suppressed plasma renin activity (PRA; normal 1–3 ng/mL per hour) indicate autonomous aldosterone secretion. Some advocate calculating an aldosterone/PRA ratio. A ratio greater than 30 and an elevated aldosterone level (above 20 ng/dL) also suggest primary hyperaldosteronism. Autonomous hyperaldosteronism may be due to a unilateral aldosterone-secreting adenoma (Conn syndrome), bilateral adrenal hyperplasia, or rarely, adrenal cancer. Radiologic evaluation often allows determination of the specific syndrome, but adrenal vein sampling is necessary in some cases. Another cause of primary hyperaldosteronism is glucocorticoid-remediable aldosteronism. This rare disorder is due to an autosomal dominant mutation, which leads to sustained synthesis and secretion of aldosterone by ACTH stimulation. Glucocorticoids suppress ACTH and reverse the clinical and biochemical abnormalities of this disorder.

Pseudohyperaldosteronism is characterized by the biochemical and clinical features of an autonomous mineralocorticoid excess state but with suppressed aldosterone levels. It may be due to secretion of a nonaldosterone mineralocorticoid. Examples include adrenal tumors secreting the mineralocorticoid deoxycorticosterone (DOC), some forms of congenital adrenal hyperplasia (17- and 11-hydroxylase deficiency), and conditions that cause glucocorticoids to develop potent mineralocorticoid properties. Glucocorticoids can normally activate the mineralocorticoid receptor. However, the enzyme 11 β-hydroxysteroid dehydrogenase type 2 is present in high concentrations at most sites where mineralocorticoid receptors exist, and inactivates the glucocorticoids. In the absence of this enzyme, physiologic levels of glucocorticoids will produce a mineralocorticoid excess state. The enzyme is congenitally absent or defective in patients with the "apparent mineralocorticoid excess (AME)" syndrome who exhibit a hyperaldosterone-like disorder of hypokalemia, metabolic alkalosis, volume expansion, and hypertension. 11 β-Hydroxysteroid dehydrogenase type 2 is also antagonized by substances such as glycyrrhetinic acid, the active ingredient in true licorice, several decongestants available in Europe, and some brands of chewing tobacco (eg, RedMan). Their excessive use results in the same clinical presentation. Also, this enzyme may be overwhelmed by the markedly elevated cortisol levels in some patients with Cushing syndrome, in particular the form due to ectopic ACTH secretion.

Liddle syndrome also has features of a mineralocorticoid excess state but all known mineralocorticoids are reduced. The disorder is caused by an autosomal dominant mutation, which causes the ENaC in the collecting duct to remain in a persistently open state in the absence of mineralocorticoid stimulation. Clinical and biochemical findings mimic a nonaldosterone mineralocorticoid excess state—volume expansion, hypertension, hypokalemia, metabolic alkalosis, and suppressed levels of renin and aldosterone.

Secondary hyperaldosteronism is a condition characterized by elevated aldosterone levels due to high renin. It occurs in patients with renal artery stenosis, but also in patients with severe hypertension whose major renal arteries are anatomically normal—blood flow in smaller vessels is likely impaired. Rarely, tumors may autonomously secrete renin and thereby cause a state of hyperaldosteronism, hypertension, and hypokalemia. These forms of secondary hyperaldosteronism are all associated with volume expansion and *hyper*tension.

Secondary hyperaldosteronism may also be associated with (and due to) reduced ECF volume and *hypo*tension. This is observed with most diuretics and several renal tubular disorders. Combining high distal renal tubule Na delivery with high aldosterone activity leads to renal K wasting, hypokalemia, and variable degrees of metabolic alkalosis. This is a common effect of loop or thiazide diuretics (acetazolamide will produce hypokalemia and metabolic acidosis due to the excretion of sodium bicarbonate). Combining a loop and thiazide diuretic generates an especially powerful kaliuretic response and the combination should be used judiciously.

Two classes of autosomal recessive genetic disorders mimic the effects of thiazide or loop diuretics. Gitelman syndrome is due to a defect of the thiazide-sensitive NaCl transporter in the early distal renal tubule. Bartter syndrome is caused by one of several generic mutations that impair the function of the Na-K-2Cl transporter in the thick ascending limb of Henle that is inhibited by loop diuretics. Both are characterized by similar clinical and biochemical abnormalities: Volume contraction, hypotension, high levels of urinary prostaglandins, renal K and NaCl wasting, and high renin and aldosterone levels. Distinguishing characteristics are reduced urine calcium excretion and severe hypomagnesemia in Gitelman syndrome patients, but hypercalciuria in those with Bartter syndrome. It is almost impossible to discern these patients from those using diuretics surreptitiously unless urine is assayed for these substances and/or specific genetic mutations are identified. While Bartter syndrome is typically a pediatric disease diagnosed early in life, the phenotype of Gitelman syndrome is often subclinical and is not diagnosed until adulthood.

In the intensive care unit, osmotic diuresis is a relatively common cause of hypokalemia and hypernatremia. It is usually due to hyperglycemia or urea in patients with highly catabolic conditions (acute illness, high-dose steroids) who are also receiving parenteral nutrition or tube feeding. Sodium delivered to the distal tubule together with the glucose or urea is reabsorbed in exchange for K and H. Infusion of mannitol can also generate this syndrome. Several nephrotoxic drugs inappropriately increase distal tubule Na delivery, generating K wasting. Some also cause magnesiuria and hypomagnesemia, which itself promotes kaliuresis. Examples include aminoglycoside antibiotics, amphotericin B, cisplatin, and foscarnet. Patients with acute myeloid or lymphoblastic leukemia may develop proximal or distal tubule dysfunction.

Hypokalemia as well as metabolic acidosis, hyponatremia, hypocalcemia, hypophosphatemia, and hypomagnesemia may result.

Na delivered to the distal nephron with a poorly reabsorbed nonchloride anion can accelerate K and H secretion. This is magnified by development of ECF contraction with high levels of renin and aldosterone (Figure 4–2). The disorder occurs in patients treated with high-dose Na-penicillin, during development and treatment of diabetic ketoacidosis (Na-β-hydroxybutyrate), with inhalation of toluene/glue (Na-hippurate), and during vomiting or nasogastric suction (when NaHCO$_3$ spills into the distal tubule and urine). By a similar mechanism, hypokalemia develops when patients with proximal renal tubular acidosis (RTA type 2) are aggressively treated with exogenous bicarbonate salts. Patients with classic distal tubular acidosis (RTA type 1) also have accelerated distal tubule Na-K exchange and hypokalemia. However, in contradistinction to proximal RTA, renal K excretion and hypokalemia *improve* with NaHCO$_3$ therapy, in part because ECF volume expands.

The colon secretes K and absorbs chloride in exchange for HCO$_3$. When urine comes in contact with the bowel wall, chloride is removed while K and HCO$_3$ are secreted. This results in hypokalemia and a hyperchloremic metabolic acidosis. Clinical situations in which this occurs include ureteral implants into the sigmoid colon and interposition of colon segments between the kidney and bladder.

▶ Treatment

The best treatment for hypokalemia is prevention. The combination of a loop and thiazide diuretic is particularly kaliuretic and should be used infrequently. Incorporating an aldosterone antagonist (spironolactone or eplerenone) or a distal tubule Na channel blocker (amiloride or triamterene) in the diuretic regimen is helpful. Angiotensin-converting enzyme inhibitors (ACEI) and angiotensin receptor blockers (ARB) also reduce K losses generated by diuretics, in part by reducing aldosterone levels.

Potassium replacement is necessary when K has been lost and total K stores are reduced. Occasionally, exogenous K is used to treat the acute clinical manifestations generated by severe K shifts into cells. However, such replacement must be done cautiously since total body K stores are normal and rebound hyperkalemia occurs. This has been described following treatment of hypokalemic periodic paralysis, and after cessation of intravenous tocolytic therapy with terbutaline for preterm labor.

Whenever possible, K should be replenished via the oral route. Potassium-rich foods (dried fruit, nuts, bananas, oranges, tomatoes, spinach, potatoes, and meat) are often less effective for replacement because their K content is relatively low compared to total calories and because food K is largely composed of organic salts (see below). K salts are required to replenish major deficits. In general, a plasma [K]

between 3 and 3.5 mEq/L represents a K deficit of 200–400 mEq, while a plasma [K] between 2.0 and 3.0 mEq/L requires 400–800 mEq.

Potassium replacement salts are divided into two broad classes: Potassium chloride (KCl) and potassium bicarbonate (KHCO$_3$). Organic K salts can be metabolized, mole for mole, to KHCO$_3$ and are therefore included in the second group. KCl is the most appropriate and effective replacement for K deficits associated with metabolic alkalosis. Conversely, alkalinizing K salts (KHCO$_3$, K-citrate, K-acetate, K-gluconate) are best for hypokalemia associated with metabolic acidosis, such as RTA, or chronic diarrhea. Alkalizing K salts are more palatable and better tolerated than oral KCl. However, organic K salts should not be used to treat hypokalemia associated with metabolic alkalosis. In this setting, alkalinizing K salts are poorly retained and less effectively reverse the K deficit and metabolic alkalosis. Table 4–2 lists the various forms of oral potassium salts.

When the oral route cannot be used, or total K deficits are severe, intravenous replacement becomes necessary. A parenteral fluid KCl concentration of 20–40 mEq/L is generally well tolerated. KCl concentrations of 60 mEq/L and greater are painful and may induce peripheral vein necrosis. When

Table 4–2. Oral potassium salts.[1]

KCl		
KCl elixir	15 mEq/20 mL	
KCl extended release tablets	8–10 mEq/tablets	Micro-K, K-Lor, Slow-K, K-Dur, Kaon-Cl, Klor-Con, Klotrix
KCl powder	20–25 mEq/pack	Kay Ciel, Klor-Con
KCl solution	20 mEq/15 mL	Kchlor, Kay Ciel, Kaon-Cl
KHCO$_3$ and K-organic salts		
KHCO$_3$ effervescent tablets	25 mEq/tablet	K-Lyte effervescent tablets, Klor-Con/EF
K citrate liquid	2 mEq/mL	Polycitra-K
K citrate tablets	5–10 mEq/tablet	Urocit-K
K gluconate liquid/tablets	6.7 mEq/5 mL 2–5 mEq/tablet	Kaon Elixir, Glu-K
KHCO$_3$/ organic anion mixtures	15 mEq/5 mL 50 mEq/tablet	Tri-K, K-Lyte DS

[1]The brand names represent the more commonly used drugs and many other brands are also available.

intravenous administration of a large volume of fluid is contraindicated, K concentrations of up to 200 mEq/L (20 mEq in 100 mL of isotonic saline) may be given via a central vein, but the administration rate should not exceed 10–20 mEq per hour. Central venous administration of very concentrated K solutions requires a rate-controlling pump. The choice of intravenous fluid must also be considered, because dextrose will increase insulin and shift K into cells, thereby potentially worsening hypokalemia!

Coca SG et al: The cardiovascular implications of hypokalemia. Am J Kidney Dis 2005;45:233-247. [PMID: 15685500]

Warnock DG: Hereditary disorders of potassium homeostasis. Best Pract Res Clin Endocrinol Metab 2003;17:505. [PMID: 14687586]

HYPERKALEMIA

 ESSENTIALS OF DIAGNOSIS

▶ Serum [K] above 5.0 mEq/L.

▶ Acute or chronic renal failure is the most common cause.

▶ Transcellular shift of K from the intracellular to the extracellular space.

▶ Inhibition of the endocrine sequence.

▶ Diagnosis & Complications

The causes of hyperkalemia, defined as a serum [K] above 5.0 mEq/L, are listed in Table 4–3. Acute or chronic renal failure is by far the most common cause or major contributor to hyperkalemia. When the kidney and the renin–angiotensin–aldosterone axis function normally, the plasma [K] is maintained in the normal range despite wide extremes in intake. Therefore, persistent or chronic hyperkalemia almost always indicates impaired renal excretion, either due to intrinsic pathology or inadequate endocrine signaling. However, rapid K shifts from cells to the ECF can generate acute hyperkalemia, despite normal renal and endocrine function. Such "shift" hyperkalemia is exacerbated by coexistent renal dysfunction and/or hormonal derangements.

Pseudohyperkalemia is an artifact related to the collection and/or preparation of the specimen or an artifact of the K measurement procedure itself. It is generally a diagnosis of exclusion and should not delay prompt intervention. Potential causes include repeated fist clenching during phlebotomy, hemolysis due to traumatic venipuncture, particularly with small gauge needles, delayed processing of the specimen (especially when placed on ice), K release from white blood cells in severe leukocytosis (usually $> 100 \times 10^3/\mu L$) or from platelets with extreme thrombocytosis (usually $> 1000 \times 10^3/\mu L$),

Table 4–3. Hyperkalemia.

Renal retention
Acute renal failure
Chronic renal failure (especially interstitial renal disease)
Drugs (see text)
Addison's disease
Renal tubular acidosis Type IV
Pseudohypoaldosteronism
Tissue release and transcellular shifts of K
Tissue breakdown (hemolysis, rhabdomyolysis, ischemia, tumor lysis)
Insulin deficiency
Hyperosmolarity
Hyperchloremic metabolic acidosis
Drugs (succinylcholine, digoxin toxicity)

and prolonged tourniquet application in some individuals. Some patients inherit a propensity to leak K from red blood cells *ex vivo* due to a membrane defect. Measurement of plasma rather than serum [K] may eliminate some of these artifacts.

A transcellular shift of K from the intracellular to the extracellular space is a common cause of acute hyperkalemia. It is often due to direct damage or destruction of cell membranes. Examples include tumor lysis related to chemotherapy, acute intravascular hemolysis due to infection, transfusion reaction or severe hemolytic anemia, hemolysis developing within a large hematoma, extensive burns, rhabdomyolysis, and intestinal ischemia/necrosis.

Excessive K efflux may also develop across intact cell membranes as a result of certain drugs, metabolic disorders, and inherited diseases. Drugs that block β-agonist activity favor K efflux from cells. The muscle relaxant succinylcholine consistently promotes cellular K efflux and many cases of profound hyperkalemia have been reported, especially in patients with an underlying neuromuscular or renal disorder. A pharmacologic dose of digitalis inhibits Na-K-ATPase in cardiac myocytes, but toxic levels inhibit these pumps in systemic muscle cells and may thereby generate extreme hyperkalemia. Potassium translocation also occurs with insulin deficiency or resistance, certain hyperosmolar conditions such as hyperglycemia, and some forms of inorganic (usually hyperchloremic) metabolic acidoses. It was previously assumed that acidemia, especially with metabolic acidosis, caused protons to move into cells with reciprocal K efflux. However, organic metabolic acidoses, such as ketoacidosis and lactic acidosis, do not generate K shifts. Although hyperkalemia may develop in these patients, it is usually the result of a pathophysiologic process and not the academia per se. Hyperkalemia does occur frequently with lactic acidosis, but is principally due to tissue ischemia/necrosis and concomitant renal insufficiency. Hyperkalemia is also a common finding in diabetic ketoacidosis due to the combination of insulin deficiency, hyperosmolarity (hyperglycemia), and decreased renal perfusion, rather than the academia per se. In contrast, the infusion of some inorganic acids, such as HCl, will directly shift K out of cells. "Shift" hyperkalemia also develops when HCl precursors are infused, such as the chloride salts of arginine or lysine. Genetic defects of cell membrane ion transporters, usually epithelial Na channels, cause the syndrome of *hyper*kalemic periodic paralysis.

Most nonphysiologic states of hypoaldosteronism (ie, not secondary to ECF expansion) generate chronic hyperkalemia because of reduced distal tubule (CCD) K secretion. This is exacerbated by concomitant renal insufficiency or markedly reduced distal tubule Na delivery. Pathologic hypoaldosteronism may be the consequence of a direct block of hormonal synthesis (a congenital or acquired enzyme defect or adrenal damage) or secondary to dysregulation of the signals mediating aldosterone synthesis and release. The most important physiologic regulator of systemic aldosterone is angiotensin II activity, and the most common form of pathologic hypoaldosteronism is due to reduced renin activity and hence angiotensin II levels. This "hyporeninemic hypoaldosteronism" often develops in patients with long standing diabetes mellitus as a result of progressive interstitial renal disease with atrophy and/or destruction of the renin-secreting cells in the juxtaglomerular apparatus. Other interstitial renal diseases, such as those associated with sickle cell disease, analgesic nephropathy, and chronic urinary outlet obstruction (especially in elderly men), may produce a state of hyporeninemic hypoaldosteronism as well. Elderly patients often have an underlying element of hyporeninemic hypoaldosteronism and are prone to develop hyperkalemia. In addition, their renal function is typically underappreciated because of low body mass.

Hypoaldosteronism slows the rate of distal tubule proton secretion. In addition, hyperkalemia inhibits renal ammonia synthesis and reduces NH_4Cl excretion. These defects combine to generate a syndrome of hyperkalemic, hyperchloremic metabolic acidosis called renal tubular acidosis type 4. Correction of the hyperkalemia often increases urine ammonia excretion and reverses the metabolic acidosis.

Inhibition of the endocrine sequence at any step will promote hyperkalemia: Renin $\longrightarrow$ angiotensin I $\longrightarrow$ angiotensin II $\longrightarrow$ aldosterone $\longrightarrow$ activation of distal tubule Na reabsorption and K (and H) secretion. Clinically important causes include the following:

1. Suppressed renin secretion by β-blockers, nonsteroidal anti-inflammatory drugs (NSAIDs), cyclosporine, and tacrolimus.

2. Impaired angiotensin II generation by ACEI.

3. Blockade of type I angiotensin II receptor by ARB.

4. Inhibition of the enzymatic sequence responsible for aldosterone synthesis by drugs such as heparin or ketoconazole.

5. Destruction of the adrenal gland as a result of autoimmune disease or infection.

6. Competitive antagonism of mineralocorticoid receptors by spironolactone or eplerenone.

7. Blockade of the cortical collecting duct epithelial sodium channels by triamterene, amiloride, trimethoprim, or pentamidine.

8. Blunted renal epithelial response to aldosterone as a result of a series of inherited disorders (the congenital pseudohypoaldosteronism syndromes)

Many other factors contribute to the hyperkalemia, which commonly develops in patients with diabetes mellitus. Autonomic sympathetic neuropathy reduces renin levels and blunts β activity, thus promoting K efflux. The multiple medications often prescribed include ACEI, ARBs, aldosterone antagonists, and NSAIDs (see below). These patients may also ingest excess K in the form of salt substitutes and their global kidney function is typically impaired. With suboptimal diabetic control, the combined effects of insulin deficiency and hyperglycemia may increase plasma [K] acutely and dramatically.

The contribution of reduced renal K excretion to the development of hyperkalemia is usually readily apparent. If not, a quantitative urine collection to measure daily K excretion is helpful. Chronic hyperkalemia will stimulate renal K excretion and the 24-hour urine should contain more than 80 mEq. If a quantitative urine collection cannot be obtained, the TTKG (described in the hypokalemia section) should be greater than 10, provided urine osmolality is above 300 mOsm/L and urinary Na excretion is above 20 mEq/L.

▶ **Treatment**

It is better to prevent hyperkalemia than to treat it. A careful review of patient medications, diet, and in particular over-the-counter drugs (NSAIDs) is mandatory. Hidden sources of K, such as herbal medicines, sports drinks, and salt substitutes, must be sought. The recent demonstration that aldosterone antagonists provide a survival benefit to patients with congestive heart failure (who are usually also taking ACEI and/or ARB drugs plus β-blockers) has generated a major increase in the prevalence of hyperkalemia among these patients.

When hyperkalemia is acute and severe, emergency intervention is necessary. Treatment options for acute and severe hyperkalemia include the following:

1. Direct reversal of cardiotoxic effects with intravenous calcium.

2. Translocating K into cells:

   a. Insulin infusion — with glucose if appropriate.

   b. β_2-Adrenergic agonists such as albuterol.

   c. $NaHCO_3$ infusion.

3. Increasing K excretion:

   a. Via the kidney by ECF volume expansion and kaliuretic diuretics.

b. Via the gastrointestinal tract by inducing diarrhea and K-binding resins.

c. Via dialysis for patients with severe acute or chronic renal failure.

If [K] is greater than 6.4 and peaked T waves are an isolated ECG abnormality, calcium should probably be infused. It is clearly indicated when a hyperkalemic patient manifests more ominous ECG abnormalities (Figure 4–3). Calcium directly antagonizes the cardiac membrane-depolarizing effects of hyperkalemia (Figure 4–4). The indication for calcium in the absence of electrocardiographic changes is unclear; however, such infusions are relatively safe in the absence of overt hypercalcemia, marked hyperphosphatemia, or digitalis toxicity. One ampule (10 mL) of 10% calcium gluconate contains 4.6 mEq of elemental calcium and is given as a slow intravenous push over 2–5 minutes. Alternatively, one ampule (10 mL) of calcium chloride 10%, containing about three times as much elemental calcium (13.6 mEq), is acceptable, but should be given more slowly and cautiously. Extravasation of either salt can produce tissue necrosis (calcium chloride is more irritating then calcium gluconate). The beneficial effect on the ECG is usually seen immediately. The dose of calcium may be repeated if ECG abnormalities persist or recur. Lidocaine is contraindicated because it can precipitate ventricular fibrillation and asystole. Importantly, calcium infusions do not directly affect the plasma [K] per se and their beneficial effects are short lived (about 1–2 hours). Therefore, this treatment must be promptly followed by other regimens that ultimately reduce plasma [K] by translocation into cells or excretion.

The three agents that drive extracellular potassium into cells are listed above. Insulin stimulates Na-K-ATPase (and the Na-H exchanger—Figure 4–1) and reliably reduces [K] by 0.5–1 mEq/L within 10–20 minutes in most patients. For a maximum K lowering effect, supraphysiologic levels of insulin are required, typically 10 units of regular insulin intravenous push. Subcutaneous or intramuscular injections and "low-dose" intravenous infusions should not be utilized because they do not produce adequate plasma insulin levels. Intravenous glucose is also administered if the patient is not already hyperglycemic. A reasonable approach is to administer one ampule (50 mL) of 50% glucose, followed by an intravenous infusion of 10% glucose at about 75 mL/hour. Hyperglycemia must be avoided because this will shift K out of cells. Infusion of glucose alone to stimulate endogenous insulin secretion in nondiabetic patients is less effective because it generates lower peak insulin levels.

The β_2-agonist albuterol also stimulates Na-K-ATPase and moves K into cells. This effect is additive to that of insulin and occurs within 30–60 minutes. The parenteral form of albuterol is not available in the United States, and the drug is given via the respiratory tract by nebulizer at a dose of 10–20 mg in 4 mL of saline. This relatively high dose is well tolerated by most patients, but contraindicated for patients with acute cardiac ischemia or severe myocardial disease. However, it is less reliable than insulin because significant numbers of patients are resistant to its K-lowering effect and therefore it should never be used alone.

Hypertonic $NaHCO_3$, 1–3 ampules (44 mEq/50 mL each) by intravenous infusion over 30–45 minutes, has been used in the treatment of hyperkalemia for many years. Overall, its potassium-lowering effect is weak and of slow onset. Hypertonic $NaHCO_3$ lowers [K] via multiple mechanisms including expansion of the ECF with dilution of [K]. Hypertonic $NaHCO_3$ does expand the ECF and should be avoided in volume overloaded patients and those with congestive heart failure.

Hyperkalemia associated with increased total K stores requires K to be removed. If kidney function is adequate, loop and thiazide diuretics (and especially in combination) markedly increase urinary K excretion. Thiazide diuretics are particularly helpful in the treatment of hyporeninemic hypoaldosteronism. Thiazides become less effective when kidney function declines, whereas high-dose loop diuretics may remain useful until renal function reaches "end stage." Occasionally, patients with hypoaldosteronism are volume contracted and the exogenous mineralocorticoid fludrocortisone is useful.

Stool potassium excretion is enhanced by administering laxatives to generate electrolyte-rich diarrhea and by binding gastrointestinal luminal K to nonabsorbable resins, such as sodium polystyrene sulfonate (Kayexalate). The resin powder is generally premixed with sorbitol (15 g suspended in 60 mL of 70% sorbitol), which speeds its transit through the gut and in itself increases fecal K loss. The usual oral dose is 30 g. The resin powder can also be ingested with other laxatives. The acute K-lowering effect of this treatment is minor and resin K binders may be more effective for chronic therapy. These resins can also be administered via enema, though this route may be less effective. A rare complication of the sodium polystyrene sulfonate in sorbitol suspension is bowel necrosis. This may be due to the hypertonic sorbitol rather than the resin itself and is more common with rectal administration.

Acute hemodialysis, generally reserved for patients with acute or chronic severe kidney failure, rapidly lowers plasma [K] and can reduce total body K stores by about 25–50 mEq per hour.

Juurlink DN et al: Rates of hyperkalemia after publication of the Randomized Aldactone Evaluation Study. N Engl J Med 2004;351:543. [PMID: 15295047]

Palmer BF: Managing hyperkalemia caused by inhibitors of the renin-angiotensin-aldosterone system. N Engl J Med 2004;351:585. [PMID: 15295051]

Perazella MA: Drug-induced hyperkalemia: old culprits and new offenders. Am J Med 2000;109:307. [PMID: 10996582]

Wiederkehr MR, Moe OW: Factitious hyperkalemia. Am J Kidney Dis 2000;36:1049. [PMID: 11054365]

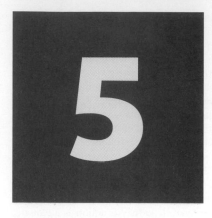

Acid–Base Disorders

John H. Galla, MD, Ira Kurtz, MD, Jeffrey A. Kraut, MD,
Gregg Y. Lipschik, MD, & Jeanne P. Macrae, MD

▼ METABOLIC ALKALOSIS

John H. Galla, MD

ESSENTIALS OF DIAGNOSIS

► Increase in plasma [HCO_3^-].
► Compensatory increase in arterial $Paco_2$.
► Increase in arterial pH.

▶ General Considerations

Metabolic alkalosis is an acid–base disorder in which a primary disease process leads to the net accumulation of base within or the net loss of acid from the extracellular fluid (ECF). When it occurs as a simple acid–base disorder, it is recognized as an increase in plasma [HCO_3^-] and a compensatory increase in arterial blood pH.

Unopposed by other primary acid–base disorders, the increase in arterial blood pH promptly and predictably depresses ventilation resulting in increased $PaCO_2$ and buffering of the magnitude of the alkalemia; an increase in $PaCO_2$ of 0.6–0.7 mm Hg for every 1.0 mEq/L increase in plasma [HCO_3^-] is predicted from empirical studies. Although a $PaCO_2$ greater than 55 mm Hg is uncommon, compensatory increases to 60 mm Hg or higher have been documented in severe metabolic alkalosis. The magnitude of the compensatory increase in $PaCO_2$ is directly related to the extent of the alkalosis and the degree of elevation of the plasma [HCO_3^-], whether or not there is an intracellular acidosis. This compensatory respiratory response is independent of hypoxia, hypokalemia, renal failure, and cause and is usually not detectable clinically because it is more dependent on a change in depth rather than the rate of ventilation.

The major clinically and pathophysiologically relevant classification is based on whether the metabolic alkalosis is dependent on Cl^- depletion. The Cl^--depletion forms, also termed the Cl^--responsive alkaloses, are more common. The other major grouping is the Cl^--resistant alkaloses, most of which are due to K^+ depletion with mineralocorticoid excess. Mixed K^+ and Cl^--depletion metabolic alkaloses also occur. Several other relatively uncommon causes constitute the balance of etiologies of metabolic alkalosis (Table 5–1).

▶ Clinical Findings

A. Symptoms and Signs

Metabolic alkalosis should be anticipated when conditions such as vomiting, diuretic use, or severe hypertension are present. Thus, a careful and complete history is vital to establishing the etiology. Although the generation and maintenance phases of metabolic alkalosis can be clearly delineated in animal models of metabolic alkalosis, in the clinical setting the genesis of the generation phase may be obscure, even after a careful history. This is especially true if the patient is concealing bulimia or diuretic or laxative abuse.

A physical examination is helpful primarily for assessing the status of body fluid volume. Both deficits and surfeits of volume can and often do accompany metabolic alkalosis depending upon etiology, but they are not causes.

Neurologic symptoms such as apathy, confusion, cardiac arrhythmias, and neuromuscular irritability are observed only when alkalosis is severe (arterial pH >7.55). Although neuromuscular irritability may be readily evident, Chvostek and Trousseau signs are uncommon.

Alkalosis per se has a mild positive inotropic effect on the heart and little or no effect on cardiac rhythm. Cardiac arrhythmias occur primarily because of hypokalemia (see Chapter 4).

Compensatory hypoventilation may contribute to hypoxia or pulmonary infection in very ill or immunocompromised patients.

Table 5–1. Classification of metabolic alkalosis by pathogenesis.

Cl⁻ depletion
Gastrointestinal losses: Vomiting or nasogastric aspiration (even with achlorhydria), congenital chloridorrhea, gastrocystoplasty, villous adenoma
Renal losses: Chloruretic diuretics, posthypercapnia, severe K⁺ depletion
Skin losses: Cystic fibrosis

K⁺ depletion
Gastrointestinal losses: Laxative abuse
Renal losses: Hyperaldosteronism, primary and secondary, other hypokalemic hypertensive syndromes, Bartter's and Gitelman's syndromes

Miscellaneous
Low glomerular filtration rate with base loading
Milk-alkali syndrome
Hypercalcemia
Nonreabsorbable antacids with cation exchange resin
Hypoalbuminemia
Recovery from starvation

Transient
Multiple blood transfusions with citrate
Infant formulas with low Cl⁻ content

Many of the clinical features of metabolic alkalosis are dependent largely on the effects of the electrolyte deficits and not on alkalosis per se. K^+ depletion may be accompanied by cardiac arrhythmias, nephrogenic diabetes insipidus, and muscle weakness. Similarly, Cl^- depletion may be associated with impaired urine concentrating ability, impaired response to loop diuretics, stimulation of renin via a macula densa mechanism, and a reduction in glomerular filtration rate (GFR).

B. Laboratory Findings

A serum electrolyte profile and an arterial blood gas are necessary to accurately diagnose metabolic alkalosis as outlined above. If the measured $PaCO_2$ is within ±3–5 mm Hg of the predicted value, a simple metabolic alkalosis is present. If not, a mixed disorder is present, respiratory acidosis if the $PaCO_2$ is higher and respiratory alkalosis if it is lower.

Disequilibrium occurs when generation of HCO_3^- and resultant elevation of plasma $[HCO_3^-]$ exceed the capacity of the renal tubule to reabsorb HCO_3^-. Transient bicarbonaturia with concomitant Na^+ or K^+ loss ensues until a new steady state is achieved and urinary HCO_3^- excretion ceases. This ushers in so-called "paradoxic aciduria" sometimes described in stable chronic metabolic alkalosis because the effects of Cl^- or K^+ depletion prevent urinary excretion of HCO_3^-.

Additional laboratory tests including serum $[Ca^{2+}]$ and osmolality and urine creatinine, $[Cl^-]$, $[K^+]$, $Na^+]$, osmolality, and Ca^{2+} for the differential diagnosis are discussed below.

▶ Differential Diagnosis

A urine $[Cl^-]$ of less than 10 mEq/L characterizes chloride depletion except when a chloruretic diuretic is present in the urine or accompanying profound K^+ depletion produces severe tubule dysfunction that induces a Cl^- leak. Cl^- depletion can be generated by losses from the gut or the kidney; in chloridorrhea, the stool $[Cl^-]$ is greater than 90 mEq/L. Fully compensated respiratory acidosis is a Cl^- depletion state that will persist after the successful treatment of chronic respiratory acidosis if Cl^- repletion has not occurred. In cystic fibrosis (in which renal Cl^- handling is normal), high sweat $[Cl^-]$ can contribute to Cl^- losses with excessive sweating.

When the urine $[Cl^-]$ is greater than 20 mEq/L, K^+-depletion alkalosis and other miscellaneous disorders are suggested. When K^+ depletion is present, the urine K^+ excretion is normally less than 20 mEq/day. Thus, in the differential diagnosis of K^+-depletion alkalosis, urine K^+ excretion greater than 30 mEq/day in the presence of hypokalemia establishes renal K^+ wasting and indicates mineralocorticoid excess or an agent that promotes renal K^+ wasting. Within this group, K^+-depletion alkalosis can be further subdivided by the status of ECF volume and blood pressure. In those diseases characterized by persistent intravascular and ECF volume expansion and consequent hypertension, such as primary aldosteronism or syndromes of apparent mineralocorticoid excess, escape from the Na^+-retaining effect of mineralocorticoids occurs but not from the K^+-wasting effects thereby promoting alkalosis. The transtubular K^+ gradient is a fast and useful test for determining the presence of renal K^+ wasting; a value of more than 4 in the setting of hypokalemia is consistent with this abnormality.

In contrast, in Bartter syndrome, Na^+ loss as well as both K^+ and Cl^- losses are associated with normotension. Gitelman's syndrome is similar but is less severe and is characterized by hypocalciuria not hypercalciuria seen in Bartter's syndrome. These uncommon syndromes could be confused with some of the commonly concealed causes of metabolic alkalosis such as diuretic or laxative abuse, bulimia, or surreptitious vomiting.

When the urine K^+ excretion is less than 20 mEq/day, K^+ depletion due solely to dietary or gut losses is established. The alkalosis in these disorders is usually mild. More severe alkalosis should suggest additional causative factors, such as concomitant Cl^- depletion or base ingestion.

Hypercalcemia, usually in the setting of suppressed parathyroid hormone such as malignancy or vitamin D excess, may uncommonly be associated with alkalosis. In milk-alkali syndrome, multiple factors likely contribute to the alkalosis including vomiting, hypercalcemia, and reduced GFR in addition to the excessive calcium intake.

Hypoalbuminemia may cause mild metabolic alkalosis because of the resultant shift in the buffering capacity of plasma. Patients can develop a metabolic alkalosis if they ingest alkali such as $NaHCO_3$ (eg, baking soda) or calcium carbonate and cannot excrete the excess HCO_3^- because of renal insufficiency. Obligate excretion of anions with preferential retention of bicarbonate putatively explains the alkalosis that has rarely been associated with some antibiotics.

Transient states of alkalosis are common but usually inconsequential. Intravenous or oral base loading may occur during the transfusion of blood or blood products with a citrate anticoagulant or with the treatment of metabolic acidosis.

▶ Treatment

A. General Principles

Specific treatment is indicated when the arterial pH is greater than 7.55 or the serum bicarbonate concentration is greater than 33 mEq/L. Existing deficits must be replaced and the continued generation of losses should be prevented or blunted to the extent possible.

B. Chloride Depletion

The Cl^- deficit must be replaced with the selection of the accompanying cation based on (1) ECF volume status, (2) the degree of associated K^+ depletion, and (3) the degree and reversibility of any depression of GFR. Because the magnitude of the loss of each of these cations is difficult to assess, an empirical clinical approach is recommended. When Cl^- and severe K^+ depletion coexist, both must be repleted to correct the alkalosis. In patients with overt signs of ECF volume contraction, administration of 3–5 L of 0.15 M NaCl at a minimum is usually necessary to correct volume deficits and metabolic alkalosis. When volume is repleted, further Cl^- repletion should be accomplished with KCl unless contraindications are present.

In the clinical setting of ECF volume overload such as congestive cardiac failure in association with Cl^- depletion alkalosis, NaCl administration is contraindicated. KCl is the preferred alternative in this setting but it too may be contraindicated or limited because of either concurrent hyperkalemia or renal insufficiency, which could precipitate hyperkalemia.

In addition to volume overload, other serious conditions such as hepatic encephalopathy, cardiac arrhythmias, digitalis cardiotoxicity, or altered mental status also may accompany severe alkalosis. No clinical studies specifically address the impact of the treatment of severe alkalosis on the outcome in these states. However, the high reported mortality of severe alkalosis suggests that to the extent that it may be a contributing factor, alkalosis should be corrected promptly. HCl (0.1 N) administration through a central venous catheter at rates up to 25 mEq/hour should be considered when either Na^+ or K^+ is not appropriate. The amount of HCl needed to correct alkalosis is calculated by the following formula: $0.5 \times$ body weight (kg) $\times$ desired decrement in plasma bicarbonate (mEq/L) with additional amounts to replace any continuing losses of acid. Plasma bicarbonate concentration should be initially restored halfway to normal.

An alternative to HCl is ammonium chloride, which may be administered via a peripheral vein at a rate of not more than 300 mEq NH_4^+/day; it should be avoided in advanced renal or hepatic insufficiency. The HCl salts of lysine or arginine are available but have been associated with severe hyperkalemia; they are not recommended. Of these agents, HCl is preferred and should be used only as noted.

In the setting of volume overload, acetazolamide 250 mg orally two or three times daily or 5–10 mg/kg intravenously may be effective if GFR is adequate. Because the distal nephron can avidly reabsorb excess Na^+ delivery promoted by acetazolamide, the carbonic anhydrase (CA) inhibitors are most effective when used in conjunction with diuretics that have more distal sites of action. Acetazolamide could also be used intermittently to avoid or decrease chloride-depletion matabolic alkalosis (CDA) in edema-forming states such as congestive heart failure treated with loop diuretics. Serum electrolyte composition should be followed serially during its administration since acetazolamide is usually associated with high urinary K^+ losses.

CA in erythrocytes and along the pulmonary capillary endothelium participates in the dehydration of bicarbonate to CO_2 and its subsequent excretion by the lung. Studies in critically ill patients have shown only minor CO_2 retention. Particularly in patients with impaired respiratory function, clinicians should be alert to this potential for CO_2 retention with CA inhibition. In such patients, the goal of treatment is the usual stable plasma bicarbonate concentration for that patient and not necessarily a normal concentration.

Other primary or adjunctive therapies should be considered. Villous adenomas require surgical removal. Congenital chloridorrhea does not respond to antidiarrheal agents and dietary repletion of fluid; Cl^- and K^+ losses are usually required. Omeprazole 20 mg twice daily may substantially decrease diarrhea and obviate the need for dietary electrolyte supplementation; the reduction in the intestinal Cl^- load by inhibition of gastric Cl^- secretion is presumably the mechanism. When continuing gastric acid losses cannot be prevented, eg, Zollinger–Ellison syndrome, omeprazole or a histamine 2-receptor blocker, eg, cimetidine or ranitidine, will reduce output. These blocking agents have also been used to augment Cl^- replacement in patients with unremitting losses due to gastrocystoplasty; on occasion, only surgical revision can correct the alkalosis in these patients.

If renal insufficiency limits the effectiveness of the above therapies or in patients on maintenance dialysis, hemofiltration with replacement infusions of NaCl, exchange of bicarbonate for high bath $[Cl^-]$ during hemodialysis, or peritoneal dialysis is an effective means for correcting metabolic alkalosis.

C. Potassium Depletion

The magnitude of K^+ depletion can be estimated from the serum $[K^+]$. The decrease in serum $[K^+]$ evoked by alkalosis per se (approximately a 0.5 mEq decrement for each 0.1 increment in arterial pH) accounts for only a modest overestimation of the K^+ deficit.

Oral replacement will often suffice unless ileus is present. Oral KCl given in the liquid form diluted with fruit juice or in the slow-release form can be given in doses of up to 40–60 mEq four or five times per day. K^+ salts such as citrate, gluconate, or bicarbonate are not appropriate.

If, however, a serious cardiac arrhythmia or generalized paralysis is present, intravenous KCl in concentrations no greater than 60 mEq/L at rates as high as 40 mEq/hour should be preferred. The downregulation of Na^+-K^+-ATPase in skeletal muscle with K^+ depletion states may slow the clearing of the K^+ load. Thus, monitoring with electrocardiograms and frequent determinations of serum $[K^+]$ are mandatory. Glucose should be omitted from infusions initially because stimulated insulin secretion may cause serum $[K^+]$ to decrease even further. However, once repletion is begun, infused glucose will facilitate cellular K^+ repletion. If chloruretic diuretics or laxatives are contributing, they should be stopped.

Correction of the K^+ deficit reverses the alkalinizing effects of K^+ depletion but blockade or removal of the source of mineralocorticoid excess is essential for definitive correction. If the source of aldosterone excess cannot be removed, K^+-sparing diuretics will blunt its effects. Amiloride 5–10 mg daily, triamterene 100 mg twice daily, or spironolactone 25–50 mg in single or divided doses daily all are useful. Restriction of Na^+ and addition of K^+ to the diet also ameliorate the alkalosis and associated hypertension.

In Bartter's syndrome, the focus of therapy is to prevent urinary K^+ loss. Converting enzyme inhibitors have been shown to be effective and are a reasonable first approach. Because of concern for hypotension, low doses should be used initially. Other interventions may also partially correct the alkalosis. The K^+-sparing diuretics mentioned above are effective but dietary K^+ supplementation is usually also needed. Spironolactone may produce unacceptable gynecomastia in men. Because renal production of prostaglandin E_2 is increased and may contribute to Na^+, Cl^-, and K^+ wasting, prostaglandin synthetase inhibitors, such as indomethacin or ibuprofen, may blunt but not completely correct the hypokalemic alkalosis. Since magnesium depletion may contribute to the increase in urinary K^+ wasting, hypomagnesemia should be corrected and magnesium stores repleted, if clinically feasible. Oral magnesium oxide in doses of 250–500 mg four times daily (12.5–25 mEq Mg^{2+}) is recommended. However, the degree to which the correction of magnesium depletion blunts the alkalosis is uncertain and magnesium salts often produce an unacceptable degree of diarrhea that can worsen electrolyte imbalance.

Several of the primary disorders of mineralocorticoid excess are treated definitively by tumor ablation or by medication when that cannot be accomplished.

D. Miscellaneous

In acute milk-alkali syndrome, cessation of alkali ingestion and the calcium sources (milk, antacids, etc.) and repletion of Cl^- and volume usually will lead to the prompt resolution of these abnormalities. The treatment of hypercalcemia is discussed in Chapter 6. For those alkaloses due to alkali loading, cessation of alkali administration and continuation of normal electrolyte intake will usually suffice.

▶ Prognosis

Data on the prevalence and outcome of metabolic alkalosis are sparse. Metabolic alkalosis is common and, when severe, is associated with high morbidity and mortality; in one study, it comprised half of all acid–base disorders. A mortality rate of 45% in patients with a pH of 7.55 and of 80% when the pH was greater than 7.65 has been recorded and confirmed in a separate study (48.5% for alkalemia greater than 7.60). While this relationship between alkalemia and mortality is not necessarily causal, severe alkalosis should be viewed with concern and should be promptly treated.

Galla JH: Metabolic alkalosis. J Am Soc Nephrol 2000;11:369. [PMID: 10665945]

▼ METABOLIC ACIDOSIS

Ira Kurtz, MD, & Jeffrey A. Kraut, MD

ESSENTIALS OF DIAGNOSIS

▶ Reduction in plasma bicarbonate concentration.

▶ Reduction in blood pH.

▶ Decreased concentration of carbon dioxide (the compensatory respiratory response).

▶ General Considerations

Metabolic acidosis is one of the four primary acid–base disorders and is caused by a reduction in plasma bicarbonate concentration. It is associated with a reduction in blood pH (termed acidemia) and a decrease in the concentration of carbon dioxide (PCO_2), termed the compensatory respiratory response.

Metabolic acidosis can result from several different mechanisms including (1) excessive systemic H^+ loads as with ketoacidosis or lactic acidosis, (2) impairment in renal

HCO_3^- generation as with renal failure, (3) extrarenal HCO_3^- loss as with gastrointestinal HCO_3^- loss with small bowel diarrhea, and (4) renal HCO_3^- loss as with proximal renal tubular acidosis (RTA).

▶ Pathophysiology

A. Normal Control of Acid–Base Balance

The plasma bicarbonate concentration is normally maintained at a constant level of 24–25 mEq/L in males and 22–23 mEq/L in nonpregnant females. Plasma bicarbonate concentration is maintained at these levels, despite ongoing H^+ production resulting from metabolism of dietary constituents, because of compensatory equimolar generation of bicarbonate by the kidney ($\sim$70 mmol/day). In addition, since the kidney filters a large quantity of bicarbonate each day, $\sim$4500 mEq, it must reclaim most of this bicarbonate to maintain a normal plasma bicarbonate concentration.

Approximately 85% of filtered bicarbonate is reclaimed in the proximal tubule. As depicted in Figure 5–1, this bicarbonate is reabsorbed indirectly via the apical sodium–hydrogen exchanger NHE3, and exits the cell via the sodium–bicarbonate cotransporter kNBC1. Membrane-bound carbonic anhydrase IV in the apical and basolateral membranes and cytoplasmic carbonic anhydrase II are necessary for efficient absorption of filtered bicarbonate from the tubular fluid to the systemic circulation.

In addition to absorbing the filtered bicarbonate load, the kidney needs to generate new bicarbonate to match the loss of HCO_3 resulting from neutralization of acid generated in the liver from the daily metabolism of dietary protein. The proximal tubule in the kidney generates the new HCO_3 primarily from the metabolism of glutamine. In addition to HCO_3, NH_4^+ is also produced. The HCO_3 is transported across the basolateral membrane of the proximal tubule cell to the systemic circulation. Were all the NH_4^+ produced in the proximal tubule transferred along with HCO_3 to the systemic circulation, the HCO_3 produced in the proximal tubule would be converted to urea in the liver and therefore would be unavailable to buffer the dietary H^+ load. As depicted in Figure 5–1, this futile cycle is prevented by intrarenal transport mechanisms that ensure that a portion of the NH_4^+ is trapped in the lumen of the collecting duct as the result of proton transport by an apically located vacuolar H^+-ATPase and possibly H^+-K^+-ATPase. Luminal proton transport by the H^+-ATPase is coupled to basolateral bicarbonate exit via the anion exchanger AE1, with the NH_4^+ subsequently excreted in the urine.

Collecting duct proton secretion by the H^+-ATPase (the primary proton transporter) is modulated by the action of aldosterone, in part by enhancing sodium reabsorption via the epithelial sodium channel (ENaC) to produce a favorable electrical gradient. The kidney generates the remaining new HCO_3 by a process called titratable acid (TA) formation/excretion. In this process, secreted H^+ (via the proximal tubule NHE3, collecting duct H^+-ATPase, and possibly H^+-K^+-ATPase transporters) bind to HPO_4^{2-} in the tubule lumen and generates intracellular HCO_3 that is transported to the systemic circulation. Clinically, the total effective new bicarbonate generated by the kidney can be quantified by measuring a parameter called net acid excretion, which is equal to the urinary excretion of $NH_4^+ + TA - HCO_3^-$. Under normal acid–base conditions, 40 mEq NH_4 and 30 mEq TA are excreted daily while HCO_3^- excretion is negligible.

B. Physiologic Response to an Increment in Acid Load or Extrarenal Bicarbonate Loss

The normal response of the body to an H^+ load or HCO_3^- loss involves four processes: (1) Extracellular buffering, (2) intracellular buffering, (3) respiratory compensation, and (4) enhanced renal HCO_3^- generation. Immediately upon an increase in an acid load, H^+ is buffered by plasma HCO_3^- followed by H^+ influx into cells (intracellular buffering). The latter process occurs more slowly, and is completed in 2–4 hours. Approximately 60% of an H^+ load is buffered intracellularly, but this can increase dramatically with more severe degrees of metabolic acidosis as bicarbonate buffers are depleted. The degree of intracellular buffering can be indirectly determined by the quantity of bicarbonate required to raise plasma bicarbonate concentration to a certain level (bicarbonate deficit $\times$ bicarbonate space). The bicarbonate space is the apparent volume of distribution of administered bicarbonate and is calculated according to the following equation: Bicarbonate space = [0.4 + (2.6/plasma bicarbonate) $\times$ lean body weight]. The bicarbonate space can increase from 50% body weight with mild to moderate metabolic acidosis (12–23 mEq/L) to more than 100% body weight with severe metabolic acidosis (plasma bicarbonate concentration <5 mEq/L).

The kidney plays the dominant role in regulating acid–base balance by increasing the quantity of new HCO_3^- generated. New HCO_3^- generation increases immediately and achieves a maximal level in approximately 4 days. The quantity of HCO_3^- generated can increase several fold and is due primarily to enhanced glutamine metabolism.

C. Respiratory Compensation

A fall in plasma bicarbonate concentration and blood pH stimulates receptors in the periphery and central respiratory center increasing alveolar ventilation. The increase in alveolar ventilation creates an inequality between mitochondrial CO_2 production and pulmonary CO_2 excretion. P_{CO_2} decreases until a new steady state is reached, a process that requires approximately 12–24 hours. The magnitude of the decrease in P_{CO_2} for any given level of sustained metabolic acidosis has been empirically determined and is given by the following relationship: For a given decrease in HCO_3 of 10 mEq/L, the P_{CO_2} decreases by approximately 12 mm Hg. When the P_{CO_2} decreases appropriately, the metabolic acidosis is called

Proximal Tubule   **Collecting Duct**

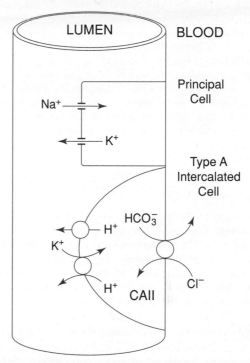

▲ **Figure 5–1.** In the proximal tubule luminal HCO_3 is absorbed across the apical cell membrane via the Na^+/H^+ exchanger NHE3. Intracellular HCO_3 is transported across the basolateral cell membrane via the electrogenic sodium bicarbonate cotransporter kNBC1 (NBCe1-A). In the collecting duct, the lumen is acidified by Type A Intercalated cells that secrete H^+ via an H^+ ATPase and possible an H^+-K^+-ATPase. Intracellular HCO_3 is transported across the basolateral cell membrane via the anion exchanger AE1. The acidification of the luminal fluid generates H_2PO_4 (titratable acid) and creates a driving force for the passive diffusion of NH_3 into the urine, thereby increasing the urinary excretion of NH_4^+. Principal cells in the collecting duct are responsible for absorbing Na^+ via the epithelial sodium channel (ENaC) and secreting K^+ via ROMK. The latter processes are stimulated by aldosterone that binds to receptors on the basolateral membrane of the principal cells.

"compensated" and a simple metabolic acidosis is said to be present. If the PCO_2 is above the predicted value, the patient has a coexisting defect in ventilation and a mixed acid–base disturbance, ie, respiratory acidosis and a metabolic acidosis. Conversely, if $PaCO_2$ falls below the expected value, the patient has a mixed metabolic acidosis and respiratory alkalosis.

SERUM ANION GAP

Metabolic acidosis is subdivided into those disorders in which the serum anion gap is normal and those in which it is elevated. The serum anion gap represents the concentration of unmeasured anions minus unmeasured cations: Na^+ + K^+ + unmeasured cations = Cl^- + HCO_3^- + unmeasured anions. Since the concentration of serum K^+ is low, it is not considered in the calculation of the serum anion gap, which is then calculated as $Na^+ - (Cl^- + HCO_3)$. The normal serum anion gap ranges between 8 and 18 mEq/L, with an average of 10–12 mEq/L. However, introduction of a new autoanalyzer method for measuring serum chloride in some clinical laboratories has resulted in a higher value of serum chloride and therefore a lower value for the mean serum anion gap (average of 6–8 mEq/L).

An increase in the serum anion gap is usually the result of retention of unmeasured anions in the blood, although rarely a decrease in the concentration of unmeasured cations can also be the cause. A decrease in the anion gap may be due to a decrease in the concentration of unmeasured anions (primarily negative charges on albumin) or an increase in unmeasured cations. An important cause of the latter is overproduction of cationic proteins seen in some cases of myeloma.

The differential diagnosis of metabolic acidosis is facilitated by examination of the serum anion gap. In certain forms of metabolic acidosis (eg, lactic acidosis, ketoacidosis) H^+ is infused into the circulation with a non-Cl^- anion such as lactate or β-hydroxybutyrate (see Table 5–2). The increase in the anion gap reflects the increase in the concentration of lactate or β-hydroxybutyrate. By contrast, in patients in whom HCO_3^- is lost from the body (eg, small bowel diarrhea, proximal RTA), the serum anion gap remains stable because the fall in plasma HCO_3 concentration is matched by an equivalent rise in serum Cl^-. C8 Metabolic acidosis associated with a high anion gap is called an elevated or high anion gap metabolic acidosis. Metabolic acidosis associated with a normal anion gap is also called hyperchloremic metabolic acidosis.

A. High Anion Gap

The disorders producing a high anion gap metabolic acidosis are shown in Table 5–2. They include renal failure, ketoacidosis, either diabetic or alcoholic, lactic acidosis, salicylate intoxication, and methanol and ethylene glycol intoxication.

A high anion gap metabolic acidosis can be observed with acute or chronic renal failure. With chronic renal failure, the acidosis is generally mild to moderate in degree, with plasma bicarbonate concentrations ranging from 12 to 22 mEq/L. Values below 12 mEq/L should raise the suspicion of superimposition of other acid–base disorders. Epidemiologic studies have indicated that the acidosis can first be detected when glomerular filtration rate (GFR) falls below 20–30 mL/minute of normal. Therefore, the presence of metabolic acidosis at higher levels of GFR should alert the physician to potential additional renal tubular disorders such as hyporeninemic hypoaldosteronism (Type IV RTA) that can cause a non-anion gap metabolic acidosis. The metabolic acidosis of chronic kidney disease remains the most common cause of chronic metabolic acidosis, ie, metabolic acidosis lasting for more than several days or weeks. Although chronic renal disease is often considered a paradigm of high anion gap metabolic acidosis, various studies have indicated that these patients can manifest a wide range of anion gap levels.

Metabolic acidosis is also frequent in oliguric acute renal failure. The severity of the metabolic acidosis in acute renal failure is dependent upon the level of residual renal function, duration of renal failure, and catabolic state of the patient. Thus, the acidosis will be more severe in catabolic patients with minimal residual renal function that has been present for several days.

Table 5–2. Causes of high anion gap metabolic acidosis.

Disorder	Anions [1]	Diagnostic clues	Comments
Renal failure[2]	Various organic and inorganic anions	GFR <30 mL/minute	Decreased renal bicarbonate generation rather than an excessive H^+ load
Lactic acidosis	Lactate	Evidence of hypotension and tissue hypoperfusion; serum lactate >5 mEq/L	Most common cause of severe metabolic acidosis
Diabetic ketoacidosis	Acetoacetate; β-hydroxybutyrate	Positive nitroprusside reaction; blood sugar elevated	Nitroprusside reaction may be trace positive or negative with coexisting lactic acidosis
Alcoholic ketoacidosis	Acetoacetate; β-hydroxybutyrate	Positive nitroprusside reaction; hypoglycemia, osmolal gap	Nitroprusside reaction may be trace positive or negative
Salicylate poisoning	Acetoacetate; β-hydroxybutyrate	Coexisting respiratory alkalosis; prolonged prothrombin time	
Methanol poisoning	Formate	Osmolal gap; optic papillitis	Osmolal gap may be absent if methanol is completely metabolized
Ethylene glycol poisoning	Glycolate; oxalate	Renal failure; oxalate crystals in urine	Osmolal gap may be absent if ethylene glycol is completely metabolized

[1]The increase in the blood concentrations of non-Cl^- anions increases the anion gap.
[2]In renal failure, the blood HCO_3 concentration decreases because of decreased new renal HCO_3 generation. In all other causes of a high anion gap metabolic acidosis the blood HCO_3 concentration decreases because of excessive H^+ influx into the blood. The mechanism for the increased anion gap in renal failure also differs from other causes of a high anion gap metabolic acidosis. Specifically, in renal failure, the decreased glomerular filtration rate (GFR) prevents various organic and inorganic anions from being excreted, whereas in the remaining diseases/poisonings in the table, the excessive organic anion load accompanying the influx of H^+ into the blood raises the anion gap.

Ketoacidosis either due to diabetes or alcohol intoxication is one of the most common causes of acute metabolic acidosis, ie, metabolic acidosis lasting a few hours to days. Diabetic ketoacidosis is detected by noting increased urinary and/or blood concentrations of ketoacids. The nitroprusside reaction detects acetoacetate and will be positive in the majority of cases of diabetic ketoacidosis. However, if diabetic ketoacidosis is complicated by lactic acidosis, or if there is alcoholic ketoacidosis, the reaction may be trace positive or even negative reflecting the predominance of β-hydroxybutyrate over acetoacetate in the body fluids. Therefore, a negative nitroprusside reaction does not exclude ketoacidosis. Most cases of diabetic ketoacidosis are associated with marked hyperglycemia. In contrast, alcoholic ketoacidosis is often characterized by a normal or low blood sugar, reflecting impaired glucose release from the liver. Another clue to the presence of alcoholic ketoacidosis is an elevated serum osmolal gap (see below). As noted with chronic renal failure, it has been recognized that patients with ketoacidosis can have a wide range of anion gap levels. However, patients with higher serum anion gap values are usually volume depleted, reflecting a decreased ability of the kidney to excrete the ketone bodies.

Lactic acidosis, another common cause of acute metabolic acidosis and possibly the most frequent cause of severe metabolic acidosis, is indicated by a blood pH <7.1 and plasma bicarbonate concentration <8–10 mEq/L. Indeed, ketoacidosis and lactic acidosis together account for more than 90% of the cases of metabolic acidosis in which the anion gap is >30 mEq/L. Type A lactic acidosis associated with tissue hypoxia is the most frequent type and can be readily suspected by the presence of hypotension and reduced tissue perfusion. The diagnosis of lactic acidosis is confirmed by a serum lactate concentration greater than 5 mEq/L.

Salicylate intoxication can cause both metabolic acidosis and respiratory alkalosis. Therefore, a high anion gap metabolic acidosis in association with respiratory alkalosis could indicate the presence of this disorder. Ketoacids accumulate and can be detected with the nitroprusside reaction. Although this acid–base disturbance has frequently been encountered in young adults trying to commit suicide, recent studies have found it in adults taking salicylates for treatment of rheumatic conditions. Another clue to its presence includes a prolonged prothrombin time. Treatment includes forced diuresis to increase urinary excretion of the salicylates and hemodialysis. The latter procedure is indicated when the serum levels of salicylates are extremely high or the patient has marked central nervous system (CNS) abnormalities.

Methanol (wood alcohol) and ethylene glycol (antifreeze) are rare, but serious causes of metabolic acidosis. Since both disorders can be rapidly lethal, it is critical to recognize their presence. Both substances are low-molecular-weight moieties and can increase serum osmolality. Therefore, measurement of serum osmolality and comparison of this value to the estimate of serum osmolality derived from consideration of the usual, osmotically active substances in blood can be of great value. Quantitatively the most important moieties contributing to serum osmolality are sodium (and its counterbalancing anions chloride and bicarbonate), glucose, and urea. Serum osmolality can rapidly be estimated using the following formula: $2 \times [Na^+] + [glucose]/18 + [BUN]/2.8$, where [glucose] and [BUN] (blood urea nitrogen) are expressed in mg/dL. An osmolal gap (defined as the difference between the measured and estimated serum osmolality) greater than 10 mOsm/kg H_2O indicates the presence in serum of additional osmotically active particles.

Alchoholic ketoacidosis is the most common cause of a high anion gap metabolic acidosis associated with an increased osmolal gap, but methanol and ethylene glycol intoxication are other important causes. A slight increase in the osmolal gap $\sim$10 mOsm/kg H_2O has been reported with lactic acidosis or chronic renal failure and might confound the diagnosis in some instances. If methanol and ethylene glycol are metabolized completely to their toxic byproducts, formic acid and glycolic acid, respectively, little or no increment in the osmolal gap might be detected. Other clues to the diagnosis of these disorders include optic papillitis in methanol intoxication and renal failure with oxalate crystals in the urine in patients with ethylene glycol intoxication. Treatments of methanol and ethylene glycol intoxication include infusion of alcohol to retard their metabolism and/or hemodialysis, which is very effective in removing these substances from the body.

In summary, rapid diagnosis of the cause of high anion gap metabolic acidosis can be facilitated by measuring serum creatinine, urine and blood ketones, serum osmolality, serum sodium, glucose, and urea nitrogen necessary for calculation of the serum osmolal gap, and serum salicylate levels. If an elevated osmolal gap is found, then measurement of methanol, ethylene glycol, and alcohol levels is warranted to detect one of these intoxications.

B. Normal Anion Gap (Hyperchloremic)

As shown in Table 5–3, disorders causing a normal anion metabolic acidosis are often subdivided into those in which serum potassium concentration is low and those in which serum potassium concentration is normal or elevated to facilitate diagnosis of the underlying cause. Alternatively, the disorders causing a normal anion gap acidosis can be categorized based on the predominant organ involved in their pathogenesis as discussed below.

1. Gastrointestinal causes—The most common cause of a normal anion gap metabolic acidosis associated with hypokalemia is diarrhea. Some studies have indicated this is more common with diarrhea emanating from the distal bowel. Other causes of gastrointestinal bicarbonate wasting include intestinal or pancreatic fistulas in which the bicarbonate-rich fluids are lost from the body. Construction of a conduit from the ureter to the sigmoid or ileal segments of the bowel is often done after removal of the bladder in patients with

Table 5–3. Causes of normal anion gap metabolic acidosis.

Disorder	Diagnostic clues	Comments
Low serum potassium		
Diarrhea	History of diarrhea	More frequent with lower bowel diarrhea
Pancreatic intestinal fistulas	History	
Ureterosigmoidostomy, ureteroileostomy		Common with use of sigmoid colon but presence with ileal conduit suggests obstruction
Proximal renal tubular acidosis (RTA)	Aminoaciduria, glycosuria; high base requirements	May be associated with less severe adverse consequences than distal RTA despite similar acidemia
Distal RTA	Decreased urine ammonium excretion; positive urine anion gap; decreased urine osmolar gap	Causes stunting of growth in children
Normal or high serum potassium		
Total parenteral nutrition (TPN) (cationic amino acids)	History of receiving TPN solution	Uncommon with balanced solutions
Hyporeninemic hypoaldosteronism	History of diabetes; urine pH <5.5	Frequent in diabetics
Aldosterone resistance	Urine pH >5.5; normal serum aldosterone values	Occurs in patients with sickle cell disease, obstructive uropathy, interstitial nephritis
Gordon's syndrome	Hypercalciuria	WNK1, WNK4 mutations
Adrenal insufficiency	Presence of salt wasting and hypotension	Metabolic acidosis detected in patients with volume depletion

bladder cancer. The former procedure is regularly accompanied by the development of hypokalemic metabolic acidosis, whereas with the latter procedure this disorder usually indicates blockage of the ileal conduit.

Administration of solutions containing amino acids that are metabolized in the liver to produce hydrochloric acid (arginine, lysine) or sulfuric acid (cysteine, methionine) can also produce a normal anion gap acidosis with hyperkalemia. In this regard, the administration of total parenteral nutrition solutions containing cationic and sulfur-containing amino acids causes a metabolic acidosis. Addition of sufficient organic anions, such as acetate, that are metabolized into HCO_3^- has eliminated or reduced the severity of this problem.

2. Renal causes—(A) PROXIMAL RENAL TUBULAR ACIDOSIS (TYPE 2)—Proximal RTA (Table 5–4) is the result of impaired reabsorption of filtered HCO_3 leading to urinary bicarbonate wasting. This can be due to selective dysfunction of proteins present in the proximal tubule essential for bicarbonate absorption such as the basolateral Na–HCO_3 cotransporter (kNBC1), defective cytoplasmic carbonic anhydrase (CAII) activity, or metabolic abnormalities that alter cellular adenosine triphosphate (ATP) production. The causes of proximal RTA are either genetic or acquired as shown in

Table 5–4. When generalized proximal tubule malabsorption is present, bicarbonate wasting may be accompanied by glycosuria, phosphaturia, aminoaciduria, and hyperuricosuria (Fanconi's syndrome).

During the generation phase of proximal RTA, an excessive amount of HCO_3 is delivered to the distal nephron (which is incapable of reclaiming it), resulting in a net renal excretion of bicarbonate. The excretion of bicarbonate causes the plasma HCO_3 to decrease, resulting in a metabolic acidosis. The decrease in plasma HCO_3 lowers the filtered load of HCO_3 (GFR $\times$ plasma bicarbonate). Once the plasma HCO_3 concentration falls below the reabsorptive threshold for the patient, the proximal tubule will again be able to reclaim the majority of the luminal HCO_3 and the excessive excretion of bicarbonate will no longer occur. A new steady state is achieved, albeit at a plasma HCO_3 concentration lower than normal.

The reabsorptive threshold in proximal RTA can vary, resulting in a steady-state plasma HCO_3 concentration ranging from 15 mEq/L to 22 mEq/L. Urinary bicarbonate wastage will also occur as bicarbonate is administered to patients to raise the plasma HCO_3 concentration. Urine pH is elevated during both the generation phase and reparative phases of proximal RTA, but is appropriately acidic during the steady state.

Table 5–4. Classification of renal tubular acidosis.

	Proximal (Type II)	Distal (Type I)	Distal (Type IV)	Distal (HDRTA)
Mechanism	Defective proximal tubule HCO_3^- absorption	Defective collecting duct H^+ secretion	Defective collecting duct H^+ secretion	Defective collecting duct H^+ secretion
$FEHCO_3^-$	↑	Normal	Normal	Normal
Urine pH	Acute >5.5 Chronic <5.5	>5.5	<5.5	>5.5
Serum K^+	↓	↓	↑	↑
Ca^{2+} excretion	↑	↑	Normal	Normal or ↑

HDRTA, hyperkalemic distal renal tubular acidosis; $FEHCO_3^-$, fractional excretion of HCO_3.

Proximal RTA is diagnosed by measuring the fractional excretion of HCO_3 ($FEHCO_3$) when the plasma HCO_3 concentration has been normalized using the following formula:

$$\frac{HCO_3 \text{ (urine)} \times \text{creatinine (plasma)} \times 100\%}{HCO_3 \text{ (plasma)} \times \text{creatinine (urine)}}$$

A value greater than 20% is diagnostic of proximal RTA. The defect in proximal tubule HCO_3 bicarbonate absorption may be mild. In this case, the $FEHCO_3$ will be less than 20%. Since the nephron segments distal to the proximal tubule normally absorb ~20% of the filtered HCO_3 load, an $FEHCO_3^-$ less than 20% does not necessarily implicate the proximal tubule as the site of defective HCO_3 absorption. Hypokalemia is prominent in proximal RTA, although it is often less severe than in distal RTA. Urinary K^+ losses are in large part associated with urinary HCO_3 and Na^+ losses, and therefore are most severe during generation and treatment of proximal RTA.

(B) DISTAL RENAL TUBULAR ACIDOSIS—Distal RTA has traditionally been divided into two types: Type I (hypokalemic) and Type IV (hyperkalemic) (Table 5–4). In both forms, there is decreased collecting duct net H^+ secretion and consequent reduced titratable acid ($H_2PO_4^{2-}$) excretion and NH_4^+ excretion leading to decreased new renal bicarbonate generation. Defective net proton transport can be due to (1) impaired hydrogen secretion from a dysfunction of one of the subunits of the H^+-ATPase and possibly the H^+-K^+-ATPase (Figure 5-1), (2) increased luminal H^+ efflux into the cells because of increased apical cellular permeability (occurring with exposure to amphotericin B), or (3) impaired hydrogen secretion because of a less favorable electrical gradient due to the abnormal function of aldosterone, decreased sodium absorption via ENaC (sodium channel), or augmented chloride entry (chloride shunt).

Type I RTA can result from genetic diseases affecting the transporters that play a role in collecting duct proton secretion or from diseases that damage the collecting duct.

Genetic causes have been ascribed to mutations in the apical H^+-ATPase and basolateral Cl–HCO_3 exchanger, AE1, and carbonic anhydrase II, which is expressed in collecting duct intercalated cells. Although many features are shared among these disorders, the clinical phenotype differs somewhat depending upon the transporter that is affected. Thus, patients with mutations in AE1 sometimes have red cell abnormalities. Type I RTA due to AE1 mutations is either autosomal dominant or autosomal negative. Some patients with mutations in specific H^+-ATPase subunits have concomitant sensorineural deafness, since the proton pump is expressed in the inner ear. Patients with carbonic anhydrase II mutations can have a combined proximal and distal RTA and bony abnormalities.

Many patients with distal RTA in addition to metabolic acidosis have hypercalciuria, nephrocalcinosis, and hypokalemia. In some patients osteomalacic bone disease can also be detected.

Although the hypercalciuria is often attributed to the metabolic acidosis and the buffering of H^+ by bone, this explanation is likely incomplete, given that many patients with Type IV RTA or patients with extrarenal causes of metabolic acidosis do not have hypercalciuria. The hypokalemia has been attributed to impaired collecting duct H^+-K^+-ATPase rather than impaired vacuolar H^+-ATPase function. This explanation may not be correct, since patients with distal RTA due to genetic defects in the vacuolar H^+-ATPase also have hypokalemia. An alternate explanation is that Na^+ wasting results in volume depletion and enhanced aldosterone secretion with subsequent increased collecting duct K^+ secretion and renal K^+ excretion. Importantly, since these disorders often appear in childhood and metabolic acidosis affects bone metabolism, stunted growth may be present.

Acquired disorders such as systemic lupus erythematosus (SLE), interstitial nephritis, and Sjögren's syndrome can injure the collecting duct and produce Type I RTA. Immunohistochemical staining of some patients with SLE have documented a decrease in H^+-ATPase pumps in the collecting duct.

Patients with distal RTA are often recognized by documenting an elevated urine pH (>5.5) in the presence of a normal anion gap metabolic acidosis in the absence of diarrhea (see below). More sophisticated studies of collecting duct proton secretion such as a urine minus blood PCO_2 difference after bicarbonate infusion or urinary acidification with sodium sulfate administration can be helpful in determining the precise mechanism of the disease, but are often not required in clinical practice.

C. Hyperkalemic Distal Renal Tubular Acidosis

Hyperkalemia associated with distal RTA was first recognized in patients with hyporeninemic hypoaldosteronism, and was designated Type IV RTA to distinguish the syndrome from Types I, II, and III RTA associated with hypokalemia. Subsequently, other causes of distal RTA associated with hyperkalemia were recognized in which a low serum aldosterone concentration was not the pathogenic mechanism. The term Type IV RTA is used when referring to patients with hyperkalemic distal RTA due to an abnormality in the renin–aldosterone axis resulting in aldosterone deficiency or aldosterone resistance (pseudohypoaldosteronism). Importantly, these patients are able to acidify their urine appropriately. Patients with distal RTA and hyperkalemia where aldosterone does not play a role (Table 5–4) are diagnosed as having hyperkalemic distal RTA (HDRTA). These patients are unable to acidify their urine appropriately.

The causes of Type IV RTA are listed in Table 5–5. It is important to realize that not all patients with Type IV RTA have hyporeninemic hypoaldosteronism. Depending on the cause, patients with Type IV RTA can have elevated aldosterone and renin levels as, for example, in genetic or acquired syndromes resulting in aldosterone resistance (Table 5–5). Furthermore, some patients with Type IV RTA have high renin and low aldosterone levels [angiotensin-converting enzyme (ACE) inhibition, adrenal abnormalities, heparin].

As shown in Table 5–6, based on the pathogenesis of the disorder patients with HDRTA are further subcategorized into those with genetic or acquired diseases that decrease ENaC activity and those with a genetic disease called Gordon's syndrome, also referred to as a chloride shunt defect. Acquired causes of decreased ENaC activity include treatment with amiloride, pentamidine, trimethoprim, or triamterene, which all bind to and block sodium absorption via ENaC. Patients with Gordon's syndrome have hypercalciuria and hypertension, distinguishing them clinically from patients with HDRTA due to decreased ENaC activity. Gordon's syndrome has recently been shown to be due to mutations in WNK1 and WNK4 kinases.

Diagnosis—Diagnosis of the cause of normal anion gap metabolic acidosis can often be made with the use of clinical information and routine laboratory studies. However, since defects in renal acidification are often prominent causes, measurement or estimates of urine NH_4^+ excretion can be helpful. In general, in patients with extrarenal metabolic acidosis, the urine NH_4^+ excretion is increased several fold. Failure to detect an appropriate increase in urine NH_4^+ excretion will implicate the kidney as the cause of the metabolic acidosis. The urine NH_4^+ concentration can be estimated from calculation of either the urine anion or osmolal gap. The former is calculated from $[Na^+] - (Cl^- + HCO_3^-)$ in a urine with

Table 5–5. Causes of type IV renal tubular acidosis.

I. Features: Elevated renin/aldosterone levels and low–normal blood pressure
Causes: Spironolactone
Pseudohypoaldosteronism Type Ib (autosomal dominant)

II. Features: Low renin/low–normal aldosterone levels and low–normal blood pressure
Causes: Congenital hyporeninemic hypoaldosteronism
Acquired hyporeninemic hypoaldosteronism: diabetic nephropathy, interstitial nephritis, multiple myeloma, renal amyloidosis, β-blockers, nonsteroidal anti-inflammatory drugs, cyclosporin A, mitomycin C

III. Features: Elevated renin/low–normal aldosterone levels and low–normal blood pressure
Causes: Angiotensin-converting enzyme inhibitor, AT_1 receptor blockers
Aldosterone synthase deficiency: Congenital: Corticosterone 18-hydroxylase/18-methyloxidase deficiency; acquired: heparin, chlorbutol Congenital adrenal hypoplasia (DAX-1 mutation)
Congenital adrenal hyperplasia: Cholesterol desmolase deficiency, 3β-hydroxysteroid dehydrogenase deficiency, 21-hydroxylase deficiency
Adrenoleukodystrophy, adrenomyeloneuropathy
Acquired adrenal insufficiency: Infectious, autoimmune, sarcoidosis, amyloidosis, mitotane, aminoglutethimide, torilostane, ketoconazole

Table 5–6. Causes of hyperkalemic distal renal tubular acidosis (HDRTA).

I. Mechanism: Decreased epithelial sodium channel (ENaC) Na^+ channel transport
Features: Low–normal blood pressure associated with elevated renin/aldosterone
Causes: Amiloride, pentamidine, trimethoprim, triamterene
Urinary tract obstruction (associated decrease in Na^+-K^+-ATPase activity)
Sickle cell disease
Pseudohypoaldosteronism Type Ib (autosomal recessive; α, β, or γ subunits)
Volume depletion (decreased collecting duct Na^+ concentration)

II. Mechanism: Enhanced NaCl absorption via the thiazide-sensitive NaCl cotransporter secondary to WNK1 or WNK4 mutations
Features: Hypertension and hypercalciuria associated with suppressed renin and low–normal aldosterone level
Cause: Gordon's syndrome (pseudohypoaldosteronism Type II or Cl^--shunt defect)

a pH <6.5, which is free of nonreabsorbable anions such as ketones. In an acidemic patient, the urine anion gap should be negative (~ -30 mEq/L). A positive urine anion gap indicates a low NH_4^+ concentration. In patients in whom there is increased excretion of unmeasured anions, such as ketones or hippurate, the urine anion gap can be positive despite ample quantities of NH_4^+ in the urine. In these rare cases, the urine osmolal gap can be calculated from the measured osmolality $- (2[Na^+ + K^+] + [\text{urea nitrogen}]/2.8 + [\text{glucose}]/18)$, where [urea nitrogen] and [glucose] are measured in mg/dL. An appropriate urine osmolal gap in an acidemic patient is greater than 150–200 mOsm/kg H_2O (the NH_4^+ concentration is half this value), whereas in patients with a decreased urine NH_4^+ concentration as in renal failure or distal RTA, the osmolal gap is usually less than 50–100 mOsm/kg H_2O.

Measurement of urine pH in patients with normal anion gap metabolic acidosis can complement the estimation of urinary ammonium excretion for further characterization of metabolic acidosis resulting from defects in renal acidification. For optimal measurement of urine pH and ammonium, a sample of urine should be obtained under oil (to prevent CO_2 loss) when the patient is acidemic. If the urine pH is below 5.5, bicarbonate is administered until the urine becomes alkaline or the serum bicarbonate returns to normal. The development of an alkaline urine (pH >6.5) prior to normalization of serum bicarbonate indicates that proximal RTA (defective proximal tubule bicarbonate absorption) is present. If urine pH is high (>6.0) and remains relatively constant despite bicarbonate administration, distal RTA is potentially present. It is necessary to be cautious in making a diagnosis of distal RTA without initially ruling out diarrhea as a cause of a non-gap acidosis and an elevated urine pH. Importantly, hypokalemia due to diarrhea can result in an inappropriately elevated urine pH that is due to a decrease in collecting duct H^+ secretion (distal RTA), but results from the fact that hypokalemia is a potent stimulus of renal NH_3 production. The excess NH_3 in the urine binds to secreted H^+, thereby elevating the urine pH despite normal tubular H^+ secretion. Importantly, when the hypokalemia is treated, NH_3 production by the kidney decreases, and the urine pH decreases appropriately. In contrast, in Type I distal RTA, correction of hypokalemia has no effect on the urine pH.

The classification of metabolic acidosis into high anion gap and normal anion gap forms is extremely useful in determining the cause of the acidosis. The reciprocal fall in serum bicarbonate, termed the (delta) ΔHCO_3, and the rise in the anion gap, termed the Δ anion gap, have also been useful in the identification of mixed forms of metabolic acidosis. It has been suggested that there is a strict 1:1 relationship between the rise in the serum anion gap and fall in serum bicarbonate concentration in patients with high anion gap metabolic acidosis. However, the ratio between the Δ anion gap and ΔHCO_3 can range between 1 and 2 and may differ with different acid–base disorders. Thus, with lactic acidosis the rise in the serum anion gap exceeds the fall in bicarbonate

concentration, reflecting in part differences in the volume of distribution of H^+ and lactate ions (H^+ is buffered in intracellular and extracellular compartments, whereas lactate anion is confined to the extracellular space). By contrast, the Δ anion gap to ΔHCO_3 ratio in diabetic ketoacidosis is $\sim 1:1$. However, irrespective of the precise nature of the relationship between the ΔHCO_3 and the Δ anion gap, the sum of the value for the Δ anion gap and the prevailing blood HCO_3 concentration allows an approximation of the basal value of the blood HCO_3 concentration existing prior to the development of the high anion gap metabolic acidosis. This concept is important both for distinguishing between a high anion gap metabolic acidosis and a mixed high and normal anion gap metabolic acidosis, and for detecting the presence of a mixed high anion gap metabolic acidosis and metabolic alkalosis.

▶ Clinical Findings

The clinical findings associated with metabolic acidosis are relatively limited and primarily related to the underlying cause. Hyperventilation reflecting the respiratory response to the metabolic acidosis might be observed. With severe degrees of metabolic acidosis organ dysfunction such as impaired cardiac output and hypotension might be apparent. With chronic metabolic acidosis, bone disease and muscle wasting may be present, which produce clinical abnormalities.

The nature of the adverse effects of metabolic acidosis depends on both the duration of the metabolic acidosis and its severity. It is valuable to consider the effects of acute and chronic metabolic acidosis separately.

A. Adverse Effects of Acute Metabolic Acidosis

The adverse effects of acute metabolic acidosis include decreased cardiac output and hypotension, impaired glucose control, decreased tissue perfusion, reduced oxygen delivery, and induction of an inflammatory state. There is a direct relationship between the severity of the acidemia and the appearance of these changes, with most appearing when the blood pH is less than 7.1–7.2. Although not definitively proven, there is a correlation between the severity of acidemia and mortality, increasing at lower values of blood pH. These findings have an important bearing on the approach to treatment taken by most clinicians (see below).

B. Adverse Effects of Chronic Metabolic Acidosis

The adverse effects of chronic metabolic acidosis are distinctly different from those of acute metabolic acidosis. Chronic metabolic acidosis has been shown to impair bone metabolism contributing to the genesis of osteomalacia and/ or osteitis fibrosa and might also play a role in the genesis of osteoporosis. Muscle wasting has been demonstrated in both experimental and clinical studies of chronic metabolic acidosis, which improves with correction of the acidosis. Similarly, chronic metabolic acidosis can contribute to the genesis of hypoalbuminemia. Insulin resistance due to impaired ligand binding may contribute to abnormal glucose tolerance. In experimental studies in animals, metabolic acidosis can exacerbate renal disease, but this remains to be shown in humans. Cardiac disease so prominent in acute metabolic acidosis has not been shown to be present by chronic metabolic acidosis, although mortality in dialysis patients was increased in the presence of acidosis. Of interest, many of these abnormalities can be seen with even mild metabolic acidosis, a finding that has important implications for treatment.

▷ Treatment

Treatment of acute metabolic acidosis remains one of the more controversial issues in clinical medicine. Although severe acidemia (blood pH <7.1 to 7.2) has been shown to have important adverse effects on organ function, base administration to raise blood pH has not been demonstrated to improve the outcome of lactic acidosis or ketoacidosis, the two disorders in which this issue has been examined. Moreover, in some studies, when bicarbonate is given, a decrease in cardiac output has been found in patients with lactic acidosis and exacerbation of cerebral edema has been noted in children with diabetic ketoacidosis. Benefits and possible adverse effects of treatment of normal anion gap metabolic acidosis have not been examined in a prospective way. These adverse effects of bicarbonate administration have been attributed in part to a bicarbonate-induced reduction in the intracellular pH rise in cellular sodium and fall in ionized calcium. We presently recommend administration of bicarbonate when blood pH is less than 7.1 as a constant infusion rather than a bolus. A calcium infusion might be indicated if ionized calcium falls. Moreover, we target a blood pH ~7.2 but not higher initially. We also recommend considering alternative bases such as tris (hydroxymethyl) aminomethane (THAM) or the use of continuous renal replacement therapy.

Treatment of chronic metabolic acidosis is less controversial because the side effects of treatment are less severe. Since even mild metabolic acidosis can contribute to abnormalities of bone and muscle metabolism, we recommend complete normalization of acid–base balance. This can be achieved with administration of either oral bicarbonate or other bases that are metabolized to produce bicarbonate, such as Shohl's solution (sodium citrate). The latter is preferred because oral bicarbonate can produce gas that patients do not tolerate well. Possible consequences of base administration include potentiation of vascular calcifications and volume excess and exacerbation of hypertension (from accompanying sodium).

▼ RESPIRATORY ACID–BASE DISORDERS

Gregg Y. Lipschik, MD, & Jeanne P. Macrae, MD

The respiratory acid–base disorders, respiratory alkalosis and respiratory acidosis, are commonly seen in intensive care units and emergency rooms, as well as in general practice. Both are caused by changes in alveolar ventilation that lead to a rise or fall in the partial pressure of CO_2 in arterial blood (PCO_2). The clinical importance of these disorders, however, is very different. While respiratory alkalosis rarely requires specific treatment, respiratory acidosis accompanies some of the most dramatic presentations of illness a physician will see.

CO_2 is produced by metabolism and eliminated by ventilation. Alveolar CO_2 concentration is conveniently measured as PCO_2. PCO_2 is inversely proportional to alveolar ventilation (V_A), so that anything that increases V_A (an increase in respiratory rate or tidal volume, or improved $\dot{V}/\dot{Q}$ matching) causes a decrease in PCO_2, and anything that decreases V_A (a decrease in respiratory rate or tidal volume, or impaired $\dot{V}/\dot{Q}$ matching leading to increased dead space) causes a decrease in PCO_2.

Understanding the diagnosis and treatment of the respiratory acid–base disorders requires knowledge of the buffer systems that serve to protect against alterations in hydrogen ion concentration and pH. As CO_2 enters the blood, it combines with H_2O to form carbonic acid (H_2CO_3), which dissociates into bicarbonate (HCO_3^-) and hydrogen ions:

$$CO_2 + H_2O \leftrightarrow H_2CO_3 \leftrightarrow HCO_3^- + H^+$$

Most of the H^+ ions produced by this addition of CO_2 to the blood combine with intracellular buffers including hemoglobin, and this tissue buffering minimizes the elevation in hydrogen ion concentration and the corresponding fall in pH.

In respiratory acid–base disturbances, a primary rise or fall in PCO_2 (respiratory acidosis or alkalosis, respectively) will result in a change in pH unless a proportional change in HCO_3^- occurs to compensate. The initial response to a primary change in PCO_2 is tissue buffering of the change with movement of intracellular HCO_3^- to or from the extracellular fluid. Subsequently, renal HCO_3^- excretion is adjusted, and serum HCO_3^- changes further to defend against pH changes.

RESPIRATORY ALKALOSIS

ESSENTIALS OF DIAGNOSIS

▶ Low PCO_2 and high pH.

▶ Acute respiratory alkalosis: HCO_3^- falls 2 mEq/L for each 10 mm Hg fall in PCO_2 (in minutes).

▶ Chronic respiratory alkalosis: HCO_3^- falls 5 mEq/L for each 10 mm Hg fall in PCO_2 (over days). pH may return to normal!

▶ If calculated compensation is too little or too much, another acid–base abnormality (a mixed disorder) must be present.

General Considerations

Respiratory alkalosis is the result of hyperventilation produced by a variety of influences. It rarely requires specific treatment, other than for the underlying condition. In fact, overly aggressive efforts to treat respiratory alkalosis itself are often fruitless or dangerous, and occasionally cause respiratory acidosis.

Pathogenesis

With hyperventilation, CO_2 is eliminated out of proportion to its production, the equilibrium described above shifts to the left, hydrogen ions are utilized, and pH rises. This decrease in P_{CO_2} (hypocapnia) and rise in pH constitute **respiratory alkalosis**.

$$\frac{CO_2 + H_2O \leftarrow H_2CO_3 \leftarrow}{HCO_3^- + H^+}$$

Acute reduction in P_{CO_2} releases H^+ from tissue buffers, titrating HCO_3^- and decreasing its concentration. Eventually, decreased P_{CO_2} also inhibits renal tubular reabsorption and generation of HCO_3^-, the serum level falls further, and pH returns toward normal.

Prevention

The only common cause of respiratory alkalosis that can be prevented occurs in a mechanically ventilated patient when the chosen ventilator settings produce too high a minute ventilation. This may be difficult to distinguish from the situation in which a ventilated patient develops a respiratory alkalosis because of dyspnea, pain, anxiety, or the underlying disease (see Treatment below).

Clinical Findings

A. Symptoms and Signs

Chronic respiratory alkalosis is generally asymptomatic, as the blood pH is near normal (Table 5–7). In acute respiratory alkalosis, patients may experience dyspnea, dizziness, anxiety, and acral or circumoral paresthesias. Symptoms are related to both decreased ionized calcium and reduced cerebral blood flow (see below).

B. Laboratory Findings

Respiratory alkalosis is diagnosed by arterial blood gas analysis showing a high pH, decreased P_{CO_2}, and variably decreased serum HCO_3^-. It must be distinguished from metabolic acidosis in which the P_{CO_2} and HCO_3^- are also decreased, but pH is low. Accurate diagnosis requires knowledge of the magnitude of the expected compensation (fall in HCO_3^-) and the duration of the abnormality. An initial decrease in HCO_3^- occurs in minutes in response to respiratory alkalosis, but full renal compensation for chronic respiratory

Table 5–7. Clinical manifestations of respiratory alkalosis.[1]

Neuromuscular
Related to cerebral vasospasm and decreased perfusion
Lightheadedness
Confusion
Syncope
Related to decreased to ionized calcium or decreased availability of calcium
Seizures (or decreased seizure threshold)
Paresthesias
Muscular cramps, tetany
Cardiovascular
Tachycardia
Ventricular arrythmias
Gastrointestinal
Nausea and vomiting
Other
Dyspnea
Anxiety
Decreased ionized calcium

[1] Most signs and symptoms are seen with acute respiratory alkalosis.

alkalosis takes days to develop. The data describing appropriate compensation for acute and chronic respiratory alkalosis come from studies of hyperventilation in normal volunteers.

1. Acute respiratory alkalosis: HCO_3^- falls 2 mEq/L for each 10 mm Hg fall in P_{CO_2} (in minutes).

2. Chronic respiratory alkalosis: HCO_3^- falls 5 mEq/L for each 10 mm Hg fall in P_{CO_2} (over days). *pH may return to normal!*

3. If calculated compensation is too little or too much, another acid–base abnormality (a mixed disorder) must be present.

C. Imaging Studies and Special Tests

Imaging studies and specialized testing are generally not helpful in the diagnosis and management of respiratory alkalosis, although such testing may be appropriate in the management of the underlying disorder.

Differential Diagnosis

Most conditions causing hyperventilation and respiratory alkalosis (with the exception of mechanical ventilation) do so via central respiratory stimulation, increasing the minute ventilation and alveolar ventilation and therefore lowering the P_{CO_2}. Table 5–8 lists the common causes.

Anxiety and pain are common causes of hyperventilation and respiratory alkalosis; the act of obtaining a blood

Table 5–8. Causes of respiratory alkalosis.

Supratentorial
Anxiety
Pain
Fever

Pulmonary
Hypoxia from all causes
    Hypoxic pulmonary or cardiac disease
    High altitude
Pulmonary disorders causing respiratory alkalosis
with or without hypoxia
    Conditions causing decreased compliance
        Pneumothorax
        Pneumonia
        Pulmonary edema
        Interstitial lung disease
        Less severe chest wall disorders
    Pulmonary embolism
    Bronchospasm
    Auto-PEEP in mechanically ventilated patients

Central nervous system
Meningitis, encephalitis
Intracranial tumors
Cerebrovascular accident
Head trauma

Drugs
Aspirin and other salicylates
Progesterone
Theophylline
Catecholamines
Thyroxine

Miscellaneous conditions
Excessive mechanical ventilation
Pregnancy
Sepsis (particularly gram-negative)
Liver disease
Exercise
Acute reversal of metabolic acidosis
Thyrotoxicosis
Alcohol withdrawal
Beri-beri

PEEP, positive end-expiratory pressure.

gas sample is likely to produce sufficient hyperventilation to demonstrate an acute respiratory alkalosis. Hypoxia in the patient with respiratory disease is also very common and often overlooked as a cause of respiratory alkalosis.

The cause of respiratory alkalosis in both liver failure and pregnancy is believed to be elevated levels of both progesterone and estradiol. Progesterone increases ventilation by acting on central nervous system progesterone receptors, while estradiol is thought to increase the number of these receptors. Increased levels of progesterone and estradiol are part of the normal physiologic milieu of pregnancy, while in liver failure they are caused by the inability of the diseased liver to metabolize free hormones.

Aspirin, although its effect in causing hyperventilation is well known, commonly causes a mixed acid–base pattern: Respiratory alkalosis and metabolic acidosis. The same pattern is seen in gram-negative sepsis. The hyperventilation seen with gram-negative sepsis, or even with fever alone, is caused by the effects of inflammatory mediators, most prominently tumor necrosis factor and the interleukins.

▶ Complications

Alkalosis directly enhances neuromuscular excitability and modestly decreases serum calcium. As mentioned above, these effects cause paresthesias, numbness, twitching, and with severe alkalosis, tetany. Severe alkalosis and hypocapnia can cause dizziness, confusion, and loss of consciousness due to cerebral vasospasm with decreased cerebral blood flow. In fact, intentional production of respiratory alkalosis (using mechanical ventilation) and subsequent cerebral vasospasm is a short-term treatment for increased intracranial pressure.

▶ Treatment

Respiratory alkalosis itself is rarely a clinically important problem. Sedation, analgesia, and antipyretics (for anxiety, pain, and fever) are often sufficient therapy.

In other cases, treating the underlying problem (oxygen for hypoxia, hemodialysis for aspirin overdose, treating infections) is necessary. In patients with respiratory alkalosis complicating mechanical ventilation, simply adjusting ventilator settings or changing the mode of ventilation [eg, to synchronized intermittent mechanical ventilation (SIMV)] should not be considered an adequate "treatment." These maneuvers can produce an apparent improvement in arterial blood gases, but at the cost of a fatigued or dyspneic patient whose reason for hyperventilation remains undiagnosed and untreated. While settings should be checked for appropriateness, a more effective approach to treating alkalosis in this setting is to search for underlying causes of hyperventilation and treat them. Typically, pain, anxiety, or dyspnea due to a concurrent or new condition (pneumonia, pulmonary edema, bronchospasm, retained secretions) is the cause of a new respiratory alkalosis in a previously stable mechanically ventilated patient.

▶ Prognosis

Prognosis in respiratory alkalosis is entirely dependent on the underlying cause; patients may recover from an episode of anxiety-related hyperventilation in minutes or remain chronically subject to increased ventilatory drive from severe lung diseases such as interstitial fibrosis.

RESPIRATORY ACIDOSIS

 ESSENTIALS OF DIAGNOSIS

▶ Low P_{CO_2} and high pH.

▶ Acute respiratory acidosis: HCO_3^- rises 1 mEq/L for each 10 mm Hg rise in P_{CO_2} (in minutes).

▶ Chronic respiratory acidosis: HCO_3^- rises 3.5 mEq/L for each 10 mm Hg rise in P_{CO_2} (over days).

▶ If calculated compensation is too little or too much, another acid–base abnormality (a mixed disorder) must be present.

▶ General Considerations

Unlike respiratory alkalosis, respiratory acidosis, particularly acute respiratory acidosis caused by severe pulmonary disease or sedative overdose, may produce dangerous hypercapnia and acidosis and often requires urgent treatment.

▶ Pathophysiology

With hypoventilation, elimination of CO_2 is unable to keep pace with its metabolic production, CO_2 is retained, and the equilibrium above shifts to the right. Excess hydrogen ions are produced, and pH falls. This rise in P_{CO_2} (hypercapnia) and fall in pH constitute **respiratory acidosis**.

$$\frac{CO_2 + H_2O \rightarrow H_2CO_3 \rightarrow}{HCO_3^- + H^+}$$

Decreased ventilation quickly results in increased P_{CO_2} because metabolic production of CO_2 is so rapid. Acutely, tissue buffering slightly raises HCO_3, limiting the pH drop. Eventually, renal acid excretion increases, HCO_3^- reabsorption is stimulated, serum HCO_3^- rises, and pH returns toward normal.

Two pathophysiologic mechanisms produce hypercapnia and respiratory acidosis: Severe ventilation–perfusion ($\dot{V}/\dot{Q}$) mismatch of the dead space (high $\dot{V}/\dot{Q}$) type and alveolar hypoventilation. Again, since P_{CO_2} is inversely proportional to V_A, any process that decreases V_A (alveolar hypoventilation or $\dot{V}/\dot{Q}$ mismatch) causes a rise in P_{CO_2}.

In patients with chronic respiratory disease and hypercapnia, excess supplemental oxygen can cause hypoventilation and $\dot{V}/\dot{Q}$ mismatch (via the release of hypoxic vasoconstriction), causing worse hypercapnia and respiratory acidosis (see Prevention and Differential Diagnosis, below).

▶ Prevention

Few of the causes of respiratory acidosis can be prevented. One exception (see Pathogenesis, above and Differential Diagnosis, below) is the iatrogenic acute respiratory acidosis that can result from overzealous oxygen administration in patients with severe, chronic respiratory disease who are adapted to hypercapnia and dependent on hypoxia to stimulate ventilation. In these patients, oxygen should be administered by low flow (nasal cannulas) or controlled dose (Venturi mask) methods to deliver the minimal FIO_2 necessary to correct hypoxemia.

In addition, extreme care should be used in administering sedative drugs to patients with underlying hypercapnic lung disease.

▶ Clinical Findings

A. Symptoms and Signs

The symptoms and signs of respiratory acidosis (Table 5–9) depend on how quickly the acidosis develops (because a rapid rise in brain P_{CO_2} is not quickly compensated for by a rise in brain HCO_3^-) and are related to its effect on brain pH. Hypercapnia lowers brain pH and produces cerebral vasodilation, increased cerebral blood flow, and increased intracranial pressure with symptoms and signs similar to the effects of narcotic agents. Early symptoms may include blurred vision, headache, restlessness, tremors, and delirium. These may progress to drowsiness, lethargy, and coma as P_{CO_2} rises and pH falls.

B. Laboratory Findings

Respiratory acidosis is diagnosed by arterial blood gas analysis showing a low pH, elevated P_{CO_2}, and variably elevated serum HCO_3^-. Respiratory alkalosis must be distinguished from metabolic alkalosis in which the P_{CO_2} and HCO_3^- are also elevated, but pH is high. When a blood gas is not immediately available, or when questioning the duration of

Table 5–9. Clinical manifestations of respiratory acidosis.[1]

Neuromuscular (presumably related to cerebral vasodilation and increased cerebral blood flow)
Headache
Drowsiness, restlessness, lethargy, coma
Delirium
Headache
Papilledema (rare)
Myoclonus
Cardiovascular
Tachycardia
Ventricular arrythmias
Other
Dyspnea
Hypoxia and related symptoms (as CO_2 replaces O_2 in the alveolus)

[1]Signs and symptoms are worse with acute or rapidly developing respiratory acidosis.

respiratory acidosis, the measured serum HCO_3^- may also be helpful. In an appropriate clinical setting, a significantly elevated serum HCO_3^- from a previous arterial blood gas (at least a few days prior) is indirect evidence of a chronic respiratory acidosis. As mentioned, an elevated serum HCO_3^- may also represent metabolic alkalosis.

As for respiratory alkalosis, accurate diagnosis requires knowledge of the magnitude of the expected compensation (rise in HCO_3^-) and the duration of the abnormality. An initial increase in HCO_3^- from tissue buffering occurs in minutes in response to respiratory acidosis, but maximal renal compensation for chronic respiratory acidosis takes days to develop. The data describing appropriate compensation for acute and chronic respiratory acidosis come from several studies of dogs, normal humans, and patients with severe underlying pulmonary disease.

1. Acute respiratory acidosis: HCO_3^- rises 1 mEq/L for each 10 mm Hg rise in P_{CO_2} (in minutes).

2. Chronic respiratory acidosis: HCO_3^- rises 3.5 mEq/L for each 10 mm Hg rise in P_{CO_2} (over days).

3. If calculated compensation is too much or too little, another process (a mixed disorder) must be present.

C. Imaging Studies and Special Tests

Imaging studies and specialized testing are generally not helpful in the diagnosis and management of respiratory acidosis, although such testing may be appropriate in the management of the underlying disorder.

▶ Differential Diagnosis

Common causes of respiratory acidosis are listed in Table 5–10.

A. Acute Respiratory Acidosis

Acute respiratory acidosis most frequently results from iatrogenic or intentional overdose of a sedative drug (opiates, benzodiazepines). These drugs suppress central respiratory drive causing alveolar hypoventilation, hypercapnia, and respiratory acidosis. Severe, acute exacerbations of any respiratory disease (eg, asthma) can also cause acute respiratory acidosis. These conditions produce severe $\dot{V}/\dot{Q}$ mismatch and a high work-of-breathing with respiratory muscle fatigue, both leading to hypercapnia and respiratory acidosis.

One important, preventable cause of acute respiratory acidosis is suppression of the hypoxic drive to breathe by administered oxygen in patients with chronic respiratory disease and hypercapnia (see Prevention and Pathogenesis, above).

B. Chronic Respiratory Acidosis

The most important and most common cause of chronic respiratory acidosis is severe emphysema [chronic obstructive pulmonary disease (COPD)]. In this condition, severe $\dot{V}/\dot{Q}$

Table 5–10. Causes of acute and chronic respiratory acidosis.

Acute
Pulmonary
  Airway problems
    Status asthmaticus
    Laryngospasm
  Parenchymal problems
    Severe pneumonia
    Severe pulmonary edema
    Any acute, severe pulmonary disease
  Other
    Excess supplemental oxygen in patients with chronic hypercapnia
    Disconnection or failure of mechanical ventilation
Nonpulmonary
  Drugs
    Anesthetics
    Sedative drugs (opiates, methadone, benzodiazepines)
    Neuromuscular blockers
    Aminoglycosides
  Flail chest
    Spinal cord injury
    Cardiopulmonary arrest

Chronic (may also cause acute acidosis)
Pulmonary
  Severe chronic obstructive pulmonary disease
  Other severe chronic lung diseases (interstitial fibrosis)
Nonpulmonary
  Obstructive sleep apnea
  Obesity hypoventilation syndrome
  Myxedema
  Neuromuscular and chest wall disease
    Brainstem infarct
    Guillain-Barré syndrome
    Myasthenia gravis
    Muscular dystrophy
    Poliomyelitis
    Kyphoscoliosis
    Diaphragmatic paralysis
    Amyotrophic lateral sclerosis

mismatch and respiratory muscle weakness/dysfunction produce hypoventilation, hypercapnia, and respiratory acidosis.

Other severe respiratory (eg, pulmonary fibrosis), neuromuscular (Guillain–Barré syndrome), and chest wall (kyphoscoliosis) diseases are less common causes of chronic respiratory acidosis. These conditions are characterized by severe $\dot{V}/\dot{Q}$ mismatch, respiratory muscle dysfunction, and/or hypoventilation, leading to hypercapnia.

C. "Acute-on-Chronic" Respiratory Acidosis

Patients with severe but compensated respiratory diseases and chronic respiratory acidosis may develop an acute

Table 5–11. Recognition, causes, and therapy of respiratory acid–base disorders.

Acid–base disorder	Primary pH change	PCO_2 change	Expected compensation	Common causes	Therapy
Acute respiratory acidosis	↓	Pco_2 ↑	HCO_3^- ↑1/↑ 10 in Pco_2	Narcotics, acute or acute- on-chronic lung	Therapy of lung disease, mechanical ventilation, specific antidotes
Chronic respiratory acidosis	↓	Pco_2 ↑	HCO_3^- ↑3.5/↑ 10 in Pco_2	Chronic lung disease	Therapy of lung disease
Acute respiratory alkalosis	↑	Pco_2 ↓	HCO_3^- ↓2/↓10 in Pco_2	Fever, pain, anxiety, mechanical ventilation	Sedation, analgesia, antipyretics
Chronic respiratory alkalosis	↑	Pco_2 ↓	HCO_3^- ↓5/↓10 in Pco_2	Chronic liver disease, pregnancy, aspirin overdose, and sepsis (with metabolic acidosis)	Therapy of underlying disease

respiratory acidosis when an acute insult (pneumonia, pulmonary embolus, flare of the underlying disease) occurs. The pathophysiologic mechanisms at work here are usually severe $\dot{V}/\dot{Q}$ mismatch due to the underlying disease and hypoventilation due to respiratory muscle fatigue and an increased work of breathing.

▶ Complications

Unlike respiratory alkalosis, respiratory acidosis is often clinically important. Severe respiratory acidosis and hypercapnia simulate the effects of opiates. They can cause hypotension, confusion and obtundation, and ultimately coma (see Table 5–11 and Symptoms and Signs above). Hypercapnia causes cerebral vasodilation, which may result in increased intracranial pressure and papilledema.

Since hyperventilation is the primary defense against metabolic acidosis, patients with chronic respiratory disease who develop metabolic acidosis are at greater risk and may need early mechanical ventilation.

▶ Treatment

Treatment is focused on improving ventilation. When chronic respiratory acidosis results from respiratory disease,

optimally treating the underlying condition (eg, COPD) will simultaneously treat the acidosis.

When acute (or acute-on-chronic) respiratory acidosis is caused by acute exacerbations of chronic respiratory disease or drug overdose, mechanical ventilation may be necessary as well as specific antidotes for the drug ingested.

Although CO_2 production is one of the determinants of alveolar and arterial Pco_2, it is rare for increased CO_2 production to play a significant role in the development of respiratory acidosis. Still, it is occasionally possible to improve hypercapnia in cases of end-stage pulmonary disease by decreasing CO_2 production with a low carbohydrate diet. This measure is rarely necessary or useful in other clinical settings.

▶ Prognosis

Prognosis in respiratory acidosis depends on the underlying etiology of the disorder. Patients may recover fully from acute acidosis associated with drug overdose or exacerbation of asthma. Patients with severe, hypercapnic obstructive lung disease generally follow an inexorably downhill course.

Laffey JG, Kavanagh BP: Hypocapnia. N Engl J Med 2002;347:43.

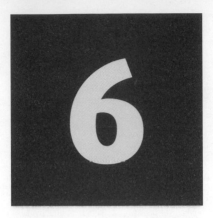

Disorders of Calcium Balance: Hypercalcemia & Hypocalcemia

Stanley Goldfarb, MD

HYPERCALCEMIA

ESSENTIALS OF DIAGNOSIS

▶ Hypercalcemia is usually manifested as a chronic but mildly elevated serum calcium level, although more severe forms that present as hypercalcemic emergencies do exist.

▶ The symptoms associated with sustained hypercalcemia are relatively nonspecific, but the constellation of symptoms often suggests the diagnosis.

▶ A combination of neuropsychiatric complaints such as depression, anxiety, cognitive dysfunction, headache, fatigue and even organic brain syndrome, renal complaints including polyuria, polydipsia, nephrogenic diabetes insipidus, nephrolithiasis, nocturia, and renal insufficiency, and gastrointestinal complaints such as constipation, peptic ulcer disease, or a diagnosis of acute pancreatitis would strongly suggest the diagnosis.

▶ Most patients with hypercalcemia are diagnosed based on data derived from laboratory screening tests.

▶ The signs and symptoms associated with the underlying disease causing hypercalcemia may dominate the clinical picture.

General Considerations

Calcium in serum exists ionized, bound to organic anions such as phosphate and citrate, and bound to proteins (mainly albumin). Of these, ionized calcium is the physiologically important form. The most common abnormality that distorts the relationship between serum calcium and ionized calcium is hypoalbuminemia. The total serum calcium is lower or higher by 0.8 mg/dL (0.2 mmol/L) for every 1.0 g/dL that the serum albumin is higher or lower, respectively, than 4 g/dL.

Thus, patients may have a normal serum ionized calcium but low total calcium if they have hypoalbuminemia due to nephrotic syndrome. Conversely, a patient can have high total calcium, with normal ionized calcium and increased total protein and/or albumin, as in states of severe dehydration.

Hypercalcemia is one of the most common metabolic disorders in malignant diseases and develops in 3–30% of such patients. Hypercalcemia of malignancy is the most common cause of hypercalcemia followed by primary hyperparathyroidism in hospital populations. The most common cause in normal populations is primary hyperparathyroidism followed by transient hypercalcemia.

▶ Pathogenesis

Hypercalcemia can result from increased bone resorption, decreased renal excretion, or increased gastrointestinal absorption. However, bone resorption and intestinal hyperabsorption of calcium are the predominant causes of hypercalcemia. Reduced renal excretion is a permissive factor in all cases of hypercalcemia as in the absence of renal conservation of calcium, any rise in serum calcium would result in the excretion of any excess in the urine and hypercalciuria but not hypercalcemia would ensue.

Typically, the mechanism underlying hypercalcemia is complex and multifactorial. In primary hyperparathyroidism, all three components come into play. High parathyroid hormone (PTH) levels induce bone resorption, increase renal tubular reabsorption, and secondarily increase gastrointestinal calcium absorption as PTH stimulates production of the most active form of vitamin D, calcitriol.

PTH is the master hormone regulating overall calcium metabolism. It is an 84-amino acid hormone that in response to a fall in serum calcium levels raises calcium levels by accelerating osteoclastic bone resorption and increasing renal tubular resorption of calcium. It also increases calcitriol, which indirectly raises serum calcium levels. PTH also induces an increased renal excretion of phosphate. This effect helps to enhance the rise in serum calcium as phosphate tends to coprecipitate with calcium and block the effects of PTH on bone and the effects of PTH on inducing the activation of vitamin D by the kidney.

In primary hyperparathyroidism, there is a fundamental dysregulation of PTH secretion. Normally, the calcium-sensing receptor on the surface of cells in the parathyroid gland senses serum calcium and the release of PTH follows a sigmoidal relationship concentration (see Figure 6–1). The "set point" of this relationship is the serum calcium concentration at which there is half-maximal inhibition of PTH secretion. As seen in Figure 6–1, this relationship is disrupted in primary hyperparathyroidism so that PTH is released even in the face of normally suppressive levels of serum calcium.

Vitamin D is a steroid hormone that may be ingested with the diet but is also produced in the skin by the action of sunlight on metabolic antecedents of vitamin D. Calcitriol, the active form of vitamin D, is derived from the hydroxylation of cholecalciferol, which is first hydroxylated in the liver to 25-hydroxyvitamin D, then in the kidneys to 1,25-dihydroxyvitamin D. Vitamin D has a plethora of actions including altering the growth dynamics of many cell types. Its actions to increase serum calcium are complex and include an increase in the transport of calcium across the gastrointestinal (GI) tract and an increase in calcium release from bone during PTH-induced bone resorption. In the absence of PTH, the GI effect in concert with adequate

dietary calcium can maintain normal serum calcium levels and with pharmacologic doses of vitamin D, even induce hypercalcemia.

PTH-related peptide (PTHrP) is the principal mediator in hypercalcemia associated with solid tumors. Patients with humoral hypercalcemia of malignancy (HHM) constitute about 80% of all patients with hypercalcemia associated with malignancy. PTHrP and PTH share the same molecular region that comprises the receptor-binding domain at the amino terminus. PTHrP binds the PTH receptor and mimics the biologic effects of PTH on bones and the kidneys. PTHrP and PTH share the same receptor, but there are some differences in actions. HHM patients have a greater degree of hypercalciuria than is generally seen in hyperparathyroidism. HHM is usually associated with low serum calcitriol levels, whereas PTH stimulates calcitriol production. Also, PTH stimulates bone resorption and formation, whereas PTHrP stimulates only bone resorption, with very low osteoblastic activity, and thus usually normal alkaline phosphatase levels.

Bone resorption is a key mechanism underlying most cases of hypercalcemia. The skeleton is continually renewed through remodeling, a sequence of events whereby old bone is replaced by new bone (bone turnover). Three types of cells produce and maintain bone. Osteoblasts act at bone surfaces by secreting osteoid, unmineralized collagen, and modulate the crystallization of hydroxyapatite and influence the activity of osteoclasts. Osteoclasts are responsible for the resorption of bone, a process that is necessary for the repair of bone surfaces and the remodeling of bone. Osteocytes are osteoblasts that have become embedded within the mineralized regions of bone.

During bone growth, formation is higher than breakdown. After peak bone mass is achieved, the rates of breakdown and formation are equal and bone mass is thought to remain constant. In hypercalcemic states associated with excess PTH, PTHrP, and other bone-active cytokines, the rate of breakdown increases and exceeds the rate at which bone is formed. If this is coupled with inadequate renal excretion, then hypercalcemia ensues.

▶ Clinical Findings

A. Primary Hyperparathyroidism

1. Symptoms and signs—Primary hyperparathyroidism, the most common cause of hypercalcemia in the outpatient setting, is usually found by routine laboratory screening, as most patients with primary hyperparathyroidism are asymptomatic. When patients are symptomatic, findings may include renal calculi, bone pain, pathologic fractures, and proximal muscle weakness, or nonspecific symptoms such as depression, lethargy, and vague aches and pains. Rarely, full blown psychiatric disorders may be seen. Occasional patients may have a family history of multiple endocrine neoplasia syndromes (type 1 or 2) or a history of preceding head and neck irradiation as a child or an adult for hyperthyroidism

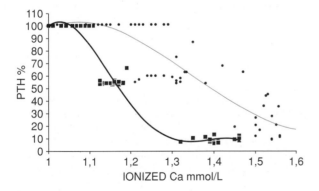

▲ **Figure 6–1.** The set point of calcium (calculated as the midpoint between maximal and minimal PTH secretion), the serum ionized calcium level at maximal PTH secretion, and the serum ionized calcium at maximal PTH inhibition are shown for individual patients affected by primary hyperparathyroidism ($n = 19$, circles) and for 14 normal subjects (squares). The sigmoidal curve is shifted to the right in primary PTH. (Reprinted with permission from Malberti F et al: The PTH-calcium curve and the set point of calcium in primary and secondary hyperparathyroidism. Nephrol Dial Transplant 1999;14:2398.)

treated with radiation modalities. Mental obtundation or coma is an infrequent but life-threatening complication of severe hypercalcemia (hypercalcemic crisis). All patients with calcium-containing renal stones should be evaluated for primary hyperparathyroidism.

2. Laboratory findings—Primary hyperparathyroidism is usually diagnosed by demonstrating persistent hypercalcemia in the presence of inappropriately normal or elevated PTH concentrations. Normally, PTH levels are suppressed in the presence of increasing serum calcium levels. Immunoassay of the intact PTH molecule is the preferred method of measurement. Primary hyperparathyroidism may present at an early stage with minimal increases in the serum calcium level in the face of normal or mildly elevated PTH levels. The intact PTH assay uses antibodies to two sites simultaneously (N- and C-terminal) to measure the intact hormone. The normal range for this assay is 18–65 pg/mL. Intact PTH is increased in 80–90% of patients with primary hyperparathyroidism while 10–20% have values in the normal range but that are inappropriately high in the face of hypercalcemia. The intact PTH assay provides good discrimination between parathyroid and nonparathyroid causes of hypercalcemia. This diagnosis should be suspected in patients with renal calculi or reduced bone density who have minimally increased PTH levels and high-normal serum calcium levels (normocalcemic primary hyperparathyroidism). Other findings include mild hypophosphatemia, hypercalciuria, and mild metabolic acidosis as PTH acts on the kidney to promote phosphate and bicarbonate excretion.

3. Imaging studies—If a parathyroid adenoma is suspected, the parathyroid glands can be imaged using nuclear medicine techniques. This procedure is based on the differential uptake between normal and abnormal parathyroid glands of the tumor-seeking compound sestamibi, labeled with ^{99m}Tc. This material is taken up by both the thyroid and parathyroids and is cleared rapidly from normal tissue but is retained in tumors of the parathyroids. Surgical exploration and the removal of the adenomatous gland constitute the treatment of choice for many patients. Preoperative imaging may not always be necessary since the success rate for parathyroid surgery has been reported to exceed 90%, even in the absence of prior imaging. Localization techniques are more useful in cases of failed primary neck exploration and in cases of postoperative persistent hypercalcemia.

B. Familial Hypocalciuric Hypercalcemia

Familial hypocalciuric hypercalcemia is characterized by benign asymptomatic hypercalcemia. It is an autosomal dominant condition in which the genetic abnormality leads to a loss of function mutation of the calcium-sensing receptor that exists on the c-cells of the parathyroid glands. This inactive receptor necessitates higher serum calcium levels in order to suppress PTH. Because the calcium-sensing receptor also exists within the kidney and regulates calcium reabsorption in the thick ascending loop of Henle, the defect in the protein structure leads to increased renal tubular calcium reabsorption and reduced excretion. Apparently many of the symptoms associated with hypercalcemia require activation of the calcium-sensing receptor as patients with this condition are remarkably free of symptoms. It is therefore important to inquire about familial hypercalcemia in any hypercalcemic patients and to assess urinary calcium excretion.

Laboratory findings—Strikingly low urinary calcium excretion (<100 mg/24 hours) is seen in the majority of patients, despite hypercalcemia and iPTH levels in the normal range in 80–85% of patients.

C. Hypercalcemia of Malignancy

Hypercalcemia of malignancy occurs in 10–20% of patients with cancer and the hypercalcemia is usually severe and of relatively short duration. The tumors that manifest in this disorder most commonly are breast, lung cancer, and multiple myeloma. The condition is induced by a number of humoral mediators: PTHrP is the most common and is found in 80–90% of cases and in both carcinomas and lymphomas. In multiple myeloma, the mediator is osteoclast-activating factor. In those patients with Hodgkin's disease and a substantial fraction of those with non-Hodgkin's lymphomas who develop hypercalcemia, high levels of calcitriol are found. The malignant cells are capable of enzymatically activating 25-hydroxyvitamin D to its more active metabolite calcitriol. In patients with osteolytic metastases, a variety of cytokines released by the tumor cells including tumor necrosis factor (TNF), interleukin (IL)-1, IL-6, and PTHrP may each lead to activation of bone resorption and, ultimately, hypercalcemia.

Laboratory findings—Generally, patients with HHM manifest higher levels of serum calcium than those with primary hyperparathyroidism. Also, serum phosphate and bicarbonate levels tend to be higher. However, specific laboratory tests are rarely required for the diagnosis of HHM since patients with malignancy almost always have other signs or symptoms of their malignancy when hypercalcemia is found. However, assays for iPTH and for PTHrP are available and finding an elevated PTHrP is specific for HHM.

D. Granulomatous Diseases

Hypercalcemia occurs in most granulomatous disorders. High serum calcium levels are seen in about 10% of patients with sarcoidosis; hypercalciuria is about three times more frequent. Tuberculosis, fungal diseases including histoplasmosis, cocidioidomycosis, and berylliosis, and some lymphomas, particularly those associated with human immunodeficiency viruses, are other conditions that are associated with disorders of calcium metabolism. These abnormalities of calcium metabolism are due to production of calcitriol by activated macrophages either in pulmonary alveoli or in granulomatous inflammation. Macrophages have the enzymatic capacity to convert 25-hydroxyvitamin D_3 to calcitriol. As this condition is associated with suppressed PTH levels, hypercalciuria is a prominent feature of this form of hypercalcemia.

E. Milk-Alkali Syndrome

The milk-alkali syndrome became rare with the advent of modern gastric ulcer therapy with antibiotics. However, the growing popularity of the use of calcium carbonate as an antacid or as calcium supplementation to prevent osteoporosis has led to a reappearance of this problem. Patients with this syndrome typically ingest massive quantities of calcium and absorbable alkali and are unaware of the toxic effects of these compounds. They present with the triad of hypercalcemia, metabolic alkalosis, and renal failure that is occasionally so severe that dialysis is necessary. The serum parathyroid hormone or calcitriol levels are appropriately decreased in response to the hypercalcemia. Since both physicians and patients are often unaware of the calcium and alkali content of many nonprescription medicines, the diagnosis of the milk-alkali syndrome, a reversible cause of renal failure, can be missed if a detailed history of such intake is not elicited.

F. Medication-Induced Hypercalcemia

Vitamin D usage is an important cause of hypercalcemia. To diagnose vitamin D intoxication, it is necessary to consider it in the differential diagnosis and obtain a history of vitamin D intake in patients with hypercalcemia, azotemia, and anemia. The renal disease is reversible if the use of vitamin D is stopped. Hypervitaminosis D is characterized by high serum levels of 25-hydroxyvitamin D, hypercalcemia, hypercalciuria, and hyperphosphatemia but normal levels of calcitriol and suppressed parathyroid hormone. The pattern of vitamin D metabolites seen is the result of unregulated production of 25-hydroxyvitamin D but inhibition of activity of the renal 1-hydroxylase enzyme in the face of suppressed PTH and hyperphosphatemia.

Thiazide diuretics increase renal calcium reabsorption and may cause mild hypercalcemia. Typically, hypercalcemia induced by thiazide diuretic therapy unmasks other underlying disorders that predispose to hypercalcemia including primary hyperparathyroidism and vitamin D usage. Lithium use can cause hypercalcemia by increasing the calcium set point for secretion of PTH requiring a higher serum calcium level to suppress PTH secretion. Large doses of vitamin A and its analogs, including Retin-A, the antiacne agent, can cause hypercalcemia, which appears to be mediated through increased bone resorption.

G. Immobilization

Immobilization leads to an increase in bone resorption. Bone mineral density tests have shown evidence of bone resorption from prolonged immobilization after a variety of diseases including spinal injury and stroke. The mechanism is unknown

and hypercalcemia usually develops after 4 weeks of immobilization. Hypercalciuria may result from the combination of hypercalcemia and suppressed PTH secretion may attenuate hypercalcemia and even maintain normocalcemia. In fact, patients can have a negative calcium balance as a result of urine calcium losses, which can last for months. If an impairment in renal function occurs, however, hypercalcemia may ensue. Children are at particular risk from this complication.

▶ Differential Diagnosis

If hypercalcemia is detected on a routine screening test, then the approach to diagnosis is to first exclude familial hypocalciuric hypercalcemia (FHH) with a careful family history looking for a pattern that has an autosomal dominant inheritance. A low urinary calcium excretion (<100 mg/24 hours in 75% of patients) and normal PTH level are typically seen. Second, the clinician must exclude hypercalcemia of malignancy. In that instance, cancer is usually clinically evident by the time it causes hypercalcemia and PTH levels are generally <25 pg/mL, unless the patient has coexistent primary hyperparathyroidism (which is somewhat increased in the setting of hypercalcemia of malignancy). If those entities are excluded, and a careful history reveals no intake of medications known to induce hypercalcemia, then a normal or elevated PTH in the face of hypercalcemia is almost certainly the result of primary hyperparathyroidism. If PTH levels are reduced upon testing, then the presence of a granulomatous disease such as sarcoidosis or tuberculosis should be considered.

▶ Treatment

A. General Principles

In patients with fairly acute, symptomatic, or severe hypercalcemia (>12 mg/dL) the initial approach is to dilute the level of extracellular calcium and enhance renal calcium excretion by correcting extracellular volume contraction with isotonic saline, thereby inhibiting tubular sodium and calcium reabsorption, and then adding a loop diuretic to inhibit thick ascending limb calcium reabsorption, after volume depletion has been corrected. Next, agents to suppress osteoclastic bone resorption should be used. They include calcitonin, a hormone with a rapid onset of action (within 2 hours) to suppress bone resorption. Unfortunately it is effective in only 60–70% of patients and even if effective, typically induces tachyphylaxis. After calcitonin infusion, pamidronate, alendronate, or zolendronic acid, drugs of the bisphosphonate class, should be used. They have a somewhat delayed onset of action (24–48 hours) but they are highly effective and will maximally reduce calcium levels in 3–4 days and have a persisting effect for up to 1 month (mean 15 days). In those patients with severe renal insufficiency, it may be necessary to remove calcium directly from the blood by hemodialysis. With chronic hypercalcemia, the specific underlying disease or cause for the hypercalcemia should also be treated or corrected if possible.

B. Primary Hyperparathyroidism

First-line treatment of symptomatic (ie, renal stones, renal insufficiency, neuromuscular symptoms, bone fractures) primary hyperparathyroidism is surgical removal of a parathyroid adenoma or removal of a large fraction of parathyroid tissue if there is diffuse parathyroid hyperplasia. In asymptomatic primary hyperparathyroidism a National Institutes of Health workshop suggested that surgery was recommended for patients with the following: (1) serum calcium >1 mg/dL (0.25 mmol/L) above the upper limit of normal, (2) urinary calcium excretion >400 mg/24 hours, (3) impaired renal function (creatinine clearance reduced by 30% from age-matched healthy patients), (4) T-score less than −2.5 (matching the World Health Organization definition of osteoporosis), and (5) age younger than 50 years. Follow-up is likely to be unreliable.

Nonsurgical treatment of primary hyperparathyroidism is less than optimal, but the following have been studied. Estrogens and bisphosphonates have been used as medical treatments for primary hyperparathyroidism. High-dose estrogen modestly reduces serum calcium levels by about 0.5 mg/dL predominantly by reducing bone resorption as opposed to a reduction in PTH. The well-known adverse effects of combined estrogen–progesterone treatment on breast cancer risk and cardiovascular disease preclude its use in most patients.

Bisphosphonates, inhibitors of osteoclastic bone resorption, have not proven to be successful in reducing hypercalcemia in primary hyperparathyroidism although treatment with alendronate for 2 years does improves bone mineral density and may therefore be indicated in patients with a clinically significant reduction in bone mass but are not candidates for surgical therapy. Failure of bisphosphonates is likely due to stimulation of further increases in PTH levels as inhibition of bone resorption tends to reduce serum calcium transiently.

Calcimimetic agents, a new class of drugs that increases the sensitivity of the calcium-sensing receptor in the parathyroid gland, have been found to be effective in controlling PTH levels and serum calcium levels in primary hyperparathyroidism in early studies. They may become a viable alternative to surgery in some patients.

C. Hypercalcemia of Malignancy

Table 6–1 presents a summary of the various treatments available for hypercalcemia associated with malignancy.

D. Granulomatous Diseases

Treatment of the hypercalcemia or hypercalciuria associated with granulomatous diseases such as sarcoidosis is aimed at reducing intestinal calcium absorption and calcitriol synthesis. Reduction of calcium absorption requires reducing intake to less than 400 mg/day and eliminating dietary sources of vitamin D. In addition, low-dose glucocorticoid therapy (10–30 mg/day of prednisone) will usually be adequate in sarcoidosis, although somewhat higher doses may be required for patients with hypercalcemia associated with lymphoma. The full hypocalcemic response usually requires 7–10 days of glucocorticoid therapy. Glucocorticoids probably act by inhibiting calcitriol synthesis by the activated macrophage cells within the granulomatous tissue.

▶ Prognosis

The outcome of treatment of hypercalcemia is dependent on the underlying disease responsible for the disorder. In all circumstances except for familial hypocalciuric hypocalcemia, long-standing hypercalcemia and hypercalciuria may lead to renal failure secondary to complications of nephrolithiasis or secondary to nephrocalcinosis. In addition, vascular calcifications may induce cardiovascular diseases such as coronary artery disease and stroke.

If hypercalcemia is caused by hyperparathyroidism, then disturbances of bone including pathologic fractures may be seen. Hypercalcemia of malignancy is often a terminal event and patients rarely survive 1 year following its onset.

HYPOCALCEMIA

ESSENTIALS OF DIAGNOSIS

▶ Hypocalcemia usually results from a failure of mobilization of calcium from bone, which typically involves a defect or deficiency in the PTH or vitamin D axis.

▶ Tissue deposition of calcium or the complexing of calcium with other ions such as phosphate can lead to hypocalcemia if these processes occur more rapidly than calcium can be mobilized from bone.

▶ Transient hypocalcemia is common in critical care medicine while sustained hypocalcemia is uncommon, with the exception of patients with chronic renal insufficiency where abnormalities of PTH and vitamin D activity are invariably found.

▶ Pathogenesis

A. Hypoparathyroidism

Hypoparathyroidism may be a primary disorder due to surgery, autoimmunity, or genetic abnormalities or it may be a functional and reversible phenomenon resulting from medications or hypomagnesemia. Postsurgical hypoparathyroidism is a rare (1–2%) but devastating complication of total thyroidectomy. It may also result from exploration of the parathyroid glands or following radical neck dissection for cancers of the head and neck. Hypocalcemia in this setting may be intermittent or permanent.

Table 6–1. Pharmacologic therapy for hypercalcemia associated with cancer.[1]

Intervention	Dose	Adverse Effect
Hydration or calciuresis		
Intravenous saline	200–500 mL/hour, depending on the cardiovascular and renal status of the patient	Congestive heart failure
Furosemide	20–40 mg intravenously, after rehydration has been achieved	Dehydration, hypokalemia
Phosphate repletion		
Oral phosphorus (if serum phosphorus ≤3.0 mg/dL)[2]	For example, 250 mg Neutraphos orally, four times daily until serum phosphorus level >3.0 mg/dL or until serum creatinine level increases	Renal failure, hypocalcemia, seizures, abnormalities of cardiac conduction, diarrhea
First-line medications		
Intravenous bisphosphonates[3]		
Pamidronate	60–90 mg intravenously over a 2-hour period in a solution of 50–200 mL of saline or 5% dextrose in water[4]	Renal failure, transient flu-like syndrome with aches, chills, and fever
Zoledronate	4 mg intravenously over a 15-minute period in a solution of 50 mL of saline or 5% dextrose in water	Renal failure, transient flu-like syndrome with aches, chills, and fever
Second-line medications		
Glucocorticoids[5]	For example, prednisone, 60 mg orally daily for 10 days	Potential interference with chemotherapy; hypokalemia, hyperglycemia, hypertension, Cushing's syndrome, immunosuppression
Mithramycin	A single dose of 25 μg/kg of body weight over a 4- to 6-hour period in saline	Thrombocytopenia, platelet-aggregation defect, anemia, leukopenia, hepatitis, renal failure[6]
Calcitonin	4–8 IU per kilogram subcutaneously or intramuscularly every 12 hours	Flushing, nausea
Gallium nitrate	100–200 mg/m^2 of body surface area intravenously given continuously over a 24-hour period for 5 days	Renal failure

[1]Many of the recommendations in this table are based on historical precedent and common practice rather than on randomized clinical trials. There are data from randomized trials comparing bisphosphonates to the other agents listed and to one another.

[2]The use of intravenous phosphorus should be avoided except in the presence of severe hypophosphatemia [serum phosphorus level <1.5 mg/dL (0.48 mmol/L)] and when oral phosphorus cannot be administered. If intravenous phosphorus is used, it should be used with extreme caution and with careful observation of the levels of serum phosphorus and creatinine. To convert values for phosphorus to millimoles per liter, multiply by 0.3229.

[3]Pamidronate and zoledronate are approved by the Food and Drug Administration. Ibandronate and clodronate are available in continental Europe, the United Kingdom, and elsewhere. Bisphosphonates should be used with caution if at all when the serum creatinine level exceeds 2.5–3.0 mg/dL (221.0–265.2 μmol/L).

[4]Pamidronate is generally used at a dose of 90 mg, but the 60-mg dose may be used to treat patients of small stature or those with renal impairment or mild hypercalcemia.

[5]These drugs have a slow onset of action compared to the bisphosphonates; approximately 4–10 days are required for a response.

[6]These effects have been reported in association with higher-dose regimens used to treat testicular cancer (50 μg/kg of body weight per day over a period of 5 days) and in patients receiving multiple doses of 25 μg/kg; they are not expected to occur with a single dose of 25 μg/kg unless preexisting liver, kidney, or hematologic disease is present.

Hypoparathyroidism induced by autoimmune mechanisms may be associated with other endocrine deficiencies termed polyglandular autoimmune syndrome type I. This condition is associated with adrenal insufficiency and mucocutaneous candidiasis, which reflect defects in thymic development. Patients may also develop anemia due to vitamin B_{12} deficiency as a result of autoantibodies to gastric parietal cells and subsequent achlorhydria. In some patients, there may be autoantibodies to the calcium-sensing receptor on the surface of parathyroid cells. These antibodies may activate the receptor and mimic the effects of calcium, thereby reducing PTH secretion.

Hypoparathyroidism on a genetic basis is a rare condition that is the result of mutations of the gene for the calcium-sensing receptor that activate the receptor at low levels of calcium, which thereby leads to reduced PTH secretion despite hypocalcemia. The condition is associated with normal but inappropriately low PTH secretion, hypercalciuria, and nephrolithiasis and nephrocalcinosis. DiGeorge's syndrome, a genetic disorder leading to maldevelopment of the third and fourth branchial pouches, is associated with absence of parathyroid glands and an associated aplasia of the thymus as well as cardiac malformations.

B. Hypomagnesemia

Hypomagnesemia results in a syndrome characterized by hypocalcemia, hypomagnesemia, and hypokalemia. It typically requires a rather severe degree of hypomagnesemia (serum magnesium <0.8 mEq/L or 1 mg/dL) for all of the manifestations to be observed. As noted, magnesium deficiency has multiple effects including reduction of PTH release, inhibition of PTH action on bone, and possibly an action to block bone resorption that may be direct and unrelated to changes in PTH. All abnormalities rapidly resolve if magnesium is infused, but calcium administration does not correct the hypocalcemia until serum magnesium levels are restored to normal.

C. Pseudohypoparathyroidism

Pseudohypoparathyroidism is a rare set of disorders characterized by normal PTH responsiveness to hypocalcemia but failure of PTH action on target-organs of bone and kidney or some combination of the two. Patients manifest the clinical features of hypoparathyroidism, but PTH levels are elevated yet hypocalcemia persists. In Type 1, binding of the PTH receptor fails to elicit the generation of cyclic AMP as there is inactivation mutation of the gene for the G protein mutation. In Type 2 pseudohypoparathyroidism, the receptor is normal but the cellular response to cyclic AMP is deficient.

D. Vitamin D Deficiency

Reduced vitamin D intake or production in skin can occur in areas in which there is minimal sun exposure or in individuals in whom exposure of the skin is minimal and whose dietary intake of vitamin D-containing foods is low, particularly if foods are not fortified with vitamin D.

Malabsorption syndromes induced by postsurgical gastrectomy state, celiac sprue, inflammatory bowel disease, cystic fibrosis, or chronic pancreatitis may be associated with either reduced absorption of dietary sources of vitamin D or defects in the enterohepatic circulation leading to decreased reabsorption of secreted calcidiol.

In addition to reduced endogenous production of vitamin D in elderly individuals, vitamin D intake is often low as it is for most Americans. This may contribute to the risk for osteoporosis. Dietary vitamin D deficiency can occur in children and results in hypocalcemia as well as abnormal bone formation and development (rickets).

Patients with chronic kidney disease are usually considered to have 1,25-dihydroxyvitamin D (calcitriol) deficiency due to reduced renal synthesis of the active hormone. Diminished availability of calcidiol in patients with severe liver disease and those taking drugs that increase the activity of P-450 enzymes that metabolize vitamin D to inactive forms, such as anticonvulsants (phenobarbital, phenytoin, carbamazepine), alcohol, isoniazid, theophylline, and rifampin, may lead to vitamin D deficiency associated with calcidiol deficiency.

E. Genetic Abnormalities of Vitamin D Metabolism

Vitamin D-dependent rickets refers to two autosomal recessive syndromes characterized by hypocalcemia, hypophosphatemia, and rickets. Type 1 vitamin D-dependent rickets, also called pseudovitamin D deficiency rickets, is characterized by an inability to produce calcitriol due to an inactivating mutation in the 1-hydroxylase gene. Type 2 vitamin D-dependent rickets is an autosomal recessive disorder due to hereditary resistance to vitamin D. It is usually caused by mutations in the gene encoding the vitamin D receptor.

In nephrotic syndrome, there may be excessive urinary loss of vitamin D-binding protein and bound vitamin D leading to vitamin D deficiency but rarely to clinically significant hypocalcemia.

F. Intravascular and Tissue Complexation of Calcium Hyperphosphatemia

Intravascular and tissue complexation of calcium hyperphosphatemia induces hypocalcemia through several mechanisms including formation of deposits of calcium phosphate in bone and soft tissue when the product of the serum calcium (mg/dL) and phosphate (mg/dL) is higher than 55 mg^2/dL^2. This may occur as phosphate infusions or oral or rectal administration for bowel cleansing or as laxatives. Also, phosphate release from cells during chemotherapy of a variety of tumors or leukemia or during rhabdomyolysis may produce the same disturbance. Intravascular precipitation may occur if the hyperphosphatemia is acute. Intravascular complexation may also occur if patients receive large amount of citrate in blood products such as may occur with plasma exchange or massive blood transfusion. In this setting, ionized calcium must be measured, as total serum calcium will include the portion bound to citrate and total calcium will be in the normal range while ionized calcium will be reduced.

"Hungry bone" syndrome refers to the rapid uptake of calcium and phosphate into bone after parathyroidectomy, particularly in patients who have had long-standing primary or secondary hyperparathyroidism and who have severe degrees of bone resorption. The syndrome typically occurs in the first few hours after parathyroidectomy and may persist for several days. A similar phenomenon may be seen in patients with certain tumors such as prostate cancer who develop osteoblastic metastasis.

Soft tissue complexation also occurs in acute pancreatitis as calcium may combine with circulating and with tissue fats and form "soap" at the sites of precipitation. Calcium may also be deposited in the damaged muscle of patients suffering from rhabdomyolysis.

G. Other Causes of Hypocalcemia

Other causes of hypocalcemia include sepsis where multiple abnormalities including hypoalbuminemia, lactic acidosis, hypomagnesemia, and a primary impairment of PTH secretion may occur. During infusions of magnesium in women treated for preeclampsia, the calcium-sensing receptor may be bound by and activated by magnesium resulting in a transient reduction in PTH secretion and hypocalcemia. Typically patients are not symptomatic from hypocalcemia because of the concurrent hypermagnesemia. Finally, cinacalcet, a drug in the new class of calcimimetic agents, will induce hypocalcemia as it acts to increase the sensitivity of the calcium-sensing receptor to calcium and thereby leads to inhibition of PTH secretion in the face of hypocalcemia.

Pseudohypocalcemia has recently been described as certain gadolinium-based contrast agents used in magnetic resonance imaging, gadodiamide and gadoversetamide, may bind to the indicator reagents used in colorimetric assays for calcium and produce a false low value. This may be a particular problem in patients with renal insufficiency receiving these agents as they are renally excreted.

▶ Clinical Findings

Symptoms and Signs

The clinical manifestations of hypocalcemia are rather specific and relate to the neuromuscular actions of hypocalcemia. Tetany is the hallmark of hypocalcemia and results from increased neuromuscular irritability after stimulation. It consists of a set of symptoms including circumoral and acral paresthesias. The signs of hypocalcemia include muscle spasms and specifically carpopedal spasm (adduction of thumb, flexion of wrists and metacarpals, and extension of fingers). The manifestations of hypocalcemia can be elicited during the physical examination and include Trousseau's sign (elicited by inflating a sphygmomanometer cuff above systolic pressure for 3 minutes and finding carpopedal spasm of the affected limb) or Chvostek's sign (twitching of facial muscles after tapping on the facial nerve anterior to the ear). While these findings are relatively specific for hypocalcemia, they are also found in hypomagnesemic patients. However, hypomagnesemia induces hypocalcemia, so

that if tetany is found, it is usually in the setting of hypocalcemia as well. These signs of neuromuscular irritability may herald grand mal seizures and therefore represent a medical emergency when seen. Cardiac abnormalities including arrhythmias, particularly in patients on digitalis, and hypotension may be seen as well, particularly in the critical care setting. These abnormalities are typically seen when patients have a serum calcium level that is 30% or greater lower than normal.

It should be noted that occasionally patients with acute, severe respiratory alkalosis will manifest tetany as the acute alkalemia itself induces neuromuscular irritability and alkalemia decreases ionized calcium by increasing the negative charges on albumin and thereby increasing albumin binding of ionized calcium.

Some patients with chronic hypocalcemia may have neuropsychiatric manifestations including dementia or mental retardation in children and other psychiatric syndromes including depression and anxiety. In addition, idiopathic hypoparathyroidism, an important cause of chronic hypocalcemia, may be associated paradoxically with intracerebral calcifications, particularly in the basal ganglia, and a Parkinsonian syndrome may result from basal ganglia damage.

▶ Differential Diagnosis

The diagnosis of hypocalcemia rests with a measurement of serum calcium as either a screening test or in response to the symptomatology described above. As the physiologically active fraction of calcium is ionized and closely regulated yet the standard measure of serum calcium includes a major fraction bound to albumin and other anions, it is important to consider the relation of total serum calcium to the bound fraction. Total serum calcium falls approximately 0.8 mg/dL for every 1 g/dL decrement in the concentration of serum albumin. Serum ionized calcium can also be measured directly by an ion electrode.

Since hypocalcemia is found only in the setting of disorders of PTH and vitamin D or as a result of tissue deposition or complexation, a variety of other assays should be made in order to diagnose the underlying disturbance. First, serum phosphate should be measured, as an elevated value might suggest kidney disease, hypoparathyroidism, or release of cellular stores of phosphate such as occurs in rhabdomyolysis or when a large tumor burden is suddenly reduced by lytic therapies such as chemotherapy for leukemia.

Serum magnesium should be measured as severe hypomagnesemia (<1 mg/dL) is associated with a failure of PTH secretion and/or a failure of bone to respond normally to circulating PTH. As chronic kidney disease reduces calcitriol levels and induces hyperphosphatemia, serum creatinine should be measured in all hypocalcemic patients.

If the diagnosis is not apparent from the patient's history, physical examination, and the above noted assays, the next step is to measure immunoreactive intact PTH levels. In diseases associated with secondary hyperparathyroidism and in defective tissue response to PTH (pseudohypoparathyroidism), the PTH level will be high in hypocalcemia. In idiopathic or postsurgical hypoparathyroidism, PTH levels will be low in hypocalcemia, although normal PTH levels may be inappropriately low if hypocalcemia is found.

If secondary hyperparathyroidism is found, then vitamin D metabolites should be measured. Low levels of 25-hydroxyvitamin D (calcidiol) suggest chronic vitamin D deficiency, usually due to decreased intake or abnormal GI absorption of vitamin D as calcidiol levels are reflective of intake and not subject to physiologic regulation. However, low or low-normal levels of calcitriol with normal calcidiol levels in hypocalcemia is a pattern seen in renal failure.

▶ Treatment

A. Symptomatic Hypocalcemia

Since there are multiple systems designed to maintain the serum calcium level and there is a large store of calcium in bone, hypocalcemia will not be successfully treated in a sustained manner by calcium infusions alone. Typically, calcium infusions may correct the symptoms of acute or chronic hypocalcemia, but sustained therapy usually requires either correction of the underlying cause of hypocalcemia or use of vitamin D supplementation.

The most appropriate treatment for patients with symptomatic hypocalcemia, either acute or chronic, is intravenous calcium, in the form of 100–200 mg (2.5–5 mmol) of elemental calcium (1–2 g of calcium gluconate) in 10–20 minutes. This should be followed by a slow infusion of calcium as the serum calcium will rapidly return to low levels under most circumstances. The dose of the slow infusion should be 1.0 mg/kg/hour as 10% calcium gluconate (90 mg of elemental calcium per 10-mL ampoule). Some postparathyroidectomy patients may require prolonged, massive calcium therapy due to hungry bone disease.

If hypomagnesemia is the cause of hypocalcemia, 2 g (16 mEq) of magnesium sulfate should be infused as a 10% solution over 10 minutes, followed by 1 g (8 mEq) in 100 mL of fluid per hour until serum magnesium remains normal. Patients with hypocalcemia and severe acute hyperphosphatemia due to tumor lysis syndrome require hemodialysis to correct hyperphosphatemia. This will typically ameliorate hypocalcemia.

B. Chronic Hypocalcemia Induced by Hypoparathyroidism

Both oral calcium and vitamin D supplementation are usually required to correct the hypocalcemia of chronic hypoparathyroidism. The target serum calcium level should be approximately 8.0 mg/dL and at that level, most patients will be asymptomatic. If serum calcium is maintained at a higher level, patients will develop hypercalciuria because of the lack of PTH to enhance calcium reabsorption across the distal nephron. Chronic hypercalciuria may lead to development of nephrocalcinosis, nephrolithiasis, and renal insufficiency.

Occasionally in mild hypoparathyroidism 2 g of oral calcium supplements will achieve normal calcium levels. If this fails, vitamin D should be added. The usual initial daily dose is 50,000 international units of ergocalciferol (vitamin D_2) or 0.25–0.5 μg of calcitriol. Appropriate doses of calcium and vitamin D are established by gradual titration. If hypercalciuria is detected, a thiazide diuretic may be added to the regimen. This will result in diminished calciuria and a further increase in the serum calcium level. Serum and urine calcium levels must be monitored carefully, as the main complications of the treatment of hypoparathyroidism are inadvertent hypercalcemia and/or hypercalciuria.

With the recent availability of a synthetic PTH preparation (1-34 PTH, teriparatide) using twice-daily subcutaneous administration has led to correction of hypocalcemia with lower risk of hypercalciuria.

C. Renal Failure

While hypocalcemia is highly prevalent in patients with chronic renal failure, symptomatic hypocalcemia is rare. The approach to hypocalcemia in renal failure is primarily to lower serum phosphorus and supplement patients with active forms of vitamin D.

Holick MF: Vitamin D for health and in chronic kidney disease. Semin Dial 2005;18:266.

Locatelli F, Rossi F: Incidence and pathogenesis of tumor lysis syndrome. Contrib Nephrol 2005;147:61.

Pecherstorfer M et al: Current management strategies for hypercalcemia. Treat Endocrinol 2003;2(4):273.

Stewart AF: Clinical practice. Hypercalcemia associated with cancer. N Engl J Med 2005;352:373.

Tfelt-Hansen J, Brown EM: The calcium-sensing receptor in normal physiology and pathophysiology: a review. Crit Rev Clin Lab Sci 2005;42:35.

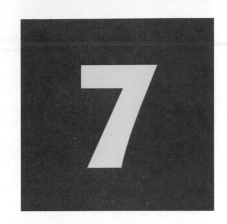

Disorders of Phosphate Balance: Hypophosphatemia & Hyperphosphatemia

Keith A. Hruska, MD

New data demonstrate that serum phosphate, similar to serum calcium, is a signaling molecule. The mechanisms for sensing serum phosphate signal transduction concentration are not understood. This chapter considers serum phosphorus in a context greater than mineral and metabolic homeostasis. The bulk of total body phosphate (85%) is in the bone as part of the mineralized extracellular matrix. This phosphate pool is accessible, albeit in a limited fashion through bone resorption. Phosphate is a predominantly intracellular anion with an estimated concentration of approximately 100 mmol/L, most of which is either complexed or bound to proteins or lipids. Serum phosphorus concentration varies with age, time of day, fasting state, and season. It is higher in children than adults. Phosphorus levels exhibit a diurnal variation with the lowest phosphate level occurring near noon. Serum phosphorus concentration is regulated by diet, hormones, and physical factors such as pH. Importantly, because phosphate moves in and out of cells under several influences, the serum concentration of phosphorus may not reflect phosphate stores.

HYPERPHOSPHATEMIA

ESSENTIALS OF DIAGNOSIS

▶ Serum inorganic phosphorus (Pi) concentration greater than 2.5–4.5 mg/dL or 0.75–1.45 mM in adults or 6 or 7 mg/dL in children.

▶ Consequence of increased intake of Pi, decreased renal excretion of Pi, or translocation of Pi from tissue breakdown into extracellular fluid.

▶ Short-term consequences are hypocalcemia and tetany.

▶ Long-term consequences are soft tissue calcification and secondary hyperparathyroidism.

Serum inorganic phosphorus (Pi) concentrations are generally maintained at 2.5–4.5 mg/dL or 0.75–1.45 mM in adults, whereas hyperphosphatemia is not present in children unless serum Pi levels are greater than 6 or 7 mg/dL. Hyperphosphatemia may be the consequence of an increased intake of Pi, a decreased excretion of Pi, or translocation of Pi from tissue breakdown into the extracellular fluid (Table 7–1). Because the kidneys are able to excrete phosphate very efficiently over a wide range of dietary intake, hyperphosphatemia most frequently results from renal insufficiency and the attendant inability to excrete Pi. However, in metabolic bone disorders such as osteoporosis and renal osteodystrophy, the skeleton is a poorly recognized contributor to serum phosphorus.

▶ Pathopysiology

A. Increased Intake

Hyperphosphatemia can be the consequence of an *increased intake* or administration of Pi. Intravenous administration of Pi during parenteral nutrition, the treatment of Pi depletion, or hypercalcemia can cause hyperphosphatemia, especially in patients with underlying renal insufficiency. Hyperphosphatemia may also result from overzealous use of oral phosphates or of phosphate-containing enemas as phosphate can be absorbed passively from the colon through paracellular pathways. Administration of vitamin D and its metabolites in pharmacologic doses may be responsible for the development of hyperphosphatemia, although suppression of parathyroid hormone (PTH) and hypercalcemia-induced renal failure are important pathogenetic factors in this setting.

B. Decreased Renal Excretion

Clinically, hyperphosphatemia is most often caused by impaired excretion due to kidney failure. During stages II and III of chronic kidney disease (CKD), phosphate balance is maintained by a progressive reduction in the fraction of filtered phosphate reabsorbed by the tubules leading to increased Pi excretion by the remaining nephrons and a maintenance of normal renal Pi clearance. In advanced kidney failure, the

Table 7–1. Causes of hyperphosphatemia.

Increased intake
Intravenous—sodium or potassium phosphate
Oral administration—Neutraphos
Rectal—Fleets phosphosoda enemas

Decreased renal excretion
Renal insufficiency/failure—acute or chronic
Pseudohypoparathyroidism
Tumoral calcinosis
Hypoparathyroidism
Acromegaly
Bisphosphonates
Childhood

Excess bone resorption
Transcellular shift from intracellular to extracellular spaces
Catabolic states
Fulminant hepatitis
Hyperthermia
Rhabdomyolysis—crush injuries or nontraumatic
Cytotoxic therapy—tumor lysis
Acute leukemia
Diabetic ketoacidosis
Hemolytic anemia
Acidosis—metabolic or respiratory

Artifactual

fractional excretion of Pi may be as high as 60–90% of the filtered load of phosphate. However, when the number of functional nephrons becomes too diminished (glomerular filtration rate usually < 20 mL/minute) and dietary intake is constant, Pi balance can no longer be maintained by reductions of tubular reabsorption, and hyperphosphatemia develops. When this occurs, the filtered load of Pi per nephron increases and Pi excretion rises. As a result, Pi balance and renal excretory rate are reestablished, but at a higher serum Pi level (hyperphosphatemia). An unresolved issue during late stages of CKD, stage IV with persistent hyperphosphatemia and elevated PTH levels, there is phosphate reabsorption. The fractional excretion may be 80%, but why isn't it 95% and balance maintained with normophosphatemia?

Defects in renal excretion of Pi in the absence of renal failure may be primary, as in *pseudohypoparathyroidism* (PHP). PHP is a term for a group of disorders characterized by hypocalcemia and hyperphosphatemia due to resistance to the renal tubular actions of parathyroid hormone. As a result of the molecular abnormalities in PHP, PTH does not decrease proximal renal tubular phosphate transport causing hyperphosphatemia.

A second primary defect in renal Pi excretion is *tumoral calcinosis*. This is usually seen in young black males with ectopic calcification around large joints and is characterized by increased tubular reabsorption of calcium and Pi and normal

responses to PTH. Familial forms of tumoral calcinosis are due to mutations in the UDP-*N*-acetyl-α-D-galactosamine: polypeptide *N*-acetylgalactosaminyltransferase 3 (GALNT3) gene and missense mutations in fibroblast growth factor (FGF)23. It has been demonstrated that besides PTH, FGF23 is a second hormonal regulator of renal phosphate transport in physiologic conditions.

Secondary tubular defects in phosphate transport include *hypoparathyroidism* and high blood levels of growth hormone in acromegaly. Finally, bisphosphonates such as Didronel (disodium etidronate), Pamidronate, or Alendronate may cause hyperphosphatemia. The mechanisms of action are unclear, but they may involve cellular phosphate redistribution and decreased renal excretion. Serum phosphorus values are normally elevated in children as compared to adults.

C. Excess Bone Resorption

Clinical and translational studies demonstrate that excess bone resorption contributes to the level of serum phosphorus, which is poorly appreciated. Even in clinical situations where bone formation is decreased (adynamic) such as osteoporosis, a variability in the serum phosphorus is produced when bone formation is stimulated (Figure 7–1). For instance, in low turnover osteodystrophy treated with a skeletal anabolic agent, if phosphorus intake is constant the serum phosphorus falls despite no change in or a decrease in phosphate excretion (Figure 7–1B).

D. Transcellular Shift

Transcellular shift of Pi from cells into the extracellular fluid compartment may lead to hyperphosphatemia, as seen in conditions associated with increased catabolism or tissue destruction (eg, systemic infections, fulminant hepatitis, severe hyperthermia, crush injuries, nontraumatic rhabdomyolysis, and cytotoxic therapy for hematologic malignancies such as acute lymphoblastic leukemia and Burkitt's lymphoma). In the "*tumor lysis syndrome*," serum Pi levels typically rise, due to release from dying cells, within 12 days after initiation of treatment. The rising serum Pi concentration is often accompanied by hypocalcemia, hyperuricemia, hyperkalemia, and renal failure. Patients with *diabetic ketoacidosis* commonly have hyperphosphatemia at the time of presentation despite total body Pi depletion. Insulin, fluid, and acid-base therapy are accompanied by a shift of Pi back into cells and the development of hypophosphatemia. In lactic acidosis, hyperphosphatemia likely results from tissue hypoxia with a breakdown of adenosine triphosphate (ATP) to adenosine monophosphate (AMP) and Pi.

E. Artifactual

Hyperphosphatemia may be *artifactual* when hemolysis occurs during the collection, storage, or processing of blood samples.

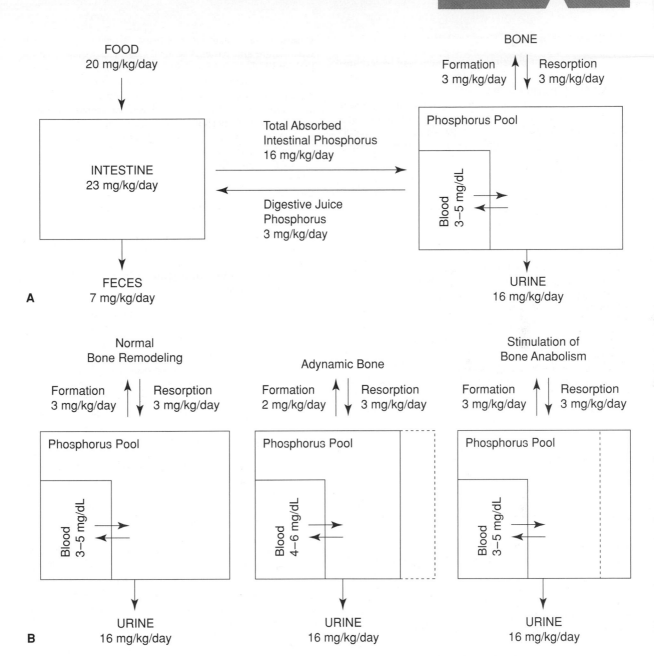

▲ **Figure 7-1.** Skeletal remodeling contributes to phosphate balance and serum phosphorus levels.
A: The phosphate balance diagram is amplified to show that the serum phosphorus is a small component of a rapidly exchangeable phosphorus pool composed of cellular phosphorus and the bone mineralization front.
B: When bone formation is decreased (adynamic bone disorders) the exchangeable pool size is diminished and intestinal absorption from food intake will produce larger fluctuations in the serum phosphorus. These fluctuations are sufficient to activate the signaling actions of the serum Pi even though the fasting serum Pi is normal. Stimulation of bone anabolism increases the exchangeable phosphorus pool size and decreases serum phosphorus fluctuations. In end-stage kidney disease, treatment of secondary hyperparathyroidism with a calcimimetic that does not affect phosphate absorption decreases serum phosphate demonstrating the role of the skeleton in hyperphosphatemia.

► Clinical Findings

The most important short-term consequences of hyperphosphatemia are hypocalcemia and tetany, which occur most commonly in patients with an increased Pi load from any source, exogenous or endogenous. By contrast, soft tissue calcification and secondary hyperparathyroidism are long-term consequences of hyperphosphatemia that occur mainly in patients with renal insufficiency and decreased renal Pi excretion.

A. Hypocalcemia and Tetany

With rapid elevations of serum Pi, hypocalcemia and tetany may occur with serum Pi concentrations as low as 6 mg/dL, a level that if reached more slowly has no detectable effect on serum calcium. Hyperphosphatemia, in addition to its effect on the calcium × phosphate ion product with resultant calcium deposition in soft tissues, also inhibits the activity of 1α-hydroxylase in the kidney, resulting in a lower circulating level of 1,25-dihydroxyvitamin D_3. This further aggravates hypocalcemia by impairing intestinal absorption of calcium and inducing a state of skeletal resistance to the action of PTH.

Phosphate-induced hypocalcemia is common in patients with acute or chronic renal failure, and usually develops slowly. Tetany is uncommon unless a superimposed acid–base disorder produces an abrupt rise in plasma pH that acutely lowers the serum ionized calcium concentration. Profound hypocalcemia and tetany are occasionally observed during the early phase of the "tumor lysis" syndrome and rhabdomyolysis.

B. Soft Tissue Calcification

Extraskeletal calcification associated with hyperphosphatemia is usually seen in patients with CKD, diabetes, severe atherosclerosis, and aging. Recent basic, translational, and clinical research studies have led to new theories concerning the pathogenesis and the consequences of this phenomenon. Several inhibitors of vascular calcification have been discovered, including osteoprotegerin, osteopontin, matrix GLA protein, the klotho gene product, and Smad6. These substances constitute an inherent defense against heterotopic mineralization, which is breached in the disease environment. In the setting of CKD, hyperphosphatemia has been identified as a major factor contributing to the forces favoring mineralization.

In contrast to the breach of defense theory of vascular calcification, there is significant evidence that vascular cells undergo osteogenesis resulting in vascular mineralization. Experimental models have demonstrated that elevated phosphate is a direct stimulus of this transformation. The finding of vascular calcification and the role of hyperphosphatemia have more than academic significance. Calcification of the neointima or the tunica media including the large blood vessels, coronary arteries, and heart valves in patients with renal failure and patients with diabetes is associated with a high morbidity and mortality from systolic hypertension, congestive heart failure, coronary artery disease, and myocardial infarction. Another manifestation of vascular calcification in more peripheral arteries, calciphylaxis, is also associated with hyperphosphatemia and carries a poor prognosis. As a result, both vascular calcification and hyperphosphatemia are independent risk factors for cardiovascular disease and mortality.

Occasionally, an acute rise in serum Pi (eg, during Pi treatment for hypercalcemia or vitamin D intoxication) may lead to soft tissue calcification in clinical settings in addition to those previously mentioned. The blood vessels, skin, cornea (band keratopathy), and periarticular tissues are common sites of calcium phosphate deposition.

C. Secondary Hyperparathyroidism and Renal Osteodystrophy

Hyperphosphatemia due to renal failure also plays a critical role in the development of secondary hyperparathyroidism and renal osteodystrophy and in mortality. Several mechanisms contribute to these complications including hyperphosphatemia-induced hypocalcemia through physicochemical interactions, expression of tumor growth factor (TGF)-α and the epidermal growth factor receptor (EGFR) in parathyroid chief cells leading to hyperplasia and increased PTH secretion and inhibition of vitamin D synthesis, and hyperphosphatemia-stimulated vascular calcification. In patients with advanced renal failure, the enhanced phosphate load from PTH-mediated osteolysis may ultimately become the dominant influence on serum phosphorus levels (Figure 7–1B). This phenomenon may account for the correlation between serum phosphorus levels and the severity of osteitis fibrosa cystica in patients maintained on chronic hemodialysis. Hyperphosphatemia also plays a critical role in the development of vascular calcification as previously discussed. There is a direct relationship between defective orthotopic mineralization (bone formation) in CKD and increased heterotopic mineralization. Data demonstrate that increasing bone formation will lower phosphate levels and diminish vascular calcification in CKD.

Finally, it should be noted that the clinical and translational data derived from the study of CKD in soft tissue calcification indicate that phosphorus is a heretofore unrecognized risk factor for cardiovascular disease.

► Treatment

Correction of the pathogenetic defect should be the primary aim in the treatment of hyperphosphatemia. When hyperphosphatemia is due solely to increased intake, discontinuation of supplemental phosphate and maintenance of adequate volume for diuresis are generally sufficient, as the kidneys will promptly excrete the excess. In the uncommon circumstance of significant hyperphosphatemia due to transcellular shift, treatment should be dictated by the underlying cause. For example, hyperphosphatemia that accompanies diabetic ketoacidosis will resolve with insulin therapy, as insulin stimulates cellular uptake of phosphate. On the other hand, hyperphosphatemia seen with tumor lysis, rhabdomyolysis, or other conditions characterized by massive cell death or injury should be treated as an excess phosphate load, albeit endogenous instead of exogenous. Limitation of phosphate intake and enhanced diuresis will generally resolve this cause of hyperphosphatemia, provided renal function is adequate.

When renal insufficiency is present, however, the most effective way to treat hyperphosphatemia is to reduce dietary Pi intake and to add phosphate-binding agents. Because Pi is present in almost all foodstuffs, rigid dietary phosphate restriction requires a barely palatable diet that few patients can accept. However, dietary Pi can be reduced to 800–1000 mg/day with modest protein restriction. A predialysis level of 4.5–5.0 mg/dL is reasonable and allows some room for removal of phosphorus with dialysis while avoiding severe postdialysis hypophosphatemia. To achieve this, the addition of phosphate binders to reduce intestinal absorption of dietary Pi is required. Calcium salts and sevelamer have replaced aluminum salts as first-line Pi binders. However, calcium salts contribute to the calcium phosphate ion product, and massive calcium intake is often required to maintain serum phosphorus in the target range.

Elevated calcium phosphorus products and the calcium load-induced increase in serum calcium contribute to the development of vascular calcification. Therefore, newer Pi binders have been introduced such as sevelamer hydrochloride and lanthanum carbonate. Sevelamer has an improved safety profile over calcium salts, and as a binding resin, it also binds cholesterol and low-density lipoprotein (LDL) leading to improved lipid profiles in patients with end-stage kidney disease (ESKD). Calcium acetate binds more Pi than equivalent amounts of calcium carbonate or citrate. Sevelamer binds calcium equally to calcium carbonate, but the large doses required to maintain serum phosphorus, the pill sizes, and gastrointestinal side effects make compliance a difficult issue with the sole use of sevelamer. In addition, the cost of the agent has limited its use in some instances. Therefore, the prescription of an effective Pi-binding regimen is a complex issue for ESKD patients. In general, treatment is started with 1 g of calcium carbonate with each meal to treat any tendency to hypocalcemia, and sevelamer is added in increasing doses until the target serum phosphorus is achieved. Calcium acetate may be preferred over calcium carbonate to limit calcium intake as an increased dose of phosphate binding is required. Either of these regimens effectively controls serum Pi in about two-thirds of patients on chronic dialysis. Calcium salts tend to increase serum calcium levels, and if hypercalcemia develops, calcium carbonate should be stopped and a switch to sevelamer, lanthanum carbonate, or a reduction in dialysate calcium should be considered. If aluminum gels are used, calcium citrate must not be taken concomitantly because citrate markedly increases the absorption of aluminum. Maximal Pi binding occurs when phosphate binder is taken with a meal rather than 2 hours afterward. Magnesium-containing antacids are also effective phosphate binders; however, their use in renal failure is limited because intestinal absorption of magnesium can lead to magnesium toxicity.

New treatments for secondary hyperparathyroidism of kidney failure besides phosphate binders discussed above and vitamin D analogs that suppress PTH gene transcription but increase intestinal Pi absorption include calcimimetics that activate the calcium sensor of the PTH gland. A calcimimetic (cinacalcet) when used in dialysis patients decreases serum phosphorus, demonstrating the role of the skeleton in the hyperphosphatemia of ESKD.

The treatment of chronic hyperphosphatemia secondary to hypoparathyroidism occasionally requires that phosphate binders be added to the other therapeutic agents.

Chertow GM et al: Long-term effects of sevelamer hydrochloride on the calcium × phosphate product and lipid profile of haemodialysis patients. Nephrol Dial Transplant 1999;14:2907.

Doherty TM et al: Calcification in atherosclerosis: bone biology and chronic inflammation at the arterial crossroads. Proc Natl Acad Sci USA 2004;100:11201.

Hruska KA et al: Bone morphogenetic proteins in vascular calcification. Circ Res 2005;97:105.

Martin DR et al: Acute regulation of parathyroid hormone by dietary phosphate. Endocrinol Metab 2005;289:E729.

HYPOPHOSPHATEMIA

 ESSENTIALS OF DIAGNOSIS

► Serum or plasma Pi concentration below 1.0 mg/dL.

► Frequently encountered in alcoholic patients.

► Consequence of decreased intestinal absorption or increased urinary losses of Pi or a shift of Pi from extracellular to intracellular compartments.

► Can result in central nervous system, red blood cell, leukocyte, platelet, and skeletal and cardiac muscle dysfunction; bone disease; and metabolic acidosis.

Hypophosphatemia is defined as an abnormally low concentration of Pi in serum or plasma. It does not necessarily indicate total body Pi depletion because only 1% of the total body Pi is found in extracellular fluids. Conversely, serious Pi depletion may exist in the presence of a normal or even elevated serum Pi concentration. Moderate hypophosphatemia, defined as a serum Pi concentration between 2.5 and 1 mg/dL, is not uncommon, and is usually not associated with signs or symptoms. Severe hypophosphatemia, defined as serum phosphorus levels below 1.0 mg/dL, is often associated with clinical signs and symptoms that require therapy. Approximately 2% of hospital patients have levels of serum Pi below 2 mg/dL according to some estimates. Hypophosphatemia is encountered more frequently among alcoholic patients and up to 10% of patients admitted to hospitals because of chronic alcoholism are hypophosphatemic.

▷ Pathogenesis

Three types of pathophysiologic abnormalities can cause hypophosphatemia and total body Pi depletion: decreased intestinal absorption of Pi, increased urinary losses of this ion, and a shift of Pi from extracellular to intracellular compartments (Table 7–2). Combinations of these disturbances are common. The causes and mechanisms of moderate hypophosphatemia are shown in Table 7–2; the clinical conditions associated with severe hypophosphatemia are shown in Table 7–3.

Table 7–2. Causes of moderate hypophosphatemia and/or phosphate depletion.

Decreased intestinal absorption
Abnormalities of vitamin D metabolism
Antacid abuse
Malabsorption
Alcoholism
Starvation—famine, anorexia nervosa, alcoholism
Increased urinary losses
Alcoholism
Hyperparathyroidism
Renal tubular defects—Fanconi, Dent's, posttransplant, hypomagnesemia, fructose intolerance
X-linked hypophosphatemia, autosomal dominant hypophosphatemia
Oncogenic osteomalacia
McCune–Albright syndrome (MAS) and fibrous dysplasia (FD)
Diabetic ketoacidosis
Metabolic or respiratory acidosis
Respiratory alkalosis
Drugs: calcitonin, diuretics, glucocorticoids, bicarbonate, agonists
Extracellular fluid volume expansion
Transcellular shift from the extracellular to the intracellular space
Respiratory alkalosis
Leukemia (blast crisis)
Recovery from metabolic acidosis, commonly diabetic ketoacidosis
Recovery from hypothermia
Nutritional repletion—refeeding syndrome
Sepsis, especially gram-negative bacteremia
Salicylate intoxication
Sugars—glucose, fructose, glycerol
Insulin therapy
"Hungry-bone" syndrome after parathyroidectomy

Table 7–3. Risk factors for severe hypophosphatemia and/or phosphate depletion.

Alcohol withdrawal
Nutritional repletion in at-risk patients
Anorexia nervosa and other eating disorders
Starvation due to famine, neglect, alcoholism, malabsorption, prisoners of war
AIDS and other chronic infections
Massive weight loss for morbid obesity
Treatment of diabetic ketoacidosis
Critical illness
Sepsis
Posttrauma
Extensive burns

A. Decreased Intestinal Absorption

1. Vitamin D deficiency (Table 7–2)—Diets deficient in vitamin D lead to the metabolic disorder known as rickets in children or osteomalacia when it appears in adults. Rickets result in severe deformities of bone because of rapid growth. These deformities are characterized by soft loose areas in the skull known as craniotabes and costochondral swelling or bending (known as rachitic rosary). The chest usually becomes flattened, and the sternum may be pushed forward to form the so-called pigeon chest. Thoracic expansion may be greatly reduced with impairment of respiratory function. Kyphosis is a common finding. There is remarkable swelling of the joints, particularly the wrists and ankles, with characteristic anterior bowing of the legs, and fractures of the "greenstick" variety may also be seen. In adults, the symptoms are not as striking and are usually characterized by bone pain, weakness, radiolucent areas, and pseudofractures. Pseudofractures represent stress fractures in which the normal process of healing is impaired because of a mineralization defect. Mild hypocalcemia may be present; however, hypophosphatemia is the most frequent biochemical alteration. This metabolic abnormality responds well to administration of small amounts of vitamin D.

Vitamin D deficiency is becoming common in Western society, especially in elderly patients who do not ingest fortified foods or get adequate sunlight exposure. It is an important problem separate from calcitriol deficiency in CKD. This is because of recent discoveries of extrarenal 1α-hydroxylase that contributes to cellular function of many organs including hematopoietic cells and the parathyroid glands.

2. Vitamin D-resistant rickets—These are recessively inherited forms of vitamin D-refractory rickets. The conditions are characterized by hypophosphatemia, hypocalcemia, elevated levels of serum alkaline phosphatase, and, sometimes, generalized aminoaciduria and severe bone lesions. Two main forms of vitamin D-dependent rickets have been characterized. Type I is caused by a mutation in the gene converting 25-hydroxyvitamin D to 1,25-dihydroxychole-calciferol, the renal 1α-hydroxylase enzyme. This condition responds to very large doses of vitamin D_2 and D_3 (100–300 times the normal requirement of physiologic doses), how-ever, 0.5–1.0 μg/day of 1,25-dihydroxycholecalciferol.

Type II is characterized by an end-organ resistance to 1,25-dihydroxycholecalciferol. Plasma levels of 1,25-dihy-droxycholecalciferol are elevated. This finding, in association with radiographic and biochemical signs of rickets, implies resistance to the target tissue to 1,25-dihydroxycholecalcif-erol. Hereditary type II vitamin D-resistant rickets is a genetic disease affecting the vitamin D receptor (VDR). Cellular de-fects found in patients with vitamin D-resistant rickets type II are heterogeneous, providing in part an explanation for the different clinical manifestations of this disorder. The treat-ment of this condition requires large pharmacologic doses of calcium, which overcome the receptor defects and maintain bone remodeling.

3. Antacid abuse and malabsorption (Table 7–2)—Severe hypophosphatemia and phosphate depletion may result from vigorous use of oral antacids, which bind phosphate, usually for peptic ulcer disease. Patients so treated may develop os-teomalacia and severe skeletal symptoms due to phosphorus deficiency. Intestinal malabsorption can cause hypophospha-temia and phosphate depletion through malabsorption of Pi and vitamin D, and through increased urinary Pi losses resulting from secondary hyperparathyroidism induced by calcium malabsorption.

4. Alcohol and alcohol withdrawal (Table 7–2 and Table 7–3)—Alcohol abuse is a common cause of hypophos-phatemia, which may be severe (Table 7–2), due to both poor intake and excessive losses. Poor intake results from dietary deficiencies, the use of antacids, and vomiting. Patients with alcoholism have also been shown to have a variety of defects in renal tubular function, including a decrease in thresh-old for phosphate excretion, which are reversible with absti-nence. Ethanol enhances urinary Pi excretion, and marked phosphaturia tends to occur during episodes of alcoholic ketoacidosis. Because such patients often eat poorly, ketonu-ria is common. Repeated episodes of ketoacidosis catabolize organic phosphates within cells and cause phosphaturia by mechanisms analogous to those seen in diabetic ketoacidosis. Chronic alcoholism may also cause magnesium deficiency and hypomagnesemia, which may, in turn, cause phosphatu-ria and Pi depletion, especially in skeletal muscle.

5. Nutritional repletion: oral, enteral, and parenteral nutrition (Table 7–3)—Nutritional repletion of the mal-nourished patient implies the provision of sufficient calo-ries, protein, and other nutrients to allow accelerated tissue accretion. In the course of this process, cellular uptake and utilization of Pi increase. When insufficient amounts of Pi are provided, an acute state of severe hypophosphatemia and intracellular Pi depletion with serious clinical and metabolic consequences can occur. This type of hypophosphatemia has been observed in malnourished patients receiving parenteral nutrition and following refeeding of prisoners of war.

B. Increased Urinary Losses

1. Hyperparathyroidism—Primary hyperparathyroidism (Table 7–2) is a common entity in clinical medicine. PTH is secreted in excess of the physiologic needs for mineral homeostasis due either to adenoma or hyperplasia of the parathyroid glands. This results in decreased phosphorus reabsorption by the kidney, and the urinary losses of phos-phorus result in hypophosphatemia. The degree of hypo-phosphatemia varies considerably because mobilization of phosphorus from stimulation of skeletal remodeling in part mitigates the hypophosphatemia. Secondary hyperpara-thyroidism associated with normal renal function has been observed in patients with gastrointestinal abnormalities re-sulting in calcium malabsorption. Such patients may have low levels of serum calcium and phosphorus. In these pa-tients, the hypocalcemia is responsible for increased release of PTH. Decreased intestinal absorption of phosphorus as a result of the primary gastrointestinal disease may contribute to the decrement in the levels of serum phosphorus. In gen-eral, these patients have urinary losses of phosphorus that are out of proportion to the hypophosphatemia, in contrast to patients with predominant phosphorus malabsorption and no secondary hyperparathyroidism in whom urinary excre-tion of phosphorus is low.

2. Renal tubular defects—Several conditions character-ized by either single or multiple tubular ion transport defects have been characterized in which phosphorus reabsorption is decreased. In Fanconi syndrome, patients excrete not only an increased amount of phosphorus in the urine but also increased quantities of amino acids, uric acid, and glucose, resulting in hypouricemia and hypophosphatemia. In Dent's disease, a proximal tubular trafficking vesicle chloride chan-nel, CLCN5, is mutated. This leads to hypercalciuria and hy-pophosphatemia. There are other conditions in which an isolated defect in the renal tubular transport of phosphorus has been found, eg, in fructose intolerance, an autosomal re-cessive disorder. Following renal transplantation, an acquired renal tubular defect is responsible for the persistence of hy-pophosphatemia in some patients. Studies in patients follow-ing transplantation demonstrate that a phosphatonin-like substance is responsible for posttransplant hypophospha-temia. The hypophosphatemia is important because recent studies implicate it in the osteoblast failure contributing to the development of osteoporosis.

3. X-Linked hypophosphatemic (XLH) rickets and autoso-mal dominant hypophosphatemic rickets (ADHR)—These hereditary disorders are characterized by hypophosphatemia, decreased reabsorption of phosphorus by the renal tubule, decreased absorption of calcium and phosphorus from the gastrointestinal tract, and varying degrees of rickets or osteomalacia. Patients with the disorders exhibit normal or reduced levels of 1,25-dihydroxycholecalciferol (which should be elevated due to the hypophosphatemia) and reduced Na-phosphate transport in the proximal tubule in the face of severe hypophosphatemia. The gene for X-linked hypophosphatemia is not the Pi transport protein itself, but a gene termed PHEX, which encodes for a neutral endopeptidase presumed to be responsible for degradation of a group of new hormones identified as systemic phosphaturic factors, "phosphatonins." The defective PHEX gene product in XLH rickets permits a phosphatonin, most likely FGF23, to inhibit renal phosphate absorption, despite persistent hypophosphatemia. FGF23, has been identified as the causal substance in ADHR.

4. Oncogenic osteomalacia—This entity is characterized by hypophosphatemia in association with mesenchymal tumors. The patients exhibit osteomalacia on histomorphologic examination of bone biopsies, renal wasting of phosphorus, and markedly reduced levels of 1,25-dihydroxyvitamin D_3. Circulating humoral factors have been identified from tumors from patients with hemangiopericytomas that inhibit renal phosphate transport and are thought to be the cause of this syndrome.

5. Diabetic ketoacidosis (Tables 7–2 and 7–3)—Patients with well-controlled diabetes mellitus do not have excessive losses of phosphate. However, in the presence of hyperglycemia, polyuria, and acidosis, Pi is lost through the urine in excessive amounts. In ketoacidosis, intracellular organic components tend to be broken down, releasing a large amount of Pi into the plasma, which is subsequently lost in the urine. This process, combined with the enhanced osmotic Pi diuresis secondary to glycosuria, ketonuria, and polyuria, may cause large urinary losses of Pi and subsequent depletion. The plasma Pi is usually normal or slightly elevated in the ketotic patient in spite of the excessive urinary losses because of the continuous large shift of Pi from the cells into the plasma. With insulin, fluids, and correction of the ketoacidosis, however, serum and urine Pi may fall sharply. Despite the appearance of hypophosphatemia during treatment, previously well-controlled patients with diabetic ketoacidosis of only a few days duration almost never have serious phosphorus deficiency. Serum Pi rarely falls below 1.0 mg/dL in these patients. Administration of Pi-containing salts does not improve glucose utilization or reduce insulin requirements or the time for recovery from ketoacidosis. Thus, Pi therapy should be reserved for patients with serum Pi concentration <1.0 mg/dL.

6. Miscellaneous urinary losses—Abnormalities in tubular handling of phosphate have also been implicated in the genesis of severe hypophosphatemia induced by systemic acidosis, hypokalemia, hypomagnesemia, hypothyroidism, and humoral hypercalcemia of malignancy. During the recovery phase from severe burns (Table 7–3), hypophosphatemia may occur secondary to massive diuresis with phosphaturia.

C. Transcellular Shift

1. Respiratory alkalosis—Intense hyperventilation for prolonged periods may depress serum Pi to values below 1.0 mg/dL. This is important in patients with alcoholic withdrawal who have attendant hyperventilation and Pi depletion. A similar degree of alkalemia induced by infusion of bicarbonate depresses Pi concentration only mildly. The combined hypophosphatemic effects of respiratory and metabolic alkalosis may be pronounced.

Severe hypophosphatemia is common in patients with extensive burns (Table 7–3). It usually appears within several days after the injury. Phosphorus is almost undetectable in the urine. Hypophosphatemia may result from transductive losses, respiratory alkalosis, or other factors.

2. Leukemia (blast crisis)—Advanced leukemia that is markedly proliferative (blast crisis) with total leukocyte counts above 100,000 has been associated with severe hypophosphatemia. This would appear to result from excessive phosphorus uptake into rapidly multiplying cells.

▶ Prevention

The most effective approach to hypophosphatemia is prevention of predisposing conditions. Patients on total parenteral nutrition should receive a daily maintenance dose of Pi amounting to 1000 mg in 24 hours, with increases as required by the clinical and metabolic states. Alcoholic patients and malnourished patients receiving intravenous fluids, particularly those containing glucose, should receive Pi supplementation, particularly if hypophosphatemia is observed.

▶ Clinical Findings

Severe hypophosphatemia with phosphorus deficiency may cause widespread disturbances. There are at least eight well-established effects of severe hypophosphatemia (Table 7–4). The signs and symptoms of severe hypophosphatemia may be related to a decrease in 2,3-diphosphoglycerate in red cells. This change is associated with increased affinity of hemoglobin for oxygen and therefore tissue hypoxia. There is also a decrease in tissue content of ATP and, consequently, a decrease in the availability of energy-rich phosphate compounds for cell function.

A. Central Nervous System

Some patients with severe hypophosphatemia display symptoms compatible with metabolic encephalopathy. They may display, in sequence, irritability, apprehension, weakness, numbness, paresthesias, dysarthria, confusion, obtundation, seizures, and coma. In contrast to delirium tremens, the syndrome does not include hallucinations. Patients with very severe hypophosphatemia may show diffuse slowing of their electroencephalogram.

Table 7–4. Consequences of severe hypophosphatemia.

Central nervous system dysfunction—encephalopathy, seizures, delirium, coma, paresthesias
Red blood cell dysfunction—hemolysis, tissue hypoxia
Leukocyte dysfunction—increased susceptibility to infection
Platelet dysfunction—thrombocytopenia, hemorrhage
Skeletal muscle dysfunction—weakness, respiratory failure, rhabdomyolysis
Cardiac muscle dysfunction—cardiomyopathy, congestive heart failure
Bone disease—osteomalacia/rickets
Metabolic acidosis

B. Hematopoietic System

A decrease in the red cell content of 2,3-diphosphoglycerate and ATP leads to increased rigidity and, in rare instances, hemolysis. Hemolysis is usually provoked by unusual stress on the metabolic requirements of the red cell, such as severe metabolic acidosis or infection. When hemolysis has occurred, ATP content has invariably been reduced. Leukocyte/macrophage dysfunction can be demonstrated *in vitro* using Pi-depleted cells. The suggestion that a predisposition to infection commonly seen in patients on intravenous hyperalimentation may be partly related to hypophosphatemia remains to be proven. Hypophosphatemia impairs granulocyte function by interfering with ATP synthesis. In experimental hypophosphatemia there is an increase in platelet diameter, suggesting shortened platelet survival and also a marked acceleration of platelet disappearance from the blood. These lead to thrombocytopenia and a reactive megakaryocytosis. In addition, there is an impairment of clot retraction and a hemorrhagic tendency, especially involving gut and skin.

C. Musculoskeletal System

1. Myopathy and rhabdomyolysis—Muscle tissue requires large amounts of high-energy bonds (ATP, creatine phosphate) and oxygen for contraction, for maintenance of membrane potential, and for other functions. Pi deprivation induces muscle cell injury characterized by a decrease in intracellular Pi and an increase in water, sodium, and chloride. An apparent relationship between hypophosphatemia and alcoholic myopathy has been observed in chronic alcoholism. The muscular clinical manifestations of Pi deficiency syndrome include myalgia, objective weakness, and myopathy with pathologic findings of intracellular edema and a subnormal resting muscle membrane potential on electromyography. In patients with preexisting Pi deficiency who develop acute hypophosphatemia, rhabdomyolysis might occur. Hypophosphatemia and phosphate deficiency may be associated with elevations in creatine phosphokinase in blood.

2. Bone—Skeletal defects have been reported in association with Pi depletion of different causes. Suffice it to say here that phosphate depletion is associated with rickets in children and osteomalacia in adults. However, the discovery of the phosphatonins, especially FGF23, demonstrates that osteomalacia is more than just hypophosphatemia decreasing mineralization, but rather impaired osteoblast function due to the actions of FGF23 or other factors that contribute directly to impaired mineralization.

D. Cardiovascular System

Severe hypophosphatemia has been associated with a cardiomyopathy characterized by a low cardiac output, a decreased ventricular ejection velocity, and an elevated left ventricular end-diastolic pressure. A decrease in myocardial content of Pi, ATP, and creatinine phosphate seems to underlie the impairment in myocardial contractibility. During phosphorus depletion, blood pressure may be low and the pressor response to naturally occurring vasoconstrictor agonists such as norepinephrine or angiotensin II is reduced.

E. Renal Effects of Hypophosphatemia and Phosphate Depletion

Severe hypophosphatemia and phosphate depletion affect the balance and serum concentrations of various electrolytes. This may produce changes in cardiovascular function as described above, as renal hemodynamics affect renal tubular transport processes and induce marked changes in renal cell metabolism. These disturbances are listed in Table 7–5.

Tubular transport

A. CALCIUM—A marked increase in urinary calcium excretion occurs during phosphate depletion proportional to the severity of phosphate depletion and the degree of hypophosphatemia.

Table 7–5. Renal effects of hypophosphatemia.

Decreased glomerular filtration rate
Metabolic abnormalities
Decreased gluconeogenesis
Insulin resistance
Hypoparathyroidism, reduced urinary cAMP
Increased production of 1,25-dihydroxyvitamin D$_3$
Transport abnormalities
Hypercalciuria
Decreased proximal tubular sodium transport
Hypermagnesiuria
Hypophosphaturia
Bicarbonaturia
Glycosuria

B. Phosphate—Dietary Pi restriction and Pi depletion are associated with enhanced renal tubular reabsorption of Pi. Urinary excretion of Pi declines within hours after the reduction in its dietary intake, and Pi almost disappears from the urine within 12 days. The changes in renal tubular reabsorption of Pi occur prior to detectable falls in serum Pi. The adaptation to a reduction in Pi supply is a direct response of the proximal tubule, rendering this nephron segment resistant to most phosphaturic stimuli, including PTH. Acutely, Pi depletion causes an increase in the apical membrane expression of sodium phosphate cotransporters likely by insertion of preexisting transporter proteins from an endosomal pool. Chronically, the increase in transporter expression is also accomplished by the synthesis of new transporter proteins. The adaptation to reduced Pi supply is independent of cellular responses to PTH. The signaling mechanisms responsible for adaptation are unknown.

C. Metabolic acidosis—Severe hypophosphatemia with Pi deficiency may result in metabolic acidosis through three mechanisms. First, severe hypophosphatemia is generally associated with a proportionate reduction of Pi excretion in the urine, thereby limiting hydrogen excretion as a titratable acid. Second, if Pi buffer is inadequate, acid secretion depends on production of ammonia and its conversion to ammonium ion. Production of ammonia is severely depressed in Pi deficiency. The third mechanism is decreased renal tubular reabsorption of bicarbonate.

▶ Treatment

The appropriate management of hypophosphatemia and Pi depletion requires identification of the underlying causes, treatment with supplemental Pi when necessary, and prevention of recurrence of the problem by correcting the underlying causes. The symptoms and signs of Pi depletion can vary, are nonspecific, and are usually seen in patients with multiple problems such as those encountered in intensive care unit settings. This makes it difficult to identify Pi depletion as the cause of clinical manifestations and Pi depletion is frequently overlooked. Mild hypophosphatemia secondary to redistribution, with plasma Pi levels higher than 2 mg/dL, is transient and requires no treatment. In cases of moderate hypophosphatemia, associated with Pi depletion (serum Pi higher than 1.0 mg/dL in adults or 2.0 mg/dL in children), Pi supplementation should be administered in addition to treating the cause of hypophosphatemia. Milk is an excellent source of phosphorus, containing 1 g (33 mmol) of Pi per liter. Skimmed milk may be better tolerated than whole milk, especially in children and malnourished patients, because of concomitant lactose or fat intolerance. Alternatively,

Neutraphos tablets (which contain 250 mg of Pi per tablet as a sodium or potassium salt) may be given. Oral Pi can be given in a dose up to 3 g/day (ie, three tablets of Neutraphos every 6 hours). The serum Pi level rises by as much as 1.5 mg/dL 60–120 minutes after ingestion of 1000 mg of Pi. A phosphosoda enema solution, composed of buffered sodium phosphate, may also be used in a dose of 15–30 mL three or four times daily.

Severe hypophosphatemia with serum levels lower than 0.5 mg/dL occurs only when there is cumulative net loss of more than 3.3 g of Pi. If asymptomatic, oral replacement with a total of 6–10 g of Pi (1–3 g of Pi per day) over a few days is usually sufficient. Symptomatic hypophosphatemia indicates that net Pi deficit exceeds 10 g. In these cases, 20 g of Pi is given spread over 1 week (up to 3 g/day). Patients with Pi deficiency tolerate substantially larger doses of oral Pi without side effects, such as diarrhea, than do normal subjects. However, patients with severe symptomatic hypophosphatemia who are unable to eat may be safely treated intravenously with 1 g of Pi delivered in 1 L of fluid over 8–12 hours. This is usually sufficient to raise serum Pi level to 1.0 mg/dL. It is unusual for hypophosphatemia to cause metabolic disturbances at serum Pi >1.0 mg/dL, so that full parenteral replacement is neither necessary nor desirable. Treatment with phosphate can result in diarrhea, hyperphosphatemia, hypocalcemia, and hyperkalemia. These side effects can be prevented by paying careful attention to phosphorus dosages.

▶ Acknowledgments

This work was supported by NIH Grants DK59602, AR41677, and DK09976 and a grant from Johnson and Johnson.

Amanzadeh J, Reilly RF Jr: Hypophosphatemia: an evidence-based approach to its clinical consequences and management. Nat Clin Pract Nephrol 2006;2(3):136.

Bellasi A et al: Phosphate binders: new products and challenges. Hemodial Int 2006;10(3):225.

Gaasbeek A, Meinders AE: Hypophosphatemia: an update on its etiology and treatment. Am J Med 2005;118(10):1094.

Kuhlmann MK: Management of hyperphosphatemia. Hemodial Int 2006;10(4):338.

Liu S et al: Emerging role of fibroblast growth factor 23 in a bone-kidney axis regulating systemic phosphate homeostasis and extracellular matrix mineralization. Curr Opin Nephrol Hypertens 2007;16(4):329.

Quarles LD: FGF23, PHEX, and MEPE regulation of phosphate homeostasis and skeletal mineralization. Am J Physiol Endocrinol Metab 2003;285:1.

Schiavi SC, Kumar R: The phosphatonin pathway: new insights in phosphate homeostasis. Kidney Int 2004;65:1.

Disorders of Magnesium Balance: Hypomagnesemia & Hypermagnesemia

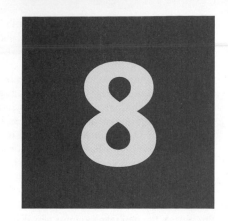

Meryl Waldman, MD, & Sidney Kobrin, MD

DISORDERS OF MAGNESIUM BALANCE

▶ General Considerations

Magnesium is the second most abundant intracellular cation and the fourth most common cation in the human body. It plays an essential role in a variety of cellular processes including enzyme activities involving adenosine triphosphate (ATP), energy metabolism, nucleic acid and protein synthesis, regulation of ion channels, and stabilization of membrane structures. The importance of magnesium in the body is reflected in the diverse clinical effects that accompany disorders of magnesium homeostasis. The average size adult contains approximately 24 g (1 mol, 2000 mEq) of magnesium. It is predominantly stored in bone (55–60%) and the intracellular compartments of muscle (20%) and soft tissues (20%) and it exchanges very slowly with extracellular magnesium. Therefore, skeletal and intracellular magnesium is an ineffective buffer in the setting of acute extracellular magnesium loss.

Approximately 1% of total body magnesium is in the extracellular fluid (ECF) and is composed of three fractions: 60–65% is free, ionized, and physiologically active; 30% is protein bound; and the balance is complexed to citrate, phosphate, and other anions. In clinical practice, magnesium status is assessed by measurement of total serum magnesium. Serum magnesium concentrations normally average 1.7–2.3 mg/dL (1.4–2.1 mEq/L). Given the intracellular nature of this cation, serum magnesium concentrations poorly reflect total body status.

Daily magnesium intake in the typical American diet averages 300–360 mg/day. Food sources of magnesium include green vegetables, nuts, and whole grains, as well as some meats and seafood. Of dietary magnesium 30–40% is absorbed in the gut, primarily by the small intestine, with smaller amounts being absorbed in the colon. There is some magnesium in intestinal secretions (approximately 20–40 mg), but under normal circumstances their contribution to overall magnesium elimination is minimal. However, these losses can become quite substantial in diarrheal states or with biliary fistulas.

The kidney is the main organ responsible for magnesium homeostasis. Approximately 70–80% (2.4 g) of the total serum magnesium is filtered by the kidneys. Under normal circumstances 95–97% is reabsorbed by the tubules. The plasma magnesium concentration is the most important determinant of renal magnesium excretion. Less than 5% (120 mg) is normally excreted in urine. However, hypomagnesemia results in conservation of magnesium by normal kidneys leading to a fractional excretion of less than 0.5% (12 mg) per day. Conversely, the kidneys increase excretion of magnesium to approximate the filtered load during periods of increased intake or excess magnesium administration.

In contrast to many of the other electrolytes (ie, Na^+, K^+, and Ca^{2+}), control of magnesium reabsorption does not appear to be tightly regulated by a specific hormone. Parathyroid hormone, calcitonin, vitamin D, glucagon, antidiuretic hormone, aldosterone, sex steroids, and β-adrenergic agonists can affect magnesium handling in experimental studies, but it is not known if these effects have an important role in humans.

While the proximal tubule is the major site of reabsorption of other ions, only a small percentage (15–25%) of the filterable magnesium is reabsorbed in this segment. Here, magnesium transport is passive, driven by bulk flow, and depends on sodium reabsorption. Factors that affect sodium reabsorption (ie, volume expansion) can also affect magnesium reabsorption. The majority of magnesium reabsorption (60–70%) occurs in the cortical thick ascending limb (TAL) of the loop of Henle. Here again, magnesium reabsorption is a passive, paracellular process and depends on sodium reabsorption. The driving force for the reabsorption of magnesium (and calcium) is the lumen-positive electrical potential generated by sodium chloride reabsorption via the $Na^+/K^+/2Cl^-$ cotransporter in concert with the coordinated activity of the basolateral $Na^+- K^+$-ATPase, a chloride channel, and an apical membrane potassium channel. Disturbances of this coordinated activity at any site (such as with loop diuretics or inherited defects/Bartter's syndrome) will abolish the lumen-positive gradient needed to drive magnesium reabsorption and, thus, result in magnesium wasting.

The potassium channel can be secondarily inhibited by the activation of the Ca^{2+}/Mg^{2+} sensing receptor (CaSR). The CaSR binds both magnesium and calcium. This accounts for the observed magnesium wasting seen in the setting of hypercalcemia that augments activation of this receptor. If the positive transepithelial gradient is ultimately generated, the paracellular reabsorption of magnesium (and calcium) occurs passively, facilitated by the tight junction protein, paracellin-1 (claudin-16). The fact that both calcium and magnesium travel in parallel through the same channel in this part of the nephron explains why disturbances resulting in hypermagnesuria will simultaneously cause hypercalciuria. The mechanism(s) of magnesium reabsorption in the distal convoluted tubule (DCT) is less well understood. Although the distal nephron accounts for only approximately 5–10% of magnesium reabsorption, it does play an important role in determining the final urinary concentration of magnesium. Reabsorption is active and transcellular and is probably mediated by Mg^{2+} selective channels and a basolateral membrane Na^+/Mg^{2+} exchanger.

HYPOMAGNESEMIA

 ESSENTIALS OF DIAGNOSIS

▸ Serum magnesium level, <1.5 mg/dL.

▸ A normal serum magnesium level does not exclude the diagnosis of total body magnesium depletion.

▸ Hypomagnesemia is a relatively common disorder, occurring in 12% of hospitalized patients and in up to 60–65% of Intensive Care Unit (ICU) patients.

▸ Evidence suggests that the presence of hypomagnesemia in the ICU patient population is associated with increased morbidity and mortality.

▸ There are conflicting data regarding the benefits of preventing hypomagnesemia, possible preventive treatment strategies, and even the level of hypomagnesemia that should prompt supplementation.

▸ Clinical Findings

A. Symptoms and Signs

The diversity of the cellular processes in which magnesium has been shown to take part is reflected by the diversity of symptoms attributed to magnesium deficiency (Table 8–1). Hypomagnesemia may be asymptomatic, particularly if it is mild and if it develops slowly. Severe hypomagnesemia,

Table 8–1. Summary of main clinical manifestations of hypomagnesemia.

General	Apathy, depression, confusion, anorexia
Cardiovascular	Cardiac arrhythmias (torsades de pointes, ventricular and supraventricular) Increased digitalis sensitivity EKG changes: widening of QRS, prolonged PR/QR intervals, T wave changes
Neuromuscular	Chvostek's and Trousseau's signs Muscle fasciculations and cramps Tetany Seizures Muscle weakness Obtundation
Electrolyte abnormalities	Hypokalemia Hypocalcemia

particularly if it develops rapidly, can be associated with signs and symptoms related to cardiovascular, neuromuscular, and central nervous system (CNS) dysfunction.

Magnesium regulates several cardiac ion channels including the calcium channel and outward potassium currents. Lowering myocardial cytosolic magnesium can lead to shortening of the action potential and an increased susceptibility to tachyarrhythmias, particularly of ventricular origin (including torsades de pointe, monomorphic ventricular tachycardia, and ventricular fibrillation). This is particularly true in acutely ill patients and in the setting of acute myocardial infarction, congestive heart failure, or after cardiopulmonary bypass surgery. Hypomagnesemia can magnify digitalis cardiotoxicity as both the cardiac glycoside and magnesium depletion reduce intracellular potassium by inhibition of the Na^+-K^+-ATPase. The EKG changes associated with hypomagnesemia include progressive widening of the QRS complex, prolongation of the PR interval, and abnormalities of T wave morphology.

Hypomagnesemia augments skeletal muscle contraction and delays muscle relaxation. Therefore, affected patients can develop signs of neuromuscular irritability including tremor, muscle twitching, Trousseau and Chvostek signs, and frank tetany. These signs may be exacerbated by a coexistent electrolyte abnormality such as hypocalcemia. Patients may also present with delirium, coma, or seizures.

Electrolyte disturbances associated with symptomatic magnesium depletion include hypokalemia and hypocalcemia, both of which can be refractory to treatment unless the underlying magnesium deficit is corrected. The hypokalemia that frequently accompanies hypomagnesemia may be due to (1) a direct effect of hypomagnesemia on potassium channels in the loop of Henle (and perhaps the cortical collecting tubule) due to impairment of the Mg-dependent Na^+-K^+-ATPase leading to renal potassium wasting; and (2) the underlying disorders (ie, diarrhea, diuretics) that simultaneously cause magnesium and potassium loss. The hypocalcemia that often accompanies severe magnesium depletion is due to the suppressive effect of hypomagnesemia on parathyroid secretion as well as skeletal resistance to parathyroid hormone (PTH). In addition, low plasma levels of calcitriol (1,25-dihydroxyvitamin D) have been noted in hypomagnesemic states and can contribute to the fall in calcium concentrations.

Normomagnesemic magnesium depletion (total body magnesium depletion in normomagnesemic patients) should be considered in patients at risk for magnesium depletion who have clinical features consistent with magnesium depletion, such as unexplained hypocalcemia or hypokalemia.

B. Laboratory Findings

The terms hypomagnesemia and magnesium deficiency tend to be used interchangeably. However, because only a small fraction of magnesium is extracellular, the serum magnesium level is not a reliable way to assess total body magnesium depletion. The total body may be markedly depleted before the serum level drops. Hence, a normal magnesium level does not rule out the possibility of a magnesium deficit. Clues to the diagnosis of true magnesium depletion despite normal measured levels include persistent, unexplained hypocalcemia or hypokalemia, which is refractory to treatment or response to empiric treatment. The magnesium retention test, which measures urinary excretion of magnesium in response to an intravenous magnesium load, has also been used to assess total body magnesium status in patients suspected of having hypomagnesemia. When magnesium stores are deficient, more of the infused magnesium will be reabsorbed and, thus, less will be excreted in the urine. If less than 50% of the infused magnesium is recovered in the urine, magnesium deficiency is likely. However, this test is not in routine use as its utility is questionable and several conditions (ie, impaired renal function and renal magnesium wasting) and drugs can lead to invalid results.

If laboratory tests confirm hypomagnesemia, the next step is to distinguish between renal and extrarenal (gastrointestinal or miscellaneous) causes of magnesium wasting. A review of the clinical history can often provide this information (ie, chronic diarrhea causing excessive gastrointestinal magnesium losses). If the cause is not readily apparent, quantitative assessment of urinary magnesium excretion with a 24-hour urine collection or the calculation of the fractional excretion of magnesium (FE_{Mg}) on a random urine specimen can provide insight. In the setting of magnesium depletion, conservation of magnesium by normal kidneys can decrease the usual fractional excretion of magnesium from 3% (approximately 100 mg) to very low levels (ie, sometimes less than 0.5% or 12 mg/day). Therefore,

Table 8-2. Differentiating renal versus nonrenal causes of hypomagnesemia.

Test	Criteria for renal magnesium wasting
24-hour urine collection for magnesium	>10–30 mg Mg/24 hours
Fractional excretion of magnesium[1] (FE_{Mg})	>2%
$\dfrac{\text{Urine Mg} \times \text{plasma Mg}}{(0.7 \times \text{plasma Mg}) \times \text{urine Cr}} \times 100$	

[1]Plasma magnesium concentration is multiplied by 0.7 since only 70% of the circulating magnesium is filtered because it is free (not bound to albumin).

demonstrating an inappropriately high rate of renal magnesium excretion in the setting of hypomagnesemia confirms the diagnosis of renal magnesium wasting. Table 8–2 summarizes the urine tests and the criteria used for renal magnesium wasting.

▶ Etiology & Differential Diagnosis

There are multiple causes of hypomagnesemia (Table 8–3). When the cause is not obvious from the clinical history and examination, it is often helpful for the clinician to try to ascertain whether the cause is due to redistribution of extracellular magnesium into the intracellular compartment, a gastrointestinal source, urinary magnesium wasting, or "complex causes."

Low measured serum magnesium is usually an indication of total body depletion. However, sometimes redistribution of extracellular magnesium into the intracellular compartment can lead to a decreased serum magnesium level. By itself, redistribution is an uncommon cause of significant hypomagnesemia, but it can unmask or exacerbate hypomagnesemia in patients with preexisting marginal stores. It can be encountered in a few settings. Sequestration of magnesium into the bone compartment may cause hypomagnesemia (in addition to profound hypocalcemia) in some patients with hyperparathyroidism and severe bone disease following parathyroidectomy. The sudden removal of excess PTH in this setting is believed to result in cessation of bone resorption with a continued high rate of bone formation. Insulin can also serve to drive magnesium (like potassium) into cells. Therefore, hypomagnesemia can be seen as part of the refeeding syndrome where overzealous administration of parenteral feeds to a malnourished patient results in a surge of endogenous insulin. Similarly, exogenous administration of insulin in the treatment of diabetic ketoacidosis can have the same effect.

Hypomagnesemia can result from chelation of the magnesium ion. This can be seen after massive blood

Table 8–3. Causes of hypomagnesemia.

High urine magnesium	Low urine magnesium

1. Polyuric states
  Diabetic ketoacidosis
  Postacute tubular necrosis
    (ATN)
  Postobstructive diuresis
  Postrenal transplant
	1. Decreased intake
	  Protein-calorie malnutrition
	  Chronic alcoholism
	  Administration of Mg-free
	    nutrition or fluids

2. Extracelluar fluid (ECF)
    volume expansion
  Aggressive intravenous
    normal saline infusion
  Primary hyperaldosteronism
	2. Gastrointestinal losses
	  Diarrhea
	  Fistulas
	  Malabsorption
	  Small bowel resection
	  Inherited defect in
	    Mg transport

3. Acquired tubular dysfunction
  Postacute tubular necrosis
  Postobstructive diuresis
  Postrenal transplant
  Chronic interstitial disease
  Hungry bone syndrome
  Acute pancreatitis
	3. Redistribution
	  Insulin effects
	  Correction of diabetic
	    ketoacidosis
	  Refeeding syndrome
	  Catecholamines
	  Chelation
	    Transfusion
	    Free fatty acids after
	      surgery
	  Foscarnet therapy
	  After thyroidectomy for
	    hyperthyroidism

4. Inherited renal Mg wasting disorders (Table 8-4)	4. Lactation

5. Medications
  Diuretics (loop and
    chronic thiazide use)
  Cisplatin
  Aminoglycosides
  Amphotericin B
  Cyclosporin
  Pentamidine
	5. Burns

6. EtOH (multifactorial)	
7. Hypercalcemia	

transfusions (ie, >10 U/24 hours) due to the chelating effects of citrate, particularly when citrate clearance is diminished by renal or hepatic disease. It also may contribute to the hypomagnesemia seen following surgery where the postsurgical increase in circulating free fatty acids chelates magnesium. Hypomagnesemia may also accompany the acute hypocalcemia seen in acute pancreatitis and is presumably due to saponification of both cations in necrotic fat. Other causes of extracellular to intracellular magnesium redistribution include metabolic alkalosis and high catecholamine states.

A. Gastrointestinal Causes

If redistribution is ruled out and the urine findings are consistent with appropriate renal magnesium conservation, the gastrointestinal tract is the usual culprit. Induction of magnesium deficiency by inadequate dietary intake is not frequent because nearly all foods contain sufficient amounts of magnesium and renal conservation is so efficient. Nevertheless, magnesium deficiency of nutritional origin can be seen in a few clinical settings. It has been described in children with protein–calorie malnutrition (although usually in combination with gastrointestinal losses such as vomiting and diarrhea). It can be seen in hospitalized patients receiving only intravenous fluids or prolonged administration of magnesium-free parenteral nutrition. Therefore, addition of 4–12 mmol of magnesium per day to total parenteral nutrition (TPN) has been recommended to prevent hypomagnesemia. This is especially true in patients with marginal magnesium stores such as those with debilitating illnesses, anorexia, or with chronic alcohol use.

Although there is only a small amount of magnesium lost (approximately 40 mg/day) in intestinal secretions on a daily basis, enteric losses of magnesium can be substantial in patients with gastrointestinal fistulas, small bowel bypass surgery, or diarrheal illnesses. This is particularly true if the chronic diarrhea is associated with fat malabsorption syndromes in which free fatty acids within the intestinal lumen may combine with magnesium, forming unreabsorbable soaps. This saponification limits magnesium absorption. Decreased intestinal absorption can also be caused by a rare inherited disorder termed *primary intestinal hypomagnesemia* in which a mutation in the magnesium ion channel leads to impaired active transport in the intestine.

B. Renal Magnesium Wasting

If redistribution and gastrointestinal causes are excluded, and renal magnesium wasting is confirmed based on laboratory findings, hypomagnesemia is due to inappropriate renal losses of magnesium.

Diuretics are a frequent cause of renal magnesium wasting. Loop diuretics, which inhibit the $Na^+/K^+/2Cl^-$ cotransporter in the loop of Henle, lead to the loss of the positive transepithelial potential difference that drives paracellular divalent cation reabsorption, thereby resulting in both magnesuria and hypercalciuria. The etiology of magnesium wasting with chronic thiazide use is not fully understood. The degree of hypomagnesemia induced by the loop and thiazide diuretics is generally mild, in part because of the associated volume contraction that tends to increase proximal sodium, water, and magnesium reabsorption.

Numerous other drugs have also been shown to cause impairment in the renal tubular reabsorption of magnesium. Cisplatin, widely used as a chemotherapeutic agent for solid tumors, causes magnesium wasting in more than 50% of treated patients and the incidence increases with the cumulative dose. Renal magnesuria continues after the cessation of the drug for several months but can persist for years. The occurrence of magnesium wasting does not correlate with cisplatin-induced acute renal failure. Aminoglycosides such as gentamicin can induce magnesuria soon after the onset of therapy. The aminoglycoside-associated magnesuria is dose dependent, and is usually reversible upon withdrawal. Cyclosporin, pentamidine, and amphotericin B also cause renal magnesium wasting.

Since the bulk of the filtered magnesium is linked to sodium chloride reabsorption, it is not surprising that factors that increase urinary excretion of sodium will also promote the urinary excretion of magnesium. Mild hypomagnesemia can occur in states of sustained ECF volume expansion as might be seen in patients receiving large amounts of intravenous normal saline. It also accounts for the hypomagnesemia that can sometimes be observed in patients with primary hyperaldosteronism. In addition, any condition that gives rise to high urine flow rates can lead to magnesium wasting. High urine flow rates can contribute to hypomagnesemia in uncontrolled hyperglycemic states with glucosuria, the recovery polyuric phase of acute tubular necrosis, postobstructive diuresis, and after renal transplantation. In the latter conditions, the residual tubule reabsorptive defects that persist from the primary renal injury likely also play an important role in inducing renal magnesium wasting.

Magnesium handling can also be affected by other electrolytes. Hypercalcemia, hypokalemia, and phosphate depletion can all lead to magnesuria by inhibiting tubular magnesium reabsorption.

Several rare hereditary renal magnesium-wasting disorders have been described and the genetic basis for many of them has recently been characterized. They represent a heterogeneous group of disorders that can usually be distinguished from each other on the basis of the clinical presentation and biochemical profile that is summarized in Table 8–4. A helpful clue to the localization of the defect is the pattern of the calcium excretion in relation to the magnesium excretion, ie, the combination of hypermagnesuria and hypocalciuria is the finding pathognomic of disturbed DCT function. Demonstrating high urinary magnesium excretion in the absence of any other apparent cause establishes the diagnosis of these inherited disorders.

C. Complex Causes

Chronic alcoholics often have hypomagnesemia due to a combination of several factors including dietary deficiency, gastrointestinal losses (diarrhea, vomiting), and renal losses. The renal losses are a direct effect of the alcohol that can induce reversible tubular dysfunction leading to inappropriate magnesium excretion that can persist for weeks after abstinence. Alcoholics are also susceptible to acute pancreatitis,

which in turn may contribute to the hypomagnesemia as a result of redistribution of magnesium as described above. Similarly, patients with insulin-dependent diabetes mellitus may have hypomagnesemia secondary to complex causes, particularly in the setting of diabetic ketoacidosis. Renal magnesium wasting accompanies the osmotic diuresis induced by hyperglycemia and rapid correction of hyperglycemia with insulin therapy drives magnesium into cells. Furthermore, magnesium deficiency may impair glucose disposal and aggravate insulin resistance.

▶ Treatment

Whenever possible the underlying cause of the hypomagnesemia should be corrected. The route and rate of magnesium repletion depend on the severity of the clinical manifestations. Since plasma magnesium is the major regulator of magnesium reabsorption in the loop of Henle, an abrupt elevation in the plasma magnesium concentration following a bolus partially removes the stimulus for magnesium reabsorption resulting in up to half of a bolus infusion being lost in the urine. In addition, uptake of magnesium by cells is slow and repletion requires sustained correction of the hypomagnesemia.

A. Severe Hypomagnesemia

If hypomagnesium is severe (<1 mEq/L) or accompanied by symptoms such as cardiac arrhythmias, neuromuscular irritability, or seizures, parenteral magnesium therapy should be administered. Magnesium sulfate 1–2 g (8–16 mEq) can be given over 15 minutes. A continuous infusion should be given after the initial bolus, ie, with $MgSO_4$ 4–6 g/24 hours (32–48 mEq). Magnesium repletion should continue for at least 1–2 days after serum magnesium normalizes because the added extracellular magnesium equilibrates slowly with the intracellular compartment.

Adverse effects associated with intravenous magnesium repletion include facial flushing, loss of deep tendon reflexes (DTR), hypotension, atrioventricular block, and hypocalcemia. Since the major route of magnesium excretion is via the kidney, the above doses should be reduced and magnesium levels should be closely monitored in patients with a decreased glomerular filtration rate (GFR) who are receiving intravenous magnesium. If the underlying cause of the hypomagnesemia persists once the acute emergency has been corrected, oral magnesium replacement may be necessary.

B. Mild Hypomagnesemia

Given that significant wasting of magnesium occurs in the setting of rapid parenteral magnesium administration, treatment with oral magnesium salts is the more efficient way to replenish magnesium stores in patients who are asymptomatic or who require maintenance therapy due to chronic magnesium losses. The slower rise in the serum

Table 8–4. Inherited disorders of magnesium handling associated with hypomagnesemia.

Disorder	Inheritance	Defect	Serum			Urine		Other
			Mg	Ca	K	Mg	Ca	
Disorders localized to the loop of Henle (thick ascending limb)								
Familial hypomagnesemia with hypercalciuria	AR	Paracellin-1, CLDN16	↓	↓	↓ or nl	↑	↑	Presents in early childhood; associated with polyuria, NDI, dRTA, nephrocalcinosis, recurrent nephrolithiasis, renal insufficiency
Bartter's syndrome	AR	Na$^+$/K$^+$/2Cl$^-$, ROMK-1, CLC-Kb, Barrtin	↓ or nl	↓	↓	↑ or nl	↑	Presents in infancy or early childhood; blood pressure normal or low; hypomagnesemia is seen in only one-third of patients due to compensatory reabsorption by other nephron segments and effects of volume depletion; Barrtin defect associated with deafness
Autosomal dominant hypoparathyroidism/ hypocalcemia	AD	Activating CaSR mutation	↓	↓	nl	↑	↑	
Disorders localized to the distal convoluted tubule (DCT)								
Gitelman's syndrome	AR	SLC12A3 gene encoding NCCT	↓	nl	↓	↑	↓	Later age of onset than Bartter's syndrome
Isolated dominant hypomagnesemia	AD	γ-Subunit of Na$^+$-K$^+$-ATPase	↓	nl	nl	↑	↓	Associated with generalized convulsions
Isolated recessive hypomagnesemia	AR	?	↓	nl	nl	↑	Nl	
Primary intestinal hypomagnesemia	AR	TRPM6 in intestinal and DCT cells	↓	↓	nl	↑ or nl	Nl	The defect is primarily associated with impaired intestinal magnesium absorption but can occasionally cause renal magnesium wasting; hypocalcemia secondary to hypomagnesemia

AR, autosomal recessive; AD, autosomal dominant; nl, normal; CaSR, calcium-sensing receptor; NDI, nephrogenic diabetes insipidus; dRTA, distal renal tubular acidosis; DCT, distal convoluted tubule; NCCT, sodium chloride cotransporter

magnesium level that results from oral therapy provides a more favorable gradient for renal magnesium reabsorption. Sustained release preparations are preferable. There are two such preparations currently available, Slow-Mag containing magnesium chloride and Mag-Tab SR containing magnesium lactate. These orally administered magnesium preparations are given in divided doses to decrease their cathartic effect. Two to four tablets daily may be sufficient for mild asymptomatic disease whereas six to eight tablets daily may be required for severe magnesium depletion. Table 8–5 summarizes some of the commonly prescribed oral magnesium preparations.

If renal magnesium wasting persists despite high dose oral magnesium replacement (as in the inherited magnesium

wasting disorders, cisplatin toxicity, etc.), addition of potassium-sparing diuretics such as amiloride may be beneficial.

Table 8–5. Magnesium preparations.

Preparation	Elemental Mg content
Mg chloride/Slo-Mag, Mag-SR (535 mg)	64 mg
Mg oxide/Uro-Mag (140 mg); Mag-Ox 400	84 mg/7 mEq; 242 mg/20 mEq
Mg gluconate/Magonate (500 mg)	27 mg/2.4 mEq

These drugs decrease magnesium excretion by increasing its reabsorption in the convoluted collecting tubule.

Prevention

Given the observed relationship between this electrolyte disorder and possible complications, it is important to recognize which patients are at increased risk of developing symptomatic hypomagnesemia and the clinical settings in which hypomagnesemia is frequently encountered. For example, patients in the ICU often have several etiologies of magnesium loss acting simultaneously, ie, poor nutrition, excessive gastrointestinal losses from diarrhea or vomiting, excessive renal losses from multiple medications such as diuretics and antibiotics, coexisting electrolyte and acid–base disturbances that exacerbate the losses, and therapeutic interventions that can redistribute magnesium. All these factors may be superimposed on a state of chronic magnesium depletion. In addition, many of these patients have underlying cardiac disease that may increase the risk of sudden death from hypomagnesemia. As such, these patients warrant more frequent monitoring of magnesium levels and systematic repletion if the disorder is discovered.

Knoers NV et al: Genetic renal disorders with hypomagnesemia and hypocalciuria. J Nephrol 2003;16(2):293.

Mouw DR et al: Clinical inquiries. What are the causes of hypomagnesemia? J Fam Pract 2005;54(2):174.

Noronha JL, Matuschak GM: Magnesium in critical illness: metabolism, assessment, and treatment. Intensive Care Med 2002;28(6):667.

Topf JM, Murray PT: Hypomagnesemia and hypermagnesemia. Rev Endocr Metab Disord 2003;4(2):195.

HYPERMAGNESEMIA

 ESSENTIALS OF DIAGNOSIS

▶ Serum magnesium concentrations >2.5 mg/dL.

▶ Occurs almost exclusively in patients with renal insufficiency and is often iatrogenic.

General Considerations

Hypermagnesemia is a relatively infrequent laboratory finding and symptomatic hypermagnesemia is even less common. However, severe hypermagnesemia is a serious and potentially fatal condition. The kidney has a remarkable capacity to increase magnesium excretion in states of body magnesium excess. This explains why hypermagnesemia primarily occurs in two settings: impaired renal function and excess magnesium intake at a rate that exceeds the renal excretion capacity.

In patients with chronic kidney disease, the serum magnesium levels are generally well maintained until the GFR falls below 20 ml/minute because the remaining functioning nephrons are able to significantly increase the fractional excretion of magnesium. At lower levels of GFR (<10 mL/minute), mild to moderate levels of hypermagnesemia may be present (2.4–3.6 mg/dL). These patients are typically asymptomatic, but are particularly vulnerable to severe and potentially fatal, symptomatic hypermagnesemia when exposed to exogenous magnesium in the form of magnesium-containing bowel preparation regimens, antacids, or laxatives, even in the usual therapeutic doses. Similarly, patients with acute renal failure are susceptible to severe hypermagnesemia.

While much less common, there are situations in which hypermagnesemia can occur in the absence of significant renal insufficiency. Hypermagnesemia is induced deliberately in pregnant women with severe preeclampsia or eclampsia to decrease neuromuscular excitability. Such regimens, with large doses given rapidly and continuously (ie, Mg sulfate loading dose of 4–6 g, maintenance 2–3 g/hour continuous infusion), can overwhelm the renal excretory capacity, achieving serum magnesium levels in the range of 6–8.4 mg/dL, or higher. Severe hypermagnesemia in the setting of normal renal function has also occasionally been described with massive oral ingestions (ie, accidental poisoning with Epsom salts in children), in chronic laxative abusers, or in patients receiving large amounts of magnesium sulfate per rectum. An elevation of serum magnesium due to ingestion of magnesium-containing medications is more likely in the presence of gastrointestinal disorders that may enhance magnesium absorption. This phenomenon has been reported in patients with active ulcer disease, gastritis, inflammatory bowel disease, and intestinal obstruction. A geographically unique cause of severe hypermagnesemia has been described in Jordan due to near drowning in the Dead Sea. The magnesium concentration in the Dead Sea averages 400 mg/dL. Interestingly, since the Dead Sea also has very high levels of calcium, the resulting hypercalcemia may be somewhat protective against the cardiac toxicity associated with hypermagnesemia.

Mild hypermagnesemia, unrelated to renal insufficiency or disorders of the gastrointestinal tract, may be seen in the a variety of clinical settings. The causes of hypermagnesemia are listed in Table 8–6.

Clinical Findings
A. Symptoms and Signs

Signs and symptoms of hyermagnesemia are generally not apparent until the serum magnesium concentration exceeds 4 mg/dL. Concomitant hypocalcemia may exacerbate the symptoms of hypermagnesemia at any level. Neuromuscular and cardiovascular manifestations dominate the clinical

Table 8–6. Causes of hypermagnesemia.

Decreased renal excretion
  Acute renal failure (oliguric)
  Chronic kidney disease [glomerular filtration rate (GFR)
    <30 mL/minute]
  Lithium intoxication
Increased magnesium load (usually in association with decreased GFR)
  Endogenous
    1. Diabetic ketoacidosis
    2. Severe tissue injury—burns
    3. Tumor lysis
    4. Rhabdomyolysis
  Exogenous
    Gastrointestinal: Mg-containing laxatives and antacids
    Parenteral: management of preeclampsia of pregnancy
    Dead Sea drowning
Increased renal magnesium absorption
  Familial hypocalciuric hypercalcemia (FHH)
  Hypothyroidism
  Mineralocorticoid deficiency/adrenal insufficiency
  Hyperparathyroidism

Table 8–7. Symptoms and signs of hypermagnesemia.

Magnesium level	Signs/symptoms
4–6 mEq/L (4.8–7.2 mg/dL)	Hyporeflexia—deep tendon reflexes disappear Nausea/vomiting/flushing
6–10 mEq/L (7.2–12 mg/dL)	Respiratory compromise/apnea Mental status changes/lethargy Hypotension EKG changes: prolonged PR, QRS, and QT intervals Hypocalcemia
>10 mEq/L (12 mg/dL)	Flaccid paralysis, complete heart block, coma, cardiac arrest/asystole

picture. High levels of magnesium decrease transmission of neuromuscular messages by inhibiting acetylcholine at the neuromuscular endplate. This ultimately leads to decreased deep tendon reflexes, muscle weakness progressing to flaccid skeletal muscle paralysis, respiratory depression, and apnea. Urinary retention and intestinal ileus due to smooth muscle dysfunction may also occur. High levels of magnesium may also cause signs and symptoms of CNS depression including drowsiness and eventually coma. Fixed dilated pupils, induced by parasympathetic blockade, and masquerading as a central brain stem herniation syndrome, has been described.

Parasympathetic blockade, vasodilation of vascular smooth muscle, and inhibition of norepinephrine release by sympathetic postganglionic nerves account for cutaneous flushing and hypotension. Hypermagnesemia also depresses the conduction system of the heart, which can manifest as lengthening of the QRS complex, PR or QT intervals, heart block, bradycardia, and eventually cardiac arrest. Hypocalcemia may be present at moderate levels of hypermagnesemia (>6 mg/dL, 5 mEq/L) due to the suppressive effects of high magnesium on PTH secretion. Hyperkalemia has been described in two hypermagnesemic patients. The mechanism is unclear, but may be related to decreased urinary excretion of potassium as a result of hypermagnesemia inducing blockade of renal potassium channels. Hypermagnesemia may decrease the anion gap, although this appears not to occur with infusion of magnesium sulfate, as retention of the anionic sulfate moiety counterbalances the unmeasured cation.

Table 8–8. Treatment of symptomatic hypermagnesemia.

Therapy	Dose	Rationale and effects
Calcium Ca chloride (central line)	5 mL of 10% solution over 5–10 minutes	If life-threatening complications are present; antagonizes effect of Mg
Ca gluconate (peripheral line)	100–200 mg elemental Ca in 150 mL D$_5$W over 10 minutes; 10 mL of 10% solution (= 1 g)	
Intravenous fluids Normal saline	1–2 L	If volume depleted and can tolerate fluids; increases Mg excretion
Loop diuretics Furosemide Bumex	40–80 mg 0.5–2 mg	Inhibits reabsorption of Mg in ascending loop of Henle
Hemodialysis or peritoneal dialysis	Low magnesium bath; 3–4 hours of hemodialysis; more prolonged course of peritoneal dialysis	In patients with renal failure; removes magnesium

The magnesium levels at which the symptoms and signs of hypermagnesemia manifest are presented in Table 8–7.

B. Laboratory Findings

Elevated serum magnesium levels above 2.5 mg/dL are usually diagnostic. Hypocalcemia may be present at moderate levels of hypermagnesemia (>6 mg/dL, 5 mEq/L).

▶ Treatment

The initial assessment should focus on identifying and discontinuing the source of exogenous magnesium. In patients with preserved renal function and mild manifestations of magnesium toxicity, cessation of exogenous magnesium administration may be the only treatment required. In the event of symptomatic, life-threatening hypermagnesemia associated with cardiovascular, neurologic, or respiratory complications, immediate administration of intravenous calcium can serve to temporarily antagonize the effects of magnesium until more definitive therapies can be initiated and take effect (Table 8–8). In patients who are not volume overloaded and in whom some renal function is preserved, volume expansion with intravenous normal saline may enhance renal magnesium excretion. The addition of loop diuretics can further augment the magnesuria by inhibiting magnesium reabsorption in the thick ascending limb of the loop of Henle. However, this therapy warrants monitoring of the calcium levels. It can result in hypercalciuria with hypocalcemia that can intensify the clinical signs of hypermagnesemia. If the aforementioned therapies are not feasible due to renal failure, hemodialysis or peritoneal dialysis against a low magnesium bath is the only way to effectively eliminate the excess body magnesium.

▶ Prevention

Most cases of symptomatic hypermagnesemia can be prevented by anticipation. It is important to avoid magnesium-containing medications in patients with acute or chronic kidney disease as well as those with active gastrointestinal diseases. Patients receiving high doses of parenteral magnesium should be closely monitored.

Birrer RB et al: Hypermagnesemia-induced fatality following Epsom salt gargles(1). J Emerg Med 2002;22(2):185.

Saris NE et al: Magnesium. An update on physiological, clinical and analytical aspects. Clin Chim Acta 2000;294(1–2):1.

Topf JM, Murray PT: Hypomagnesemia and hypermagnesemia. Rev Endocr Metab Disord 2003;4(2):195.

Touyz RM: Magnesium in clinical medicine. Front Biosci 2004;9:1278.

Acute Kidney Injury

9

Muhammad Sohail Yaqub, MD, & Bruce A. Molitoris, MD

ESSENTIALS OF DIAGNOSIS

▶ Acute increase in blood urea nitrogen (BUN) and serum creatinine.

▶ May be associated with oliguria or normal urine output.

▶ Symptoms and signs depend on cause.

General Considerations

Acute kidney injury (AKI) is a life-threatening disease process occurring in approximately 5% of all hospitalized patients and accounting for up to 30% of the admissions to intensive care units. AKI is preferred to acute renal failure as both kidney and injury are more patient-appropriate terms. Patients with AKI, regardless of their associated comorbid conditions, have a greater than 5-fold increased mortality rate. AKI is characterized by a reduction in the glomerular filtration rate (GFR) resulting in retention of nitrogenous wastes (creatinine, BUN, and other molecules that are not routinely measured). Early in the course of AKI patients are often asymptomatic and the condition is diagnosed only by observed elevations of BUN and serum creatinine levels or oliguria. An initial rise in serum creatinine of 0.5 mg/dL or a 25% increase in serum creatinine is often used to define AKI, although there is no definitive definition.

Oliguria (urine output less than 400 mL per 24 hours or 15 mL per hour) occurs commonly in AKI and may be an important indicator of renal dysfunction. However, urine output cannot be the only measure of kidney function. Patients with nonoliguric AKI usually have a better prognosis primarily due to less severe injury and/or a higher incidence of nephrotoxic-induced AKI in the nonoliguric group. Unfortunately, there has been little improvement in survival from AKI since the advent of hemodialysis and the mortality remains greater than 50% in many studies.

Schrier RW et al: Acute renal failure: definitions, diagnosis, pathogenesis, and therapy. J Clin Invest 2004;114(1):5.

▶ Definition

The RIFLE criteria consists of various graded levels of kidney injury based upon percent rise in serum creatinine, urine output and outcome measures.

Risk: 1.5-fold increase in the serum creatinine or GFR decrease by 25 percent or urine output <0.5 mL/kg per hour for six hours

Injury: Twofold increase in the serum creatinine or GFR decrease by 50 percent or urine output <0.5 mL/kg per hour for 12 hours

Failure: Threefold increase in the serum creatinine or GFR decrease by 75 percent or urine output of <0.5 mL/kg per hour for 24 hours, or anuria for 12 hours

Loss: Complete loss of kidney function (eg, need for renal replacement therapy) for more than four weeks

ESRD: Complete loss of kidney function (eg, need for renal replacement therapy) for more than three months

The AKIN (Acute Kidney Injury Network) criteria are a modification of the RIFLE criteria and include both diagnostic and staging system.

Stage 1. Increase in serum creatinine ≥0.3 mg/dl or 1.5 to 2 fold increase from baseline or urine output less than 0.5 mL/kg per hour for more than 6 hours

Stage 2. Increase in serum creatinine >2-3 folds from baseline or urine output less than 0.5 mL/kg per hour for more than 12 hours

Stage 3. Increase in serum creatinine >3 fold from baseline or serum creatinine of ≥4.0 mg/dl with an acute rise of at least 0.5 mg/dl or urine output less than 0.3 mL/kg per hour for 24 hours or anuria for 12 hours.

Bellomo R; Ronco C; Kellum JA; Mehta RL; Palevsky P: Acute renal failure – definition, outcome measures, animal models, fluid therapy and information technology needs: the Second International Consensus Conference of the Acute Dialysis Quality Initiative (ADQI) Group. Crit Care. 2004 Aug;8(4): R204-12. Epub 2004 May 24.

Mehta RL; Kellum JA; Shah SV; Molitoris BA; Ronco C; Warnock DG; Levin A: Acute kidney injury network: report of an initiative to improve outcomes in acute kidney injury. Crit Care. 2007 Mar 1;11(2):R31.

▶ Pathogenesis

The etiology of AKI is best divided into prerenal, intrarenal, and postrenal causes.

A. Prerenal Azotemia

Prerenal azotemia, the most common cause of AKI, accounting for 30–50% of all cases, is characterized by a diminished renal blood flow, primarily due to decreased effective arterial blood flow (Table 9–1). By definition, prerenal azotemia is a rapidly reversible process if recognized early and the underlying cause of reduced renal blood flow is corrected. Prerenal azotemia occurs when there is a reduction

Table 9–1. Causes of prerenal azotemia.

Etiology	Mechanism	Extracellular fluid volume

Hemorrhage
Burns
Diuretics
Dehydration
Gastrointestinal losses
  Vomiting
  Diarrhea
  Pancreatitis
  Nasogastric suctioning
  Enteric fistula
	True intravascular volume depletion	Reduced

Congestive heart failure Cardiac tamponade Aortic stenosis Cirrhosis with ascities Nephrotic syndrome	Decreased effective circulating volume	Increased

Angiotensin-converting enzyme
  inhibitors
Nonsteroidal anti-inflammatory
  drugs
Renal artery stenosis
Renal vein thrombosis
	Impaired renal blood flow	Normal

Sepsis Vasodilatory drugs Anesthetic agents	Systemic vasodilation	Normal

in the effective arterial blood flow to the kidney, either from an absolute reduction in the volume of extracellular fluid (eg, hypovolemia) or in conditions in which the effective circulating volume is reduced despite a normal total extracellular fluid volume (eg, congestive heart failure). Effective arterial blood flow is the amount of arterial blood perfusing vital organs. The determinants of effective arterial blood flow include the actual arterial volume, cardiac output, and vascular resistance. It is important to realize that the extracellular fluid (ECF) volume and/or venous volume may have no relationship to effective arterial volume. Although venous and ECF volumes can be accessed by careful physical examination, effective arterial volume cannot. Therefore, in certain circumstances clinicians must rely on additional information beyond the physical examination to ascertain a measure of organ perfusion. Invasive cardiac monitoring and determination of the renal fractional excretion of Na^+ (FE_{Na^+}) are the useful estimates of effective arterial circulatory volume.

The fractional excretion of sodium is calculated as follows:

$$FE_{Na^+} = \frac{\text{Urine sodium/Serum sodium}}{\text{Urine creatinine/Serum creatinine}}$$

An FE_{Na^+} of less than 1%, in the setting of an increasing serum creatinine or BUN, is generally indicative of prerenal azotemia as the reduced, renal blood flow results in a sodium avid state. In patients with prerenal azotemia, proximal tubule cells are undamaged and continue to function appropriately to avidly reabsorb Na^+ and water. Due to increased proximal reabsorption of Na^+ there is decreased distal delivery of Na^+ leading to increased renin secretion. This mediates enhanced aldosterone synthesis resulting in increased distal Na^+ reabsorption. The end result is a low FE_{Na^+} (<1%). Exceptions to this rule, resulting in a high FE_{Na^+} with prerenal azotemia, include use of diuretics within the previous 24 hours, glucosuria, metabolic alkalosis with high urinary bicarbonate, obligatory loss of Na^+, and chronic kidney disease with a high baseline Na^+ excretion. A low FE_{Na^+} is also seen in the early stages of acute glomerulonephritis, urinary obstruction, pigment nephropathy, and AKI induced by radiocontrast agents.

Low effective arterial volume states also stimulate release of antidiuretic hormone (ADH), leading to increased distal urea and water reabsorption. A low fractional excretion of urea nitrogen (<35%) can be especially useful in states of high urinary flow when prerenal azotemia occurs as in cases of high solute administration, such as in burn and trauma patients. The BUN to serum creatinine ratio, which is usually 10:1, also increases (>20:1) as filtered urea is reabsorbed and creatinine is excreted in prerenal azotemia.

The primary pharmacologic agents causing prerenal azotemia include angiotensin-converting enzyme (ACE) inhibitors, angiotensin receptor blockers (ARBs), and nonsteroidal anti-inflammatory drugs (NSAIDs) including Cox-2 inhibitors. ACE inhibition results in a decreased GFR due to dilation of the efferent arteriole and reduction in glomerular filtration pressure. In certain patients (eg, those with bilateral renal artery stenosis) the GFR is particularly dependent on the effects of angiotensin II. If these patients take an ACE inhibitor, their GFR decreases even though renal blood flow is not reduced. NSAIDs cause prerenal azotemia by blocking the intrarenal vasodilatory effect of prostaglandins. They should be avoided in patients with reduced effective arterial volume including patients with congestive heart failure, liver disease, nephrotic syndrome, and preexisting renal dysfunction.

B. Intrarenal Acute Kidney Injury

Intrinsic AKI is subdivided into four categories: tubular disease, glomerular disease, interstitial disease, and vascular disease (Table 9–2).

1. Acute tubular necrosis—Acute tubular cell injury is the most common cause of intrinsic AKI, accounting for approximately 90% of all hospital acquired AKI. Acute tubular necrosis (ATN) is the common term used for this type of AKI, which is usually induced by ischemia, sepsis, or toxins. Acute tubular dysfunction resulting from tubular cell injury is far more common than true cellular necrosis. ATN is usually reversible unless the ischemia was severe enough to cause cortical necrosis, which is associated with severe oliguria or anuria and is rare.

Tubular cell injury and death are important contributors to alterations in GFR following ischemic injury through several mechanisms. Figure 9–1 outlines the pathophysiology and clinical phases of ischemic AKI. In the initiation phase

Table 9–2. Common causes of intrinsic acute kidney injury.

Etiology	Examples
Tubular ischemia and inflammation (moderate to severe)	Shock, sepsis, bypass surgery
Nephrotoxins	Aminoglycosides, cisplatin, heme pigments, radiocontrast agents, nonsteroidal anti-inflammatory drugs, cyclosporine A
Small vessel vasculitis	Pauci-immune glomerulonephritis, hemolytic uremic syndrome
Acute glomerular nephritis	Rapidly progressive glomerulonephritis, infective endocarditis
Interstitial nephritis	Methicillin, any drug
Tubular obstruction	Uric acid, methotrexate, acyclovir, sulfonamides

of AKI there is ATP depletion resulting in proximal tubule, endothelial, and smooth muscle injury and apoptosis. The extension phase of AKI occurs with persistent ischemia, vascular congestion, and ongoing hypoxia. Endothelial damage and activation result in an imbalance in vasoactive mediators and persistent vasoconstriction, particularly in the outer medulla. These mediators and endothelial damage lead to an increase in permeability, which increases interstitial pressure and decreases capillary blood flow. This results in continued hypoxia during reperfusion and enhanced tubular cell injury and death via apoptosis in this area. The end result of these various pathophysiologic processes is further worsening of the GFR. The extension phase is followed by a prolonged maintenance phase in which BUN and creatinine continue to rise. If there is no further injury the recovery phase begins in 1–2 weeks. Apoptosis occurs in all phases leading to remodeling of injured tubules and facilitating their return to a normal structural and functional state. Most cells recover by cellular repair. However, some epithelial cells dedifferentiate, replicate, and migrate to fill the epithelial defect. Thereafter they spread out, become attached to the tubular membrane, and reestablish their polarized differentiated structure.

A. ACUTE KIDNEY INJURY AND SEPSIS—AKI occurs in approximately 20-25% of patients with sepsis and 51% with septic shock. The combination of AKI and sepsis is associated with a 70% mortality, as compared with a 45% mortality among patients with AKI alone. Thus, the combination of sepsis and AKI constitutes a particularly serious medical problem. There is experimental evidence that early in sepsis-related AKI the predominant pathogenetic factor is renal vasoconstriction with intact tubular function, as demonstrated by increased reabsorption of tubular sodium and water. Thus, intervention at this early stage may prevent progression to AKI and cell injury. Renal vasoconstriction in sepsis seems to be due, at least in part, to the ability of tumor necrosis factor to release endothelin. Endothelial damage, endotoxemiageneration of oxygen radicals, complement pathway activation, and disseminated intravascular coagulation may all contribute to the pathophysiology of ischemic AKI.

Since the early vasoconstrictor phase of sepsis and AKI is potentially reversible, it should be an optimal time for intervention. However, clinical studies performed in patients up to 72 hours after admission to the intensive care unit, in which attempts were made to optimize hemodynamics and monitor the patients with a pulmonary artery catheter, not only were negative but showed increased mortality among patients with sepsis. In contrast, a randomized study of over 200 patients showed that early goal-directed therapy during the first 6 hours after admission was effective. In patients treated with this approach, the multiorgan dysfunction score and in-hospital mortality was decreased significantly compared with four patients who received standard care. The goal-directed approach included early volume expansion and administration of vasopressors to maintain mean blood

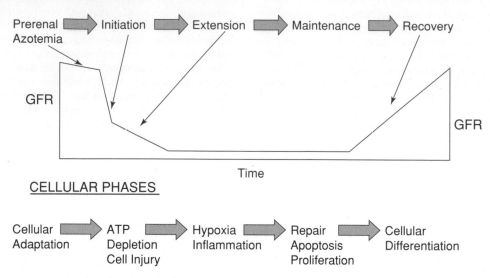

CLINICAL PHASES

Prerenal Azotemia ➡ Initiation ➡ Extension ➡ Maintenance ➡ Recovery

GFR

Time

CELLULAR PHASES

Cellular Adaptation ➡ ATP Depletion Cell Injury ➡ Hypoxia Inflammation ➡ Repair Apoptosis Proliferation ➡ Cellular Differentiation

▲ **Figure 9–1.** Phases of acute kidney injury. GFR, glomerular filtration rate.

pressure at or above 65 mm Hg and transfusion of red cells to increase the hematocrit to 30% or more if central venous oxygen saturation was less than 70%. If these interventions failed to increase central venous oxygen saturation to greater than 70%, therapy with dobutamine was instituted.

B. NEPHROTOXINS—Nephrotoxins induce tubular cell injury by several primary mechanisms including direct cellular injury, vasoconstriction, and tubular obstruction.

(1) Exogenous nephrotoxins
(a) Antibiotics—Nephrotoxins such as aminoglycosides, amphotericin, heavy metals, foscarnet, pentamidine, and cis-platin cause direct tubular cell injury. The most important manifestation of aminoglycoside nephrotoxicity is AKI secondary to ATN, which occurs in 10–20% of patients receiving aminoglycosides. Maintaining blood levels in the therapeutic range reduces but does not eliminate the risk of nephrotoxicity. Risk factors for developing nephrotoxic nephropathy include use of high or repeated doses or prolonged therapy, advanced age, volume depletion, a reduced effective arterial volume, and the coexistence of renal ischemia or other nephrotoxins. Again, patients with a reduced effective arterial volume are at a markedly increased risk for nephrotoxin-induced AKI. This synergistic interaction may raise the incidence of AKI from a nephrotoxin by as much as a factor of ten.

AKI caused by aminoglycosides is usually nonoliguric. It is manifested by an increase in BUN and creatinine after about 1 week of therapy, although in patients with concurrent renal hypoperfusion it can occur within 48 hours. Patient may de-

velop polyuria and hypomagnesemia. Once-daily dosing of aminoglycosides is as effective as more frequent dosing and may result in less nephrotoxicity, but should not be used in patients with chronic kidney disease (CKD).

Cyclosporin and tacrolimus nephrotoxicity is usually dose dependent. High blood levels may help to predict renal failure. In many cases a kidney biopsy may be necessary to distinguish between toxicity and other causes. Renal function usually improves after decreasing the dose or discontinuing the drug.

(b) Radiographic contrast media—Radiocontrast agents cause both vasoconstriction and direct cellular injury. Contrast nephropathy typically presents as an acute decline in GFR within 24–48 hours following administration. Individuals with reduced baseline kidney function, diabetic nephropathy, severe cardiac failure, volume depletion, and advanced age, as well as those receiving a large dose of contrast and concomitant exposure to other nephrotoxins appear particularly vulnerable and should be volume expanded prior to the study.

(c) Intratubular obstruction—AKI may occur in patients with malignancies with a high rate of tumor cell turnover (tumor lysis syndrome). Such cell turnover may occur either spontaneously or after chemotherapy. There may be an increase in uric acid production and hyperuricosuria, causing uric acid nephropathy. The peak uric acid level is often greater than 20 mg/dL. Prevention of AKI involves establishing a urine output greater than 3–5 L/24 hours and initiating treatment with allopurinol before institution of chemotherapy. Allopurinol blocks uric acid production by inhibiting xanthine oxidase. Urinary alkalization also increases the solubility of xanthine and enhances its excretion. More rapid declines in uric acid levels are seen following the intravenous administration of urate oxidase (uricase, rasburicase), which converts uric acid to allantoin, a much more soluble metabolite.

Tubular obstruction has been implicated as a central event in the pathophysiology of ATN induced by some therapeutic agents such as acyclovir, sulfonamides, methotrexate, triamterene, ethylene glycol, and myeloma light chains. To minimize possible nephrotoxicity from these agents, hydration and a high urine flow rate should be obtained in these patients.

(d) Ethylene glycol—Ingestion of ethylene glycol, usually in the form of antifreeze, produces severe metabolic acidosis with an elevated anion gap and osmolar gap. Ethylene glycol is metabolized by alcohol dehydrogenase to glycolic and oxalic acid, which are toxic to the renal tubules. Hypocalcemia is a prominent feature that occurs as a result of the deposition of calcium oxalate in multiple tissues. Calcium oxalate crystals are typically found in the urine sediment. Aggressive intervention with intravenous sodium bicarbonate to increase excretion of glycolate through ion tapping along with intravenous ethanol or fomepizole to block the metabolism of ethylene glycol should be done. In many cases emergent hemodialysis is needed to remove ethylene glycol and glycolate and to correct metabolic acidosis.

(2) Endogenous nephrotoxins—Myoglobinuria as a consequence of rhabdomyolysis is a frequent cause of AKI. The release of large amounts of myoglobin from necrotic muscle tissue in the setting of volume depletion results in ATN. Patients with rhabdomyolysis will frequently complain of muscle pain and have elevated levels of creatine phosphokinase. In addition to trauma, other metabolic derangements that can cause rhabdomyolysis include hypokalemia and hypophosphatemia. Cocaine use, neuroleptic malignant syndrome, and the use of hydroxymethylglutaryl coenzyme A (HMG-CoA) reductase inhibitors in the treatment of hypercholesterolemia also contribute or cause rhabdomyolysis. The urine will appear dark brown. The urine dipstick, even in the absence of red blood cells, will be positive for blood because of the presence of myoglobin. Hyperkalemia, hyperphosphatemia, hyperuricemia, and hypocalcemia, followed by hypercalcemia, are other clinical features associated with rhabdomyolysis. The most important aspect of management is rapid volume repletion. Experience from recent disasters has shown that early aggressive hydration and urinary alkalinization are capable of preventing myoglobinuric AKI.

Massive intravascular hemolysis can be seen in severe transfusion reactions and snake bites and may cause significant hemoglobinuria and ATN. The renal injury in this setting is due to the obstruction by intratubular heme pigment casts and concurrent volume depletion and renal ischemia. In contrast to other forms of acute tubular necrosis, the fractional excretion of sodium is often less than 1%, a finding that may reflect the primacy of tubular obstruction rather than tubular necrosis.

2. Glomerular disease—Glomerulonephritis is characterized by hypertension, proteinuria, and hematuria. Glomerulonephritis that causes AKI is referred to as rapidly progressive glomerulonephritis (RPGN). RPGN can occur in systemic lupus nephritis, Wegener's granulomatosis, polyarteritis nodosa, Goodpasture's syndrome, Henoch–Schönlein purpura, immunologic glomerulonephritis due to infection, and hemolytic uremic syndrome. Together these account for less than 5% of AKI cases.

3. Interstitial nephritis—Many drugs can induce interstitial nephritis by an idiosyncratic immune-mediated mechanism. This is often associated with fever, maculopapular rash, and eosinophils in the urine. Many drugs can cause acute interstitial nephritis but the most common are NSAIDs, penicillins, cephalosporins, sulfonamides, diuretics, and allopurinol. In the hospital setting AKI is usually multifactorial and it is very important to carefully analyze the hospital course and the medication history of every patient.

4. Vascular disease—Atheroembolic disease is another important cause of AKI, especially in elderly patients. It may present 1 day to several weeks after undergoing an invasive vascular procedure or major trauma. Patients classically present with lower extremity rash, livedo reticularis, and eosinophils in the urine. Unfortunately, there is no specific treatment. The patient's blood pressure should be controlled and further intra-arterial procedures should be limited.

C. Postrenal Acute Kidney Injury

The primary causes of postrenal AKI include benign prostatic hypertrophy, prostate cancer, cervical cancer, retroperitoneal fibrosis, retroperitoneal lymphoma, metastatic carcinoma, and nephrolithiasis. Blood clots within the urinary tracts can also present with obstruction. Hydronephrosis detected on renal ultrasound examination is the major signal that obstruction is present. False-negative ultrasound examinations can occur if the obstruction is very early or retroperitoneal fibrosis is present.

Allison RC, Bedsole DL: The other medical causes of rhabdomyolysis. Am J Med Sci 2003;326(2):79.

Landry DW, Oliver JA: The pathogenesis of vasodilatory shock. N Engl J Med 2001;345(8):588.

Schrier RW, Wang W: Acute renal failure and sepsis. N Engl J Med 2004;351(2):159.

▶ Prevention

The underlying principles of identification of high-risk patients, use of preventative measures, and aggressive surveillance are of key importance. Prevention of AKI is of paramount importance. Certain risk factors that have been identified to enhance the likelihood of AKI are listed in Table 9–3. These include volume depletion or hypoperfusion, preexisting renal failure, and exposure to vasoconstricting drugs such as NSAIDs.

Prevention of AKI primarily involves recognition of the high risk patient and correction of volume depletion. Persistent volume depletion leads to a prolonged "extension phase" resulting in worsening ATN. Aggressive restoration of intravascular volume dramatically reduces the incidence of ATN after major surgery or trauma. The mortality of AKI is higher if it develops in the hospital. Therefore, it is imperative to prevent AKI, particularly if it is associated with nephrotoxic drugs and interventional procedures. Correction of hypovolemia (normalizing the effective arterial volume) before radiocontrast administration, surgical procedures, and nephrology consultation in patients with even minimally decreased renal function may decrease the frequency of AKI. For the prevention of contrast-induced nephropathy, prophylactic infusion of saline (1 mL/kg for 12 hours before and after the procedure) appears more effective in preventing AKI than other commonly used agents such as mannitol and furosemide. *N*-Acetylcysteine and sodium bicarbonate infusion may also be beneficial in the prevention of contrast-induced nephropathy. Finally, since many cases of ischemic or nephrotoxic AKI result from sepsis or use of nephrotoxic antibiotics, respectively, limiting infection and careful monitoring for infections are important strategies.

Merten GJ et al: Prevention of contrast-induced nephropathy with sodium bicarbonate: a randomized controlled trial. JAMA 2004;291(19):2328.

▶ Clinical Findings

A. Symptoms and Signs

Unfortunately, the signs and symptoms are limited, nondiagnostic, and often go unrecognized. The symptoms of AKI include those related to azotemia generally and those due to underlying cause. Suggestive symptoms include a decrease in urine output and dark and cola-colored urine. Azotemic patients often complain of anorexia, nausea, malaise, metallic

Table 9–3. Patients at risk.

Elderly patients
Diabetes mellitus
Volume depletion
Vascular surgery
Chronic renal failure
Multiple antibiotics
Multiple insults

taste in the mouth, itching, confusion, fluid retention, and hypertension. Physical examination may reveal signs of volume overload, pericardial friction rub, or asterixis. This is why aggressive laboratory surveillance in high-risk patients is necessary.

▶ B. Laboratory Findings

The diagnosis of AKI is made by documenting elevations of the BUN and serum creatinine. Serum cystatin C is also a useful marker of AKI, and may detect AKI 1–2 days earlier than serum creatinine. Cystatin C is a 13-kDa endogenous cysteine protease inhibitor produced by nucleated cells at a constant rate. It is freely filtered at the glomerulus, reabsorbed, and catabolized, but it is not secreted by tubules.

Classifying intrinsic AKI into one of the histologic sites is in large part dependent upon the urinanalysis. For example, in ischemic or nephrotoxin-induced AKI the urinalysis shows mild proteinuria and often pigmented granular casts. However, in acute glomerulonephritis there is a higher degree of proteinuria, white blood cells, erythrocytes, and cellular casts. In interstitial nephritis, urinalysis shows mild to moderate proteinuria, leukocytes, erythrocytes, and eosinophils. The presence of heme positivity on the urine dipstick in a freshly voided sample and no erythrocytes suggest the presence of myoglobin or free hemoglobin, indicating either rhabdomyolysis or hemolysis. The presence of eosinophils is suggestive of acute interstitial nephritis, but can also be seen in renal atheroembolism or pyelonephritis. Specific urinary crystals can also be indicative of causes of AKI. For example, calcium oxalate crystals are seen in cases of ethylene glycol ingestion, and uric acid crystals are seen in cases of tumor lysis syndrome. Urinary diagnostic indices should be sent in any case in which prerenal azotemia is in the differential diagnosis. Glomerulonephritis and acute interstitial nephritis require kidney biopsy for diagnosis. Table 9–4 lists the urine findings suggestive of specific etiologies of AKI.

It is important to remember that a very high serum creatinine does not preclude the diagnosis of prerenal azotemia. A low FE_{Na^+}, less than 1%, is generally indicative of prerenal azotemia as the etiology of AKI. If the patient had existing CKD, prior to developing AKI, a high FE_{Na^+} may not indicate ATN. In CKD patients adaptation to volume depletion may take days, not hours, and FE_{Na^+} may be falsely high. An ultrasound is done to evaluate for obstruction. If the clinical situation dictates evaluation of renal vasculature with isotope scans, Doppler flow studies or angiography should be utilized. Figure 9–2 outlines the clinical approach to the common causes of AKI.

▶ Complications

A. Hyperkalemia

In patients with AKI the serum potassium rises rapidly, especially in the presence of cell lysis such as occurs with

Table 9–4. Urinary findings in acute kidney injury.

Etiology	Sediment	FE_{Na^+}	Fe-urea	Proteinuria
Prerenal azotemia	Few hyaline casts	<1	<35	None or trace
Ischemia	Epithelial cells, muddy-brown casts, pigmented granular casts	>2	>50	Trace to mild
Acute interstitial nephritis	White blood cells (WBC), WBC cast, eosinophilis, red blood cells (RBC), epithelial cells	>1		Mild to moderate
Acute glomerulonephritis	Dysmorphic RBCs, RBC cast	<1 early		Moderate to severe
Postrenal	Few hyaline casts, possible RBC	<1 early		None or trace
		>1 late		
Tumor lysis	Uric acid crystals			None or trace
Arterial/venous thrombosis	RBCs			Mild to moderate
Ethylene glycol	Calcium oxalate crystals			Trace to mild

muscle injury, hemolysis, gastrointestinal ischemia, tumor lysis syndrome, high fever, or blood transfusions. Hyperkalemia is further aggravated by metabolic acidosis as potassium is shifted from the intracellular to the extracellular compartment. The serum potassium concentration can be temporarily lowered by the administration of glucose and insulin, bicarbonate, inhaled β_2-agonists, and potassium-binding resins. However, if renal failure persists hyperkalemia will continue to reoccur and will ultimately respond only to renal replacement therapy (RRT). As AKI patients are more prone to the cardiotoxic side effects of hyperkalemia,

the serum potassium level should be lowered to nontoxic levels as soon as possible. Potassium is a small molecule and is easily dialyzable. Even at a blood flow of 200 mL/minute, dialysate potassium concentration of 1 mmol/L, and starting serum potassium concentration of 6 mmol/L, about 60 mmol of potassium is removed per hour.

B. Metabolic Acidosis

The severity of metabolic acidosis cannot usually be explained by the normal production rate of 1 mEq/kg/day of hydrogen ions. Patients with AKI are often in a hypercatabolic state

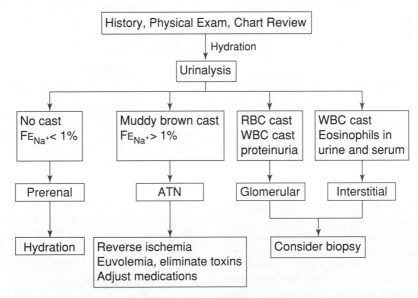

▲ **Figure 9–2.** Stepwise approach to the common causes of acute kidney injury. FE_{Na^+}, fractional excretion of Na^+; RBC, red blood cells; WBC, white blood cells; ATN, acute tubular necrosis.

(fever, trauma, sepsis) and, in addition, lactic acidosis may also occur because of anaerobic metabolism (hypoperfusion). The addition of respiratory acidosis, secondary to CO_2 retention, to metabolic acidosis can result in severe acidemia (pH <7.1) that may have severe negative inotropic and metabolic effects. Correction of a metabolic acidosis with administration of intravenous sodium bicarbonate is limited by the risk of hypervolemia and/or hypernatremia. Since bicarbonate is the commonly used buffer in hemodialysis dialysate, dialysis will result in reasonable control of metabolic acidosis and removal of organic acids. Continuous forms of dialysis have also been shown to be effective in the correction of severe acidosis.

C. Volume Overload

Volume overload is a major problem in oliguric AKI (urine output <400 mL/day). Critically ill patients are at high risk of developing hypervolemia, as fluid restriction is not always feasible because of the need for intravenous administration of drugs, nutrition, blood, and blood products. In addition, patients often receive aggressive fluid resuscitation in the early phase of their illness. This may result in pulmonary and peripheral edema when this fluid is redistributed later during their illness.

The most useful therapy for volume overload is loop diuretics. Furosemide or other loop diuretics can be given intravenously as a bolus or by continuous infusion. If started in the early stages of AKI this intervention, along with fluid restriction, can be very beneficial in preventing or minimizing volume overload. When using diuretics it is important to avoid volume depletion as the lack of renal autoregulation during AKI leaves the kidney vulnerable to additional hypotensive insults.

Hemofiltration, both by hemodialysis or continuous renal replacement therapy (CRRT), removes fluid and small-molecular-weight solute by convection and is the treatment modality of choice for fluid removal in hemodynamically unstable patients. In oliguric patients with a degree of fluid overload, who are about to receive large amounts of fluids for therapeutic purposes, RRT should be initiated early with the aim of preventing clinically important pulmonary edema. Episodes of hypotension should be avoided as renal functional recovery may be retarded because of recurrent ischemia and cell injury.

D. Hyponatremia

Hyponatremia is usually associated with volume overload. The clinical manifestations of hyponatremia are primarily neurologic in nature. Symptomatic hyponatremia should be treated aggressively but also with caution as rapid correction of low sodium levels can lead to central pontine myelinolysis if the duration of electrolyte imbalance has been longer than 48 hours. The targeted range of change of sodium level should be 1–2 mEq/L/hour until symptoms resolve or until the serum sodium level increases to 120 mEq/L.

E. Anemia

Anemia is very common in patients with AKI. Several mechanisms are involved. The most common cause of anemia associated with AKI is inadequate production of erythropoietin and decreased responsiveness to erythropoietin plays a role. There is also an increase in the rate of destruction of red blood cells as a result of increased erythrocyte fragility. Furthermore, patients with AKI have an increased tendency to bleed from various sites due to platelet dysfunction secondary to azotemia.

F. Hyperphosphatemia

Hyperphosphatemia is common in patients with AKI. The main mechanism is a decrease in renal excretion, tissue destruction, and shifts from intracellular to extracellular space. If patients can ingest food, hyperphosphatemia should be treated with phosphate binders such as calcium carbonate, calcium acetate, sevelamer HCl, or lanthanum carbonate. If the calcium $\times$ phosphorous product is high (>70) or the phosphate concentration exceeds 5.5 mEq/L a non-calcium-based binder such as sevelamer or lanthanum should be used.

G. Other Electrolyte Imbalances

Hypocalcemia, although common, rarely requires treatment. The factors responsible for hypocalcemia include hypomagnesemia, hyperphosphatemia, resistance to parathyroid hormone, lack of active vitamin D, calcium sequestration in tissues, use of blood products that have been stored in citrate, and use of sodium bicarbonate infusions. Rarely patients may have hypercalcemia if the underlying disorder is malignancy or multiple myeloma. Hypercalcemia can also occur in AKI due to rhabdomyolysis.

▶ Treatment

A. Prerenal Azotemia

By definition, prerenal azotemia is rapidly reversible on restoration of renal perfusion. Hypovolemia caused by hemorrhage is ideally corrected with packed red blood cells if the hematocrit is dangerously low. In the absence of active bleeding isotonic saline may suffice. The routine use of colloids has recently been associated with adverse outcomes and this has been called into question. Serum potassium and acid–base status should be monitored in all subjects. Cardiac failure may require aggressive management with positive inotropes, preload- and or afterload-reducing agents, and mechanical aids such as an intraaortic balloon pump. Fluid management is particularly challenging in patients with cirrhosis, requiring careful monitoring to avoid increased ascites formation.

B. Acute Tubular Necrosis

Management of ATN is usually supportive. Attempts to convert oliguric to nonoliguric AKI may be attempted by giving a loop diuretic such as furosemide. However, volume depletion as a result of the diuretic must be avoided. Use of mannitol should be avoided as it may precipitate congestive heart failure due to intravascular volume expansion if urine output remains low. In oliguric AKI, management consists of restricting fluids to match measurable insensible losses, potassium restriction, and limitation of phosphorous intake.

There are no prospective clinical data to support the use of low-dose dopamine for the protection or improvement of renal function in patients with ATN or AKI. Dopamine has not found to improve survival or eliminate the need for dialysis in AKI.

C. Role of Renal Replacement Therapy in Acute Kidney Injury

Dialysis is the only Food and Drug Administration-approved treatment of AKI. Although hemodialysis is the standard modality in hemodynamically stable patients with AKI, both continuous renal replacement therapy (CRRT) and peritoneal dialysis are also used in selected cases. The determining factors of which modality is chosen include the catabolic state, hemodynamic stability, and whether the primary goal is solute removal (uremia, hyperkalemia), fluid removal, or both.

1. Indications for dialysis—The indications for RRT in patients with AKI include refractory fluid overload, hyperkalemia, severe metabolic acidosis, azotemia, signs of uremia, such as pericarditis, neuropathy, or an otherwise unexplained decline in mental status, and overdose with a dialyzable drug/toxin.

In an attempt to minimize morbidity, dialysis should generally be started prior to the onset of complications due to renal failure. Nephrologists often initiate RRT even in the absence of the above-mentioned indications when the BUN reaches 60–80 mg/dL to prevent complications from AKI. Currently, peritoneal dialysis (PD) is rarely performed in adults as a treatment modality for AKI. This modality can be used in selective patient populations with access difficulties, contraindication to anticoagulation, or patients who are hemodynamically unstable.

2. Hemodialysis—Frequent hemodialysis is required to control metabolic abnormalities and volume status in AKI. Hypercatabolic patients require more aggressive dialysis to maintain acceptable or optimal steady-state or time-averaged concentrations of solutes. Daily hemodialysis may result in better control of uremia, fewer hypotensive episodes during hemodialysis, and more rapid resolution of AKI than conventional (every other day) hemodialysis.

3. Continuous renal replacement therapies—Continuous renal replacement therapies (CRRTs) involve either dialysis (diffusion-based solute removal) or filtration (convection-based solute and water removal) treatments that operate in a continuous mode. The various forms of CRRTs include Continuous venovenous hemofiltration (CVVH), Continuous venovenous hemodialysis (CVVHD), Continuous arteriovenous hemodialysis (CAVHD), Continuous venovenous hemodiafiltration (CVVHDF), Slow continuous ultrafiltration (SCUF) and sustained low efficiency dialysis (SLED).

CRRTs have several theoretical advantages over intermittent hemodialysis in critically ill patients with AKI. These include accurate continuous control of volume, increased delivered dose of dialysis, hemodynamic stability, the ability to provide aggressive nutritional support, gradual and continuous removal of fluid and solutes and a possible anti-inflammatory effect. Patients with multi-organ failure or sepsis require large amounts of volume in the form of blood products, vasopressors, and parentral nutrition. In these settings, continuous therapies provide an ability to remove fluid, which in most patients achieves an optimal volume balance. The possible elimination of inflammatory mediators is another advantage of CRRT. Many proposed mediators of sepsis have a molecular weight below the cutoff point of hemofilters and thus are filterable. CRRT may also be more beneficial in patients with increased intracranial pressure and combined fulminant hepatic failure and AKI. However, the superiority of CRRT in terms of patient outcomes is still controversial.

Several studies have attempted to assess the optimal dose of continuous renal replacement therapy in acute kidney injury. In one study, patients were randomized to three doses (assessed as effluent flow rate) of continuous venovenous hemofiltration (CVVH): 20 ml/kg per hr, 35 ml/kg per hr, and 45 ml/kg/hr. Although there was a significant improvement in survival with the intermediate dose (35 ml/kg per hour) as compared to the lower dose (25 ml/kg per hour), in nonseptic patients there was no added benefit associated with the highest dose (45 ml/kg per hr) of therapy. In another study, CVVH at an average effluent flow rate of 25 ml/kg per hour was compared to continuous venovenous hemodiafiltration (CVVHDF) at an average total effluent flow rate of 42 ml/kg per hour (25 ml/kg per hr ultrafiltration and 18 ml/kg per hour dialysate flow). The higher dose of therapy, delivered as CVVHDF was associated with improved survival. These results suggest that the benefit associated with increased solute clearance can be achieved by either increasing convection (hemofiltration) or adding a diffusive (hemodialysis) component. Thus, an effluent flow rate during CRRT of at least 35 ml/kg per hour is supported by the current data as associated with improved survival as compared to lower doses of therapy. However, no additional survival benefit has been established with higher doses of therapy.

Intensive renal support in critically ill patients with acute kidney injury did not decrease mortality, improve recovery of kidney function, or reduce the rate of non-renal organ failure as compared with less-intensive therapy involving a defined dose of intermittent hemodialysis three times per week and continuous renal-replacement therapy at 20 ml per kilogram per hour.

CRRT also has some disadvantages. Transport of patients for technical investigations becomes far more complicated and many times a new set of disposable tubing have to be used to restart dialysis. Anticoagulation is needed on a continuous basis during CRRT and thus the risk of bleeding is greater in CRRT than HD.

Ronco C, Bellomo R, Homel P, Brendolan A, Dan M, Piccinni P, La Greca G: Effects of different doses in continuous veno-venous hemofiltration on outcomes of acute renal failure: a prospective randomized trial. *Lancet* 356:26–30, 2000

Saudan P, Niederberger M, De Seigneux S, Romand J, Pugin J, Perneger T, Martin PY: Adding a dialysis dose to continuous hemofiltration increases survival in patients with acute renal failure. *Kidney Int* 70:1312–1317, 2006

Palevsky PM. Zhang JH. O'Connor TZ. Chertow GM. Crowley ST. Choudhury D. Finkel K. Kellum JA. Paganini E. Schein RM. Smith MW. Swanson KM. Thompson BT. Vijayan A. Watnick S. Star RA. Peduzzi P. Intensity of renal support in critically ill patients with acute kidney injury. VA/NIH Acute Renal Failure Trial Network New England Journal of Medicine. 359(1):7–20, 2008 Jul 3

D. Nutrition in Acute Kidney Injury

Recent evidence indicates more attention should be paid to the nutritional aspect of patients with both chronic renal failure and AKI. Excessive catabolism caused by shock, sepsis, burns, or rhabdomyolysis is common. During sepsis cytokines, including interleukins and tumor necrosis factor, are stimulated and, in turn, increase skeletal muscle breakdown. Severe net protein catabolism may accelerate the rate of rise in plasma concentrations of potassium, phosphorous, nitrogenous metabolites, and non-nitrogen-containing acids. Acute uremia is associated with increased gluconeogenesis and protein degradation as well as reduced protein synthesis. Insulin resistance, secondary hyperparathyrodism, increased glucagon concentrations, and metabolic acidosis also contribute to the malnutrition in AKI.

Renal replacement therapy (RRT) itself can cause increased metabolism through several mechanisms. Inevitable losses of nutrients during RRT also cause increased catabolism. If high flux membranes are used the losses of amino acids increase by 30% as compared to low-flux membranes. The losses of amino acids may range between 7 and 50 g/day with CRRT. This unavoidable removal of nutrients predisposes the AKI patient to negative nitrogen balance. In addition to increased catabolism, AKI patients also have a diminished utilization of available nutrients. Abnormalities in the growth hormone insulin-like growth factor 1 (IGF-1) axis prevent optimal utilization of available nutrients. Although the plasma concentration of growth hormone increases in renal failure, there is growth hormone resistance at the cellular level. Also, many patients are unable to eat adequately because of anorexia or vomiting. Malnutrition is a predictor of outcome in AKI patients.

Protein intake should be around 1.2–1.4 g/kg and 20–25% of daily calories should be provided by lipids. Glucose is usually administered in a 70% solution. The estimated energy requirements for patients with AKI usually fall between 30 and 40 kcal/kg normal body weight/day. Vitamin and mineral requirements have not been well defined for patients with AKI. However, water-soluble vitamins should be supplemented, as these are lost during RRT. Controlled studies are needed as nutrition requirements for HD versus CRRT may be different.

Augustine JJ et al: A randomized controlled trial comparing intermittent with continuous dialysis in patients with AKI. Am J Kidney Dis 2004;44(6):1000.

Chan LN: Nutritional support in acute renal failure. Curr Opin Clin Nutr Metab Care 2004;7(2):207.

Friedrich JO et al: Meta-analysis: low-dose dopamine increases urine output but does not prevent renal dysfunction or death. Ann Intern Med 2005;142(7):510.

Schiffl H et al: Daily hemodialysis and the outcome of acute renal failure. N Engl J Med 2002;346(5):305.

▶ Prognosis

The outcome of patients with AKI has consistently remained at a 50% survival rate despite improved technology. The prognosis for hospitalized patients with AKI depends largely on the site (ICU or ward). In hospitalized patients with AKI caused by ATN, the oliguric phase of ATN typically lasts for 1–2 weeks, but it can persist for 4–6 weeks. It is followed by a diuretic phase. Although uremia and volume overload can be controlled with dialysis, AKI and its complications worsen patient outcomes. Survival after AKI is dramatically influenced by the severity of the underlying illnesses and number of failed organs. The mortality rate of patients with AKI on a ventilator is about 80% and the mortality dramatically increases with an increasing number of failed nonrespiratory organs. Oliguric AKI, developing in a surgical setting or in older patients, carries a higher mortality than other forms of AKI. It has been noted that after discharge from a hospitalization that included AKI, a substantial fraction of patients required RRT in long-term care facilities.

In summary, AKI remains a medical challenge to clinicians and researchers. Recognition of patients at risk, institution of preventive measures and aggressive surveillance, and early treatment of acute kidney injury will be much more effective than treatment of established AKI with RRT.

Mehta RL et al: Spectrum of acute renal failure in the intensive care unit: the PICARD experience. Kidney Int 2004;66(4):1613.

Hepatorenal Syndrome

Florence Wong, MD, FRACP, FRCP(C)

10

ESSENTIALS OF DIAGNOSIS

▶ Renal failure in patients with advanced liver failure (acute or chronic) in the absence of any identifiable causes of renal pathology.

▶ All other causes of renal failure, functional or organic, have been excluded.

▶ General Considerations

Renal dysfunction is a common and serious problem in patients with advanced liver disease, estimated to occur in 10% of hospitalized patients with cirrhosis. It is a syndrome characterized by (1) oliguria, severe renal sodium retention, and rapidly progressive azotemia, (2) circulatory instability with marked systemic arterial vasodilation and activation of vasoactive systems, and (3) a very poor prognosis. Without treatment, the median survival for type 1 hepatorenal syndrome patients is on the order of 1–2 weeks, while that for type 2 hepatorenal syndrome is about 20% at 1 year. However, hepatorenal syndrome has always been considered to be a form of functional renal failure, as kidneys from patients with hepatorenal syndrome, when transplanted into someone with renal failure, regain their normal function. Similarly, renal function also improves in patients with end-stage cirrhosis following liver transplantation, although the renal function can remain abnormal for quite sometime in the postoperative period.

Hepatorenal syndrome is defined as the development of renal failure in patients with advanced liver failure (acute or chronic) in the absence of any identifiable causes of renal pathology. It is a diagnosis of exclusion, when all other causes of renal failure, functional or organic, have been excluded. The International Ascites Club further defines the criteria for the diagnosis of hepatorenal syndrome, as detailed in Table 10–1. It must be emphasized that urinary parameters are supportive, but not essential for the diagnosis of hepatorenal

syndrome. For example, urinary volume is usually <500 mL/day, but there are nonoliguric forms of hepatorenal syndrome. Urinary sodium excretion is usually <10 mEq/day in hepatorenal syndrome. However, cases of well-documented hepatorenal syndrome with urinary sodium of >10 mEq/day have been reported. Finally, although the urinary osmolality is higher than the plasma osmolality in most patients with hepatorenal syndrome, a decrease in urinary osmolality may occur as renal failure progresses.

The Internal Ascites Club divided hepatorenal syndrome into type 1 and type 2. Type 1 hepatorenal syndrome is characterized by a rapid decline in renal function defined as a doubling of serum creatinine to a level greater than 220 μmol/L or a halving of the creatinine clearance to less than 20 mL/minute within 2 weeks. The clinical presentation is that of acute renal failure. The patient is usually very sick, with marked jaundice and severe coagulopathy. In type 2 hepatorenal syndrome, renal function deteriorates more slowly with the serum creatinine increasing to greater than 133 μmol/L or a creatinine clearance decreasing to less than 40 mL/minute over the course of weeks to months. The clinical presentation is that of gradual renal failure in a patient with cirrhosis and refractory ascites.

▶ Pathogenesis

The pathophysiology of hepatorenal syndrome is complex. The hallmark of hepatorenal syndrome is renal hypoperfusion, which is due to a reduction in the renal perfusion pressure as well as to active renal vasoconstriction. This leads to a decrease in the renal blood flow and a reduction in the glomerular filtration rate. Many pathophysiologic factors are involved in the development of hepatorenal syndrome in patients with end-stage cirrhosis.

A. Hemodynamic Changes in Cirrhosis

Liver cirrhosis and portal hypertension are characterized by an increased cardiac output and decreased systemic vascular

Table 10-1. Diagnostic criteria for hepatorenal syndrome.

Cirrhosis with ascites
Serum creatinine >133 μmol/L (1.5 mg/dL)
No improvement of serum creatinine (decrease to a level of ≤133 μmol/L) after at least 2 days of diuretic withdrawal and volume expansion with albumin; the recommended dose of albumin is 1 g/kg body weight/day up to a maximum of 100 g/day
Absence of shock
No current or recent treatment with nephrotoxic drugs
Absence of parenchymal kidney disease as indicated by proteinuria >500 mg/day, microhematuria (>50 red blood cells per high power field), and/or abnormal renal ultrasonography

Reproduced with permission from Salerno F et al: Diagnosis, prevention and treatment of hepatorenal syndrome in cirrhosis. Gut 2007;56:1310.

resistance, the so-called hyperdynamic circulation. The basis for the hyperdynamic circulation is systemic arterial vasodilation. This occurs mainly in the splanchnic circulation, a result of both increased resistance to portal flow due to the cirrhosis and to the presence of excess vasodilators and/or decreased responsiveness of the vasculature to endogenous vasoconstrictors. Clinically, this is manifested as systemic hypotension, tachycardia, wide pulse pressure, and warm peripheries. The homeostatic response is the activation of various vasoconstrictor systems, including the renin–angiotensin system, the sympathetic nervous system, and arginine vasopressin. These will counteract the vasodilatory effects of the vasodilators and direct the kidneys to retain sodium and water in order to maintain hemodynamic stability. As cirrhosis progresses, systemic hypotension worsens as the systemic arterial vasodilation increases, and at some point in time the renal perfusion pressure will fall. When combined with increasing levels of the systemic vasoconstrictors, total renal blood flow gradually falls. When the production of endogenous vasodilators cannot keep pace with the fall in renal blood flow, renal failure ensues (Figure 10–1).

B. The Role of Mesangial Contraction

Not all cirrhotic patients with similarly reduced renal blood flow will develop hepatorenal syndrome. Therefore, other factors must also play a pathogenetic role. In addition to reduced renal blood flow, various vasoconstrictors, in particular, endothelin-1 and leukotrienes, may also cause mesangial contraction, thereby reducing the glomerular ultrafiltration coefficient and further decreasing the glomerular filtration rate.

C. The Role of Portal Hypertension

Portal hypertension is associated with a reduction of renal blood flow and may play a role in the pathogenesis of hepatorenal syndrome. The connection between portal hypertension and renal hemodynamics may be the sympathetic nervous system.

D. The Role of Hepatic Dysfunction

Renal hypoperfusion, due to a reduction of renal vasodilators, in cirrhosis could also be related to liver dysfunction. However, the mechanism whereby liver dysfunction could directly induce a reduction in renal vasodilators is unclear. It

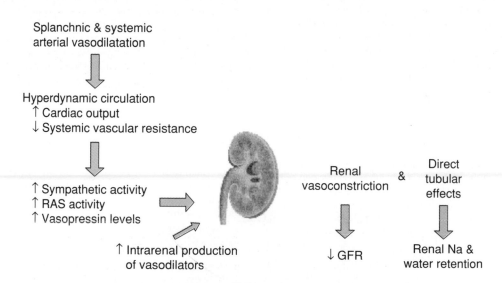

▲ **Figure 10-1.** Pathophysiology of hepatorenal syndrome GFR, glomerular filtration rate; RAS, renin–angiotensin system.

is possible that the liver is involved in the synthesis or release of renal vasodilators such as nitric oxide. The severe jaundice associated with liver failure can sensitize the renal vasculature to the vasoconstrictive effects of norepinephrine, resulting in greater renal vasoconstriction with any given level of circulating norepinephrine. High levels of bile acids observed in cholestasis can cause arterial vasodilation, thereby exaggerating the hemodynamic instability. That is, hepatic dysfunction "makes a bad situation worse." In patients with severe jaundice (bilirubin >510 μmol/L), there is direct bilirubin nephrotoxicity.

E. Precipitating Factors

At least 50% of patients with hepatorenal syndrome arrive in the hospital with near normal renal function. Therefore, it is what clinicians do to these patients that frequently precipitates hepatorenal syndrome. These precipitating events cause a further reduction in the filling of the effective arterial circulation, exaggerating the hemodynamic instability, resulting in further renal hypoperfusion and a decrease in the glomerular filtration rate.

1. Diuretic therapy—Cirrhotic patients with refractory ascites (Table 10–2) experience a reduction in their effective arterial blood volume and do not respond well to diuretic therapy. Diuretic therapy, by decreasing the intravascular volume, further exaggerates the reduction in effective arterial blood volume, and predisposes the patient to the development of hepatorenal syndrome. Clinicians have a tendency to increase the diuretic doses when there is an inadequate diuretic and natriuretic response, despite rising serum creatinine levels. Cirrhotic patients with refractory ascites typically excrete only approximately 500 mL of urine per day even in the presence of a "normal" serum creatinine level. Therefore, when increasing doses of diuretics do not result in an increased urine volume or urinary sodium excretion, further increases in the diuretic doses will increase the likelihood of developing hepatorenal syndrome in these patients. Conversely, decreasing the diuretic doses in a patient with refractory ascites and rising serum creatinine may reverse the renal dysfunction.

Table 10–2. Definition of refractory ascites.[1]

Weight loss ≤1.5 kg/week while on
400 mg of spironolactone
or
30 mg of amiloride   ⎫ ≥1 week, while on
plus   ⎬
160 mg of furosemide daily ⎭
Dietary sodium restriction ≤50 mmol/day

[1]Patients who are intolerant of diuretic therapy because of the development of complications are also regarded as having refractory ascites.

2. Large volume paracentesis—Large volume paracentesis leads to an exaggeration of the hyperdynamic circulation. The systemic circulation becomes more vasodilated about 24 hours after a large volume paracentesis. The subsequent further activation of the vasoconstrictor systems predisposes the patient to the development of hepatorenal syndrome. Reducing the rate of paracentesis could potentially prevent deleterious hemodynamic consequences and reduce the risk of developing hepatorenal syndrome.

3. Spontaneous bacterial peritonitis—It is estimated that at least 30% of patients with spontaneous bacterial peritonitis will develop hepatorenal syndrome despite adequate treatment of their infection. It has been postulated that sepsis in cirrhosis induces an increased production of various cytokines and endotoxins, which in turn stimulates the production of nitric oxide and other vasodilators, causing further arterial vasodilation. Therefore, spontaneous bacterial peritonitis exaggerates the reduction in the effective arterial blood volume and increases the risk of further deterioration of the systemic hemodynamics, leading to decreased renal function.

4. Gastrointestinal bleeding—Acute blood loss with acute blood volume contraction usually leads to acute tubular necrosis and not hepatorenal syndrome. However, patients with decompensated cirrhosis and gastrointestinal bleeding can develop a systemic inflammatory response syndrome, manifesting as an increase in temperature, tachycardia, tachypnoea, and leukocytosis with or without an infection, associated with the activation of many cytokines. Once again, these cytokines can stimulate the production of nitric oxide and other vasodilators. Thus, the patient with gastrointestinal bleeding is also predisposed to further exaggeration of the systemic arterial vasodilation, due to the fact that the accompanying inflammatory response will yield more vasodilators, aggravating the effective arterial underfilling. Gastrointestinal bleeding also predisposes the cirrhotic patient to the development of infection, which in turn predicts rebleeding after control of the initial bleeding episode. The presence of infection in a cirrhotic patient with gastrointestinal bleeding adds to the inflammatory response and to cytokine production, further exaggerating the hemodynamic instability and increasing the likelihood of developing hepatorenal syndrome. To support this hypothesis, the routine use of prophylactic antibiotics in cirrhosis with gastrointestinal bleeding has led to a significant reduction in the incidence of hepatorenal syndrome associated with the bleeding episode.

5. Cholestasis—Acute biliary obstruction is associated with the development of renal impairment, leading to the suggestion that increased production of F_2-isoprostanes in cholestasis was responsible for the development of renal failure, since F_2-isoprostanes are potent renal vasoconstrictors, and the administration of antioxidants that reduced

F_2-isoprostane levels was associated with improvement of renal function. Cholestasis per se appears to be detrimental to the systemic circulation. It is not surprising that when cholestasis is superimposed on cirrhosis and portal hypertension, the circulatory changes are likely to worsen, predisposing the patient to the development of hepatorenal syndrome.

6. Nephrotoxic agents—The use of nonselective nonsteroidal anti-inflammatory drugs (NSAIDs) in cirrhosis is associated with a reduction in renal perfusion and glomerular filtration rate, secondary to an inhibition of the renal production of vasodilatory prostaglandins. In addition, NSAIDs impair renal sodium and water excretion, and these effects are independent of the deterioration in renal hemodynamics. These effects are particularly pronounced in cirrhosis with ascites, as these patients are dependent on the intrarenal production of prostaglandins to counteract the effects of various vasoconstrictors. Therefore, ascitic cirrhotic patients should not receive NASIDs in order to avoid the precipitation of hepatorenal syndrome. Cirrhotic patients are dependent on the activated renin–angiotensin system to maintain systemic blood pressure. Therefore, the use of angiotensin-converting enzyme inhibitors and angiotensin II antagonists can result in arterial hypotension and precipitate renal failure in these patients.

The pathogenesis of hepatorenal syndrome can be best summed up by the 2-hit theory (Figure 10–2). The cirrhotic patient with advanced liver disease and massive ascites has a compromised circulatory state (the first hit). The activation of various compensatory mechanisms maintains the circulation. Further progression of liver disease with deterioration of the circulation will lead to the development of hepatorenal syndrome (nonprecipitated cases). Alternatively, the presence of a precipitating factor will lead to rapid deterioration of the systemic circulation and to the development of the hepatorenal syndrome (second hit).

▶ Clinical Findings

A. Type 1

Type 1 hepatorenal syndrome is characterized by a rapid and progressive deterioration of renal function. The patient is usually ill with severely decompensated liver cirrhosis, jaundice, and hyponatremia. Oliguria and rising creatinine develop over the course of a few days. In about half the patients, there is no obvious precipitating cause. In the other half, the onset of hepatorenal syndrome follows some clear precipitating event such as infection, major gastrointestinal hemorrhage, or overaggressive diuresis or large volume paracentesis (>5 L) without replacement of the intravascular volume. On examination, these patients usually have florid signs or stigmata of liver failure. There may be evidence of encephalopathy with asterixis and hyperreflexia, but patients usually do not lapse into coma until the final stages.

Clinically, the patient may appear hypovolemic with a low jugular venous pressure. There is an obvious hyperdynamic circulation with bounding tachycardia, low normal blood pressure, or frank hypotension, and a precordial systolic flow murmur. The ascites is often massive with or without associated leg edema.

Over the years, several factors have been found to be associated with a greater risk for the development of type 1 hepatorenal syndrome (Table 10–3). These parameters are all related to severe hemodynamic instability and marked renal sodium and water retention.

B. Type 2

Patients with type 2 hepatorenal syndrome have a relatively stable serum creatinine that gradually climbs over a period of months. They are usually stable Child–Pugh Class B patients with relatively preserved liver function, but with a history of diuretic-resistant ascites. Jaundice is mild, and the patient

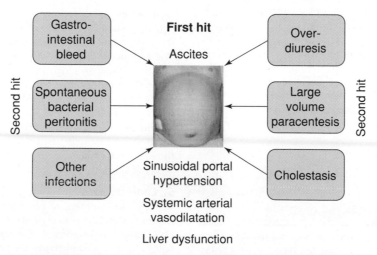

▲ **Figure 10–2.** The pathogenesis of hepatorenal syndrome.

Table 10–3. Factors associated with a greater risk for the development of type 1 hepatorenal syndrome.

Low arterial pressure

Glomerular filtration rate of <50 mL/minute

Serum creatinine >133 μmol/L

Blood urea nitrogen >21 mmol/L

Hyponatremia

Hyperkalemia

Low urinary sodium excretion

Low plasma osmolality

High urinary osmolality

Reduced free water excretion after water load

High plasma renin activity

High plasma norepinephrine

usually has some degree of coagulopathy. Hepatic encephalopathy is usually absent. Urine output is maintained over the course of weeks to months and only slowly diminishes as the serum creatinine climbs.

▶ Differential Diagnosis

The clinician needs to recognize that renal dysfunction may be present despite a normal serum creatinine. This may be due to two factors: (1) cirrhotic patients are often wasted with a reduced muscle mass and hence lower normal serum creatinine levels and (2) a high bilirubin level may interfere with the creatinine assay. A creatinine >88 μmol/L in a patient with cirrhosis should alert the clinician to the presence of renal dysfunction.

Hepatorenal syndrome represents only a small portion of all causes of renal failure in decompensated cirrhotic patients with ascites. It is a diagnosis of exclusion. To arrive at a diagnosis of hepatorenal syndrome, the circulation of the patient has to be full and there has to be no evidence of intrinsic (organic) kidney disease.

A. Prerenal Renal Failure

Patients with decompensated cirrhosis and ascites and hemodynamic instability are poised to develop renal impairment if their circulation is further compromised. Therefore, events that tend to reduce the intravascular volume further such as gastrointestinal bleed, large volume paracentesis, or overzealous diuresis are likely to lead to renal failure. It follows that patients who have evidence of significant arterial vasodilation clinically, such as low arterial blood pressure and tachycardia, should be assessed to receive intravascular volume replacement for their large volume paracentesis. Likewise, resuscitation following gastrointestinal bleeding should be as complete as possible. It is very tempting to increase the diuretic doses in patients who have large ascites and an inadequate urine output. The end result may be further reduction in renal function as the intravascular volume is further compromised. Often, by reducing or eliminating the diuretic doses, the serum creatinine may decrease, accompanied by an improved urine output. A low urinary sodium excretion cannot be used as a guide to the presence of prerenal failure, as patients with hepatorenal syndrome have a reduced effective arterial blood volume and therefore will also have a low urinary sodium excretion. Rather, patients with decompensated cirrhosis, ascites, and renal failure should be challenged with a fluid load, with their central venous blood pressure filled up to 10 cm of water. Colloid solutions are preferred, as crystalloids tend to be distributed directly to the peritoneal cavity as ascites and not be retained in the circulation. If the patient has prerenal renal failure, the serum creatinine should slowly decrease as the circulation is gradually refilled.

B. Organic Renal Disease

Patients with decompensated cirrhosis can also develop organic renal disease. In fact, many organic renal diseases occur as a result of the liver disease (Table 10–4). Alternatively, there are many systemic diseases that can affect the liver and the kidney simultaneously (Table 10–5). Intrinsic or structural renal disease can be excluded by inactive urinary sediment, a urinary protein excretion of <500 mg/day, and a normal ultrasound examination of both kidneys. Differentiating hepatorenal syndrome from acute tubular necrosis is often difficult. Distinguishing the two is important when considering therapy and for prognostication. Typically, urine sodium of <10 mmol/L occurs in hepatorenal syndrome, while a urine sodium of >20 mmol/L is typical for acute tubular necrosis due to impaired reabsorption of sodium from damaged renal tubules. However, this distinction is not always reliable, especially in the late stages of hepatorenal syndrome.

Table 10–4. Primary liver diseases complicated by renal diseases.

Liver Disease	Kidney Disease
Alcoholic hepatitis	IgA nephropathy
Hepatitis B	Glomerulonephritis Polyarteritis nodosa Cryoglobulinemia
Hepatitis C	Glomerulonephritis Cryoglobulinemia
Obstructive jaundice	Acute renal failure
Primary biliary cirrhosis	Renal tubular acidosis Interstitial nephritis
Wilson's disease	Renal tubular acidosis

Table 10–5. Systemic diseases affecting both liver and kidney.

Drugs		
Acetaminophen	Liver failure	Acute/chronic renal failure
Aspirin	Acute hepatitis Reye's syndrome	Papillary necrosis
Pregnancy	HELLP Hepatic rupture	Preeclampsia
Cysts	Polycystic liver disease	Polycystic kidney disease
Sarcoidosis	Liver granulomas Portal hypertension	Renal stones
Diabetes	Steatohepatitis	Diabetic nephropathy
Amyloidosis	Hepatomegaly	Nephrotic syndrome
Sickle cell anemia	Hyperbilirubinemia Gallstonews Cholecystitis Secondary hemochromatosis	Hematuria Renal infarct
Paroxysmal nocturnal hemoglobinuria	Budd–Chiari syndrome Portal vein thrombosis	Hemoglobinuria
Shock	Ischemic hepatitis	Acute tubular necrosis

Acute tubular necrosis can also occur. This should be considered when renal failure develops abruptly following hypovolemia, septic shock, or exposure to nephrotoxins.

▶ Treatment

In patients with cirrhosis and acute or chronic liver failure who present with a serum creatinine of >133 μ mol/L (1.5 mg/dL), a thorough workup should be done to exclude other causes of renal disease. In addition, patients should be initially challenged with fluid to assess response and to treat subclinical hypovolemia. All precipitants of hepatorenal syndrome should be sought and corrected. A careful assessment of the patient's history should identify preceding events such as gastrointestinal bleeding, overdiuresis, or aggressive paracentesis. Sepsis should be suspected in any cirrhotic patient with renal deterioration even in the absence of symptoms. Fever and leukocytosis may not be present. A full septic workup should be done and cultures should be obtained, including examination of the ascitic fluid to rule out spontaneous bacterial peritonitis. Recent exposure to nephrotoxins such as NSAIDs or aminoglycosides prior to the increase in serum creatinine should be ruled out. In contrast to the general belief, the use of radiocontrast dye has not been shown

to be detrimental to renal function in cirrhosis. If proteinuria and/or hematuria are present, additional investigations should be undertaken to rule out renal parenchymal diseases. Renal biopsy should be considered if there is a strong suspicion for glomerulonephritis. Finally, an abdominal ultrasound should be performed to determine if the patient has postobstructive renal failure.

Once the diagnosis of hepatorenal syndrome is firmly established, the treatment options are aimed at correcting different aspects of the pathophysiology of hepatorenal syndrome. Patients should be supported until liver recovery or transplantation.

A. Pharmacology

The aim of pharmacotherapy is to improve systemic hemodynamics. This can be achieved by increasing either systemic or splanchnic vasoconstriction. The former improves renal perfusion pressure, while the latter redistributes part of the splanchnic volume to the systemic circulation, thereby improving the systemic arterial blood volume, with consequent improved renal perfusion and glomerular filtration.

1. Dopamine—Low-dose dopamine is a renal vasodilator. Despite this, it has not been shown to be effective in improving the glomerular filtration rate in either cirrhotic patients with refractory ascites but no hepatorenal syndrome or in cirrhotic patients with established hepatorenal syndrome. Furthermore, in cirrhotic patients with refractory ascites but without hepatorenal syndrome, dopamine has been shown to decrease arterial pressure and accentuate portal hypertension. Therefore, it should not be used in cirrhotic patients with refractory ascites or hepatorenal syndrome.

2. Norepinephrine—Although the use of intravenous norepinephrine (0.5–3 mg/hour) in combination with intravenous albumin and furosemide resulted in the reversal of hepatorenal syndrome in a small study, until the results of randomized controlled trials are available the routine use of norepinephrine for hepatorenal syndrome cannot be recommended.

3. Vasopressin analogues

A. Ornipressin—Ornipressin is a nonselective agonist of the V1 vasopressin receptors. It preferentially causes vasoconstriction of the splanchnic vasculature, thus increasing systemic pressure and renal perfusion pressure. While treatment with ornipressin and albumin has improved renal function in cirrhotic patients with hepatorenal syndrome, there is an increased risk of serious, life-threatening, ischemic complications associated with the use of ornipressin. Therefore, the use of this agent for hepatorenal syndrome is rather limited, and it is no longer commercially available.

B. Terlipressin—Terlipressin is a synthetic analogue of vasopressin with intrinsic vasoconstrictor activity. It is also a nonselective V1 vasopressin agonist but has a lower incidence of ischemic complications than vasopressin or ornipressin. It also has the advantage over vasopressin of a longer half-life, allowing administration as a 4 hourly bolus. The infusion of terlipressin at a dose of 0.5–2 mg/4–6 hours intravenously up to 15 days is associated with improved renal function, although usually not to normal, with suppressed plasma renin activity and aldosterone levels, increased atrial natriuretic factor levels, and some improvement of urinary sodium excretion, without serious side effects in the majority of patients. It is not clear whether treatment beyond 15 days would result in further improvement of renal function. Terlipressin is not available in North America, but is the first-line therapy for hepatorenal syndrome in Europe.

4. Midodrine and octreotide—Midodrine is an oral α-adrenergic agonist that improves systemic blood pressure and hence improves renal perfusion pressure. Octreotide is a long-acting analogue of somatostatin that antagonizes the action of various splanchnic vasodilators and reduces the mismatch between the extent of arterial vasodilation and the intravascular volume. The use of midodrine or octreotide alone has not proved useful for patients with hepatorenal syndrome. However, when midodrine is combined with plasma volume expansion and octreotide, there is often a significant improvement in both the systemic and renal hemodynamics and urinary sodium excretion, along with a partial improvement in renal function. The use of this combination is popular in North America because of the nonavailability of terlipressin. However, its place in the treatment of hepatorenal syndrome still awaits the results of larger randomized controlled trials.

5. Endothelin receptor antagonists—Endothelin has been postulated to be a mediator of intrarenal vasoconstriction in hepatorenal syndrome, and treatment with endothelin receptor antagonists has been associated with dose-related increases in both the glomerular filtration rate and renal plasma flow. However, based on personal experience, the use of a nonselective endothelin receptor antagonist in cirrhotic patients with hepatorenal syndrome resulted in both decreased renal function and urinary volume (unpublished data). Therefore, such agents should be used only in a clinical trial setting.

6. Pentoxifylline—Pentoxifylline is a phosphodiesterase inhibitor with antitumor necrosis factor activity. While use of pentoxifylline in patients with acute alcoholic cirrhosis has resulted in a significant reduction in the incidence of hepatorenal syndrome, there are no studies assessing the use of pentoxifylline as a treatment for established hepatorenal syndrome.

B. Extracorporeal Albumin Dialysis

Extracorporeal albumin dialysis is a system that uses a cell-free, albumin-containing dialysate that is recirculated and perfused through charcoal and anion exchange columns. One such extracorporeal albumin dialysis device is the molecular absorbent recirculating system (MARS). During dialysis, a closed loop dialysate circuit allows the transfer of albumin-bound toxins from plasma onto a permeable polysulfone-saturated membrane. The membrane-bound albumin plus toxin is recycled by continuous deligandization. Water-soluble toxins can then be removed with the use of charcoal columns and ion-exchange resins as the adsorbents (Figure 10–3). The system is very efficient in removing molecules with a molecular weight of less than 50 kDa. The rationale for using MARS as a treatment for hepatorenal syndrome is that it can remove many cytokines such as tumor necrosis factors and interleukin 6, which have been implicated in the production of various vasodilators. Therefore, by reducing the levels of vasodilators, the expected result is improved systemic hemodynamics and hence better renal perfusion and renal function.

MARS dialysis reduces serum bilirubin and creatinine levels and has been ssociated with a small prolongation of survival. It is not clear at present whether the reduction in serum creatinine with MARS treatment is maintained after withdrawal of MARS. It is also not clear how long MARS treatment should be given before sustained improvement in renal function can be achieved. Therefore, MARS should not be used in the treatment of patients with hepatorenal syndrome, except in the context of a clinical trial.

C. Transjugular Intrahepatic Portosystemic Stent Shunt (TIPS)

TIPS is prosthesis that bridges a branch of the portal vein with a branch of the hepatic vein (Figure 10–4), effectively functioning as a side-to-side portal caval shunt. It is very effective in reducing portal pressure. Since sinusoidal portal hypertension plays a pivotal role in the control of renal hemodynamics, it is not surprising that the insertion of TIPS, especially in cirrhotic patients with refractory ascites and some degree of renal dysfunction, is associated with improvement in both the glomerular filtration rate and renal blood flow. In addition, TIPS returns a significant portion of the splanchnic volume into the systemic circulation, leading to suppression of various vasoactive neurohormones, resulting in better renal perfusion. The successful treatment of type 2 hepatorenal syndrome in cirrhotic patients with refractory ascites can also result in elimination of ascites. It must be emphasized that TIPS often leads to improvement in but cannot normalize renal function.

Attempts have been made to combine various treatment options to correct several aspects of the pathophysiology of hepatorenal syndrome. One such combination is the use of pharmacotherapy followed by TIPS for patients with type 1 hepatorenal syndrome. For instance, midodrine, octreotide, and albumin followed by TIPS insertion in those who responded to treatment and were deemed to be suitable to receive a TIPS has been associated with maintenance of normal renal function and eventual elimination of ascites with improvement in survival. The challenge is how to select the most appropriate combination therapy for each individual patients.

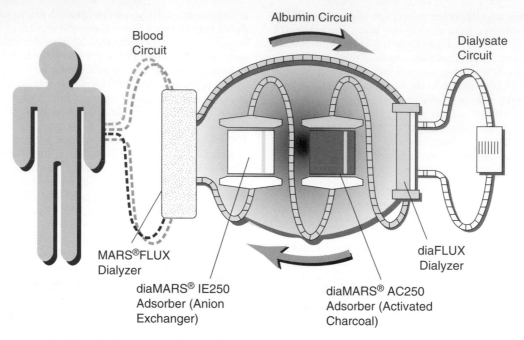

▲ Figure 10–3. Molecular adsorbent recirculating system.

D. Liver Transplantation

Liver transplantation remains the only effective permanent treatment for hepatorenal syndrome, as it corrects liver dysfunction and eliminates portal hypertension. Renal function improves in patients with hepatorenal syndrome after transplantation, associated with a reduction in plasma levels of vasoactive factors, although the glomerular filtration rate generally remains subnormal. Hepatorenal syndrome patients who are transplanted have a lower probability of both graft and patient survival after liver transplantation, compared to patients without hepatorenal syndrome. Furthermore, patients with hepatorenal syndrome require a longer stay in intensive care units, longer hospitalization, and more dialysis treatments after liver transplantation. In patients whose hepatorenal syndrome is treated prior to liver transplantation, the posttransplantation clinical outcome is significantly improved, being similar to transplanted patients without hepatorenal syndrome. Therefore, in patients with end-stage cirrhosis awaiting liver transplantation, every attempt should be made to improve renal function in order to maximize the posttransplantation outcome.

▶ Prevention

The most important aspect of management of hepatorenal syndrome is to prevent its occurrence. This is achieved by avoiding or minimizing further deterioration in liver and circulatory functions and renal hypoperfusion.

A. Judicious Use of Diuretics

Diuretic-induced renal impairment occurs in 20% of patients with ascites. This happens when the rate of diuresis exceeds the rate of ascites reabsorption resulting in a reduction in effective arterial blood volume. The renal failure is usually reversible with cessation of the diuretics. Patients with ascites and no edema are able to mobilize maximally only 700 mL of ascitic fluid per day. Any diuresis of more than 700 mL/day will occur at the expense of plasma volume contraction

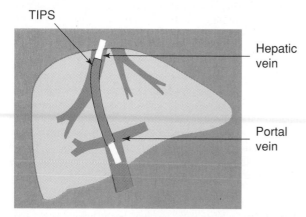

▲ Figure 10–4. Schematic picture of a transjugular intrahepatic portosystemic stent shunt (TIPS) *in situ*.

and the risk of renal insufficiency. Patients with peripheral edema appear to be protected from these effects because of the preferential mobilization of edema and may safely undergo diuresis at a more rapid rate (greater than 2 kg/day) until the edema disappears.

B. Avoidance of Nephrotoxic Agents

NSAIDs should not be given to cirrhotic patients with ascites because the incidence of renal failure with their use is much higher than in the general population. They inhibit the formation of intrarenal prostaglandins, which are vasodilatory compounds that counteract the effects of various vasoconstrictors on the renal circulation. Patients with cirrhosis and ascites are predisposed to acute tubular necrosis with the use of aminoglycosides and thus these should be avoided. Angiotensin-converting enzyme inhibitors and angiotensin II blockers result in arterial hypotension and predispose cirrhotic patients to the development of renal failure. They therefore should also be avoided.

C. Prophylaxis Against the Development of Bacterial Infections

Cirrhotic patents with gastrointestinal bleeding have a high incidence of infection, especially spontaneous bacterial peritonitis. Since infections, whether occult or proven, are the trigger for renal failure in cirrhosis, patients with gastrointestinal bleeding should be given antibiotic prophylaxis. Short-term antibiotic prophylaxis has been shown to increase the survival rate in cirrhotic patients with gastrointestinal bleeding. However, it is unclear as to how long prophylactic antibiotics should be given during any episode of gastrointestinal bleeding.

D. Prophylaxis in Cases of Established Bacterial Infections

Once an infection is established, the release of various cytokines and endotoxins associated with the inflammatory response will trigger the production of many vasodilators. The resultant systemic arterial vasodilation will exaggerate the imbalance between the vascular capacitance and the intravascular volume in the cirrhotic patient, thereby predisposing the patient to the development of renal failure. Albumin infusions have been shown to reduce the incidence of renal failure and improve mortality compared to antibiotics alone in patients with spontaneous bacterial peritonitis. There is still much resistance to the use of albumin in certain parts of the world because of the concern of transmitting unknown diseases. Furthermore, albumin is expensive. It is also not clear whether fluid support with crystalloids or other colloids in patients who did not receive albumin would have produced the same results. Until the results of further trials are available, it seems prudent to give albumin to prevent renal failure in episodes of infection.

E. Prophylaxis against Circulatory Dysfunction

Large volume paracentesis of >5 L is associated with the deterioration of systemic hemodynamics, with a reduction in systemic vascular resistance and hence vasodilation, the so-called postparacentesis circulatory dysfunction. Therefore, it may be prudent to use vasoconstrictor agents such as terlipressin to limit the arterial vasodilation and prevent the circulatory changes that occur in patients undergoing large volume paracentesis.

It has been suggested that pentoxifylline be administered as a prophylaxis against the development of hepatorenal syndrome in patients with alcoholic hepatitis as it has been shown to reduce the incidence of hepatorenal syndrome. Since it is a relatively harmless drug, and the cost is not prohibitive, it may be administered to patients with alcoholic hepatitis until the results of randomized control trials are available.

▶ Prognosis

Hepatorenal syndrome is a dreaded complication of cirrhosis with a dismal outcome. Untreated patients with type 2 hepatorenal syndrome have a slightly better prognosis than patients with type 1 hepatorenal syndrome, with a median survival of months rather than weeks (Figure 10–5). However, their survival is still shorter than that of cirrhotic patients with ascites but no renal dysfunction. Patients without precipitating factors of hepatorenal syndrome tend to survive slightly longer, while those who develop hepatorenal syndrome as a result of sepsis tend to do worse. With a better understanding of the pathophysiology and more effective treatment of hepatorenal syndrome, there has been significant improvement in the outcome of these patients. Since there is a worldwide shortage of donor organs available

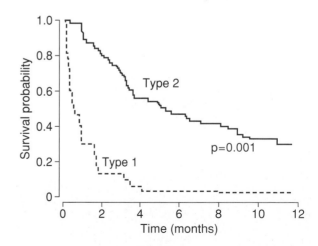

▲ **Figure 10–5.** Survival of patients with hepatorenal syndrome. (Adapted with permission from Gines P et al: Hepatorenal syndrome. Lancet 2003;362:1819.)

for liver transplantation, the strategy may be to use either pharmacotherapy, or TIPS, or a combination of both as a bridge to liver transplantation.

Significant strides have been made in the treatment of hepatorenal syndrome, which used to carry a mortality rate of almost 100%. Based on sound pathophysiologic principles with the reversal of factors causing extreme but potentially reversible renal vasoconstriction, we now have a therapeutic armamentarium to deal with hepatorenal syndrome. The diagnosis of hepatorenal syndrome is no longer synonymous with a death sentence, but rather a therapeutic challenge involving a team approach of intensivists, hepatologists, nephrologists, interventional radiologists, and transplant surgeons to continue to improve the prognosis of these patients. The onus is on us as the treating physicians to recognize the onset of hepatorenal syndrome and to initiate prompt treatment before these patients spiral down the inevitable path of liver failure.

Angeli P: Prognosis of hepatorenal syndrome—has it changed with current practice? Aliment Pharmacol Ther 2004; 20(Suppl. 3):44.

Cardenas A: Hepatorenal syndrome: a dreaded complication of end-stage liver disease. Am J Gastroenterol 2005;100:460.

Cassinello C et al: Effects of orthotopic liver transplantation on vasoactive systems and renal function in patients with advanced liver cirrhosis. Dig Dis Sci 2003;48:179.

Gines P et al: Hepatorenal syndrome. Lancet 2003;362:1819.

Gines P et al: Pharmacological treatment of hepatorenal syndrome. Aliment Pharmacol Ther 2004;20(Suppl. 3):57.

Moreau R et al : Terlipressin in patients with cirrhosis and Type 1 hepatorenal syndrome: a retrospective multicenter study. Gastroenterology 2002;122:923.

Salerno F et al: Diagnosis, prevention and treatment of hepatorenal syndrome in cirrhosis. Gut 2007;56:1310.

Sherman DS et al: Assessing renal function in cirrhotic patients: problems and pitfalls. Am J Kidney Dis 2004;41:269.

Rhabdomyolysis

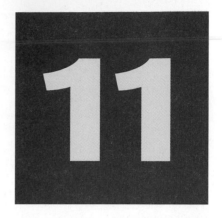

James P. Knochel, MD

ESSENTIALS OF DIAGNOSIS

▶ Muscular pain, tenderness, or weakness.
▶ Elevated creatine kinase MM.

General Considerations

Rhabdomyolysis is a disorder resulting from an injury or a metabolic defect in the skeletal muscle cell (myocyte) resulting in lysis of the cell membrane (sarcolemma) and leakage of its contents (myoglobin, enzymes, phosphorus, potassium) into the blood. Myoglobin is readily filtered by the glomerulus and when it appears in the urine it defines the term myoglobinuria. Although some patients experience few symptoms, most demonstrate muscular pain, tenderness, stiffness, and weakness. Serum creatine kinase (CK) of the MM isoform is nearly always elevated. A rare exception is diabetic myonecrosis, in which painful infarction of skeletal muscle, usually in the thigh, often occurs in the absence of a significant elevation in CK.

Table 11–1 shows a general classification for the causes of rhabdomyolysis.

Pathogenesis

Normal subjects can develop modest rhabdomyolysis after intense exertion. Violent, repetitive activities or a grand mal seizure are good examples. Presumably, exhaustive exercise not only may directly injure structural components of muscle cells, but may also deplete energy stores, which lowers the normal threshold for injury. Other factors that lower the threshold for injury include poor physical condition or preexistent injury, typified by alcoholic myopathy. For any given unit of work, women unexplainably show much less rhabdomyolysis than men. Volume depletion and exercise

in the heat, perhaps by causing overheating of muscle and reduced blood flow, are potentiating factors. Eccentric muscle contractions (running downhill) are more likely to cause rhabdomyolysis than concentric contractions (running uphill). Fasting lowers the threshold presumably by limiting substrates for muscle contraction. Severe trauma and crush injury commonly cause rhabdomyolysis and the related acute renal failure often contributes to the mortality of these conditions. Direct muscle injury during surgery may cause modest elevations of muscle enzymes.

A. Inherited Metabolic Myopathies

A number of specific enzyme derangements are responsible for exertional rhabdomyolysis by impairing energy metabolism. Classic examples are myophosphorylase deficiency (McArdle's syndrome) and carnitine palmityltransferase deficiency.

B. Acquired Metabolic Myopathies

Potassium deficiency is a typical example. Potassium deficiency impairs glycogen synthesis in muscle. Since glycogen is a major energy substrate during anaerobic work, physical work performed by a potassium-deficient individual can result in rhabdomyolysis. Potassium deficiency also interferes with the normal increase of muscle blood flow with exercise. This can impose damage by ischemia. Phosphorus deficiency may also cause rhabdomyolysis. This is most frequently seen in severe alcoholics and/or in patients being refed after severe weight loss.

C. Hypoxia/Ischemia

Carbon monoxide poisoning, by causing hypoxia due to carboxyhemoglobin formation, is a recognized cause of acute rhabdomyolysis. Severe congestive heart failure may cause modest rhabdomyolysis.

Table 11–1. Causes of rhabdomyolysis.

Exertion and physical trauma
  Direct trauma
    Crush syndrome
    Prolonged pressure with coma
    Electrical shock
    Thermal burns
    Freezing

  Excessive exercise
    Athletic injury
    Convulsive seizures
    Punitive exercise

  Hereditary myopathies
    Myophosphorylase deficiency
      (McArdle's disease)
    Carnitine palmitoyltransferase deficiency

  Acquired metabolic disorders
    Hyperthyroidism
    Diabetic ketoacidosis
    Potassium deficiency
    Phosphorus deficiency with acute hypophosphatemia
    Alcoholism
    Acute hyponatremia

  Hypoxia and ischemia
    Carbon monoxide poisoning
    Vascular occlusion
    Atheromatous embolism
    Compartment syndrome

  Drugs
    Cocaine
    Ephedra compounds
    Amphetamine derivatives
    3-Hydroxy-3-methylglutaryl coreductase inhibitors
      (statins)
    Lipid-lowering drugs

  Infectious disorders
    Bacterial
      Clostridial infection
      Legionella
      Streptococcal infection
      Staphylococcal infection
      Pneumococcal pneumonia

    Viral
      Influenza
      Coxsackie
      HIV

    Toxins
      Snake venom
      Poisonous mushrooms
      Quail fed on sweet parsley seeds
      Fish poisoning (Haff disease)

    Miscellaneous
      Malignant hyperthermia
      Neuroleptic malignant syndrome

D. Drugs

Many drugs cause rhabdomyolysis. Although hundreds have been implicated anecdotally, those of major concern include cocaine and amphetamine derivatives. Recent studies have shown that experimentally, ephedrine and ecstasy (3,4-methylenedioxymethamphetamine, MDMA) stimulate β_3-adrenergic receptors in skeletal muscle resulting in overproduction of heat and myocyte injury, thus explaining the combination of rhabdomyolysis and hyperthermia observed in these cases.

The 3-hydroxy-3-methylglutaryl coenzyme A (HMG-CoA) reductase inhibitors (statins) are common causes of rhabdomyolysis. This adverse reaction may occur with statin monotherapy but is potentiated by simultaneous use of a number of drugs including fibric acid derivatives, cyclosporine, nicotinic acid, or erythromycin. These drugs and the statins are metabolized by the same enzyme system (P4SO3A4) in muscle or liver, thus increasing statin concentration to toxic levels. Prevention of rhabdomyolysis in patients using legitimate medications known to increase the risk of myocyte injury is a more difficult issue. Some patients show a modest increase in CK levels during statin therapy but have neither complaints nor clinically adverse effects. However, it is recommended that anyone developing symptoms or showing a 10-fold rise in CK levels (to 2500 IU/L) or more should stop the drug.

E. Infections

Viral infections, especially influenza, coxsackievirus, and HIV, may be directly myopathic causing severe rhabdomyolysis. Certain bacterial infections including pneumococcal pneumonia, gas gangrene, systemic streptococcal infections, and *Legionella* are also well known causes.

F. Special Causes

A number of substances are directly myotoxic. Severe rhabdomyolysis has occurred following snake bites due to the proteolytic enzymes in venom. It has also been caused by a myotoxin that accumulates in skeletal muscle after consuming quail that have eaten sweet parsley seeds. Hypothyroidism consistently causes elevated CK and sometimes causes frank rhabdomyolysis. Acute dermatomyositis may rarely cause rhabdomyolysis. Finally, moderate elevations in creatine kinase, muscle type (CKMM) occur in a variety of serious illnesses including hypoxia, congestive heart failure, and sepsis.

Malignant hyperthermia is a rare inherited abnormality of the ryanodine receptor in skeletal muscle that presents as acute attacks of muscular rigidity, hypoxia, increased CO_2 production, metabolic and respiratory acidosis, hyperthermia, and rhabdomyolysis. It usually occurs during general anesthesia and is provoked by succinylcholine and volatile anesthetics. It is often fatal unless promptly recognized and prevented or treated with dantrolene.

Neuroleptic malignant syndrome is a condition characterized by muscular rigidity, dystonia, and in some cases, fever. It occurs as an adverse reaction to a variety of neuroleptic drugs. Severe rhabdomyolysis may be a complication.

▶ Prevention

Most persons who have undergone serious physical fitness programs have developed painful and stiff muscles during the first few days. They may show modestly elevated CK activity (up to 10,000 IU/L) and in this sense, most of us have experienced rhabdomyolysis. Physical training elevates the threshold of injury. Some believe that exercise-induced muscle injury is a necessary component of myocyte remodeling and hypertrophy during the training process. Perhaps an element of rhabdomyolysis is physiologic, representing the trainer's concept of "no pain, no gain." Extreme violent and repetitive exercise such as squat thrusts or pull ups to the point of exhaustion may have serious consequences. Thus, in untrained persons, a more gradual increase in the tempo and duration of such activities will allow them to become trained safely. Work in the heat, electrolyte and water depletion, and use of drugs purported to enhance physical performance such as amphetamine derivatives, ephedra compounds, and cocaine should be avoided.

▶ Clinical Findings

The symptoms and physical findings in rhabdomyolysis are usually sufficiently characteristic to make a diagnosis. Muscular pain, tenderness, edema, stiffness, weakness, and impaired mobility are common. It is risky to assume that this clinical presentation is merely a "back sprain" or "fibromyalgia." It is necessary to consider rhabdomyolysis and rule it in or out by measuring CK levels.

The CKMM is the dominant isoform in skeletal muscle and the most sensitive test to confirm the diagnosis. Without ongoing necrosis, CK peaks at 12–36 hours after muscle injury and has a $t_{1/2}$ of about 48 hours. The creatine kinase, myocardial bound (CKMB) isoform, commonly employed to detect myocardial injury, may comprise 5% of total CK in skeletal muscle of highly trained athletes. Total CK levels seldom exceed 5000 IU/L in myocardial infarction. Any level higher than 5000 IU/L should lead to a suspicion of acute rhabdomyolysis. In rhabdomyolysis of clinical importance, elevations of this enzyme commonly reach levels of 100,000 IU/L or more. In extreme cases, CK may approach 3 million IU/L. Elevations of other muscle enzymes in rhabdomyolysis such as aldolase, lactic dehydrogenous, or transaminases provide no additional useful information. Elevations of γ-glutamyltransferase (GGT) do not occur as a result of muscle injury and, accordingly, this test is useful to exclude hepatic injury.

A transient elevation of serum creatinine disproportionate to the elevation of blood urea nitrogen (BUN) is common in early acute rhabdomyolysis. Presumably, this results from release of creatine from injured muscle, which is spontaneously dehydrated to creatinine. The usual ratio of urea nitrogen to creatinine in serum is 10:1. Ratios of 5 or less shortly after onset suggest acute rhabdomyolysis. Uric acid in serum may exceed 40 mg/dL. Purines released from injured muscle are converted to urate in the liver. Hyperuricemia of this magnitude is seldom seen in other conditions, even acute tumor lysis induced by chemotherapy. Leukocytosis is common in rhabdomyolysis of any etiology. Hypoalbuminemia, especially when associated with hemoconcentration, is an ominous sign and implies major capillary damage with leakage of plasma components out of the vascular space. On rare occasions, capillary damage may be so extensive that erythrocytes also escape into interstitial tissues. This results in shock with an acute reduction of hematocrit in the absence of bleeding or hemolysis. In oliguric patients, a urine sodium concentration above 20 mEq/L suggests tubular injury. However, the urine sodium concentration may be low in cases of myoglobinuria and, accordingly, this finding in pigment nephropathy may be less helpful than in other oliguric settings. Hyperkalemia is often observed as a consequence of release of potassium from damaged muscle cells. Profound hypocalcemia, with serum calcium values below 3.0 mg/dL, may result from hyperphosphatemia and trapping of calcium in injured muscle. Hypercalcemia may occur later, especially during the diuretic phase of acute renal failure. Usually, this is seen in patients who have been given calcium salts earlier in the illness.

▶ Differential Diagnosis

There are fundamental differences between the fate of hemoglobin and myoglobin after their release into plasma. Free hemoglobin in plasma saturates haptoglobin at a concentration of approximately 100 mg/dL. Because the hemoglobin–haptoglobin complex is a large molecule, it is not filtered by the glomerulus. Accordingly, hemoglobin will not appear in the urine until plasma haptoglobin becomes saturated and total hemoglobin exceeds 100 mg/dL. Both hemoglobin and myoglobin become visible in serum or urine at a concentration of 100 mg/dL. In contrast to hemoglobin, myoglobin has no quantitatively important binding protein in plasma. Myoglobin has a molecular weight of about 16,000 Da, and has a fractional clearance (compared to that of inulin) of 75%. Thus, any myoglobin entering plasma is readily filtered by the glomerulus. Therefore, the presence of stained serum suggests hemolysis, not rhabdomyolysis. Accordingly, if heme pigment is present in the urine, a clear serum suggests rhabdomyolysis and myoglobinuria. Discoloration of both serum and urine suggests hemoglobinuria. Because dipstick tests are exquisitely sensitive for detection of heme pigment in the urine, there is no practical need to perform more sophisticated and expensive tests to either detect or differentiate myoglobin or hemoglobin in either plasma or urine. Classic findings of a pigmented urine that has a positive dipstick test for blood in the absence of significant hematuria is of help diagnostically. However, this complex of findings may be lacking unless checked early in the course. Since myoglobin is rapidly excreted, it may be easily missed. Glycosuria in the absence of hyperglycemia is another common laboratory finding early in the cause of myoglobinuria. It may reflect proximal tubular injury.

The classic pathologic findings in pigment nephropathy include proximal tubular necrosis and distal tubular obstruction by pigmented casts. The mechanisms underlying acute renal failure have been explored in detail. Heme pigments are intense vasoconstrictors and can cause renal ischemia. Once the myoglobin or hemoglobin molecule is filtered by the glomerulus and enters the proximal tubular fluid, a portion enters the proximal tubular cell. Inside the cell, the molecule releases elemental iron and iron compounds, forming toxic products that injure or kill the proximal tubular cell. The remaining unabsorbed pigment passes to the distal nephron. If the tubular urine has an acid pH, the pigment will interact with Tamm–Horsfall proteins, form a gel, and obstruct flow. Once this occurs, the concentration of pigment in the tubule above that level rises, augmenting proximal tubular absorption and toxicity.

▶ Treatment

When acute renal failure complicating crush injury was described shortly after World War II, it was recognized that when pigmenturia occurs in a setting of hypotension, decreased renal perfusion, and an acid urine, acute tubular necrosis is likely to follow. Subsequent experimental studies showed that if arterial volume, blood pressure, and renal perfusion were intact before the event, infusion of crude muscle extracts, myoglobin, or hemoglobin had no adverse effects on renal function. Experimental studies also showed that infusion of saline, bicarbonate solutions, or mannitol before pigmenturia was induced protected against acute renal failure.

The foregoing principles form the basis for early treatment of rhabdomyolysis and myoglobinuria. Severe cases should be managed in critical care units where staffing and dialysis facilities are available. Aggressive and urgent volume replacement to maintain organ perfusion is critical. Alkalinization of the urine with bicarbonate infusions to prevent obstructive cast formation is recommended but not always achievable in severe cases. If the urine remains acid despite overcorrection of serum bicarbonate levels, acetazolamide might be considered. Caution must be taken to avoid volume overload and pulmonary edema. Since myoglobin is a direct toxin to the kidney, it seems sensible to enhance its clearance by employing mannitol. Infusion of 25 g of mannitol may increase urine flow and clearance of myoglobin, thereby at least theoretically reducing myoglobin toxicity.

After rising for several days, serum CK levels should begin to fall. If there is a secondary rise in CK, a compartment syndrome should be considered. There is some evidence that early employment of intravenous mannitol may forestall this complication. Respiratory failure due to diaphragm weakness may occur in severe cases. Careful and frequent observation for hyperkalemia is mandatory. Hyperkalemia may not be controllable by glucose and insulin infusions alone because of extensive muscle cell injury. Frank potassium cardiotoxicity may occur with serum potassium concentrations in the vicinity of 6.5 mEq/L in those patients who are severely hypocalcemic. This means that monitoring for hyperkalemic toxicity is best done by electrocardiographic changes and not only serum potassium levels. If electrocardiographic changes suggestive of hyperkalemia despite only modest hyperkalemia appear, a test dose of calcium salts will cause temporary reversal of these changes without affecting serum potassium values. Frequent and sometimes nearly constant hemodialysis may be necessary in such cases. Hypocalcemia per se is usually not treated unless necessary because infused calcium salts tend to precipitate in injured muscle. These precipitates become mobilized later in the diuretic stage and may cause serious hypercalcemia. Nonetheless, calcium salt infusions may be lifesaving for temporary reversal of hyperkalemic cardiotoxicity while preparing a patient for dialysis. Infection and volume overload are also important complications. In severe cases, coagulopathy consequent to liver injury or disseminated intravascular coagulation is a common complication.

▶ Prognosis

Patients who survive acute extensive rhabdomyolysis are at risk for permanent disability due to muscle fibrosis. Others appear to recover completely, thus making it difficult to predict outcome for any given case. Any patient who suffers repeated episodes of rhabdomyolysis should be considered for specific testing to determine if there is a cause such as McArdle's disease or other metabolic disorders. In cases provoked by combinations of statins and medications preventing their metabolism (eg, fibrates), patients may often resume statin monotherapy safely but must be observed carefully when this decision is made.

Bywaters EGL, Beall D: Crush injuries with impairment of renal function. Republished with comments by E.G. Bywaters and J.P. Knochel: Milestones in nephrology. J Am Soc Nephrol 1998;9:322. [PMID: 9527411]

Grundy SM: The issue of statin safety. Where do we stand? Editorial. http://www.circulationaha.org. DOI:10.1161/Circulation AHA. 105.557652. [PMID: 15911705]

Vanholder R et al: Rhabdomyolysis. J Am Soc Nephrol 2000; 11:1553. [PMID: 10906171]

Contrast-Induced Nephropathy

12

Steven Brunelli, MD, & Michael R. Rudnick, MD, FACP

ESSENTIALS OF DIAGNOSIS

▶ Rise of serum creatinine of ≥0.5 mg/dL or 25% above baseline within 48 hours after parenteral contrast administration.

▶ Majority of cases are nonoliguric.

▶ Peak in serum creatinine usually occurs within 3–5 days with complete resolution in 7–10 days for most patients.

▶ Oliguria and need for dialysis are unusual and are primarily seen in patients with diabetes with severe chronic kidney disease.

▶ General Considerations

Contrast-induced nephropathy (CIN) is a common cause of hospital-acquired acute renal failure. Although the incidence of CIN is low, the number of patients receiving intravenous contrast media is enormous and is expected to rise as the population ages and greater numbers of patients will be subjected to diagnostic and therapeutic procedures requiring intravascular contrast.

Observational retrospective studies have demonstrated that patients incurring CIN had significantly higher in-hospital mortality than counterparts who did not develop CIN, particularly so if they went on to need dialysis. Multivariate regression analysis, adjusting for baseline differences in comorbidities, strongly suggests that CIN is, in fact, an independent predictor of mortality.

Various patient and procedural factors influence the likelihood of developing CIN. Among patient-related factors, preexisting chronic kidney disease (CKD) is regarded as the most potent risk factor. Nearly 60% of patients developing CIN have baseline CKD, and the incidence of CIN parallels the severity of prestanding renal impairment. Diabetes

mellitus also confers increased risk of developing CIN, but only in patients with CKD. Thus the risk of CIN is greatest in patients with CKD and diabetes, lower in nondiabetic patients with CKD, and lowest in patients without preexisting CKD regardless of their diabetic status. Similarly, patients with CKD and diabetes are at the highest risk of developing oliguric acute renal failure and of requiring dialysis. Patients with CIN who require dialysis have a very high in-hospital mortality.

Volume depletion, congestive heart failure, older age, and hypotension have all been cited as risk factors for CIN but are probably primarily markers for a low glomerular filtration rate (GFR), the true risk factor. Concomitant use of nephrotoxins such as nonsteroidal anti-inflammatory agents also increase the risk for CIN.

Multiple myeloma has traditionally been considered a risk factor for CIN. However, recent studies using modern contrast agents indicate that patients with multiple myeloma are not at a greater risk, provided that they are volume replete at the time of contrast exposure.

Procedure-related factors will also influence the likelihood of CIN. Most studies, although not all, suggest that exposure to larger volumes of parenteral contrast causes greater predisposition to CIN. In addition, the type of contrast material (specifically its osmolality) influences the development of CIN. Contrast media formulations occur in three types: High-osmolar contrast media (also termed ionic), which have an osmolality of approximately 2000 mOsm/L, low-osmolar contrast media (also termed nonionic), which have an osmolality of 600–900 mOsm/L, and iso-osmolar contrast media (also a nonionic composition), which have an osmolality of 300 mOsm/L (Figure 12–1). Multiple studies in high-risk patients with CKD have demonstrated that low-osmolar contrast media results in less CIN than high-osmolar contrast media, and there is some evidence that iso-osmolar contrast media may be less nephrotoxic than low-osmolar contrast media.

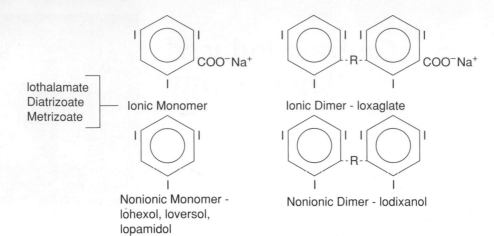

▲ Figure 12–1. Chemical structure of contrast agents.

▶ Pathogenesis

Several mechanisms have been proposed to explain the pathogenesis of CIN. Measures aimed to prevent CIN (see Prevention below) are based on these pathogenetic mechanisms. Renal ischemia is currently considered the primary mechanism for CIN. It is known that the outer renal medulla has an extremely low oxygen tension (PO_2 10–20 mm Hg), as the result of countercurrent oxygen exchange and removal between vasa rectae and utilization of oxygen by active tubular transport by the ascending loop of Henle. Administration of contrast media has been shown to selectively further reduce oxygen tension in this area of the kidney by a two-pronged mechanism. The first is reduction in renal blood flow, mediated by release of vasoconstrictive compounds such as endothelin and adenosine, an effect that is magnified by blockade of vasodilatory compounds such as nitric oxide and prostaglandins. The second is increased oxygen utilization caused by increased work of active transport in response to an osmotic diuresis induced by contrast media in the renal tubule. A summary of these effects is depicted in Figure 12–2.

Hyperosmolarity may itself be etiologic in the development of CIN. Intratubular hyperosmolality may activate tubuloglomerular feedback or increase intratubular hydrostatic pressure, either of which could reduce glomerular filtration. Hyperosmolality may also increase tubular cell apoptosis.

There is also evidence to suggest that generation of oxygen free radicals contributes to the pathogenesis of CIN. This theory would explain the possible ability of N-acetylcysteine (NAC), a free radical scavenger, and sodium bicarbonate, which inhibits the enzymatic formation of free radicals, to prevent CIN (see Prevention below).

Finally, there is evidence to suggest that contrast media cause direct cellular toxicity. Contrast media have been shown to cause proximal tubule cell vacuolization, interstitial inflammation, and cellular necrosis both in experimental animals and in isolated nephron segments.

▶ Prevention

Multiple preventive strategies for CIN have been studied (Table 12–1). A number of these have been proven to be ineffective in well-designed, randomized control trials. Among this group are diuretics, mannitol, dopamine, atrial natriuretic peptide, endothelin receptor antagonists, and fenoldopam. Other strategies have proven more successful and are discussed below.

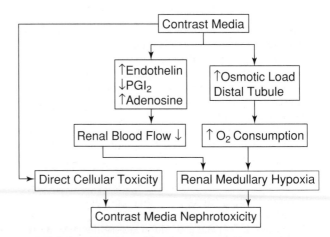

▲ Figure 12–2. Mechanism for contrast-induced nephropathy. (Adapted with permission from Heyman SN et al: Radiocontrast nephropathy: a paradigm for the synergism between toxic and hypoxic insults in the kidney. Exp Nephrol 1994;2:153.)

Table 12–1. Strategies for the prevention of contrast-induced nephropathy.

Strategies that do not work
  Mannitol
  Furosemide
  Dopamine
  Atrial natriuretic factor
  Fenoldopam
  Hemodialysis
Strategies that may work
  Calcium channel blockers
  Theophylline
  N-Acetylcysteine
  Hemofiltration
  Sodium bicarbonate
  Ascorbic acid
  Iso-osmolar contrast media
Current recommended strategies
  Employ noniodinated contrast studies
  Avoid nonsteroidal anti-inflamatory agents
  Space between contrast administrations
  Minimize contrast volume
  Hydration
  Low osmolar contrast media

Extracellular fluid (ECF) volume expansion has traditionally been considered the primary therapeutic intervention to prevent CIN. Correction of volume contraction with ECF expansion is expected to diminish vasoconstrictive responses that contribute to renal ischemia and decrease contact time and concentration of contrast media within the renal tubules. Early clinical studies using historic controls suggested a beneficial role for ECF expansion. Following these studies, volume expansion quickly became the standard of care, although no prospective, randomized, placebo-controlled studies have been conducted to evaluate its efficacy, probably for ethical concerns. Subsequent studies have attempted to delineate the best protocol for prophylactic ECF expansion, but to date, no consensus has been reached due to variability among studies in quality, size, subject selection, and endpoint definition. The limited literature suggests that intravenous volume expansion is superior to oral, that longer courses of parenteral fluid administration are superior to shorter courses, and that isotonic fluids are superior to hypotonic fluids.

NAC was first reported in the late 1990s to be a viable prophylactic strategy for CIN. The most commonly employed dose of NAC is 600 mg by mouth twice daily the day prior to and the day of contrast administration. Initially, this finding was greeted with widespread enthusiasm and the use of NAC quickly became common in clinical practice. Subsequent studies of its efficacy have been mixed, as have meta-analyses of those studies. To date, it remains uncertain if NAC is an effective preventative measure, but it is nonetheless often used in clinical practice, based on its safety, simplicity, and low cost.

Theophylline may also be effective in the prevention on CIN. Several studies have demonstrated that theophylline blunts the decrement in GFR following contrast exposure, possibly by inhibiting adenosine-induced renal vasoconstriction. However, none of these studies included high-risk patients nor has clinically significant CIN been observed in theophylline-treated subjects or controls. Therefore no conclusions can be made about its efficacy. It should be noted that theophylline carries the risk of precipitating ventricular arrhythmias, seizures, and other adverse effects, and these drawbacks must be factored into any decision regarding its use in CIN prophylaxis.

Reduction in contrast volume and osmolality are well-established and reliable means of diminishing the occurrence of CIN in high-risk azotemic patients. With regard to osmolality, clinical trials have established the superiority of low-osmolar over high-osmolar contrast media. Although initial clinical reports demonstrate lower nephrotoxicity with iso-osmolar versus at least one low-osmolar contrast media, the relative nephrotoxicity of iso-osmolar contrast media is still under investigation.

Although hemodialysis has largely been proven not to be an efficacious means of CIN prophylaxis, hemofiltration has been suggested to be effective. Unfortunately, limitations in study design do not allow the value of hemofiltration in this setting to be known for certain. Given the high cost and logistic difficulty associated with providing hemofiltration, this modality is unlikely to gain widespread clinical acceptance for CIN prophylaxis unless additional and better designed studies demonstrate its effectiveness.

Although initial reports showed a superiority of sodium bicarbonate over saline in the prevention of CIN, more recent publications suggest that the two modalities have equivalent prophylactic value. Additional studies are ongoing which may further clarify the question of whether sodium bicarbonate has any advantage compared to isotonic saline in this setting.

▶ Clinical Findings

A. Symptoms and Signs

In the vast majority of patients with CIN, there are no symptoms or signs that would indicate the presence of this complication. In a smaller subset of affected patients, symptoms of oliguria with or without symptoms or physical findings of fluid overload may be present. Rarely, a patient with CIN may present with symptoms and signs of uremia.

B. Laboratory Findings

In the majority of patients with CIN, the serum creatinine value begins to rise within 24–48 hours after contrast media exposure, peaks within 3–5 days, and returns to baseline levels within 7–10 days. The majority of patients are nonoliguric and often have low urine sodium concentration.

In more severe cases of CIN, the serum creatinine may not peak until 5–10 days and may be accompanied by oliguria and a requirement for dialysis. Severe cases of CIN are more often (though not exclusively) seen in patients with advanced CKD, particularly those with coexisting diabetes mellitus.

The urinalysis in patients with CIN typically demonstrates coarse granular casts, renal tubular epithelial cells, and amorphous debris, findings characteristic of acute tubular necrosis.

C. Imaging Tests

Renal imaging is not helpful in confirming the diagnosis of CIN, but may be undertaken to exclude other causes of acute renal failure (ie, renal ultrasound to obstructive nephropathy).

► Differential Diagnosis

Renal atheroembolism as a cause of acute renal failure following contrast exposure needs to be distinguished from CIN. This complication may arise in any patient who receives contrast media through an arterial route, regardless of whether the contrast was administered for a diagnostic procedure or for an interventional therapeutic indication. Renal atheroembolism is suggested when the rise in serum creatinine begins more than 48 hours after contrast exposure but can also present within 48 hours following contrast administration. On physical examination, the physician should look for livedo reticularis, digital ischemia (purple/blue toe syndrome), retinal embolization (Hollenhorst plaque), or other signs of systemic embolization, which would suggest atheroembolism. Patients with atheroembolism may demonstrate urine or peripheral blood eosinophilia and/or hypocomplementemia on laboratory analysis, abnormalities not found with CIN.

Since contrast media are commonly administered to hemodynamically unstable patients, the possibility of ischemic acute tubular necrosis in the differential of acute renal failure following contrast exposure must be considered. Clinically, acute renal failure from ischemia may be difficult to impossible to distinguish from CIN.

Other diagnoses to consider are allergic interstitial nephritis (since many contrast-exposed patients will be hospitalized and receive new medications), which usually presents with some combination of fever, rash, peripheral blood eosinophilia and sterile pyuria, and obstructive nephropathy, which is suggested by absent to low urine output and hydronephrosis seen on renal imaging.

► Treatment

There is no specific therapy for CIN once it occurs. The best strategy is one of prevention. Preemptive nephrologic consultation to ensure that optimal prophylactic strategies are provided may be of value in certain high-risk azotemic patients.

Once a patient develops CIN, care should be taken to judiciously manage fluid and electrolytes and adjust medications that are renally eliminated. Regular monitoring of electrolytes, blood urea nitrogen (BUN), and creatinine is recommended since it is not possible to predict which patients with CIN will have a short, transient, and asymptomatic course of acute renal failure or demonstrate more clinically severe acute renal failure. Patients developing oliguria, severe electrolyte or acid–base abnormalities, or volume overload may require hemodialysis. Patients with advanced CKD, particularly those with diabetes mellitus, are most likely to require dialytic support.

► Prognosis

Complete recovery of renal function usually occurs in patients affected with CIN. A small minority of patients may go on to require chronic renal replacement therapy while others may be left with residual renal injury but not require dialysis. Patients in the former group invariably have severe CKD prior to contrast administration. The proportion of patients who develop sustained, subclinical decrements in GFR is unknown.

In recent years, multiple studies have suggested that in-hospital mortality is significantly higher in patients developing CIN after contrast exposure than those without this complication. Mortality appears to be highest in those patients with CIN who require hemodialysis. Methodologic limitations of these studies do not allow a definitive conclusion as to whether the higher mortality seen in these patients is due to CIN per se or other comorbidities more commonly seen in the patients affected with CIN.

Aspelin P et al for the Nephric Study Investigators: Nephrotoxic effects in high-risk patients undergoing angiography. N Engl J Med 2003;348:491.

Bader BD et al: What is the best hydration regimen to prevent contrast media-induced nephrotoxicity? Clin Nephrol 2004;62:1.

Brar SS et al: Sodium bicarbonate vs sodium chloride for the prevention of contrast medium-induced nephropathy in patients undergoing coronary angiography: a randomized trial. JAMA. 2008 3;300:1038.

Durham JD et al: A randomized controlled trial of N-acetylcysteine to prevent contrast nephropathy in cardiac angiography. Kidney Int 2002;62:2202.

Marenzi G et al: The prevention of radiocontrast-agent-induced nephropathy by hemofiltration. N Engl J Med 2003;349:1333.

Merten GJ et al: Prevention of contrast-induced nephropathy with sodium bicarbonate. A randomized controlled trial. JAMA 2004;291:2328.

Pannu N et al: Systematic review of the impact of N-acetylcysteine on contrast nephropathy. Kidney Int 2004;65:1366.

Trivedi HS et al: A prospective randomized trial to assess the role of saline hydration on the development of contrast nephrotoxicity. Nephron Clin Pract 2003;93:c29.

Tumor Lysis Syndrome

13

Brian Stephany, MD, & Martin Schreiber, Jr, MD

ESSENTIALS OF DIAGNOSIS

▶ Hyperuricemia, hyperkalemia, hyperphosphatemia, hypocalcemia, often accompanied by azotemia and oliguric acute renal failure.

▶ Caused by the rapid release of the intracellular contents of tumor cells into the systemic circulation.

▶ Most commonly seen following treatment of hematologic malignancies of high cellular burden and chemosensitivity, such as lymphomas and leukemias.

General Considerations

First described in 1929, tumor lysis syndrome (TLS) defines a well-established constellation of potentially fatal metabolic derangements that can occur most commonly following chemotherapy for certain hematologic malignancies such as acute lymphoblastic leukemia or high-grade non-Hodgkin's lymphoma (NHL) (Table 13–1). Less commonly, TLS complicates the treatment of other hematologic malignancies such as chronic lymphocytic leukemia, acute myeloid leukemia, plasma cell disorders including multiple myeloma or isolated plasmacytomas, Hodgkin's lymphoma, and low- or intermediate-grade NHL. Finally, TLS has been reported anecdotally in the setting of solid tumors such as testicular cancer, breast cancer, and lung cancer. Although usually seen after the administration of cytoreductive chemotherapy, TLS can occur spontaneously prior to initiation of any treatment and also may be seen following other therapies such as radiation, corticosteroids, interferon-α, rituximab, and tamoxifen.

This oncologic emergency is characterized by the acute onset of hyperuricemia, hyperkalemia, hyperphosphatemia, and hypocalcemia, often associated with acute renal failure (ARF). TLS results from the rapid release of the intracellular contents of tumor cells (ie, uric acid, phosphate, potassium) into the systemic circulation that overwhelms physiologic metabolic pathways that maintain homeostasis. Not all patients with cancer develop TLS, and the incidence varies depending on the patient population studied and exact definition of TLS used. Factors associated with an increased risk of developing TLS include bulky tumors of high cellular burden and rapid proliferation kinetics (such as Burkitt's lymphoma or acute lymphocytic leukemia), extensive bone marrow involvement, lactate dehydrogenase levels above 1500 IU/mL (a surrogate marker of tumor cellular burden), and tumors with exquisite sensitivity to chemotherapy or radiation.

The clinical consequence of TLS is dependent on the degree of organ damage inflicted by these metabolic derangements, most notably acute kidney, cardiovascular, and neurologic complications. ARF as evidenced by worsening azotemia (usually defined as an increase in serum creatinine greater than 30–50% of baseline) is a serious but potentially reversible entity that commonly accompanies TLS. Renal replacement therapy may be required in up to 30% of cases of ARF associated with TLS. The etiology of ARF as part of this syndrome is multifactorial, but primarily is due to acute obstruction of urine flow by precipitated uric acid crystals within the renal tubules as well as acute nephrocalcinosis with interstitial and tubular damage from calcium–phosphorus complex deposition.

Risk factors associated with ARF accompanying TLS include preexisting chronic kidney disease, volume depletion with a concentrated urine, concomitant nephrotoxic medication use, and an acidic urine pH that can facilitate uric acid crystal formation. ARF is not only a consequence of TLS, but also can exacerbate the metabolic derangements and limit the efficacy of medical therapies to correct it. If left untreated, TLS associated with ARF may lead to dangerous disturbances in potassium, phosphorus, and calcium and lead to severe, life-threatening cardiac arrhythmias, seizures, muscle paralysis, and death.

Table 13–1. Characteristic laboratory abnormalities encountered in tumor lysis syndrome and their clinical consequences.

Electrolyte		Pathophysiology	Clinical consequence	Treatment options
Potassium	↑	Rapid expulsion of intracellular potassium into the circulation due to cell lysis	Adverse muscle (skeletal and cardiac) and neurologic manifestations: Muscle cramps/weakness, paresthesias, ventricular arrhythmia	Calcium gluconate, insulin/glucose, sodium bicarbonate, inhaled β-agonist, potassium-binding resins, dialysis
Phosphate	↑	Release of intracellular phosphate with cell lysis (compounded by reduced renal phosphorus clearance) leads to a rapid rise in phosphorus and drop in calcium due to the precipitation of calcium–phosphorus complexes	Muscle cramps, tetany, arrhythmias, seizures; exacerbation of acute renal failure through calcium–phosphorus complex deposition in renal interstitium and tubules (ie, acute nephrocalcinosis)	Phosphate binders, dialysis
Calcium	↓			Calcium gluconate (only in symptomatic patients exhibiting neuromuscular irritability)
Uric acid	↑	Cell lysis leads to increased levels of purine nucleotides into the circulation that are metabolized to uric acid	Renal failure (uric acid nephropathy)	Hydration, alkalization of urine, xanthine oxidase inhibitors, urate oxidase, dialysis
Creatinine	↑	Decreased GFR from urate crystal tubular obstruction, acute nephrocalcinosis, ± concomitant ATN or volume depletion	Oligoanuria, uric acid crystalluria, urine uric acid/creatinine ratio >1, radiographic hydronephrosis (rare)	Force diuresis with intravenous fluids and/or diuretics, increased uric acid solubility, decreased uric acid production, dialysis

GFR, glomerular filtration rate; ATN, acute tubular necrosis.

▶ Prevention

Although spontaneous cases of TLS occur where preemptive therapy is not possible, the majority of cases of TLS can be predicted based on both tumor and patient-specific risk factors. Thus, imperative in the management of TLS is early and aggressive initiation of preventive measures that may both attenuate the severity of electrolyte disturbances and hopefully prevent any kidney damage as tumor cells begin to lyse.

▶ Clinical Findings

A. Symptoms, Signs, and Laboratory Findings

The clinical presentation of patients with TLS is varied and depends on the extent of metabolic derangements present and type of end-organ damage caused by the released intracellular products. A heightened clinical suspicion for TLS should be maintained in those patients with known malignancies associated with high-risk features, especially following tumor reduction therapy.

1. Hyperkalemia—Hyperkalemia (ie, potassium level >5 mEq/L) develops commonly in TLS and may be seen as early as 6 hours postchemotherapy. The predominant mechanism is a shift of large intracellular stores of potassium into the extracellular fluid (ECF) compartment as tumor cells lyse. In addition, a further shift of potassium

out of viable tumor and host cells may occur if metabolic acidosis due to renal failure is present. Finally, the presence of chronic kidney disease prior to TLS and/or ARF developing as a result of TLS impairs renal clearance of this potassium load to the ECF, thereby exacerbating the severity of hyperkalemia and limiting the efficacy of attempts at medical management.

As the ratio of intracellular to extracellular potassium is important in the maintenance of the normal resting membrane potential, the symptoms associated with hyperkalemia most commonly reflect altered neuronal and muscular excitability. Mild elevations in serum potassium can manifest as lethargy, muscle weakness, muscle cramps, and paresthesias. Unfortunately, concomitant hypocalcemia often seen in TLS can further exacerbate the hyperkalemia-induced membrane excitability and neuromuscular symptoms. More progressive hyperkalemia is worrisome due to its effect on the cardiac conduction system, as can be seen during electrocardiogram (ECG) monitoring by peaked T waves, PR and QRS interval prolongation, various atrioventricular blocks, and eventual asystole and cardiac standstill.

In general, serum potassium levels >6.0 mEq/L associated with neuromuscular manifestations or ECG changes require immediate correction. However, one important caveat to consider is pseudohyperkalemia, which is frequently encountered in hematologic malignancies with significant elevations in white blood cell counts (ie, >100,000/mm³). The elevated potassium results from its release from leukocytes mechanically lysed during phlebotomy or as a result of shift following coagulation of blood within the vial. In such cases, the potassium levels returned by the laboratory, sometimes significantly elevated, do not reflect the level *in vivo* and are not associated with neuromuscular symptoms or ECG changes. By not using tourniquets and measuring plasma (instead of serum) values, potassium values that reliably reflect *in vivo* levels can be obtained.

2. Hypocalcemia and hyperphosphatemia—Disturbances in calcium and phosphorus are common in TLS, and following cytoreductive therapy typically occur within 24–48 hours. The massive phosphorus load to the extracellular compartment as tumor cells lyse can overwhelm the maximal renal phosphaturic threshold thus leading to levels above 4.5 mg/dL, sometimes of great severity (ie, >15 mg/dL). Hypocalcemia, ie, a total calcium level <8.5 mg/dL corrected for albumin or an ionized calcium level <1.08 mmol/L, develops in the setting of hyperphosphatemia as calcium complexes with rising phosphorus levels. These calcium–phosphorus complexes are insoluble at physiologic conditions and precipitate in various tissues and can result in end-organ damage seen in TLS (ie, acute nephrocalcinosis). To a lesser degree, sustained hypocalcemia may also be a result of less 1,25-dihydroxyvitamin D_3 (ie, calcitriol) synthesis.

Patients with TLS and disturbances of calcium and phosphorus typically manifest with neuromuscular signs or symptoms related to the hypocalcemia. In particular, patients can present with paresthesias, muscle cramps, tetany (eg, Chvostek's sign or carpopedal spasm), or seizures. Cardiac manifestations may also accompany significant hypocalcemia, most notably prolongation of the QT interval on ECG and depression of cardiac contractility leading to hypotension.

3. Hyperuricemia—Uric acid is produced in hepatocytes as a byproduct of purine nucleotide catabolism [guanylic acid (GMP), inosinic acid (IMP), and adenylic acid (AMP)] (Figure 13–1). The rate-limiting and final reaction involves the conversion of xanthine to uric acid, driven by the enzyme xanthine oxidase. Further metabolism of uric acid in humans does not occur as the enzyme responsible for its conversion to allantoin, urate oxidase, was lost due to a nonsense mutation during human evolution. The major route of clearance of excessively produced uric acid is through the kidney. In the case of TLS a sudden load of purine nucleotides released from lysed tumor cells results in an acute rise in uric acid production that overwhelms the normal excretory capacity leading to a rise in serum uric acid levels above 7–8 mg/dL, with severe hyperuricemia >15 mg/dL being common. As will be discussed in the following section, the presenting clinical symptoms and signs of hyperuricemia associated with TLS are those associated with oliguria and ARF, which it can induce.

4. Azotemia and acute renal failure—As stated earlier, a common and potentially serious complication of TLS is acute renal failure. Usually presenting as oliguria associated with a progressive rise in serum creatinine and urea nitrogen, the etiology of ARF is multifactorial. A major mechanism is acute uric acid nephropathy. With a pK_a of 5.5, urate is soluble as the ionized form in the blood at a physiologic pH of 7. However, in the distal nephron where the glomerular effluent is acidified to a pH <5.5, under appropriate conditions urate can become protonated and precipitate, especially in the setting of low urine flow rates. When the uric acid load is high enough, such precipitation can lead to intratubular crystal formation and obstruction of urine flow. As a result of this obstruction, the glomerular filtration rate (GFR) drops and clinical ARF ensues. Although rare, the intratubular obstruction can be severe enough to cause collecting system dilation as evidenced by bilateral hydronephrosis on renal ultrasound. Another likely mechanism leading to ARF with TLS is acute nephrocalcinosis. As stated earlier, the precipitous rise in serum phosphorus levels results in the acute formation of calcium–phosphorus complexes, which deposit in tissues. In the kidney this deposition results in tubular toxicity and interstitial inflammation, which further exacerbate the reduction in GFR.

Patients with ARF associated with TLS can present along a spectrum of severity, from asymptomatic azotemia to severe anuria with uremia and volume overload. Particular attention should be paid to volume status (ie, depletion or overload) and electrolyte anomalies (especially potassium and calcium) as disturbances of these can be immediately life threatening and dictate the initial plan of therapy.

B. Other Studies

Although most often identified in the appropriate clinical setting with compatible laboratory findings, other studies may assist the clinician in the diagnosis of TLS and guide appropriate therapy.

1. Electrocardiogram—As alluded to earlier, a serious yet treatable complication of TLS is hyperkalemia with associated cardiac conduction defects and arrhythmias. All patients with TLS and laboratory evidence of hyperkalemia should have an ECG performed. Attention should particularly be focused on changes typically indicative of elevated serum potassium levels on cardiac myocyte conduction: T wave peaking, prolongation of the PR and QRS complex, flattened or absent P waves, and atrioventricular blocks or ventricular arrhythmias. The presence of any of these dictates the immediate need for intervention to stabilize the myocardium and lower the serum potassium level.

2. Urinalysis—As part of an initial evaluation of patients with ARF due to TLS the urinalysis (UA) is indispensable in guiding the clinician to the correct diagnosis. Although their presence does not firmly rule in or their absence rule out

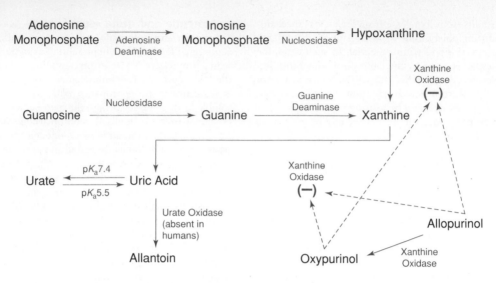

▲ **Figure 13–1.** Purine catabolism metabolic pathway.

TLS, uric acid crystals may be seen on microscopic examination of the urine sediment. These appear as rhomboid or rosette-shaped crystals of yellow or brown color under light microscopy. Other aspects of the UA can aid the clinician during the evaluation of ARF, and, although not specific for TLS, provide useful information. These include an elevated specific gravity indicative of a concentrated urine from concomitant volume depletion, microscopic hematuria, and minimal if any proteinuria in the absence of other renal disease.

3. Renal ultrasound—As described above, a major pathophysiologic mechanism of ARF associated with TLS is obstruction of tubular fluid flow by uric acid crystal formation. Although rare, bilateral hydronephrosis has been reported due to presumed extensive tubular obstruction. However, a renal ultrasound can also provide valuable information to help differentiate ARF from TLS from other causes in patients with known malignancies, most notably obstructive uropathy from extrinsic compression of ureters by solid tumors.

4. Urine uric acid/creatinine ratio—Although quite sensitive, elevated serum uric acid levels in the setting of ARF are not specific for TLS. Although rarely extremely high, mild to moderate elevations in serum uric acid levels can be seen in ARF from various causes due to impaired renal clearance of normally produced quantities of uric acid as GFR falls. In these cases the uric acid found in the urine results mostly from tubular secretion. Thus the sum total of uric acid excreted is less than normal. This is in contrast to uric acid nephropathy associated with TLS where uric acid

production and excretion are greatly increased. Despite the presence of impaired GFR, as long as anuria is not present the net amount of uric acid excreted is higher than the basal state. As such, by measuring the concentration of uric acid in the urine and dividing this value by the urine creatinine concentration to control for the degree of urinary concentration, it is possible to help differentiate ARF due to TLS from other causes. While one study reported that a urinary uric acid/creatinine ratio of >1 was specific for cases of ARF associated with TLS, and a ratio <0.6–0.75 was found in cases of ARF due to other causes, the utility of the urine uric acid/creatinine ratio has not been confirmed in other studies.

▶ **Differential Diagnosis**

The evaluation of electrolyte disturbances and/or ARF can be complex in patients with newly diagnosed malignancies, especially in the setting of recent chemotherapy or radiation treatments. As such it is imperative for the clinician to be mindful of confounding conditions that may mimic TLS, as definitive therapies may be different. Statistically the most common reasons for ARF in hospitalized patients are prerenal azotemia from volume depletion and acute tubular necrosis (ATN). Patients with malignancies are prone to dehydration due to poor oral intake, high gastrointestinal losses of fluid from vomiting or diarrhea, and febrile illnesses with increased rates of insensible fluid loss. However, volume depletion often accompanies TLS. Therefore clinical evidence of prerenal azotemia does not rule out TLS. Regardless, as will be discussed further, intravenous hydration is appropriate and indicated in either scenario.

Hospitalized patients with malignancies are often afflicted by infectious processes requiring evaluations and/or therapies that may be potentially nephrotoxic such as contrast dye, aminoglycoside antibiotics, and amphotericin B. Additionally, significant hypotension may accompany these infections. As a result, ATN from toxins or ischemia is frequently responsible for ARF in this patient population. Although not universally sensitive, dense granular casts on microscopic examination of the urine sediment in cases of ATN can help distinguish it from TLS. Although less common, obstructive uropathy related to direct compression of the ureters and/or urethra by tumors themselves must be part of the differential diagnosis and radiologic evaluation for hydronephrosis is appropriate. Finally, other rare etiologies of ARF in patients with malignancies include acute interstitial nephritis, glomerulonephritis, and microangiopathic hemolytic anemias. However, as these usually present with urine findings not typically seen in TLS (ie, pyuria or significant proteinuria), their differentiation from TLS is not difficult.

Any of these etiologies of ARF can result in electrolyte disturbances as a result of a drop in GFR, including hyperkalemia, hyperphosphatemia/hypocalcemia, and hyperuricemia. However, it is the constellation of all these anomalies together, particularly with very high phosphorus and uric acid levels, in the appropriate clinical setting that clues the clinician toward the correct diagnosis of TLS.

▶ Treatment

In cases where preventive therapies are not possible and/or when clinically significant TLS develops despite their institution, further treatments may be indicated.

A. Eliminate Potential Nephrotoxins or Confounders

In situations in which TLS may occur it is prudent to avoid or eliminate any agents that may exacerbate the condition. Most notably the clinician should discontinue any medications that may promote hyperkalemia such as oral or parenteral supplements, β-blockers, and inhibitors of the renin–angiotensin–aldosterone axis [ie, angiotensin-converting enzyme (ACE) inhibitors, angiotensin receptor blockers, potassium-sparing diuretics, and heparin]. Similarly, exogenous phosphate should be avoided, eg, oral supplements and fleets phosphosoda enemas. Given the potential for kidney damage with TLS it is prudent to avoid when possible other potential nephrotoxins including nonsteroidal anti-inflammatory agents, radiocontrast dye, amphotericin-B, and aminoglycoside antibiotics. Finally, prior to chemotherapy patients at risk for TLS should have all uricosuric agents stopped that otherwise impair tubular reabsorption of uric acid and potentially could promote crystallization

even further. Such agents include probenecid, aspirin, and thiazide diuretics.

B. Hydration

As volume depletion can exacerbate the clinical effects of TLS in many different ways, intravenous hydration (eg, 3 L/m^2/day) should be initiated 48 hours prior to administration of chemotherapy or as soon as possible if TLS is already present. The goals of this volume expansion are to decrease uric acid, phosphorus, and potassium concentrations in the extracellular compartment. This volume expansion also results in an increased renal blood flow and GFR, thereby inducing a brisk diuresis (>100–150 mL/m^2/hour), which can inhibit intratubular uric acid crystallization and obstruction. Forced diuresis with loop diuretics may be necessary if urine flow rates are not high enough with hydration alone, as long as volume depletion is corrected first. Patients should be monitored for signs of volume overload, especially those with established ARF or known preexisting cardiomyopathy. Controversy exists over the type of crystalloid that should be used. As urate is more soluble in the ionized form at physiologic pH, an alkaline diuresis using intravenous sodium bicarbonate (eg, 50–100 mEq of sodium bicarbonate diluted in 1 L of D$_5$ 0.45% saline) to maintain a urine pH >7.0–7.5 should help prevent ARF beyond its ability to expand the extracellular volume. However, ARF in TLS is also caused by acute nephrocalcinosis, where calcium-phosphate precipitation is facilitated at a higher pH. Thus bicarbonate administration should be used judiciously and may not offer significant advantages over volume expansion with isotonic saline alone.

C. Hyperkalemia

Hyperkalemia as part of TLS can be a medical emergency requiring immediate therapy. When cardiac effects of hyperkalemia are present based on ECG findings, membrane stabilization can be temporarily achieved with administration of intravenous calcium (ie, 10% calcium gluconate). Repeat doses may be required if potassium levels cannot be reduced within 15–30 minutes. Simultaneous expansion of the extracellular volume should be initiated to decrease the potassium concentration by dilution. Attempts to shift intracellular potassium are indicated as well by using intravenous insulin with or without glucose, intravenous or inhaled β-agonists, and intravenous bicarbonate. With regard to the latter, caution should be used given the potential for volume overload, exacerbation of hypocalcemia, and facilitation of calcium-phosphate precipitation as mentioned above. Finally, total body potassium can be effected through saline and diuretic-induced kaliuresis, gastrointestinal exchange resins (ie, sodium polystyrene sulfate), and dialysis if needed.

D. Hyperphosphatemia and Hypocalcemia

Attempts to correct hypocalcemia are contraindicated unless the patient is experiencing neuromuscular symptoms thought to be due to low calcium concentrations. Intravenous calcium administration may potentially facilitate precipitation of calcium and phosphate as long as phosphate levels remain high. The main goal is to correct the underlying hyperphosphatemia as this usually results in concomitant normalization of calcium levels. Beyond expansion of the extracellular volume space, which helps to increase renal phosphate excretion, short courses of non-calcium-containing oral phosphate binders may be initiated such as aluminum hydroxide or carbonate. Dialysis may be necessary for calcium and phosphate correction if these more conservative therapies are not effective and/or if significant ARF is present.

E. Hyperuricemia

A major focus in the management of TLS is decreasing the elevated serum and urine uric acid concentrations. This may be achieved in different ways. First, volume contraction exacerbates the condition by concentrating the uric acid in the urine, which promotes crystallization. Therefore, volume expansion itself is an effective means of attenuating hyperuricemia. Urine alkalinization to a pH >7 promotes urate to exist almost completely in its ionized form, further decreasing urine crystallization. Although necessary, volume expansion and urine alkalinization are usually not sufficient.

The amount of purine nucleotide precursors released by the lysed tumor cells is not controllable, but it is possible to decrease the conversion of these compounds to uric acid. This is achieved by targeting xanthine oxidase. Allopurinol, along with its active metabolite oxypurinol, acts as a competitive inhibitor of xanthine oxidase. Studies have shown that in cancer patients administered allopurinol at a dose of up to 800 mg daily (usually 200–400 mg/m^2/day, intravenous or oral divided two or three times a day), approximately 70% will normalize and 90% will decrease their uric acid levels by at least 1 mg/dL. Intravenous administration is the preferred route, especially if the patient has limited ability to tolerate oral medications, and should be started 24–48 hours prior to chemotherapy if possible along with intravenous hydration. As allopurinol does not affect the amount of uric acid already produced, any decrease in uric acid levels is usually slow due to dependence on renal clearance. An initial effect can be seen within 72 hours of initiation of allopurinol with maximal effect by 7–10 days. As the drug allopurinol and its metabolite oxypurinol are renally cleared, its dose needs to be lowered by over 50% in cases of renal failure.

Finally, newer agents have become available that convert uric acid into the more soluble allantoin, which is easily excreted. Urate oxidase, the enzyme absent in most higher primates including humans, has been utilized since 1975 in Europe in the prophylactic treatment of cancer patients at risk for TLS. Recently a recombinant form of urate oxidase, rasburicase (Elitek, Sanofi-Synthelabo, Inc.), has been approved in the United States. Suggested dosing is 0.05–0.20 mg/kg intravenously each day at the onset of chemotherapy for up to 5 days. In general, given that this enzyme degrades already formed uric acid and is not dependent on renal clearance, uric acid levels decrease quickly within 4 hours of dose administration and to lower levels (ie, <1 mg/dL) compared to allopurinol. No data exist as to whether rasburicase is more effective at preventing ARF associated with TLS. Common side effects of rasburicase include rash and hemolytic anemia due to the generation of hydrogen peroxide during its metabolism. Due to the latter, it is contraindicated in patients with glucose-6-phosphate dehydrogenase deficiency. Potential advantages of rasburicase over allopurinol include a more rapid decline in uric acid levels, which would limit exposure of kidney tissue to high plasma and urine uric acid levels. However, a major drawback to rasburicase is its cost, which is significantly more than allopurinol.

F. Acute Renal Failure: Role of Renal Replacement Therapy

Renal replacement therapy is indicated in cases of TLS when conservative measures fail to correct the associated metabolic disturbances, when volume overload limits the aggressiveness of conservative measures and/or adversely affects the patient (eg, pulmonary edema), or when patients become symptomatic from uremia. Dialytic therapies not only are capable of restoring metabolic equilibrium, but also offer the advantage of clearing compounds (ie, uric acid and phosphorus) that may otherwise continue to inflict damage on the kidneys. In general, clearance of uric acid and phosphate is greater with hemodialysis compared to peritoneal dialysis, which makes the former the modality of choice when possible.

However, despite high clearance of these solute and volume derangements during each hemodialysis treatment, the limited time exposed to dialysis and the rapid reaccumulation of these compounds and volume excess after the treatment ends may dictate repeated sessions every 12–24 hours. Conversely, although less efficient per unit time, continuous renal replacement therapy over extended periods of hours to days has also proven efficacious in restoring metabolic and volume control in patients with TLS, especially those who are hemodynamically unstable and would not tolerate the intermittent form.

▶ Prognosis

The clinical outcome of patients with TLS varies with the severity of the presentation, the degree to which preventive measures can be instituted, and the extent of the underlying malignant disease. Use of the prophylactic and therapeutic maneuvers described can significantly improve the short-term outcome and prevent fatal complications. In general, ARF associated with TLS is reversible assuming the ability to control the metabolic derangements and limit further renal insults, although renal replacement therapy may be required for a short time.

Cairo MS: Prevention and treatment of hyperuricemia in hematological malignancies. Clin Lymphoma 2002;3 (Suppl 1):S26.31.

Cairo MS, Bishop M: Tumour lysis syndrome: new therapeutic strategies and classification. Br J Haematol 2004;127(1):3.

Davidson MB et al: Pathophysiology, clinical consequences, and treatment of tumor lysis syndrome. Am J Med 2004;116(8):546.

Jeha S: Tumor lysis syndrome. Semin Hematol 2001; 38 (4 Suppl 10):4.

Navolanic PM et al: Elitek-rasburicase: an effective means to prevent and treat hyperuricemia associated with tumor lysis syndrome, a Meeting Report, Dallas, Texas, January 2002. Leukemia 2003;17(3):499.

Ribeiro RC, Pui CH: Recombinant urate oxidase for prevention of hyperuricemia and tumor lysis syndrome in lymphoid malignancies [see comment]. Clin Lymphoma 2003;3(4):225.

Yarpuzlu AA: A review of clinical and laboratory findings and treatment of tumor lysis syndrome. Clin Chim Acta 2003;333(1):13.

Yim BT et al: Rasburicase for the treatment and prevention of hyperuricemia. Ann Pharmacother 2003;37(7–8):1047.

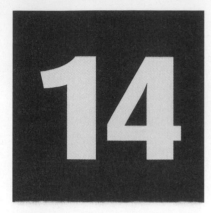

Acute Renal Failure from Therapeutic Agents

Ali J. Olyaei, PharmD, & William M. Bennett, MD

▶ Acute renal failure occurs in 4.9% of hospitalized patients with renal insufficiency.

▶ Fifty percent of patients experience nonoliguric acute renal failure.

▶ Antibiotics, analgesics, nonsteroidal anti-inflammatory drugs, contrast media, and angiotensin-converting enzyme inhibitors are the most common causes of acute renal failure.

▶ Impaired renal function, decreased volume status, exposure to contrast media, and aminoglycosides account for 79% of all cases of renal failure.

▶ General Considerations

Although most therapeutic agents infrequently cause community-acquired renal failure, a number of diagnostic and therapeutic agents can produce renal injury and renal failure among hospitalized patients. These renal injuries may be caused either directly or indirectly by drugs or metabolites of these agents in critically ill patients. Recent data suggest that renal adverse effects caused by pharmaceutical agents may contribute to approximately 30% of acute renal failure (ARF) incidents in hospitalized patients. Antibiotics, analgesics, nonsteroidal anti-inflammatory drugs (NSAIDs), contrast media, and angiotensin-converting enzyme (ACE) inhibitors were the most commonly reported causes of ARF (see Figure 9–2).

A number of factors make the kidneys more susceptible to drug toxicity. First, the kidneys receive a high fraction (20–25%) of cardiac output relative to their weight, so drugs transit to the kidneys in large amounts. The kidneys represent only 0.4% of the body weight but receive 25% of resting cardiac output; therefore kidneys are exposed to a significant concentration of therapeutic agents. Second, blood flow to the kidneys is rich in oxygen, and the kidneys are very sensitive to reduction in blood perfusion and oxygen deprivation. Third, the renal countercurrent concentrating mechanism for water also concentrates drugs and chemicals within the filtered tubular fluid. Thus, local concentrations of these substances in contact with renal epithelia may exceed that in peripheral blood. Finally, most drug-induced renal failure occurs in patients with subclinical preexisting renal dysfunction.

Renal failure associated with drug-induced nephropathy can be classified into six categories based on pathophysiologic injuries. These injuries include prerenal failure, acute tubular necrosis (ATN), acute tubulointerstitial disease (ATID), tubular obstruction (crystal-induced ARF), hypersensitivity (glomerulonephritis), and thrombotic microangiopathy. A list of common therapeutic agents associated with each of these injuries is provided in Table 14–1.

Histologically, acute interstitial nephritis (AIN), most commonly known as tubulointerstitial disease, is differentiated from other injuries by infiltration and proliferation of inflammatory cells within the interstitium. The most frequent etiologies of AIN include drug-induced AIN, infection, and autoimmune hypersensitivity reactions. Patients with drug-induced AIN usually present with nonspecific symptoms. A sudden oliguria, increase in serum creatinine, and decrease in renal function are usually present. Nausea and vomiting, malaise, and/or anorexia should be expected over 5–10 days of exposure to nephrotoxins. However, patients with NSAID-induced AIN usually present with renal dysfunction 8–12 months following exposure. In addition, decreased inflammation and tubulitis may be present.

The clinical features of AIN include a low grade fever, rash, and eosinophilia. In AIN, the reduction of renal function appears as a result of infiltration of inflammatory cells within the renal interstitium. Accumulation of proteins and

Table 14–1. Classification of various drugs based on pathophysiologic categories of acute renal failure.

1. Prenal failure
    NSAIDs, ACE inhibitors, cyclosporine, norepinephrine, angiotensin receptor blockers, diuretics, interleukins, cocaine, mitomycin C, tacrolimus, estrogen, quinine
2. Acute tubular necrosis
    Antibiotics: Aminoglycosides, cephaloridine, cephalothin, amphotericin B, rifampicin, vancomycin, foscarnet, pentamide
    NSAIDSs, contrast media, acetaminophen, cyclosporine, cisplatin, intravenous immunoglobulin, dextran, maltose, sucrose, mannitol, heavy metals
3. Acute interstitial nephritis
    Antibiotics: Ciprofloxacin, methicillin, penicillin G, ampicillin, cephalothin, oxacillin, rifampicin
    NSAIDs, contrast media, sulfonamides, thiazides, phenytoin, furosemide, allopurinol, cimetidine, omeprazole, phenindione
4. Tubular obstruction
    Sulfonamides, methotrexate, methoxyflurane, triamterene, acyclovir, ethylene glycol, protease inhibitors
5. Hypersensitivity reaction
    Penicillin G, ampicillin, sulfonamides
6. Thrombotic microangiopathy
    Mitomycin C, cyclosporine, oral contraceptives

NSAIDs, nonsteroidal anti-inflammatory drugs; ACE, angiotensin-converting enzyme; ADA, adalimumab.

fibronectin is thought to be the major cause of reduced renal function. Although fibrosis is not very common initially, patchy fibrotic lesions will ultimately develop in the renal cortex and medullocortical sections. The most common causes of drug-induced AIN include NSAIDs, penicillins and cephalosporins, rifampin, sulfonamides (including medications that include sulfa moieties such as furosemide, bumetanide, and thiazide-type diuretics), cimetidine, allopurinol, ciprofloxacin, 5-aminosalicylates (eg, mesalamine), and, to a lesser degree, other quinolone antibiotics. There is strong evidence that suggests hypersensitivity and immunologically mediated mechanisms play an important role in the etiology of drug-induced AIN. The presence of cytotoxic T cells, helper T cells, T cell-mediated cell injury, and B cell involvement suggests activation of an immune cascade following exposure to an offending agent. Clinically, these histopathologic reactions are often accompanied by fever, skin rash, eosinophilia, and arthralgia. Supportive care, withdrawal of nephrotoxins, and discontinuation of any suspected offending agents are the initial steps in the treatment of AIN. Drug-induced AIN is often reversible and patients usually improve without any long-term sequalae. In more serious cases, systemic corticosteroid therapy leads to rapid improvement.

Crystal nephropathy defines a prototype of renal injury associated with crystal deposition and tubular obstruction in the kidneys. Drugs that may cause crystal nephropathy include acyclovir, sulfonamides, methotrexate, and indinavir. Risk factors for drug-induced crystal nephropathy include age, renal impairment, volume depletion from nausea and vomiting, liver failure, and decreased effective circulating volume. The patient's risk factors influence renal blood flow and ultimately drug tubular flow. Many cases of drug-induced crystal nephropathy have occurred after prolonged administration of causative agents or large doses without adjustment of the dose for impaired renal function. Certain drugs (methotrexate, sulfonamides, and triamterene) are eliminated more readily in an alkaline environment and lowering of the urine pH may place these patients at a higher risk of crystal nephropathy. In contrast, the severity of crystal nephropathy by indinavir is influenced by alkaline urine.

The mechanism of drug-induced glomerulonephritis involves several different pathways. In most cases, the exact pathway is unknown but several theories have been proposed. Drugs that have been reported to cause drug-induced glomerular disease are listed in Table 14–1. Drugs that induce glomerular disease can be classified according to the immunologic reaction they induce or by acting as a hepatan and activating antigen–antibody complex formation. Some agents have a dose-dependent effect on glomerular structures. Although the signs and symptoms of drug-induced glomerular disease are highly variable, most patients with glomerular disease usually present with sudden loss of GFR and proteinuria.

Cheng HF, Harris RC: Renal effects of non-steroidal anti-inflammatory drugs and selective cyclooxygenase-2 inhibitors. Curr Pharm Des 2005;11:1795.

Izzedine H et al: Antiviral drug-induced nephrotoxicity. Am J Kidney Dis 2005;45:804.

Markowitz GS, Perazella MA: Drug-induced renal failure: a focus on tubulointerstitial disease. Clin Chim Acta 2005;351:31.

Perazella MA: Drug-induced renal failure: update on new medications and unique mechanisms of nephrotoxicity. Am J Med Sci 2003;325:349.

▼ ANTIBIOTICS & ANTIINFECTIVE AGENTS

AMINOGLYCOSIDES

Incidence & Risk Factors

Aminoglycosides have important antibacterial properties for the treatment of gram-negative infections in clinically unstable patients. These agents have shown a concentration-dependent bactericidal property against most gram-negative bacteria. The major dose and duration-limiting factors related to toxicity of aminoglycosides are nephrotoxicity and ototoxicity. Although a single large dose may cause reversible renal dysfunction, most studies correlate nephrotoxicity with prolonged use in patients at risk for aminoglycoside toxicities. According to a number of studies, the incidence of aminoglycoside-induced nephrotoxicity is in the range of 5–15%. Patients over 70 years of age and patients with preexisting renal impairment, intravascular volume depletion, hepatorenal syndrome, and septic patients have a higher incidence of renal dysfunction following exposure to aminoglycosides. Even with aggressive monitoring and when peak and trough serum concentrations are kept within the desired therapeutic range, aminoglycoside-induced renal dysfunction is still a possibility in high-risk populations. Various risk factors that predispose to the development of aminoglycoside nephrotoxicity have been identified.

Aminoglycoside-induced nephrotoxicity manifestations have varied from asymptomatic, to a mild and reversible increase in blood urea nitrogen (BUN) and serum creatinine, to serious but infrequent end-stage renal disease (ESRD) requiring life-long dialysis. The onset of aminoglycoside-induced nephrotoxicity is usually after 7–10 days of therapy. However, a rapid onset of nephrotoxicity after even one dose of aminoglycosides has been reported. In most patients, serum creatinine and BUN return to normal levels 2–3 weeks after discontinuation of aminoglycosides. Nonoliguric renal insufficiency is the most common manifestation of aminoglycoside nephrotoxicity. Less common manifestations include various isolated tubular syndromes, eg, nephrogenic diabetes insipidus, Fanconi syndrome, and renal potassium or magnesium wasting. Fortunately, severe oliguric renal failure requiring dialysis is rare from aminoglycosides alone. A drug-induced concentrating defect characterized by polyuria and secondary thirst stimulation precedes the detectable rise in BUN and serum creatinine and occurs in as many as 30% of hospitalized patients given >5–7 days of aminoglycoside treatment. Granular casts and mild proteinuria occur frequently but are not of diagnostic assistance. In addition, in patients who satisfy the clinical criteria for aminoglycoside nephrotoxicity, cellular autophagocytosis has been observed with electron microscopy.

Loading doses should be sufficient to achieve high peak levels to maximize bacterial killing. Because the elimination half-life of aminoglycosides, is markedly prolonged as renal function falls, maintenance-dose intervals should be carefully adjusted in patients with existing renal dysfunction when aminoglycosides are required. Extending the interval between doses is safer than reducing the size of individual doses in patients with renal insufficiency. Correctable risk factors should be minimized. Among the clinically available aminoglycosides, the spectrum of nephrotoxicity is gentamicin > tobramycin > amikacin > netilmicin. Monitoring of peak serum levels will ensure efficacy, whereas elevation of the trough level, showing drug accumulation, will often precede a rise in the less-sensitive serum creatinine measurements. Once-daily aminoglycoside dosing may be less nephrotoxic for a given total daily dose.

▶ Pathogenesis

A number of mechanisms have been proposed for nephrotoxicity of aminoglycosides. Most data suggest that aminoglycosides accumulate in the renal cortex. These findings have been reported in animal and human studies. Megalin is an endocytotic receptor expressed and located at the brush-border membrane. Following binding to this receptor, aminoglycosides are taken up into the proximal tubular cells. The concentration of aminoglycosides in the proximal tubule is approximately 10- to 100-fold higher than the plasma concentration. At this concentration, aminoglycosides may interfere with protein synthesis in proximal tubular cells and lead to ATN.

Once-a-day gentamicin dosing or once every 36-hour dosing has become common in recent years. This method is particularly common when patients are at risk of nephrotoxicity or ototoxicity. A number of meta-analyses of randomized clinical trials and single-center reports with the use of a once-a-day dosing schedule suggest a reduced incidence of aminoglycoside nephrotoxicity. Compared to conventional three times a day administration, once-daily dosing may result in a 10–50% lower incidence of serious adverse reactions. This paradoxic finding can be explained in part by the saturable nature of aminoglycoside transport across the brush-border membrane of proximal tubular cells. During once-daily dosing, only a limited quantity (15 mg/dL) of aminoglycosides can cross during the initial high plasma concentration. This method of administration allows for a prolonged exposure to a low plasma concentration of aminoglycosides below the saturable threshold.

▶ Prevention & Treatment

Therapeutic drug monitoring plays an important role in the treatment of serious infections with aminoglycosides. Several studies have demonstrated that therapeutic drug monitoring with appropriately applied pharmacokinetic principles reduces the nephrotoxicity and other adverse drug reactions related to usage of aminoglycosides. Table 14–2 provides dosing recommendations for the use of aminoglycosides in the treatment of various infections.

Aminoglycoside nephrotoxicity may occur despite therapeutic drug monitoring, use of once-daily dosing, and/or short-term treatment. Progression of nephrotoxicity can occur after discontinuation of the last dose. Most patients recover but it may take several months before recovery is complete. Renal dysfunction may be prolonged and require up to a year for function to return to normal. Permanent renal impairment requiring dialysis may occur.

Table 14–2. Adult once-a-day aminoglycoside (gentamicin and tobramycin) dosing guidelines.

Dosing
For dosing weight, use adjusted ideal body weight (IBW)

Use IBW to calculate dose
Male = 50 kg + 2.3(height in inches − 60)
Male = 45.5 kg + 2.3(height in inches − 60)
Obese = IBW + 0.4(actual BW − IBW)

A. Calculate creatinine clearance (CrCl)
Males: [(140 − Age) × IBW]/[SrCr × 72]
Female: [(140 − Age) × IBW]/[SrCr × 72] × 0.85

B. Gentamicin/tobramycin dosing
Dose according to estimated CrCl
CrCl ≥ 60 mL/minute = 5 mg/kg/24 hours
CrCl 40–60 mL/minute = 5 mg/kg/36 hours
CrCl 40–20 mL/minute = 1–1.5 mg/kg/q12h or consult pharmacist
CrCl <20 mL/minute ARF = consult clinical pharmacist

Round dose to the nearest 25 mg. For patients <35 kg, do not need to round.

Labs
For once daily dosing, please order serum creatinine/BUN every day or every 2 days.

Random level (12 hours before the next dose). Note: Level should not be drawn from the same line from which it is administered. Repeat every 5 days or as needed while in hospital.

Dosage increases
If random level (drawn 12 hours before the next dose) is undetectable, consider increasing the aminoglycoside dosage to 7 mg/kg/day. Repeat random level on new dosage.

If random level is >3, check a 24-hour level; if it is >0.5 mg/dL consider extending the dosing interval. Repeat random level on new dosage.

BW, body weight; ARF, acute renal failure; BUN, blood urea nitrogen.

Darko W et al: Mississippi mud no more: cost-effectiveness of pharmacokinetic dosage adjustment of vancomycin to prevent nephrotoxicity. Pharmacotherapy 2003;23:643.

Olsen KM et al: Effect of once-daily dosing vs. multiple daily dosing of tobramycin on enzyme markers of nephrotoxicity. Crit Care Med 2004;32:1678.

VANCOMYCIN

Incidence & Risk Factors

Vancomycin is a commonly used antibiotic for the treatment of gram-positive bacterial infections resistant to penicillin and cephalosporines. The reported incidence of vancomycin-induced nephrotoxicity varies widely depending on the criteria used to define nephrotoxicity and generally ranges between 0 and 35%.

The relationship between therapeutic plasma monitoring (trough) of vancomycin and nephrotoxicity is uncertain.

Since vancomycin is excreted mainly through the kidneys, renal dysfunction would predispose patients to elevated serum vancomycin concentrations. It is not clear whether high serum vancomycin levels and nephrotoxicity are linked.

Pathogenesis

Most histologic examinations of the kidneys indicate that vancomycin might cause marked destruction of proximal tubules. The hallmark of vancomycin-induced renal dysfunction is destruction of glomeruli and necrosis of proximal tubules. It has been suggested that oxidative stress is the underlying pathogenesis of vancomycin-induced nephrotoxicity.

Prevention & Treatment

Vancomycin-induced nephrotoxicity is a largely unpredictable event. However, if patients are at risk for renal dysfunction, a number of measures can be taken to prevent overt renal failure. When treating a serious bacterial infection, all therapeutic options should be considered. Vancomycin should be utilized only when medically necessary. In patients who require vancomycin treatment consideration should be given to volume status, renal function, prolonged treatment course (over 10 days), concomitant use of aminoglycosides and/or other nephrotoxic agents, and advanced age. Frequent monitoring of renal function is highly recommended, particularly in patients with preexisting renal dysfunction. If renal toxicity is observed, the vancomycin dose should be adjusted according to renal function (Table 14–3). A doubling of the baseline serum creatinine is indicative of serious nephrotoxicity.

ACYCLOVIR

Incidence & Risk Factors

Over the past decade, there has been an increased usage of antiviral agents to treat local and severe systemic viral infections in immunocompromised patients. Most antiviral agents appear to be safe and do not cause nephrotoxicity. Acute renal failure is an important dose-limiting toxicity of acyclovir.

Acyclovir is primarily eliminated through the kidney with a small amount being metabolized in the liver. Many cases of acyclovir nephrotoxicity have been reported in the medical literature over the past 15 years. These reports have increased awareness and concern of acyclovir's nephrotoxic potential. Renal dysfunction most commonly occurs within the first few days of initiation of intravenous acyclovir therapy. Patients who receive high-dose bolus intravenous therapy, those who are volume depleted, and patients with preexisting renal insufficiency are at the greatest risk of developing renal injury. ARF has been reported in 5% of patients who receive high-dose bolus intravenous therapy but is rare in patients receiving oral therapy. The most common symptoms include

Table 14–3. Initial and adjusted vancomycin dose determination in adults.

Initial maintenance dose[1]	
Estimated CrCl (mL/minute)	Initial dosing regimen
Continuous renal eplacement (eg, CVVH, CVVHD)	1000 mg intravenously q24h
<20 and/or intermittent hemodialysis	1000 mg intravenously q72h
20–29	1000 mg intravenously q48h
30–39	1500 mg intravenously q48h or 750 mg intravenously q24h
40–55	1000 mg intravenously q24h
56–99	1000 mg intravenously q12h
100–120, age >65	1000 mg intravenously q12h
100–120, age <65	1250 mg intravenously q12h
≥120 and/or hypermetabolic state[2]	1000 mg intravenously q8h

[1]Consider loading doses in obese patients: Obese = actual body weight >120% ideal body weight. Give 1500 mg loading dose for obese patients weighing 85–109 kg. Give 2000 mg loading dose for obese patients weighing >110 kg.
[2]Hypermetabolic states include trauma and burn patients.
CVVH, continuous venovenous hemofiltration; CVVHD, continuous venovenous hemodialysis.

Adjusted dose		
Trough serum concentration[1]	Dose adjustment recommended	Follow-up/monitoring[2]
<3.5 mg/L	Shorten dose interval to next standard interval: If q48h → q24h If q24h → q12h If q12h → q8h If q8h → q6h	Draw trough level 30 minutes prior to third dose of new dosing regimen
3.5–4.9 mg/L	Increase dose by 250 to 500 mg at same time interval; if improvement in renal function,[3] consider shortening interval	Draw trough level approximately 30 minutes prior to third dose of new dosing regimen
5–15 mg/L	No change in therapy[4]	No further trough levels to be drawn unless Duration of therapy is >7 days; if therapy >7 days, check trough level every 5–7 days Patient status declines Serum creatinine in increases >0.5 mg/dL from baseline
15.1–19.9 mg/L	Decrease dose by 250 mg at same time interval	Draw trough level approximately 30 minutes prior to third dose of new dose regimen therapy
≥20 mg/L and dose ≥1000 mg	Decrease dose by 500 mg at same time interval or If decline in renal function,[3] hold dose(s) and check another level in 12–24 hours; when trough is therapeutic, restart at lower dose and/or extend interval, based on patient-specific clearance	Draw trough level approximately 30 minutes prior to third dose of new dose regimen therapy

Table 14–3. *Continued*

Trough serum concentration[1]	Dose adjustment recommended	Follow-up/monitoring[2]

≥20 mg/L and dose <1000 mg	Extend dose interval to next standard interval:
	    If q6h → q8h
	    If q8h → q12h
	    If q12h → q24h
	    If q24h → q48h
	or
	If decline in renal function,[3] hold dose(s) and check another level in 12-24 hours; when trough is therapeutic, restart at lower dose and/or extend interval, based on patient-specific clearance
		Draw trough level approximately 30 minutes prior to third dose of new dose regimen therapy

[1]Higher trough concentrations may be necessary for some types of patients/infections. Examples include, but are not limited to, meningitis, endocarditis, and osteomyelitis.
[2]Serum creatinine levels should also be monitored daily in patients with decreased renal function and/or increased risk of nephrotoxicity.
[3]Changes in serum creatinine of ±50% from baseline may signify change in renal function.
[4]Maximum serum trough level in patients with increased risk for nephrotoxicity is 12 mg/L, particularly patients on concomitant nephrotoxins (eg, aminoglycosides, amphotericin B, cisplatin, cyclosporin, foscarnet, ganciclovir, loop diuretics, nonsteroidal anti-inflammatory drugs, radiocontrast dye, tacrolimus, vasopressors).

nausea, vomiting, abdominal pain, and/or back pain. Patients may, however, be asymptomatic. A moderate rise (1–3 mg/dL) in serum creatinine from baseline should be expected while oliguria is uncommon. Urinalysis may show trace proteinuria, pyuria, and microscopic hematuria. Birefringent needle-shaped crystals may be seen free or within white blood cells in the urine sediment.

Pathogenesis

The pathogenesis of acyclovir-induced ARF is unclear and may involve an obstructive nephropathy from intratubular precipitation of acyclovir and/or immune hypersensitivity reaction. Acyclovir is moderately insoluble in the urine. The maximum solubility of acyclovir is 2.5 mg/mL. Low urine output and fast intravenous infusion of a large dose (500 mg/mm^2) of acyclovir may lead to intratubular precipitation.

Prevention & Treatment

The most effective means of preventing acyclovir nephrotoxicity is to administer adequate intravenous fluid [normal saline (NS) 0.9%] to induce a urinary output of 100–150 mL/hour. Acyclovir-induced nephropathy may also be prevented by avoiding rapid bolus infusion. Acyclovir should be administered at a rate of 60 minutes for every 500-mg dose. Approaches to treatment of acyclovir-induced nephropathy are similar to those caused by other agents. Discontinuation of acyclovir therapy, increased hydration, or dose reduction/interval extension allows most patients to return to normal renal function within a few days to 2 weeks. Temporary dialysis is usually unnecessary, however, for severe complications of renal failure associated with acyclovir, hemodialysis could be utilized to remove 40–60% of plasma acyclovir.

FOSCARNET

▶ Incidence & Risk Factors

Foscarnet is a virostatic agent used in HIV-infected and other immunocompromised patients to prevent or treat serious cytomegalovirus (CMV) infections and acyclovir-resistant mucocutaneous herpes simplex infections. Foscarnet exhibits poor oral absorption necessitating intravenous therapy. As foscarnet is a phosphate analog, it can chelate calcium and be deposited in bone. Biotransformation does not occur and up to 28% is excreted unchanged in the urine. Foscarnet induces a rather unique form of renal failure in a majority of patients. Renal impairment occurs in varying degrees in the majority of patients. The exact incidence of foscarnet-induced nephropathy is not known. The rates of ARF from foscarnet vary in patients from 27% to 66%. Risks for renal failure have not been well defined but include impaired renal function, age, concomitant administration with other nephrotoxic agents, and dehydration.

▶ Pathogenesis

The pathogenesis of foscarnet-induced renal failure remains speculative with a number of hypotheses being suggested. ARF appears to be caused by the formation of a foscarnet/ionized calcium complex that precipitates in renal glomeruli causing a crystalline glomerulonephritis. The salt crystals may also precipitate in renal tubules causing tubular necrosis. Fluid and electrolyte imbalances have been reported with foscarnet therapy. Polyuria, nephrogenic diabetes insipidus, hypokalemia, hypomagnesemia, hypophosphatemia or hyperphosphatemia, and hypocalcemia have been observed in patients treated with foscarnet. Hypocalcemia is the most frequently encountered and most serious imbalance. Although the total calcium levels remain unaffected, the ionized calcium decreases substantially. Patients with low ionized calcium levels may experience paresthesias, tingling, numbness, seizures, and death. Foscarnet therapy has been able to be resumed in some patients after restoration of electrolyte or mineral abnormalities. Ionized hypocalcemia may primarily be a result of foscarnet complexing with ionized calcium. However, renal dysfunction may also contribute to these electrolyte abnormalities.

Prevention & Treatment

Minimization of foscarnet-induced nephrotoxicity can be accomplished through vigorous hydration prior to therapy. Use of foscarnet with other nephrotoxins increases the likelihood of developing ARF. Intermittent infusion, as opposed to continuous infusion, may reduce foscarnet-induced nephrotoxicity. ARF is usually reversible, however, recovery may be gradual. Azotemia may worsen and last for several days before resolving. Continuation of foscarnet in patients who develop mild azotemia may be possible with reduced doses. Temporary dialysis may be necessary. Patients with preexisting renal insufficiency may require several months to recover full renal function following discontinuation of foscarnet.

Berns JS et al: Antivirial agents. In: *Clinical Nephrotoxins.* De Broe ME et al: (editors). Kluwer, 2004:249.

CIDOFOVIR, ADEFOVIR, & TENOFOVIR

Incidence & Risk Factors

Cidofovir, adefovir, and tenofovir belong to a newer class of antiviral agents structurally described as acyclic nucleoside phosphonates. Cidofovir is an analog of the monophosphate of cytosine. When activated, these agents appear to interfere with synthesis and/or degradation of cellular membrane phospholipids. Cidofovir exhibits broad activity against the herpes viruses. It is primarily used to treat CMV retinitis in patients who have failed other treatments. Adefovir is an analog of adenine that interferes with a variety of ATP-dependent processes once it undergoes phosphorylation within cells. It is used to treat active or chronic hepatitis B infections in patients intolerant to other antiviral therapies. Tenofovir, a newer nucleotide analog, is a reverse-transcriptase inhibitor approved to treat HIV infection. Nephrotoxicity is a major dose-dependent and dose-limiting toxicity of both cidofovir and adefovir. In clinical trials, approximately 25% or more of patients receiving intravenous cidofovir 3 mg/kg or more developed ARF related to renal proximal tubular injury. Associated abnormalities included proteinuria, increased serum creatinine, Fanconi syndrome with tubular proteinuria, and evidence of proximal tubular injury including glucosuria, hypophosphatemia, urinary bicarbonate wasting, and, rarely, chronic interstitial nephritis and nephrogenic diabetes insipidous. Upon discontinuation of cidofovir, renal function parameters return toward baseline. Proximal tubular injury was reported in 22–50% of HIV-positive patients infected with hepatitis B virus receiving doses of adefovir at greater than 30 mg/day for 72 weeks. The role of adefovir at doses of 10 mg/day inducing any renal or tubular dysfunction is rare and no case reports were found in a recent literature search. Toxicity appeared to be mild to moderate and accompanied by changes in serum potassium, bicarbonate and uric acid levels, proteinuria, and glucosuria. The incidence of these abnormalities appeared to be dose related.

Pathogenesis

Cidofovir and adefovir (>30 mg/day) have been noted to have significant nephrotoxicity. These potent drugs cause injury to proximal tubular epithelia. Proximal tubular cells express an organic anion transporter that actively takes up a variety of acyclic nucleotide analogs, including cidofovir and adefovir. These agents concentrate in tubular cells, interfere with various cell processes, and are then actively secreted into the tubular lumen. Renal clearance of these agents exceeds creatinine clearance suggesting that active tubular secretion contributes to renal clearance. Probenecid, an inhibitor of organic anion transport, decreases renal toxicity of these agents by reducing cellular uptake. A spectrum of injuries ranging from isolated proximal tubular defects (Fanconi-like syndrome) to severe ATN requiring renal replacement therapy has been observed with cidofovir and adefovir. Tenofovir, like cidofovir and adefovir, appears to accumulate in proximal tubular epithelial cells. However, based on clinical trials to date, tenofovir appears to have a low nephrotoxic potential. Only four case reports of renal dysfunction following exposure to tenofovir have been cited.

Prevention & Treatment

The following guidelines should be employed to reduce or avoid renal injury caused by cidofovir and adefovir. Pretreatment intravascular volume expansion with intravenous fluids, appropriate dosing for the level of renal function exhibited prior to therapy, avoidance in patients with significant renal dysfunction, avoidance of administration with recent use of any potentially nephrotoxic drug, and coadministration with probenecid.

Recent use of other nephrotoxic agents, preexisting renal impairment, and the development of proteinuria or other proximal tubular abnormalities during treatment may result in severe ARF. Renal failure may require dialysis. Despite drug discontinuation proximal tubular damage and resulting renal failure may be partially reversible or irreversible.

INDINAVIR

Incidence & Risk Factors

Several protease inhibitors have been approved by the U.S. Food and Drug Administration (FDA). Protease inhibitors share common adverse drug reaction profiles. Each agent, however, has its own unique toxicity. Compared with other protease inhibitors, a lower incidence of nausea, vomiting, abdominal discomfort, and taste disturbances have been reported with the use of indinavir. Indinavir is considered safe, although 4% of patients experienced flank pain with or without hematuria associated with nephrolithiasis during phase II/III clinical studies. However, it was not clear that indinavir or its metabolites were responsible for the formation of crystals in the urine. Nephrolithiasis or crystal precipitation has not been associated with other protease inhibitors.

Two distinct patterns of crystalluria have been reported in HIV-positive patients: Symptomatic and asymptomatic crystalluria. Asymptomatic crystalluria is more common than actual nephrolithiasis with symptomatic renal colic. In addition to nephrolithiasis, some patients develop crystalluria and dysuria with evidence of intrarenal sludge.

Several risk factors may influence the incidence of indinavir-induced urolithiasis. The incidence of first episode or recurrence of urolithiasis may increase during warmer temperatures. This finding may correlate with a higher incidence of dehydration or lack of compliance with fluid replacement during high environmental temperatures. HIV-positive patients with hepatitis C virus (HCV) coinfection and hemophilia or receiving trimethoprim-sulfamethoxazole (TMP/SMX) may incur greater risk of indinavir-associated urolithiasis.

Pathogenesis

Indinavir stones are considered radiolucent. These stones include calcium oxalate and calcium phosphate. Therefore, they may present as partly radiopaque. Renal biopsy documentation of acute indinavir-induced interstitial nephritis and obstructive ARF has been described in several HIV-positive patients. Renal biopsy showed evidence of interstitial nephritis/fibrosis and tubular atrophy. The medullary collecting tube was filled with crystals associated with histiocytes and giant cells. The exact mechanism of indinavir-induced ARF has not been elucidated. A high incidence of asymptomatic crystalluria or urolithiasis suggests the possibility of intrarenal obstruction due to precipitation of indinavir and/or its metabolites in the urinary collecting system.

Prevention & Management

Management and prevention in patients with indinavir-induced renal dysfunction may include discontinuation of indinavir, dose reduction, and hydration. Most patients can be treated for indinavir-associated nephrolithiasis with aggressive hydration and pain control. Patients should be advised to ingest at least 48 oz of fluid throughout the day. The urine output should be 1500 mL/day to limit indinavir urine concentrations less than 0.2–0.3 mg/mL. Patients with indinavir stones may be treated with hydration, but surgical

intervention may be needed for the treatment of both obstruction and pain.

Daudon M, Jungers P: Drug-induced renal calculi: epidemiology, prevention and management. Drugs 2004;64:245.

INTRAVENOUS IMMUNOGLOBULIN & HYDROXYETHYLSTARCH

Incidence & Risk Factors

Intravenous immunoglobulin (IVIG) is used to treat a variety of autoimmune disorders. Since IVIG is prepared from pooled plasma from thousands of donors, it contains a range of antibodies. The majority of the antibodies are unmodified immunoglobulin (Ig)G (95%). The pharmacologic effect of IVIG includes blockade of macrophage Fc receptor, anti-inflammation by inhibiting the generation of membrane attack complex, neutralization of autoantibody, inhibition of cell proliferation, and regulation of apotosis. The side effects of IVIG include infusion reaction (fever, chills, and facial flush), tachycardia, palpitation, anaphylaxis ARF, thrombosis, and aseptic meningitis. The FDA has received over 100 reports of adverse renal events related to IVIG use. Most of these serious adverse events have occurred in older patients with diabetes with previous renal impairment. Renal dysfunction usually occurs within 7 days of IVIG administration, with mean peak serum creatinine levels in the range of 6.2 mg/dL. Approximately 40% of patients required dialysis and 15% mortality was reported despite renal replacement therapy. The mean time to recover renal function in surviving patients is 10 days. Histologic evidence of extensive vacuolation of the proximal tubules has been reported in patients with IVIG-induced renal dysfunction. This histologic finding is consistent with osmotic nephrosis associated with administration of a high load of sucrose. Since 90% of the cases were reported in patients receiving sucrose-containing IVIG, sucrose was thought to be the culprit in IVIG-induced nephrotoxicity. Renal failure has been reported in a small number of patients exposed to hydroxyethylstarch following surgery. Osmotic nephrosis has been reported in these patients, however, a number of studies have refuted these findings.

Pathogenesis

IVIG-induced nephrotoxicity is largely related to the preparation of the product. Factors such as volume load, sugar, and sodium content, and osmolarity of the product should be considered. Sugar, such as sucrose, is often used as a stabilizer to prevent the aggregation of IgG. Sucrose is a disaccharide of glucose and fructose. It is reabsorbed in the proximal convoluted tubule (PCT) after being filtered. Unfortunately, the human kidney lacks the enzyme to hydrolyze sucrose. The accumulation of sucrose inside the PCT cells increases the osmolarity and draws the fluid into the cells. Renal failure occurs as a result of cell swelling, vacuolization, and tubular luminal occlusion from swollen tubular cells.

Different preparations contain varied amounts of sucrose. The incidence of ARF does not seem to correlate with the amount of sucrose, so it has been proposed that small amounts of sucrose may be sufficient to induce renal impairment or IVIG itself may be contributing to or causing renal failure.

Prevention & Management

Patients should be adequately hydrated prior to IVIG administration. The concurrent use of IVIG, NSAIDs, metformin, and radiocontrast agents should be avoided because of the synergistic effect on renal function. For sucrose-containing products, the infusion rate should not exceed 3-mg sucrose/kg/minute. Baseline serum creatinine, BUN, and urine output should be obtained and monitored closely during the course of IVIG therapy. In patients at an increased risk of ARF, use of non-sucrose-containing IVIG products is highly recommended.

AMPHOTERICIN B

Incidence & Risk Factors

Amphotericin B is a polyene antibiotic with activity against a broad spectrum of fungi. However, renal function becomes impaired in approximately 80% of patients given amphotericin B. This nephrotoxicity is dose related and probably inevitable when the cumulative dose exceeds 3 g in adults. Patients at high risk include elderly patients, particularly those with depleted extracellular volume.

Pathogenesis

The usual clinical presentation of amphotericin B nephrotoxicity is characterized by defects in renal tubular function. Occasionally, this condition will progress to nonoliguric renal failure. Modest proteinuria associated with a relatively normal urinary sediment is the initial finding. Frank azotemia is preceded by hypokalemia, renal tubular acidosis, and impaired urinary concentrating capacity. In addition, the presence of a magnesium-wasting syndrome is a prominent feature of amphotericin nephrotoxicity. Repetitive courses of amphotericin B may cause permanent impairment of renal function.

Histologic changes associated with the administration of amphotericin B are surprisingly minimal. These changes are seen in the glomerulus and renal tubule. Amphotericin B has been shown to cause acute renal vasoconstriction and damage to the distal tubular epithelium. Although the exact mechanism causing nephrotoxicity is unclear, amphotericin B may bind to membrane sterols in renal vasculature cells and renal tubular epithelial cells altering membrane permeability. This event may initiate a sequalae of other events that alter renal function. These events may include activation of second messengers, activation of renal homeostatic mechanisms, and/or release of mediators. Frequent monitoring of serum creatinine is recommended. If toxicity occurs, the amphotericin dosage can be reduced to the previous level, interrupted for 2 days, or a double dose can be given on alternate days. A doubling of the baseline serum creatinine is indicative of serious nephrotoxicity.

Prevention & Treatment

Sodium supplementation in the form of intravenous saline can be used as a safe and effective means of reducing the risk of amphotericin nephrotoxicity to approximately 10%. Sodium (150 mEq/day) can be administered as follows: 500 mL NS 30 minutes before amphotericin B administration and a second 500 mL given during the 30 minutes after completion of the amphotericin infusion. The goal is to achieve a urinary sodium excretion of 250–300 mmol/day. Liposomal amphotericin B may allow for larger doses to be administered with a higher therapeutic index. Several different lipid-based amphotericin B preparations have been introduced in the market recently. These formulations have a lower rate of nephrotoxicity when compared to the standard formulation of amphotericin B. Administration-associated adverse drug reactions (fever, chills) are significantly lower with lipid-based amphotericin B. Among all lipid-based amphotericin B formulations, liposomal amphotericin (AmBisome) is significantly less nephrotoxic. Fewer patients require a dose reduction/discontinuation with Ambisome for the treatment of invasive mycoses due to adverse drug reactions when compared to other lipid-based amphotericin B formulations (ABLC, Abelcet, and ABCD, Amphotec).

Patients should be premedicated with diphenhydramine 25 mg intravenously/orally and acetaminophen 650 mg orally before receiving amphotericin to minimize infusion-related reactions. To protect the kidneys, patients should be well hydrated and should receive sodium loading. This can easily be accomplished by administering an intravenous 250–500 mL 0.9% saline bolus before and after infusion of amphotericin.

Voriconazole is pharmacokinetically and therapeutically superior to amphotericin B in many respects and should be substituted for amphotericin for the treatment of disseminated *Candida* and invasive aspergillosis infections. It is a potent inhibitor of cytochrome P450-3A4 hepatic metabolism. Therefore, plasma concentrations of cyclosporine/tacrolimus should be monitored closely to avoid potential toxicities.

Boucher HW et al: Newer systemic antifungal agents: pharmacokinetics, safety and efficacy. Drugs 2004;64:1997.

ACE INHIBITORS & ANGIOTENSIN RECEPTOR BLOCKERS

Incidence & Risk Factors

ACE inhibitors and ARBs are frequently used in the treatment of hypertension. Emerging evidence suggests that treatment of hypertension and concomitant lowering of intraglomerular

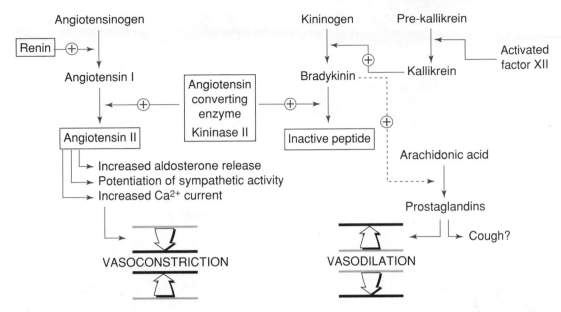

▲ **Figure 14–1.** Inhibition of the angiotensin-converting enzyme or kinase II.

pressure has a renoprotective effect in patients with diabetes and non-diabetic nephropathy. ACE inhibitors have become the antihypertensive therapeutic class of choice when the first evidence of microalbuminuria is detected in patients with diabetes.

ACE inhibitors and ARBs selectively dilate the efferent arteriole affecting renal hemodynamics. Dilation of the efferent arteriole rarely compromises the glomerular filtration rate (GFR) in patients with normal renal perfusion. However, acute renal dysfunction can occur if atherosclerotic vascular disease is present in major renal arteries, when high-grade bilateral renal artery stenosis or stenosis in a single kidney (renal transplant recipients) exists, or in any condition or drug-induced condition in which renal hemodynamics maintained by the renin/angiotensin system is altered.

Pathogenesis

Several conditions including volume depletion from diuretic therapy, concomitant administration with agents that cause vasoconstriction (NSAIDs, cyclosporine), chronic renal insufficiency of any cause [eg, congestive heart failure (CHF), hypertension], or during development of illnesses that decrease circulatory volume (vomiting, diarrhea, worsening CHF) put patients at greater risk of renal impairment. These patients depend on efferent arteriolar vasoconstriction to maintain adequate glomerular filtration. Initiation of ACE inhibitors or ARBs may result in a rapid fall in the GFR and a rise in serum creatinine. This usually occurs within 2 weeks of initiation of these agents and can be more pronounced in patients with documented risk factors. Clinicians should

ensure that patients are not hypovolemic and therapy should begin with a low dose that is slowly titrated. A chemistry panel should be obtained on all patients prior to and within 5–7 days of initiation of drug therapy. This is critical, especially in elderly patients and those with known preexisting risk factors. Patients at risk of developing ARF with initiation of ACE inhibitors or ARBs can be identified early in therapy if cautious monitoring occurs (Figure 14–1).

▶ Prevention & Treatment

ARF caused by ACE inhibitors is usually reversible. If renal dysfunction occurs, dosage reduction or reduction in the dosage of any concomitantly administered diuretic usually results in improved renal hemodynamics. Restoration of fluid and electrolyte balance, withdrawal of any interacting drugs, and, if necessary, temporary dialysis may be indicated. Substitution with an ARB almost always elicits the same effect and should be avoided.

Hyperkalemia is often present with ACE inhibitor-induced ARF, especially in elderly patients with chronic renal disease or patients receiving selective aldosterone inhibitors. The rise in plasma potassium concentration is usually modest. Often, ACE inhibitors offset hypokalemia, which occurs with many diuretics. Concomitant administration with potassium-sparing diuretics or potassium supplements increases the risk of developing hyperkalemia. If potassium levels above 6 mEq/L do not decline upon restoration of fluid balance, treatment with sodium polystyrene sulfonate may be indicated. Substitution with an ARB may reduce the incidence of hyperkalemia if potassium is less than 5.5 mEq/L.

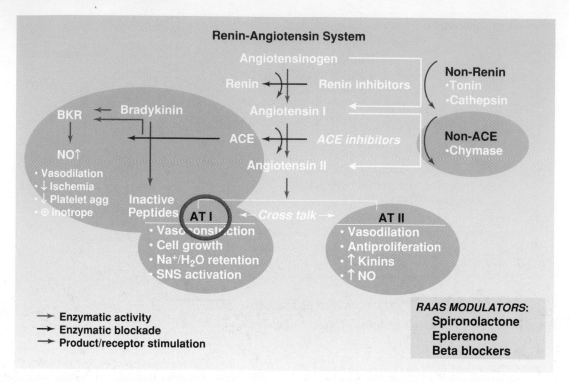

▲ **Figure 14–2.** The renin–angiotensin–aldosterone system (RAAS). ACE, angiotensin-converting enzyme; SNS, sympathetic nervous system.

Mortality secondary to ACE inhibitor or ARB therapy is low. Upon discontinuation of ACE inhibitors/ARBs renal function usually improves within a few days provided tubular damage has not occurred. Correction of risk factors for developing ACE inhibitor/ARB-induced ARF may allow continuation of therapy unless renal vascular disease or chronic renal insufficiency is the cause of ACE inhibitor/ARB-associated ARF. In patients with chronic renal insufficiency, up to a 20% rise in serum creatinine can be anticipated. This rise indicates that the drug is exerting its desired effect, reversing glomerular hyperfiltration. If the rise in serum creatinine does not exceed 20%, the ACE inhibitor or ARB should be continued. As surviving nephrons adapt, stabilization of serum creatinine usually ensues. A 50% dosage reduction can be attempted when serum creatinine rises above 30%. If the rise in serum creatinine does not stabilize within 4 weeks the ACE inhibitor or ARB should be discontinued (Figure 14–3).

CISPLATIN AND CARBOPLATIN

▷ Incidence & Risk Factors

Cisplatin and carboplatin are among the most widely used antineoplastic agents. Both agents exhibit a dose-related effect against a variety of solid tumor types. Cisplatin inhibits DNA synthesis through formation of DNA intrastrand cross-links, denatures the double helix, binds covalently to DNA bases, and disrupts DNA function. It also binds to RNA and proteins. Nephrotoxicity is the primary dose-limiting toxicity of cisplatin. Carboplatin was subsequently developed to avoid the nephrotoxicity of cisplatin while maintaining the antitumor effect. Carboplatin has since been shown to possess nephrotoxicity comparable to cisplatin. The epidemiology of nephrotoxicity varies between different cancer treatment regimens. Loss of 30–50% of GFR is a common reported adverse reaction with the use of platins. Use of other nephrotoxic agents, volume depletion, larger doses, coadministration with other nephrotoxic agents, and/or diuretics increased the risk of nephrotoxicity following exposure to platin analogs.

▷ Pathogenesis

The majority of cisplatin is excreted largely unchanged in the urine. Platinum binds extensively to plasma proteins. Unbound cisplatin is freely filtered at glomeruli and may be secreted. Excreted platinum is mutagenic and may be responsible for second malignancies that arise after cisplatin therapy. Cisplatin accumulates in renal tubular cells via transport or binding to components of the organic base transport system.

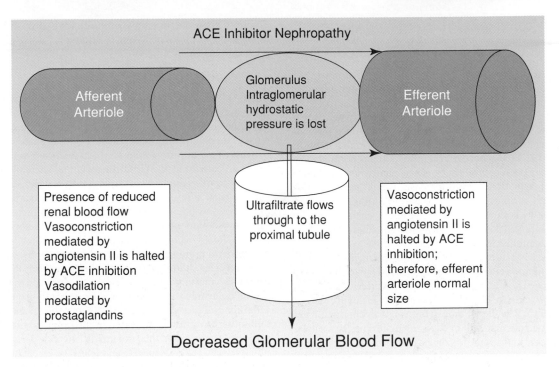

ACE Inhibitor Nephropathy

Afferent Arteriole

Glomerulus Intraglomerular hydrostatic pressure is lost

Efferent Arteriole

Presence of reduced renal blood flow Vasoconstriction mediated by angiotensin II is halted by ACE inhibition Vasodilation mediated by prostaglandins

Ultrafiltrate flows through to the proximal tubule

Vasoconstriction mediated by angiotensin II is halted by ACE inhibition; therefore, efferent arteriole normal size

Decreased Glomerular Blood Flow

▲ **Figure 14–3.** Angiotensin-converting enzyme (ACE) inhibitor nephropathy.

Autoradiographic studies have shown that radiolabeled cisplatin accumulated primarily in the S3 segment of proximal tubules, which is also the site of cisplatin-induced renal cell toxicity. The pathogenesis of cisplatin-induced cytotoxicity has been studied. Several suspected intracellular targets have been identified, including those involved in renal tubule energy production and DNA synthesis. Upon entry into renal cells, cisplatin undergoes biotransformation. Cisplatin binds cell macromolecules while a large portion of total cell platinum exists in a form with a molecular weight below 500 Da and exhibits a different chromatographic behavior than cisplatin.

Polyuria, reduced glomerular filtration, and electrolyte disturbances are frequently observed in cisplatin-treated patients. Polyuria occurs in two phases. During the first 24–48 hours after administration, urine osmolality falls while the GFR remains unchanged. Early polyuria often improves spontaneously. A second phase of polyuria occurs between 72 and 96 hours following cisplatin administration. This phase is accompanied by a disruption of glomerular filtration. A 20–40% sustained reduction in the GFR is common. Cisplatin-induced alteration of cellular respiration may lead to an incomplete distal tubule acidosis causing disturbances in magnesium, potassium, hydrogen, and calcium balance. Hypomagnesemia is a frequent complication of treatment with cisplatin. Repletion of serum magnesium levels and magnesium supplementation reduce the risk of adverse effects from

hypomagnesemia. ATN and AIN have been reported with cisplatin treatment.

▶ **Prevention & Management**

Several strategies have been employed to reduce cisplatin-induced nephrotoxicity. Prehydration with hypertonic salts may reduce cisplatin-induced ARF. A high urinary chloride concentration following saline-based hydration may reduce conversion of cisplatin to toxic aquated metabolites. Diuretics (furosemide) have also been utilized to decrease cisplatin transit time thorough renal tubules and to maintain adequate urinary output during vigorous hydration therapy. Although diuresis is commonly used, several clinical studies have shown it to be of no clinical benefit. Administering cisplatin as a continuous infusion or divided daily dose over 3–5 days is as effective therapeutically as a bolus dose. Avoidance of a large bolus dose decreases the intensity of renal drug exposure and may reduce cisplatin-induced nephrotoxicity. Coadministration with mannitol is thought to confer a protective effect by dilution of cisplatin within renal tubules due to urine volume expansion. Coadministration with nephrotoxic drugs such as aminoglycosides, NSAIDs, or iodinated contrast media should be avoided. Cisplatin and carboplatin should be used with caution in patients at risk for renal dysfunction.

Arany I, Safirstein RL: Cisplatin nephrotoxicity. Semin Nephrol 2003;23:460.

LITHIUM

▶ Incidence & Risk Factors

Lithium was discovered in 1817 and has been used since 1949 for the treatment of bipolar disorder. Following oral administration, lithium is absorbed completely from the gastrointestinal (GI) tract. Lithium is not protein bound and distributes in all human tissues. It is eliminated largely unchanged through renal excretion without any metabolism. A higher lithium half-life has been reported in bipolar patients compared to others. The most common side effects reported with lithium are renal toxicities, thyroid toxicosis, weight gain, somnolence, and cardiovascular abnormalities. Lithium-induced nephropathy is slow but progressive and is characterized by chronic interstitial nephritis including fibrosis, tubular atrophy, cystic tubular lesions, and glomerular sclerosis.

The true incidence of lithium-induced nephropathy is largely unknown. Renal dysfunction secondary to exposure to lithium occurs in up to 20% of the patients receiving lithium for any psychiatric disorder. The reported incidence ranged from 1% to 30%. Renal biopsy information obtained from psychiatric patients without exposure to lithium have shown similar renal injuries and histologic patterns. This finding suggests that renal injury can be from other etiologic processes independent of exposure to lithium. The prevalence, incidence, and severity of lithium-induced renal failure depend on the plasma concentration as well as the patient's renal function.

▶ Pathogenesis

Lithium toxicities appear to be dose and concentration dependent. Serum concentrations between 1 and 1.5 mEq/L will most likely cause impaired concentration, lethargy, irritability, muscle weakness, tremor, slurred speech, and nausea. Plasma concencerations greater than 2.5 mEq/L have been associated with renal failure. At therapeutic plasma concentrations lithium impairs the acidification ability of distal collecting tubules, which leads to renal tubular acidosis but not systemic metabolic acidosis. In the collecting tubule, lithium inhibits production of cyclic AMP (cAMP), downregulates the aquaporin-2 channel, decreases antidiuretic hormone (ADH) receptor density, and leads to ADH resistance and impairment of collecting duct concentrating capacity, which leads to polyuria, polydipsia, and nephrogenic diabetes insipidus. Because of the need for long-term lithium therapy in bipolar patients, chronic renal disease manifesting as chronic tubulointerstitial nephropathy (CTIN) is often seen. Renal biopsy reveals tubular atrophy and interstitial fibrosis either associated with cortical and medullary tubular cysts and dilation. CTIN is predominantly found in the distal and collecting tubule. Lithium also directly affects the glomerulus. Focal segmental glomerulosclerosis and global glomerulosclerosis are also seen, and tend to parallel in severity the underlying tubulointerstitial disease. This finding explains the reduced GFR and proteinuria in patients with chronic

lithium therapy. Despite the discontinuation of the lithium, many patients who had serum creatinine >2.5 mg/dL progressed to ESRD.

▶ Prevention & Management

Bipolar patients usually require long-term lithium treatment. Lithium has a narrow therapeutic range (1–1.5 mEq/L during acute episode therapy and 0.6–1.2 mEq/L during maintenance therapy). Chronic and acute poisoning can occur in patients whose lithium dosage has been increased or in those with a decreased effective circulating volume. Therefore, close monitoring of serum levels is important to prevent acute and chronic renal failure. Patients should be instructed to drink 8–12 glasses of liquid every day during lithium therapy. Because low sodium intake could promote lithium reabsorption, patients should maintain a regular non-low-salt diet. To avoid dehydration, prolonged exposure to the sun is discouraged and physicians should be contacted immediately if fever, diarrhea, or vomiting develops. Diuretics, especially thiazides, should be avoided with lithium concomitantly if possible. Thiazide diuretics contract extracelluar volume; therefore, lithium reabsorption is increased in the proximal tubule. In addition, medications that potentially increase serum lithium levels such as cyclosporine and NSAIDs (except low dose aspirin) or drugs with nephrotoxic properties such as aminoglycosides should be avoided (Table 14–4).

Table 14–4. Drug interactions with lithium.

Drug	Effect on Serum Lithium Concentration
Thiazide diuretics	Increase
Acetazolamide and other carbonic anhydrase inhibitors	Decrease[1]
Osmotic diuretics	Decrease
K+ sparing diuretics	Minimal decrease or no effect
Methyl xanthine inhibitors	Decrease
Loop diuretics	Decrease[1]
ACE inhibitors	Increase
NSAIDs Indomethacin Ibuprofen Mefenamic acid Naproxen Sulindac	 Increase Increase Increase Increase No effect
Aspirin	No effect

[1]When given acutely for lithium intoxication.
ACE, angiotensin-converting enzyme; NSAIDs, nonsteroidal anti-inflammatory drugs.

Fluid restoration is essential to manage lithium-induced nephrotoxicity. Acute renal insufficiency usually occurs in association with severe dehydration, and adequate fluid replacement rapidly restores kidney function. Loop diuretics can acutely abolish the lithium reabsorption process in the loop of Henle and increase lithium excretion; hence, furosemide (up to 40 mg/hour) can be used in case of lithium toxicity. However, such treatment cannot take place unless a large volume of fluids will be used to replace the loss of sodium and water induced by furosemide. In addition, lithium retention can occur following the discontinuation of furosemide due to its short duration of action and the reestablishment of intra- and extracellular lithium equilibrium. Acetazolamide combined with sodium bicarbonate can also be used instead of furosemide because acetazolamide inhibits the reabsorption of lithium by the proximal tubules.

Electrolyte supplements, especially sodium and potassium, should be given at the same time as management of lithium-induced nephrotoxicity because hyponatremia and hypokalemia are often seen in these patients. When patients cannot be managed medically or when renal function is severely impaired, hemodialysis is the most efficient way to decrease lithium levels because lithium is entirely dialyzable. Lithium leaves the cells rather slowly and serum levels can rebound if hemodialysis stops too soon. Therefore, hemodialysis should take place for a longer period or at frequent intervals (Table 14–5).

NONSTEROIDAL ANTI-INFLAMMATORY DRUGS

▶ Incidence & Risk Factors

NSAIDs are frequently used to treat chronic inflammatory conditions and for amelioration of acute and chronic pain. Widespread access and over-the-counter availability of these agents lead to the frequent impression that these drugs are safe and relatively devoid of toxicity. Unfortunately, NSAIDs or even aspirin use can pose a substantial risk to a large number of patients, especially when used chronically. Renal toxicity of the NSAIDs is discussed in Chapter 15.

Table 14–5 Management of lithium intoxication.

1. Protect oral airway if consciousness is impaired
2. Volume resuscitation
3. Gastric lavage, whole bowel irrigation with polyethylene glycol to prevent continued absorption of lithium
4. Lithium removal

   Serum lithium level >3.5–4 mEq/L: Most patients require hemodialysis

   Serum lithium level 2–4 mEq/L: Unstable patients and patients with severe nephrologic signs of renal insufficiency require hemodialysis

   Serum lithium level 1.5–2.5 mEq/L:

   Hemodialysis indicated for patients with renal failure or if patient fails to reach a lithium level below 1 mEq/L

   Fluid therapy or forced diuresis treatment should be recommended in patients with early signs of lithium intoxication and normal renal function, and when it is known that lithium levels have been elevated for only a few days

Aspelin P et al for the Nephric Study Investigators: Nephrotoxic effects in high-risk patients undergoing angiography. N Engl J Med 2003;348:491.

Bader BD et al: What is the best hydration regimen to prevent contrast media-induced nephrotoxicity? Clin Nephrol 2004;62:1.

Durham JD et al: A randomized controlled trial of N-acetylcysteine to prevent contrast nephropathy in cardiac angiography. Kidney Int 2002;62:2202.

Marenzi G et al: The prevention of radiocontrast-agent-induced nephropathy by hemofiltration. N Engl J Med 2003;349:1333.

Merten GJ et al: Prevention of contrast-induced nephropathy with sodium bicarbonate. A randomized controlled trial. JAMA 2004;291:2328.

Pannu N et al: Systematic review of the impact of N-acetylcysteine on contrast nephropathy. Kidney Int 2004;65:1366.

Trivedi HS et al: A prospective randomized trial to assess the role of saline hydration on the development of contrast nephrotoxicity. Nephron Clin Pract 2003;93:c29.

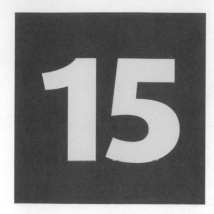

NSAIDs & the Kidney: Acute Renal Failure

Mark A. Perazella, MD

▶ Nonsteroidal anti-inflammatory drug (NSAID)-associated acute renal failure (ARF) develops predominantly in patients with underlying risk factors.

▶ Clinical presentations can be asymptomatic or associated with uremic symptoms, edema (pulmonary and peripheral), hypertension, or electrolyte and acid–base disturbances.

▶ Elevated blood urea nitrogen (BUN) and serum creatinine (Cr) concentrations are present.

▶ An elevated BUN/Cr ratio (> 20) is often noted.

▶ Hyponatremia (serum $[Na^+] < 135$ mEq/L), hyperkalemia (serum $[K^+] > 5.5$ mEq/L), and non-anion gap metabolic acidosis (serum $[HCO_3^-] < 20$ mEq/L) are common.

▶ Urine $[Na^+] < 10–20$ mEq/L and $Fe_{Na^+} < 1.0\%$ characterize NSAID-associated ARF.

▶ ARF is generally reversible with discontinuation of NSAIDs and treatment of concurrent disease processes.

▶ Severe ARF from NSAIDs may require dialysis.

▶ General Considerations

A. Epidemiology of Nonsteroidal Anti-inflammatory Drug Use

NSAIDs are employed widely to treat pain, fever, and inflammation. Other potential uses for these drugs include treatment and prevention of colonic polyposis and Alzheimer-type dementia. The first NSAID discovered was sodium salicylate in 1763. In 1950, phenylbutazone was introduced into clinical practice. It was efficacious but its use faded due to bone marrow toxicity. Subsequently, indomethacin entered the market in the 1960s. More than 20 NSAIDs from seven major classes,

including the selective cyclooxygenase (COX)-2 inhibitors (Table 15–1), are available in the United States. In addition to prescription NSAIDs, a large percentage of the general population consumes over-the-counter NSAIDs. Annually, more than 50 million patients ingest these drugs on an intermittent basis, while some 15–25 million people in the United States use an NSAID on a regular basis. Importantly, the elderly who are at risk for multiple complications of NSAID therapy, constitutes a growing population that has a prevalence of NSAID use as high as 15%.

B. Epidemiology of Nonsteroidal Anti-inflammatory Drug-Associated Acute Renal Failure

Unfortunately, the price paid for these therapeutic benefits include a number of gastrointestinal (GI) complications and, to a lesser degree, adverse renal effects. It has been estimated that from 5% to 7% of admissions to the hospital occur due to toxicity of NSAIDs, with the major organs involved being the GI tract, kidneys, and nervous system. The nephrotoxicity of NSAIDs, in particular hemodynamic ARF, is a relatively uncommon but important problem. It has been estimated that anywhere from 1% to 5% of patients who ingest NSAIDs will develop nephrotoxicity. Some calculations approximate that 500,000 persons are likely to develop some form of NSAID-associated adverse renal impairment (Table 15–2). Exposure to NSAIDs has been noted to double the risk of hospitalization for ARF in patients with chronic kidney disease (CKD). Patients with a history of heart failure and hypertension, as well as those treated with diuretics are at greatest risk of NSAID-induced ARF. The effect also appeared to be dose related with ARF occurring with higher NSAID dose. Hospitalized patients are at even higher risk. Of the cases of drug-induced ARF that develop in the hospital, it is estimated that nearly 16% are due to NSAID therapy.

As will be discussed in more detail, the healthy general population is at less risk for ARF as compared with patients

Table 15–1. Classes of nonsteroidal anti-inflammatory drugs.

Class	Trade name	Total dose/day (dosing interval)
Carboxylic acids		
Aspirin	Aspirin	2.4–6.0 g (qid)
Salsalate	Disalcid	1.5–3.0 g (bid)
Choline magnesium	Trilisate	1.5–3.0 g (bid-tid)
Diflunisal	Dolobid	0.5–1.5 g (bid)
Acetic acids		
Indomethacin	Indocin	75–150 mg (bid-qid)
Tolmetin	Tolectin	400–2400 mg (bid-tid)
Sulindac	Clinoril	200–400 mg (bid)
Diclofenac	Voltaren, Cataflam	100–150 mg (bid)
	Arthrotec	100 mg (bid)
Etodolac	Lodine	400–1200 mg (bid-qid)
Ketorolac	Toradol	Oral 40 mg (qid)
		Intravenous 60–120 mg (qid)
Propionic acids		
Ibuprofen	Motrin, Rufen	800–3200 mg (qid)
Naproxen	Naprosyn, Anaprox	500–1000 mg (bid)
	Alleve	450 mg (bid)
Ketoprofen	Orudis	225 mg (tid)
Flurbiprofen	Ansaid	200–300 mg (bid-tid)
Fenoprofen	Nalfon	1200–2400 mg (qid)
Oxaprozin	Daypro	1200 mg (qd)
Enolic acids		
Piroxicam	Feldene	10–20 mg (qd)
Phenylbutazone	Butazolidin	300–600 mg (tid)
Fenamates		
Mefenamic acid	Ponstel	1000 mg (qid)
Meclofenamate	Meclomen	150–400 mg (tid-qid)
Naphthylkanones		
Nabumetone	Relafen	1000–1500 mg (bid-tid)
COX-2 inhibitors		
Celecoxib	Celebrex	100–400 mg (qd-bid)
Valdecoxib	Bextra	10 mg (qd)
Rofecoxib[1]	Vioxx	12.5–50 mg (qd)

[1]Withdrawn from the market.

who possess multiple risk factors associated with NSAID nephrotoxicity. The majority of adverse renal effects are attributable to inhibition of renal prostaglandins by NSAIDs.

Table 15–2. Renal syndromes associated with nonsteroidal anti-inflammatory drugs.

Acute renal failure
Metabolic disturbances
   Hyponatremia
   Hyperkalemia
   Metabolic acidosis
Hypertension
Edema
Acute interstitial nephritis
Chronic interstitial nephritis
Papillary necrosis
Uroepithelial malignancy

The selective COX-2 inhibitors (celecoxib, valdecoxib, rofecoxib) appear to have a renal profile similar to other NSAIDs. Therefore, the term NSAIDs will refer to both nonselective NSAIDs and the selective COX-2 inhibitors. Electrolyte and acid–base disorders that occur with these drugs (hyperkalemia, hyponatremia, metabolic acidosis), hypertension that develops or is exacerbated by NSAIDs, and disturbances in sodium balance (edema formation, exacerbation of heart failure) will also be reviewed briefly in the context of ARF.

▶ Pathogenesis

A. Prostaglandin Synthesis

It is essential to review the pathway of prostaglandin (PG) production to facilitate an understanding of NSAID efficacy and toxicity. PGs, the major products of COX enzyme metabolism, are produced throughout the body and act at the local organ level in an autocrine and paracrine fashion. The initial step in PG synthesis is the liberation of arachidonic acid from cell membrane phospholipids. This reaction is mediated by phospholipase A_2, which is triggered by a number of hormones and mechanical factors. Arachidonic acid is the substrate for COX. Following synthesis, PGs promptly exit the cell to bind PG receptors found on parent or neighboring cells, thereby modulating cellular functions (Figure 15–1).

Two isomers of COX, COX-1 and COX-2, catalyze the synthesis of PGs. These isomers share a similar amino acid sequence and catalytic function. Differences in gene regulation between the COX isomers provide a molecular basis for their purported roles as "constitutive" (COX-1) and "inducible" (COX-2) enzymes. These labels accurately describe the synthesis of COX in most tissues, where COX-1, but not COX-2 is expressed in appreciable levels at baseline. In contrast, abundant expression of COX-2 is demonstrated in macrophages and other cell types in response to inflammatory mediators. However, it is now known that COX-2 is also constitutively expressed and upregulated in the kidney and plays an important role in renal physiologic processes. It is probable that the nephrotoxicity of selective and nonselective NSAIDs results from the inhibition of COX-2 rather than COX-1.

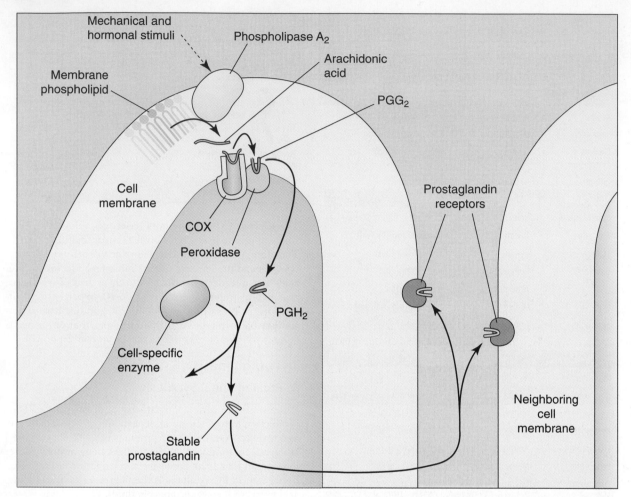

▲ **Figure 15–1.** Pathway of prostaglandin biosynthesis. Arachidonic acid is released from membrane phospholipids, modulated by cyclooxygenase (COX) and cell specific enzymes to form prostaglandins (PGs). Prostaglandins then produce their effect by binding receptors on parent and neighboring cells. (Reproduced with permission from Perazella MA: COX-2 inhibitors and the kidney. Hosp Pract 2001;36:43.)

B. Role of Prostaglandins in Renal Physiology

PG synthesis is of minimal importance in the kidney of healthy individuals with normal volume status. As such, it is not a primary regulator of renal function. Rather, eicosanoids locally modulate the effects of both systemic and locally produced vasoconstrictor hormones. A variety of PGs are synthesized within distinct anatomic locations in the kidney, including PGI_2, PGE_2, thromboxane A_2 (TXA_2), and $PGF_{2\alpha}$ (Figure 15–2). PGI_2 and PGE_2 are the predominant mediators of physiologic activity in the kidney. Functionally, PGI_2 and PGE_2 induce vasodilation in interlobular arteries, afferent and efferent arterioles, and glomeruli.

In the loop of Henle and distal nephron, PGE_2 decreases cellular transport of sodium chloride in thick ascending limb cells and collecting duct cells, respectively. An increase in

renal sodium excretion and a decrease in medullary tonicity are the direct result of PGE_2 action in these nephron segments. PGE_2 and PGI_2 also stimulate renin secretion in the juxtaglomerular apparatus, ultimately leading to increased angiotensin II and aldosterone synthesis, enhancing sodium retention and potassium excretion in the distal nephron. Finally, PGE_2 and PGI_2 also inhibit cyclic-AMP synthesis and oppose the action of antidiuretic hormone (ADH), facilitating water excretion.

C. Risk Factors for Nonsteroidal Anti-inflammatory Drug-Associated Acute Renal Failure

Since basal PG production is low in healthy persons, the risk of NSAID-associated ARF is negligible. There are, however,

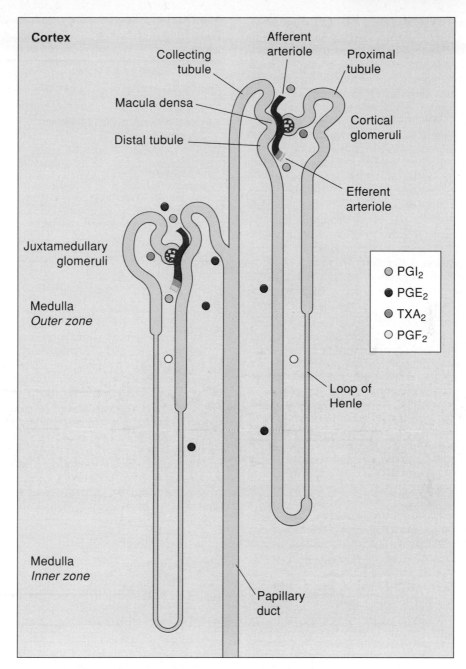

▲ **Figure 15–2.** Anatomic locations of prostaglandin (PG) synthesis within the kidney and their sites of action. TXA_2, thromboxane A_2. (Reproduced with permission from Perazella MA: COX-2 inhibitors and the kidney. Hosp Pract 2001;36:43.)

risk factors (Table 15–3) that render the kidney PG dependent and, therefore, place patients at risk for the development of ARF when they use NSAIDs. PGs have their major role in the preservation of renal function when pathologic states supervene and compromise physiologic kidney processes. The development of "true" intravascular volume depletion, as seen with vomiting, diarrhea, and diuretic therapy, stimulates PG synthesis to optimize renal blood flow. "Effective" decreases in renal blood flow as seen with congestive heart failure (CHF), cirrhosis, and nephrotic syndrome also stimulate compensatory PG production. PGI_2 and PGF_2 antagonize the local effects of circulating angiotensin II, endothelin, vasopressin, and catecholamines that would normally maintain systemic blood pressure at the expense of the renal circulation. Specifically, these eicosanoids preserve glomerular filtration rate (GFR) by antagonizing arteriolar vasoconstriction and blunting mesangial and podocyte contraction induced by these endogenous vasopressors. A significant reduction in GFR can occur following administration of an NSAID to a patient with any of these underlying disease states (Figure 15–3).

Table 15–3. Risk factors for NSAID-associated acute renal failure.

"True" intravascular volume depletion
Vomiting
Diarrhea
Diuretics
"Effective" intravascular volume depletion
Congestive heart failure
Cirrhosis
Nephrotic syndrome
Kidney disease
Acute renal failure
Chronic kidney disease
Medications
Angiotensin-converting enzyme inhibitors
Angiotensin receptor blockers
Old age

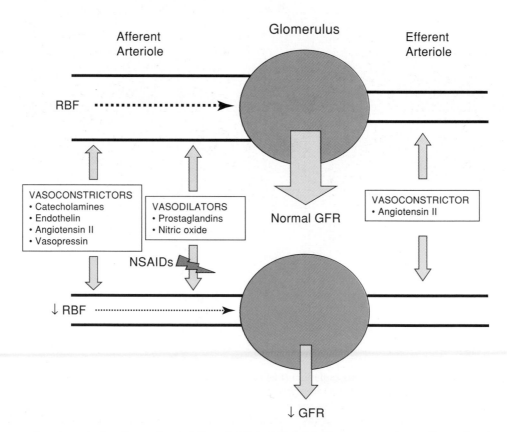

▲ **Figure 15–3.** Renal prostaglandins maintain RBF and GFR by balancing the vasoconstrictor effects of various endogenous factors during "true" or "effective" volume depletion. NSAIDs blunt prostaglandin production and tip the balance in favor of vasoconstriction, resulting in reduced RBF and GFR, manifesting clinically as acute renal failure. NSAIDs, nonsteroidal anti-inflammatory drugs; RBF, renal blood flow; GFR, glomerular filtration rate.

PG production is also increased in CKD. Upregulation of PG synthesis in CKD is induced by intrarenal mechanisms activated to increase perfusion of remnant nephrons. As a result, impairment of PG production with an NSAID is associated with acute reductions in renal blood flow and GFR. Certain medications, such as drugs that antagonize the renin–angiotensin–aldosterone system (RAAS) such as angiotensin-converting enzyme (ACE) inhibitors and angiotensin receptor blockers (ARBs), increase the risk for ARF when an NSAID is administered. This is typically a problem in patients with true or effective intravascular volume depletion or underlying CKD. In the absence of underlying kidney disease, ARF rarely develops when these patients are euvolemic. Finally, the elderly are at risk for ARF because of unrecognized CKD, intravascular volume depletion, and hypoalbuminemia (which increases levels of free NSAID in the circulation).

▶ Clinical Findings

A. Symptoms and Signs

In the absence of severe ARF, most patients with NSAID-associated prerenal azotemia are asymptomatic. The underlying risk factor that predisposes the patient to ARF often determines the clinical presentation. For example, patients with "true" intravascular volume depletion will present with uremic manifestations such as anorexia, nausea and vomiting, weakness, fatigue, inability to concentrate, and possibly GI dyspepsia (from NSAID gastropathy). They will not be hypertensive or edematous. In contrast, patients with "effective" intravascular volume depletion such as CHF, cirrhosis, or nephrotic syndrome will manifest volume overload. In the CHF patient, this can manifest as lung crackles, elevated jugular venous pulsations, and an S3 cardiac gallop from pulmonary edema, as well as peripheral pitting edema. Increased abdominal girth from ascites and worsened peripheral edema can develop in the patient with cirrhosis. Increased peripheral edema and anasarca may develop in the patient with nephrotic syndrome. Patients with CHF and nephrosis will often be hypertensive, whereas the patient with cirrhosis does not develop an increase in blood pressure. Patients with underlying hypertension, especially when under therapy with antihypertensive medications, will often manifest a destabilization of blood pressure and present with worsened hypertension. The patient with CKD will develop acute uremia, severe hypertension, increased peripheral edema, and CHF. Muscle weakness and cardiac arrhythmias (from hyperkalemia) can occur in CKD patients who receive NSAIDs. In addition, patients treated with medications that impair potassium homeostasis (ACE inhibitors, ARBs, spironolactone, eplerenone, calcineurin inhibitors, heparin) may also develop these adverse effects when an NSAID is added to their regimen. The elderly patient can present with any number of these clinical symptoms and signs.

B. Laboratory Findings

ARF associated with NSAIDs is hemodynamic and, therefore, the laboratory parameters typically reflect a "prerenal" state. Both serum and urine tests support this. BUN and serum Cr concentrations are both elevated, however, the BUN concentration typically increases more than the serum Cr concentration. In general, the BUN/Cr ratio is greater than 20, although this does not occur in all patients. Not uncommonly, several electrolyte disturbances may also be present. They include hyponatremia (serum $[Na^+]$ <135 mEq/L) from impaired renal water excretion and hyperkalemia (serum $[K^+]$ >5.5 mEq/L) with or without a non-anion gap metabolic acidosis. NSAID-induced hyporeninemic hypoaldosteronism underlies the hyperkalemia and non-anion gap metabolic acidosis. Importantly, these electrolyte and acid–base disturbances can develop even with minimal ARF as they are caused via direct effects of the NSAID on various tubular segments in the nephron.

Urine testing also points to a prerenal state of ARF. The urine specific gravity (SG) is typically greater than 1.015. Urine $[Na^+]$ is often less than 10–20 mEq/L. Calculation of the fractional excretion of sodium (FE_{Na^+} = [urine Na^+ × serum Cr] ÷ [serum Na^+ × urine Cr]) reveals a value less than 1.0% (Table 15–4). This contrasts with a value greater than 3.0%, which would characterize acute tubular necrosis (ATN). Rarely, the specific gravity and FE_{Na^+} may be suggestive of ATN (SG ≤1.015, FE_{Na^+} >3.0%) in patients with NSAID-associated ARF. This represents a situation in which some level of ischemic ATN developed, probably due to hypotension and severe renal hypoperfusion. Hyperkalemia is evaluated by calculating the transtubular potassium gradient (TTKG). TTKG is calculated as follows: TTKG = [urine K^+ ÷ (urine osmolality/serum osmolality)] ÷ serum K^+. A TTKG <6 in the setting of hyperkalemia reflects impaired renal potassium excretion due to hypoaldosteronism and is consistent with a diagnosis of NSAID nephrotoxicity.

Table 15–4. Urine findings noted in NSAID-associated acute renal failure and acute tubular necrosis.

SG	Urine $[Na^+]$	FE_{Na^+}	Sediment
NSAID >1.020	<10–20 mEq/L	<1.0%	Bland, acellular, hyaline casts
ATN ± 1.015	>20 mEq/L	>3.0%	RTE cells, RTE cell casts, granular casts
AIN ± 1.015	>20 mEq/L	>3.0%	WBCs, RBCs, rare eosinophils, WBC casts

NSAID, nonsteroidal anti-inflammatory drug; SG, specific gravity; ATN, acute tubular necrosis; AIN, acute interstitial nephritis; RTE, renal tubular epithelial; WBCs, white blood cells; RBCs, red blood cells.

Microscopic examination of the urine in patients with NSAID-associated ARF generally reveals a bland sediment with no cellular elements and sometimes a few hyaline casts. This is consistent with the prerenal azotemia that develops in this setting. Rarely, a few renal tubular epithelial (RTE) cells, RTE cell casts, and granular casts may be present if ischemic tubular injury has also developed. It is uncommon to view red blood cells, white blood cells, or casts containing these cellular elements unless another renal disease coexists. Their presence suggests superimposition of NSAID nephrotoxicity on another renal process, such as acute interstitial nephritis (AIN).

Imaging tests are normal in the absence of another concurrent disease process in the kidneys. Renal ultrasonography reveals normal sized kidneys with normal echotexture and no evidence of hydronephrosis. Computerized tomography (CT) scan and magnetic resonance imaging (MRI) are also normal in pure NSAID-associated ARF. An ACE inhibitor renal perfusion scan would show bilateral decreased uptake of tracer by the kidneys, consistent with prerenal azotemia.

▶ Differential Diagnosis

ARF that develops in the setting of NSAID therapy needs to be differentiated from other prerenal states, as well as various intrinsic renal processes such as ATN and AIN. As with other causes of ARF, obstructive uropathy also needs to be considered in the differential diagnosis.

Since both "true" and "effective" intravascular volume depletion cause prerenal ARF and also are risk factors for NSAID-associated ARF, it is very difficult to ascribe renal injury to either alone. This is because the addition of an NSAID can potentially worsen underlying CHF and cirrhosis, making them appear as poorly compensated disease states. Regardless, discontinuation of the drug and therapy directed at the underlying clinical disease are required. Ischemic ATN can develop from the underlying clinical problem (ie, hypotension, sepsis) as well as from the effect of NSAID on renal hemodynamics, which further worsens renal perfusion and GFR in these settings. The urine data distinguish NSAID-associated ARF from ATN as an SG ≤ 1.015, urine [Na^+] >20 mEq/L, FE_{Na^+} >3%, and urine sediment with RTE cells, RTE cell casts, and granular casts characterize ATN.

ARF from AIN may also develop from an NSAID. Patients who do not recover within several days of stopping the NSAID should be evaluated for AIN. Although not always the case, AIN usually is associated with eosinophilia, tubular proteinuria (<1 g/day), pyuria (± eosinophiluria), and hematuria (Table 15–4). AIN from NSAIDs, however, is often devoid of the classic findings of AIN and can present with a bland urine sediment. Finally, ARF from partial urinary tract obstruction can be confused with NSAID-associated ARF because the urine sediment can also be unremarkable. However, the urine SG and electrolytes more often reflect tubular injury and are similar to those seen with ATN.

▶ Complications

As with any drug that induces ARF, a number of uremic, metabolic, and intravascular volume-related complications can develop. Severe ARF may be associated with several uremia-related problems. These include central nervous system dysfunction (confusion, agitation, seizure), bleeding from platelet dysfunction, increased infection risk, malnutrition from a catabolic state, and inflammation of serosal surfaces (pericarditis, pleuritis). Hyponatremia, hyperkalemia, and metabolic acidosis can develop from ARF or from direct effects of the NSAID. Hyperkalemia can be more severe than expected for the level of renal dysfunction due to the state of hyporeninemic hypoaldosteronism promoted by the NSAID. Volume overload with pulmonary edema and peripheral edema can complicate NSAID-associated nephrotoxicity in cardiac patients. Precipitation of hepatorenal syndrome is a potentially devastating complication of NSAID therapy in cirrhotic patients. Also, diuretic resistance can develop in patients with CHF and nephrotic syndrome. Recently, increased risk for adverse cardiovascular events has been noted with both selective and nonselective NSAIDs.

▶ Treatment

The mainstay of therapy is discontinuation of the NSAID. Additional measures include correction of the underlying process that predisposed to nephrotoxicity. In some cases, intravenous normal saline rapidly repairs volume status and facilitates renal recovery in patients with intravascular volume depletion. High-dose intravenous diuretics, sometimes in combination, may be required in cardiac patients with ARF complicated by CHF and in nephrotic patients with severe edema and anasarca. Life-threatening hyperkalemia mandates intravenous calcium gluconate (stabilize cardiac tissue), intravenous insulin plus glucose, high-dose nebulized β_2-agonists to shift K^+ into cells, and diuretic therapy to enhance renal excretion in patients who maintain reasonable kidney function. It is unusual for metabolic acidosis to be severe enough to warrant sodium bicarbonate administration. Severe ARF complicated by advanced uremia or other life-threatening complications (pulmonary edema, metabolic disturbances) that does not recover within a few days of stopping NSAID therapy requires renal replacement therapy.

▶ Prognosis

Fortunately, discontinuation of the NSAID is often associated with recovery of renal function. In general, renal function returns to baseline within 2–5 days, however, recovery may be delayed in patients with decompensated heart disease, cirrhosis, and underlying CKD. It is extremely unusual that a patient does not recover kidney function. The failure to do so should elicit an evaluation for other causes of ARF such as ATN, AIN, and obstructive uropathy.

Bouvy ML et al: Effects of NSAIDs on the incidence of hospitalizations for renal dysfunction in users of ACE inhibitors. Drug Safety 2003;26(13):983. [PMID: 1458372]

Eras J, Perazella MA: NSAIDs and the kidney revisited: are selective cyclooxygenase-2 inhibitors safe? Am J Med Sci 2001;321:181. [PMID: 11269794]

Gambaro G, Perazella MA: Adverse renal effects of anti-inflammatory agents: evaluation of selective and non-selective cyclooxygenase inhibitors. J Intern Med 2003;253:643. [PMID: 12755960]

Huerta C et al: Nonsteroidal anti-inflammatory drugs and risk of ARF in the general population. Am J Kidney Dis 2005;45(2):531. [PMID: 15754275]

Perazella MA, Tray K: Selective COX-2 inhibitors: a pattern of nephrotoxicity similar to traditional nonsteroidal anti-inflammatory drugs. Am J Med 2001;111:64. [PMID: 11448662]

Perazella MA: Drug-induced hyperkalemia: old culprits and new offenders. Am J Med 2000;109:307. [PMID: 10996582]

Sturmer T et al: Nonsteroidal anti-inflammatory drugs and the kidney. Curr Opin Nephrol Hypertens 2001;10:161. [PMID: 11224688]

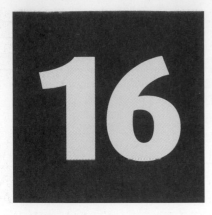

Obstructive Uropathy

Beckie Michael, DO

▶ Urinary tract obstruction, not an uncommon problem, can occur at any age.

▶ It can be acute or chronic, partial or complete, with unilateral or bilateral renal involvement.

▶ The diagnosis of obstructive uropathy usually requires the presence of hydronephrosis (dilation of the renal pelvis and calyces), hydroureter, and/or bladder distention.

General Considerations

Patients presenting with unexplained acute or chronic kidney disease, with or without obstructive symptoms, should be evaluated for the possibility of obstructive uropathy. Chronic obstruction can result in chronic tubulointerstitial disease. Bladder outlet obstruction is common in older males due to prostatic hypertrophy or carcinoma. Urinary retention can be seen in both genders postoperatively and as a complication of urinary tract infection.

Prevention

Patients complaining of voiding dysfunction including hesitancy, decreased force of stream, interruption in stream, or postvoid dribbling should be evaluated for the presence of urinary retention. These symptoms are usually due to prostate disease, urethral stricture, or neurogenic bladder. Medications can often be used to treat many of these symptoms and prevent complications. Patients with bladder spasticity can benefit from anticholinergic agents such as oxybutinin and propantheline bromide. Patients with bladder outlet problems can be treated with α-antagonists, which act by relaxing the smooth muscle of the bladder neck and prostate. Patients with severe bladder atony may require intermittent bladder catheterization.

Clinical Findings

A. Symptoms and Signs

Patients with obstruction of a solitary kidney or bilateral obstruction present with acute oligoanuric renal failure. Incomplete obstruction can result in fluctuating urine output. Pain is related to the location, duration, and severity of obstruction. Acute obstruction can result in severe pain due to distention of the collecting system or renal capsule. Renal colic due to calculi is often sudden and severe, with pain beginning in the flank and radiating into the ipsilateral groin. This can be accompanied by nausea and vomiting. Patients with renal colic prefer to be in motion, compared to patients with peritonitis, whose pain is worsened with movement.

A distended bladder on physical examination or the presence of a flank mass is suggestive of obstruction. Hypertension can be seen in obstructive uropathy due to volume expansion and activation of the renin–angiotensin–aldosterone system.

B. Laboratory Findings

Table 16–1 lists the common laboratory abnormalities in obstructive uropathy. The kidneys lose their ability to concentrate the urine early in obstruction. Later, they cannot concentrate or dilute urine well (isosthenuria). Defects in distal urinary acidification result in a hyperchloremic metabolic acidosis (distal renal tubular acidosis). This can be accompanied by hyperkalemia. Patients will have renal insufficiency if there is bilateral obstruction or obstruction to a solitary functioning kidney. Often the ratio of blood urea nitrogen to serum creatinine will be greater than 10:1 due to increased urea reabsorption throughout the collecting system. Patients with a partial obstruction can have nephrogenic diabetes insipidus (resistance to antidiuretic hormone) and develop hypernatremia. Patients may have polycythemia due to excess erythropoietin production, or may be anemic with more advanced renal impairment. Urinary stasis can result in urinary tract infection with urea splitting bacteria like

Table 16–1. Common laboratory findings in obstructive uropathy.

Elevated serum creatinine (Cr)
Elevated blood urea nitrogen (BUN)
Ratio of BUN:Cr >10:1
Normal anion gap metabolic acidosis (distal renal tubular acidosis)
Normal or hyperkalemia
Hematuria and/or pyuria

Proteus and *Staphylococcus*. This results in an alkaline urine pH and is associated with struvite (magnesium, ammonium, phosphate) calculi.

C. Imaging Studies

1. Abdominal x-ray—Abdominal x-ray is useful in identifying radiopaque calculi. However, it is often omitted as part of the evaluation for obstructive uropathy because spiral computed tomography (CT) without contrast is often performed as part of the initial evaluation.

2. Ultrasound—Ultrasound is 90% sensitive and specific for detecting hydronephrosis. It can be falsely negative in the presence of an early obstruction, volume depletion, or if the ureters are encased due to a retroperitoneal process. Ultrasound of the bladder reveals a thickened bladder wall with trabeculations in chronic bladder outlet obstruction. Duplex Doppler can also be performed. A high resistive index is seen from increased vascular resistance in obstruction.

3. Spiral computed tomography—Spiral CT (noncontrast) has become the radiographic study of choice to evaluate a patient for stone disease. It is a very short procedure that is highly sensitive for detecting renal and ureteric calculi.

4. Magnetic resonance urography (MRU)—MRU is available at some centers and can be performed without the use of contrast agents. Although T_2-weighted MRU can determine the severity and location of obstruction, it has a sensitivity of only 70% for detecting calculi. This fact combined with its cost will likely limit the utilization of MRU.

5. Radioisotope renography—Radioisotope renography with the administration of furosemide can be used to differentiate mechanical from functional obstruction.

6. Intravenous pyelography (IVP)—IVP should be avoided in patients with renal insufficiency due to the risk of radiocontrast-induced acute renal injury. It may be used in patients in whom ultrasound or noncontrast spiral CT has been unable to determine the exact location of obstruction, and is helpful in diagnosing papillary necrosis. However, the use of IVP has been largely replaced by contrast-enhanced CT, which has been found to be more sensitive than IVP in determining the cause of obstruction.

D. Special Examinations

Documenting postvoid residual urine by bladder catheterization or ultrasound is an integral part of the initial evaluation of a patient with suspected obstructive uropathy. Patients may also need rectal and/or pelvic examinations to determine the presence of a mass (cervix, rectal, prostate) and the size of the prostate. Cystoscopy with retrograde ureterograms and percutaneous nephrostomy with antegrade ureteropyelograms are diagnostic and therapeutic procedures done to determine the site of and potentially relieve the obstruction.

▶ Differential Diagnosis

As mentioned earlier, obstructive uropathy should be included in the differential diagnosis of acute or chronic renal failure. Table 16–2 lists the common causes of obstructive uropathy according to location. In men, bladder outlet obstruction due to prostate disease or urethral stricture is the most common cause of lower tract obstruction and is easily diagnosed by the assessment of postvoid residual urine (by catheter or ultrasound). In women, cervical cancer, uterine prolapse, and pregnancy are common causes of obstructive uropathy. Stones often cause unilateral upper tract obstruction. Urine flow is usually obstructed due to the presence of stones at one of the three places: The ureteropelvic junction, where the ureter crosses over the iliac vessels, and at the

Table 16–2. Etiologies of obstructive uropathy.

Upper tract obstruction
Intrinsic
    Stone
    Papillary necrosis
    Blood clot
    Transitional cell carcinoma
    Valve/polyp
Extrinsic
    Retroperitoneal fibrosis
    Aortic aneurysm
    Retroperitoneal or pelvic malignancy
    Masses of uterus/ovary
    Endometriosis
Other
    Ureter ligation
Lower tract obstruction
Urethral stricture
Prostate disease (benign, malignant)
Bladder, cervix, colon cancer
Bladder stones
Blood clot
Neurogenic bladder

ureterovesicular junction. An ultrasound often reveals hydro-ureter and/or hydronephrosis. Papillary necrosis occurs when there is sloughing of renal papillae due to ischemia or toxins. This can be complicated by ureteric obstruction. These patients often have gross or microscopic hematuria.

Pathologic processes in the retroperitoneal space (radiation injury, trauma, infection, granulomatous diseases, fibrosis) can cause ureteric obstruction. Retroperitoneal fibrosis can result in obstructive uropathy without evidence of obstruction on ultrasound. Retroperitoneal fibrosis is an insidious process resulting from a local or systemic inflammatory process. Intravenous pyelography reveals external compression of the ureters.

Urinary tract dilation can occasionally be seen without obstruction. A classic example is pregnancy, where there is a progesterone-mediated decrease in ureter peristalsis and hydroureter, more commonly involving the right collecting system. Other examples include a dilated extrarenal pelvis and hydroureter due to vesiculoureteral reflux.

▶ Complications

Obstruction results in decreased renal blood flow, decreased glomerular filtration rate, and impaired tubular function. There is some controversy as to the duration of complete obstruction after which correction will result in substantial renal recovery. Complete obstruction for greater than 1 week will likely result in some permanent renal damage. Complete obstruction for greater than 8–12 weeks is unlikely to result in renal recovery. Obstruction may be complicated by urinary tract infection, which requires emergent relief of obstruction.

Postobstructive diuresis can occur after relief of obstruction. This large volume of urine output after relief of obstruction can result in volume and electrolyte (potassium, sodium, and magnesium) depletion. Urine output should be measured hourly. Intravenous fluids (IVF) are required if the patient has evidence of volume depletion (orthostatic hypotension, tachycardia), is unable to maintain adequate oral intake, or has urine output greater than 200 mL/hour. Urine and serum electrolytes can be measured every 6 hours to determine the IVF composition, but 0.5 normal saline solution (NSS) with KCl and sodium bicarbonate if needed is often most appropriate. Urine output should be replaced 0.5 mL IVF/mL urine output unless the patient is volume depleted. This will prevent continued diuresis due to IVF administration.

▶ Treatment

Obstruction should be relieved as indicated by its location. Obstructive uropathy complicated by acute renal failure and hyperkalemia requires emergent intervention. Bladder outlet obstruction can be relieved with a transurethral or suprapubic catheter. Ureteric obstruction can be relieved via cystoscopy with retrograde ureteroscopy and stent placement or with percutaneous nephrostomy. Stones that are less than 5–6 mm usually pass spontaneously and can be observed. These patients are treated with increased fluid intact and analgesic medications. Stones larger than 7 mm are unlikely to pass spontaneously. Stones in the distal ureter can be treated with ureteroscopic stone extraction. Extracorporeal shock wave lithotripsy (ESWL) can also be performed.

Some patients may require intermittent straight catheterization or a chronic indwelling Foley catheter. Careful technique must be used to prevent urinary tract infection with bladder instrumentation. If possible, definitive therapy should be performed to limit the use of catheters.

Abo El-Ghar ME et al: Contrast enhanced spiral computerized tomography in patients with chronic obstructive uropathy and normal serum creatinine: a single session for anatomical and functional assessment. J Urol 2004;172:985.

Grotegut CA: Ureteral obstruction in pregnancy. N Engl J Med 2004;351:pe14.

Shokeir AA et al: Diagnosis of ureteral obstruction in patients with compromised renal function: the role of noninvasive imaging modalities. J Urol 2004;171:2303.

Chronic Renal Failure & the Uremic Syndrome

17

Gregorio T. Obrador, MD, MPH

ESSENTIALS OF DIAGNOSIS

▶ Abnormally elevated serum creatinine for 3 or more months.

▶ Calculated glomerular filtration rate (GFR) ≤60 mL/minute/1.73 m² for 3 or more months.

▶ Clinical manifestations of the uremic syndrome in patients with advanced kidney failure.

▶ General Considerations

The National Kidney Foundation–Kidney Disease Outcomes Quality Initiative (NKF-K/DOQI) has defined chronic kidney disease (CKD) as (1) kidney damage for 3 or more months, as defined by structural or functional abnormalities of the kidney, with or without decreased GFR, manifested by either pathologic abnormalities or markers of kidney damage, including abnormalities in the composition of the blood or urine or in imaging tests; or (2) GFR ≤60 mL/minute/1.73 m² for 3 or more months, with or without markers of kidney damage. The NKF-K/DOQI recommends using the equation derived from the Modification of Diet in Renal Disease (MDRD) to estimate GFR from the serum creatinine (eGFR) and has proposed a classification of CKD based on level of eGFR (Table 17–1).

CKD with decreased GFR (stages 2 through 5 of the NKF-K/DOQI classification), also known as chronic renal failure or chronic renal insufficiency in the literature prior to the NKF-K/DOQI classification, is a clinical syndrome that results from progressive decline of the GFR, typically over months to years, and is due to irreversible destruction of nephrons independent of the cause. In stage 2, the only manifestation of CKD may be a persistently decreased eGFR. As the GFR continues to decline (stages 3 and 4), other laboratory abnormalities begin to appear. The uremic syndrome refers to a constellation of symptoms and signs that occurs in patients with advanced kidney failure (typically GFR <10–15 mL/minute/1.73 m²) and reflects generalized organ dysfunction (stage 5). At this stage, kidney replacement therapy with dialysis or transplantation becomes necessary to sustain life. End-stage renal disease (ESRD) is an administrative term based on conditions for payment of health care by the Medicare ESRD program for patients treated by dialysis and/or transplantation in the United States.

It has been estimated that 8.3 million Americans have an eGFR ≤60 mL/minute/1.73 m². Moreover, in the year 2002 alone, 100,359 patients began kidney replacement therapy and 431,284 were under active care in the United States. The prevalence and incidence rates of treated ESRD were 333 and 1435 cases per million population, respectively. Diabetes mellitus is the most common cause of ESRD, accounting for nearly 45% of cases; systemic hypertension is the second leading cause, and together with diabetes accounts for over two-thirds of the cases of ESRD. African-Americans are more susceptible to ESRD secondary to diabetes or hypertension.

▶ Pathogenesis

The progressive nephron and GFR loss associated with progressive CKD leads to (1) abnormalities in water, electrolyte, and pH balance, (2) accumulation of waste products that are normally excreted by the kidney, and (3) abnormalities in the production and metabolism of certain hormones (ie, erythropoietin, active vitamin D). Fortunately, as the GFR declines, a number of compensatory mechanisms are activated, of which the most important is glomerular hyperfiltration in the remaining functioning nephrons. Due to this compensatory mechanism, a patient may be totally asymptomatic despite having lost 70% of kidney function. However, glomerular hyperfiltration is associated with the development of glomerulosclerosis in the remaining functioning nephrons, which contributes to further nephron loss. Other factors that contribute to nephron loss include (1) ongoing activity of the primary cause of CKD, (2) proteinuria, (3) development of

Table 17–1. Classification of chronic kidney disease and management recommendations.[1]

Stage	Description	GFR (mL/minute/1.73 m^2)	Management
	At increased risk	>90 (CKD risk factors)	Screening CKD risk reduction
1	Kidney damage with normal or ↑ GFR	>90	Diagnosis and Rx CVD risk reduction
2	Mild ↓ GFR	60–89	Estimating progression
3	Moderate ↓ GFR	30–59	Evaluating and treating complications
4	Severe ↓ GFR	15–29	Preparation for kidney replacement therapy
5	Kidney failure	<15 or dialysis	Replacement, if uremia is present

[1]Recommendations by the National Kidney Foundation–Kidney Disease Outcomes Quality Initiative (NKF-K/DOQI). GFR, glomerular filtration rate; CKD, chronic kidney disease; CVD, cardiovascular disease.

Reproduced with permission from *Am J Kid Dis.* 2002;39(Suppl):S46.

tubulointerstitial lesions, (4) hyperlipidemia, and (5) acute superimposed renal insults (ie, contrast nephropathy, aminoglycoside toxicity, etc.).

▶ **Prevention**

Aggressive glucose and blood pressure control in diabetic and/or hypertensive patients reduces the risk of developing CKD. Screening individuals at high risk for CKD, particularly those with diabetes, hypertension, or a family history of diabetes, hypertension, or kidney disease, allows for early detection and implementation of interventions that prevent or slow the progression of CKD. Appropriate screening tests include a urinalysis, a first morning or a random "spot" urine sample for albumin or protein to creatinine ratio, serum creatinine level for estimation of GFR using an accepted prediction equation, and blood pressure measurement.

▶ **Clinical Findings**

A. Symptoms and Signs

Patients are usually asymptomatic until kidney failure is advanced. When the GFR falls to approximately 10–15 mL/minute, nonspecific symptoms such as general malaise, weakness, insomnia, inability to concentrate, and nausea and vomiting begin to appear. Eventually other symptoms and signs that reflect generalized organ dysfunction develop as part of the uremic syndrome (Table 17–2).

Table 17–2. Clinical and laboratory manifestations of the uremic syndrome.

System	Clinical Manifestations
Skin	Paleness and hyperpigmentation Echymosis and hematomas Pruritus Skin necrosis (calciphylaxis) Bullous lesions
Cardiovascular	Volume overload and systemic hypertension Accelerated atherosclerosis and ischemic heart disease Left ventricular hypertrophy Heart failure Rhythm disturbances Uremic pericarditis
Neurologic	Cerebrovascular accidents Encephalopathy Seizures Peripheral and autonomic neuropathy
Gastrointestinal	Anorexia Nausea and vomiting Malnutrition Uremic fetor Inflammatory and ulcerative lesions Gastrointestinal bleeding
Hematologic	Anemia Leukocyte and immune system dysfunction (tendency to infections) Platelet dysfunction (bleeding diathesis)
Bone	Renal osteodystrophy Growth retardation in children Muscle weakness Amyloid arthropathy secondary to β_2-microglobulin deposition
Endocrine	Sexual dysfunction Infertility in women Glucose intolerance due to insulin resistance Hyperlipidemia
Laboratory	Hyponatremia (if excessive water intake) Hyperkalemia Hyperphosphatemia Hypocalcemia Hypermagnesemia Hyperuricemia Metabolic acidosis

1. Skin manifestations—The skin is often pale (due to anemia) and hyperpigmented [due to increased production of β-melanocyte-stimulating hormone (β-MSH) and retention of carotenes and urochromes]. Pruritus is common and can be accompanied by scratching lesions. Ecchymoses and hematomas are often seen as a result of bleeding diathesis. Uremic frost is a fine white powder visible on the skin surface that results from crystallization of urea after sweat evaporates; it is now uncommon because of earlier initiation of dialysis. Other infrequent but clinically important abnormalities include skin necrosis due to vessel calcification (calciphylaxis) and bullous lesions.

2. Cardiovascular manifestations—Cardiovascular manifestations are the most common cause of morbidity and mortality among patients with progressive CKD and include volume overload, edema, systemic hypertension, ischemic heart disease, left ventricular hypertrophy, heart failure, rhythm disturbances, and uremic pericarditis. Systemic hypertension is primarily due to volume overload; other contributing factors are hyperreninemia and erythropoietin therapy. Patients with chronic kidney failure (CKF) have accelerated atherosclerosis due to a high prevalence of "traditional" (ie, hypertension and hyperlipidemia) and "nontraditional" risk factors (those associated with the hemodynamic and metabolic abnormalities of CKF, such as volume overload, anemia, glucose intolerance, and hyperparathyroidism). Left ventricular hypertrophy is seen in 65–75% of patients with advanced CKF, and both arterial hypertension and anemia contribute to its development. Heart failure is usually multifactorial, with volume overload, hypertension, anemia, ischemic heart disease, and uremic cardiomyopathy as the main contributing factors. Rhythm disturbances are often precipitated by electrolyte abnormalities, metabolic acidosis, calcification of the conduction system, ischemia, and myocardial dysfunction. Uremic pericarditis occurs in 6–10% of patients with advanced uremia, just before initiation of dialysis or immediately after; it is associated with high blood urea levels (>60 mg/dL) and hemorrhagic pericardial effusion is seen in at least 50% of cases.

3. Neurologic manifestations—Cerebrovascular accidents are common in these patients due to accelerated atherosclerosis. Uremic encephalopathy occurs in patients with advanced uremia and is characterized by insomnia, sleep pattern changes, inability to concentrate, memory loss, confusion, disorientation, emotional lability, anxiety, depression, and occasionally hallucinations. Without treatment, the encephalopathy progresses to generalized seizures, coma, and death. Other manifestations may include dysarthria, tremor, and myoclonic movements, and in advanced stages, hyperreflexia, clonus, and the Babinsky sign. The electroencephalogram shows diffuse slowing of cortical activity. Dialysis improves most of the manifestations of uremic encephalopathy. Another complication is peripheral neuropathy, which typically presents insidiously as a mixed symmetric polyneuropathy of the lower extremities. It may also affect the upper extremities but only after the lower extremities have been involved. Sensory abnormalities include the restless leg syndrome and a burning sensation on the feet, which may be severe enough to prevent ambulation. Motor abnormalities occur after the sensory abnormalities and include extremity weakness, unsteady gate, decreased deep tendon reflexes, and occasionally paraparesis and even paralysis. Autonomic nerves can also be affected, which may result in orthostatic hypotension, sweating abnormalities, impotence, and an abnormal response to the Valsalva maneuver.

4. Gastrointestinal manifestations—Anorexia, nausea, and vomiting are typical manifestations of advanced kidney failure. Anorexia usually occurs earlier, can be intermittent, and is occasionally referred to some types of food such as meat. Nausea initially presents predominantly in the morning. The combination of these symptoms together with abnormalities in protein and energy metabolism, other comorbid conditions (ie, gastroparesis in diabetic patients), and side effects of medications often leads to malnutrition. Uremic fetor is a uriniferous odor of the breath that results from the breakdown of urea to ammonia in saliva and is often associated with an unpleasant metallic taste sensation. Other manifestations include a higher frequency of inflammatory and/or ulcerative lesions at all levels of the digestive tract and of gastrointestinal bleeding.

5. Hematologic manifestations—A normochromic, normocytic anemia almost invariably develops in patients with CKF. It is mainly due to deficiency in the production of erythropoietin by the diseased kidneys. Other factors may also contribute, including hyporesponsiveness of progenitor cells to erythropoietin, accelerated hemolysis secondary to uremia, vitamin deficiencies (ie, folic acid), and iron losses associated predominantly with gastrointestinal bleeding. The white blood cell count is usually normal and increases in response to infections; however, leukocyte and immune system functions are abnormal, which predisposes to more frequent and severe infections. The platelet count is also normal, but function is abnormal, which results in a prolonged bleeding time and a tendency to bleed.

6. Bone manifestations—The term renal osteodystrophy refers to various types of bone lesions that occur in patients with progressive CKD as a result of abnormalities in calcium and phosphorus metabolism. The lesions include secondary hyperparathyroidism, osteomalacia, adynamic bone disease, and growth retardation in children. Subcutaneous, vascular, joint, and visceral calcifications are also seen in patients with poorly controlled calcium-phosphate product. Although secondary hyperparathyroidism is the most common type of renal osteodystrophy, patients often have a predominant lesion or a combination of mixed lesions. Although close to 100% of patients have abnormalities in bone biopsy, radiologic abnormalities are found in only 40% of patients, and clinical manifestations, such as bone pain or fractures, in less than 10% of patients. Renal osteodystrophy can be prevented or attenuated with appropriate management of calcium and phosphate metabolism.

7. Endocrine and metabolic manifestations—Sexual dysfunction is common in patients with progressive CKD. Impotence, infertility, and decreased libido occur as a result of primary hypogonadism. Hyperprolactinemia also contributes to amenorrhea and galactorrhea in women. Total T_4 and T_3 and free T_3 may be low, but free T_4, reverse T_3, and thyroid-stimulating hormone (TSH) are normal, suggesting a normal thyroid state. In early CKD, there is insulin resistance and glucose intolerance (azotemic pseudodiabetes), whereas in advanced CKD hypoglycemic episodes are common due to the longer half-life of insulin secondary to decreased renal catabolism and to decreased renal gluconeogenesis. Lipid abnormalities include elevated triglycerides and very low-density lipoprotein (VLDL) and decreased high-density lipoprotein (HDL); total cholesterol is normal and lipoprotein A may be elevated. Abnormalities of protein metabolism include decreased synthesis and increased catabolism.

B. Laboratory Findings

In addition to an elevated blood urea nitrogen (BUN) and serum creatinine, which are a reflection of a decreased GFR, patients with progressive CKD develop other laboratory abnormalities, particularly if they do not comply or are not given appropriate dietary instructions as the GFR declines. Typical abnormalities include hyponatremia (due to excessive water intake), hyperkalemia, hyperphosphatemia, hypocalcemia, hypermagnesemia, and hyperuricemia. Metabolic acidosis, usually with an elevated anion gap, is also common (Table 17–2). With the exception of hypocalcemia, these fluid and electrolyte disturbances result from an imbalance between intake and output by the progressively diseased kidneys.

C. Imaging Studies

Renal ultrasound is particularly helpful for diagnosing some cases of CKD [ie, polycystic kidney disease (PKD), obstructive uropathy] and for distinguishing acute from chronic kidney disease. The presence of symmetrically small (<8.5 cm) kidneys supports the diagnosis of CKD, whereas the occurrence of normal-sized kidneys favors an acute rather than a chronic process. There are exceptions, however, as some causes of CKD are associated with normal-sized or even enlarged kidneys, including diabetes, PKD, and amyloidosis. Other imaging studies may help determine the cause of CKD. Duplex Doppler ultrasound of the renal arteries, renal scintigraphy, and magnetic resonance angiography are useful in patients in whom renovascular ischemic disease is suspected. Voiding cystourethrography is helpful to rule out reflux nephropathy. Computed tomography allows for assessment of kidney stone activity and for evidence of papillary necrosis.

D. Special Tests

Kidney biopsy should be reserved for patients with near-normal kidney size, in whom a clear-cut diagnosis cannot be made by less invasive means, and when a potentially treatable cause is suspected.

▶ Treatment

Conservative treatment, usually with diet and medications, is indicated in all CKD stages. Kidney replacement therapy with dialysis or transplantation eventually becomes necessary in CKD stage 5. The goals of conservative treatment are to (1) treat the cause of CKD if possible and also to detect and treat any reversible cause of decreased kidney function, such as volume depletion, urinary tract infection, obstructive uropathy, use of nephrotoxic agents, accelerated or uncontrolled hypertension, and reactivation or flare of the original underlying etiologic disease process, (2) implement interventions to prevent or slow progression of CKD, (3) prevent or treat complications of CKD, (4) prevent or treat complications associated with other comorbid conditions, particularly diabetes and cardiovascular disease, and (5) prepare the patient and family for kidney replacement therapy (Figure 17–1). In addition, frequent review of medications is recommended; nephrotoxic agents should be avoided and dose adjustments should be made for drugs that are excreted by the renal route. Patients with CKD should be referred to a nephrologist when the eGFR is <30 mL/minute (stage 4), as this allows enough time for adequate preparation for kidney replacement therapy; for earlier stages of CKD, joint management between the primary care physician and the nephrologist is appropriate.

A. Interventions to Slow Progression of CKD

It has been shown that certain interventions slow the progression of CKD, including blood pressure control, use of angiotensin-converting enzyme (ACE) inhibitors and/or angiotensin receptor blockers (ARBs), and glycemic control in diabetic patients. These interventions are most effective if they are implemented early in the course of CKD. Blood pressure control is essential not only to delay progression of CKD, but to reduce the risk of developing coronary artery disease and left ventricular hypertrophy. Treatment includes a low salt diet and antihypertensive medications. ACE inhibitors and ARBs are the antihypertensive agents of choice because they reduce glomerular hypertension by a dual mechanism: Lowering of systemic blood pressure and predominant vasodilation of the efferent arteriole; in addition, they improve glomerular membrane permeability and decrease production of fibrogenic cytokines. ARBs have fewer side effects than ACE inhibitors, such as cough or hyperkalemia; however, due to their higher cost, they are usually recommended for patients who do not respond to or tolerate ACE inhibitors. Recent studies suggest that the combination of ACE inhibitors and ARBs may be more effective to slow the progression of CKD than either agent alone. The recommended target blood pressure is <130/80 in patients with proteinuria of <1 g/day and <125/75 in those with proteinuria of >1 g/day. ACE inhibitors and ARBs have also been shown to be

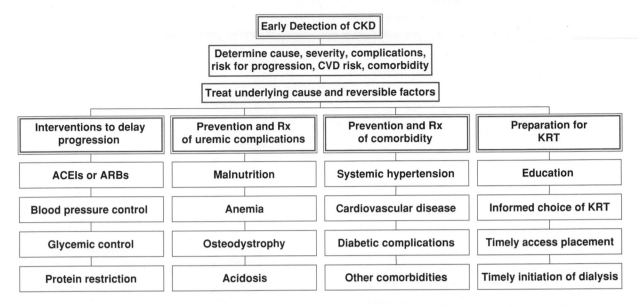

▲ **Figure 17–1.** Early detection of chronic kidney disease (CKD). CVD, cardiovascular disease; ACEIs, angiotensin-converting enzyme inhibitors; ARBs, angiotensin receptor blockers; Rx, treatment; KRT, kidney replacement therapy.

renoprotective in patients with normal blood pressure and proteinuria, particularly those with type 1 diabetes. Strict glycemic control is another intervention that reduces the risk of developing nephropathy, particularly if it is initiated early in the course of diabetes and/or of diabetic nephropathy (stage of normoalbuminuria or microalbuminuria). The benefit of strict glycemic control in patients with diabetes and overt nephropathy (proteinuria >300 mg/day) is less clear. Lastly, dietary protein restriction is another intervention that slows the progression of CKD.

B. Prevention and Treatment of Uremic Complications

As CKD becomes more severe, appropriate dietary changes must be made to prevent or treat water, electrolyte, and acid–base disorders. A low salt diet (2–3 g of sodium per day) and loop diuretics are recommended for volume overload. Thiazide diuretics are ineffective when the GFR is <30 mL/minute. Hyponatremia can be avoided by reducing water intake (for example, to 1.5 L/day). To prevent hyperkalemia, a low potassium diet (40–60 mEq/day) is recommended; in addition, exogenous sources of potassium should be avoided, including blood transfusions, salt substitutes, and certain medications (nonsteroidal anti-inflammatory drugs and potassium-sparing diuretics). Although ACE inhibitors and ARBs may cause hyperkalemia and acute kidney failure, they can be used in patients with progressive CKD because of their renoprotective effect, but with careful monitoring of serum potassium and creatinine. Hyperuricemia rarely leads

to symptomatic gout, and thus treatment of this complication with low-dose allopurinol is not necessary unless it becomes a recurrent problem. To reduce the risk of developing hypermagnesemia, magnesium-containing antacids and cathartics should be avoided. Lastly, serum bicarbonate should be maintained at ≥22 mEq/L with administration of sodium bicarbonate, particularly in symptomatic patients and to prevent growth retardation in children.

Regarding cardiovascular complications, management of volume overload and hypertension includes a low salt diet, loop diuretics, and antihypertensive agents (see above). Risk factors for atherosclerotic complications should be aggressively treated. Uremic pericarditis is an indication for initiation of dialysis; a short course of nonsteroidal anti-inflammatory drugs is sometimes needed for pain control; pericardiocentesis is indicated if tamponade is present. Neurologic complications such as encephalopathy are an indication for initiation of dialysis; neuropathy also improves with dialysis and more consistently with kidney transplantation. Gastrointestinal complications such as anorexia, nausea, and vomiting improve with dialysis; in the evaluation of nausea and vomiting it is important to exclude nonuremic causes, for example, diabetic gastroparesis, peptic ulcer disease, or side effects of medications. Follow-up by a qualified dietician is recommended to avoid malnutrition; a protein and energy intake of 0.75 g/kg/day and 30–35 kcal/kg/day, respectively, is generally recommended. Treatment of platelet dysfunction is indicated in patients with active bleeding and before a surgical procedure; appropriate measures include (1) correction of anemia with erythropoietin or blood transfusion, (2) administration of desmopressin or cryoprecipitate for rapid correction, (3) conjugated estrogens for long-term correction, and (4) reduction of azotemia with dialysis if indicated.

C. Prevention and Treatment of Comorbid Conditions

Since cardiovascular complications are the main cause of death in patients with CKD, appropriate management of risk factors and of established cardiovascular disease is of the utmost importance. Diabetic complications should also be managed appropriately.

D. Preparation for Kidney Replacement Therapy

An adequate preparation for kidney replacement therapy includes (1) information on the different treatment modalities, (2) education regarding preservation of forearm veins for future vascular access placement for hemodialysis, (3) referral to social services to assess transportation needs to the dialysis unit, continuation of work in some cases, rehabilitation, and participation in support groups, and (4) placement of a permanent vascular access, preferably an arteriovenous fistula, when the creatinine clearance is <25 mL/minute, the serum creatinine is >4 mg/dL, or the estimated time before initiation of dialysis is 12 months; peritoneal dialysis catheters should be placed 2–4 weeks before dialysis initiation.

▶ Prognosis

CKD is associated with high morbidity and mortality. Compared to the general population, the number of hospitalizations and of days spent in the hospital per year are three times higher in patients with CKD stages 2–4, and six to seven times higher in patients with ESRD receiving dialysis. One-, two-, and five-year survival for dialysis patients are 80, 65, and 38%, respectively. The expected remaining lifetimes of white dialysis patients are only one-fourth to one-sixth those of the general population. Lastly, cardiovascular mortality is 10–30 times higher in ESRD patients treated by dialysis compared with those in the general population. These poor outcomes underscore the importance of early detection and appropriate management of CKD long before dialysis is required.

Levey AS: Nondiabetic kidney disease. N Engl J Med 2002;347:1505.

Levey AS et al: National Kidney Foundation Practice Guidelines for Chronic Kidney Disease: Evaluation, Classification and Stratification. Ann Intern Med 2003;139:137.

Menon V, Sarnak MJ: The epidemiology of chronic kidney disease stages 1 to 4 and cardiovascular disease: a high risk combination. Am J Kidney Dis 2005;45:223.

National Kidney Foundation: K/DOQI Clinical Practice Guidelines for Chronic Kidney Disease: Evaluation, Classification and Stratification. Am J Kidney Dis 2002;39:S122.

Remuzzi G et al: Nephropathy in patients with type 2 diabetes. N Engl J Med 2002;346:1145.

St Peter WL et al: Chronic kidney disease: issues and establishing programs and clinics for improved patient outcomes. Am J Kidney Dis 2003;41:903.

WEB SITES

United States Renal Data System: http://www.usrds.org. Provides epidemiologic data on CKD and ESRD in the United States.

National Kidney Foundation-Kidney Disease Outcomes Quality Initiative (NKF-K/DOQI): http://www.kidney.org/professionals/kdoqi/index.cfm. Provides access to the GFR calculator and the NKF-K/DOQI Clinical Practice Guidelines.

End-stage Renal Disease (ESRD) Program: http://www.cms.hhs.gov/esrd/3.asp. Provides information on the Medicare ESRD Program.

Anemia & Chronic Kidney Disease

18

Robert Provenzano, MD, FACP

ESSENTIALS OF DIAGNOSIS

▶ Anemia is a comorbidity of progressive chronic kidney disease (CKD).

▶ Anemia of CKD results from the inability of the kidney to produce significant quantities of erythropoietin.

▶ Decreased red blood cell survival and iron deficiency are cofactors.

General Considerations

Since the initial observations by Richard Bright in 1836 on the relationship of anemia to renal inefficiency, anemia has remained as an ever-present comorbidity of progressive chronic kidney disease (CKD). The Kidney Disease Outcomes Quality Initiatives (K/DOQI) clinical practice guidelines for chronic kidney disease first published in 2002 helped focus attention on chronic kidney disease and its comorbidities, specifically anemia.

Recent data support the direct relationship of anemia to cardiovascular disease and to patient mortality in end-stage renal disease (ESRD). Anemia of CKD is generally caused by the inability of the kidneys to produce significant quantities of erythropoietin, but other factors are frequently involved including decreased red blood cell survival and iron deficiency. Despite the clinical introduction of recombinant human erythropoietin (rHuEPO) in 1989, there is still an estimated 1.5 million individuals with anemia in the United States. Additionally, anemia (hemoglobin <12 mg/dL) is present in greater than 75% of dialysis patients.

The availability of rHuEPO revolutionized our understanding of uremia and quickly became a major tool in the armamentarium of nephrologists to improve symptoms previously thought to be due to the "uremic syndrome." Correction of anemia in these patients resulted in an improved sense of well being, improved energy levels, a significant improvement in sleep disturbances, improved cognitive function, and an improvement in the ability to perform tasks of daily living. More significantly, improved hemoglobin levels in CKD patients have been correlated with decreased left ventricular hypertrophy (LVH) and improved cardiovascular outcomes.

Although debate continues on the proper "target" hemoglobin, the days of accepting hemoglobins less than the K/DOQI guideline recommended of 11–12 g have passed. Clinical research identifying cardiovascular events as a leading cause of mortality in CKD, ESRD, and transplant patients has made a critical understanding of the management of anemia essential to the practice of nephrology.

Pathogenesis

Under normal homeostatic conditions, the kidney very precisely regulates plasma volume through the reabsorption or excretion of salt and water. Hemoglobin levels are maintained in response to the production of erythropoietin to tissue hypoxia.

Erythropoietin is known to be a multifunctional tropic factor with effects on not only the bone marrow but on the central nervous system where studies have shown both neurotrophic and neuroprotective functions. Its primary target although is the pluripotent hematopoietic stem cells of the bone marrow. This cell line is capable of forming erythrocytes, leukocytes, and megakaryocytes. Erythropoietin is produced by specialized fibroblasts in the interstitium of the kidney in response to hypoxia (Figure 18–1).

As renal function declines, anemia becomes more common. The majority of patients with a GFR less than 60 mL/minute/1.73 m^2 (K/DOQI stage 3) have insufficient erythropoietin production to maintain hemoglobin >12 g/dL. This results in the typical normochromatic normocytic anemia present in CKD and ESRD. However, anemia of CKD often has etiologies other than insufficient erythropoietin levels.

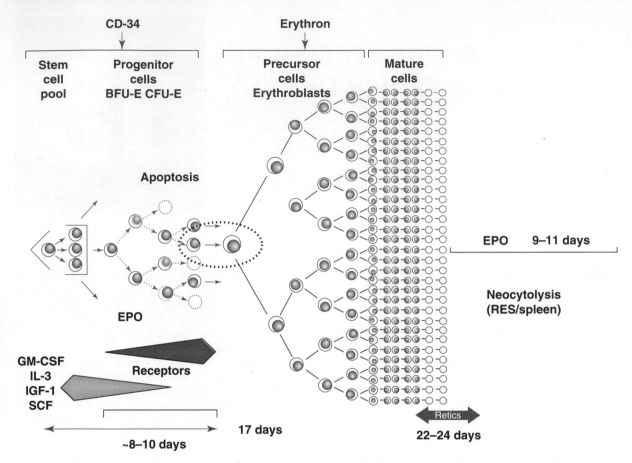

▲ **Figure 18–1.** Erythropoiesis is divided into two stages. Erythropoietin (EPO) is needed in the first stage (from multipotential to progenitor cells in the burst-forming unit erythroid) but not in the second precursor cell stage. The site of action of EPO and other growth factors is shown. Dashed circles indicate potential apoptosis of progenitor cells. (Adapted with permission from Erslev AJ et al: Erythropoietin in the pathogenesis of the anemia of chronic renal failure. Ersler AJ et al: Kidney Int 1997;51:623.)

▷ Treatment

A. Historical Perspective

Prior to the clinical introduction of cloned erythropoietin (rHuEPO) in 1989, the world of nephrology was very different. There was no focus on CKD, little focus on treating anemia, but considerable focus on improving the adequacy of dialysis (delivered amount of dialysis). The continued evolution of dialysis equipment including volumetric dialysis machines and dialyzer membrane biocompatibility with improvement of uremic symptoms was of paramount importance. Our ability to more accurately measure the amount of delivered dialysis added to these endeavors.

Anemia was managed in two ways: Severe anemia with hemoglobins less than 8 g/dL was treated with blood transfusions. Less critical management of anemia, viewed as "maintenance management," involved the use of anabolic steroids. Iron deficiency was rarely a problem; indeed, iron overload from frequent blood transfusions was a much greater problem occasionally resulting in secondary hemachromatosis.

The introduction of erythropoietin and the correction of anemia resulted in the elimination of many symptoms previously thought to be due to uremia. The avid production of new red blood cells consumed the additional iron stores and secondary hemachromatosis soon became a historical footnote along with the use of steroids and their inherent side effects.

B. Cardiovascular Disease and Anemia

See Chapter 19, on cardiovascular disease.

C. Current Management of Anemia of CKD

Although anemia of CKD has a direct impact on cardiovascular mortality and the availability of recumbent erythropoietin, only approximately 30% of patients with CKD are treated with erythropoietin. The mean hematocrit of this treated population remains below K/DOQI guidelines at 30.2% (recommended 33–36%). Although there is great debate about why so many patients remain untreated (barriers by insurers, fragmentation of care, late referrals, etc.), studies looking at the logistics of management of anemia in nephrology offices suggest that a lack of an organized methodology to treat anemia is still missing in most nephrology clinical settings.

An organized methodology of identification, evaluation, treatment, and maintenance of anemia has now become a critical requirement in all nephrology practices. Although this will vary from practice to practice, algorithms (Figure 18–2) help define the minimum steps necessary to identify the majority of patients with anemia and guide them toward treatment solutions.

Providing all patients upon introduction to the CKD clinic with information on anemia and the fact that they may become anemic is critical. Checking their hemoglobin at each visit will ensure a focus on one of the major comorbidities of their disease.

1. Iron supplementation—The K/DOQI guidelines recommend baseline iron studies prior to initiation of erythropoietin therapy (serum iron, transferrin, and ferritin levels).

Although some controversy exists as to the best methods of continually accessing adequate iron stores and iron delivered to the bone marrow, the most universally available test remains transferrin saturation and serum ferritin. If iron deficiency is identified, an appropriate workup including evaluation for gastrointestinal sources of blood loss (gastritis or malignancy) must be initiated.

The USRDS Dialysis Morbidity and Mortality (UDMM) Study showed that up to 50% of patients receiving epoetin were iron deficient, making this the most common cause of "erythropoietin resistance." Although multiple normograms exist for the replacement of iron, two important points need to be made concerning oral iron. First, oral iron can rarely be given in doses high enough to compensate for iron requirements in patients receiving erythropoietin therapy. Second, oral iron is rarely well tolerated and can cause gastric upset, which can easily be misidentified as uremic symptoms. The use of oral iron with gastrointestinal upset may further

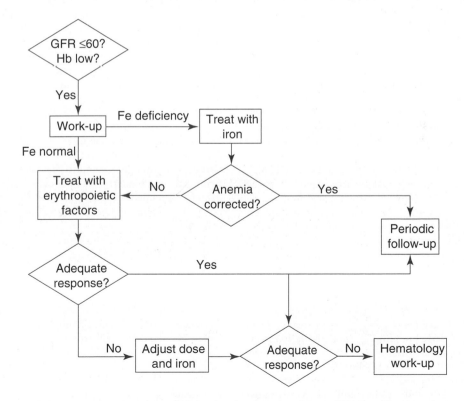

▲ **Figure 18–2.** Anemia assessment flowchart. (Adapted with permission from National Kidney Foundation: K/DOQI clinical practice guidelines for anemia of chronic kidney disease. Am J Kidney Dis 2001;37:S182.)

Table 18-1. Administration of intravenous iron.[1]

Iron compound	Maximum single dose	Recommended dosage
Iron dextran	1000 mg	100 mg × 10 doses
Iron gluconate	125 mg	125 mg × 8 doses
Iron sucrose	100 mg	100 mg × 10 doses

[1]One gram of iron is required to increase the hematocrit from 25% to 35% and to maintain iron stores over a 3-month period. The recommended dose is ≤1 g.

Reproduced with permission from National Kidney Foundation: K/DOQI clinical practice guidelines for anemia of chronic kidney disease. Am J Kidney Dis 2000;37:S182 and Van Wyck D et al: Safety and efficacy of iron sucrose in patients sensitive to iron dextran: clinical trial. Am J Kidney Dis 2000;36:88.

demoralize patients and dissuade them from compliance with other medications important to their care, which they may believe to be the cause of their gastric upset. Therefore in the United States the standard route for iron replacement remains the intravenous route.

Most protocols established for iron repletion are predicated on the iron requirements of ESRD patients. The goals, however, remain the same, achieving a TSAT of greater than 20% and a ferritin >100 ng/mL. Approximately 1 g of iron is required to increase the hematocrit 10% over a 3-month period. Currently available commercial iron products are listed in Table 18-1. It should be noted that intravenous iron dextrin (INFeD) has been associated with fatal anaphylactic reactions and must be preceded by a test dose. Newer preparations such as iron gluconate (Ferrlecit) and iron sucrose (Venofer) have substantially lower rates of anaphylactic reactions and do not require test dosing. Recently Venofer has been approved by the U.S. Food and Drug Administration (FDA) for use in CKD patients. Rapid administration of high doses of iron (>500 mg) has recently been made possible by the introduction of ferumoxytol. As compared to currently available iron formulations, this product is isotonic and has very low free iron levels which may account for its very low incidence of anaphylactoid reactions.

During active administration of erythropoietin most protocols recommend reevaluating iron stores every three months as patients vary in their ability to utilize iron.

2. Erythropoietin therapy—There are currently two commercially available erythropoietic agents to treat anemia: Epoetin-alfa and darbepoetin-alfa. Epoetin-alfa is manufactured and sold under two brand names, Epogen (Amgen, Inc.) and Procrit (Ortho-Biotech, Johnson & Johnson). Both these products are biologically and structurally identical.

Epoetin-alfa is immunologically and biologically indistinguishable from endogenous erythropoietin. Darbepoetin-alfa (AraNESP) structurally differs from endogenous erythropoietin by having additional oligosaccharide chains and a rearranged amino acid sequence. It has a higher molecular weight then epoetin-alfa resulting in a longer half-life, estimated to be approximately three times that of epoetin-alfa (8 hours versus 25 hours).

Although there have been no randomized controlled studies comparing the efficacy of each of these products to the other, they have both been shown to effectively treat anemia of chronic kidney disease. Drug selection is predicated upon the comfort level of the clinical nephrologist and cost. Although darbepoetin-alfa has a prolonged half-life and its labeling allows for dosing every 2 weeks, evidence has accumulated that both darbepoetin-alfa as well as epoetin-alfa can be dosed as infrequently as once every 4 weeks. Initial dosing of epoetin-alfa is generally 10,000 units per week subcutaneously. Depending on the protocol used, once the desired hemoglobin range is achieved (11–12 g/dL) most physicians will double the administered dose and double the administrative time (10,000 units once a week becomes 20,000 units every 2 weeks and then 40,000 units every 4 weeks). Once a convenient time interval is reached for the patient, ie, once-a-month dosing, titration of the dose up or down is used to maintain the target hemoglobin.

As mentioned, darbepoetin-alfa has a significantly longer half life and is typically started at 0.45–0.60 µg/kg/week subcutaneously. It too can be titrated by increasing the dose and increasing the time interval to reach an administrative schedule convenient for the patient.

Although higher initial doses of erythropoietic agents may result in a more rapid increase in hemoglobin, this is rarely necessary (rapid correction) and should be avoided as higher costs and potential target hemoglobin overshoots will result.

Recent studies, CHOIR and CREATE, have suggested that targeting higher hemoglobin levels (generally >12.5 g/dL) may result in higher cardiovascular events. Reanalysis of the CHOIR data though, has linked these adverse events to patients receiving higher doses of epoetin-alfa and not reaching their target hemoglobins. Those patients achieving higher target hemoglobins did not show increased risk of cardiovascular events.

Until the debate on appropriate hemoglobin targets is settled; NKF KDOQI guidelines recommend a target range of 11-12 g/dL and avoidance of targets >13 g/dL.

3. Adverse effects associated with epoetin-alfa—The common side effects from the use of epoetin-alfa and darbepoetin-alfa are generally mild and transient. Approximately 5% of patients will experience flu-like symptoms and 12–15% will experience headaches. The relationship between administration of epoetin-alfa and hypertension has been well documented and occurs in approximately 23% of patients. Therefore, increases in blood pressure should be closely monitored following initiation of therapy. This hypertension appears to be related to an imbalance between endothelin and proendothelin resulting in increased responsiveness to the vasoconstricting actions of norepinephrine and decreased responsiveness to the vasodilatory affects of nitric oxide. This affect (hypertension) is seen most frequently when the route of administration is intravenous.

Recently approximately 100 cases of pure red blood cell aplasia have been reported in Europe. This has been linked to the European formulation of epoetin-alfa (Eprex), with patients producing neutralizing antiepoetin antibodies. This appears to be linked to a different immunogenicity of Eprex. No cases of red cell aplasia have been reported to date in patients using darbepoetin-alfa.

4. Resistance to epoetin—Resistance to epoetin-alfa is seen primarily in patients with ESRD receiving dialysis, but is now being observed in CKD patients. Resistance is defined as the need for >150 units/kg of epoetin-alfa three times per week or the development of refractiveness to a previous stable dose allowing the hemoglobin level to fall below the targeted hemoglobin range. Although reports vary, approximately 5–10% of all patients with ESRD can be categorized as resistant. It is not known how many patients with CKD fall into this category. However, the numbers may be higher due to the persistent chronic "inflammatory" state in which these patients exist.

D. Resistance to Erythropoietin

1. Iron deficiency—Iron deficiency is the most common cause of resistance as previously mentioned. Serum iron saturation, ferritin, and transferrin should be checked frequently to avoid this condition. Ensuring adequate iron stores also allows epoetin-alfa to be administered in a cost-effective manner.

2. Infection and inflammation—Infection and inflammation are the second most common conditions resulting in hyporesponsiveness to epoetin-alfa. Mediators of inflammation [tumor necrosis factor (TNF) and interleukin-1 (IL-1) directly cause hyporesponsiveness to epoetin. Patients should be carefully scrutinized for conditions that result in chronic inflammatory processes.

3. Hyperparathyroidism—Although a much less common cause of resistance in the era of multiple vitamin D analogs and cinacalcet (Sensipar) availability, severe untreated hyperparathyroidism can result in fibrosis of the bone marrow. Unfortunately, the relationship between serum PTH levels does not directly correlate with the required epoetin dose and resistance.

4. Hemoglobinopathies—Sickle cell disease accounts for the majority of patients with resistance who have a hemoglobinopathy. High-dose epoetin-alfa therapy has mixed results with this disorder, often not reaching target hemoglobin goals.

5. Thalassemia—Thalassemia accounts for the remainder of resistant hemoglobinopathies and does respond to high-dose epoetin-alfa therapy.

6. Cofactor deficiency and malnutrition—Cofactor deficiency and malnutrition should cause close scrutiny on the part of the physician, who should then consider the initiation of dialytic therapy, particularly in the elderly who may downplay their uremic symptoms. Anorexia is an early, subtle, symptom of uremia. Falling serum albumin levels and/or the development of folate or vitamin B_{12} deficiencies necessitate close observation and treatment (dialysis) as they are directly related to dialytic mortality.

▶ Prognosis

As expectations of care continue to evolve on both the payer and patient side, closer scrutiny will be made of those disorders whose treatment results in improved outcomes. The more actionable a treatment parameter, the more likely physicians will be held accountable for its identification and management. There is considerable literature concerning the relationship of anemia to CKD, the growing population of patients with CKD and anemia, and the relationship of anemia to cardiovascular mortality. This knowledge, coupled with the availability of highly effective erythropoietic-stimulating factors and dosing strategies, makes the identification and treatment of anemia in CKD of paramount importance in the management of this at-risk population.

Bonomini M et al: Uremic toxicity and anemia. J Nephrol 2003;16:21.

Provenzano R et al: Extended epoetin alfa dosing as maintenance treatment for the anemia of chronic kidney disease: the PROMPT study. Clin Nephrol 2005;64:113.

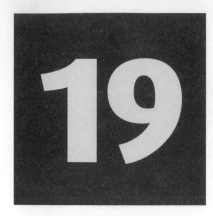

Cardiovascular Disease in Chronic Kidney Disease

Nadia Zalunardo, MD, FRCPC, & Adeera Levin, MD, FRCPC

ESSENTIALS OF DIAGNOSIS

- ▶ Cardiovascular disease (CVD) is highly prevalent among patients with chronic kidney disease (CKD) and is the most common cause of death in this population.
- ▶ The manifestations of CVD in CKD are variable and include left ventricular hypertrophy, ischemic heart disease, heart failure, and peripheral vascular disease.
- ▶ Traditional and nontraditional (or "uremia-related") cardiac risk factors are common in CKD.
- ▶ Clinicians should maintain a high index of suspicion for the presence of CVD in patients with CKD, even when the presentation is atypical.
- ▶ An aggressive approach to diagnosis and treatment of CVD is recommended in patients with CKD.

General Considerations

CVD is highly prevalent among patients with CKD and is the most common cause of death in this population. Importantly, patients with impaired kidney function are more likely to die than to progress to end-stage renal disease (ESRD) requiring renal replacement therapy and those who do reach dialysis have a staggering mortality rate of about 20% per year. In dialysis patients of all ages, the mortality rate from CVD far exceeds that observed in the general population (Figure 19–1). Dialysis has the greatest impact on younger patients, whose mortality rate from CVD is more than 100 times greater than that of their counterparts with normal kidney function.

The burden of CVD begins to accumulate long before patients reach ESRD. For example, left ventricular (LV) hypertrophy (LVH) increases in prevalence with declining renal function and is present in 75% of patients beginning dialysis treatment. Ischemic heart disease (IHD) and heart failure also develop early, and are present in 40% and 35% of incident dialysis patients, respectively. Recent publications have

demonstrated a profound impact of a reduced glomerular filtration rate (GFR) below 60 mL/minute on cardiovascular event rates.

In recent years both the National Kidney Foundation (NKF) and the American Heart Association (AHA) have recommended that patients with CKD be placed in the highest risk group for the development of CVD. However, while recognition of their high-risk status has improved, evidence from clinical trials evaluating the benefit of interventions aimed at reducing CVD risk in the CKD population is still largely lacking.

Recommendations by the NKF for the evaluation and treatment of CVD in dialysis patients were published in April 2005. The key to these guidelines is the recommendation that an aggressive approach to diagnosis and treatment is warranted in patients with ESRD due to the high risk of CVD in this patient group.

The spectrum of CVD in CKD is wide, and includes abnormalities of the heart and blood vessels, such as LVH, congestive heart failure (CHF), valvular heart disease, pericarditis, cardiac arrhythmias, IHD, and peripheral vascular disease (PVD). Those disorders that are most common and account for the majority of the morbidity and mortality in patients with CKD will be the focus of this chapter: LVH, IHD, heart failure, and PVD. In this chapter, the term CKD is used generically to refer to patients with all degrees of kidney dysfunction, including those on dialysis. Comments pertaining to a particular subgroup of patients (for example, predialysis patients or ESRD patients) are specified as such.

Go AS et al: Chronic kidney disease and the risks of death, cardiovascular events, and hospitalization. N Engl J Med 2004;351:1296. [PMID: 15385656]

Keith DS et al: Longitudinal follow-up and outcomes among a population with chronic kidney disease in a large managed care organization. Arch Intern Med 2004;164:659. [PMID: 15037495]

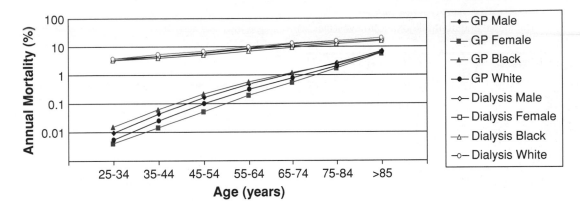

▲ **Figure 19–1.** Cardiovascular disease mortality for patients on dialysis, by age, gender, and race, in comparison to the general population. (Reproduced with permission from Foley RN et al: The clinical epidemiology of cardiovascular disease in chronic renal disease. Am J Kidney Dis 1998;32:S112.)

Kidney Disease Outcomes Quality Initiative (K/DOQI) Group: K/DOQI clinical practice guidelines for cardiovascular disease in dialysis patients. Am J Kidney Dis 2005;45(4 Suppl 3):S16. [PMID: 15806502]

Manjunath G et al: Level of kidney function as a risk factor for cardiovascular outcomes in the elderly. Kidney Int 2003;63:1121. [PMID: 12631096]

Sarnak MJ et al: American Heart Association Councils on Kidney in Cardiovascular Disease, High Blood Pressure Research, Clinical Cardiology, and Epidemiology and Prevention. Kidney disease as a risk factor for development of cardiovascular disease: a statement from the American Heart Association Councils on Kidney in Cardiovascular Disease, High Blood Pressure Research, Clinical Cardiology, and Epidemiology and Prevention. Circulation 2003;108:2154. [PMID: 14581387]

▶ Pathogenesis

A. Cardiovascular Risk Factors in Chronic Kidney Disease

Traditional and nontraditional risk factors have been discussed in the literature as contributors to the high rate of CVD in CKD (Table 19–1). Certainly, traditional cardiac risk factors are highly prevalent in these patients. These include advanced age, diabetes mellitus, hypertension, low high-density lipoprotein (HDL), and LVH. However, the complexity of the relationship between some traditional cardiovascular risk factors and overall mortality in ESRD must be appreciated. For example, a "reverse epidemiology" or "U-shaped" mortality curve has been observed whereby ESRD patients with low cholesterol and low blood pressure paradoxically have an increased mortality. This increase in mortality is hypothesized to reflect underlying malnutrition and/or inflammation (in the case of low cholesterol) and advanced cardiomyopathy (in the case of low blood pressure). Thus, the benefits of strategies traditionally used to combat CVD in the general population, such as lowering of cholesterol and

blood pressure, may be questioned in the setting of kidney disease.

Furthermore, there is accumulating evidence that a reduced GFR per se is an independent risk factor for CVD. It may be that lower GFR is associated with, or marks for, nontraditional or "uremic" risk factors. These nontraditional risk factors, outlined in Table 19–1, include anemia, abnormalities of calcium and phosphate metabolism, inflammation, prothrombotic factors, oxidative stress, and perhaps also hyperhomocysteinemia, and elevated levels of lipoprotein (a). However, despite strong associations between these factors and CVD in epidemiologic studies, a causal relationship has not been proven, nor have interventional studies been conducted that demonstrate changes in outcomes with treatment of these abnormalities.

In patients with residual kidney function (ie, those not yet on dialysis), the issue of proteinuria and cardiovascular risk merits specific comment. First, microalbuminuria is associated with an increased risk of cardiovascular events in both diabetic and nondiabetic subjects, even in the absence of renal insufficiency. While patients with microalbuminuria often have an increased prevalence of traditional cardiac risk factors, it is also thought that microalbuminuria may be a marker of generalized endothelial dysfunction or inflammation. Second, individuals with the nephrotic syndrome are known to have an increased risk of myocardial infarction (MI). Among the potential explanations for this are that hyperlipidemia, hypercoagulability, and hypertension are common in the nephrotic syndrome and these may contribute to the increased risk of IHD. In addition, recent publications describe clear associations between proteinuria and increased rates of CVD at all levels of kidney dysfunction.

Given the documented burden of CVD in CKD, the association with adverse outcomes in patients where the two coexist, and the biologically plausible explanations as to the impact of traditional and nontraditional risk factors in CKD

Table 19–1. Traditional and nontraditional cardiovascular risk factors in chronic kidney disease.

Traditional risk factors	Nontraditional factors
Older age	Albuminuria
Male gender	Homocysteine
Hypertension	Lipoprotein (a) and apo (a) isoforms
Higher LDL cholesterol	Lipoprotein remnants
Lower HDL cholesterol	Anemia
Diabetes	Abnormal calcium/phosphate metabolism
Smoking	Extracellular fluid volume over-load
Physical inactivity	Electrolyte imbalance
Menopause	Oxidative stress
Family history of cardiovascular disease	Inflammation (C-reactive protein)
Left ventricular hypertrophy	Malnutrition
	Thrombogenic factors
	Sleep disturbances
	Altered nitric oxide/endothelin balance

LDL, low-density lipoprotein; HDL, high-density lipoprotein.

Reproduced with permission from Sarnak MJ et al: American Heart Association Councils on Kidney in Cardiovascular Disease, High Blood Pressure Research, Clinical Cardiology, and Epidemiology and Prevention. Kidney disease as a risk factor for development of cardiovascular disease: a statement from the American Heart Association Councils on Kidney in Cardiovascular Disease, High Blood Pressure Research, Clinical Cardiology, and Epidemiology and Prevention. Circulation 2003;108:2154.

populations, it is important for the practicing clinician to understand the complexity of this area, what is known and where gaps in our knowledge base exist.

B. Left Ventricular Hypertrophy

The work performed by the LV in each cardiac cycle is equal to the product of the ventricular pressure and stroke volume. In kidney disease, the work of the LV is increased due to both pressure and volume overload. Hypertension, arteriosclerosis, and aortic stenosis contribute to pressure overload, while volume overload occurs as a result of factors such as anemia, increased extracellular fluid volume, and the presence of arteriovenous fistulas. These and potentially other factors, such as hyperparathyroidism and the "uremic milieu," contribute to the development of LVH, an independent risk

factor for mortality in all CKD patients, independent of dialysis status.

The LVH that occurs intitially as an adaptive response to physiologic stimuli (pressure or volume) eventually becomes maladaptive. At the cellular level, the metabolically active myocytes begin to experience an energy deficit, partly due to ischemia, resulting in cell death. In addition, cardiac fibroblasts proliferate, expanding the extracellular matrix of the myocardium and causing myocardial fibrosis. From a functional point of view, the hypertrophied ventricle becomes stiff, impairing relaxation and resulting primarily in diastolic dysfunction, at least initially. These changes may partially explain the high prevalence of heart failure in this patient group.

C. Heart Failure

Heart failure is common in CKD and is present in about one-third of incident dialysis patients. Patients may have systolic dysfunction, diastolic dysfunction, or both. The pathogenesis of heart failure is multifactorial with contributions from LVH, IHD, valvular heart disease, and other abnormalities specific to the uremic state such as chronic extracellular fluid volume expansion, disturbances in divalent ion metabolism, anemia, and the presence of arteriovenous (AV) fistulas.

D. Vascular Disease: Atherosclerosis and Arteriosclerosis

There are two general types of arterial vascular disease in CKD: Atherosclerosis and arteriosclerosis. Atherosclerosis is a disease of the intima and is characterized by plaques and vessel occlusion. The most common vessels affected are the medium-sized arteries, such as the coronary, femoral, and carotid arteries. There are many contributors to atherosclerosis, including the high prevalence of cardiac risk factors such as advanced age, dyslipidemia, hypertension, and the metabolic syndrome.

Patients with CKD also have a high prevalence of arteriosclerosis, or stiffening of the arteries; this may occur in the presence or absence of significant atherosclerosis. Although it normally occurs with aging, the process appears to be accelerated in kidney disease. The intima and media of the large, elastic arteries such as the aorta and the common carotid are affected in particular. The vessel wall is remodeled and becomes thickened and stiff, reducing compliance. These stiff vessels contribute to hemodynamic changes, including an increase in systolic blood pressure, a decrease in diastolic blood pressure, and as a result, a widened pulse pressure and increased pulse wave velocity. The raised systolic blood pressure increases LV afterload and contributes to the development of LVH, while the reduced diastolic pressure compromises coronary artery perfusion and contributes to myocardial ischemia. Recent data from both dialysis and predialysis patients have confirmed the association among an elevated pulse pressure, a clinical manifestation of arterial stiffness, and adverse outcomes.

A contributor to the arterial stiffening in kidney disease that has recently been given some attention is calcification of the intimal and medial layers of these vessels. It has been observed that this calcification is a key feature of the arterial disease in CKD, especially in ESRD. The calcification is more extensive and is observed much earlier in ESRD than in the general population. Abnormalities of bone mineral metabolism, including elevations in serum phosphorus, calcium, and calcium × phosphorus product, among other factors, are intimately involved in promoting vascular calcification.

This unique contribution of specific factors to arterial calcification and measured arterial stiffness, in conjunction with anemia (also common in CKD), may explain in part the high prevalence of CVD in CKD patients.

Giachelli CM: Vascular calcification: in vitro evidence for the role of inorganic phosphate. J Am Soc Nephrol 2003;14(9 Suppl 4): S300. [PMID: 12939385]

Giachelli CM: Vascular calcification mechanisms. J Am Soc Nephrol 2004;15:2959. [PMID: 15579497]

London GM: Cardiovascular calcifications in uremic patients: clinical impact on cardiovascular function. J Am Soc Nephrol 2003;14(Suppl 4):S305. [PMID: 12939386]

London GM: Cardiovascular disease in chronic renal failure: pathophysiologic aspects. Semin Dial 2003;16:85. [PMID: 12641870]

Moe SM et al: Uremia induces the osteoblast differentiation factor Cbfa1 in human blood vessels. Kidney Int 2003;63:1003. [PMID: 12631081]

▶ Clinical Findings

A. Symptoms and Signs

1. Left ventricular hypertrophy—LVH may be asymptomatic or patients may present with diastolic dysfunction, which is discussed in further detail in the next section.

On physical examination, hypertension is common. Particular attention should be paid to the pulse pressure as a surrogate measure of arterial stiffness, where "normal values" are <40–60 mm Hg. Precordial palpation may reveal a left ventricular heave and a sustained and diffuse cardiac apical impulse. On auscultation, a fourth heart sound may be heard.

Due to the lack of sensitivity of symptoms and physical examination findings, echocardiography is usually used for diagnosis and clinical follow-up of patients with LVH.

2. Heart failure—Heart failure may occur as a result of systolic dysfunction, diastolic dysfunction, or both. It may be asymptomatic or patients may present with shortness of breath, orthopnea, paroxysmal nocturnal dyspnea, reduced exercise tolerance, and progressive extracellular fluid volume expansion. In addition, patients with LV dysfunction on hemodialysis often tolerate dialysis treatments poorly and episodes of intradialytic hypotension may occur.

On physical examination, the signs of heart failure include pulmonary vascular congestion such as jugular venous distention and crackles due to pulmonary edema. LVH is the most common cause of diastolic dysfunction in CKD and these patients would be expected to have the cardiac findings discussed under that section. However, findings in patients with predominantly systolic heart failure include cardiomegaly, manifested by an inferiorly and laterally displaced apical pulsation, and the presence of a third heart sound on auscultation.

Due to the insensitivity of the physical examination, echocardiography is usually used for the diagnosis of heart failure. In addition to evaluating left ventricular function and geometry, echocardiography also has the advantage of providing other useful information, such as the presence of valvular heart disease, which may also contribute to left ventricular dysfunction.

3. Ischemic heart disease—The main symptom of cardiac ischemia is angina, which may be accompanied by symptoms of CHF. In CKD, the high proportion of patients with a concomitant diagnosis of diabetes mellitus means that atypical presentations of cardiac ischemia, such as shortness of breath without chest pain, may occur. In addition, patients with CKD may experience episodes of silent cardiac ischemia. For example, asymptomatic ST segment depression has been observed during hemodialysis treatments.

Findings on physical examination of acute cardiac ischemia may be relatively few. Signs of left and/or right heart failure may be observed depending on the size and location of the vascular territory affected. In general, the diagnosis of an acute coronary syndrome (ACS) relies on laboratory findings, including serial cardiac enzyme determinations and an electrocardiogram (ECG).

In the CKD population, a number of factors may interfere with the timely diagnosis of IHD, including diabetes, atypical presentations, and the relative lack of utility of specific tests in dialysis patients. Thus, a high index of suspicion in patients at high CVD risk is imperative.

4. Peripheral vascular disease—PVD, also a result of the atherosclerotic process, is common in CKD. The symptoms and signs depend on the vascular territory affected. Carotid artery disease causes neurologic changes during a transient ischemic attack or stroke. When the arteries supplying the lower extremities are affected, intermittent claudication with exertion may result. However, given the poor tolerance to exercise in the CKD population in general, this symptom probably lacks sensitivity. Chronic ischemia of the legs results in skin changes, hair loss, and muscle atrophy. Other signs include pallor, reduced or absent pulses, and bruits. Without treatment, skin ulceration and gangrene can occur when ischemia becomes critical.

The key to the diagnosis of PVD is serial assessment of peripheral arterial function through clinical examination and laboratory investigations. Reluctance to evaluate PVD in a timely manner may have led to an increase in morbidity and mortality in this particular cohort of patients.

B. Laboratory Findings

1. Cardiac disease

A. CARDIAC TROPONINS—Troponins comprise part of the contractile apparatus of myocytes in both cardiac and skeletal muscle. They consist of three subunits: Troponin C, troponin T, and troponin I. While cardiac and skeletal troponin C are identical, cardiac troponin T (cTnT) and I (cTnI) are encoded by genes different from their skeletal counterparts, and the molecules are also different. The assays currently in use for detection of cTnT and cTnI are specific for troponin released from the heart muscle. They are also highly sensitive to even small amounts of myocardial damage. The degree of troponin elevation in patients presenting with a suspected ACS provides important prognostic information, even in the presence of renal dysfunction. For these reasons, cTnT and cTnI are the preferred markers for the diagnosis of acute cardiac injury.

Interpretation of cardiac troponin concentration in the setting of ESRD is complicated by the fact that the levels, particularly of cTnT, may be elevated in apparently asymptomatic individuals. The reasons for elevations in troponin in the absence of cardiac symptoms and the significance of the levels are still debated, but the finding of an elevated troponin concentration in a patient with ESRD cannot necessarily be dismissed as a false-positive result even if unaccompanied by cardiac symptoms.

What is even less clear is why asymptomatic troponin elevations in ESRD are observed more frequently with cTnT than with cTnI. Proposed explanations for this include differences in release patterns from damaged cardiac myocytes, circulating half-life, and dialyzability, in addition to the particular characteristics of the assays themselves.

Despite these controversies and uncertainties, patients with renal failure suspected of having an ACS should be followed with serial cardiac troponin assessments. A troponin level rising over time suggests an acute injury, especially if accompanied by other cardiac symptoms or ECG changes. A positive but unchanging level may not indicate acute damage, but it has prognostic implications in ESRD patients nonetheless. On the other hand, obtaining serial "normal" or "negative" results has an excellent negative predictive value and is therefore useful for excluding an ACS.

B. CARDIAC IMAGING STUDIES

(1) *Electrocardiography*—All patients suspected of having an ACS should be evaluated with an ECG. However, the interpretation can be complicated by preexisting abnormalities on the baseline tracing. In the absence of acute cardiac ischemia, ST-T segment morphology can be altered by LVH, electrolyte disturbances, and medications such as digoxin. In a patient presenting with possible cardiac ischemia, obtaining an old ECG for comparison can be extremely helpful. Aside from abnormalities of the baseline study, ischemic changes are expected to have an appearance the same as in individuals without kidney disease.

(2) *Exercise treadmill testing*—In screening for coronary artery disease (CAD), detection of exercise-induced ischemia with exercise treadmill testing is of limited utility in renal failure. Patients are often unable to attain their target heart rate for reasons that include poor exercise tolerance, autonomic neuropathy, and use of medications that impair the chronotropic response to exercise, such as β-blockers and calcium channel blockers. Abnormalities of the resting ECG further compromise the sensitivity and specificity of this test. For these reasons, pharmacologic stress testing is generally preferred in renal failure.

(3) *Echocardiography*—Two-dimensional echocardiography has multiple uses in the renal failure population. It can be used to assess for abnormalities of cardiac structure, such as LVH and valvular heart disease, and also provides a good estimate of systolic and diastolic LV function. Ideally, patients on dialysis should be as close to their estimated dry weight as possible at the time of this study or at least have studies performed at the same time in their dialysis cycle for comparison purposes.

Dobutamine stress echocardiography (DSE) can be used as a noninvasive screening test for ischemic heart disease. Studies in the renal failure population are limited in number and comparisons between studies are difficult because of inconsistencies in methodology. Overall, DSE appears to be a useful, but imperfect, screening test for CAD in CKD.

(4) *Nuclear scintigraphy*—Nuclear scintigraphy has uses similar to echocardiography in patients with kidney disease: Assessment of ventricular function, screening for CAD, and prediction of future cardiac events.

To screen for myocardial ischemia, a radionuclide is injected and fixed or reversible perfusion defects are detected by comparing cardiac single-photon emission computed tomography (SPECT) images at rest and following stress (exercise or pharmacologic). Dipyridamole is a pharmacologic agent that acts by blocking the cellular reuptake of adenosine, thereby increasing its levels and causing vasodilation. In patients with markedly impaired kidney function, baseline levels of adenosine are increased, thus a reduced vasodilatory response to exogenously administered dipyridamole may occur, thereby potentially producing a false-negative result.

Several studies have evaluated the use of nuclear scintigraphy in patients with renal failure; however, the reported results are variable, likely due to inconsistencies in methodology. Like DSE, nuclear scintigraphy appears to be a moderately useful but suboptimal screening test for CAD in this group of patients.

Both thallium scintigraphy and DSE have prognostic implications in the renal failure population. In a recent meta-analysis of these myocardial perfusion studies for stratifying cardiac risk among patients with ESRD who were candidates for kidney or kidney–pancreas transplantation, compared to patients with negative test results, patients with positive tests had a relative risk of myocardial infarction of 2.73 and of cardiac death of 2.92 following transplantation.

Currently, there is no literature to guide the choice between nuclear scintigraphy and DSE in screening for CAD in CKD, as there are no studies directly comparing the two modalities. Therefore, it is reasonable to consider local expertise, availability, and cost to guide test selection.

(5) Computerized tomography scanning—Electron beam computerized tomography (EBCT) and helical CT scanning methods can be used to assess the degree of coronary artery calcification (CAC). In the general population, where calcification occurs in the intima in association with atherosclerotic deposits, CAC scores have been found to correlate with angiographic plaque burden and to predict future cardiac events. However, their utility in CKD populations is less clear.

Vascular calcification of both the intimal and medical layers is common in renal failure. The CAC scores of ESRD patients in particular are often several times greater than those found in the general population. However, CT scanning cannot distinguish between intimal and medial calcification, and there are conflicting reports as to whether there is a correlation between CAC scores and atherosclerotic plaque burden. Furthermore, while data demonstrate an association between higher CAC scores and mortality in ESRD, debate still exists as to the utility of this test in routine clinical care or as an endpoint in clinical trials. Until the appropriate long-term and interventional studies are undertaken, CT scanning is not recommended as a screen for CAD in the CKD population.

(6) Percutaneous coronary angiography—While IHD is most commonly a result of atherosclerotic CAD, a substantial proportion of patients with CKD experience cardiac ischemia without significant coronary artery stenosis. It is likely that these patients, particularly those with LVH, have microvascular insufficiency that limits myocardial perfusion and causes ischemia.

The gold standard for diagnosis of CAD is angiography; however, the cost and the potential for morbidity make it impractical as a screening test. In general, it is reserved for patients whose noninvasive screening tests are positive, those who present with an ACS, or those with known CAD who have developed recurrent symptoms despite optimal management.

In predialysis patients, angiography may worsen renal function by causing contrast nephropathy or cholesterol embolization. Invasive examinations should be undertaken only after careful consideration of their necessity, and whether the results will alter patient management. Contrast nephropathy generally produces a transient and reversible decline in renal function and in the modern era, with low osmolality contrast dyes, improved technology, and some evidence of renoprotective effects of specific agents, the risk may be lower than previously described. On the other hand, the decline in renal function caused by cholesterol emboli is usually permanent and can render patients with earlier stages of CKD dialysis dependent.

2. Peripheral vascular disease—In general, the initial approach to investigating PVD is with noninvasive testing, as is done in the general population. An ankle–brachial index (ABI)(at rest plus or minus postexercise) is a simple test that can be performed in the physician's office to confirm the suspicion of PVD. An ABI of <0.90 suggests PVD and further investigations with segmental limb pressures, plethysmography, and various ultrasound techniques or magnetic resonance angiography are indicated.

Conventional angiography is generally performed in patients with significant ischemia as part of the workup for a revascularization procedure in suitable candidates.

Aviles RJ et al: Troponin T levels in patients with acute coronary syndromes, with or without renal dysfunction. N Engl J Med 2002;346:2047. [PMID: 12087140]

Beciani M et al: Cardiac troponin I (2nd generation assay) in chronic haemodialysis patients: prevalence and prognostic value. Nephrol Dial Transplant 2003;18:942. [PMID: 12686669]

deFilippi C et al: Cardiac troponin T and C-reactive protein for predicting prognosis, coronary atherosclerosis, and cardiomyopathy in patients undergoing long-term hemodialysis. JAMA 2003;290:353. [PMID: 12865376]

Haydar AA et al: Coronary artery calcification is related to coronary atherosclerosis in chronic renal disease patients: a study comparing EBCT-generated coronary artery calcium scores and coronary angiography. Nephrol Dial Transplant 2004;19:2307. [PMID: 15213315]

Lamb EJ et al: The significance of serum troponin T in patients with kidney disease: a review of the literature. Ann Clin Biochem 2004;41(Pt 1):1. [PMID: 14713380]

Moe SM et al: Natural history of vascular calcification in dialysis and transplant patients. Nephrol Dial Transplant 2004;19:2387. [PMID: 15252163]

Rabbat CG et al: Prognostic value of myocardial perfusion studies in patients with end-stage renal disease assessed for kidney or kidney-pancreas transplantation: a meta-analysis. J Am Soc Nephrol 2003;14:431. [PMID: 12538744]

Saw J et al: Coronary artery disease in chronic kidney disease patients: assessing the evidence for diagnosis, screening and revascularization. Can J Cardiol 2004;20:807. [PMID: 15229763]

Sharples EJ et al: Coronary artery calcification measured with electron-beam computerized tomography correlates poorly with coronary artery angiography in dialysis patients. Am J Kidney Dis 2004;43:313. [PMID: 14750097]

▶ Prevention & Treatment

A. Left Ventricular Hypertrophy

LVH is an independent predictor of morbidity and mortality in patients with ESRD. LV growth begins early in CKD and is associated with a number of potentially modifiable risk factors, such as anemia and hypertension. Partial regression of LVH has been associated with reduced mortality in observational studies, but randomized studies have yet to convincingly demonstrate this. It may be that primary prevention of LVH by earlier treatment of risk factors is a better approach; however, there is a paucity of randomized data supporting this as well. The following sections will outline the current evidence for the prevention and treatment of LVH with a focus on treatment of anemia and hypertension.

1. Anemia—In observational studies, declining hemoglobin, particularly <10–11 g/dL, is associated with the development of LVH and increased cardiovascular mortality. Uncontrolled studies have also shown that treatment of anemia is associated with partial regression of LVH and reduced mortality. Unfortunately, the data available from randomized controlled trials are less convincing. Although quality of life and exercise capacity certainly improve, there is no conclusive evidence that hemoglobin levels >10–11 g/dL improve LVH and other important clinical outcomes such as cardiovascular events and mortality.

Early randomized trials focused on the progression of LV structural abnormalities in the ESRD population with pre-existing asymptomatic cardiac disease. The findings suggest that normalization of hemoglobin does not lead to regression of established LVH; however, prevention of LV dilation may occur with normalization of hemoglobin.

The predialysis population has also been evaluated for changes in cardiac dimensions with treatment of anemia. At the end of the 2-year follow-up period in the major study in this regard, there was no difference between the two groups with respect to the primary outcome, change in LVMI. It has been hypothesized that perhaps the development and progression of LVH were not clearly affected because the actual observed difference in hemoglobin between the two groups was relatively small. However, another study with a similar design demonstrated similar findings: A lack of change in LVMI with control of hemoglobin and other parameters. Additional clinical trials are ongoing to further explore the effects of various degrees of anemia correction on cardiac structure in CKD patients not yet on dialysis.

2. Hypertension—In the general population with essential hypertension, lowering blood pressure is associated with a regression of LVH. A meta-analysis evaluating the relative efficacy of various antihypertensive agents found that the reduction in LVMI was greatest with angiotensin II receptor blockers (ARBs), followed by angiotensin-converting enzyme (ACE) inhibitors and calcium channel blockers. Diuretics and β-blockers were least effective. In addition, it has recently been shown that ARBs can reduce the myocardial fibrosis observed in LVH, indicating that these medications have a direct effect on the myocardium, beyond their ability to lower blood pressure.

Data are limited in kidney disease, but some small studies support regression of LVH when hypertension is treated with pharmacologic inhibition of the rennin–angiotensin–aldosterone system (RAAS), although this has not been an entirely consistent finding. In most studies, it is difficult to ascertain how much of the effect is due to blood pressure reduction per se and how much is related to a specific effect of RAAS blockade. Nonetheless, because of the clinical and basic science evidence demonstrating that ACE inhibitors and ARBs are associated with delay of progression of kidney disease and fibrotic processes as well as other cardiovascular benefits, they are recommended as first-line antihypertensives in the CKD population.

Finally, blood pressure control has been associated with regression of LVH in observational studies of hemodialysis patients receiving either nocturnal or short daily hemodialysis compared to standard three times weekly hemodialysis.

B. Ischemic Heart Disease

1. Primary prevention—There have been few randomized controlled trials conducted in the CKD population addressing primary prevention of ischemic heart disease. In addition, elevated serum creatinine is often a criterion for exclusion from interventional studies of the general population, which further contributes to the scarcity of data in patients with kidney disease. Nonetheless, given that CKD patients are in the highest risk group for development of CVD, it seems reasonable to apply the same general treatment recommendations applied for other patients at similar CV risk. This includes lifestyle modification, such as smoking cessation, exercise, and maintenance of ideal body weight. Glycemic control in diabetic patients and treatment of hypertension to a target blood pressure of <130/80 mm Hg (<140/90 mm Hg predialysis in hemodialysis patients) are also recommended by the Kidney Disease Outcomes Quality Initiative (K/DOQI) group for CV risk reduction in CKD.

Aspirin has been recommended for primary prevention of myocardial infarction in the general population when CVD risk is high. However, these recommendations are based on the CV benefits outweighing the risk of major (intracranial or gastrointestinal) bleeding events. Although individuals with CKD have a propensity for bleeding, in the recently published First United Kingdom Heart and Renal Protection (UK-HARP-1) Study only an increased risk of minor, not major, bleeding episodes was observed with use of low-dose aspirin in CKD. However, patients with severe renal failure, who would be expected to be at highest risk of bleeding complications, represented a minority of patients in this study. Well-conducted clinical trials in heterogeneous populations of both dialysis and predialysis populations need to be conducted before aspirin can be adopted into clinical practice on a routine basis.

3-Hydroxy-3-methylglutaryl coenzyme A (HMG-CoA) reductase inhibitors (statins) appear to be safe and effective in reducing LDL cholesterol levels in renal failure; however, the evidence regarding their benefit in CKD populations is conflicting, particularly in primary prevention of CVD.

From subgroup and post hoc analyses, it appears that statin therapy may be of benefit in primary prevention in patients with mild to moderate CKD. While these analyses are encouraging, it is difficult to draw firm conclusions without corroborative data from well-designed prospective studies.

In fact, one prospective randomized trial of statin therapy for primary prevention of CVD in kidney transplant recipients yielded somewhat less optimistic results with the use of Lescol in renal transplant patients.

Data from ongoing prospective trials should help to clarify the question of whether statin use is of benefit in primary prevention of CVD in CKD. Until data from these studies become available, recommendations for treatment of dyslipidemia are taken from trials performed in the general population and summarized in K/DOQI guidelines for the treatment of dyslipidemias. As for other very high risk patients, treatment to a target LDL of <100 mg/dL (2.59 mmol/L) is recommended. The potential benefit of even further reductions in LDL levels has not yet been evaluated in CKD.

Although there are some reports that CKD increases the risk of statin toxicity, recently published studies do not confirm this. An initial dose reduction is generally recommended in severe renal failure (creatinine clearance <10 mL/minute) and caution is required in renal transplant recipients given the potential for drug interactions that may result in increased toxicity.

2. Acute coronary syndromes—CKD patients presenting with an ACS should be managed in the same way as the general population, recognizing that patients with severe renal insufficiency have generally been excluded from most trials of therapy. There are some important caveats with respect to the use of low-molecular-weight heparin (LMWH) and GPIIb-IIIa antagonists in CKD. Unlike unfractionated heparin, the clearance of LMWH is primarily renal, therefore elimination is slower and less predictable, and bleeding complications may be increased. Thus, unfractionated heparin is generally preferred in patients with significant renal insufficiency. There are some reports of an increased risk of bleeding with the use of GPIIb-IIIa antagonists; however, their use is still generally recommended in appropriate individuals. Dose adjustments may be necessary for some of the preparations as their excretion is partially renal.

3. Secondary prevention—Because of a lack of evidence specific to the renal failure population, patients with CKD should receive the same secondary prevention measures employed in the general population. This includes lifestyle modification (smoking cessation, exercise, and maintenance of ideal body weight), aspirin, β-blockers, statins, ACE inhibitors, and revascularization procedures in suitable candidates.

Anemia can contribute to exercise-induced ischemia and exacerbation of angina in CKD. The target hemoglobin currently recommended by K/DOQI is 11–12 g/dL in patients with IHD. While there may be theoretical benefits to achieving a "normal" hemoglobin level, one well-known prospective randomized study in hemodialysis patients with a history of IHD or CHF showed that a more normal hematocrit (~40%) was associated with an increased risk of nonfatal MI and death compared to the group with a lower target hematocrit (~30%).

Coronary revascularization with percutaneous coronary intervention (PCI) or coronary artery bypass grafting (CABG) is sometimes necessary in suitable candidates with CAD. When CKD patients are compared to the general population with CAD, patients with renal failure are more likely to experience postprocedure hemorrhagic complications, and they have higher rates of in-hospital mortality as well as poorer long-term survival with both PCI and CABG. In addition, PCI restenosis rates appear to be increased with angioplasty alone, but are likely improved if accompanied by stenting. The role of drug-eluting stents in renal failure is not yet well known. Finally, while there are no prospective randomized studies guiding the choice of revascularization method in CKD, a retrospective analysis of data from the United States Renal Data System (USRDS) favors CABG over PCI in dialysis patients, particularly in those with diabetes. Ideally, prospective studies are needed to answer this question.

In general, the decision for revascularization must be individualized and assessed on a case-by-case basis. Unfortunately, current decision making often reflects a pervasive therapeutic nihilism on the part of the general medical community toward patients with renal failure, which may lead to a postponement of testing and interventions and ultimately adversely impact the long-term outcomes of this group of patients.

C. Heart Failure

The two variants of heart failure, diastolic and systolic, can coexist in patients with CKD. Those CKD patients with predominantly diastolic heart failure often have significant LVH. In this case, attention should be focused on potentially modifiable contributing factors, which include hypertension and anemia.

Systolic heart failure has been studied extensively in the general population, but much less so in CKD patients. Thus studies in the general population are the only basis upon which to guide treatment in CKD. Salt restriction and diuresis are the mainstays of therapy to attain euvolemia. While loop diuretics are the diuretics of choice, a thiazide may be added to potentiate diuresis in resistant patients. Drug dose modification is often necessary in those with GFR <60 mL/minute. The dose of loop diuretics must often be increased while medications that rely on renal excretion, including certain β-blockers (eg, atenolol) and digoxin, require a dose reduction. Close follow-up is required for potentially dangerous complications that may be more common in CKD, such as hyperkalemia with the use of ACE inhibitors, ARBs, or aldosterone antagonists, and cardiac toxicity with digoxin. In addition, sotalol has been recognized as a particularly problematic anti-arrythmic in CKD patients and should probably be avoided.

While patients with CKD are underrepresented in studies of heart failure, recent observational studies seem to indicate that patients with CHF and mild to moderate CKD derive a mortality benefit from medications including ACE inhibitors and β-blockers.

Finally, while correction of anemia to a target of 11–12 g/dL is important, current evidence suggests that further normalization of hemoglobin may be associated with adverse outcomes, at least in hemodialysis patients with CHF.

D. Peripheral Vascular Disease

PVD is a significant source of morbidity in CKD patients. The medical management of PVD generally focuses on treatment of cardiovascular risk factors such as sedentary lifestyle, smoking, diabetes, hypertension, and dyslipidemia. Revascularization, either with percutaneous intervention or with bypass surgery, is often required and amputations are common.

Given that calcification is a key feature of the vascular pathology of CKD, attempts to reduce this should theoretically be of benefit in attenuating the progression of vascular disease. This is currently an area of active research. Perhaps rigorous attention to bone mineral metabolism and maintenance of appropriate levels of serum calcium, phosphorus, and parathyroid hormone through judicious use of calcium and non-calcium-containing phosphate binders, vitamin D, and calcimimetics will attenuate the progression of vascular calcification and improve clinical outcomes in CKD.

Baigent C et al: Study of Heart and Renal Protection (SHARP). Kidney Int Suppl 2003;84:S207. [PMID: 12694346]

Baigent C et al: First United Kingdom Heart and Renal Protection (UK-HARP-I) study: biochemical efficacy and safety of simvastatin and safety of low-dose aspirin in chronic kidney disease. Am J Kidney Dis 2005;45:473. [PMID: 15754269]

Ciulla MM et al: Different effects of antihypertensive therapies based on losartan or atenolol on ultrasound and biochemical markers of myocardial fibrosis: results of a randomized trial. Circulation 2004;110:552. [PMID: 15277331]

Coletta AP et al: Clinical trials update from the European Society of Cardiology Heart Failure meeting: SHAPE, BRING-UP 2 VAS, COLA II, FOSDIAL, BETACAR, CASINO and meta-analysis of cardiac resynchronisation therapy. Eur J Heart Failure 2004;6:673. [PMID: 15302018]

Frank H et al: Effect of erythropoietin on cardiovascular prognosis parameters in hemodialysis patients. Kidney Int 2004;66:832. [PMID: 15253740]

Furuland H et al: A randomized controlled trial of haemoglobin normalization with epoetin alfa in pre-dialysis and dialysis patients. Nephrol Dial Transplant 2003;18:353. [PMID: 12543892]

Holdaas H et al: Assessment of Lescol in Renal Transplantation (ALERT) Study Investigators. Effect of fluvastatin on cardiac outcomes in renal transplant recipients: a multicentre, randomised, placebo-controlled trial. Lancet 2003;361:2024. [PMID: 12814712]

Kidney Disease Outcomes Quality Initiative (K/DOQI) Group: K/DOQI clinical practice guidelines for management of dyslipidemias in patients with kidney disease. Am J Kidney Dis 2003;41(4 Suppl 3):S1. [PMID: 12671933]

Kidney Disease Outcomes Quality Initiative (K/DOQI): K/DOQI clinical practice guidelines on hypertension and antihypertensive agents in chronic kidney disease. Am J Kidney Dis 2004;43(5 Suppl 1):S1. [PMID: 15114537]

McAlister FA et al: Renal insufficiency and heart failure: prognostic and therapeutic implications from a prospective cohort study. Circulation 2004;109:1004. [PMID: 14769700]

McMahon LP et al: Slimheart Investigators Group. Development, prevention, and potential reversal of left ventricular hypertrophy in chronic kidney disease. J Am Soc Nephrol 2004;15:1640. [PMID: 15153576]

Pinkau T et al: Coronary revascularization in patients with renal insufficiency: restenosis rate and cardiovascular outcomes. Am J Kidney Dis 2004;44:627. [PMID: 15384013]

Roger SD et al: Effects of early and late intervention with epoetin alpha on left ventricular mass among patients with chronic kidney disease (stage 3 or 4): results of a randomized clinical trial. J Am Soc Nephrol 2004;15:148. [PMID: 14694167]

Suzuki H et al: Comparison of the effects of angiotensin receptor antagonist, angiotensin converting enzyme inhibitor, and their combination on regression of left ventricular hypertrophy of diabetes type 2 patients on recent onset hemodialysis therapy. Ther Apher Dial 2004;8:320. [PMID: 15274684]

Tonelli M et al: Veterans' Affairs High-Density Lipoprotein Intervention Trial (VA-HIT) Investigators. Gemfibrozil for secondary prevention of cardiovascular events in mild to moderate chronic renal insufficiency. Kidney Int 2004;66:1123. [PMID: 15327407]

Tonelli M et al: Effect of pravastatin on cardiovascular events in people with chronic kidney disease. Circulation 2004;110:1557. [PMID: 15364796]

Wanner C et al: Deutsche Diabetes-Dialyse-Studie (4D) Study Group. Randomized controlled trial on the efficacy and safety of atorvastatin in patients with type 2 diabetes on hemodialysis (4D study): demographic and baseline characteristics. Kidney Blood Press Res 2004;27:259. [PMID: 15316128]

▶ Prognosis

The prognosis for CKD patients with CVD is uniformly poor. The mortality rate of dialysis patients is an astounding 20% per year, with CVD representing the most common cause. LVH is an independent risk factor for mortality in ESRD. Declining GFR is associated with increased mortality following an acute myocardial infarction. In a recent study, patients with an estimated GFR >75 mL/minute had a 3-year mortality rate from MI of 14% compared to almost 46% in patients with an estimated GFR <45 mL/minute. The outcome for patients with CHF and/or PVD in conjunction with lower GFR is also much worse than that observed in the general population.

The evidence base for treating CVD in CKD is far from complete. However, it now appears that patients with concurrent CKD and CVD likely benefit from many of the interventions implemented in individuals with CVD alone. In addition, most of these interventions can be used safely with appropriate monitoring in the CKD setting. Nonetheless, it has been consistently demonstrated that patients with CKD are less likely to receive these potentially beneficial therapies than their counterparts with normal kidney function. This has been termed "therapeutic nihilism" by some and may represent a further contribution to the poor outcomes observed with CVD in CKD.

In summary, CVD in patients with CKD is prevalent, and is likely due to a combination of both traditional and non-traditional risk factors. These factors are present to variable extents and for varying durations over the lifespan of patients with reduced GFR, and their effects are likely multiplicative rather than additive. Current data describing methods of investigation and treatment fail to give adequate direction to physicians caring for patients throughout the entire spectrum of CKD. Nonetheless, this chapter attempts to synthesize the current state of knowledge, identify gaps in the evidence base, and describe reasonable strategies based on the data available.

Given the increasing recognition of CKD as a risk factor for CVD, ongoing trials will need to explore more completely the mechanisms by which lower GFR or dialysis therapies impact the natural history of CVD. Therapeutic strategies will then be evaluated in the context of a more complete understanding of the complexity of this disease.

Anavekar NS et al: Relation between renal dysfunction and cardiovascular outcomes after myocardial infarction. N Engl J Med 2004;351:1285. [PMID: 15385655]

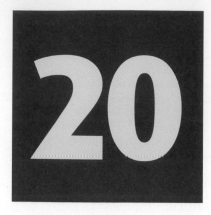

Renal Osteodystrophy

William G. Goodman, MD

The kidneys play a crucial role in the regulation of mineral metabolism by serving both excretory and endocrine functions. Each of these components becomes compromised as renal function declines. In the broadest sense, the term renal osteodystrophy encompasses all of the disorders of bone and mineral metabolism that are associated with chronic kidney disease (CKD). Often, however, the term is used more narrowly to describe the various skeletal disorders and their histologic manifestations among patients with renal dysfunction.

Disturbances in calcium, phosphorus, and vitamin D metabolism, alterations in the regulation of parathyroid hormone (PTH) synthesis and secretion, and factors that lead to the development of parathyroid gland hyperplasia are key components in the pathogenesis of renal bone disease. Additional pathogenic factors include systemic acidosis, aluminum retention, and the accumulation of β_2-microglobulin (β_2M) in bone and joints. The skeletal manifestations of renal bone disease in individual patients are determined ultimately by the interplay among one or more of these causative factors.

ESSENTIALS OF DIAGNOSIS

▶ Disorder of bone and mineral metabolism associated with chronic renal disease.

▶ Skeletal disorders associated with renal dysfunction.

▶ Disturbances in calcium, phosphorus, and vitamin D metabolism.

▶ Parathyroid gland hyperplasia.

▶ Systemic acidosis, aluminum retention, accumulation of β_2M in bone and joints.

▶ Pathogenesis

The renal bone diseases represent a spectrum of skeletal disorders ranging from high-turnover lesions arising predominantly from excess PTH secretion to low-turnover lesions of diverse etiology that are typically associated with normal or reduced plasma PTH levels (Figure 20–1). Transitions among histologic subtypes are determined by one or more dominant pathogenic factors. Such changes can be documented by bone biopsy and quantitative bone histology, which represent the definitive method for the diagnosis of renal osteodystrophy. Because plasma PTH levels are a major determinant of bone formation and turnover among patients with CKD, alterations in parathyroid gland function play a key role in the pathogenesis and evolution of renal osteodystrophy. Other factors, however, including diabetes, age-related bone loss, postmenopausal osteoporosis, gender, and race have been recognized increasingly as potentially important additional modifiers of skeletal metabolism and bone turnover among patients undergoing dialysis regularly. Such considerations are particularly relevant given the evolving demographics of the dialysis population in the United States, which is composed increasingly of persons older than 65 years of age and those with diabetes.

A. High-Turnover Renal Bone Disease

Secondary hyperparathyroidism—Several factors contribute to sustained increases in plasma PTH levels and, ultimately, to the development of high-turnover skeletal lesions in patients with chronic renal failure. Among these are hypocalcemia, impaired renal calcitriol, or 1,25-dihydroxyvitamin D, production, skeletal resistance to the calcemic actions of PTH, alterations in the regulation of prepro-PTH gene transcription, reductions in vitamin D receptor (VDR) and calcium-sensing receptor (CaSR) expression in the parathyroids, and hyperphosphatemia due to diminished renal phosphorus excretion.

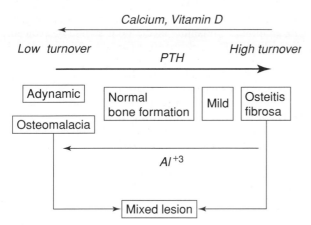

▲ **Figure 20–1.** Spectrum of the renal bone diseases. PTH, parathyroid hormone.

Because blood ionized calcium levels represent the most immediate stimulus for PTH secretion, disturbances that lead to hypocalcemia in patients with kidney disease promote excess PTH secretion. Renal 1,25-dihydroxyvitamin D production serves to maintain serum calcium levels by promoting active intestinal calcium absorption, by facilitating calcium release from bone, and by enhancing renal tubular calcium reabsorption. Serum calcitriol levels fall progressively, however, as renal function declines with wide-ranging effects on mineral homeostasis. Although serum 1,25-dihydroxyvitamin D levels vary considerably at any given level of renal function, the proportion of patients with subnormal values increases as renal failure worsens. Such changes account, at least in part, for impaired intestinal calcium absorption and for moderate reductions in serum calcium concentration in many patients with moderate to advanced renal failure. Diminished VDR expression in intestinal epithelial cells may contribute to this disturbance.

Skeletal resistance to the calcemic actions of PTH further compromises the ability to maintain serum calcium levels in those with advanced renal disease. As a result, higher serum PTH levels are required to elicit equivalent biologic responses in patients with chronic renal failure. Abnormalities in vitamin D metabolism and alterations in VDR expression may contribute to this abnormality.

Because calcitriol is a potent inhibitor of cell proliferation, disturbances in renal 1,25-dihydroxyvitamin production and/or reductions in VDR expression have been thought traditionally to contribute to the development of parathyroid hyperplasia in CKD. Vitamin D receptor expression is markedly reduced in parathyroid tissues that exhibit a nodular pattern of tissue hyperplasia, whereas decreased reductions occur in glands with diffuse chief-cell hyperplasia. Moreover, the extent of glandular enlargement is generally greater in the nodular form of parathyroid hyperplasia.

The development and progression of parathyroid gland hyperplasia are a critically important components of renal secondary hyperparathyroidism. Once established, parathyroid enlargement is difficult to reverse because the rate of apoptosis in parathyroid tissue is quite low and the half-life of parathyroid cells has been estimated to exceed 30 years. Clinical assessments of parathyroid gland function demonstrate that differences in functional parathyroid gland size account largely for wide variations in basal plasma PTH levels among patients with advanced renal failure. The secretion of PTH from massively enlarged parathyroid glands may ultimately become uncontrolled due to the ongoing nonsuppressible component of calcium-regulated PTH release thus leading to hypercalcemia and progressive bone disease in patients with advanced CKD.

Phosphorus retention and hyperphosphatemia have been recognized for many years as important factors in the pathogenesis of secondary hyperparathyroidism. The disorder can be prevented in experimental animals with chronic renal failure when dietary phosphorus intake is reduced in proportion to glomerular filtration rate (GFR). Dietary phosphate restriction also lowers plasma PTH levels in patients with moderate renal failure.

Phosphorus retention and hyperphosphatemia appear to aggravate secondary hyperparathyroidism in several ways. Marked elevations in serum phosphorus concentration may lead to the formation of soluble complexes of calcium and phosphorus in plasma, lower blood ionized calcium concentrations, and thus stimulate PTH secretion. Phosphorus abundance impairs renal 1α-hydroxylase activity directly and reduces 1,25-dihydroxyvitamin D synthesis. Either phosphorus retention or renal failure per se may affect posttranscriptional events that influence PTH mRNA stability and hormone synthesis. Finally, phosphorus retention can aggravate parathyroid gland hyperplasia by altering the expression of factors involved in cell cycle regulation and parathyroid cell proliferation.

The skeletal manifestations of hyperparathyroidism are often more pronounced in patients with secondary as compared to those with primary hyperparathyroidism, probably because of the very high plasma PTH levels that occur in renal failure. Values are typically 5- to 10-fold above the upper limit of normal among patients with secondary hyperparathyroidism due to advanced CKD, and they may reach levels that are 20–40 times higher than normal. By contrast, plasma PTH levels in most patients with primary hyperparathyroidism are only 2- to 3-fold above the upper limit of normal.

Unlike those with advanced renal disease who are treated with dialysis, patients with moderate renal insufficiency often have overt histologic evidence of secondary hyperparathyroidism when PTH levels are only modestly elevated. The disparity in disease severity despite markedly different plasma PTH levels between patients with moderate and advanced renal failure is probably attributable to differences in skeletal resistance to the biologic actions of PTH and/or to disturbances in vitamin D metabolism.

B. Low-Turnover Renal Bone Disease

Adynamic bone and osteomalacia: In the past, secondary hyperparathyroidism developed almost invariably in untreated patients with progressive renal disease. More recently, however, fewer patients have markedly elevated plasma PTH levels when regular dialysis is begun. Many have bone biopsy evidence of adynamic renal osteodystrophy, which is characterized by subnormal rates of bone formation and turnover. As mentioned previously, changes in the demographics of the dialysis population may account for this change.

Adynamic renal osteodystrophy currently accounts for most cases of low-turnover bone disease in patients undergoing dialysis regularly. Osteomalacia is seen much less often. Approximately 40% of those treated with hemodialysis and more than 50% of those receiving peritoneal dialysis have plasma PTH levels that are only modestly elevated or that fall within the normal reference range. Such values are typically associated with reduced rates of bone formation and turnover without evidence of defective skeletal mineralization.

In the 1970s and 1980s, aluminum retention and bone aluminum accumulation accounted for most cases of adynamic bone and osteomalacia among patients with CKD. Two distinct patterns of aluminum exposure were described. One was due to inadequate water purification during the preparation of dialysis solutions, which led to inadvertent parenteral aluminum loading. The other was due to the long-term ingestion of aluminum-containing, phosphate-binding agents, which led to gradual aluminum loading from intestinal aluminum absorption. Bone aluminum deposition was a prominent finding both in patients with adynamic bone and in those with osteomalacia. Bone and muscle pain, proximal myopathy, and skeletal fracture were common. Bone histology improved and bone formation increased when aluminum overload was treated effectively.

Aluminum has diverse effects on bone and mineral metabolism. It inhibits the proliferation and the differentiated function of osteoblasts, reduces collagen synthesis, and suppresses PTH secretion. Accordingly, adynamic bone due to aluminum retention may arise both through direct inhibitory actions of aluminum on osteoblasts and through indirect effects on bone cell activity that are mediated by reductions in parathyroid gland function and low plasma PTH levels. Aluminum also interferes directly with skeletal mineralization to cause osteomalacia.

Risk factors for aluminum-related bone disease include previous parathyroidectomy, a history of renal transplantation and graft failure, bilateral nephrectomy, and diabetes mellitus. By promoting the formation of soluble complexes with aluminum, citrate markedly enhances intestinal aluminum absorption, and the use of citrate-containing

compounds in patients with renal failure who are also ingesting aluminum-containing medications should be avoided. High plasma PTH levels appear to partially offset the adverse skeletal effects of aluminum. This may account for the somewhat greater risk of aluminum-related bone disease among diabetic patients and those who have undergone parathyroidectomy previously, conditions associated with low plasma PTH levels.

Fortunately, aluminum-related bone disease is now uncommon. Diabetes, corticosteroid therapy, and increasing age account for adynamic lesions in many patients. In this regard, the proportion of diabetic and elderly patients in the dialysis population continues to increase. Many of the histologic features of adynamic renal osteodystrophy are indistinguishable from those of osteoporosis from any of a variety of causes. The possibility of osteoporosis from causes other than renal bone disease must be considered when reductions in trabecular bone volume or cortical thinning are prominent histologic features in patients with CKD because such changes are not integral components of adynamic renal osteodystrophy.

The widespread use of large doses of oral calcium as a phosphate-binding agent and the use of large doses of active vitamin D sterols to treat secondary hyperparathyroidism may account for the increased prevalence of adynamic bone among patients receiving dialysis. Both interventions can lead to sustained reductions in plasma PTH levels. Calcitriol may also diminish osteoblastic activity directly when given in large intermittent doses to patients undergoing regular dialysis.

The long-term consequences of adynamic renal osteodystrophy, when not due to aluminum toxicity, remain uncertain. Some studies suggest that the risk of skeletal fracture may be greater among patients with relatively low plasma PTH levels, although the data are not conclusive. The prevalence and extent of arterial calcification have been reported to be greater among adult dialysis patients with adynamic skeletal lesions than in those with hyperparathyroidism. Episodes of hypercalcemia, which occur more often in those with adynamic renal osteodystrophy, may be contributory. In prepubertal children, adynamic skeletal lesions have been reported to be associated with reductions in linear growth.

For patients with osteomalacia, aluminum toxicity must be excluded if there is a history of sustained aluminum ingestion or if there are concerns about the adequacy of water purification procedures in dialysis facilities. Evidence of inadequate vitamin D nutrition, which is common among patients with CKD, should be sought by measuring serum 25-hydroxyvitamin D levels, and vitamin D nutrition should be restored by the administration of cholecalciferol or ergocalciferol if values are below 30 ng/mL. Long-term treatment with phenytoin and/or phenobarbital can lead to osteomalacia in nonuremic persons, and a higher prevalence of symptomatic bone disease has been reported in dialysis patients receiving these drugs. Persistent hypocalcemia and/or hypophosphatemia can lead to osteomalacia in some patients, but the disorder is seen much less frequently now that aluminum-containing medications are used sparingly and more attention has been given to maintaining adequate calcium and vitamin D nutrition among patients with CKD.

C. Mixed Lesion of Renal Osteodystrophy

Some patients with CKD have histologic features of both osteitis fibrosa and osteomalacia, a disorder known as the mixed lesion of renal osteodystrophy. There is biochemical evidence of secondary hyperparathyroidism, but other factors account for defects in skeletal mineralization. Persistent hypocalcemia and/or hypophosphatemia are found in some patients, and nutritional vitamin D deficiency is present in others. Mixed lesions of renal osteodystrophy can be seen in patients with osteitis fibrosa who are in the process of developing aluminum-related bone disease or in those with aluminum-related osteomalacia who respond favorably to treatment with deferoxamine (DFO) with increases in bone formation. Mixed renal osteodystrophy can thus represent a transitional state between the high-turnover lesions of secondary hyperparathyroidism and the low-turnover disorders of osteomalacia or adynamic bone.

Eknoyan G et al: Bone metabolism and disease in chronic kidney disease. Am J Kidney Dis 2003;42:1.

London GM et al: Arterial calcifications and bone histomorphometry in end-stage renal disease. J Am Soc Nephrol 2004;15:1943.

▶ Clinical Findings

The signs and symptoms of renal bone disease are rather nonspecific. Both the extent of various laboratory abnormalities and the severity of certain radiographic changes often fail to correspond to the clinical manifestations. Many patients report few symptoms despite striking disturbances in biochemical and x-ray parameters, but subtle complaints of musculoskeletal discomfort are common when sought by specific inquiry. Bone pain and muscle weakness are common. Skeletal deformities can develop in advanced cases, and extraskeletal calcifications are frequent.

A. Bone Pain

Bone pain is often present in patients with renal osteodystrophy. The onset is insidious with symptoms progressing gradually over many months or years. Pain is diffuse and nonspecific, and it is often aggravated by bearing weight and by changes in posture. When localized, the lower back, hips, and legs are affected most often. Pain in the heels or ankles may be a prominent complaint. Some patients experience an acute arthritis or periarthritis that is unrelieved by massage or the application of heat locally. Severe bone pain is more common in patients with aluminum related bone disease than in those with osteitis fibrosa, and it is a prominent clinical feature of bone aluminum toxicity. Nevertheless, some patients with advanced secondary hyperparathyroidism are incapacitated substantially. Physical examination is generally unremarkable unless skeletal fractures have occurred or unless bony deformities have developed.

B. Muscle Weakness

Proximal myopathy occurs in some patients with advanced renal failure. Symptoms appear slowly, and weakness and aching of the muscles are the most common manifestations. The physiologic basis of this disorder is not understood. Favorable clinical responses have been noted in some patients after treatment with calcitriol or 25-hydroxyvitamin D, following parathyroidectomy, after successful renal transplantation, or during treatment of aluminum-related bone disease with DFO. The role of abnormal vitamin D metabolism in the pathogenesis of uremic myopathy remains uncertain, but a careful evaluation must be done to exclude severe secondary hyperparathyroidism or bone aluminum toxicity. An empirical therapeutic trial of calcitriol or 25-hydroxyvitamin D is warranted in patients with persistent complaints of muscle pain and weakness.

C. Skeletal Deformities

In patients with aluminum-related bone disease, skeletal deformities are confined predominantly to the axial skeleton and include lumbar scoliosis, kyphosis, and distortion of the thoracic cage. Some persons with severe osteitis fibrosa develop rib deformities and pseudoclubbing.

D. Extraskeletal Manifestations

Several types of soft tissue calcification can be detected by radiographic examination. The most common are tumoral or periarticular calcifications. These are due mostly to amorphous deposits of calcium and phosphorus that sometimes are associated with acute periarticular inflammation and acute arthritis. Such calcifications commonly develop when serum phosphorus levels are markedly elevated or when the calcium–phosphorus ion product in serum is extremely high. They can resolve almost completely if serum phosphorus levels become better controlled. Although extraskeletal calcifications are more common with advancing age, they can occur at any age among those with CKD including children.

Visceral calcifications are rather infrequent, and their chemical composition may differ from those of other soft-tissue calcifications. The lungs, heart, kidneys, skeletal muscle, and stomach are involved most often. Pulmonary calcification can cause restrictive lung disease that may be progressive, and the disorder can persist even after successful kidney transplantation or parathyroidectomy.

Vascular calcification, specifically arterial calcification, is common among patients with CKD. The disorder is now recognized as an integral component of renal osteodystrophy, and it represents a risk factor for morbidity and mortality, predominantly from cardiovascular causes, among those undergoing dialysis.

Arterial calcifications among patients with CKD involve the medial layer of small- and medium-sized arteries predominantly, a lesion known as Monckerberg's sclerosis. Calcifications occur diffusely along the course of the vessel within the arterial wall, typically in associated with elastic collagen fibrils. Medial calcification is common in diabetic patients, and the radiographic appearance differs from the irregular, intermittent pattern that characterizes calcified intimal plaques due to atherosclerosis. It is best detected by lateral views of the ankle or anterior–posterior views of the hands or feet using magnification techniques with macroradioscopy. Imaging techniques such as electron beam computed tomography may be useful for detecting calcification in the coronary arteries or cardiac valves.

Medial wall calcification is usually asymptomatic, but the palpation of peripheral pulses and blood pressure measurements may be rendered difficult in affected limbs. Reductions in vascular compliance due to medial wall calcification adversely affect cardiovascular hemodynamics by raising systolic blood pressure, widening pulse pressure, and increasing pulse wave velocity. Such hemodynamic changes have been associated with worse cardiovascular outcomes.

It is now apparent that vascular calcification in patients with CKD is associated with serious adverse clinical outcomes including cardiovascular disease and high mortality rates from cardiovascular causes. In part, vascular calcification in such patients is related to disturbances in mineral metabolism such as phosphorus retention and hyperphosphatemia. Indeed, high serum phosphorus levels and elevated serum calcium concentrations have been identified as independent risk factors for death in adults undergoing regular hemodialysis. Episodes of hypercalcemia and calcium retention due to the use of large amounts of calcium as a phosphate-binding agent and from the administration of large doses of vitamin D sterols may also contribute.

Although soft-tissue and vascular calcification in end-stage renal disease (ESRD) has traditionally been thought to represent dystrophic calcification due predominantly to passive, physicochemical processes, there is now considerable evidence that vascular calcification is a regulated process that may be modulated by various genes and proteins normally involved in bone and mineral metabolism.

In some patients with extensive vascular calcification, ischemic necrosis of the skin, muscle, and/or subcutaneous tissues can develop. The condition is known variously as calciphylaxis or calcific uremic arteriolopathy (CUA). Its pathogenesis is not understood, but the disorder has been described in patients with CKD, in those receiving regular dialysis, and in renal transplant recipients. Most cases in early studies had advanced secondary hyperparathyroidism with markedly elevated PTH levels. Reports of clinical improvement after parathyroidectomy suggested that very high PTH levels played a pathogenic role. It is now evident, however, that CUA can occur in patients with adynamic renal osteodystrophy when plasma PTH levels are not substantially elevated.

Morbidity is severe and mortality rates are extremely high. Risk factors identified from various studies include female gender, increasing age, obesity, large doses of calcium-containing medications, and the use of the anticoagulant warfarin. It is quite possible that disturbances in the regulation of tissue-specific inhibitors of vascular calcification play a role in the pathogenesis of CUA.

Blacher J et al: Aortic pulse wave velocity index and mortality in end-stage renal disease. Kidney Int 2003;63:1852.

Ketteler M et al: Association of low fetuin-A (AHSG) concentrations in serum with cardiovascular mortality in patients on dialysis: a cross-sectional study. Lancet 2003;361:827.

▶ Complications

A. Amyloidosis

Most patients who are treated with dialysis for more than 7–10 years develop deposits of a unique amyloid protein that is derived from β_2M, a normal plasma constituent. Patients present with multiple bone cysts, pathologic fractures, carpal tunnel syndrome, scapulohumeral arthritis, and spondyloarthropathy. Involvement of the musculoskeletal system with bone pain and articular symptoms makes it difficult to separate dialysis-related amyloidosis from other forms of renal osteodystrophy.

The fibrils of β_2M have a molecular weight of approximately 12,000 Da and are produced by many cells, particularly those of lymphoid tissue and other cells with high rates of turnover. The protein serves to stabilize the structure of the MHC class I antigen on cell surfaces, but it is released into the circulation when the complexes are shed from the cell membrane. Approximately 180–250 mg of β_2M is generated normally each day. Nearly all β_2M is filtered at the glomerulus and catabolized subsequently by renal tubular epithelial cells. It accumulates in plasma, however, in patients with advanced renal failure, and levels reach values 50 times greater than normal in dialysis patients with little or no residual renal function.

Histologically, β_2M amyloid fibrils have an appearance that is similar to amyloid AA, but deposits of β_2M occur predominantly in bones and joints, leading to musculoskeletal manifestations. Both the slow rate of appearance and the predilection for bone and articular structures suggest that elevated serum β_2M levels do not fully account for the clinical syndrome observed in patients with chronic renal failure. Increases in age-related glycosylation products, certain specific proteases, and inhibitors of other proteases have each been suggested as factors that contribute to the deposition of β_2M amyloid in bone and synovial tissues. Much less often, β_2M amyloid deposits occur systemically, and these may be fatal.

The clinical features of amyloid deposition rarely appear before 5 years of dialysis therapy, and the disorder is more common among patients who start regular dialysis after the age of 50 years. Carpal tunnel syndrome is the most frequent clinical feature, but shoulder pain, other arthritic complaints, and cystic bone lesions are common. Deposits of β_2M are found in periarticular structures, joints, bone, and tendon sheaths. Far less commonly, the liver, spleen, rectal mucosa, or blood vessels are involved.

Skeletal manifestations include generalized arthritis, erosive arthritis, and joint effusions. Scapulohumeral involvement with shoulder pain is a common clinical presentation. Generalized arthritis can lead to pain and stiffness, decreased joint mobility, joint effusions, and deformities. Pain is characteristically worse at night or when patients sit quietly for several hours during dialysis sessions. Motion of affected joints or activity provides temporary relief. Erosive arthritis can involve the metacarpophalangeal and interphalangeal joints, shoulders, wrists, and knees, sometimes with joint effusions. The cervical spine is the most common site of destructive spondyloarthropathy.

On skeletal radiographs, bone cysts are located most commonly at the ends of long bones, particularly in the femoral head and proximal humerus, but they may also occur in the metacarpal and carpal bones. Multiple cystic lesions are common, and sequential radiographs often demonstrate cyst enlargement over time. Cysts containing deposits of β_2M may resemble the brown tumors of osteitis fibrosa, but their location and the presence of multiple rather than solitary cysts suggest that amyloid deposition is responsible. Cystic changes most commonly occur at sites of tendon insertions, and pathologically these may represent "amyloidomas" that have replaced trabecular bone. Fractures sometimes occur at these sites, and hip fractures in dialysis patients commonly arise at sites of β_2M deposition. Examinations of the shoulder by ultrasound are a simple noninvasive method to assess progressive tendon involvement with β_2M amyloid deposits.

The fraction of patients afflicted with amyloidosis increases progressively with the duration of dialysis therapy; thus, 70–80% of adult patients treated with hemodialysis for 10 or more years will have clinical features of β_2M amyloidosis. The distinction between this disorder and either severe secondary hyperparathyroidism or aluminum-related bone disease can be difficult, and thorough clinical, biochemical, and radiographic evaluations are required. Amyloidosis due to β_2M accumulation can coexist with either high-turnover or low-turnover skeletal lesions of renal osteodystrophy.

The clinical management of amyloidosis among patients undergoing dialysis has proven unsatisfactory. The carpal tunnel syndrome may respond to surgical correction, but it often reoccurs. The use of highly permeable dialysis membranes can moderately lower the serum levels of β_2M, but there is no evidence that this intervention alters disease progression. The appearance of certain clinical features of dialysis amyloidosis may be delayed in patients treated from the onset of renal replacement therapy with dialysis membranes composed of polyacrylonitrile (PAN) membranes as compared to those treated with conventional cellulosic dialyzers. Successful renal transplantation is followed by symptomatic relief in most patients, but there is no evidence that β_2M amyloid deposits in bone or other soft tissues actually regress after renal transplantation.

B. Biochemical Features

Serum calcium levels often are within the lower range of normal or modestly reduced in untreated patients with renal failure. After beginning treatment with dialysis, values usually rise and they may return to normal. The magnitude of the increase in serum calcium levels is in part related to the calcium concentration utilized in dialysis solutions. In patients treated with continuous ambulatory peritoneal dialysis (CAPD) who are not receiving vitamin D sterols, serum calcium levels are often within the normal range.

After calcium-containing, phosphate-binding agents were introduced as an alternative to aluminum-containing phosphate-binding medications, hypocalcemia became a less frequent problem in patients with CKD. Indeed, normal or high serum calcium levels are not uncommon among patients undergoing dialysis even in those who are not receiving vitamin D sterols. Such findings emphasize the importance of passive, vitamin D-independent intestinal calcium transport as a determinant of net intestinal calcium absorption when sufficiently large amounts of calcium are given orally to patients with renal failure.

The development of hypercalcemia in patients undergoing regular dialysis warrants prompt and thorough investigation. Common causes include marked hyperplasia of the parathyroid glands due to severe secondary hyperparathyroidism, adynamic renal osteodystrophy, treatment with calcitriol or other active vitamin D sterols, and the administration of large oral doses of calcium. Less frequent causes are aluminum-related bone disease, immobilization, malignancy, and granulomatous disorders such as sarcoidosis or tuberculosis where there is unregulated 1,25-dihydroxyvitamin D production by monocytes in granulomatous tissue. Basal serum calcium levels are generally higher and episodes of hypercalcemia occur more often in patients with adynamic bone than in persons with other skeletal lesions of renal osteodystrophy. Because skeletal calcium uptake is limited in the adynamic lesion, calcium entering the extracellular fluid from dialysate or following intestinal absorption cannot adequately be buffered in bone, and serum calcium levels rise. Lowering the doses of calcium-containing, phosphate-binding agents and decreasing temporarily the concentration of calcium in dialysate usually correct the hypercalcemia in such cases.

When the GFR falls below 15–20% of normal, hyperphosphatemia may develop. Phosphate-binding agents and dietary phosphorus restriction are usually required to avoid overt phosphate retention. Because the efficiency of phosphorus removal is limited during hemodialysis and peritoneal dialysis procedures, such measures are needed to adequately maintain serum phosphorus levels in most patients undergoing dialysis regularly without regard to the underlying type of renal bone disease.

In advanced renal failure, serum magnesium levels rise due to diminished renal magnesium excretion. Values are normal or slightly elevated when the concentration of magnesium in dialysate is kept between 0.5 and 0.8 mEq/L. The use of magnesium-containing laxatives or antacids can abruptly raise serum magnesium levels in patients with renal failure, and these medications should generally be avoided. It is prudent to monitor serum magnesium levels regularly if and when magnesium-containing medications are used.

Serum alkaline phosphatase values are fair markers of the severity of secondary hyperparathyroidism in patients with renal failure. Osteoblasts express large amounts of one isoenzyme of alkaline phosphatase, and serum levels are elevated when osteoblastic activity and bone formation are increased. High levels generally correspond to the extent of histologic change in patients with high-turnover lesions of renal osteodystrophy, and values frequently correlate with plasma PTH levels. Serum total alkaline phosphatase measurements may also be useful for monitoring the skeletal response to treatment with vitamin D sterols in patients with osteitis fibrosa. Values that decrease progressively over several months usually indicate histologic improvement.

Plasma aluminum levels are usually markedly elevated in patients with renal failure who have ongoing exposure to aluminum-containing medications or to inadequately purified dialysate. As such, plasma aluminum levels should be monitored regularly in patients undergoing maintenance dialysis, particularly in those who continue to use aluminum-containing, phosphate-binding medications. Plasma aluminum levels do not, however, serve as a reliable indicator of the extent of aluminum retention in tissues. Serum levels fall substantially within a few months after aluminum-containing medications are discontinued despite persistent aluminum retention in tissues. For these reasons, DFO infusions are a more reliable indicator of aluminum retention in tissues and provide useful information about the extent of tissue aluminum accumulation in patients undergoing dialysis.

Plasma PTH levels differ markedly according to type of renal bone disease, but double antibody immunometric assays generally provide reliable and reproducible results in patients with advanced renal failure. Indeed, plasma PTH measurements using first-generation immunometric assays are used widely for the initial diagnosis of renal osteodystrophy and to monitor therapy. The reference range of normal for these assays is generally in the range of 10–65 pg/mL, or 1–6 pM. Plasma PTH values are more useful than other serum biochemical markers for distinguishing between patients with secondary hyperparathyroidism and those with adynamic skeletal lesions. In untreated patients and in those receiving small daily oral doses of calcitriol, bone biopsy evidence of secondary hyperparathyroidism is found when plasma PTH levels exceed 250–300 pg/mL, or 25–30 pM. In contrast, values below 150 pg/mL, or 15 pM, and particularly levels below 100 pg/mL, or 10 pM, are typical for patients with adynamic renal osteodystrophy. Plasma PTH levels in the range of 150–300 pg/mL, or 2- to 4-fold higher than the upper limit of normal, generally correspond to normal rates of bone formation as documented by bone histomorphometry.

In contrast to the findings summarized previously for patients undergoing dialysis, plasma PTH levels that exceed the upper limit of normal are often associated with overt histologic evidence of secondary hyperparathyroidism in patients with earlier stages of CKD. Guidelines different from those that apply to patients treated with dialysis are thus required for patients with less advanced renal failure.

Until recently, the first-generation immunometric PTH assays that have been used widely in clinical chemistry for the past 15–20 years were thought to detect either predominantly or exclusively full-length PTH(1–84). It is now apparent, however, that these assays cross-react with other large amino-terminally truncated PTH fragments. In contrast, recently introduced second-generation immunometric PTH assays detect PTH(1–84) exclusively. When measured by second-generation assays, plasma PTH concentrations are on average 40–45% lower than values obtained using first-generation assays both in subjects with normal renal function and in those with ESRD. Several studies indicate, however, that values obtained with each assay are highly correlated.

The proper interpretation of PTH measurements in patients with renal failure depends largely on the extent to which values reflect bone histology as documented by bone biopsy. These relationships have been established for first-generation immunometric PTH assays, but only limited information is available using second-generation assays. It remains to be determined whether second-generation immunometric PTH will serve as better predictors of bone histology in patients with CKD.

▶ Treatment

The management of renal bone disease requires specific interventions that address selected pathogenic factors while limiting recognized risks. Key aspects of treatment include efforts to maintain serum calcium and phosphorus levels within the normal range and the judicious use of vitamin D sterols, calcimimetic agents, and phosphate-binding compounds. Additional considerations include the prevention of extraskeletal calcification, the avoidance of exposures to toxic agents such as aluminum and iron, and the selective use of chelating agents such as DFO to manage aluminum toxicity.

A. Diet

Adequate control of serum phosphorus levels is important for preventing soft-tissue calcification and for effectively managing secondary hyperparathyroidism in patients with advanced renal failure. The dietary intake of phosphorus ranges normally from 1.0 g/day to 1.3 g/day in healthy adults, but it must be reduced to 400–800 mg/day to prevent hyperphosphatemia in patients undergoing dialysis. Such diets are generally unpalatable, and long-term compliance is difficult to achieve. Consequently, phosphate-binding agents are usually employed together with dietary phosphorus restriction to control serum phosphorus levels when GFRs decrease to 15–20% of normal.

To diminish dietary phosphorus content effectively, the intake of dairy products must be curtailed. Phosphorus-restricted diets thus contain limited amounts of elemental calcium, often only 500–600 mg. As a result, many patients with CKD who abide strictly with current dietary recommendations ingest amounts of calcium that are insufficient to satisfy daily nutritional requirements. Modest dietary calcium supplementation is needed to achieve daily calcium intakes that approach 1200 mg as recommended by the World Health Organization. Concurrent therapy with calcium-containing or calcium-free phosphate-binding agents must be considered, however, when assessing overall calcium intake and the adequacy of calcium nutrition among patients with CKD.

B. Phosphate-Binding Agents

Phosphate-binding agents diminish intestinal phosphate absorption by forming insoluble complexes with phosphorus in the intestinal lumen. In the past, aluminum-containing medications were used widely, but these should now be employed sparingly, if at all, to avoid aluminum loading and aluminum toxicity. If they are used, the duration of treatment should be limited to a few months, and doses should be kept as low as possible. The concurrent administration of citrate-containing compounds must be avoided, and plasma aluminum levels should be monitored regularly.

Calcium carbonate and calcium acetate are the two most widely utilized phosphate-binding medications. They have similar efficacy. Calcium citrate can also be used as a phosphate-binding agent, but citrate enhances intestinal aluminum absorption in patients receiving aluminum-containing medications and should thus be used with caution. Calcium-containing agents, like all phosphate-binding compounds, are most effective when ingested with meals to maximize binding with phosphorus within the intestinal lumen. Such a dosing strategy also reduces the amount of unbound calcium that remains available for transport across the intestinal epithelium. Although reasonably effective for controlling serum phosphorus levels, very large amounts of elemental calcium are required to control hyperphosphatemia in patients undergoing dialysis regularly. The total daily intake of elemental calcium usually exceeds 1500–2000 mg among patients who use calcium-containing phosphate-binding medications exclusively, and it may reach 4–6 g or more. Episodes of hypercalcemia thus represent a major treatment-related side effect.

The use of very large does of calcium as a phosphate-binding agent has been associated with evidence of soft-tissue and vascular calcification among patients undergoing dialysis regularly. As a result, alternative phosphate-binding strategies that limit cumulative calcium intake to 1500–2000 mg/day from both dietary and medicinal sources have been recommended. Because of the limited efficacy of calcium salts as phosphate-binding agents, the feasibility of such strategies is dependent largely on the availability of calcium-free, phosphate-binding agents. Several are available currently including sevelamer and lanthanum carbonate.

Sevelamer hydrochloride, or hydrogel of cross-linked polyallylamine hydrochloride (RenaGel), is an ion-exchange polymer that was designed specifically as a phosphate-binding agent. It does not contain calcium or aluminum. In short-term clinical trials, sevelamer has been shown to be as effective as calcium acetate for controlling serum phosphorus levels with a substantially lower incidence of episodes of hypercalcemia. In studies of longer duration, total daily doses averaging 5–6 g were sufficient to maintain serum phosphorus levels at approximately 5.8–6.0 mg/dL, or 1.8–2.0 mM, among patients undergoing hemodialysis. Interestingly, the serum levels of total cholesterol and low-density lipoprotein (LDL) cholesterol decreased by 20–30% during treatment, whereas high-density lipoprotein (HDL) cholesterol levels rose. In patients with chronic renal failure who do not require dialysis, modest reductions in serum carbon dioxide levels, which reflect decreases in plasma bicarbonate concentrations, may occur during treatment with sevelamer. The change is probably due to the release of protons from the resin during phosphate binding.

Lanthanum carbonate is another calcium-free, phosphate-binding agent that is now available for use clinically. Its capacity to bind phosphorus in vitro is equivalent to that of aluminum hydroxide and exceeds that of both calcium carbonate and calcium acetate. Moreover, variations in pH have much less effect on the phosphate-binding capacity of lanthanum carbonate in vitro than on calcium-containing compounds. In large clinical trials, lanthanum carbonate has been shown to be an effective phosphate-binding agent among patients undergoing long-term dialysis.

Although lanthanum absorption from the gastrointestinal tract was thought originally not to occur, a small percentage of ingested lanthanum is absorbed. As compared to aluminum, the fractional absorption of lanthanum is several orders of magnitude lower. Nevertheless, lanthanum is detectable in plasma and low levels of the metal are found in bone among patients treated for as long as 2 years. Serial assessments of bone biopsies from such patients have thus far revealed no untoward effects on bone histology, skeletal mineralization, or bone cell activity.

Magnesium carbonate has been reported to be an effective phosphate binder when used together with magnesium-free dialysate in patients undergoing regular hemodialysis. Unfortunately, gastrointestinal side effects, particularly diarrhea, occur often when magnesium-containing compounds are used regularly as phosphate-binding agents.

C. Vitamin D Sterols

Despite efforts to control phosphorus retention and hyperphosphatemia and to optimize calcium nutrition, many patients who require ongoing treatment with dialysis develop secondary hyperparathyroidism. Until the introduction of calcimimetic agents, vitamin D sterols represented the only definitive pharmacologic intervention to treat the disorder. Although calcifediol, or 25-hydroxyvitamin D_3, 1α-hydroxyvitamin D_3, and dihydrotachysterol have all been shown to be effective therapeutically, calcitriol and other recently introduced vitamin D sterols such as paricalcitol and doxercalciferol are used much more widely for treating secondary hyperparathyroidism among patients undergoing dialysis regularly.

Daily oral doses of calcitriol are effective in many patients with symptomatic renal bone disease due to secondary hyperparathyroidism. Treatment is started using a dose of 0.25 μg/day and daily doses are adjusted upward periodically if serum calcium and phosphorus levels remain within acceptable limits. Bone pain diminishes, muscle strength and gait-posture improve, and osteitis fibrosa frequently resolves either partially or completely. When measured using reliable assays, PTH levels decrease in those who respond favorably to treatment. Similar findings have been reported in patients given daily oral doses of 1α-hydroxyvitamin D_3, or alfalcidol, which undergoes 25-hydroxylation in the liver to form calcitriol.

Doses of oral calcitriol in most clinical trials have ranged between 0.25 and 1.5 μg/day. Hypercalcemia is the most common side effect of treatment, but most adult patients tolerate daily doses of 0.25–0.50 μg without marked increases in serum calcium levels. Pediatric patients may require somewhat larger daily doses per unit of body weight. Growth velocity has been reported to increase during calcitriol therapy in children with severe renal bone disease.

Oral calcitriol therapy is now used relatively infrequently in patients treated with regular hemodialysis because vitamin D sterols can be given conveniently by the intravenous route during three times a week dialysis procedures. Parenteral dosing strategies ensure patient compliance, and they produce very high plasma sterol levels shortly after intravenous doses, which have been suggested to enhance the suppressive actions of vitamin D on PTH synthesis. Evidence from clinical studies to support this contention is limited. Intermittent as opposed to daily vitamin D administration may, however, decrease the effect of vitamin D to promote intestinal calcium transport. Calcitriol, paricalcitol, and doxercalciferol are all available as preparations that can be given intravenously.

Large intermittent oral doses of calcitriol have been used to treat secondary hyperparathyroidism in patients undergoing peritoneal dialysis where repeated parenteral dosing is impractical. When given two or three times per week, the cumulative weekly dose of calcitriol that can be achieved is somewhat greater than with daily therapy. Dosage regimens have ranged from 0.5–1.0 μg to 3.5–4.0 μg three times a week or from 2.0 to 5.0 μg twice weekly. Small doses should be used initially for reasons of safety, but upward adjustments to the dose can be made subsequently if serum calcium and phosphorus levels remain controlled adequately. It is not yet known whether intermittent calcitriol therapy is more effective than treatment with daily oral doses of calcitriol for managing secondary hyperparathyroidism among patients undergoing peritoneal dialysis.

The development of hypercalcemia during calcitriol therapy may be helpful in judging the status of bone remodeling among patients with renal osteodystrophy. When hypercalcemia occurs after several months of treatment and when previously elevated serum PTH and alkaline phosphatase levels have returned toward normal, it is likely that osteitis fibrosa has improved and that bone remodeling has diminished substantially. In contrast, episodes of hypercalcemia occurring during the first few weeks of treatment with calcitriol suggest either preexisting low-turnover bone disease, which in some cases is due to bone aluminum deposition, or severe secondary hyperparathyroidism. Bone biopsy and measurements of bone aluminum content may be needed to exclude aluminum-related bone disease. If there is biochemical evidence of progressive or advanced secondary hyperparathyroidism, parathyroidectomy is required.

In adult hemodialysis patients, the intravenous administration of calcitriol three times a week effectively lowers serum PTH levels in those with mild to moderate secondary hyperparathyroidism. As mentioned previously, somewhat larger cumulative weekly doses of calcitriol are achievable using intermittent parenteral dosage regimens as compared to daily oral dosing.

Increases in serum calcium and phosphorus levels often limit the doses of calcitriol that can be given safely to patients undergoing dialysis, particularly in those who are also ingesting large oral doses of calcium as a phosphate-binding agent. Because of ongoing concerns about the possibility of aggravating soft-tissue and vascular calcification during the medical management of secondary hyperparathyroidism with vitamin D sterols, the use of intravenous calcitriol has been superceded largely by treatment with new analogs of vitamin D such as paricalcitol and doxercalciferol. Both are vitamin D_2 derivatives. Each has been shown to effectively lower plasma PTH levels by 50–60% over 12–16 weeks of treatment in hemodialysis patients with secondary hyperparathyroidism, whereas serum calcium and phosphorus concentrations increased only modestly. It is possible therefore that paricalcitol and doxercalciferol provide a wider margin of safety in managing calcium and phosphorus metabolism during the treatment of secondary hyperparathyroidism among patients with CKD. Indeed, results from one comparative study of 12 months duration indicate that the frequency of persistent episodes of hypercalcemia and hyperphosphatemia was modestly lower among patients receiving paricalcitol compared to those treated with calcitriol.

Reductions in plasma PTH levels are used most often to assess the therapeutic efficacy of vitamin D sterols in patients with secondary hyperparathyroidism. Although serum PTH levels generally reflect the severity of bone disease in untreated patients and in those receiving small daily oral doses of calcitriol, similar relationships may not apply during the treatment of secondary hyperparathyroidism with large intermittent doses of vitamin D sterols given twice or three a week. Bone formation and turnover have been shown to fall strikingly during intermittent calcitriol therapy, and a substantial proportion of patients develops adynamic renal osteodystrophy. In some, adynamic lesions occur after plasma PTH levels fall substantially. In others, however, decreases in bone formation can occur as documented by bone histomorphometry despite persistent elevations in plasma PTH levels. Such findings suggest that large intermittent doses of calcitriol diminish osteoblastic activity and lower bone formation rates directly by PTH-independent mechanisms. Accordingly, plasma PTH levels should be monitored regularly during intermittent calcitriol therapy, and the dose of calcitriol should be reduced when serum PTH levels fall to values four or five times the upper limit of normal to diminish the risk of suppressing PTH values excessively and inducing adynamic bone. It is not known whether new vitamin D analogs affect osteoblastic activity and lower bone formation in a manner similar to that described during intermittent calcitriol therapy. Interval changes in bone histology after treatment with paricalcitol and doxercalciferol have yet to be reported.

D. Calcimimetic Agents

Calcimimetic agents are small organic molecules that function as allosteric activators of the CaSR. In parathyroid cells, they lower the threshold for receptor activation by extracellular calcium ions and diminish PTH secretion. When given orally to patients with secondary hyperparathyroidism, plasma PTH levels decline abruptly within 1–2 hours after drug administration. Calcimimetic compounds thus represent a novel way of altering parathyroid gland function. They represent a new class of therapeutic agents for secondary hyperparathyroidism with a mechanism of action that differs fundamentally from that of the vitamin D sterols, and they provide a second, previously unavailable, pharmacologic intervention for managing the disorder among patients with CKD.

Clinical trials have demonstrated that the calcimimetic agent cinacalcet hydrochloride effectively lowers plasma PTH levels without increasing serum calcium or phosphorus concentrations in patients with secondary hyperparathyroidism who are managed with either hemodialysis or peritoneal dialysis. Indeed, serum calcium and phosphorus concentrations and values for the calcium–phosphorus ion product in serum often decrease as plasma PTH levels decline during treatment. The ability of cinacalcet to lower plasma PTH levels without increasing serum calcium and phosphorus levels is noteworthy for several reasons.

First, considerable evidence has accumulated to suggest that persistent elevations in serum calcium and phosphorus levels are associated with adverse clinical outcomes in general and with cardiovascular events in particular among patients undergoing long-term dialysis. Second, recent guidelines for managing bone disease and mineral metabolism among patient with CKD set more stringent limits, which differ substantially from previous recommendations, with respect to the upper limits for serum calcium and phosphorus levels that are considered to be acceptable among patients who require renal replacement therapy. Such recommendations are based largely upon concerns about the long-term safety of various therapeutic interventions for secondary hyperparathyroidism, which include the use of large intravenous doses of vitamin D sterols and large oral doses of calcium as a phosphate-binding agent. Within this context, the use of vitamin D sterols becomes quite challenging, and many patients with secondary hyperparathyroidism are precluded from treatment because calcium and phosphorus metabolism cannot be controlled adequately to permit their safe therapeutic use.

E. Parathyroidectomy

Parathyroid surgery may be required to control secondary hyperparathyroidism in many patients undergoing long-term dialysis. The likelihood of parathyroidectomy increases progressively as a function of the number of years of treatment with dialysis, and annual parathyroidectomy rates among those undergoing dialysis regularly have not changed appreciably over the past 10–15 years. Severe secondary hyperparathyroidism should be documented thoroughly by biochemical, radiographic, and bone histologic criteria, if necessary, before surgery is undertaken. The diagnosis of aluminum-related bone disease must be considered and excluded before proceeding with parathyroidectomy because the disorder may worsen after surgery.

Specific indications for parathyroidectomy include persistent hypercalcemia together with persistently elevated plasma PTH levels, intractable pruritus that does not respond to intensive dialysis or to other medical interventions, worsening extraskeletal calcifications and/or persistent hyperphosphatemia despite the continued use of dietary phosphorus restriction and phosphate-binding agents, severe bone pain or fractures, and the development of calciphylaxis with biochemical evidence of ongoing excess PTH secretion. Other causes of hypercalcemia such as sarcoidosis, malignancy, or the intake of excessive amounts of calcium or vitamin D must be considered and excluded.

Uncertainties persist about the use of subtotal versus total parathyroidectomy among patients with secondary hyperparathyroidism due to CKD. The disorder reoccurs in 15–30% of those who undergo subtotal parathyroidectomy, which is likely due to ongoing hyperplasia in remnant parathyroid tissue. This observation together with the ability to effectively manage postoperative hypocalcemia with calcitriol and other vitamin D sterols renders total parathyroidectomy a viable approach to long-term management. For patients who may subsequently undergo renal transplantation, however, the better preservation of calcium metabolism in general and the lower risk of persistent hypocalcemia after renal function is restored favor subtotal rather than total parathyroidectomy.

It is generally not advisable to implant remnant parathyroid tissue into subcutaneous tissue in the forearm or other sites in an effort to preserve parathyroid gland function after surgery. Such grafts may exhibit autonomous secretory behavior, and they occasionally spread locally into surrounding tissues and cause recurrent hyperparathyroidism. Adequate surgical resection can be difficult.

F. Management of Aluminum Intoxication

The clinical manifestations and histologic features of aluminum-related bone disease improve during treatment with DFO in patients undergoing regular dialysis. Aluminum removal during hemodialysis and peritoneal dialysis increases substantially after DFO is given either intravenously or subcutaneously before dialysis procedures. Clinical benefit has been reported in a large proportion of patients with severe bone disease after 4–10 months of treatment.

Biochemical changes during DFO treatment include reductions in serum calcium levels and increases in serum alkaline phosphatase values, findings consistent with improvements in skeletal mineralization and osteoblastic activity. Plasma PTH levels rise modestly in many patients, but it is not known whether this change is due to aluminum removal from the parathyroid glands or to a fall in serum calcium concentrations. Sequential bone biopsies generally show increases in bone formation and improvements in mineralization. The amount of surface stainable aluminum in bone decreases in most patients who improve with treatment, but patients who have undergone previous parathyroidectomy respond less well or not at all.

Serious, often lethal, infections with *Rhizipus* and *Yersinia* spp. can develop in dialysis patients given DFO. The chelation of iron by DFO enhances iron delivery to certain organisms, increasing their pathogenic potential. As such, DFO should be used cautiously and judiciously in the treatment of aluminum intoxication among patients undergoing dialysis.

DFO should be given only to patients with symptomatic aluminum intoxication, and evidence of tissue toxicity should be documented fully before treatment is begun. Doses of DFO should not exceed 0.5–1.0 g/week, and plasma aluminum levels should be monitored regularly. Subcutaneous administration avoids the high serum levels of ferrioxamine that can occur after intravenous doses, and this therapeutic approach may limit the risk of developing opportunistic infections. In asymptomatic patients who have evidence of bone aluminum deposition, bone histology and bone formation often improve solely by withdrawing aluminum-containing medications and using calcium-containing compounds to manage phosphorus retention.

Chertow GM et al: Sevelamer attenuates the progression of coronary and aortic calcification in hemodialysis patients. Kidney Int 2002;62:245.

Finn WF et al: Efficacy and safety of lanthanum carbonate for reduction of serum phosphorus in patients with chronic renal failure receiving hemodialysis. Clin Nephrol 2004;62:193.

Foley RN et al: The fall and rise of parathyroidectomy in U.S. hemodialysis patients, 1992 to 2002. J Am Soc Nephrol 2005;16:210.

Joy MS, Finn WF: Randomized, double-blind, placebo-controlled, dose-titration, phase III study assessing the efficacy and tolerability of lanthanum carbonate: a new phosphate binder for the treatment of hyperphosphatemia. Am J Kidney Dis 2003;42:96.

Sprague SM et al: Paricalcitol versus calcitriol in the treatment of secondary hyperparathyroidism. Kidney Int 2003;63:1483.

This work was supported in part by USPHS Grant DK-60107.

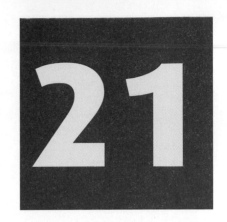

Chronic Renal Failure & the Uremic Syndrome: Nutritional Issues

Kamyar Kalantar–Zadeh, MD, PhD, MPH, &
Joel D. Kopple, MD

ESSENTIALS OF DIAGNOSIS

- ▶ Decline in the glomerular filtration rate.
- ▶ Diminished appetite or anorexia.
- ▶ Abnormalities in intestinal absorption of some minerals and vitamins.
- ▶ Abnormalities in urinary, intestinal, and dermal excretion of nutrients.
- ▶ Disorders of nutrient metabolism.

▶ General Considerations

In patients with chronic kidney disease (CKD), as the glomerular filtration rate (GFR) declines, numerous *nutritional and metabolic disorders* develop, and the *dietary requirements* for many nutrients are altered. These disorders and alterations include (1) diminished appetite or anorexia; (2) abnormalities in intestinal absorption of certain minerals (eg, calcium) and other nutrients including some trace elements (eg, iron and possibly zinc) and vitamins (eg, riboflavin); (3) abnormalities in urinary, intestinal, and dermal excretion of nutrients; and (4) disorders of nutrient metabolism.

Patients with renal insufficiency also are prone to accumulate toxins that normally are eaten in small amounts and would readily be excreted by the kidneys, such as aluminum. There are alterations in the concentrations and/or composition of certain lipoproteins, with an abnormal proportion of individual lipids and altered structure of some apolipoproteins. Potentially toxic oxidants and reactive carbonyl compounds accumulate in plasma and tissues. Deficiencies of antioxidants, including vitamins C and E and possibly selenium, may increase oxidative stress. Oxidative stress, along with the occurrence of inflammation

in renal insufficiency, increases the risk of endothelial injury and atherosclerosis, leading to cardiovascular disease and higher death rates usually observed in patients with advanced CKD.

▶ Pathogenesis

A. Malnutrition

Patients with advanced CKD (stages 4 and 5) frequently suffer from *protein–energy malnutrition*. Protein–energy malnutrition is defined as a state of decreased body protein mass with or without fat depletion or a state of diminished functional capacity due to protein–energy depletion, which is usually caused at least partly by inadequate nutrient intake relative to nutrient demand and/or which is improved by nutritional repletion. In CKD, several conditions may contribute to protein–energy malnutrition or wasting. Because these conditions may be caused by factors in addition to inadequate nutrient intake, the term "wasting" (or protein–energy wasting) can also be used instead of protein–energy malnutrition. It is important to recognize that in advanced chronic renal insufficiency (CRI), ie, stages 4–5 CKD, there are other types of wasting or malnutrition. This is particularly likely to occur for calcium, iron, zinc, and vitamins C, B_6, folic acid, and 1,25-dihydroxycholecalciferol.

Approximately one-third to one-half of patients with advanced CKD including those undergoing maintenance dialysis have mild to moderate malnutrition and 5–10% more have severe malnutrition. In malnourished CKD patients, *decreased* relative body weight or body mass index (BMI, body weight (kg) divided by the square of body height in meters^2), skinfold thickness (an estimate of body fat), arm muscle diameter area (a reflection of muscle mass), total body nitrogen and potassium, and *increased* total body water and extracellular water (Table 21–1) are usually observed. Malnutrition is also manifested by decreased concentrations of many serum proteins including

Table 21–1. Manifestations of protein–energy malnutrition in patients with chronic kidney disease.

Decreased food intake

Low body weight (body mass index or standardized height for weight)

Decreased total body fat percent and skinfold thickness

Decreased muscle mass and arm circumference

Low growth rate in children

Decreased total body nitrogen

Increased levels of acute phase proteins and proinflammatory cytokines

Decreased levels of albumin, prealbumin, transferrin, and cholesterol

Decreased levels of plasma amino acids

albumin, prealbumin, and transferrin. Serum lipoprotein concentrations including total cholesterol may also be reduced. Low growth rates are observed in children with advanced CKD. Increased levels of proinflammatory cytokines occur frequently.

The Modification of Diet in Renal Disease (MDRD) Study indicated that the dietary protein and energy intake and the nutritional status begin to decline when the GFR is about 25–38 mL/minute/1.73 m². In a cross-sectional analysis of the baseline data obtained in over 1700 individuals with stage 3–5 CKD, a gradual but persistent decline in serum transferrin and albumin concentrations (Figure 21–1), body weight, mid-arm muscle circumference, and percent body fat was observed parallel to the reduction in the GFR. Decreased energy intake was also observed when the GFR was reduced below about 25–35 mL/minute/1.73 m².

B. Causes of Malnutrition and Wasting

Table 21–2 lists potential causes of malnutrition in chronic renal insufficiency.

1. Inadequate nutrient intake—*Anorexia*, a salient manifestation of CRI, worsens as CKD progresses and is thought to be engendered by uremic toxins. Levels of serum leptin, a hormone known to induce anorexia, are also elevated in uremia. Several studies describe an inverse relationship between serum leptin and dietary protein intake or a direct relationship between serum leptin and weight loss in patients on dialysis. Elevated serum leptin levels in CKD can be caused by impaired degradation by the diseased kidney and possibly also by insulin stimulation of leptin synthesis in CRI patients who are often hyperinsulinemic. *Inflammation*, which is commonly present in renal insufficiency, is associated with increased levels of proinflammatory cytokines, including interleukin-1 (IL-1), interleukin-6 (IL-6), and tumor necrosis factor α (TNF-α), each of which is known to induce anorexia.

Other reasons for inadequate food intake include the debilitating effects of renal failure and underlying illnesses (eg, diabetes mellitus, lupus erythematosus), the impact of the progressive illness on the patient's ability to eat, and emotional disorders. Also, the fact that physicians and dietitians usually recommend a low protein diet for CKD patients plays a role. Moreover, imposing restrictions on intake of potassium and phosphorus may lead to nutrients that are less palatable to the patient and more difficult to prepare.

2. Increased losses of nutrients—The dialysis procedure itself may promote wasting by removing nutrients. During routine hemodialysis there are losses of about 6–10 g of free amino acids when patients are postabsorptive (fasting) and about 8–10 g when they are postprandial. Approximately 2–3 g of peptides or bound amino acids is also removed. The use of high flux polysulfone hemodialyzers may lead to greater losses of amino acids. During peritoneal dialysis, about 2–3.5 g of free amino acids, 8–9 g of total protein, and 5–6 g of albumin are lost into the dialysate per day. With mild peritonitis, the quantity of protein removed increases to an average of 15 g/day. Peritoneal protein losses as high as 100 g/day have been reported in severe peritonitis. Protein losses fall rapidly with antibiotic therapy but may remain elevated for many days to weeks.

Water-soluble *vitamins* and other bioactive compounds are also removed by both hemodialysis and peritoneal dialysis. Although these vitamin losses can be theoretically replaced from the diet or by multivitamin supplementations, these measures may be suboptimal in patients with poor nutrient intake due to a myriad of clinical, social, or financial barriers.

Finally, many CRI patients often lose substantial quantities of blood secondary to occult gastrointestinal bleeding, frequent blood sampling for laboratory testing, and the sequestration of blood in the hemodialyzer. Since blood is rich in protein, these blood losses may contribute to additional protein wasting. For example, a person with a hemoglobin of 12 g/dL and a serum total protein of 7 g/dL will lose approximately 16.5 g of protein in each 100 mL of blood removed.

3. Increased net catabolism—CKD patients usually suffer from additional concurrent *comorbid conditions*, which often induce a hypercatabolic state and also may physically prevent ingestion, gastrointestinal absorption, or assimilation of foods (eg, pancreatitis, gastrointestinal surgery). Hemodialysis per se can enhance *net protein breakdown* and promote negative nitrogen balance. More bio*in*compatible hemodialysis membranes, such as cuprophane, are more likely to stimulate the release of interleukins and promote net protein degradation than are more biocompatible membranes. The accumulation of endogenously formed *uremic toxins* might engender wasting more directly. In renal failure, there are increased plasma or tissue concentrations of probably hundreds

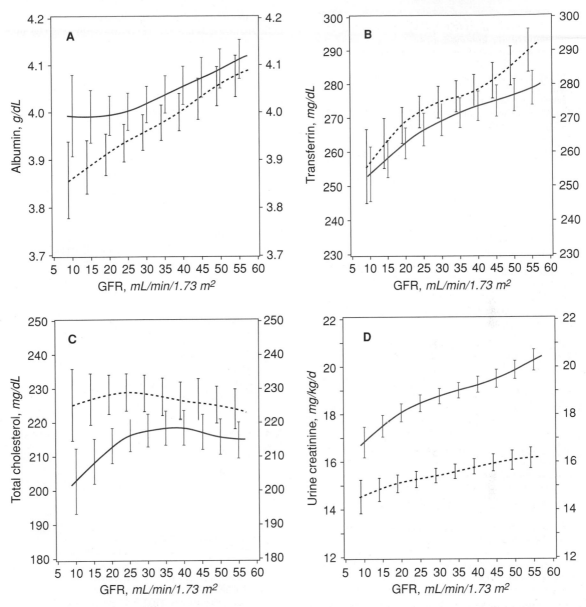

▲ **Figure 21–1.** Mean levels of biochemical measures of nutritional status as a function of glomerular filtration rate (GFR) in the Modification of Diet in Renal Disease (MDRD) Study. The estimated mean levels with 95% confidence limits of biochemical nutritional markers are shown as a function of GFR (males, solid line; females, dashed line) controlling for age, race, and use of protein and energy–restricted diets. In men, the slope of the relationship was greater at GFR = 12 than GFR = 55 mL/minute/1.73 m² for serum total cholesterol ($p = 0.014$). **A:** Males, $N = 1065$ ($p = 0.004$); females, $N = 698$ ($p < 0.001$). **B:** Males, $N = 1065$ ($p < 0.001$); females, $N = 698$ ($p < 0.001$). **C:** Males, $N = 1063$ ($p = 0.052$); females, $N = 694$ ($p = 0.63$). **D:** Males, $N = 1017$ ($p < 0.001$); females, $N = 664$ ($p < 0.001$). (Reprinted with permission from Kopple J et al: Relationship between nutritional status and the glomerular filtration rate: results from the MDRD Study. Kidney Int 2000;57:1688.)

Table 21–2. Causes of protein–energy malnutrition in patients with chronic kidney disease.

A. Inadequate nutrient intake
  1. Anorexia[1]
     Caused by uremic toxicity
     Caused by impaired gastric emptying
     Caused by inflammation with or without comorbid conditions[1]
     Caused by emotional and/or psychologic disorders
  2. Dietary restrictions
     Prescribed restrictions: Low-potassium, low-phosphate dietary regimens
     Social constraints: Poverty, inadequate dietary support
     Physical incapacity: Inability to acquire or prepare food or to eat

B. Sources of nutrient loss in dialysis patients
  1. Loss through hemodialysis membrane into hemodialysate
  2. Adherence to hemodialysis membrane or tubing
  3. Loss into peritoneal dialysate

C. Hypercatabolism caused by comorbid illnesses
  1. Cardiovascular diseases[1]
  2. Diabetic complications
  3. Infection and/or sepsis[1]
  4. Other comorbid conditions[1]

D. Hypercatabolism associated with dialysis treatment
  1. Negative protein balance
  2. Negative energy balance

E. Endocrine disorders of uremia
  1. Resistance to insulin
  2. Resistance to growth hormone and IGF-1
  3. Increased serum level of and sensitivity to glucagons
  4. Hyperparathyroidism
  5. Other endocrine disorders

F. Acidemia with metabolic acidosis
G. Concurrent nutrient loss with frequent blood losses
H. Inflammation

[1]The given condition may also be associated with inflammation. IGF–1, insulin–like growth factor 1.
Adapted with permission from Kalantar-Zadeh K et al: Appetite and inflammation, nutrition, anemia and clinical outcome in hemodialysis patients. Am J Clin Nutr 2004;80:299.

of metabolic products. Some of these compounds are bioactive and may have catabolic or antianabolic actions.

Acidemia enhances decarboxylation of branched chain amino acids and engenders protein catabolism in skeletal muscle, bone reabsorption, and negative nitrogen balance. The *endocrine disorders* of uremia may also promote wasting. Resistance to the actions of insulin and insulin-like growth factor-1 and hyperglucagonemia may promote protein wasting. Parathyroid hormone increases hepatic gluconeogenesis, and may lead ultimately to protein wasting. The findings that 1,25-dihydroxycholecalciferol has pervasive effects on calcium metabolism, that vitamin D deficiency may cause a proximal myopathy, and that 25-hydroxycholecalciferol

stimulates muscle protein synthesis *in vitro* suggest that deficiency of 1,25-dihydroxycholecalciferol might be another cause of muscle protein wasting.

Exogenously derived uremic toxins may cause debility (eg, aluminum) and possibly wasting. Finally, since the kidney synthesizes or degrades many biologically active compounds including certain amino acids, peptide hormones, other peptides, glucose, and fatty acids, it is possible that loss of these metabolic activities of the kidney in renal failure may disrupt the body's metabolism and promote protein–energy wasting.

4. Inflammation—Advanced CKD and the dialysis treatment process may sustain inflammation and an associated acute phase response with elevation of serum acute phase proteins and reduction in negative acute phase proteins. Potential causes of inflammation in CKD patients are listed in Table 21–3. In patients on maintenance dialysis, indicators of

Table 21–3. Possible causes of inflammation in CKD and ESRD patients.[1]

Causes of inflammation due to CKD or decreased GFR
  1. Decreased clearance of proinflammatory cytokines
  2. Volume overload[2]
  3. Oxidative stress (eg, oxygen radicals)[2]
  4. Carbonyl stress (eg, pentosidine and advanced glycation end-products)
  5. Decreased levels of antioxidants (eg, vitamin E, vitamin C, carotenoids, selenium, glutathione)[2]
  6. Deteriorating protein–energy nutritional state and food intake[2]

Coexistence of comorbid conditions
  1. Inflammatory diseases with kidney involvement (SLE, HIV, etc)
  2. Increased prevalence of comorbid conditions (CVD, DM, advanced age, etc)[2]

Additional inflammatory factors related to dialysis treatment
Hemodialysis
  1. Exposure to dialysis tubing
  2. Dialysis membranes with decreased biocompatibility (eg, cuprophane)
  3. Impurities in dialysis water and/or dialysate
  4. Back-filtration or back-diffusion of contaminants
  5. Foreign bodies (such as PTFE) in dialysis access grafts
  6. Intravenous catheter

Peritoneal dialysis
  1. Episodes of overt or latent peritonitis[2]
  2. PD catheter as a foreign body and its related infections
  3. Constant exposure to PD solution

[1]CKD, chronic kidney disease; ESRD, end-stage renal disease; GFR, glomerular filtration rate; SLE, systemic lupus erythematosus; HIV, human immune deficiency virus; CVD, cardiovascular disease; DM, diabetes mellitus; PTFE, polytetrafluoroethylene; PD, peritoneal dialysis.
[2]The given factor may also be associated with protein–energy malnutrition.

inflammation are correlated with anorexia, wasting, and malnutrition. These findings, together with the known catabolic effects of some proinflammatory cytokines, have bolstered the conclusion that inflammation promotes wasting. With inflammation, serum concentrations of negative acute phase proteins decrease; these include albumin, transferrin, retinol binding protein, transthyretin (prealbumin), and certain lipoproteins. Most surveys suggest that the serum concentration of C-reactive protein (CRP), a marker of inflammation, is increased in about 30–50% of American and European patients on dialysis and perhaps in a lower proportion of Asian patients. It has been argued that these elevated cytokines may promote protein–energy wasting in CKD patients both by inducing anorexia and also by engendering protein catabolism, eg, by activation of proteolytic enzymes released from granulocytes, or by suppressing protein synthesis. Indeed, albumin synthesis is often suppressed when serum CRP is elevated.

Both biocompatible as well as bioincompatible hemodialysis membranes, hemodialysis tubing and filters, both functioning and old thrombosed arteriovenous synthetic grafts, other vascular accesses and peritoneal dialysis catheters, hemodialysate and possibly peritoneal dialysate solutions, and low grade infections, such as caused by *Chlamydia*, may stimulate the inflammatory response in CKD patients by activating monocytes and/or macrophages. These inflammatory cells then release the cytokines (eg, IL-1, IL-6, and TNF-α) that stimulate the acute phase response. Finally, both *oxidants* and *carbonyl* compounds, as well as a deficiency of antioxidants, may cause tissue injury and inflammation and possibly engender a catabolic state.

C. Malnutrition–Inflammation Complex and Clinical Outcome

Nutritional status is a powerful predictor of morbidity and mortality and quality of life in CKD patients. Low dietary protein intake, decreased body weight for a given height such as BMI, and low serum concentrations of albumin, transthyretin, urea, creatinine, cholesterol, bicarbonate, and phosphorus are also associated with a higher death risk in patients on dialysis. Serum albumin is probably the strongest predictor of mortality in patients on maintenance dialysis (Figure 21–2). Some of these measurements such as daily protein intake [as determined by the normalized protein equivalent of total nitrogen appearance (nPNA)] and serum concentrations of cholesterol, phosphorus, and bicarbonate have a "J" or "U" curve relationship with mortality, in that both low and very high values are associated with a poor survival.

Since obesity and hypercholesterolemia are paradoxically associated with better survival and lower cardiovascular

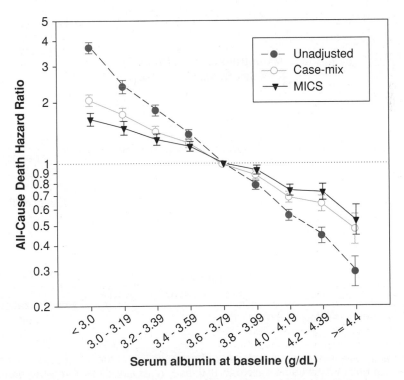

▲ **Figure 21–2.** Association between serum albumin and mortality. MICS, malnutrition–inflammation complex syndrome.

death in patients on maintenance dialysis, a *reverse epidemiology* of cardiovascular risk factors has been described. This phenomenon is believed to be mostly due to the overwhelming effect of malnutrition and inflammation, both of which are common in CRI. Indeed, according to some investigators, the strong association observed between malnutrition and mortality in CKD patients is the result of the atherogenetic role of inflammation. Because the causes and consequences of malnutrition and inflammation overlap considerably and many of the clinical manifestations of malnutrition and inflammation are identical, the term *malnutrition–inflammation complex syndrome* (MICS) has been suggested to indicate the close associations between malnutrition and inflammation in CKD patients and their link to clinical outcome (Figure 21–3).

The occurrence of measures indicating the presence of either malnutrition or inflammation in CKD patients or patients on maintenance dialysis has become of great concern to researchers and clinicians, because there is a strong association between the markers of MICS such as hypoalbuminemia, hypocholesterolemia, and underweight, and an increased risk of death. This issue is of particular importance because in patients on maintenance dialysis in the United States the mortality rate, especially due to cardiovascular disease, has remained inappropriately high, over 20% per year, and because traditional cardiovascular risk factors such as hypertension, hypercholesterolemia, and obesity not only do not appear to be associated with this high death risk, but paradoxically show a protective effect, ie, the reverse epidemiology. The time discrepancy between competing risk factors may play a role; it

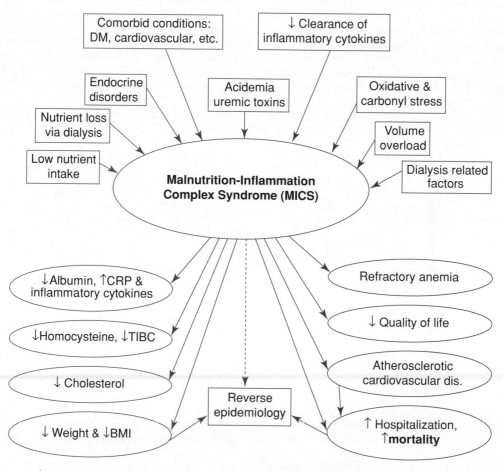

▲ **Figure 21–3.** Schematic representation of the causes and consequences of the malnutrition–inflammation complex syndrome or malnutrition–inflammation–atherosclerosis. BMI, body mass index; CRP, C–reactive protein; DM, diabetes mellitus, TIBC, total iron–binding capacity.

is possible that the deleterious effects associated with undernutrition can be manifested within a much shorter period of time when compared to the consequences of overnutrition, which usually requires a longer time to become manifest. According to this theory, many patients on dialysis may die prematurely of undernutrition before they can experience the cardiovascular consequences of overnutrition.

Garibotto G et al: Protein and amino acid metabolism in renal disease and renal failure. In: *Nutritional Management of Renal Disease*, ed 2. Kopple J, Massry S (editors). Lippincott, Williams & Wilkins, 2004, pp 1–24.

Himmelfarb J et al: The elephant in uremia: oxidant stress as a unifying concept of cardiovascular disease in uremia. Kidney Int 2002;62:1524.

Kalantar-Zadeh K et al: Reverse epidemiology of cardiovascular risk factors in maintenance dialysis patients. Kidney Int 2003;63:793.

Kalantar-Zadeh K et al: Malnutrition–inflammation complex syndrome in dialysis patients: causes and consequences. Am J Kidney Dis 2003;42:864.

Kalantar-Zadeh K et al: Appetite and inflammation, nutrition, anemia and clinical outcome in hemodialysis patients. Am J Clin Nutr 2004;80:299.

Mitch WE: Insights into the abnormalities of chronic renal disease attributed to malnutrition. J Am Soc Nephrol 2002;13(Suppl 1):S22.

Pupim LB et al: Protein homeostasis in chronic hemodialysis patients. Curr Opin Clin Nutr Metab Care 2004;7:89.

Stenvinkel P et al: IL-10, IL-6, and TNF-alpha: central factors in the altered cytokine network of uremia—the good, the bad, and the ugly. Kidney Int 2005;67:1216.

▶ Clinical Findings

A. Assessment of Nutritional Status

Classically, three major lines of inquiries, ie, dietary intake, biochemical measurements, and body composition, are used to assess the protein–energy nutritional status in CKD patients. Composite scores based on assessment measures within these categories are also utilized. These include subjective global assessment (SGA) of nutrition and malnutrition inflammation score (MIS). More technologically based nutritional measures that have been used in CKD patients include dual energy x-ray absorptiometry (DEXA), total body nitrogen or potassium measurements, underwater weighing, bioelectrical impedance analysis, and near infrared interactance. These four categories of nutritional assessment tools are described in Table 21–2. As indicated in Table 21–4, many of these also respond to inflammation and provide a measure of its severity. Hence, the overlap between malnutrition and inflammation exists both at the diagnostic and at the etiologic level. Currently, no uniform approach has been agreed upon for rating the severity of malnutrition in CRI patients.

The National Kidney Foundation Kidney Disease Outcomes Quality Initiative (K/DOQI) Clinical Procedure

Table 21–4. Systematic classification of the assessment tools for evaluation of protein–energy malnutrition (PEM) in patients on maintenance dialysis.[1]

Nutritional intake
1. Direct: Diet recalls and diaries, food frequency questionnaires[2]
2. Indirect: Based on urea nitrogen appearance: nPNA (nPCR)[2]

Body composition
1. Weight-based measures: BMI, weight-for-height, edema-free fat-free weight[2]
2. Skin and muscle anthropometry via caliper: Skinfolds, extremity muscle mass[2]
3. Total body elements: Total body potassium
4. Energy-beam-based methods: DEXA, BIA, NIR[2]
5. Other energy-beam-related methods: Total body nitrogen
6. Other methods: Underwater weighing

Scoring systems
1. Conventional SGA and its modifications (eg, DMS, MIS, CANUSA-version)[2]
2. Other scores: HD-PNI, others (eg, Wolfson, Merkus, Merckman)[2]

Laboratory values
1. Visceral proteins (negative acute phase reactants): Albumin, prealbumin, transferrin[2]
2. Lipids: Cholesterol, triglycerides, other lipids and lipoproteins[2]
3. Somatic proteins and nitrogen surrogates: Creatinine, SUN
4. Growth factors: IGF-1, leptin
5. Peripheral blood cell count: Lymphocyte count

[1]nPNA, normalized protein nitrogen appearance; nPCR, normalized protein catabolic rate; BMI, body mass index; DEXA, dual-energy x-ray absorptiometry; BIA, bioelectrical impedance analysis; NIR, near infrared interactance; SGA, subjective global assessment of nutritional status; DMS, dialysis malnutrition score; MIS, malnutrition inflammation score; CANUSA, Canada–USA study-based modification of the SGA; HD-PNI, hemodialysis prognostic nutritional index; SUN, serum urea nitrogen; IGF-1, insulin-like growth factor 1; CRP, C-reactive protein; IL, interleukin (eg, IL-1 and IL-6); TNF-α, tumor necrosis factor α; SAA, serum amyloid A.
[2]The given tool may also be altered by inflammation.

Guidelines on Nutrition in Chronic Renal Disease and Renal Failure recommends that nondialyzed CKD patients with a GFR less than 20 mL/minute undergo periodic nutritional assessments by serial measurements of a panel of markers including at least one measure from each of the following clusters: (1) serum albumin, (2) edema-free actual body weight and% standard body weight, (3) SGA, and (4) the nPNA or dietary interviews and diaries.

B. Assessment of Dietary Protein Intake

In CKD patients *dietary protein intake* can be estimated by both dietary interviews and diaries and the nPNA, ie, protein equivalent of total nitrogen appearance normalized to the volume of distribution of urea or some other function of body mass; this measure is also known as the normalized protein catabolic rate (nPCR) in patients on dialysis. Since the control of protein intake is central to the nutritional management of patients with renal insufficiency, it is important to accurately monitor nitrogen intake.

A simple and practical method to evaluate the compliance of patient's actual protein intake with the prescribed dietary protein intake is the following formula:

$$\text{Estimated protein intake} = 6.25 \times (\text{UUN} + 30 \text{ mg/kg} \times \text{BW})$$

where UUN is urine urea nitrogen measured in a 24-hour urine collection. If the patient's proteinuria is 5 g/day or higher, this quantity needs to be added to the estimated protein intake.

C. Role of Dietary Protein Intake

Different methods to slow the rate of progression of chronic renal insufficiency in CKD patients are discussed in Chapter 22. Low protein diets are one method. In recent years, three types of low nitrogen diets have primarily been used for the treatment of patients with CRI: (1) A low protein diet providing about 0.55–0.60 g protein/kg body weight/day; (2) a very low protein diet providing approximately 16–20 g/day of protein of miscellaneous quality (ie, about 0.28 g protein/kg/day) supplemented with about 10–20 g/day of the nine essential amino acids; and (3) a similar 16–20 g protein diet generally supplemented with four essential amino acids—histidine, lysine, threonine, and tryptophan—and the ketoacid or hydroxyacid analogs of the other five essential amino acids sometimes with a few other amino acids added.

Several meta-analyses indicate that low protein diets are effective is slowing the rate of progression of CKD to renal replacement therapy (maintenance dialysis or renal transplantation). On average, this effect, although clearcut, is not dramatic and often requires many months of treatment to become evident.

An unresolved issue is whether a low protein diet will retard the progression of renal failure in patients receiving angiotensin-converting enzyme inhibitors (ACEIs) and/or angiotensin receptor blockers (ARBs). Since dietary protein restriction exerts many of the same hemodynamic and other physiologic effects on the kidney as do ACEIs and ARBs, it is possible that the renal-protective effects of a low protein diet, when combined with ACEIs and ARBs, are replicative, rather than additive.

For CKD stages 1 and 2 (GFR >60 mL/minute) there is almost no information concerning the most desirable dietary protein and phosphorus prescription. Currently protein intake is usually not restricted for these patients except possibly to 0.80–1 g protein and 1200–1400 mg phosphorus/kg/day unless there is evidence that renal function is continuing to decline. Under these circumstances, the patient is treated as indicated below.

For CKD stage 3, low protein, low phosphorus diets may retard progression. A diet providing about 0.60–0.75 g protein/kg/day, of which at least 0.35 g/kg/day is high biologic value protein, is needed to ensure a sufficient intake of the essential amino acids.

For CKD stage 4 and 5, the potential advantages to using a low protein, low phosphorus diet are more compelling. A low protein diet will generate less nitrogenous compounds that are potentially toxic both systemically and to the kidney itself. In addition, it generally contains less phosphorus and potassium, reductions of which are usually imperative at this advanced stage of renal failure. Patients should be prescribed 0.60 g protein/kg/day or, if this is not feasible, up to 0.75 g protein/kg/day. This diet will generally maintain a neutral or positive nitrogen balance as long as the energy intake is not deficient. At least 50% of the protein intake with these low protein diets should be of high biologic value. The protein content of this diet should be increased by 1 g/day of high biologic value protein for each gram of protein excreted in the urine each day. However, only 10–20% of individuals with chronic renal disease are willing and able to adhere to diets providing 0.60 g protein/kg/day or essential amino acid-supplemented very low protein diets.

D. Dietary Protein Requirements in Patients on Maintenance Dialysis

Some current guidelines including the K/DOQI recommend a nutritional indicator for inaugurating renal replacement therapy. Indeed in patients with stage 5 CKD (GFR <15 mL/minute) who are not undergoing maintenance dialysis, if protein–energy malnutrition develops or persists despite vigorous attempts to optimize protein and energy intake and there is no apparent cause for malnutrition other than low nutrient intake, initiation of maintenance dialysis or a renal transplant is recommended.

Studies in nitrogen balance suggest that most patients on maintenance hemodialysis require more than 1 g protein/kg/day to maintain both protein balance and normal total body protein. The high protein requirement can be due to the fact that patients on maintenance dialysis have increased dietary protein requirements because of the removal of amino acids and peptides by the dialysis procedure and possibly because hemodialysis appears to stimulate protein catabolism by engendering an inflammatory, catabolic response. The K/DOQI Clinical Practice Guidelines currently recommend 1.2 g protein/kg body weight/day for clinically stable patients undergoing maintenance hemodialysis and 1.2–1.3 g protein/kg/day for patients undergoing chronic peritoneal dialysis (PD). At least 50% of the dietary protein should be of high biologic value. It is possible that PD patients who are protein depleted may become more anabolic when they ingest up to 1.4 g protein/kg/day. A recent study showed that the lowest mortality is associated with a protein intake (nPNA) between 0.9 and 1.4 g protein/kg/day (Figure 21–4).

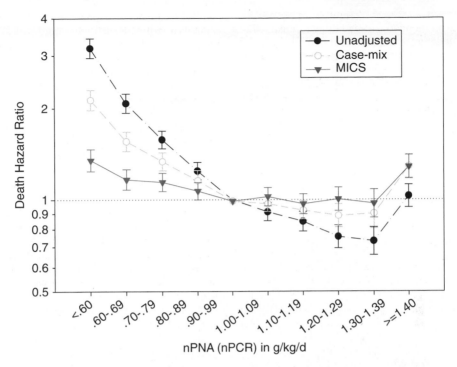

▲ **Figure 21–4.** Protein intake and survival in patients on maintenance hemodialysis. MICS, malnutrition–inflammation complex syndrome; nPNA, normalized protein nitrogen appearance; nPCR, normalized protein catabolic rate.

E. Energy Intake

In nondialyzed CKD patients and patients undergoing maintenance dialysis, energy expenditure, measured by indirect calorimetry, appears to be normal during resting and sitting, following ingestion of a standard meal, and with defined exercise. Studies in nitrogen balance in nondialyzed stage 5 CKD patients ingesting 0.55–0.60 g protein/kg/day indicate that the amount of energy intake necessary to ensure neutral or positive nitrogen balance is approximately 35 kcal/kg/day. However, most studies of the dietary habits of nondialyzed stage 4 and 5 CKD patients and patients on dialysis indicate that their mean energy intakes are lower than this level, usually about 24–27 kcal/kg/day.

The K/DOQI Clinical Practice Guidelines currently recommend that the energy intake for nondialyzed patients with advanced CKD (GFR <25 mL/minute) and for patients on maintenance dialysis should be 35 kcal/kg/day for individuals who are less than 60 years of age and 30–35 kcal/kg/day for those who are 60 years of age or older, who are usually more sedentary (Table 21–5). The same energy intakes are recommended for people with stage 3 or 4 CKD (ie, GFR <60 mL/minute/1.73 m^2).

Since energy (and protein) intake seems to decrease when the GFR falls to about 35–50 mL/minute/1.73 m^2, to prevent malnutrition, it is important to monitor dietary intake and to treat inadequate intakes, even in clinically stable healthy appearing adults, when the GFR decreases to this level. This low level of GFR may be associated with a serum creatinine as low as 1.5–2.5 mg/dL in some adult patients.

Caglar K et al: Therapeutic effects of oral nutritional supplementation during hemodialysis. Kidney Int 2002;62:1054.

Fouque D: Influence of dietary protein intake on the progression of chronic renal insufficiency. In: *Nutritional Management of Renal Disease*, ed 2. Kopple J, Massry S (editors). Lippincott, Williams & Wilkins, 2004, pp 261–286.

Pupim L et al: Assessment of protein–energy nutritional status. In: *Nutritional Management of Renal Disease*, ed 2. Kopple J, Massry S (editors). Lippincott, Williams & Wilkins, 2004, pp 223–240.

▶ Complications

A. Management of Other Nutritional Factors

The number and magnitude of the changes in the dietary intake for CKD patients are so great that if they were all presented to the patient at one time, the patient could become demoralized and lose the motivation to comply with the diet. It is therefore necessary to prioritize goals for dietary treatment.

Table 21–5. Recommended dietary nutrient intake for adult patients undergoing maintenance hemodialysis.

Macronutrients and fiber	Recommended intake
Dietary protein intake (DPI)[1]	1.2 g/kg body weight/day for clinically stable MHD patients (at least 50% of the dietary protein should be of high biologic value) ≥1.2-1.3 g/kg/day for acutely ill patients
Daily energy intake (DEI)[1,2]	35 kcal/kg body weight/day for those who are less than 60 years of age and 30–35 kcal/kg body weight/day for individuals 60 years or older
Fat intake[3]	30% of total energy intake
Total fat[3,4]	30% of total energy intake
Saturated fat[3]	Up to 10% of total energy intake
Polyunsaturated–saturated fatty acids[3]	Up to 10% of total calories
Monounsaturated fatty acids[3]	Up to 20% of total calories
Carbohydrate[3-5]	Rest of nonprotein calories
Total fiber[6]	20–25 g/day

[1]According to K/DOQI guidelines
[2]Refers to percent of total energy intake (diet plus dialysate).
[3]Although atherosclerotic vascular disease constitutes a common and serious problem for patients on maintenance hemodialysis (MHD), these recommendations are often hard to adhere to. Moreover, there is no prospective interventional study indicating these dietary modifications are beneficial for patients on MHD, although, reasonably, the potential benefits of these modifications seem valuable. They are strongly recommended only if patients adhere closely to more critical aspects of the diet (eg, sodium, water, potassium, phosphorus, protein, and energy intake), and have expressed a particular interest in these modifications or have a specific disorder that may respond to their medications.
[4]Refers to percent of total energy intake; if triglyceride levels are very high, the percentage of fat in the diet may be increased to about 35% of total calories; otherwise, 25–30% of total calories is preferable. Intake of fatty acids should be kept low because they raise low-density lipoprotein cholesterol (see text).
[5]Should be primarily complex carbohydrates.
[6]Less critical to adhere to for the typical MHD patient.

Usually the importance of controlling the protein, phosphorus, sodium, energy, potassium, and magnesium intake and the need to take calcium and vitamin supplements should be emphasized. However, unless the patient has a lipid disorder or other risk factors that indicate there is a high odds ratio for adverse cardiovascular events, the recommended quantity and types of dietary carbohydrate, fat, and fiber are discussed with the patient, but adherence to these dietary guidelines are not as strongly emphasized. If the patient has complied well with the other, more critical elements of dietary therapy, has a specific lipid disorder that may benefit from dietary therapy, or has expressed an interest in modifying fat, carbohydrate, or fiber intake, then modifications of the dietary intake of these latter nutrients should be explored more intensively.

1. Lipids—Elevated serum triglyceride levels are common in stage 4–5 CKD. Hypertriglyceridemia is caused primarily by impaired catabolism of triglyceride-rich lipoproteins. The reduced catabolic rate leads to increased quantities of apolipoprotein B (apoB)-containing triglyceride-rich lipoproteins in intermediate-density lipoproteins (IDL) and very low-density lipoproteins (VLDL) and reduced concentrations of high-density lipoproteins (HDL). Since diets for patients with renal failure are usually restricted in protein, sodium, potassium, and water, it is often difficult to provide sufficient energy without resorting to intakes of purified sugars that may increase triglyceride production. In patients on peritoneal dialysis, the glucose load in the peritoneal fluid appears to further increase serum triglycerides and cholesterol. Low serum HDL cholesterol, a common phenomenon in CKD patients, appears to be an independent risk factor for adverse coronary artery disease. Most clinicians recommend treatment of lipid abnormalities in dialysis patients in a manner similar to that used for the general population.

Low fat diets and lipid-lowering medicines retard the rate of progression of renal failure in animal models. In humans, some research suggests that taking supplements rich in omega-3 fatty acid may lower the progression of renal failure in renal transplant patients. A preponderance of studies suggests that omega-3 fatty acids given as fish oil may retard the rate of progression of immunoglobulin A (IgA) nephropathy.

Abnormal carnitine metabolism (see below) has also been implicated as a cause of hypertriglyceridemia in CKD. However, the many studies of treatment of hypertriglyceridemia with carnitine in CKD patients are divided between substantial numbers that show carnitine lowers serum triglycerides and substantial numbers that show no change or, rarely, a rise in serum triglycerides.

At present, there is no consensus as to what dietary fat constellation is the most appropriate for CKD patients. We recommend a Therapeutic Lifestyle Changes (TLC) diet for those with mild to moderate CKD not on maintenance dialysis treatment (Table 21–6). We treat hypertriglyceridemia by dietary modification only when serum triglycerides are greatly elevated (>200 or 300 mg/dL). In this situation, dietary fat intake should not be above 40% of total calories. A high proportion of dietary carbohydrates should be complex. These modifications often lower the palatability of the diet; therefore, the patient's total energy intake must be monitored closely to ensure that it does not fall. With high serum triglyceride values that are unresponsive to dietary therapy,

Table 21–6. Nutrient composition of the Therapeutic Lifestyle Changes (TLC) diet.

Nutrient	Recommended intake
Saturated fat[1]	<7% of total calories
Polyunsaturated fat	Up to 10% of total calories
Monounsaturated fat	Up to 20% of total calories
Total fat	25–35% of total calories
Carbohydrate[2,3]	50–60% of total calories
Fiber	20–30 g/day
Protein[3]	Approximately 15% of total calories
Cholesterol	<200 mg/day
Total calories[4]	Balance energy intake and expenditure to maintain desirable body weight/prevent weight gain

Trans-fatty acids are another low-density lipoprotein-raising fat that should be kept at a low intake.
[2]Carbohydrates should be derived predominantly from foods rich in complex carbohydrates including grains, especially whole grains, fruits, and vegetables.
[3]Dietary content of proteins and, hence, carbohydrates should be modified according to the specific needs of patients on maintenance hemodialysis (ie, 1.20 g protein/kg/day) (see text).
[4]Daily energy expenditure should include at least moderate physical activity (contributing approximately 200 kcal/day).
Reprinted with permission from Executive Summary of The Third Report of The National Cholesterol Education Program (NCEP) Expert Panel on Detection, Evaluation, and Treatment of High Blood Cholesterol in Adults (Adult Treatment Panel III). JAMA 2001;285:2486.

a fibrate (eg, femofibrate) may be tried. L-Carnitine, about 500–1000 mg/day, or for patients on hemodialysis L-carnitine, 10–20 mg/kg/day at the end of each dialysis three times weekly, may be tried if hypertriglyceridemia is severe and unresponsive to these treatments.

2. Homocysteine—Plasma homocysteine is increased in CKD patients. The mechanism for this increase is unclear but may involve impaired remethylation of homocysteine back to methionine. In the general population, elevated plasma homocysteine is associated with a high incidence of cardiovascular disease. In CRI patients and patients on dialysis, there are contradictory observations pertaining to the association between hyperhomocysteinemia and risk of cardiovascular disease. Most recent studies do not show any association between hyperhomocysteinemia and death in both CRI patients and patients on dialysis.

Vitamin B$_6$ is a cofactor for cystathionine synthetase, which catalyzes the conversion of methionine to cystathionine, and for cystathionase, which converts cystathionine

to cysteine. Pyridoxine, given as pyridoxine HCl, a form of vitamin B$_6$, generally does not lower plasma homocysteine in CKD patients. The folate metabolite tetrahydrofolic acid is necessary for the remethylation of homocysteine to reform methionine, and folic acid or folinic acid supplements may decrease plasma homocysteine concentrations in CKD patients, although usually not to normal values.

3. Carnitine—Carnitine is a naturally occurring compound that is essential for life. It is both synthesized in the body and ingested. Carnitine facilitates the transfer of long-chain (>10 carbon) fatty acids into muscle mitochondria. Since fatty acids are the major fuel source for skeletal and myocardial muscle at rest and during mild to moderate exercise, this activity is considered necessary for normal skeletal and cardiac muscle function.

Patients undergoing maintenance dialysis not infrequently have low serum free carnitine and in some but not all studies, low skeletal muscle free and total carnitine levels. Carnitine deficiency could be due to impaired synthesis of carnitine *in vivo*, reduced dietary intake of carnitine, and removal of carnitine by dialysis. The weekly loss of free carnitine by dialysis is reported to be approximately equal to the normal weekly urinary excretion of carnitine. However, the finding that serum free carnitine is normal in nondialyzed patients with stage 5 CKD and is low in patients on maintenance dialysis is consistent with the thesis that dialysis of L–carnitine is the major cause of low serum carnitine in patients on maintenance dialysis.

A number of clinical trials in patients with CRI, particularly those undergoing maintenance dialysis therapy, suggest that L-carnitine may provide clinical benefits including (1) increased physical exercise capacity, (2) reduced interdialytic symptoms of skeletal muscle cramps or hypertension, (3) improvement in overall global sense of well being or various symptoms often found in CRI patients, (4) improved response of anemia to erythropoietin treatment, (5) decreased predialysis serum urea, creatinine, and phosphorus, and (6) increased midarm muscle circumference. However, not all clinical trials confirm these findings.

The K/DOQI recommends that L-carnitine can be administered to patients on MHD or PD who suffer from disabling or very bothersome skeletal muscle weakness or cardiomyopathy, skeletal muscle cramps, or hypotension during hemodialysis treatment, severe malaise, or anemia refractory to erythropoietin therapy, and in whom the above conditions do not respond to more standard treatment. The patient can then be given a 3- to 6-month trial of L-carnitine (up to 9 months for refractory anemia). L-Carnitine may be administered orally, intravenously, or into dialysate. Oral L-carnitine is less expensive, but its intestinal absorption may be somewhat unpredictable. A dose of 20 mg/kg at the end of each hemodialysis, three times weekly, can be prescribed.

4. Sodium and water—In both normal individuals and people with CKD, about 1–3 mEq/day of sodium is excreted in the feces. In the absence of visible sweating, only a few milliequivalents per day of sodium is lost through the skin. Because both the glomerular filtration and the fractional reabsorption of sodium fall parallel to each other as renal insufficiency progresses in CKD patients, most patients with renal failure are able to maintain sodium balance with a normal sodium intake if they do not have heart or liver failure. Patients with advanced renal failure who receive large loads of sodium, particularly as sodium chloride, may be unable to excrete the quantity of sodium ingested, and they may develop edema, hypertension, and congestive heart failure. This syndrome is particularly likely to occur in stage 4 and 5 CKD. In these patients, hypertension often is more easily controlled when they are sodium restricted, and may be accentuated by an increased sodium intake, probably because of expanded extracellular fluid volume and possibly due to altered intracellular electrolyte composition within arteriolar smooth muscle cells that increase contractility. Moreover, the antiproteinuric effects of ACE inhibitors and probably ARBs are substantially abrogated by even moderate sodium intakes; as urinary sodium excretion rises above about 100 mEq/day, the antiproteinuric effects abate.

In most nondialyzed patients with advanced renal failure, a daily intake of 1000–3000 mg (40–130 mEq) of sodium and 1500– 2000 mL of fluid will maintain sodium and water balance. The requirement for sodium and water varies markedly, and each patient must be managed individually. Patients undergoing maintenance dialysis frequently are oliguric or anuric. For patients on hemodialysis, sodium and total fluid intake generally should be restricted to 1000–1500 mg/day and 700–1500 mL/day, respectively. Since sodium and water can be removed easily and continuously with peritoneal dialysis, a more liberal salt and water intake is usually allowed. Indeed, by maintaining a larger dietary sodium and water intake, the quantity of fluid removed from the patient on chronic peritoneal dialysis (CPD) and hence the daily dialysate outflow volume can be increased. This may be advantageous, since with CPD the daily clearance of small- and middle-sized molecules is directly related to the volume of dialysate outflow. Thus for some CPD patients, a higher sodium and water intake (eg, 6–8 g/day of sodium and 3 L/day of water) may enable the patient to use more hypertonic or hyperoncotic dialysate to increase the dialysate outflow volume, thereby increasing dialysate clearances and, if hypertonic glucose is used, energy uptake from the dialysate.

In nondialyzed CKD patients or patients undergoing maintenance dialysis who are not anuric and who have excessive sodium or water retention despite attempts at dietary restriction, a potent loop diuretic, such as furosemide or bumetanide, may be tried to increase urinary sodium and water excretion.

5. Potassium—Approximately 90% of daily potassium intake is excreted through the kidneys. Potassium excretion occurs mostly in the cortical collecting duct and is regulated by aldosterone and distal nephron sodium delivery. Because of the relative state of fluid overload and the frequent suppression of the renin–angiotensin–aldosterone axis, due to volume expression, diabetes mellitus and/or ACE inhibitors, ARB and aldosterone blockers, potassium tends to be retained in advanced CKD. This is accentuated by diminished distal nephron sodium delivery in the setting of low GFR.

Fecal excretion of potassium is increased due to its enhanced intestinal secretion, and dietary restriction and anorexia can decrease intake. Nonetheless, hyperkalemia is rather universal in patients with advanced CKD not undergoing dialysis, and amounts of urine output prevail. Factors promoting hyperkalemia in CKD include (1) excessive intake of potassium; (2) acidemia; (3) worsening oliguria, eg, due to superimposed acute renal failure; (4) catabolic stress or tissue degradation; (5) possibly hypoinsulinism or hyperglycemia (solvent drag) in patients with diabetes; (6) use of medicines such as ACE inhibitors, aldosterone receptor blockers (eg, spironolactone, epherenone), nonsteroidal anti-inflammatory drugs, and β-receptor blockers.

Patients with stage 4 or 5 CKD (ie, GFR less than 30 mL/minute), including those undergoing MHD, should generally receive no more than 70–75 mEq (about 3 g) of potassium per day. Those with frequent hyperkalemia (>5.5 mEq/L) should restrict their potassium to 1–2 g/day if possible. However, it is important to note that many types of fresh fruits and vegetables and other healthy food contain substantial amounts of potassium. Their restriction by rigid dietary regimens deprive CKD patients, who already have a high risk of cardiovascular disease, from important sources of antiatherogenic foods and neutraceuticals. Patients on peritoneal dialysis are an exception, since they tend to develop hypokalemia due to potassium losses in their peritoneal fluid.

6. Magnesium—In CKD patients, the difference between dietary intake and fecal excretion of magnesium (net absorption) amounts to about 40–50% of ingested magnesium. Since the absorbed magnesium is excreted primarily by the kidney, hypermagnesemia may occur in CRI. Magnesium also commonly accrues in bone in renal failure and may play a causal role in renal osteodystrophy. The restricted diets of stage 4 or 5 CKD patients are low in magnesium (usually about 100–300 mg/day for a 40-g protein diet). The patients' serum magnesium levels are therefore usually normal or only slightly elevated unless the patient takes substances that are high in magnesium content, such as magnesium-containing antacids and laxatives. Nondialyzed patients with stage 5 CKD require about 200 mg/day of magnesium to maintain neutral magnesium balance. The optimal dietary magnesium allowance for patients on maintenance dialysis has not been well defined. Experience suggests that when the magnesium content is about 1.0 mEq/L in hemodialysate or 0.50–0.75 mEq/L in peritoneal dialysate, a dietary magnesium intake of 200–300 mg/day will maintain the serum magnesium at normal or only slightly elevated levels.

7. Phosphorus—Renal osteodystrophy and the management of bone disease in CKD are discussed in Chapter 20. Chapter 20 reviews the rationale for controlling dietary phosphorus and the use of gastrointestinal binders of phosphate, hyperphosphatemia, the serum calcium–phosphorus product, calcium phosphate deposition in soft tissue, and hyperparathyroidism. The dietary phosphorus intake and the use of phosphate binders therefore will be discussed here only briefly.

There are inconclusive data concerning the optimal level of phosphorus restriction for retarding progressive renal failure or for minimizing hyperparathyroidism. For both nondialyzed and dialyzed CKD patients, the morning fasting serum phosphorus concentrations should always be maintained at or above 2.5 mg/dL. Lower serum phosphorus levels usually indicate severe malnutrition and have been shown to correlate with high risks of death in patients on maintenance dialysis even after extensive multivariate adjustments for other markers of malnutrition.

Since there is a rough correlation between the protein and phosphorus content of the diet, it is much easier to reduce phosphorus intake if a lower protein diet is used. One approach for patients with moderate CKD (stages 3, 4, and 5) is to maintain phosphorus intake at about 10–15 mg/kg/day. This quantity of phosphorus intake is not overly difficult to attain by patients who are ingesting a 0.60–0.75 g protein/kg/day diet.

The K/DOQI guidelines recommend maintaining serum phosphorus between 3.5 and 5.5 mg/dL in advanced stages of CKD including patients on maintenance dialysis. This often requires the patients to ingest a low phosphorus diet intake of about 800–1000 mg/day, particularly when CKD patients have elevated serum phosphorus concentrations and especially if they have moderate or severe hyperparathyroidism. However, there is the risk that protein–energy malnutrition and hypoalbuminemia also exist with such low amounts of protein intake, especially among patients on maintenance dialysis. Serum phosphorus levels should be monitored monthly following the initiation of dietary phosphorus restriction to ensure that serum phosphorus remains within the target range of each CKD stage.

Without phosphate binders, there is a net intestinal phosphate absorption (diet minus fecal phosphorus) of roughly 60% of the phosphorus intake. Therefore, this level of dietary phosphorus restriction usually will not maintain normal serum phosphorus levels in patients with stage 5 CKD (GFR <15 mL/minute), even with a substantial reduction in the renal tubular reabsorption of phosphorus. Hence, binders of gastrointestinal phosphate are also employed. The recommended phosphorus intake for patients on maintenance dialysis is about 12–15 mg/kg/day or less. This higher upper limit was chosen because with their greater protein intakes, patients on dialysis cannot readily ingest less phosphorus without making the diet too restrictive. Patients on maintenance dialysis almost always require phosphate binders to prevent hyperphosphatemia. Different types of phosphorus binders and their effects on serum phosphorus levels, bone disease, and cardiovascular risk are discussed in Chapter 20.

8. Calcium—The role of calcium in CKD-associated renal osteodystrophy and the management of bone disease are discussed in detail in Chapter 20. Stages 4 and 5 CKD patients who do not undergo maintenance dialysis usually have an increased dietary requirement for calcium, because they have vitamin D deficiency and resistance to the actions of vitamin D. The risk of calcium deficiency in these patients is enhanced because the diets prescribed for uremic patients are almost always reduced in calcium. Foods high in calcium content are usually high in phosphorus (eg, dairy products) and are therefore restricted for CRI patients. For example, a 40 g protein diet generally provides only about 300–400 mg/day of calcium, whereas the recommended dietary allowances for healthy, nonpregnant, nonlactating adults are about 800–1200 mg/day. Balance studies indicate that nondialyzed stage 5 CKD patients not receiving calcitriol (1,25-dihydroxycholecalciferol) or other vitamin D compounds usually require about 1200–1600 mg/day of calcium for neutral or positive calcium balance.

Low protein diets prescribed to CKD patients may need to be supplemented with approximately 600–1000 mg of elemental calcium daily. Supplemental calcium should not be given unless the serum phosphorus concentration is normal (2.5–5.5 mg/dL) to reduce the risk of calcium phosphate deposition in soft tissues. In addition, frequent monitoring of serum calcium is important because hypercalcemia may develop, particularly if serum phosphorus falls to low-normal or low levels. This is especially likely to occur if the patient also has hyperparathyroidism, a common complication of chronic renal failure.

An adjusted serum calcium range of 8.4–9.5 mg/dL is recommended for CKD stage 5 according to the current K/DOQI guidelines. To calculate the adjusted serum calcium, for each g/dL decrement of serum albumin below 4.0 g/dL, 0.8 mg/dL is subtracted from the measured serum calcium. Treatment with vitamin D analogs will decrease the daily calcium requirement by enhancing intestinal calcium absorption. This will reduce the total daily calcium load for the patient on dialysis who is taking calcium binders of phosphate.

B. Trace Elements

Trace elements are elements that are present in the body at concentrations <50 mg/kg. Recent advances in analytic methodology allow accurate measurements of trace element levels in body fluids. The main source of body trace elements levels is diet. However, the blood and tissue levels of these elements may be affected by nondietary factors, including renal excretory function, environmental and occupational exposure, duration of renal failure, the concentrations in the fresh dialysate and in flow, and possibly the mode of dialytic therapy. Also, many trace elements are largely protein bound.

Table 21-7. Recommended dietary intake of trace elements for adult patients with advanced chronic kidney disease (CKD).

Macronutrients	Daily requirement in chronic renal insufficiency	Toxicity reported with excessive intake
Iron[1]	Dependent on erythropoietin treatment and other factors	Yes
Zinc	15 mg/day	
Selenium	Not known	No data available in CKD
Copper	Not known	Yes
Aluminum	Not known	Yes

[1]Iron requirements vary according to the dose of administered erythropoietin.

In CRI, there may be altered serum levels of binding protein levels or increased serum concentrations of compounds that compete for binding sites on these proteins; such factors may also cause a major alteration in serum trace element concentrations independently of the body burden or nutritional needs for these elements. The malnutrition–inflammation complex syndrome in CKD patients may lead to low serum protein concentrations and may be one of the causes of low serum zinc, manganese, and possibly selenium and nickel in CKD patients.

Because many trace elements are present in minuscule amounts in the plasma and are protein bound, losses during dialysis may be minimal. However, substantial amounts of bromide and zinc are removed during hemodialysis because a large proportion of the serum concentrations is not protein bound and because the levels in fresh dialysate are quite low. Conversely, the presence in the dialysate of even minute quantities of certain trace elements may lead to uptake by the body because of the avidity with which some trace elements bind to proteins. This phenomenon has been observed for lead, copper, and zinc. Table 21–7 gives the dietary recommendations for some trace elements in patients on maintenance dialysis.

1. Zinc—Serum zinc levels are often low, but erythrocyte zinc is often high–normal or elevated in CKD patients. Low levels of serum zinc may be related to removal by dialysis, inadequate dietary intake, and possibly reduced intestinal absorption. Although levels of serum zinc tend to rise at the end of dialysis, this can be attributed entirely to the rise in concentration of carrier proteins due to hemoconcentration. Dysgeusia and impotence in males have been reported to be ameliorated with zinc supplements, but not all studies confirm these findings. Until more definitive studies are conducted concerning

dietary zinc requirements, it is recommended that patients on dialysis should receive the recommended dietary allowance for zinc, which is 15 mg/day. Intestinal zinc absorption is not affected by vitamin D metabolites.

2. Selenium—Selenium is an antioxidant; it is required for the activity of the enzyme glutathione peroxidase. Several studies have indicated low serum levels of selenium in patients with CRI. MICS and its associated poor energy and protein intake along with the restricted diet of CRI patients and patients on dialysis may play a major role in the development of selenium deficiency, especially since meat and fish are rich in selenium. In patients on maintenance dialysis, an association between selenium deficiency and increased oxidative stress has been noted.

3. Copper—Copper is essential for the activity of many enzymes including cytochrome oxidase and superoxide dismutase. In CKD patients, hypercupremia has been reported more often than copper deficiency. Excessive intake or absorption of copper, especially due to copper tubing used in heating coil for dialysate fluid, has caused hemolytic anemia (also known as Heinz-body-associated anemia) in patients on hemodialysis. The required intake and recommended dietary allowances (RDA) for copper in dialysis patients are currently not known.

4. Aluminum—Until about a decade ago, aluminum intake was often excessive in patients on dialysis, who regularly took aluminum-containing phosphorus binders such as aluminum hydroxide. Another source of aluminum in patients on hemodialysis is poorly treated fresh dialysate water. In patients on maintenance dialysis, refractory anemia (ie, erythropoietin hyporesponsiveness), osteodystrophy, myopathy, and neurologic disturbances including dementia have been attributed to aluminum toxicity. When nonaluminum-containing phosphorus binders became available, aluminum toxicity was encountered less frequently.

5. Iron—Iron deficiency is common in patients on maintenance dialysis and is discussed in Chapter 18. The causes include binding of iron to the dialyzer membrane, frequent blood drawing, sequestration of blood in the dialyzer at the termination of a hemodialysis procedure, and intestinal blood loss. Treatment with recombinant human erythropoietin (EPO) may reduce the nonhemoglobin-bound iron stores by enhancing erythropoiesis unless adequate iron supplementation is given. Iron deficiency can be determined by measuring serum iron and total iron binding capacity (TIBC), calculating their ratio, known as transferrin saturation, and assessing serum ferritin levels. Serum TIBC may be affected by the presence of the MICS, since TIBC is a negative acute phase reactant. Hence, its serum level is usually decreased in the setting of MICS. Thus, in CKD patients with evidence of inflammation or malnutrition, the iron saturation ratio (ie, serum iron divided by TIBC) may be erroneously normal or high if the denominator (TIBC) is decreased. Serum ferritin is a positive acute phase reactant and may increase due to non-iron-related factors, such as the MICS.

C. Vitamin Requirements

CKD patients are at increased risk for deficiencies of several vitamins. The causes for vitamin deficiencies include (1) reduced total food intake due to anorexia; (2) prescription of low-phosphorus, low-potassium diets that restrict intake of nutritionally valuable foods such as fresh fruits and vegetables, dairy products, and other items that are high in vitamins; (3) altered metabolism, as is the case for pyridoxine and possibly folate; (4) impaired synthesis (eg, for 1,25-dihydroxyvitamin D); (5) resistance to the actions of vitamins (eg, vitamin D and possibly folate); (6) decreased intestinal absorption (eg, decreased intestinal absorption of riboflavin, folate, and vitamin D have been described in rats with chronic renal insufficiency); and (7) dialysate losses of water-soluble vitamins.

In some studies, CRI patients who did not receive vitamin supplements generally did not develop signs of vitamin deficiency when followed longitudinally. Based on these findings, the need for vitamin supplementation for patients on maintenance dialysis has been questioned. However, recent reports continue to show that many CKD patients ingest a vitamin intake that provides less than the recommended dietary allowances, and there is a small but persistent prevalence of deficiencies for some water-soluble vitamins (as well as for 1,25-dihydroxyvitamin D) in CRI patients not taking vitamin supplements. At present, it does not seem feasible to identify, a priori, those patients who will develop vitamin deficiencies. Since the intake of water-soluble vitamins at the proposed levels appears to be safe, we propose that these vitamins be supplemented. Table 21–8 shows the dietary recommendations for various vitamins in patients on maintenance dialysis. The RDAs that are proposed for each of the water-soluble vitamins and for vitamin A are similar to those of normal individuals except for higher doses of pyridoxine HCl (10 mg/day, 8.2 mg/day of pyridoxine) and folic acid (about 1 mg/day). Vitamin C is recommended only at the daily allowance levels (70 mg/day) because of the risk of increased oxalate formation at higher intakes. Some studies indicate that vitamin E has an antioxidant effect in patients on chronic dialysis and may protect against cardiovascular events. However, a recent study showed that individuals with no apparent kidney disease who were randomized to receive a vitamin E supplement of 400 units/day had an increased risk of developing heart failure. However, given positive results in CKD patients with CRI, we currently encourage vitamin E administration to all patients with renal insufficiency.

1. Water-soluble vitamins—Some reports indicate that *vitamin C* supplementation may promote intestinal iron absorption and reduce the incidence of iron deficiency anemia in CKD patients. Serum homocysteine concentrations, a cardiovascular risk factor in the general population, are

Table 21–8. Recommended dietary intake of selected vitamins for adult patients with advanced chronic kidney disease.

Macronutrients	Daily requirement	Toxicity reported with excessive intake
Vitamin B[1] (thiamine)	1.1-1.2 mg/day	
Vitamin B[2] (riboflavin)	1.1-1.3 mg/day	
Pantothenic acid	5 mg/day	
Biotin	30 μg/day	
Niacin	14-16 mg/day	
Vitamin B[6] (pyridoxine)	10 mg/day	
Vitamin B[12]	2.4 μg/day	
Vitamin C	75-90 mg/day	Yes
Folic acid[1]	1-10 mg/day	
Vitamin A	See text	Yes
Vitamin D	See text	Yes
Vitamin E[2]	400-800 IU (optional, see text)	
Vitamin K[3]	See text	

[1]At least 1 mg/day of folic acid should be given, but up to 10 mg/day may be administered to reduce elevated plasma homocysteine levels.
[2]Vitamin E, 300 or 800 IU/day, may be given to reduce oxidative stress and prevent cardiovascular disease, but the value of these supplements is controversial (see text).
[3]Vitamin K supplements may be needed for patients who are not eating and who receive antibiotics.

significantly increased in patients on maintenance dialysis and pharmacologic doses of *folic acid* may lower plasma total homocysteine levels. However, some recent data indicate that patients on dialysis with a higher plasma homocysteine concentration may paradoxically have a better survival, a phenomenon also known as reverse epidemiology.

Erythrocyte or serum levels of riboflavin (vitamin B_2), thiamine (vitamin B_1), niacin, pantothenic acid, and biotin are usually normal in CRI patients. However, case reports of Wernicke's encephalopathy in patients on maintenance dialysis due to thiamine deficiency are occasionally described. Pyridoxine (vitamin B_6) is removed by hemodialysis; this factor, and probably also altered vitamin B_6 metabolism, may account for the increased daily requirement for this vitamin. Vitamin B_6 participates in the metabolism of homocysteine, although pyridoxine supplements have not been consistently shown to decrease plasma homocysteine in patients with renal failure.

2. Lipid-soluble vitamins—The lipid-soluble vitamins are D, K, A, and E. Vitamin D is discussed in detail in Chapter 20. *Vitamin K* levels are usually normal in CKD patients. Administration of a pharmacologic dose of vitamin K (45 mg/day orally) for 1 year was found to prevent loss of bone mass in patients on maintenance dialysis with bone disease characterized by low bone turnover. Several reports describe a relationship between high plasma vitamin K levels and ectopic soft tissue calcification in patients on maintenance dialysis. Since CKD patients generally do not have vitamin K deficiency, vitamin K supplements are not recommended for routine use. However, patients may be at increased risk for vitamin K deficiency if they are not eating, are not given vitamin K by parenteral administration, and are receiving antibiotics that suppress the intestinal bacteria that synthesize vitamin K. Under these conditions, vitamin K supplements should be considered.

There are inconsistent reports about the levels of serum and erythrocyte *vitamin E* (α-tocopherol) in patients on dialysis. The dialysis procedure does not remove significant amounts of α-tocopherol. These findings may reflect either increased consumption of tocopherol, possibly due to oxidative stress, or a defect in the HDL-mediated transfer of α-tocopherol from plasma to the red blood cell membrane. Since patients on maintenance dialysis often have oxidant stress, several studies have examined the effects on oxidant stress of vitamin E supplementation given orally, during HD treatment utilizing vitamin E-coated dialyzer membranes, or through dialysate (hemolipodialysis). Since chronic renal failure is clearly associated with increased oxidant stress and increased cardiovascular risk, and since vitamin E appears to be rather safe and may be beneficial, it is not unreasonable to consider prescribing a supplement of 400–800 IU/day of vitamin E.

Serum *vitamin A* concentrations are generally increased in CRI patients, especially among long-term dialysis survivors. Patients on maintenance dialysis who are binephrectomized are reported to have serum retinol levels higher than other CKD patients; this probably reflects the loss of the renal contribution to the degradation of retinal-binding protein (RBP), the carrier protein for vitamin A. Hemodialysis treatment does not change vitamin A levels except possibly by hemoconcentration; indeed losses of vitamin A into dialysate would not be expected because of the relatively large size of the vitamin A–RBP–transthyretin (prealbumin) complex and because vitamin A is lipid soluble. However, β-carotene, ubiquinol, and lycopene have been found to be lower in CKD patients than in individuals without renal insufficiency, and β-carotene and ubiquinol are reported to fall further after a single hemodialysis. It is possible that lipid metabolism may also affect serum vitamin A levels. Evidence suggests that vitamin A may promote erythropoiesis.

Patients with advanced CKD appear to be particularly vulnerable to *vitamin A toxicity*. Hypercalcemia and elevated serum alkaline phosphatase levels have been described in patients on maintenance dialysis ingesting as little as 7500–15,000 units/day of vitamin A. Therefore, it is recommended that the daily vitamin A intake from foods and supplements combined should not exceed the recommended dietary allowance of 800–1000 μg/day.

D. Acid–Base Management in Renal Insufficiency

CKD patients with moderate to advanced renal failure frequently develop metabolic acidosis. This is usually associated with a mild to moderate increase in anion gap because of impairment in the ability of the kidney to excrete acidic metabolites. In the earlier stages of renal insufficiency, and occasionally with advanced renal failure, hyperchloremic (nongap) metabolic acidosis may also be caused by excessive renal losses of bicarbonate. Ingestion of low protein diets may prevent or decrease the severity of the acidosis because the endogenous generation of acidic products of protein metabolism will be reduced. Metabolic acidemia may engender oxidation of branched chain amino acids and protein catabolism, impair albumin synthesis, increase β_2-microglobulin turnover, cause bone loss, possibly predispose to inflammation, and cause symptoms of weakness and lethargy. The acidemia-induced increased proteolysis in skeletal muscle appears to be caused by enhanced activity of the ATP-dependent ubiquitin–proteosome pathway. Conversely, correction of acidosis has been associated with decreased protein degradation rates and increased plasma branched chain amino acids, serum albumin, body weight, and midarm circumference. It is important to note that epidemiologic studies have shown that in MHD patients, lower predialysis serum bicarbonate and/or higher serum anion gap are associated with a paradoxically greater survival. This is considered to be due to the association of greater appetite and higher protein intake in healthier patients, leading to more acid generation during the interdialytic period.

The K/DOQI Clinical Practice Guidelines for both nutrition in chronic renal failure and bone disease recommend that serum bicarbonate levels should be measured once monthly in all patients on maintenance dialysis and that the predialysis or stabilized serum bicarbonate level should be maintained at or above 22 mmol/L. Because of the safety of giving bicarbonate and the potential advantages of completely eradicating acidemia, serum bicarbonate levels should be maintained in the 23–25 mEq/L range and arterial blood pH should be at 7.36 or higher. A similar recommendation concerning the threshold for treating low serum bicarbonate levels would seem appropriate for nondialyzed patients with any level of renal function.

Since in clinically stable CRI patients, the rate of acid production is usually normal or below normal, alkalinizing medicines are usually very effective for preventing or treating the acidemia. Hence, 35 mg of sodium bicarbonate tablets (4 mEq alkali) or Shohls solution or bicitra (1 mEq alkali/mL) may be given, eg, 650–1300 mg of sodium bicarbonate or citrate twice daily. If the nondialyzed chronically uremic patient is not oliguric and is not likely to develop edema, sodium is usually readily excreted when it is given as sodium bicarbonate or citrate. Since protein metabolism yields acidic products, a low protein diet (eg, 0.60 g protein/kg/day) will also reduce acid production and acidemia. Such a diet can be nutritious for nondialyzed stage 3, 4, and 5 CKD patients, but patients on maintenance dialysis will require more dietary protein (see above). Calcium carbonate may correct mild acidosis, provide needed calcium, and reduce intestinal phosphate absorption. However, the risk of soft tissue and particularly arterial calcification limits the amount of calcium that can be given to CKD patients (see above). However, the non-calcium-containing phosphate binder sevelamer hydrochloride may aggravate acidosis, although there is currently no evidence that this aspect of the medication may be harmful. If the acidosis is more severe, sodium bicarbonate or citrate may be administered intravenously. If acidemia is severe and not controlled by the foregoing measures, hemodialysis or peritoneal dialysis may be employed.

Chazot C, Kopple J: Vitamin metabolism in renal disease. In: *Nutritional Management of Renal Disease*, ed 2. Kopple J, Massry S (editors). Lippincott, Williams & Wilkins, 2004, pp 315–356.

Falkenhain ME et al: Nutritional management of water, sodium, potassium, chloride, and magnesium in renal disease and renal failure. In: *Nutritional Management of Renal Disease*, ed 2. Kopple J, Massry S (editors). Lippincott, Williams & Wilkins, 2004, pp 287–298.

Kalantar-Zadeh K, Kopple JD: Trace elements and vitamins in maintenance dialysis patients. Adv Ren Replace Ther 2003;10:170.

Kalantar-Zadeh K, Kopple J: Nutritional management of hemodialysis patients. In: *Nutritional Management of Renal Disease*, ed 2. Kopple J, Massry S (editors). Lippincott, Williams & Wilkins, 2004.

Moe SM: Calcium, phosphorus and vitamin D metabolism in renal disease and chronic renal failure. In: *Nutritional Management of Renal Disease*, ed 2. Kopple J, Massry S (editors). Lippincott, Williams & Wilkins, 2004, pp 41–62.

Vanholder R et al: Trace elements metabolism in renal failure. In: *Nutritional Management of Renal Disease*, ed 2. Kopple J, Massry S (editors). Lippincott, Williams & Wilkins, 2004, pp 299–314.

Wanner C: Altered lipid metabolism and serum lipid in renal disease and renal failure. In: *Nutritional Management of Renal Disease*, ed 2. Kopple J, Massry S (editors). Lippincott, Williams & Wilkins, 2004, pp 41–62.

▶ Treatment

A. Protein–Energy Malnutrition and Inflammation

There are four goals for the dietary treatment of CKD patients: (1) To maintain good nutritional status, (2) to reduce the risk of cardiovascular disease and to improve survival, (3) to prevent or ameliorate uremic toxicity and the metabolic disorders of renal failure, and (4) if possible, to retard the progression of renal failure. The latter two may appear to contradict the first two goals, since low protein intake is not infrequently recommended to slow the rate of progression of renal insufficiency. Dietary restrictions may remove important sources of antioxidant vitamins such as fresh fruits and vegetables, due to their rich potassium and phosphorus content; the consequences of such limitations are not yet known. Adherence to specialized diets is often a difficult and frustrating endeavor for patients and their families. Patients usually must make fundamental changes in their patterns of behavior. Often, the patients must procure special foods, prepare special recipes, forego or severely limit their intake of favorite foods, or eat foods that they may not like. Demands are made on the patient's time and daily activities and on the emotional support system of the family or close associates. Therefore, it is incumbent on the physician not to prescribe radical changes in the patient's diet unless there is good reason to believe that these modifications may be beneficial.

A number of different modalities have been employed to improve the nutritional or inflammatory status in patients on dialysis, as shown in Table 21–9. A recent study in animal models raises the possibility that protein–energy wasting may lead to inflammation. If this is confirmed in humans, dietary interventions may mitigate inflammation in CKD, as shown in several recent clinical trials in the general population.

Table 21–9. Classification of nutritional/antiinflammatory interventions in patients on dialysis.

1. Oral interventions
   Increasing food intake
   Oral supplements
2. Enteral interventions
   Tube feeding
3. Parenteral interventions
   IDPN
   Other parenteral interventions
4. Hormonal interventions
   Androgens
   Growth factors/hormones
5. Nonhormonal medications
   Antiinflammatory agents (see Table 21-10)
   Antioxidants (see Table 21-10)
   Appetite stimulators (see Table 21-11)
   Carnitine
   Bicarbonate
6. Dietary counseling
   Incenter supervision/counseling
7. Dialysis treatment related
   Dialysis dose and frequency
   Membrane compatibility

IDPN, intradialytic parenteral nutrition.

1. Nutritional supplements—Among more intensive interventions, *tube feeding* has been reported to be an effective modality, particularly in pediatric, elderly, or disabled individuals. However, according to some, this modality is a cumbersome option that cannot be used in the average (stable and functional) CKD outpatient. Experience with tube feeding in adults with CRI is still limited, probably because many patients and doctors are reluctant to use it.

Parenteral interventions such as intradialytic parenteral nutrition (IDPN) are quite costly and can be employed only during dialysis treatment. Several studies have examined the role of IDPN in improving nutritional status and outcomes in patients on dialysis, and have shown inconsistent results. The cost and strict regulatory criteria of IDPN might have restricted clinical access to these methods. Some retrospective analyses suggest that in patients on dialysis with protein–energy wasting, IDPN may reduce mortality. However, because of these reasons, enthusiasm for providing intensive nutrition modalities such as tube feeding and IDPN is currently limited.

Among simple interventions, *hormonal* medications may be associated with many side effects such as virilism or the potential for worsening atherosclerosis seen with androgens. However, some other medications, especially appetite stimulants and anti-inflammatory/antioxidant agents, show some promise (see below). Moreover, an increase in energy or protein intake without the concurrent provision of anti-inflammatory or antioxidant nutrients may not be optimally effective and an increased protein intake above 1.4 g/kg/day may be paradoxically associated with decreased survival in MHD patients (see Figure 21–4). Therefore, it is unlikely, although not impossible, to find one single medication to correct MICS. However, oral supplements, especially if they contain a combination of several nutritional and antiinflammatory agents, are practical and promising treatment modalities.

2. Anti-inflammatory and antioxidant modalities— Although epidemiologic evidence strongly links inflammation and oxidative stress to each other and to poor outcome in CKD patients, there have been only a few randomized trials that indicate an improvement in outcome with anti-inflammatory or antioxidant treatment. Other treatments (Table 21–10) have been proposed for reducing inflammation or oxidative stress in patients on dialysis but the data supporting the efficacy of these modalities are still inconclusive. One example is the administration of vitamin E, which may be associated with a decreased risk of cardiovascular mortality in patients on dialysis according to some but not all reports (see above).

Statins have been shown to decrease CRP levels irrespective of their effects on lipids, and may be associated with reduced mortality in patients on hemodialysis. However, the issue of worsening hypocholesterolemia in patients on hemodialysis as a result of statins is not resolved.

Table 21–10. Potential antiinflammatory and antioxidant agents for patients with chronic kidney disease.[1]

Antioxidant vitamins
Vitamin E
Vitamin C
Vitamin A/carotenoids
Other antioxidants
Eicosanoids (fish oil)
γ-Linolenic (borage oil)
Megestrol acetate
Pentoxifylline
Steroids/adrenocorticotropic hormone
Nonsteroidal antiinflammatory drugs
Anti-TNF-α agents
Thalidomide
HMG-CoA reductase inhibitors (statins)
Angiotensin-converting enzyme inhibitors
Erythropoietin
N-Acetylcysteine
Glitazones
Others: Dialysis technique

[1]TNF, tumor necrosis factor; HMG-CoA, 3-hydroxy-3-methylglutaryl coenzyme A.

ACE inhibitors may have anti-inflammatory properties both in the general population with diabetes or hypertension and in those with stage 2–5 CKD including patients on maintenance dialysis. However, many patients on dialysis who already receive these agents continue to have poor outcomes. Acetylcysteine may reduce adverse cardiovascular events in patients on maintenance dialysis. Glitazones are another group of drugs that has been shown to inhibit the activation of inflammatory response genes and promote an immune deviation away from T helper type 1 to T helper type 2 cytokine production. The optimization of dialysis treatment, ultrapure dialysate fluid, and more biocompatible dialysis membranes may improve the inflammatory status in patients on hemodialysis. However, the HEMO Study did not confirm such effects. As discussed above, it is possible that one single agent will not correct MICS, and a combination of nutritional, anti-inflammatory, and antioxidant interventions is needed to do so.

3. Correction of anorexia—It has been argued that CRI–associated anorexia is an integral component of the systemic inflammatory response as well as of other factors (see above). Anorexia can be induced by proinflammatory cytokines such as IL-6 and TNF-α and is correlated with all-cause and cardiovascular mortality in patients on dialysis. Consequently,

Table 21–11. Potential appetite stimulants (orexigenic agents) for patients with chronic kidney disease.

Steroids
   Glucosteroids
   Anabolic steroids
Megestrol acetate
Medroxyprogesterone
Cyproheptadine
Pentoxifylline
Dronabinol
Melanocortin blocker
Cannaboids

an exploration of the interaction between energy and protein-regulatory mechanisms and proinflammatory cytokines may lead to an effective treatment for MICS-associated anorexia.

Several appetite stimulants have been studied clinically (Table 21–11). Megestrol acetate (MA) is by far the most utilized and best-studied agent. MA, at a dose of 800 mg/day, has been shown to increase appetite and food intake in patients with anorexia due to cancer or AIDS. However, at this dose, it may be associated with side effects, including venous thrombosis, vaginal bleeding, altered liver function, and adrenal insufficiency. The pharmacokinetics of MA have not been evaluated in patients with renal impairment. In addition to improving appetite and food intake, MA has also been found to have significant anti-inflammatory properties (see Table 21–10). MA downregulates the synthesis and release of proinflammatory cytokines and relieves the symptoms of the anorexia–cachexia syndrome based on the modulation of cytokines. There are very few studies concerning MA in patients on dialysis. Our experience with a lower dose of MA (400 mg/day) has been encouraging.

Another potential orexigenic agent for CKD patients is pentoxifylline, which downregulates the local proinflammatory cytokine-mediated nitric oxide synthase pathway, inhibits TNF-α production, and decreases body weight loss and muscle protein wasting in acutely ill patients. There is indirect evidence that pentoxifylline may be an effective treatment for MICS and its clinical consequences including anorexia and erythropoietin resistance. Further research will be necessary to define the role for these agents as therapies for individuals with stage 3–5 CKD.

B. Nutritional Management of Renal Transplant Patients

Patients who undergo successful renal transplantation often develop normal or even supranormal appetite. Gain in body weight and fat is common. During the first year after transplantation, women may be particularly likely to increase dietary energy and protein intake and gain fat and lean body mass. Several nutritional disorders appear to be related to other factors associated with renal transplantation. These include obesity, insulin resistance and diabetes mellitus, impaired growth in children, protein wasting, altered serum lipid and homocysteine concentrations, and abnormalities in bone, mineral, and vitamin metabolism. Many of these complications are of particular concern because cardiovascular disease is the major cause of morbidity and mortality in renal transplant recipients. Indeed, unlike patients on dialysis, in whom obesity confers survival advantages (reverse epidemiology), obesity has been shown to have a strong association with increased mortality in transplanted patients, hence a so-called "reversal of the reverse epidemiology" is observed.

1. Lipids—Renal transplant patients often have increased serum triglyceride, VLDL triglyceride, small dense low-density lipoprotein (LDL) cholesterol, and total LDL cholesterol concentrations. HDL cholesterol is often low, and the LDL/HDL cholesterol ratio may be increased. Serum triglyceride levels correlate with the daily dose of prednisone, degree of obesity, and severity of renal insufficiency. These findings are of particular concern because several studies have found a correlation between increased serum lipids and the risk of cardiovascular disease, graft failure, and fatality in renal transplant recipients. Causes of increased serum triglycerides and cholesterol include excessive fat and energy intake, obesity, treatment with glucocorticoids, diuretics, calcinerin inhibitors or rapamycin, nephrotic-range proteinuria, and underlying diseases (eg, diabetes mellitus).

A low cholesterol, high fiber diet with a polyunsaturated:saturated fatty acid ratio greater than 1.0 may lower serum total cholesterol and LDL cholesterol levels in renal transplant recipients. However, the altered lipoprotein pattern may not be affected. A combination of a similar diet with regular exercise may improve the plasma lipid pattern. Fish oil providing 3 g/day of omega-3 fatty acids for 3 months decreased serum triglycerides and VLDL cholesterol in hyperlipidemic renal transplant recipients. However, the effects of diet on the improvement in the serum lipid pattern tend to be modest, and combining dietary therapy with serum 3-hydroxy-3-methylglutaryl coenzyme A (HMG-CoA) reductase inhibitors (statins) is generally far more effective in reducing serum total and LDL cholesterol.

The observation that a diet low in carbohydrates and modestly restricted in calories may reduce the cushingoid appearance suggests that such individuals may be given a low carbohydrate intake (1 g/kg/day), which is limited to 28–30 kcal/kg/day. If such a low carbohydrate, moderately restricted energy intake is employed in renal transplant recipients, it should be limited to short periods of time when the prednisone dosage is very high (eg, greater than 40 mg/day). This level of energy intake may not minimize the catabolic response during acute illness and may lead to further wasting. However, the higher protein intake with such diets (eg, 2 g protein/kg/day) may reduce protein malnutrition.

Also, given the abnormalities in lipid metabolism in renal transplant recipients, such a high fat diet should not be continued for long periods of time. In general, renal transplant patients should be encouraged to ingest a National Cholesterol Education Program TLC diet as described above for CKD patients. Patients should be encouraged to exercise regularly and to maintain a normal or desirable body weight. For transplant recipients with superimposed catabolic illnesses, 30–40 kcal/kg/day may be prescribed. Other maneuvers to correct abnormal serum lipids are as described for the nontransplant renal failure patient (see above). For renal transplant recipients with serum LDL cholesterol levels above about 70 mg/dL, the TLC diet should be supplemented with statins.

2. Hyperhomocysteinemia—In patients on maintenance dialysis who have had a successful kidney transplant, plasma homocysteine decreases but remains greater than in nontransplanted individuals with similar levels of renal function. The causes of hyperhomocysteinemia include reduced GFR, which appears to be the most important determinant, low serum folate levels, and possibly calcineurin inhibitor therapy. Folic acid may decrease plasma homocysteine levels in renal transplant recipients, and pyridoxine HCl, 50 mg/day, and vitamin B_{12}, 0.4 mg/day, may also be added to folic acid, 5 mg/day, to potentiate the treatment.

3. Vitamins after renal transplantation—Low serum folate levels were observed in transplant patients as long as 6 years after transplantation. Serum thiamine and vitamin B_{12} levels are generally normal in renal transplant patients. After successful renal transplantation, serum vitamin A often remains elevated for extended periods of time and may not fall to normal levels in some patients for several years.

4. Other nutritional issues—Calcineurin inhibitors (cyclosporine A and tacrolimus) as well as sirolimus may increase serum cholesterol, and cause potassium retention with hyperkalemia and urinary magnesium wasting with hypomagnesemia. Moreover, hypophosphatemia is relatively common during the first few months after successful renal transplantation and may occur because of a condition similar to hungry bone syndrome. Hence, judicious phosphorus and magnesium supplementation is imperative to avoid the deleterious effects of hypomagnesemia and hypophosphatemia, which can be profound. Low levels of zinc in plasma and hair and hyperzincuria have also been reported often within 12 months after successful renal transplantation. However, patients who have a functioning renal transplant for more than 12 months after the surgery usually have normal plasma, hair, and urine zinc and normal taste detection and recognition thresholds.

Foulks CJ: Intradialytic parenteral nutrition. In: *Nutritional Management of Renal Disease*, ed 2. Kopple J, Massry S (editors). Lippincott, Williams & Wilkins, 2004, pp 467–476.

Heimburger O et al: Nutritional effects and nutritional management of chronic peritoneal dialysis. In: *Nutritional Management of Renal Disease*, ed 2. Kopple J, Massry S (editors). Lippincott, Williams & Wilkins, 2004, pp 477–512.

Kalantar-Zadeh K et al: Malnutrition-inflammation complex syndrome in dialysis patients: causes and consequences. Am J Kidney Dis 2003;42:864.

Kasiske B et al: Clinical practice guidelines for managing dyslipidemias in kidney transplant patients: a report from the Managing Dyslipidemias in Chronic Kidney Disease Work Group of the National Kidney Foundation Kidney Disease Outcomes Quality Initiative. Am J Transplant 2004;4(Suppl 7):13.

Kasiske BL, Adeva-Andany M: Nutritional management of renal transplantation. In: *Nutritional Management of Renal Disease*, ed 2. Kopple J, Massry S (editors). Lippincott, Williams & Wilkins, 2004, pp 513–526.

Yamamoto S et al: The impact of obesity in renal transplantation: an analysis of paired cadaver kidneys. Clin Transplant 2002;16:252.

Slowing the Progression of Chronic Kidney Disease

22

Maarten W. Taal, MBChB, MD

ESSENTIALS OF DIAGNOSIS

▶ Estimated glomerular filtration rate (GFR) <60 mL/minute/1.73 m².

▶ Proteinuria or hematuria.

▶ Hypertension.

▶ Focal and segmental sclerosis and tubulointerstitial fibrosis on renal biopsy.

General Considerations

End-stage renal disease (ESRD) represents a major challenge to health care providers around the globe. It is estimated that in 2001 there were approximately 1.1 million people receiving dialysis worldwide and this number is projected to rise by 7% per year to over 2 million by 2010. The financial costs of dialysis provision are considerable and projected worldwide expenditure on dialysis treatment for the decade 2000–2010 is expected to exceed US$ 1 trillion. Whereas chronic dialysis does prolong life in ESRD, it is associated with an annual mortality of approximately 20%, representing a survival rate worse that many common forms of cancer. Renal transplantation does offer improved survival and quality of life, but the majority of patients are not medically suitable for transplantation and a universal shortage of donor organs continues to restrict the number of transplants performed.

Against this background it is critical to appreciate that the majority of cases of ESRD result from the slow progression of chronic kidney disease (CKD) over many months or years. There is therefore an opportunity to intervene in the course of CKD to slow the rate of decline in renal function and thereby reduce the number of patients requiring renal replacement therapy. In this chapter we review the mechanisms that contribute to CKD progression as well as clinical aspects and interventions that are effective in slowing the rate of decline in renal function.

Lysaght MJ: Maintenance dialysis population dynamics: current trends and long-term implications. J Am Soc Nephrol 2002;13: S37. [PMID: 11792760]

Pathogenesis

CKD should be viewed as a clinicopathologic syndrome (defined above) that ensues after renal injury resulting from a wide range of kidney pathologies. This suggests that the progressive decline in renal function that is characteristic of CKD results from a common set of mechanisms that is largely independent of the initiating renal pathology. Intensive research over the past three decades has identified several interacting mechanisms that together produce a vicious cycle of progressive nephron loss resulting in ESRD (Figure 22–1).

A. Glomerular Hemodynamic Factors

Studies in animal models of CKD reported that when the nephron number was severely reduced by surgical ablation, marked hemodynamic changes were observed in the remaining glomeruli, characterized by a substantial increase in the filtration rate of each glomerulus (single nephron glomerular filtration rate, SNGFR) that resulted in part from an increase in glomerular capillary hydraulic pressure (P_{gc}). Whereas these adaptations initially allowed partial compensation for nephron loss, further studies indicated that they were associated with structural injury to glomerular cells and subsequent glomerulosclerosis. In subsequent experiments, treatment with an angiotensin-converting enzyme inhibitor (ACEI) normalized P_{gc} without abrogating the adaptive increase in SNGFR and prevented glomerulosclerosis, suggesting that increased P_{gc} (also termed glomerular capillary hypertension) was the hemodynamic factor most likely responsible for glomerular injury. These observations suggested that adaptive hemodynamic changes in glomeruli after substantial nephron loss result in further glomerular damage and nephron loss, thereby establishing a vicious cycle of progressive renal injury.

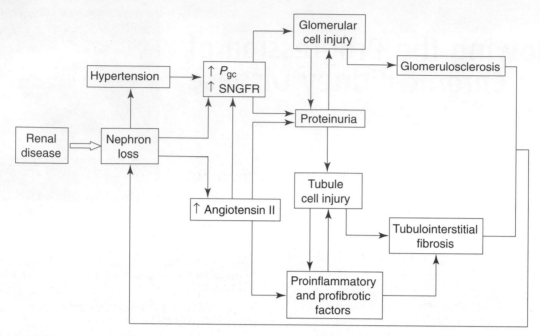

▲ **Figure 22–1.** The role of multiple interacting mechanisms that contribute to renal injury and establish a vicious cycle of progressive nephron loss.
P_{gc}, glomerular capillary hydraulic pressure; SNGFR, single nephron glomerular filtration rate.

B. Angiotensin II

Angiotensin II is a potent vasoconstrictor peptide that has been identified as an important mediator of the glomerular hemodynamic adaptations observed after nephron loss. Whereas systemic levels of angiotensin II are normal or decreased in CKD, experimental studies have confirmed that intrarenal angiotensin II levels are elevated. Additionally, recent research has identified multiple nonhemodynamic effects of angiotensin II that may contribute to progressive renal injury. These include effects on glomerular permeability resulting in exacerbation of proteinuria, plasminogen activator inhibitor-1 production by endothelial and vascular smooth muscle cells, mesangial cell proliferation and transforming growth factor (TGF)-β expression, macrophage activation, and adrenal production of aldosterone, recently identified as a mediator of renal fibrosis. Taken together, it is clear that angiotensin II plays a central role in the pathogenesis of progressive renal injury through multiple hemodynamic and nonhemodynamic mechanisms. Inhibition of the production or actions of angiotensin II therefore represents a single intervention that may abrogate many of these mechanisms and would be expected to be effective in slowing the progression of CKD.

C. Proteinuria

Proteinuria is usually a result of disordered permselectivity of the glomerular filtration barrier and is therefore the hallmark of glomerulopathy as well as a marker of disease severity. Additionally, research over the past decade has produced evidence that the presence of abnormal amounts of plasma proteins in glomerular ultrafiltrate may contribute directly to further renal damage. In the normal kidney small amounts of low-molecular-weight proteins are present in the tubular fluid and are reabsorbed by proximal tubule cells. *In vitro* experiments have found that culturing renal tubule cells in the presence of high concentrations of plasma proteins induces expression of a range of proinflammatory cytokines. Moreover, in animal models of renal disease this enhanced expression is evident on the basolateral aspect of tubule cells. It therefore seems likely that these proinflammatory molecules are secreted into the peritubular interstitium where they contribute to the development of interstitial inflammation and fibrosis. Thus, proteinuria provides a mechanistic link between glomerular and tubulointerstitial pathology. Further experimental evidence indicates that abnormally filtered plasma proteins also accumulate within podocytes where they may contribute to glomerular injury.

▶ Prevention

CKD results from a wide range of renal pathologies, many of which occur sporadically; it is therefore difficult to devise an effective strategy for primary prevention of CKD. One important exception to this principle, however, is diabetic nephropathy, the most common cause of CKD in many developed countries. In this case the "at-risk" population may be readily identified and at least two interventions have been shown to reduce the incidence of diabetic nephropathy. Following the landmark Diabetes Control and Complications Trial (DCCT) it became clear that the level of glycemic control is critical in determining the risk of microvascular complications, including nephropathy. Among patients in the intensive diabetic control group, significantly lower hemoglobin A_{1C} (HbA_{1C}) levels versus conventional therapy (7.2% versus 9.1%) were associated with a 34% reduction in the risk of developing microalbuminuria. Second, treatment with an ACEI may reduce the risk of developing microalbuminuria. One small study found some beneficial effect (absolute risk reduction of 12.5%) of ACEI treatment among normotensive, normoalbuminuric patients with type 2 diabetes and recently a large randomized trial (BENEDICT) that included 1204 patients with type 2 diabetes and hypertension reported a significantly lower incidence of microalbuminuria among patients treated with trandolapril (6.0%) or trandolapril plus verapamil (5.7%) versus those treated with verapamil (11.9%) or placebo (10%). Thus tight glycemic control (HbA_{1C} <7%) and treatment of hypertension with an ACEI should be regarded as essential interventions for preventing nephropathy in patients with diabetes.

For other forms of CKD the most critical factor for improving outcomes is early detection to allow intervention with measures that slow the rate of decline in renal function. Appropriate tests for CKD screening will vary according to circumstances and available resources. As most forms of CKD are associated with urinary abnormalities, the simplest form of detection is urinalysis with standard urinary dipsticks. Some forms of CKD may not cause urinary abnormalities and screening should therefore also include an estimate of renal function based on a measurement of serum creatinine. Diagnostic tests and further investigations are discussed in more detail below.

As CKD is relatively uncommon in the general population, it would be expensive and inefficient to screen entire populations. On the other hand, epidemiologic studies indicate that substantial numbers of patients have undiagnosed CKD. Focused screening of "at-risk" patients would therefore increase the detection of early stage CKD and facilitate early intervention to preserve renal function. Factors that place patients at risk for CKD vary in different countries, but general categories of patients who should be considered for screening are listed in Table 22–1. The optimal interval for screening remains to be determined but annual screening in high-risk groups is recommended.

Coresh J et al: Chronic kidney disease awareness, prevalence, and trends among U.S. adults, 1999 to 2000. J Am Soc Nephrol 2005;16:180. [PMID: 15563563]

Ruggenenti P et al: Preventing microalbuminuria in type 2 diabetes. N Engl J Med 2004;351:1941. [PMID: 15516697]

Table 22–1. Characteristics of patients for whom annual screening for chronic kidney disease (CKD) is recommended.

1. **Medical conditions associated with increased risk of developing CKD**
   Diabetes mellitus
   Hypertension
   Atherosclerotic vascular disease
   Cardiac failure

2. **Urologic conditions associated with increased risk of CKD**
   Bladder outlet obstruction or neurogenic bladder
   Renal calculi
   Urinary diversion surgery

3. **Multisystem disorders that may cause renal pathology**
   Systemic lupus erythematosis
   Vasculitis
   Rheumatoid arthritis
   Multiple myeloma
   Amyloidosis

4. **Chronic treatment with potentially nephrotoxic drugs**
   Nonsteroidal anti-inflammatory drugs and other analgesics
   Gold, penicillamine
   Calcineurin inhibitors
   Lithium carbonate
   Aminosalicylates

5. **First degree relatives of patients with CKD stage 3–5**
6. **Age >65 years**

▶ Clinical Findings

A. Symptoms and Signs

CKD is often asymptomatic until moderate to severe renal failure has developed. Nocturia due to a failure of urine-concentrating mechanisms may be an early symptom of CKD, but this is often attributed to prostatism and rarely prompts patients to seek medical attention. If severe proteinuria is present, peripheral edema may be the first symptom to develop. Patients with advanced renal failure may present with malaise, breathlessness, pruritis, loss of appetite, nausea, and vomiting.

Similarly, abnormal clinical signs are often lacking in patients with CKD. Hypertension is almost universally present and is often the first detectable sign. It is thus critical that all patients with newly diagnosed hypertension be screened for CKD. Peripheral edema may be present in patients with severe proteinuria or more advanced renal failure. Clinical pallor due to anemia may be observed in patients with CKD stage 3–5. Most (but not all) patients with CKD have urinary abnormalities detectable with standard dipstick testing. Proteinuria is the hallmark of CKD and may be accompanied by hematuria.

B. Laboratory Findings

Laboratory investigations are essential for the diagnosis of CKD. As discussed previously, the diagnosis rests on the detection of urinary abnormalities (usually proteinuria) and impaired renal function.

1. Assessment of proteinuria—The measurement of protein or albumin concentration in a 24-hour urine collection represents the most accurate method for assessment of proteinuria, but clinical utility is limited by inconvenience to patients and variable success in achieving a complete collection. Whereas protein or albumin concentration in a random urine specimen is of limited use due to variations in urine osmolality, the urine protein or albumin-to-creatinine ratio provides a reliable measure of proteinuria. Moreover, the urinary protein-to-creatinine ratio expressed in milligrams/milligram correlates closely with 24-hour urinary protein excretion expressed in grams/day and is thus convenient for patients as well as being easy to interpret. Some authorities prefer to use the albumin-to-creatinine ratio. Due to diurnal variations in the urinary protein excretion rate the assessment should be performed on an early morning specimen of urine.

2. Assessment of renal function—Determining the optimal method for the assessment of GFR depends upon finding a method with the best compromise between accuracy and reproducibility as well as patient convenience. Radioisotope clearance studies represent the most accurate method, but these require a hospital attendance of several hours as well as some radiation exposure and are therefore not suitable for serial monitoring of renal function. Creatinine clearance studies based on 24-hour urine collections were widely used until recently, but are inconvenient for patients and results may be significantly affected by undercollections or overcollections of urine. These difficulties prompted the development of a variety of formulas for estimating GFR based on serum creatinine concentration. Comparison with radioisotope clearance studies has shown that a four-variable equation [GFR = $1.86.3 \times (P_{cr}$ in mg/dL$)^{-1.154} \times$ (age)$^{-0.203} \times$ 1.212 (if black) $\times$ 0.742 (if female)] derived from the Modification of Diet in Renal Disease (MDRD) Study provides the most accurate estimate of GFR and is more accurate than creatinine clearance. Variations in the creatinine assays used by different laboratories have been overcome by the use of standardised assays and a modified MDRD formula. Many laboratories now report an estimated GFR with each creatinine result. It should be noted, however, that the MDRD formula was derived from the data of patients known to have CKD. It therefore tends to underestimate GFR in patients with normal serum creatinine values. Thus, patients with moderately reduced estimated GFR ($>$60 mL/minute/1.73 m^2) may not necessarily have CKD. On the other hand, normal estimated GFR does not necessarily exclude CKD as increases in single nephron GFR may compensate for nephron loss in the early stages. It is therefore critical that urinalysis remain a part of the screening process. Finally it should be noted that the four-variable equation does not account for body size and may not be reliable at extremes of body habitus. Further validation is required in ethnic groups other than African-American.

C. Special Examinations

Patients with CKD should be investigated to establish a specific diagnosis and to identify possible etiologic factors. This is important to facilitate the use of disease-specific therapies to limit the initial renal insult and reduce the risk of progressive renal injury. A detailed description of the diagnostic approach to specific renal diseases is beyond the scope of this chapter and is discussed in other sections of this book. Additionally, cardiovascular risk should be assessed with a fasting lipid profile and electrocardiograph.

▶ Complications

A progressive decline in renal function and the risk of developing ESRD are the obvious complications of CKD that form the focus of this chapter. It should be noted, however, that CKD is associated with a marked increase in the risk of cardiovascular disease that in many patients exceeds the risk of ESRD. Additional complications of CKD include anemia, renal osteodystrophy, and malnutrition.

▶ Treatment

A. Nonpharmacology

1. Modification of lifestyle—Patients with CKD should be encouraged to adopt a healthy lifestyle to reduce their cardiovascular risk. Whereas large randomized trials of lifestyle modification in CKD have not been conducted, there is evidence that some of the measures recommended may also slow the rate of CKD progression. If overweight, patients should be encouraged to lose weight as obesity per se is associated with glomerular hyperfiltration and proteinuria. Dietary salt should be restricted to assist with blood pressure control, particularly in patients prescribed an ACEI or angiotensin receptor blocker (ARB). Physical exercise should be encouraged and swimming in particular may reduce proteinuria. Smoking cessation is critical for cardiovascular risk reduction; in addition, there is growing evidence that smoking is associated with worse outcomes in diabetic and nondiabetic CKD.

2. Dietary protein restriction—The role of dietary protein restriction in renoprotective strategies remains controversial. Whereas experimental studies reported clear renoprotective benefits in animals assigned to a low protein diet, these findings have not been duplicated in humans. In the largest clinical trial to investigate this issue, the MDRD Study, the conclusion was to recommend protein restriction of 0.6 g/kg/day for patients with GFR $<$25 mL/minute/1.73 m^2. Two meta-analyses also support a role for dietary protein restriction. However, it is not clear whether these benefits accrue to patients who are already receiving optimal ACEI or ARB treatment and there are concerns regarding the risk of malnutrition. A recent consensus statement from the International Society of Nephrology recommends dietary protein restriction to 0.8 g/kg/day in all patients and consideration of further restriction to 0.6 g/kg/day if renal function continues to decline or proteinuria persists despite ACI or ARB treatment.

B. Pharmacology

1. Control of hypertension—The treatment of hypertension remains fundamental to therapeutic interventions for slowing the progression of CKD. Early clinical studies found that even modest reductions in blood pressure result in substantial attenuation of the rate of decline in renal function. These observations raise two important questions: What level of blood pressure control is required for optimal preservation of renal function? What antihypertensive drugs afford the most effective renoprotection?

A. LEVEL OF BLOOD PRESSURE CONTROL—It is increasingly being recognized that lower therapeutic goals for blood pressure reduction are associated with better outcomes with respect to cardiovascular disease. Two large prospective randomized studies have sought to examine this issue in patients with CKD but unfortunately have failed to provide clear answers. Despite the equivocal results of randomized studies, other evidence supports the notion that lower blood pressure targets are associated with slower rates of decline in GFR. Analysis of data from nine long-term clinical trials involving patients with diabetic and nondiabetic forms of CKD found lower rates of GFR decline among patients with lower blood pressure. The extent of consensus on this point is reflected by the fact that several professional bodies including the American Diabetes Association, National Kidney Foundation, Joint National Committee on Prevention, Detection and Treatment of High Blood Pressure, and the International Society of Nephrology now recommend that blood pressure should be lowered to <130/80 mm Hg in all patients with CKD. It should be noted that aggressive treatment of hypertension may be associated with an increased risk of hypotension in patients with autonomic neuropathy, labile blood pressure, or arteriosclerosis (resulting in decreased vascular compliance), all of which were excluded from the MDRD Study.

B. CHOICE OF ANTIHYPERTENSIVE DRUG—Whereas some studies, including the Antihypertensive and Lipid-Lowering Treatment to Prevent Heart Attack Trial (ALLHAT) study, have found no differences in outcomes between different classes of antihypertensive agents among hypertensive patients, other evidence shows that when the hypertension is associated with CKD, some drugs may produce specific benefits or adverse effects. As discussed in detail below, ACEIs and ARBs afford significant renoprotective benefit beyond that attributable to their antihypertensive effects and should

be regarded as first-line therapy in patients with CKD unless contraindicated. Diuretics are generally not effective as monotherapy in patients with renal failure, but may produce a substantial additional decrease in blood pressure if added to ACEI or ARB therapy. However, nondihydropyridine calcium channel blockers (CCB) may produce undesirable effects in patients with CKD. We therefore recommend that in patients with CKD, non-dihydropyridine CCB should be used only in combination with an ACEI or ARB.

2. Inhibition of the renin–angiotensin system—Several randomized prospective trials published over the past two decades have established a firm evidence base to support the use of ACEI or ARB therapy as the single most effective intervention for slowing the rate of progression of CKD.

A. DIABETIC NEPHROPATHY—Diabetic nephropathy is the most common underlying cause of end-stage renal failure in many developed countries and is projected to increase worldwide over the next two decades. This topic is comprehensively discussed in Chapter 54 and here we will review only specific aspects relevant to the treatment of CKD. Whereas the pathogenesis of diabetic nephropathy is similar in type 1 and type 2 diabetes, the populations affected by these two forms of diabetes are quite distinct and have different associated comorbidities. Therapeutic trials have therefore included either one or the other and are reviewed separately.

(1) Microalbuminuria—Microalbuminuria (urinary albumin excretion of 30–300 mg/day) represents the earliest manifestation of diabetic nephropathy and identifies patients at risk for developing overt nephropathy as well as a progressive decline in renal function. Among patients with type 1 diabetes, several small trials have shown benefits from treatment with an ACEI. A meta-analysis that combined the results of 12 such studies (689 patients) found that ACEI treatment was associated with a significant reduction in the risk of progression to overt nephropathy (odds ratio 0.38) and three times the incidence of complete normalization of the microalbuminuria. Among patients with type 2 diabetes, several studies have reported a reduction in microalbuminuria or a decrease in the number of patients progressing from microalbuminuria to overt nephropathy (risk reduction 24–67%) with ACEI treatment. Importantly, subgroup analysis in the HOPE Study also reported cardiovascular benefits associated with ACEI treatment. Among patients with type 2 diabetes treated with an ACEI, there was a 25% reduction in the combined primary endpoint of myocardial infarction, stroke, or cardiovascular death. However, one relatively large study found no renoprotective benefit of ACEI over β-blocker treatment among patients with hypertensive type 2 diabetes with normoalbuminuria or microalbuminuria.

Two studies have reported a clear benefit associated with ARB treatment of microalbuminuria in patients with type 2 diabetes. Among 590 patients randomized to irbesartan treatment (at 300 or 150 mg/day) versus placebo there was a significant, dose-dependent reduction in the incidence of overt proteinuria (5.2% versus 9.7% versus 14.9%). In a similar study 332 patients were randomized to treatment with valsartan or amlodipine and doses were adjusted to achieve equivalent blood pressure control. Valsartan treatment was associated with significantly lower levels of albuminuria and more patients receiving valsartan reverted to normoalbuminuria (29.9% versus 14.5%).

The benefits observed with ACEI or ARB treatment suggest that there may be additional benefit with combination ACEI and ARB therapy. In the candesartan and lisinopril microalbuminuria (CALM) study 199 hypertensive patients with type 2 diabetes with microalbuminuria were randomized first to ACEI or ARB therapy and then, after 12 weeks, to combination therapy or continued monotherapy. Whereas combination therapy afforded greater reductions in blood pressure and, to some extent, albuminuria than continued monotherapy, the study was only of 24 weeks duration and did not examine the relative incidence of overt nephropathy in different groups.

In summary, there is evidence that ACEI treatment decreases the risk of overt nephropathy associated with microalbuminuria in type 1 and 2 diabetes and that ARB treatment has a similar effect in type 2 diabetes. Importantly, the irbesartan study found a substantial dose-dependent effect and treatment should therefore be escalated to the maximum recommended dose. At present there are insufficient data to support the use of combination ACEI and ARB therapy in patients with microalbuminuria. Finally, the HOPE Study findings provide important evidence that ACEI treatment also reduces cardiovascular risk in patients with diabetes with microalbuminuria.

(2) Overt diabetic nephropathy—Evidence of the benefit of ACEI treatment in patients with type 1 diabetes and overt nephropathy was provided by a landmark study that was the first large trial to show renoprotection attributable to ACEI treatment in human CKD. Four hundred and nine patients with proteinuria >0.5 g/day and serum creatinine <2.5 mg/dL were randomized to either captopril or placebo treatment. Additional antihypertensive treatment was added as required to achieve a blood pressure goal of <140/90 mm Hg. After a median follow-up of 3 years, captopril treatment was associated with a 48% reduction in the risk of a doubling of serum creatinine and a 50% reduction in the incidence of the combined endpoint of death, dialysis, and renal transplantation. Blood pressure control was similar in the two groups, implying that the additional renoprotection was not due only to the antihypertensive effects of captopril.

Among patients with type 2 diabetes with overt nephropathy evidence for the use of ACEI treatment is less clear, with only one study reporting benefit. However, two large randomized studies have reported renoprotective effects with ARB therapy. In summary, available data provide good

evidence for renoprotective efficacy with ACEI treatment in patients with overt nephropathy and type 1 diabetes as well as ARB treatment in type 2 diabetes. There are currently no data from large long-term studies regarding the use of combination ACEI and ARB therapy in overt diabetic nephropathy.

B. NONDIABETIC CKD—The clear benefits of ACEI treatment in diabetic nephropathy prompted further trials to examine potential renoprotective effects in nondiabetic patients with CKD. In the REIN Study, 352 patients with nondiabetic CKD were randomized to treatment with ACEI, ramipril, or placebo. Other antihypertensive drugs were added to achieve a diastolic blood pressure of <90 mm Hg in both groups. Among patients with pretreatment proteinuria of ≥3 g/day, the study was stopped prematurely after an interim analysis found a significantly slower rate of decline in GFR in patients receiving ramipril (0.53 versus 0.88 mL/minute/month). Further analysis showed a significant reduction in the risk of the combined endpoint of a doubling of serum creatinine or ESRD in the ramipril group (risk ratio = 1.91 for the placebo group). Among patients with pretreatment proteinuria of 1–3 g/day, ramipril treatment also significantly reduced the incidence of ESRD (relative risk for placebo group = 2.72), particularly among those with a GFR of <45 mL/minute at baseline. Similarly in the AASK Study, African-American patients randomized to treatment with ramipril evidenced a lower incidence of the composite outcome (reduction in GFR by 50% or more, ESRD, or death) than those receiving amlodipine or metoprolol (risk reduction 38% and 22%, respectively). This is an important observation because ACEIs are often not prescribed in African-American patients due to decreased antihypertensive efficacy, a problem that can readily be overcome by combination with a diuretic. One randomised study has confirmed that ACEI treatment slows CKD progression even in patients with advanced CKD. The findings of these studies were confirmed by a meta-analysis of 11 studies of nondiabetic CKD that included 1860 patients. ACEI treatment was associated with greater reductions in blood pressure and proteinuria than other antihypertensive treatments, but even after statistical adjustment for these factors, ACEI treatment afforded a lower risk of reaching ESRD (relative risk = 0.69; CI 0.51–0.94). Few studies have examined the benefits of ACEI treatment in patients with a single form of nondiabetic CKD. In one such study of 44 patients with IgA nephropathy and >0.5 g/day of proteinuria, ACEI treatment was associated with a reduction in proteinuria and a significantly lower incidence of the primary endpoint, a 50% increase in serum creatinine concentration.

One large randomized study has examined the role of combination ACEI and ARB therapy in nondiabetic CKD. This trial was halted prematurely after an interim analysis revealed a substantial difference in outcomes, such that combination therapy was associated with significantly greater reductions in proteinuria (−75.6% versus −42.1% and −44.3%) and a lower incidence of the primary endpoint, doubling of serum creatinine or ESRD (hazard ratio 0.4 versus monotherapy groups). Close matching of blood pressure between the groups ensured that these benefits could be attributed specifically to combination therapy. There were no significant differences in outcomes between the monotherapy groups. Thus, although this study was not designed to compare ACEI and ARB monotherapy, it does provide some evidence that they provide similar renoprotection in nondiabetic CKD.

In summary, there is now clear evidence that ACEI treatment affords renoprotection in patients with nondiabetic CKD and proteinuria. There are no data from large randomized studies regarding ARB monotherapy in nondiabetic CKD, but the COOPERATE study results suggest that ARB treatment is associated with renoprotection similar to ACEI treatment. Finally, the COOPERATE Study reported significant additional renoprotection with combination ACEI and ARB therapy. Further studies are required to clarify the role of combination therapy, but pending these we recommend that it should be considered when therapeutic goals for blood pressure control or reduction of proteinuria are not achieved with monotherapy.

C. ANGIOTENSIN-CONVERTING ENZYME INHIBITORS VERSUS ANGIOTENSIN RECEPTOR BLOCKERS—Whereas ACEI and ARB both inhibit the renin–angiotensin system, they act on different elements of the system and may not necessarily produce equivalent therapeutic effects. ACEIs inhibit angiotensin-converting enzyme (ACE) and therefore block conversion of the inactive peptide angiotensin I to the potent vasoconstrictor angiotensin II. Additionally, ACE catalyzes the breakdown of bradykinin and thus ACEI treatment is associated with elevated bradykinin levels that may mediate some of its effects. However, ARBs bind to and inhibit the angiotensin subtype 1 receptor. Loss of feedback inhibition results in elevated angiotensin II levels that may exert effects via other subtypes of angiotensin receptor. Despite these considerations, experimental studies of CKD have generally found no differences in the efficacy of ACEI versus ARB treatment. Few clinical trials have directly compared the renoprotective effects of ACEI and ARB in CKD patients. Nevertheless, available data suggest that ACEI and ARB treatments probably do afford similar renoprotection.

Randomized trials have shown ACEI treatment to be renoprotective in type 1 diabetes with microalbuminuria or overt nephropathy and type 2 diabetes with microalbuminuria as well as in nondiabetic CKD. However, ARB treatment has proven renoprotective effects in type 2 diabetes with microalbuminuria or overt nephropathy. Despite the lack of specific data, an ARB should be considered as alternative therapy in patients who are ACEI intolerant, most often due to a cough that may affect up to 20%.

D. DIRECT RENIN INHIBITORS—Direct renin inhibitors (DRI) represent novel treatments for inhibiting the RAS. One randomised trial of aliskerin, the first DRI in clinical use, reported additional albuminuria reduction when aliskerin was combined with ARB therapy in patients with type 2 diabetes and diabetic nephropathy.

E. SAFETY CONSIDERATIONS—Despite the proven renoprotective benefits of ACEI and ARB treatment, some physicians remain reluctant to prescribe them in patients with CKD due to concerns about their potential adverse effects in patients with renal failure. The two principal areas of concern are hyperkalemia and exacerbation of renal failure, but the risk of each can be minimized by the application of simple precautions.

(1) Hyperkalemia—In large randomized trials of ACEI or ARB treatment in CKD, the risk of hyperkalemia is reported to be low and resulted in discontinuation of therapy in only 0–4% of patients. A higher risk can be anticipated in patients with more advanced renal failure and in diabetic nephropathy. The mainstay of prevention is comprehensive counseling to reduce dietary potassium intake and avoidance of potassium supplements as well as potassium-sparing diuretics. Serum potassium should be measured prior to initiation of therapy and again 3–5 days after the first dose as well as after any dose increase.

(2) Exacerbation of renal failure—As discussed above, ACEI and ARB treatment results in lowering of glomerular capillary hydraulic pressure and can therefore be expected to produce an initial reduction in GFR, evidenced by a rise in serum creatinine. Analysis of data from 12 randomized trials found that, paradoxically, the extent of the reduction in renal function associated with the initiation of ACEI treatment was inversely correlated with the subsequent rate of decline in renal function over time. Thus an initial increase in serum creatinine should not prompt the discontinuation of ACEI or ARB treatment, provided the increase is not progressive and is less than 30% over the first 2 months. We recommend that serum creatinine should be monitored 3–5 days after initiation of ACEI treatment and after each dose increase. Additional measures that may reduce the risk of a decline in renal function include ensuring adequate hydration, omitting or reducing diuretic treatment for 1 or 2 days prior to starting the ACEI or ARB, avoidance of nonsteroidal anti-inflammatory drugs, and starting ACEI or ARB treatment at a low dose. ACEI and ARB treatments are contraindicated in patients with bilateral renal artery stenosis and should be used with caution in patients with extensive vascular disease who may have undiagnosed renovascular disease.

3. Reduction of proteinuria—Evidence that abnormal urinary excretion of protein may contribute directly to progressive renal injury has focused attention on the relationship between renal outcomes and proteinuria. It has been recognized for many years that the extent of proteinuria is a marker of disease severity and in several studies, baseline proteinuria showed a positive correlation with the subsequent

rate of decline in GFR. Recent analyses have found that residual proteinuria on therapy is also a powerful predictor of outcomes. The importance of residual proteinuria has been confirmed by a meta-analysis of data from 1860 patients with nondiabetic CKD that found a 5.56-fold increase in the risk of reaching a combined endpoint of doubling of serum creatinine or onset of ESRD for each 1.0 g/day increase in extent of proteinuria after initiation of treatment. One randomised trial has confirmed that titrating ACEI or ARB treatment to the maximum antiproteinuric dose affords greater renoprotection than standard doses. Thus proteinuria is regarded as an independent, modifiable risk factor for CKD progression and a clinically useful surrogate marker of the success of renoprotective interventions. Moreover, albuminuria is also predictive of cardiovascular risk and in the RENAAL Study each 50% reduction in albuminuria over the first 6 months was associated with an 18% reduction in cardiovascular risk as well as a 27% reduction in the risk of heart failure. Based on these data we recommend that treatment with ACEI or ARB should be escalated until proteinuria is reduced to <1 g/day and combination ACEI and ARB therapy should be considered if this goal is not achieved. Even lower proteinuria goals of <0.3 g/day have been recommended, but data regarding the optimal target for proteinuria reduction are currently lacking.

4. Treatment of dyslipemia—Dyslipemia characterized

by elevated triglyceride-rich lipoproteins and reduced high-density lipoprotein (HDL) cholesterol is commonly associated with CKD and probably contributes to the attendant increased cardiovascular risk. Moreover, experimental evidence suggests that lipid abnormalities may also contribute to progressive renal injury. In several animal models, treatment of hyperlipidemia has been associated with attenuation of CKD progression. To date only small prospective studies have been conducted in humans. A meta-analysis of 13 such studies reported a significantly slower rate of GFR decline among CKD patients receiving lipid-lowering therapy. Several large randomized trials are underway to test the hypothesis that treatment of dyslipemias contributes to renoprotection and results should be available within 2–3 years. Until these data are published it is possible to recommend active treatment of dyslipemias on the basis of cardiovascular risk alone. It should be noted that standard cardiovascular risk estimates probably underestimate the risk in CKD patients, who were excluded from the studies used to derive the estimates. Thresholds and targets for treatment as well as the relative efficacy of different drugs all remain to be determined. The Kidney Disease Outcome Quality Initiative (K/DOQI) Guidelines currently recommend that patients with CKD stage 1–4 should be considered to be in the highest cardiovascular risk group and managed according to guidelines published by the National Cholesterol Education Program. Low-density lipoprotein (LDL) cholesterol should be reduced to <100 mg/dL and

additional treatment should be considered if triglyceride levels are >200 mg/dL.

5. Treatment of Anemia—Anemia due to decreased renal

production of erythropoietin is a common complication of CKD and may have a major impact on patients' quality of life. Replacement therapy with recombinant human erythropoietin allows correction of the anemia and results in improvement in quality of life as well as a decrease in hospital admissions. Additionally, correction of anemia may contribute to slowing the rate of GFR decline in CKD. Analysis of data from the RENAAL Study found that baseline hemoglobin was a significant predictor of the subsequent development of ESRD such that each 1 g/dL decrease in hemoglobin was associated with an 11% increase in the risk of ESRD. Moreover, one randomized study that included 88 patients with nondiabetic CKD has shown that early treatment (started when hemoglobin <11.6 g/dL) with erythropoietin alpha was associated with a 60% reduction in the risk of doubling serum creatinine, ESRD, or death versus delayed treatment (started when hemoglobin <9.0 g/dL). It should be noted, however, that ACEI and ARB treatments were discontinued prior to entry into this trial and it is therefore not clear whether these benefits would occur in patients receiving ACEIs or ARBs. On the other hand, the CREATE trial reported more rapid progression to ESRD among CKD patients receiving erythropoietin treatment and randomised to a target haemoglobin of 13.0–15.0 g/dL versus those randomised to a target haemoglobin of 10.5–11.5 g/dL. There are insufficient data available at present to allow recommendations regarding thresholds for treatment or therapeutic goals. K/DOQI currently recommends treatment to achieve a hemoglobin of 11.0–12.0 g/dL in CKD patients not requiring dialysis.

6. Glycemic control—As discussed above, there is good evi-

dence that tight glycemic control reduces the risk of developing microalbuminuria in patients with type 1 and type 2 diabetes. Among patients who already have microalbuminuria data are conflicting with some but not all studies reporting a lower risk of progression to proteinuria in patients with better glycemic control. In patients with established diabetic nephropathy there are no data regarding the effect of glycemic control. Nevertheless, a study that found regression of early diabetic nephropathy lesions after pancreatic transplantation suggests that improved glycemic control does confer renoprotective benefit. Moreover, patients with diabetes with nephropathy remain at risk for other microvascular complications and tight glycemic control (HbA$_{1C}$ <7%) should therefore remain a treatment goal. It should be noted however that in some patients, attempts to achieve tight glycemic control may be associated with adverse consequences. In the ACCORD trial patients with type 2 diabetes randomised to a low target HBA$_{1C}$ of <6.0% evidenced increased mortality.

ACCORD Study Group. Effects of intensive glucose lowering in type 2 diabetes. N Engl J Med 2008;358:2545–59.

Barnett AH et al: Angiotensin-receptor blockade versus converting-enzyme inhibition in type 2 diabetes and nephropathy. N Engl J Med 2004;351:1952. [PMID: 15516696]

Coordinators for the ALLHAT Collaborative Research Group: Major outcomes in high-risk hypertensive patients randomized to angiotensin-converting enzyme inhibitor or calcium channel blocker vs diuretic: The Antihypertensive and Lipid-Lowering Treatment to Prevent Heart Attack Trial (ALLHAT). JAMA 2002;288:2981. [PMID: 12479763]

de Zeeuw D et al: Proteinuria, a target for renoprotection in patients with type 2 diabetic nephropathy: lessons from RENAAL. Kidney Int 2004;65:2309. [PMID: 15149345]

de Zeeuw D et al: Albuminuria, a therapeutic target for cardiovascular protection in type 2 diabetic patients with nephropathy. Circulation 2004;110:921. [PMID: 15302780]

Drüeke TB et al: Normalization of hemoglobin level in patients with chronic kidney disease and anemia. N Engl J Med 2006;355:2071–84.

Gouva C et al: Treating anemia early in renal failure patients slows the decline of renal function: a randomized controlled trial. Kidney Int 2004;66:753. [PMID: 15253730]

Hou FF, Xie D, Zhang X et al: Renoprotection of optimal antiproteinuric doses (ROAD) study: a randomized controlled study of benazepril and losartan in chronic renal insufficiency. J Am Soc Nephrol. 2007; 18:1889–1898.

Hou FF, Zhang X, Zhang GH et al: Efficacy and safety of benazepril for advanced chronic renal insufficiency. N Eng J Med 2006; 354:131–140.

Jones M et al: Impact of epoetin-alfa on clinical end points in patients with chronic renal failure: a meta-analysis. Kidney Int 2004;65:757. [PMID: 14871396]

Li PK et al: A report with consensus statements of the International Society of Nephrology 2004 Consensus Workshop on Prevention of Progression of Renal Disease, Hong Kong, June 29, 2004. Kidney Int Suppl 2005;94:S2. [PMID: 15752234]

Mohanram A et al: Anemia and end-stage renal disease in patients with type 2 diabetes and nephropathy. Kidney Int 2004;66:1131. [PMID: 15327408]

Nakao N et al: Combination treatment of angiotensin-II receptor blocker and angiotensin-converting-enzyme inhibitor in nondiabetic renal disease (COOPERATE): a randomised controlled trial. Lancet 2003;361:117. [PMID: 12531578]

Parving HH et al: Aliskiren combined with losartan in type 2 diabetes and nephropathy. N Engl J Med 2008; 358:2433–2446.

Pechter U et al: Regular low-intensity aquatic exercise improves cardio-respiratory functional capacity and reduces proteinuria in chronic renal failure patients (letter). Nephrol Dial Transplant 2003;18:624. [PMID: 12584298]

Praga M et al: Treatment of IgA nephropathy with ACE inhibitors: a randomized and controlled trial. J Am Soc Nephrol 2003;14:1578. [PMID: 12761258]

Ruggenenti P et al: Retarding progression of chronic renal disease: The neglected issue of residual proteinuria. Kidney Int 2003;63:2254. [PMID: 12753315]

Viberti G, Wheeldon NM: Microalbuminuria reduction with valsartan in patients with type 2 diabetes mellitus: a blood pressure-independent effect. Circulation 2002;106:672. [PMID: 12163426]

Wright JT Jr et al: Effect of blood pressure lowering and antihypertensive drug class on progression of hypertensive kidney disease: results from the AASK trial. JAMA 2002;288:2421. [PMID: 12435255]

▶ Prognosis

Clinical trials have identified several interventions that are effective in slowing the rate of GFR decline in CKD. Whereas each affords benefit, none is able to arrest progression of CKD in the majority of patients. Thus, many will still progress to ESRD, albeit at a slower rate. Factors shown to be predictive of a worse prognosis include severity of proteinuria, serum creatinine, serum albumin, and hemoglobin. In light of these data it seems logical to combine effective interventions directed at different aspects of CKD progression into a comprehensive strategy for maximizing renoprotection. One study has shown that application of intensive combination therapy in patients with type 2 diabetes and microalbuminuria was associated with a 53% reduction in risk of cardiovascular disease and an approximately 60% reduction in risk of microvascular complications. Additionally, it is helpful to apply the concept of "remission" to CKD such that treatment is escalated until the major manifestations of CKD have been brought under control. The interventions that comprise such a strategy and therapeutic goals that define remission are summarized in Table 22–2. It should be noted that the

Table 22–2. Interventions and therapeutic goals for a comprehensive strategy to maximize renoprotection in patients with chronic kidney disease.

Intervention	Therapeutic goal
1. ACEI or ARB treatment[2]	Proteinuria <1.0 g/day
2. Additional antihypertensive therapy[1]	BP <130/80 mm Hg
3. Dietary protein restriction	0.8 g/kg/day
4. Tight glycemic control	HbA$_{1c}$ <7%
5. Lipid lowering therapy	LDL cholesterol <100 mg/dL
6. Treatment of anemia	11.0–12.0 g/dL
7. Lifestyle modification	Smoking cessation, weight loss

[1]Consider combination therapy if goals are not achieved with monotherapy.
ACEI, angiotensin-converting enzyme inhibitor; ARB, angiotensin receptor blocker; BP, blood pressure; HbA$_{1c}$, hemoglobin A$_{1c}$; LDL, low-density lipoprotein.

treatments and tests required for monitoring are relatively inexpensive and are widely available. Application of this approach should therefore be possible across a wide range of healthcare systems and may substantially reduce the number of patients dependent on renal replacement therapy worldwide. Achieving this goal is arguably the greatest challenge facing nephrologists today.

Gaede P et al: Multifactorial intervention and cardiovascular disease in patients with type 2 diabetes. N Engl J Med 2003;348:383. [PMID: 12556541]

Keane WF et al: The risk of developing end-stage renal disease in patients with type 2 diabetes and nephropathy: the RENAAL study. Kidney Int 2003;63:1499. [PMID: 12631367]

WEB SITES

Kidney Disease Improving Global Outcomes: www.kdigo.org. Provides links to several major national and international treatment guidelines.

National Kidney Foundation: www.kidney.org/professionals/kdoqi/ guidelines. Provides access to all K/DOQI treatment guidelines as well as updates. The Web site also offers online calculation of estimated GFR and CKD stage-specific treatment plans. Many features are available for downloading.

Nephrotic Syndrome versus Nephritic Syndrome

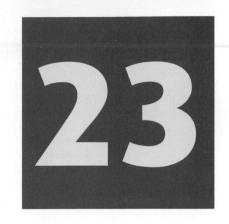

Isaac Teitelbaum, MD, & Laura Kooienga, MD

Glomerulonephropathies are disorders that primarily affect the structure and function of the renal glomerular apparatus. Frequently encountered in clinical practice, glomerulopathies are usually suspected from the history and the urinary findings of hematuria, red cell casts, or proteinuria. The many different causes of glomerular disease can be generally classified into one of three major syndromes: Nephrotic syndrome, nephritic syndrome, and asymptomatic renal disease. However, there may be considerable overlap in their clinical presentation with some diseases presenting with components of both syndromes.

NEPHROTIC SYNDROME

 ESSENTIALS OF DIAGNOSIS

▶ Proteinuria >3.5 g/1.73 m²/24 hours (40–50 mg/kg/day).
▶ Hypoalbuminemia.
▶ Edema.
▶ Hyperlipidemia.
▶ Lipiduria.

▶ General Considerations

Nephrotic syndrome may appear as a primary (idiopathic) renal disease or occur in association with any of a number of systemic conditions and hereditary diseases. The most common primary glomerular diseases include membranous nephropathy, focal segmental glomerular sclerosis, minimal change, and membranoproliferative glomerulonephritis (MPGN). In the United States, diabetes mellitus is the most common cause of nephrotic syndrome. Approximately one-third of patients with both type 1 and type 2 diabetes mellitus of at least a 25-year duration will develop nephrotic syndrome, predictably leading to renal failure. Other systemic diseases that may lead to the nephrotic syndrome include systemic lupus erythematous (SLE), amyloidosis, and leukemia.

▶ Pathogenesis

Nephrotic syndrome generally reflects noninflammatory damage to the glomerular capillary wall. The underlying glomerular disease results in proteinuria, which occurs from alterations in the charge or size selectivity of the glomerular capillary wall. This increases glomerular permeability to plasma proteins. Albumin is the principal urinary protein lost, but other plasma proteins lost in the urine include hormone-carrying proteins such as vitamin D-binding protein, transferrin, and clotting inhibitors.

▶ Prevention

We do not know how to prevent primary nephrotic syndrome. Secondary nephrotic syndromes can often be improved and sometimes completely reversed by treating and controlling the underlying disease.

▶ Clinical Findings

A. Symptoms and Signs

Nephrotic syndrome can present with a spectrum of findings ranging from asymptomatic proteinuria to the most common presentation of edema. Edema occurs initially in areas of high intravascular hydrostatic pressure such as in the feet and ankles as well as in areas in which tissue hydrostatic pressure is lowest such as the periorbital and scrotal areas. If the edema is severe and generalized it can present as anasarca.

B. Laboratory Findings

1. Urinalysis—Urine dipstick often demonstrates 3+ to 4+ protein and 24-hour urine collection with >3.5 g protein/1.73 m². Proteinuria can also be estimated from a single urine specimen by calculating the ratio of total urine protein in mg/dL to urine creatinine in mg/dL. This ratio approximates the actual 24-hour protein excretion in grams per day per 1.73 m² body surface area. Typically the urine sediment has few cells or casts. Urinary lipid may be present in the sediment. It may be entrapped in casts, free in the urine, or enclosed in the plasma membrane of degenerated epithelial cells known as oval fat bodies. Under polarized light, the lipid in oval fat bodies appears as "Maltese crosses" (Figure 23–1).

2. Blood chemistries—Fundamental laboratory abnormalities in nephrotic syndrome include decreased serum albumin (<3 g/dL), decreased total serum protein (<6 g/dL), and hyperlipidemia. Patients may have elevations in their blood urea nitrogen (BUN) and creatinine, but the glomerular filtration rate (GFR) can be normal. Some patients may also manifest anemia, elevated erythrocyte sedimentation rate (ESR), hypocalcemia, and vitamin D deficiency. Other less common laboratory tests may be indicated depending on the patient's clinical presentation. These may include serum protein electrophoresis (SPEP) and urine protein electrophoresis (UPEP) to evaluate for myeloma or amyloidosis, and antinuclear antibody (ANA) to evaluate for SLE. Other tests might include hepatitis serologies, syphilis serology, HIV, complements, cryoglobulins, and thyroid function tests.

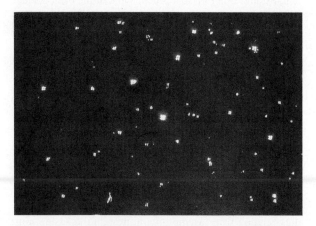

▲ **Figure 23–1.** Polarized anisotropic fat droplets. Note the "Maltese-cross" formation. (Reproduced with permission from Graff L: *A Handbook of Routine Urinalysis.* J.B. Lippincott Company, 1983.)

C. Special Tests

Indications for and benefits of a renal biopsy remain controversial. Nevertheless, it is the standard procedure for determining the cause of proteinuria in adults. Biopsy is often recommended when the etiology of nephrotic-range proteinuria is in doubt, prior to beginning cytotoxic drugs, when the presence of multiple diseases contributing to the clinical picture confounds the diagnosis, or if the patient's clinical course differs from the expected. In general, renal biopsy may be used to aid in management decisions, for example, whether to discontinue therapy because of lack of salvageable renal parenchyma.

▶ Differential Diagnosis

The differential diagnosis in nephrotic syndrome can be narrowed significantly based on the patient's age, race, and urine evaluation. For example, minimal change accounts for the majority of cases in children. In adults worldwide, membranous nephropathy and focal glomerulosclerosis are among the commonest causes of primary nephrotic syndrome. In adults over the age of 50 years, membranous nephropathy is the most common cause of idiopathic nephrotic syndrome while focal glomerulosclerosis is the most common cause in African-Americans. Overall, about 50% of patients with nephrotic syndrome have a secondary cause, with the majority of these being secondary to diabetic nephropathy.

▶ Complications

A. Hyperlipidemia

Numerous alterations in lipid profiles occur in the nephrotic syndrome as a result of increased synthesis and decreased catabolism of individual lipid fractions. These include hypercholesterolemia, hypertriglyceridemia, and increased low-density protein (LDL) and very low-density protein (VLDL). These abnormalities may possibly contribute to accelerated atherosclerosis.

B. Thrombosis

Several abnormalities of the coagulation system occur in nephrotic syndrome. These abnormalities include urinary losses of antithrombin III, proteins C and S, and factors IX, XI, and XII. In addition, plasma fibrinogen, tissue plasminogen activator, and platelet aggregability are all increased. These aberrations lead to an increased incidence of venous and arterial thromboemboli, especially deep venous thrombosis, pulmonary embolism, and renal vein thrombosis. Renal vein thrombosis is most common in membranous nephropathy, with as many as 20–40% of patients affected.

C. Vitamin D Deficiency and Hypocalcemia

Vitamin D-binding protein is a relatively small protein (59 kDa) that is readily filtered and hence lost in the urine. 25-Hydroxyvitamin D, which is bound to vitamin D-binding protein, is also lost in the urine in nephrotic syndrome.

D. Infection

Patients with nephrotic syndrome have urinary losses of immunoglobulins and defects in the complement cascade. This results in a higher susceptibility to infection, especially with encapsulated organisms such as *Streptococcus pneumoniae*. In addition, the immunosuppressive medications often used to treat the underlying glomerulopathy contribute to the increased risk of infection in these patients.

E. Hypoalbuminemia

Serum levels of albumin are low in hypoalbuminemia secondary to both losses in the urine and increased albumin catabolism.

F. Malnutrition

Prolonged and massive proteinuria may culminate in malnutrition as a result of negative nitrogen balance with loss of lean body mass.

G. Anemia

Urinary losses of erythropoietin (30 kDa) and transferrin may lead to an iron-resistant microcytic hypochromic anemia. If renal function deteriorates to the point of chronic kidney disease decreased erythropoietin production may play a role as well.

▶ Treatment

A. Underlying Systemic or Renal Disease Immunosuppressive Medications

Medications such as corticosteroids may be used for diseases such as minimal change disease and focal glomerular sclerosis. Other treatments may consist of antimicrobial agents such as those for the treatment of secondary syphilis, chemotherapy or tumor resection for nephrotic syndrome associated with malignancy, or simply discontinuing an offending medication such as nonsteroidal anti-inflammatory drugs (NSAIDs) or phenytoin.

B. Complications of the Nephrotic Syndrome

1. Hyperlipidemia—Premature atherosclerosis and anincreased incidence of myocardial infarction have been reported in patients with the nephrotic syndrome. In addition, hyperlipidemia is likely a separate risk factor for both atherosclerotic cardiovascular disease as well as for the progression of renal disease. Hyperlipidemia typically improves after the resolution of the nephrotic syndrome. All lipid-lowering medications have been used in nephrotic syndrome to help reduce the rate of adverse coronary events. The most potent agents are the 3-hydroxy-3-methylglutaryl coenzyme A (HMG-CoA) reductase inhibitors alone or in combination with bile acid sequestrants such as cholestyramine.

2. Edema—Nephrotic syndrome results in primary renal sodium retention. This may result in peripheral and periorbital edema and, if severe and generalized enough, may result in anasarca with serous effusions. Goals of treatment include salt restriction and use of loop diuretics to achieve slow resolution of edema; rapid diuresis can result in hypovolemia and hypotension. Occasionally, thiazide diuretics must be added to the loop diuretics in order to block sodium reabsorption at multiple sites in the nephron.

3. Thrombosis—Anticoagulation is indicated in patients with nephrotic syndrome and documented thrombotic events. Anticoagulation is usually continued until the patient experiences resolution of the nephrotic syndrome. Prophylactic anticoagulation and antiplatelet therapy in patients with nephrotic syndrome remain controversial. However, in patients with idiopathic membranous nephropathy the benefits of anticoagulation may outweigh the risks.

4. Treatment of proteinuria

A. ANGIOTENSIN-CONVERTING ENZYME INHIBITORS (ACEI) AND ANGIOTENSIN II RECEPTOR BLOCKERS (ARB)—These agents work by lowering intraglomerular capillary hydrostatic pressure and preventing the development of hemodynamically mediated focal segmental glomerulosclerosis. ARBs also decrease the formation of tumor growth factor (TGF)-β 1, which has been shown to play a role in progressive renal fibrosis.

B. NSAIDs—NSAIDs probably work by altering glomerular hemodynamics or glomerular basement membrane permeability, but their benefits must be balanced against the risk of inducing acute renal failure, salt and water retention, and hyperkalemia.

C. Low protein diet—A low-fat soy-protein diet that provides 0.7 g protein/kg/day has been demonstrated to be beneficial in decreasing urinary protein excretion and lipid profiles. However, protein-restricted diets in general may lead to malnutrition, which is a known potent predictor for death in end-stage renal disease (ESRD) patients.

Prognosis

The prognosis in nephrotic syndrome is typically worse in patients with heavy proteinuria, renal insufficiency, and severe hypertension. The overall prognosis depends on etiology and is related to histology. For example, minimal change disease can have spontaneous remissions and is highly steroid responsive with an excellent prognosis. In contrast, spontaneous remission of primary focal segmental glomerulosclerosis (FSGS) is rare and the renal prognosis is relatively poor.

NEPHRITIC SYNDROME

ESSENTIALS OF DIAGNOSIS

- ▶ Hematuria.
- ▶ Red blood cell (RBC) casts.
- ▶ Variable proteinuria.
- ▶ Renal insufficiency.
- ▶ Salt retention [hypertensive nephropathy (HTN) and edema].

General Considerations

Glomerulonephritis is characterized by an intraglomerular inflammatory process and renal dysfunction. It can be acute, subacute, or chronic and may or may not progress to ESRD. The nephritic syndrome may be caused by an intrinsic renal disease or may be part of a systemic disease process. Classic causes of the nephritic syndrome include postinfectious glomerulonephritis, immunoglobulin A (IgA) nephropathy, and lupus nephritis. IgA is the most common cause of glomerulonephritis worldwide. A subset of acute glomerulonephritis, known as rapidly progressive glomerulonephritis (RPGN), can present with severe and progressive renal failure. Examples of RPGNs include Goodpasture's disease, polyarteritis nodosum, and Wegener's granulomatosis.

Pathogenesis

The nephritic syndrome is characterized by an inflammatory process. The degree of glomerular inflammation in part determines the severity of renal dysfunction and associated clinical manifestations. Immunologic perturbations underlie many of the glomerulopathies. Two basic mechanisms of antibody-mediated glomerular injury exist. The first involves antibodies that bind to a structural component or other material implanted in the glomeruli. For example, circulating antibodies may form and be directed against the glomerular basement membrane (GBM) as in Goodpasture's disease. The second mechanism involves formation of circulating antigen--antibody complexes that escape the reticuloendothelial system and are then deposited in the glomerulus. Examples include DNA-nucleosome complexes in SLE and cryoglobulins in hepatitis C-related MPGN.

Other diseases, such as poststreptococcal glomerulonephritis, involve deposition of an antigen in the glomeruli with subsequent activation of complement. This can result in direct tissue injury or result in an inflammatory reaction, with proliferation of the intrinsic glomerular cells such as the mesangial, endothelial, and epithelial cells. In severe cases, obliteration of the glomerular capillary lumens can occur in addition to rupture of the glomerulus into Bowman's space resulting in crescent formation.

Prevention

It is not yet known how to guard against intrinsic renal diseases or systemic diseases that cause the nephritic syndrome such as IgA nephropathy or SLE. Hence, the focus in this area is aimed at early recognition with prompt diagnosis and therapy so as to prevent irreversible loss of renal function.

Clinical Findings

A. Symptoms and Signs

Nephritic syndrome can present with edema, oliguria, or uremic symptoms. Many patients have hypertension, which may even be malignant in some cases. Other physical examination findings depend on the underlying disorder. For example, a malar rash and oral ulcers may be found in SLE, whereas palpable purpura is found in Henoch–Schönlein purpura and cryoglobulinemia.

B. Laboratory Findings

1. Urinalysis—Patients may present with macroscopic hematuria often described as tea- or cola-colored urine. Microscopic urine examination often reveals RBCs. These are classically dysmorphic or misshapen as a result of the osmotic and chemical stress they incur as they pass through the nephron. Urinary RBCs with membrane blebs or "bubble-like" projections (acanthocytes) are strong evidence of a glomerular cause of hematuria. RBC casts may also be found. Urinary protein excretion varies widely in nephritic syndromes, but is generally less than 3 g of protein per day. Proteinuria can be quantified by either a 24-hour urine collection or can be estimated based on a single urine specimen.

2. Serum chemistries—A chemistry profile should be obtained to assess electrolyte status and to estimate the GFR in order to document the degree of renal dysfunction. A complete blood count (CBC) will often demonstrate anemia as well as possibly thrombocytopenia or leukopenia as seen in SLE. Additional useful tests depend on the patient's history and physical examination. These may include blood cultures if a fever or heart murmur is heard, streptozyme and anti-streptolysin O (ASO) titers if a sore throat is present, or a hepatitis panel and cryoglobulins if a history of intravenous drug abuse (IVDA) is obtained or hepatomegaly palpated. Other helpful tests might include complement levels, anti-neutrophilic cytoplasmic antibodies (ANCAs), anti-GBM, and immune complex disease markers such as ANA and anti-DNA. It is important to note that up to 10% of patients with heavy proteinuria may have negative serologic findings at presentation due to loss of antibody in the urine or tissue deposition.

C. Imaging Studies

Chest x-ray may demonstrate pulmonary edema or findings suggestive of Wegener's granulomatosis or Goodpasture's disease. An echocardiogram may identify a pericardial effusion or endocarditis. Renal ultrasound is frequently obtained when a decreased GFR is present in order to evaluate for kidney size. A kidney size of <9 cm may suggest extensive renal scarring with a low likelihood of reversibility.

D. Special Tests

Renal biopsy is often used for definitive diagnosis and is helpful in distinguishing between primary and secondary causes of renal disease as well as subtypes in SLE. It can allow rapid diagnosis in cases of RPGNs where prompt diagnosis and treatment are essential in preserving renal function. Renal biopsy can also yield information regarding the level of inflammation, extent of fibrosis, and overall prognosis.

▶ Differential Diagnosis

The differential diagnosis of nephritic syndromes requires distinguishing between a primary renal disease and one that occurs as a result of a systemic disease process. A useful clinical approach can be based on the results of serum complement levels, serologies, and immunofluorescence findings on renal biopsy.

▶ Complications

Nephritic syndrome can lead to fluid retention with resulting edema and HTN. Renal insufficiency also occurs and can

require both short- and long-term renal replacement therapy. Anemia may occur as a result of resistance to erythropoietin or decreased production.

▶ Treatment

A. Underlying Renal or Systemic Disease

1. Immunosuppressive agents—For primary renal diseases such as IgA nephropathy treatment often involves corticosteroids. Fish oil in doses of 6–12 g/day has been employed to possibly prevent or slow the rate of loss of renal function.

2. Cytotoxic agents—Diseases such as Gooodpastures's disease, Wegener's granulomatosis, and certain subtypes of SLE may require treatment with cytotoxic agents such as cyclophosphamide, mycophenolate mofetil, and azathioprine.

3. Plasmapheresis—Plasmapheresis is used to remove circulating pathogenic autoantibodies seen in diseases such as Goodpasture's disease and occasionally in pauci-immune crescentic glomerulonephritis and cryoglobulin-related MPGN.

4. Others—Successful treatment of infections such as hepatitis B with lamivudine, hepatitis C with interferon-α and ribavirin, or HIV with HAART may lead to substantial improvement in renal dysfunction. On the other hand, treatment of poststreptococcal glomerulonephritis is only supportive, as the use of antimicrobial agents does not prevent or attenuate its course. However, they should be given to prevent the spread of organisms to other susceptible hosts.

▶ B. Complications of Nephritic Syndrome

1. Edema—Salt and water restriction in conjunction with diuretics may occur.

2. HTN—Antihypertensive treatment is usually achieved with ACEI and ARBS as these have the added antiproteinuric benefits via reduction in the intraglomerular capillary hydrostatic pressure.

3. Renal insufficiency—If renal failure is severe or progressive renal replacement therapy will often be necessary.

▶ Prognosis

Prognosis of the nephritic syndrome depends on the underlying etiology of the disease. In cases of poststreptococcal glomerulonephritis the prognosis is excellent with spontaneous recovery of renal function occurring in 70–85% of adults.

However, in diseases such as MPGN the prognosis is generally unfavorable. Spontaneous remissions are infrequent, and at least 50% of patients with >10 g of proteinuria per day develop ESRD within 7 years after diagnosis. Other diseases such as Wegener's granulomatosis and Goodpasture's disease may be fatal if left untreated. However, with treatment with steroids and cytotoxic agents a dramatic recovery may be achieved.

Crew RJ et al: Complications of the nephrotic syndrome and their treatment. Clin Nephrol 2004;62:245.

Donadia JV, Grande JP: The role of fish oil/omega-3 fatty acids in the treatment of IgA nephropathy. Semin Nephrol 2004;24:225.

el-Agroudy AE et al: Effect of angiotensin II receptor blocker on plasma levels of TGF-beta 1 and interstitial fibrosis in hypertensive kidney transplant patients. Am J Nephrol 2003;23:300.

Minimal Change Disease

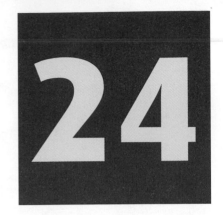

Elaine S. Kamil, MD

Minimal change disease (MCD) is a term used to describe the pathologic findings in a group of patients who present with heavy proteinuria, typically leading to nephrotic syndrome. On renal biopsy the findings include apparently normal glomeruli on light microscopy, negative immunofluorescence, and diffuse podocyte foot process effacement on electron microscopy. While occasionally MCD may be secondary to another condition such as lymphoma, in the majority of cases MCD is one of the idiopathic renal diseases. Because MCD is most likely to be the diagnosis in children presenting with the nephrotic syndrome, the majority of children do not undergo a kidney biopsy, but receive empiric treatment without one. Seventy percent of children with MCD present before age 5 years, and 20–30% of adolescents who present with nephrotic syndrome have MCD. Nevertheless, MCD is the third commonest finding in adults with nephrotic syndrome, after membranous nephropathy and focal, segmental glomerulosclerosis. The typical patient with MCD responds to therapy but experiences recurrent relapses.

 ESSENTIALS OF DIAGNOSIS

▶ Heavy proteinuria, typically leading to nephrotic syndrome.

▶ Renal biopsy with minimal changes on light microscopy, negative immunofluorescent microscopy, and podocyte foot process effacement on electron microscopy (Figure 24–1).

▶ Usually there is no known etiology, although secondary MCD may be associated with neoplastic disease, toxic or allergic reactions to drugs, infections, autoimmune disorders, or other miscellaneous disorders.

▶ General Considerations

MCD is the most common cause of nephrotic syndrome in children and the third most common cause of nephrotic syndrome in adults. In children the incidence of nephrotic syndrome is two to seven cases per 100,000 children and the prevalence is nearly 16 cases per 100,000. While most patients with MCD respond to therapy and have a good long-term prognosis, they are at risk for developing serious complications such as infection and thrombosis, and they are at risk for complications from therapy. The treatment of the MCD patient who is resistant to or dependent on corticosteroid therapy remains a challenge, despite the several therapeutic options available.

▶ Pathogenesis

Since first postulated by Shaloub in the 1970s, the pathogenesis of MCD has been associated with the presence of a circulating factor capable of inducing proteinuria. Presumably, the circulating factor is secreted by lymphoid cells and functions as a vascular permeability factor or directly affects the function of the podocyte. The induction of remission by immunosuppressive medications further strengthens the argument that the circulating factor is secreted by immune cells whose function is inhibited by these agents. In addition, patients who develop end-stage renal disease from MCD or focal, segmental glomerulosclerosis (FSGS) are at risk for recurrent disease occurring rapidly after transplant. To date, the most promising candidate factors include hemopexin, interleukin (IL)-4, vascular endothelial growth factor (VEGF), low-molecular-weight (<100 kDa) non-Ig permeability factors, and heparanase. The isolation and identification of the pathogenic circulating factors currently remains a "Holy Grail" in nephrotic syndrome research.

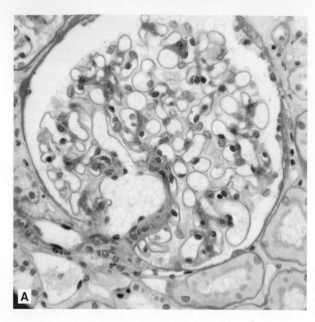 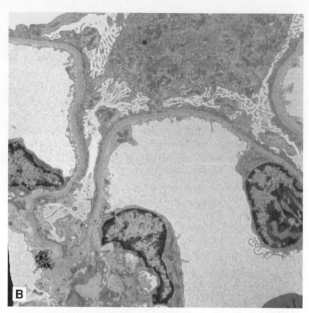

▲ **Figure 33–1. A:** Light microscopy (PAS stain) shows a completely normal looking glomerulus. **B:** Electron microscopy is normal except for the characteristic foot process effacement. (Photomicrographs courtesy of Arthur Cohen, MD.)

▶ Clinical Findings

A. Symptoms and Signs

The symptoms of MCD are related to the presence of nephrotic syndrome including peripheral swelling, abdominal discomfort from ascites, occasionally diarrhea from edema of the bowel wall, and, in extreme cases, pain from scrotal swelling and shortness of breath because of pleural effusions. Patients may experience oliguria, rarely leading to acute renal failure because of renal hypoperfusion. Because of an increased susceptibility to infection, especially from encapsulated bacteria, patients may present with signs of peritonitis or septic shock. They are also at an increased risk for thromboembolic phenomena, which may present with signs of deep venous thrombosis, flank pain and hematuria from renal venous thrombosis (rare), or a central nervous system catastrophe from a sagittal sinus thrombosis (also rare). An occasional patient has only minimal swelling.

B. Laboratory Findings

Urinalysis in patients with MCD shows dipstick positive proteinuria (3+ to 4+); about 15% of patients with MCD also have microscopic hematuria. The urinary protein-to-creatinine ratio (in milligrams/milligram) is ≥3.5 and can be obtained on a random sample, alleviating the need for a 24-hour urine collection. As a consequence of the heavy proteinuria the patient develops hypoalbuminemia. The magnitude of proteinuria in MCD tends to be much greater than that

seen in other glomerular diseases, leading to more profound hypoalbuminemia. Hypogammaglobulinemia may also be seen secondary to urinary losses of IgG or due to impaired immunoglobulin G (IgG) production and/or IgG catabolism in MCD. Children with MCD who have low IgG levels also have elevated IgM levels, changes in γ-globulins that may persist during periods of remission.

Renal function is typically normal, although there might be a minor increase in creatinine as a consequence of intravascular volume contraction. In severe cases, the hemoglobin and hematocrit will also be elevated from volume contraction, and platelets may also be elevated. Serum cholesterol and triglycerides are elevated and return to normal slowly after the induction of a remission. It is appropriate to draw a C3 complement level and an antinuclear antibody to rule out other causes of nephrotic syndrome; these will be normal in MCD.

C. Imaging Studies

Renal ultrasound is not necessarily indicated in nephrotic syndrome, but patients with MCD tend to have enlarged kidneys on ultrasound along with ascites fluid. A chest radiograph will be normal or may show pleural effusions.

D. Special Tests

Adults with nephrotic syndrome are diagnosed with MCD following a percutaneous renal biopsy that is

Table 24–1. Selected secondary causes of minimal change disease.

Neoplasia: Hodgkin's disease, non-Hodgkin's lymphoma, leukemia, thymoma, renal cell carcinoma, mesothelioma, bronchogenic carcinoma, colon carcinoma, pancreatic carcinoma, urothelial cancer, prostate carcinoma, renal oncocytoma

Drugs: Gold, antimicrobials, nonsteroidal antiinflammatory drugs (NSAIDs), trimethadione, paramethadione, lithium, interferon (α, γ), methimazole, tamoxifen, enalapril, penicillamine, provenecid, immunizations

Infections: Syphilis, human immunodeficiency virus, mycoplasma, ehrlichiosis, echinococcus, schistosomiasis

Atopy: Pollen, cow's milk, house dust, pork, bee stings, poison oak/ivy

Superimposed on another renal disease: IgA nephropathy, systemic lupus erythematosus, diabetes mellitus (type 1), autosomal dominant and recessive polycystic kidney disease, HIV-associated nephropathy

Miscellaneous: Sclerosing cholangitis, sclerosing mesenteric inflammation, vigorous exercise, acute decompression sickness, sarcoidosis, Grave's disease, thyroiditis, vasculitis, partial lipodystrophy, myasthenia gravis, renal artery stenosis, bis-albuminemia, Guillain-Barré syndrome, dermatitis herpetiformis

Adapted with permission from Glassock R: Secondary minimal change disease. Nephrol Dial Transplant 2003;18(Suppl 6):vi52.

usually performed with ultrasound or computed tomography (CT) guidance. Since the vast majority of young children with nephrotic syndrome have MCD, they do not undergo a biopsy at presentation unless they have features suggesting a diagnosis other than MCD such as age <1 year, positive family history of nephrotic syndrome, extrarenal disease (eg, arthritis, rash, anemia), symptoms due to intravascular volume expansion, renal failure, or an active urine sediment. Children will undergo a renal biopsy, however, if they follow a steroid-resistant or steroid-dependent course. It is important to have the biopsy tissue studied by immunofluorescent and electron microscopy in addition to light microscopy. The presence of mesangial IgM on biopsy may portend a more therapy-resistant course.

A search for diseases leading to secondary MCD should be considered in adults with MCD (Table 24–1).

Differential Diagnosis

The differential diagnosis of a patient with nephrotic syndrome and minimal to no hematuria includes MCD, FSGS, and membranous nephropathy. These lesions are differentiated on renal biopsy, although early FSGS may look like MCD since only some of the glomeruli show segments of sclerosis, and the sclerotic lesions, which tend to appear first in the deep, corticomedullary glomeruli, can be missed in a superficial biopsy.

Complications

The complications of MCD are the complications seen with nephrotic syndrome, including infection, thromboembolic phenomenon, and cardiovascular disease, in addition to the potential side effects of therapy. The increased susceptibility to infections, especially infections from encapsulated organisms, is multifactorial. Patients with MCD exhibit defective opsonization of bacteria secondary to low levels of factor B and I, and experience low levels of total IgG, and IgG subclass deficiencies. Treatment with immunosuppressive medications enhances the susceptibility to infections that can be life threatening. The most common infections include peritonitis (especially pneumococcal), cellulitis, and pneumonia. Patients with nephrotic syndrome should receive pneumococcal vaccine, preferably during remission and when they are off immunosuppressive medications. Varicella immune status should be assessed in all patients with MCD, with prompt administration of varicella-zoster immune globulin to non-immune patients after exposure to an active case of varicella infection. Treatment with acyclovir may be lifesaving in a patient with MCD on immunosuppressive medication who develops a varicella infection. Varicella vaccine given during remission while off steroid therapy appears to be safe and effective in children with MCD. Patients with MCD should also receive yearly influenza vaccine.

Children with MCD appear to be at a lower risk of thrombotic events than adults with MCD, but still may experience life-threatening thrombosis such as sagittal sinus thrombosis, pulmonary artery thrombosis, or inferior vena caval thrombosis, while nephrotic adults are more prone to deep vein or renal vein thrombosis. The hypercoaguable state in nephrotic syndrome is due to several factors including increased clotting factor synthesis (fibrinogen, II, V, VII, IX, X, XIII), urinary losses of anticoagulants (antithrombin III), platelet abnormalities (thrombocytosis, increased aggregability), hyperviscosity, and hyperlipidemia.

Most patients with MCD experience periods of remission during which their lipid profiles eventually return to normal. However, adults with nephrotic syndrome have a higher incidence of coronary heart disease and children with therapy-resistant MCD or steroid dependency may well be at an increased risk of cardiovascular complications. Corticosteroid treatment and hypertension undoubtedly add to the cardiovascular risk.

Other complications include a risk of acute renal failure secondary to renal hypoperfusion during relapse, iron deficiency anemia secondary to loss of iron binding proteins during relapse, and vitamin D deficiency, also due to loss of vitamin D-binding proteins during relapse.

Treatment

The first line-therapy in MCD is corticosteroids. Children with MCD are highly likely to experience a prompt (75% are in remission by 2 weeks), complete remission with steroid therapy (>95%) while adults seem to be less responsive. Several studies in children have shown that prolonged induction therapy with corticosteroids will lead to a lower incidence of frequent relapses, and once-a-day therapy is equally as effective as divided-dose therapy. A recent randomized, controlled trial of two steroid regimens in children compared the protocol from the Arbeitsgemeinschaft für Pädiatrische Nephrologie consisting of 6 weeks of 60 mg/m^2 of prednisone daily for 6 weeks followed by 40 mg/m^2 every other day for 6 weeks with a second regimen of 60 mg/m^2 daily for 4 weeks followed by 60 mg/m^2 every other day for 4 weeks, with tapering by 10 mg/m^2 every 4 weeks for an additional 20 weeks. Both regimens were equally as effective in inducing remission, but children under age 4 in the group treated with a longer taper had a lowered incidence of frequent relapses compared to the younger children treated with the 12-week course of therapy.

Adults with MCD require a more prolonged course of steroids to achieve a complete remission. One study from Japan showed that only 45% of adults over 50 years old were in remission after 4 weeks of treatment and many required >8 weeks of treatment to achieve remission. Adults, however, are less likely than children to experience relapses after a steroid-induced remission.

The majority of steroid-sensitive children, and some adults, with MCD experience relapses that typically follow an infection, and remain responsive to treatment with steroids. Relapses are treated with shorter courses of prednisone; prolonged treatment of a relapse does not influence the subsequent frequency of relapses. However, most of these patients with frequent relapses will develop steroid-induced side effects such as hypertension, Cushingoid appearance, hyperactive behavior (in the younger children), and poor growth. Some patients will do well on a prolonged course of low-dose, alternate-day prednisone therapy.

Other therapies should be considered for MCD patients with frequent relapses and steroid toxicity. A course of treatment with alklylating agents such as cyclophosphamide or chlorambucil has been shown to lead to a prolonged remission in children who are frequent relapsers. Cyclophosphamide (2 mg/kg) for 12 weeks is more commonly used and may induce remission lasting several years. Patients must be monitored for bone marrow toxicity with weekly complete blood counts and prompt treatment with varicella-zoster immune globulin if they are not immune to varicella infection. Courses longer than 12 weeks may lead to gonadal toxicity. In practice, many patients begin cyclophosphamide therapy while on alternate day steroids, which are weaned gradually over the course of 3–6 months. If patients resume a frequently relapsing course after receiving a course of cyclophosphamide, alternate day steroid therapy, levamisole (unavailable in the United States) or a course of cyclosporine may be tried. Levamisole has been shown to reduce the incidence of relapses in children with frequent relapses but not

in children with steroid dependence. If the patient has not yet had a kidney biopsy, most pediatric nephrologists will perform one prior to using cyclosporine. Cyclosporine has been shown to be useful therapy in the patient with frequent relapsing, steroid- dependent, and probably even steroid-resistant MCD. Because of its toxicity profile, cyclosporine should be prescribed only by physicians who are experienced in its use. Side effects of treatment include hirsuitism, gingival hyperplasia, hypertension, hypomagnesemia, and nephrotoxicity. The usual starting dose is 5–6 mg/kg/day divided in two doses with close monitoring of cyclosporine levels (target trough levels of 50–125 ng/mL), renal function, and magnesium levels. The typical course of therapy is 1–2 years, followed by a slow taper. Many patients experience relapses after discontinuation of cyclosporine; if continued therapy is needed, kidney biopsies should be performed to monitor for nephrotoxicity. Many patients also require alternate day steroid therapy in conjunction with cyclosporine. Tacrolimus, also a calcineurin inhibitor, also shows some promise for therapy of patients with therapy-resistant nephrotic syndrome. Recent reports have suggested that mycophenolate mofetil (MMF), a purine synthesis inhibitor, may be useful in the treatment of children with steroid-dependent nephrotic syndrome.

The majority of patients with steroid resistance are likely to have FSGS. Patients with secondary MCD may experience a remission after successful treatment of the disease inducing the MCD. Angiotensin-converting enzyme (ACE) inhibition or angiotensin receptor blockade is a useful adjunct for patients with steroid resistance even in the absence of hypertension. All patients with MCD should follow a no added salt diet during periods of relapse. Children with marked anasarca, pleural effusions, or signs of renal hypoperfusion associated with sepsis should benefit from the cautious use of intravenous albumin (25%) —1 g/kg given over 2 hours followed by a 1 mg/kg dose of furosemide. The albumin infusion can be repeated up to every 12 hours to achieve a sustained diuresis. However, the patient's urine output must be closely monitored. A patient who has acute tubular necrosis as a complication of renal hypoperfusion may not respond to the albumin and furosemide infusions and is thus at risk for developing pulmonary edema. Intravenous γ-globulin (IVIg) may be useful acutely in a nephrotic patient with hypogammaglobulinemia experiencing sepsis or once monthly in a chronically nephrotic patient to reduce the incidence of sinus infections or bacteremia.

▶ Prognosis

The outcome in MCD is largely based on the patient's response to steroid therapy. In children, prompt remission within 7–9 days of therapy, absence of microhematuria, and age greater than 4 years at presentation predict fewer relapses. By 10 years from diagnosis, only 16% of children are still experiencing relapses. Many children will "outgrow" their disease by or during puberty, although some continue to experience relapses into adulthood. During periods of relapse, patients remain vulnerable to life threatening infections and thrombotic events. The long-term cardiovascular risk in children with MCD who have experienced long periods of steroid therapy and periods of hyperlipidemia and hypertension is largely unknown. Adults with MCD may have an increased risk of coronary artery disease. Patients with MCD who become resistant to steroids later in their course are likely to have FSGS with its high risk for end-stage renal disease.

Alpay H et al: Varicella vaccination in children with steroid-sensitive nephrotic syndrome. Pediatr Nephrol 2002;17:181. [PMID: 11956856]

Bagga A et al: Mycophenolate mofetil and prednisone in children with steroid-dependent nephrotic syndrome. Am J Kidney Dis 2003;42:1114. [PMID: 14655181]

Brenchley PEC: Vascular permeability factors in steroid-sensitive nephrotic syndrome and focal, segmental glomerulosclerosis. Nephrol Dial Transplant 2003;18:vi21. [PMID: 12953037]

Eddy AA et al: Nephrotic syndrome in childhood. Lancet 2003;362:629. [PMID: 12944064]

Filler G: Treatment of nephrotic syndrome in children and controlled trials. Nephrol Dial Transplant 2003;18:vi75. [PMID: 12953047]

Glassock RJ: Secondary minimal change disease. Nephrol Dial Transplant 2003;18:vi52. [PMID: 12953043]

Hiraoka M et al: West Japan Cooperative Study Group of Kidney Disease in Children: a randomized study of two long-course prednisolone regimens for nephrotic syndrome in childhood. Am J Kidney Dis 2003;41:1155. [PMID: 12776266]

Howie AJ: Pathology of minimal change nephropathy and segmental sclerosing glomerular disorders. Nephrol Dial Transplant 2003;18:vi33. [PMID: 12953040]

Iijima K et al: Risk factors for cyclosporine-induced tubulointerstitial lesions in children with minimal change nephrotic syndrome. Kidney Int 2002;61:1801. [PMID: 11967030]

Loeffler K et al: Tacrolimus therapy in pediatric patients with treatment resistant nephrotic syndrome. Pediatr Nephrol 2004;19:281. [PMID 14758528]

Mathieson PW: Immune dysregulation in minimal change nephropathy. Nephrol Dial Transplant 2003;18:vi26. [PMID: 12953038]

Tse KC et al: Idiopathic minimal change nephrotic syndrome in older adults: steroid responsiveness and pattern of relapses. Nephrol Dial Transplant 2003;18:1316. [PMID: 12808168]

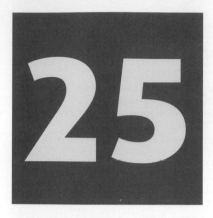

Focal Segmental Glomerulosclerosis

Debbie S. Gipson, MD, MSPH, & Howard Trachtman, MD

► Focal segmental glomerulosclerosis (FSGS) can be primary or secondary.

► Diagnosis requires the presence of the characteristic histopathologic lesion.

► Genetic abnormalities in podocyte proteins may account for 25% of primary FSGS.

► The presenting complaint is usually proteinuria or nephrotic syndrome.

► Nearly 50% of cases progress to end-stage renal disease (ESRD) over 5–10 years and disease recurs in 30% of those who receive a kidney transplant.

► Failure to respond to corticosteroid treatment is a poor prognostic sign and there is no proven therapy in these patients.

General Considerations

A. Epidemiology

FSGS is an important glomerulopathy because it has a high risk of progression to ESRD. It is not a distinct disease but rather represents a pattern of response to injury that probably originates in the podocyte. FSGS occurs in all ethnic groups, both genders, and all geographic locales. Recent data indicate that the incidence of FSGS is rising, especially in black patients. This has been confirmed in reviews of renal biopsy findings in the United States and Canada that demonstrate a 2- to 3-fold increase in the incidence of FSGS over the period from 1984 to 2002. In addition, according to the North American Pediatric Renal Transplant Collaborative Study, FSGS is the most frequent form of acquired renal disease necessitating renal replacement therapy in pediatric patients. Similarly, it is the most common cause of idiopathic nephrotic syndrome in adults and is a major cause of ESRD.

B. Presenting Complaints

FSGS usually presents with asymptomatic proteinuria or overt nephrotic syndrome. In those patients who are diagnosed with isolated proteinuria, the abnormality is usually detected on a routine urinalysis. The clinical picture in those who present with nephrotic syndrome is almost indistinguishable from those with minimal change nephrotic syndrome (MCNS). Hematuria, evidence of tubular dysfunction such as glycosuria, hypertension, and mild azotemia, may be present in 15–30% of patients with new-onset nephrotic syndrome and these features may increase the clinical suspicion that a patient has FSGS. However, the key feature that prompts further investigation to establish the diagnosis of FSGS is failure to respond to a standard course of corticosteroids. It is this clinical finding that triggers the performance of a diagnostic renal biopsy; however, the utilization and timing of this procedure may differ among those who care for children or adults. Although the prognosis may be better in patients who present with subnephrotic-range proteinuria versus nephrotic syndrome, this difference has not been confirmed in patients of all ages.

C. Pathologic Findings

The diagnosis of FSGS requires histopathologic evidence of segmental glomerular sclerosis and hyalinosis. The lesion often manifests in juxtamedullary nephrons during the early stages of disease and it can be associated with periglomerular scarring, tubular atrophy, and interstitial fibrosis in the vicinity of the affected glomerulus (Figure 25–1). Generally, immunofluorescence studies are unrevealing. Electron microscopy demonstrates foot process effacement, the absence of immune deposits, and mesangial sclerosis.

In view of the widely divergent clinical course that patients with FSGS may follow, an attempt has been made to classify FSGS into distinct histologic subcategories. A scheme that has been proposed includes five variants: Perihilar, tip, cellular, collapsing, and not otherwise specified. Additional

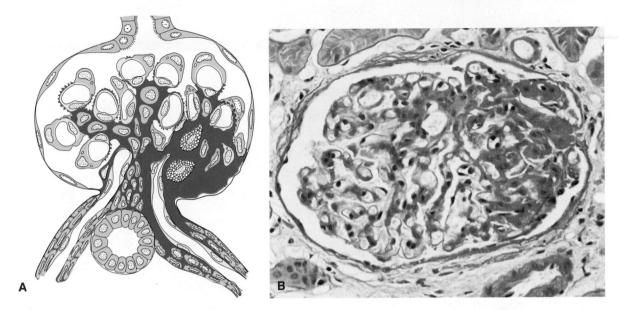

▲ **Figure 25–1. A:** Focal segmental glomerulosclerosis with a segmental scar shown from 4 to 6 o'clock. (Courtesy of J. C. Jennette, MD.) **B:** Human glomerulosclerosis with a segmental scar shown from 12 to 5 o'clock.

studies are necessary to determine whether this categorization provides information that can be used to guide treatment or clarify the long-term prognosis.

▶ Pathogenesis

A. Primary Focal Segmental Glomerulosclerosis

This form has also been called idiopathic FSGS. Based on clinical evidence of variable response to immunosuppressive medications, the presumption has been that primary FSGS reflects a disturbance in the immune system. However, unlike MCNS, no consistent abnormality has been demonstrated except for altered synthesis and release of tumor necrosis factor (TNF)–α in peripheral blood leukocytes. In addition, various circulating factors including hemopexin, and immunoglobulin-like molecules have been isolated from the sera of patients with FSGS. Removal of these circulating factors, using plasmapheresis or immunoadsorption columns, has been associated with disease remission and infusion into animals has resulted in glomerular proteinuria. Further work on the nature of these substances may help identify the cause of proteinuria in FSGS and define better treatments.

Exciting findings over the past 10 years underscore the pivotal role of the podocyte in maintaining the integrity of the glomerular permselective barrier. A number of proteins have been identified that are components of the cell membrane or actin cytoskeleton of the podocyte. These include nephrin, α-actinin-4, podocin, CD2AP, Wilms tumor suppressor (WT1), and TRPC6 (Figure 25–2). Mutations in the genes for these proteins, occurring in autosomal dominant and recessive patterns, have been associated with steroid-resistant nephrotic syndrome and biopsy-proven FSGS (Table 25–1). Recent series suggest that up to 25% of familial and sporadic cases of steroid-resistant nephrotic syndrome in Europe are related to these genetic abnormalities. Moreover, the response to standard immunosuppressive medications and the risk of recurrent disease after transplantation may be markedly lower in patients with a genetic basis for FSGS. Clarification of these issues is imperative in designing an optimal approach to the evaluation and treatment of patients with FSGS.

B. Secondary Focal Segmental Glomerulosclerosis

The FSGS lesion represents a nonspecific response to podocyte injury and can arise in a variety of disease states. These include infections with viral agents including HIV and parvovirus B19. A variety of medications including lithium, pamidronate, and illicit drugs such as heroin have been associated with FSGS. Reduced renal mass secondary to surgical ablation (eg, surgery, trauma), reflux nephropathy, and low birth weight can lead to FSGS. Finally, secondary FSGS can occur in patients with a normal renal mass but who have obesity, sickle cell anemia, or cyanotic congenital heart disease (Table 25–2). Identification of these causes and treatment of reversible conditions leads to regression of the FSGS lesions.

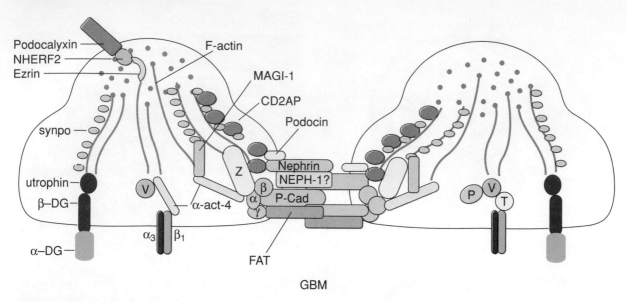

▲ **Figure 25–2.** Podocyte architecture.
GBM, glomerular basement membrane; synpo, synaptopodin; DG, dystroglycan; α-act-4, α-actinin-4; P-Cad, P-cadherin; P, paxillin; V, vinculin; T, talin. (Reproduced with permission from Mundel P, Shankland SJ: Podocyte biology and response to injury. J Am Soc Nephrol 2002;13:3005.)

▶ **Clinical Findings**

A. Symptoms and Signs

The presentation of FSGS can be subtle with few or no presenting symptoms or may be apparent with the typical findings of nephrotic syndrome. Overtly nephrotic patients may manifest edema, ascites, and weight gain secondary to fluid retention. Edema is typically dependent in the lower extremities when upright and in the periorbital and presacral areas when supine. Edema of the scrotum and labia may also be present. Hypertension is found in approximately 60% of patients at presentation even among the nonedematous patients. Freshly voided urine may be foamy secondary to the effects of significant proteinuria.

Table 25–1. Genetic mutations associated with focal segmental glomerulosclerosis.

Gene Product	Gene	Chromosome	Inheritance
Podocin	NPHS2	1q25–31	AR
α-Actinin-4	ACTN4	19q13	AD
CD2AP	CD2AP	6p12	AD
WT-1	WT-1	11p13	AD or AR
TRPC6	TRPC6	11q21–22	AD

AR, autosomal recessive; AD, autosomal dominant.

B. Laboratory Findings

1. Urine—The urine contains from 1 to over 20 g of protein in a 24-hour collection. Determination of proteinuria can be screened with a simple urinalysis but should be verified

Table 25–2. Secondary causes of focal segmental glomerulosclerosis.

Drugs
  Adriamycin
  Heroin
  Interferon-α
  Lithium
  Pamidronate

Infections
  HIV
  Malarial nephropathy
  Parvovirus B19
  SV40 virus
  Schistosomiasis

Malignancies
  Hodgkin's lymphoma
  Non-Hodgkin's lymphoma

Nephron loss
  Reflux nephropathy
  Surgical ablation
  Low birth weight

with a measurement of urine protein as either a single voided specimen or 24-hour timed urine collection for quantification of protein and creatinine. Proteinuria of 1 g/day/1.73 m^2 or a urine protein-to-creatinine ratio of 1 or more is considered a level suggestive of a glomerular lesion. Microscopic hematuria is found in approximately 20%, but gross hematuria is rare. Oval fatbodies and hyaline casts are commonly found when proteinuria is >3 g/day/1.73 m^2.

2. Blood—Blood chemistries may reveal the typical findings of hypoalbuminemia and dyslipidemia in patients with frank nephrotic syndrome. Serum albumin may be less than 1.0 g/dL. Serum cholesterol, triglycerides, and very low-density lipoproteins are elevated in patients with severe hypoalbuminemia. Total serum calcium is low because of the hypoalbuminemia; however, the ionized calcium is not reduced proportionately. Serum sodium may be low due to water retention. However, pseudohyponatremia secondary to hyperlipidemia is no longer a concern because automated serum chemistry analyzers use an ion selective electrode. At diagnosis FSGS patients may have an elevated serum creatinine representing a loss of kidney function that may be acute or chronic.

Hematocrit may be elevated in patients with volume contraction or depressed in the patient with chronic loss of kidney function. Platelet counts may be significantly elevated as are coagulation factors V, VII, VIII, X and fibrinogen. Antithrombin III and factors XI and XII may be decreased. These changes in clotting factors are related to the severity of the proteinuria and contribute to the risk of thrombosis in the grossly nephrotic patient.

The laboratory evaluation of a patient with FSGS may aid in the diagnosis of a primary or secondary lesion. Secondary forms of FSGS may be identified or confirmed by laboratory tests specific to the primary disease such as serology for HIV-associated FSGS. Although an unusual etiology, parvovirus B19 or SV40 can be confirmed by polymerase chain reaction (PCR).

C. Imaging Studies

Radiographic procedures such as renal ultrasound or computerized tomography may serve to exclude secondary or alternative conditions. For example, the patient with vesicoureteral reflux nephropathy may have evidence of hydronephrosis, hydroureter, or renal parenchymal scarring suggesting a urinary tract abnormality. Any patient with advanced glomerular sclerosis, whether from FSGS or from an alternative cause, may have small kidneys with a pattern of increased echogenicity in the kidney ultrasound.

D. Special Tests

The assessment of genetic markers of familial FSGS is not universally available. In 2006 the only gene test associated with FSGS available in commercial laboratories in the United States was the NPHS2 (podocin). Research laboratories make other candidate gene testing available in a limited fashion but not for clinical use.

E. Special Examinations

The diagnosis of FSGS is based on the kidney biopsy finding of glomerular scaring in portions (segmental) of some (focal) of the glomeruli. Indeed, the finding of a single glomerulus with a segmental scar may be adequate to establish the diagnosis. Immunofluorescence staining is minimal and electron microscopy shows only foot process effacement. The pattern of scarring lesions has been used to classify FSGS into five subtypes. Using either the traditional classification or the newest classification scheme, the pattern of collapsing FSGS with glomerular capillary collapse and visceral epithelial cell hyperplasia has been associated with the worst prognosis among patients with primary FSGS. Collapsing FSGS has also been associated with HIV infection. All patients with FSGS should be evaluated for HIV as the treatment considerations differ according to etiology. The FSGS tip lesion has been considered the subtype most likely to respond to corticosteroid therapy with reduction or normalization of urine protein excretion and long-term kidney survival.

▶ Differential Diagnosis

Distinguishing primary from secondary FSGS has important therapeutic and prognostic implications. Primary FSGS is defined by confirmation by biopsy of the kidney pathology; the medical history, serology, and imaging studies confirm the absence of an alternative cause.

Disease entities such as Alport's syndrome or immunoglobulin A (IgA) nephropathy may be associated with the finding of focal glomerulosclerosis on kidney biopsy but additional findings of glomerular basement membrane abnormalities on electron microscopy in Alport's syndrome or IgA staining on immunofluorescence microscopy will identify the primary pathologic entity.

Although controversy exists, C1q nephropathy is considered a distinct pathologic entity wherein patients may present with nephrotic-range proteinuria, nephritis with cellular casts and proteinuria, or hematuria alone. Although kidney tissue from patients with C1q nephropathy may not have a focal sclerosing lesion, those with an FSGS lesion will also have C1q dominant staining on immunofluorescence microscopy, which ensures the distinct diagnosis of this secondary lesion. Other investigators do not distinguish primary FSGS based on the presence or absence of C1q deposits. Further study is required to clarify this issue.

Obesity-related glomerulopathy is an entity that causes glomerulomegaly in addition to focal sclerotic lesions. Patients with obesity-related glomerulopathy tend to have a nonedematous body mass index of 40 kg/m^2 or greater. These patients may demonstrate a resolution of proteinuria with significant weight loss and, even without effective weight loss programs, tend to have a better long-term prognosis compared to those with the primary FSGS lesion. Immunosuppression therapy is not warranted in this obesity-induced lesion.

▶ Complications

A. Infection

Bacterial infections causing spontaneous bacterial peritonitis, sepsis, and cellulitis may complicate nephrotic syndrome from FSGS. Episodes of peritonitis typically manifest with abdominal pain, rebound tenderness, guarding, and anorexia with or without fever. The diagnosis can be confirmed by performing a paracentesis, which demonstrates leukocytosis of the peritoneal fluid with a predominance of neutrophils and a positive peritoneal fluid culture. The most common causes of peritonitis in patients with nephrotic syndrome are *Streptococcus pneumoniae*, *Escherichia coli*, and a variety of Gram-negative rods. The exclusion of alternate abdominal pathology is critical as a ruptured appendix, for example, may also present with abdominal pain, rebound tenderness, and guarding.

B. Thrombosis

Venous and arterial thrombosis and thromboemboli occur in <2% of patients with significant proteinuria. The increased risk of formation of thrombus is thought to be secondary to the urinary loss of factors responsible for inhibition of coagulation such as antithrombin III, protein S, and protein C. Increased platelet activation and a reduction in plasmin-mediated fibrinolysis may also play a role. Additional risk factors may relate to decreased mobility in the grossly edematous patient.

C. Acute Kidney Failure

Acute renal failure may be present at diagnosis or with episodes of severe volume contraction. The restoration of circulating volume is the treatment of choice in these cases. Chronic renal failure may be present at the time of diagnosis of FSGS. Kidney biopsy may assist in determining the likelihood for renal function recovery based on the severity of the glomerular and tubulointerstitial fibrosis.

▶ Treatment

A. Corticosteroids

The course of untreated FSGS is generally one of persistent proteinuria and progressive kidney failure. Less than 5% of patients experience a spontaneous remission. The therapy of FSGS remains controversial because there are few randomized trials to support an evidence-based practice. Use of

corticosteroids as initial therapy in pediatric and adult aged patients is common for primary disease. The treatment course is typically between 6 weeks and 6 months with increasing response rates of 25–40% and diminishing relapse rates as the steroid treatment duration increases. Regional differences have been reported in steroid responsiveness, which may relate to duration of corticosteroid administration or varying prevalence of underlying genetic or other etiologic factors.

Persistent proteinuria after a course of corticosteroids is observed in the majority of patients with FSGS. The selection of a second-line therapy may include immunosuppressive agents, agents to control symptoms alone such as diuretics, antifibrotic therapy, and plasmapheresis (Table 25–3).

B. Calcineurin Inhibitors

Cyclosporine is the standard second-line therapy for patients with steroid-resistant FSGS. A 50% or greater reduction in urinary protein excretion with preservation of kidney function is expected in approximately 70% of patients treated

Table 25–3. Treatment options in patients with steroid-resistant focal segmental glomerulosclerosis.

Immunosuppressive agents
Calcineurin inhibitors
Cyclosporine
Tacrolimus
Cyclophosphamide
Mycophenolate mofetil
Conservative therapy
Diuretics
Antifibrotic therapy
Angiotensin-converting enzyme inhibitors
Angiotensin receptor blockers
Aldosterone antagonists
Lipid-lowering drugs
Antioxidants
Plasmapheresis
Genetic/familial
Alport's syndrome
Branchiootorenal syndrome
Charcot–Marie–Tooth disease
Partial lecithin-cholesterol acyltransferase deficiency
Spondylometaphyseal dysplasia
Miscellaneous
Cyanotic congenital heart disease
Eclampsia
Healed focal proliferative nephritis
Obesity
Sarcoidosis
Sickle cell nephropathy
Systemic sclerosis
Type I glycogen storage disease

with cyclosporine. The risk for relapse after discontinuation of the treatment may be related to the duration of therapy and the degree of control of the proteinuria. The desire to continue therapy to maintain a remission is offset by the risk for cyclosporine-induced nephrotoxicity, which may be severe and depend on duration of drug exposure. In short-term studies, kidney function was better preserved in those treated with cyclosporine. Generalization of this response to the other calcineurin inhibitor, tacrolimus, has theoretical merit but is without sufficient supporting evidence.

C. Cyclophosphamide

A nonrandomized study using combined high-dose corticosteroids and cyclophosphamide suggested improved control of proteinuria compared with historical controls. In a randomized trial of cyclophosphamide plus alternate day steroids versus alternate day steroids alone, cyclophosphamide was not found to improve renal survival or control proteinuria better than the steroid-only group.

D. Mycophenolate Mofetil

Anecdotal reports of mycophenolate mofetil have suggested that this agent may improve proteinuria and preserve renal function in steroid-dependent or -resistant nephrotic syndrome. At present an ideal approach to immunomodulatory therapy for FSGS has not been identified.

E. Diet and Diuretics

Sodium-restricted diet is the mainstay of therapy to control edema in a patient with hypoalbuminemia and edema. Even with sodium restriction, additional therapy with diuretic agents may be required until proteinuria excretion is controlled.

F. Antihypertensive Agents

Angiotensin-converting enzyme inhibitors and angiotensin receptor blockade are part of the standard regimen in steroid-resistant FSGS patients. In isolation or combination, these agents have been shown to reduce proteinuria up to 50% from baseline and lower the risk for progression to kidney failure in diabetic and nondiabetic kidney disease. Monitoring should include assessment of serum potassium to allow early identification of a need for potassium restriction and measurement of serum creatinine to ensure preservation of the glomerular filtration rate. A small rise in serum creatinine is expected on these agents but the change should be less than 20% and should be reversible if the agent(s) are discontinued. Despite a mild increase in serum creatinine, the agents are to be continued with the goal of long-term preservation of kidney function. If therapy with angiotensin-converting enzyme inhibitors and angiotensin receptor blockade does not control hypertension, additional antihypertensive agents should be prescribed. Aldosterone antagonists may reduce proteinuria and prevent renal fibrosis, although this effect has not been evaluated specifically in patients with FSGS.

G. Lipid Control

Lipid-lowering agents have been included in the nephrotic syndrome armamentarium to control hyperlipidemia. Hypercholesterolemia in animal models has been shown to cause glomerulosclerosis. Therapy with the 3-hydroxy-3-methylglutaryl coenzyme A (HMG-CoA) reductase inhibitors, statins, diminishes the effects of lipemia on the kidney even with persistent hypercholesterolemia in animal and human investigation.

H. Vitamin E

Vitamin E is also considered a means of controlling proteinuria and progressive kidney disease through the antioxidant mechanism. One open-label pilot study reported a 50% reduction in protein excretion in 11 children with FSGS, while others have found no beneficial effect. Controversy continues to exist regarding the efficacy of vitamin E.

In general, a combination therapy approach may be resorted to for corticosteroid-resistant FSGS patients. Cyclosporine, angiotensin-converting enzyme inhibitor, angiotensin receptor blockade, and statin combination are commonly used.

I. Plasmapheresis

The patient with FSGS-induced rapid progression to kidney failure has a 30% risk of FSGS recurrence in the kidney transplant and an 18% risk of graft failure from recurrent disease. In an effort to diminish the risk for recurrent disease and to preserve the survival of the transplanted organ, plasmapheresis may be used in the peritransplant period as a preventive therapy or in response to rapid return of proteinuria. The success of this approach is apparently better in children than adults. Occasionally, long-term plasmapheresis has been used to sustain a response.

▶ Prognosis

Nearly 50% of cases of FSGS progress to ESRD over 5–10 years. Those at greatest risk to progress to kidney failure include those who show resistance to therapy with continued proteinuria and those with collapsing variant FSGS. For patients with progression to kidney failure, dialysis and transplant support are options for therapy. Unfortunately, those who receive a kidney transplant may have a recurrence of FSGS in the transplanted kidney. Patients with FSGS who present with azotemia or progress rapidly to ESRD are more susceptible to disease recurrence in a kidney transplant. The impact of age, ethnicity, and donor type is controversial. The presence of a genetic mutation has been associated with a diminished, but not absent, risk for FSGS recurrence in the kidney transplant recipient.

Buemi M et al: Statins in nephrotic syndrome: A new weapon against tissue injury. Med Res Rev 2005;25:587.

Cattran DC et al: Mycophenolate mofetil in the treatment of focal segmental glomerulosclerosis. Clin Nephrol 2004;62:405.

Chun MJ et al: Focal segmental glomerulosclerosis in nephrotic adults: presentation, prognosis, and response to therapy of the histologic variants. J Am Soc Nephrol 2004;15:2169.

Crook ED et al: Effects of steroids in focal segmental glomerulosclerosis in a predominantly African-American population. Am J Med Sci 2005;330:19.

Gohh RY et al: Preemptive plasmapheresis and recurrence of FSGS in high-risk renal transplant recipients. Am J Transplant 2005;5:2907.

Hodson EM et al: Corticosteroid therapy for nephrotic syndrome in children. Cochrane Database Syst Rev 2005;CD001533.

Huang K et al: The differential effect of race among pediatric kidney transplant recipients with focal segmental glomerulosclerosis. Am J Kidney Dis 2004;43:1082.

Rodriguez MM et al: Comparative renal histomorphometry: a case study of oligonephropathy of prematurity. Pediatr Nephrol 2005;20:945.

Ruf RG et al: Patients with mutations in NPHS2 (podocin) do not respond to standard steroid treatment of nephrotic syndrome. J Am Soc Nephrol 2004;15:722.

Troyanov S et al: Focal and segmental glomerulosclerosis: definition and relevance of a partial remission. J Am Soc Nephrol 2005;16:1061.

Valdivia P et al: Plasmapheresis for the prophylaxis and treatment of recurrent focal segmental glomerulosclerosis following renal transplant. Transplant Proc 2005;37:1473.

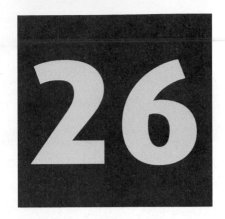

Membranous Nephropathy

26

Fernando C. Fervenza, MD, PhD, &
Daniel C. Cattran, MD, FRCP(C)

ESSENTIALS OF DIAGNOSIS

- ▶ The clinical features of nephrotic syndrome are present.
- ▶ The glomeruli are not inflamed.
- ▶ The glomerular capillary basement membrane appears thickened.
- ▶ There is an absence of glomerular inflammation.
- ▶ Idiopathic membranous nephropathy (MN) is relatively common and remains the leading cause of nephrotic syndrome in white adults. It is diagnosed by ruling out secondary causes.
- ▶ Secondary MN forms may account for up to one-third of cases and are associated with autoimmune diseases.
- ▶ Malignancy increases with increasing age.

General Considerations

Sixty years ago E.T. Bell coined the term membranous glomerulonephritis to describe the renal pathology of a group of patients with the clinical features of nephrotic syndrome in whom the glomeruli were not inflamed but in whom the glomerular capillary basement membrane appeared thickened. The synonymous terms extramembranous nephropathy and epimembranous glomerulonephritis have also been used to describe the disease. The word glomerulonephritis is, however, misleading as one of the main features of the condition is the absence of glomerular inflammation; because of this the word nephropathy is more often employed.

Idiopathic MN is a relatively common immune-mediated glomerular disease and remains the leading cause of nephrotic syndrome in white adults. In the majority of cases, the etiologic agent is unknown, and the disorder is termed idiopathic. Secondary MN forms may account for up to one-third of cases and are associated with autoimmune diseases (eg, systemic lupus erythematosus, SLE), infections (eg, hepatitis B and C), medications [eg, nonsteroidal anti-inflammatory drugs (NSAIDs), D-penicillamine, gold], and neoplasias (eg, colon cancer, kidney cancer) (Table 26–1). The association with malignancy increases with age, reaching up to 20% in patients over the age of 60 years. Since idiopathic and secondary forms have similar clinical presentations, the designation of idiopathic is made by ruling out secondary causes by a careful history, physical examination, and laboratory evaluation of the patient. The disease is rare in children, and when it does occur, is commonly associated with an immunologically mediated disorder such as SLE.

Pathogenesis

There is considerable evidence to support the hypothesis that idiopathic MN is an autoimmune disease. However, the pathogenic mechanisms that cause immune deposits of immunoglobulin G (IgG) and complement to localize predominantly or exclusively on the subepithelial surface of the glomerular basement membrane (GBM) and the subsequent development of proteinuria are not fully understood. The Heymann model of experimental MN in rats, which closely mimics the histologic features of human disease, suggests that the podocyte is the target of injury. The antigenic targets of the antibody response in this experimental model have been localized to the clathrin-coated pits of the podocyte foot processes. They are, specifically, a 515-kDa glycoprotein called megalin, a polyspecific receptor related to the low-density lipoprotein receptor family that functions as a multiligand receptor for the uptake of a variety of macromolecules (eg, aminoglycosides, advanced glycation end products, vitamin D) and a second 44-kDa protein, know as RAP (receptor-associated protein), that is closely related to megalin and is an additional target antigen in the model. Binding of the antibody to the antigen results in activation of the complement with insertion of C5b-9 (membrane attack complex) to the podocyte membrane. Because the antigen–antibody binding

Table 26–1. Secondary membranous nephropathy.

Infections: Hepatitis B and C,[1] syphilis (congenital and secondary), leprosy, filariasis, hydatid cyst disease, hepatosplenic schistosomiasis, echinococcus, post-streptococcus infection, malaria

Neoplasias: Carcinomas,[1] leukemia, lymphoma, pheochromocytoma, carotid body tumor

Autoimmune: SLE,[1] thyroiditis, rheumatoid arthritis, mixed connective tissue disease, sarcoidosis, angiolymphoid hyperplasia with eosinophilia (Kimura disease), primary biliary cirrhosis, Sjögren's syndrome, ankylosing spondylitis, dermatitis herpetiformis

Drugs: NSAIDs (diclofenac[1]), gold, D-penicillamine, mercury, captopril, formaldehyde, thiola, probenecid, bucillamine, tiopronin

Other: *de novo* renal transplant, sickle-cell disease, Gardner–Diamond syndrome, Guillain–Barré syndrome, graft-versus-host disease following bone marrow transplant, diabetes mellitus

[1]Most common causes, accounting for approximately 85% of secondary forms.
SLE, systemic lupus erythematosus; NSAIDs, nonsteroidal anti-inflammatory drugs.

and subsequent complement cascade activation occurs on the urinary side of the GBM, and thus away from the circulation, the cellular inflammatory response is blunted, and this accounts for the absence of inflammatory cells in the glomeruli on light microscopy. Although the insertion of C5b-9 to the podocyte membrane is insufficient to cause cell lysis, it does induce podocyte activation and signal transduction, resulting in an increased production of a number of potentially cytotoxic molecules (eg, cytokines, toxic oxygen radicals, proteases, vasoactive substances) that will ultimately damage the underlying GBM. The result is excessive synthesis of GBM, increased glomerular permeability, development of nonselective proteinuria, and effacement of the foot processes. The reduction in the glomerular filtration rate (GFR) results from progressive thickening of the GBM and reduced glomerular hydraulic permeability coefficient (Kf) whereas the effects of proteinuria on tubular cell differentiation and cytokine release engender progressive tubulointerstitial fibrosis. Megalin, however, is not present in human glomeruli, and except for rare cases secondary to hepatitis B or thyroiditis, where the specific antigen has been found as part of the immune complex, and a well-documented case of congenital MN due to passive transfer of a maternal antibody against a neutral endopeptidase present on the infant's glomerular podocyte, the nature of the antigen involved in the majority of cases of idiopathic MN remains unknown.

It is quite likely that a number of different antigen-antibody combinations may cause MN. Some antigens may be endogenous, while others may be exogenous. The electrical charge of the antigens, antibodies, and/or circulating immune complexes, as well as their size, may play a role in determining whether an immune complex will form in a subepithelial

position. There is an increased risk for MN in white patients with HLA-DR3 and in Japanese patients with HLA-DR2. The rare occurrence of MN in more than one family member suggests that genetic factors may be involved in the pathogenesis related either to a predisposition for developing the disease or its progression.

▶ Pathogenesis

The diagnosis of MN is made by renal biopsy. In very early cases of MN, the glomeruli appear normal by light microscopy (hematoxylin and eosin), although abnormalities may be seen in silver preparations and by immunofluorescence and electron microscopy. Capillary loops are widely patent and the glomeruli show no increase in cellularity and there is no nuclear crowding. As the number and size of subepithelial immune complexes increase, the GBM develops a diffuse and uniform thickening on light microscopy. These changes affect all the glomeruli. Thin sections examined by the periodic-silver-methenamine stain demonstrate the classical "spike" pattern on the epithelial side of the basement membrane reflecting the increased synthesis and deposition of GBM-like material around the immune deposits (Figure 26–1). As the disease progresses, thickening of the capillary wall becomes pronounced, the capillary lumen narrows, and eventually sclerosis and hyalinization of the glomerular tuft develop.

Proximal tubules are remarkable for the lipid vacuoles in the cytoplasm and numerous proteinaceous casts in the lumen. In the initial stages the interstitium is often normal, but with progression of the disease fibrosis and lymphocyte

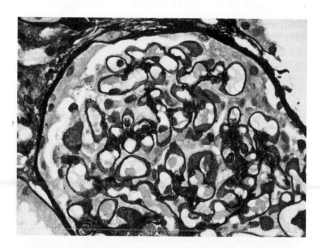

▲ **Figure 26–1.** Membranous nephropathy (stage II). Thicken the glomerular basement membarane (GBM) with spikes and remodeling. Silver stain (×800) (Courtesy of Dr. Donna Lager, Department of Pathology, Mayo Clinic, Rochester, MN.)

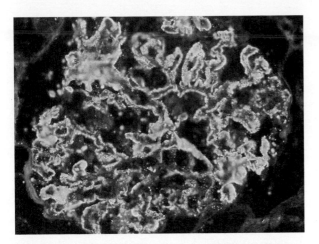

▲ **Figure 26–2.** Immunofluorescence staining showing intense diffuse finely granular IgG deposition along glomerular capillary walls (×600). (Courtesy of Dr. Donna Lager, Department of Pathology, Mayo Clinic, Rochester, MN.)

infiltrates are present. Immunofluorescence microscopy shows a very characteristic and uniform deposition of IgG and C3 in a granular pattern along the epithelial side of the GBM (Figure 26–2). IgG (with IgG4 being the predominant IgG subclass) is present in >95% of cases, but C3 may be seen in only 30–50% of cases of idiopathic MN. It has been suggested that positive C3 staining represents active, ongoing

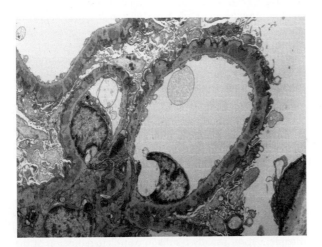

▲ **Figure 26–3.** Electron micrograph showing regularly distributed subepithelial deposits with well-developed glomerular basement membarane (GBM) spikes and marked foot process effacement (×9600). (Courtesy of Dr. Donna Lager, Department of Pathology, Mayo Clinic, Rochester, MN.)

immune deposit formation and complement activation at the time biopsy was performed, whereas the absence of C3 reflects cessation of the immunopathologic process. Electron microscopy demonstrates that the typical electron-dense deposits are localized in the subepithelial space together with effacement of the foot processes (Figure 26–3). Deposits usually have a synchronous, homogeneous electron-dense appearance, but a heterogeneous type with dense deposits at various stages of formation can also be found. A four-stage (I–IV; Table 26–2) classification system has been developed based on their specific localization. Unfortunately the clinical and laboratory correlation with these stages is poor.

Secondary forms on MN have histologic features similar to idiopathic MN. However, the presence of deposits of immunoglobulins other then IgG (ie, IgA and IgM), particularly in the mesangium, small subendothelial deposits, tubular basement membrane deposits, and intense C1q deposition are more suggestive of membranous nephropathy secondary to SLE, hepatitis B, or drugs (gold, D-penicillamine).

▶ Clinical Findings

The disease affects patients of all ages and races, but is more common in men than women by about a 3:1 ratio. Idiopathic MN is most often diagnosed in middle age, with the peak incidence during the fourth and fifth decades of life, and is relatively uncommon in patients under 20 years. At presentation 60–70% of patients will have the nephrotic syndrome (NS) and its associated features: edema, hypoalbuminemia, and hyperlipidemia. The remaining 30–40% of patients present with subnephrotic range proteinuria (<3.5 g/24 hours), most commonly found at the time of routine examination in an otherwise asymptomatic patient. Proteinuria is nonselective. The presence of microscopic hematuria is common

Table 26–2. Clinical features.[1]

Rare in children: <5% of total cases of NS
Common in adults: 15–50% of total cases of NS, depending on age; increasing frequency after age 40 years
Males > females in all adults groups
Whites > Asians > African-Americans > Hispanics
NS in 60–70%
Normal or mildly elevated BP at presentation
"Benign" urinary sediment
Nonselective proteinuria
Tendency to thromboembolic disease (DVT, RVT, PE)

[1]Secondary causes are covered more extensively in Table 26–1. NS, nephrotic syndrome; BP, blood pressure; DVT, deep venous thrombosis; RVT, renal vein thrombosis; PE, pulmonary embolism.

Table 26–3. The Ehrenreich and Churg "staging" of glomerular morphology in membranous nephropathy.[1]

Stage I or early stage: Light microscopy shows a normal glomeruli or slightly thickened capillary walls. There is no evidence of "spike-like" projections or only very scattered. Few and small, superficially placed, subepithelial electron-dense deposits on EM. Fusion of foot processes in the region of the deposits.

Stage II or fully developed lesion: Diffuse, uniform thickening of capillary walls on light microscopy. Prominent, "spike-like" projections along the GBM. Numerous, larger, and more confluent deposits cover the entire capillary loop on EM.

Stage III or advanced lesion: Highly irregular and thickened capillary walls ("moth-eaten" appearance). EM shows deposits (electron dense and lucent) have been encircled by the GBM ("domes") and become intramembranous.

Stage IV or late stage: Deposits become more lucent or absent, and fewer in numbers with numerous electron-lucent vacuolated areas seen within a markedly thickened GBM ("swiss cheese"). Glomerular collapse and fibrosis are found on light microscopy.

[1]The stages are based on the sequence of events observed primarily by electron microscopy. The extent to which individual patients will exhibit these sequential stages will vary according to the duration and the severity of the pathologic process. EM, electron microscopy; GBM, glomerular basement membrane.

(30–40%), but macroscopic hematuria and red cell casts are rare and suggest a different histopathology. In patients with idiopathic MN serum C3 and C4 complement levels are always normal. At the time of diagnosis, the majority of patients are normotensive; only 10–20% are hypertensive. Renal function is normal in the majority of patients at presentation, with only a small fraction (<10%) exhibiting renal insufficiency (Table 26–3) Additional complications related to the disease include a variety of abnormalities in the lipid profile, which probably contribute to the increased cardiovascular risk seen in these patients, and a high prevalence of thromboembolic events including renal vein thrombosis in 10–40% of patients.

▶ Differential Diagnosis

The differential diagnosis includes other causes of NS such as minimal change disease, focal segmental glomerulosclerosis, membranoproliferative glomerulonephritis type I and II, amyloidosis, light chain deposition disease, and diabetic nephropathy. It is important to exclude secondary causes of MN, particularly, hepatitis B, SLE, malignancy, and drugs. In patients less than 16 years of age secondary MN is most commonly due to viral infection or SLE, while in adults >60 years, secondary MN is usually due to malignancy or drugs (Table 26–4). In patients with MN, ruling out secondary causes, apart from a thorough history and physical examination, should involve appropriate laboratory evaluation including

Table 26–4. Secondary causes of membranous nephropathy according to age.

	Children <16 Years	Adults >60 Years
SLE[1]	27%	1%
Viral infection	53%	2%
Neoplasia	<1%	54%
Drugs	3%	38%
Other	17%	5%

[1]SLE, systemic lupus erythematosus.

complement profile, hepatitis serology, antinuclear antibodies, a chest x-ray, testing for occult blood in the stools, a mammogram in women, and prostate-specific antigen testing in men.

In a biopsy series from patients with SLE, MN histology accounts for 8–27% of cases of lupus nephritis. Patients with "pure" membranous lupus nephropathy often have no clinical symptoms that could suggest SLE and serologic markers of lupus activity, such as serum complement and anti-dsDNA levels, are frequently normal and do not correlate with disease activity. Hepatitis B-associated MN occurs frequently in hepatitis B- prevalent areas of the world and affects both adults and children who are chronic carriers of hepatitis B virus [positive hepatitis B surface antigen (HbsAg), hepatitis B core antigen (HbcAg), and usually hepatitis B early antigen (HBeAg)], with or without a history of overt liver disease. In children with hepatitis B-associated MN the nephrotic syndrome usually has a benign course, but progressive renal insufficiency is common in adults.

Hypocomplementemia is present in approximately 50% of the reported cases. Solid tumors (eg, carcinoma of the lung, colon, or kidney) are the most common underlying malignancy involved in cases of tumor-induced MN. It is hypothesized that antigen(s) derived from the tumor are deposited in the glomeruli where they trigger an antibody response and activation of the complement cascade, leading to disruption of the GBM integrity and podocyte injury. In some patients proteinuria resolves with removal or adequate treatment of the tumor. There are, however, well-described cases in which no improvement or remission of the proteinuria occurred following removal of the tumor.

In cases of MN secondary to drugs, discontinuation of the offending agent usually results in complete remission of the nephrotic syndrome. Although resolution of the proteinuria may occur as early as 1 week following discontinuation of the offending drug (eg, NSAIDs), it is not unusual for proteinuria to persist and in certain types associated with the use of gold or D-penicillamine it may take up to 3 years for remission of the proteinuria to occur (mean: 9–12 months). A number of glomerular pathologies have been reported to occur in association with or superimposed upon MN. Such diseases include IgA nephropathy, focal and segmental glomerulosclerosis, crescentic glomerulonephritis (anti-GBM disease, ANCA vasculitis), acute interstitial nephritis, and diabetic nephropathy. In some diabetic patients, MN is thought to occur as a consequence of the development of antiporcine insulin antibodies against porcine insulin deposited along the GBM.

► Complications

The clinical course is characterized by great variability in the rate of disease progression. Even the natural course is difficult to assess, in part due to the criteria used by the local nephrologists to select patients for biopsy. Historically, spontaneous remissions occur in up to 30% of cases, but this percentage is much lower when patients are selected with higher grades of proteinuria at presentation, eg, proteinuria >8 g/24 hours. In untreated patients the reported 10-year kidney survival has varied from 50% to 70%, although many of these studies have included patients with proteinuria <3.5 g/24 hours producing a bias for a more favorable prognosis. For example, a 72% renal survival at 8 years for 100 untreated patients with MN has been reported. However, 37% of patients were nonnephrotic (proteinuria <3.5 g/day) and in 56% of patients proteinuria was <5 g/day. Furthermore, the median follow-up was 39 months and deaths were excluded from the analysis. Even when these exceptions and the "benign" characteristics of the patients are taken into consideration, 25% reached end-stage renal disease (ESRD) at the end of 8 years. In the majority of the more severely affected patients, the disease progresses, albeit slowly, with up to 40–60% of patients eventually developing ESRD over a 15–20-year span. However, because of its high incidence rate, MN remains the second or third leading cause of ESRD among the primary types glomerulonephritis. Cardiovascular and thromboembolic events are increased in this population, especially in patients who remain nephrotic. When loss of renal function occurs more quickly than expected or there is an unexpected acceleration of the disease, a superimposed condition (eg, interstitial nephritis, anti-GBM disease, renal vein thrombosis) should be considered.

A. Predictors of Poor Outcome

An accurate predictor of outcome of patients with idiopathic MN would allow more specific targeting of immunosuppressive treatment to those who are at high risk of developing ESRD. However, finding useful markers that predict this group has been difficult. Both age and gender influence outcome, with male sex and increasing age associated with a higher risk for renal failure. As well, the degrees of glomerulosclerosis, tubulointerstitial fibrosis, and vascular disease seen on renal biopsy have all been associated with a poor prognosis. More recently, the percent of glomeruli with focal segmental sclerosis and the configuration of the immune deposits (synchronic/single stage or heterogeneous/multistage) on electron microscopy have been suggested to be predictors of both outcome and treatment response. Neither of these last two indicators has been validated in prospective studies. The degree of renal impairment (creatinine clearance) at presentation is also correlated with long-term renal survival. However, renal function at presentation is widely variable and may be independent of disease severity. A better and more sensitive predictor of long-term prognosis is the ongoing rate of renal function loss as measured by the decline of creatinine clearance over time.

Thus far, the best model for the identification of patients at risk was developed with data derived from the Toronto Glomerulonephritis Registry. This model takes into consideration the initial creatinine clearance, the slope of the creatinine clearance, and the lowest level of proteinuria during a 6-month observation period. This risk score assessment has good performance characteristics and to date is the only one validated in two geographically diverse MN populations, one from Italy and the other from Finland. In the validity data sets the sensitivity of the model varied from 60% to 89%, the specificity from 86% to 92%, and the overall accuracy from 79% to 87%. Based on data using this model, patients who present with a normal creatinine clearance, proteinuria ≤4 g/24 hours, and stable renal function over a 6-month observation period have an excellent long-term prognosis, and conservative treatment only is recommended. Since even in this group the natural history may rarely include worsening of renal function, these patients need to continue to be monitored. Patients whose creatinine clearance remains unchanged during 6 months of observation, but continue to have proteinuria >4 g but <8 g/24 hours, have a 55% probability of developing chronic renal insufficiency and patients with persistent proteinuria >8 g/24 hours, independent of the degree of renal dysfunction, have a 66–80% probability of progression to chronic renal failure within 10 years (Table 26–5).

Most recently, certain levels of elevation of the urinary excretion of α_1-microglobulin, β_2-microglobulin, IgM, and IgG have also been found to be strong predictors of outcome in MN, but these parameters have yet to be validated.

Table 26–5. Risk of progression categories.

Low risk:	Normal serum creatinine and creatinine clearance plus proteinuria <4 g/day over 6 months of observation
Medium risk:	Normal or near normal creatinine clearance and persistent proteinuria ≥4 g/day to ≤8 g/day over 6 months despite maximum conservative treatment
High risk:	Deteriorating renal function and/or persistent proteinuria ≥ 8 g/day in <6 months of observation

B. Relapse after Complete or Partial Remission

About 30% of MN patients will relapse subsequent to a complete remission (CR). The majority who do, however, will relapse only to a subnephrotic range of proteinuria and will have stable long-term function. In the two largest studies of patients with MN who achieved CR, only a few developed, over a long observation period, mild renal insufficiency and none progressed to ESRD. We recently reviewed our data on 350 nephrotic patients with MN and found that the 10-year renal survival was 100% in the CR group, 90% in the partial remission (PR) group, and 45% in the no remission group. Thus, both CR and PR appear to be excellent predictors of long-term renal survival.

▶ Treatment

A. Nonimmunosuppressive Therapy

Conservative management is directed at control of edema, treatment of high blood pressure and hyperlipidemia, dietary protein intake, and reduction of proteinuria through inhibition of the renin–angiotensin system. Blood pressure control is important to protect against the cardiovascular risk of hypertension, to reduce proteinuria, and to slow the progression of the renal disease. In the Modification of Diet in Renal Disease (MDRD) study, patients with proteinuria >1 g/day had a significantly better outcome if their blood pressure was reduced to 125/75 mm Hg. Thus, in patients with proteinuric renal disease, including MN, the current target for blood pressure is ≤125/75 mm Hg.

The selection of an antihypertensive agent has been controversial. Numerous studies have shown that angiotensin-converting enzyme inhibitors (ACEI) and/or angiotensin II receptor blockers (ARBs) are cardioprotective and can reduce proteinuria and slow progression of renal disease in both diabetic and nondiabetic chronic nephropathy patients. These classes of drugs reduce glomerular intracapillary pressure and protein ultrafiltration, improve glomerular barrier size selectivity, and have been shown to be renoprotective in experimental models of renal diseases and in both diabetic and nondiabetic renal disease in humans. A recent meta-analysis of some large renal protection trials with ACEI showed that the degree of protection is related to the degree of reduction of proteinuria; if proteinuria is not lowered, the benefit is substantially attenuated. The most recent data from the RENAAL study shows that the renal protective effect of angiotensin II blockade was nearly fully explained by its antiproteinuric effect. Some studies have attempted to address this issue in patients with MN, but they have been small, with a limited follow-up. In some, the use of ACEI has been associated with a significant improvement in the glomerular filtration barrier in patients with MN, but in others the efficacy of ACEI in reducing proteinuria appears to be modest at best (<30% reduction in proteinuria). In those with a positive outcome the antiproteinuric effect of these agents is almost always

early (within 2 months of initiation of therapy). Patients at low risk for progression (proteinuria <4 g/24 hours) should be treated with ACE ±ARB since this may further reduce their proteinuria and offer additional renal protection with little chance of significant adverse effects. It is worth noting patients need to be instructed to follow a low salt diet since a high salt intake (eg, 200 mm NaCl/day or 4.6 g sodium/day) can significantly impair the beneficial effects of angiotensin II blockade. Therefore, although these drugs should be tried first, achieving CR in patients with proteinuria >5 g/24 hours using conservative treatment with ACEI and/or ARBs alone appears unlikely, even when these are used at their highest recommended dosages.

Dietary protein intake should be restricted to 0.8 g/kg ideal body weight per day of high-quality protein. Although dietary protein restriction may reduce proteinuria (15–25%) and slow the progression of renal disease somewhat, it has never been shown to induce complete remission of the NS. Proteinuria is also an independent risk factor for cardiovascular (CV) morbidity and mortality. Proteinuric patients have elevated cholesterol and triglycerides and markedly elevated CV risk, as illustrated by the almost 6-fold increase in the incidence of myocardial infarction in this population. It is likely that the lipid abnormalities associated with proteinuria are important players in the high CV risk in these patients, and thus provide an important target for treatment.

Statins have been effective in improving the lipid profile and in reducing CV morbidity and mortality in hyperlipidemic and hypertensive patients and in patients with chronic renal failure. These agents are also effective in reducing serum levels of total cholesterol and low-density lipoprotein (LDL)-cholesterol in nephrotic patients and their use is appropriate in patients with hyperlipidemia. Although no study to date has been conducted to demonstrate that reducing cholesterol lowers the risk of CV events in nephrotic patients, the evidence derived from other studies strongly supports this concept. If the proteinuria persists at >3 g/day even these agents may not completely normalize the lipid profile. The adverse risk profile with these agents in the nephrotic syndrome is similar to the normal population with the exception of an increased incidence of rhabdomyolysis when used in conjunction with high-dose cyclosporine. Apart from the proven efficacy of statins in improving the lipid profile, experimental data together with a number of small, controlled trials have suggested that 3-hydroxy-3-methylglutaryl coenzyme A (HMG-CoA) reductase inhibitors have a synergistic antiproteinuric effect when combined with ACEI. The antiproteinuric effect of statins is small, and is mainly observed in patients with nonnephrotic range proteinuria. These results are in stark contrast to the reports indicating that proteinuria (albuminuria) may be a complication of statin treatment. These findings have been corroborated by recent phase III studies showing the development of proteinuria (albuminuria) in some patients with the use of high-dose rosuvastatin.

Renal proximal tubule cells are responsible for the reabsorption of proteins present in the tubular lumen. Receptor-mediated endocytosis is the process that is responsible for albumin uptake in proximal tubular cells, a process that requires prenylated GTP-binding proteins. HMG-CoA reductase inhibitors reduce intracellular levels of isoprenoid pyrophosphates that are required for the prenylation and normal function of GTP-binding proteins. Recent studies have demonstrated that statins, as a class, inhibit protein uptake by tubular cells by reducing prenylation of proteins involved in endocytosis and thus inhibit receptor-mediated endocytosis in both animal and human kidney proximal tubular cell lines. These data may help to explain the occurrence of proteinuria in some patients treated with high statin doses. Patients with severe NS are at increased risk for thromboembolic complications. Prophylactic anticoagulation has been shown to be beneficial in reducing fatal thromboembolic episodes in nephrotic patients with MN without a concomitant increase in the risk of bleeding. Although no consensus has emerged as to whether prophylactic anticoagulation should be used in this disease, the majority of physicians would consider using it for patients at high risk of a thromboembolic event. No laboratory test can help predict which patient is in this high-risk category, although thromboembolic events are more common in patients who are severely nephrotic (proteinuria >10g/day and serum albumin <2.5 g/day). Both heparin and low-molecular-weight heparin reduce proteinuria, but this effect has not been routinely employed in the care of patients with MN.

NSAIDs are antiproteinuric but can cause acute renal failure and should be avoided in patients with kidney disease. However, in severe untreatable nephrotic syndrome, NSAIDs can reduce proteinuria by 30–50%, are additive to the effects of ACEI, and can provide symptomatic relief. The combined use of NSAIDs and ACEI/ARBs should be carefully monitored, especially in elderly patients and in those with hypertension and renal insufficiency. In rats with 5/6 nephrectomy, pentoxifylline, a tumor necrosis factor (TNF)-α-suppressing agent, can prevent progression of proteinuria and renal diseases, possibly by suppression of mitogenic and profibrotic genes. In patients with MN, there is increased production of TNF-α in the glomeruli, and urinary excretion of this cytokine correlates with proteinuria. In a pilot study, 10 patients with MN were treated with pentoxifylline (1200 mg/day) for 6 months. Proteinuria decreased from 11 g/day (range 4.6–27) to 1.8 g/day (0–10.9) ($p = 0.001$), whereas serum albumin concentration increased from 17 g/L to 39 g/L. Complete remission was achieved in five patients. The results are encouraging but are very preliminary.

Lipid peroxidation has been involved in the pathophysiology of proteinuria in Heymann's nephritis model and was the rationale behind using probucol, a lipid peroxidation scavenger, in patients with MN. Treatment with probucol, 1 g/day orally for 3 months, had a modest antiproteinuric effect

[proteinuria 6.4 (3.8–9.1) versus 4.7 (1.3–16) g/day pretreatment versus posttreatment (median, range), respectively]. In Heymann's nephritis model, intraperitoneal injection of immune globulin reduced proteinuria by over 50%, accompanied by a reduction in glomerular C5-9 and C3 staining and urinary C5-9 excretion. In humans, intravenous high-dose immune globulin therapy has been beneficial in the treatment of a number of antibody-mediated diseases including idiopathic thrombocytopenic purpura, IgA nephropathy, and ANCA vasculitis. A multitude of mechanisms are thought to be involved in mediating the therapeutic effects of intravenous immune globulin in immune complex-mediated diseases and involve, among others, the blocking of Fc receptors, antiidiotype inhibition of pathogenic immunoglobulin, and the regulation of the complement cascade by preventing the binding of activated C3 to antibody-coated targets, eg, the glomeruli, thus reducing complement-mediated glomerular injury. In patients with idiopathic MN, a short-term low-dose (100–150 mg/kg/day for 6 consecutive days; total dose 600–900 mg/kg) course of intravenous immune globulin was capable of inducing early remission of the nephrotic syndrome (within 6 months), although the benefit was seen mainly in a subgroup of patients with homogeneous type synchronous electrodense deposits on electron microscopy, and long-term renal outcome was unaffected.

B. Immunosuppressive Therapy

Several treatment strategies, including a variety of immunosuppressive agents, have been shown to be at least partially successful in reducing proteinuria in MN. Many questions about this type of therapy do remain as follows: (1) How long should conservative therapy be extended, and how long should you wait for a spontaneous remission before initiating immunosuppressive therapy, (2) which patients with MN should receive this type of treatment, (3) which of the various drugs available should be used, ie, which are the most effective and safest, and (4) how long should the drug be used before considering it a failure. We will briefly review the available evidence.

1. Corticosteroids—The early U.S. collaborative study of adult idiopathic nephrotic syndrome reported that a 2–3-month course of high-dose alternate-day prednisone (100–150 mg), when compared to placebo, resulted in a significant reduction in the progression to renal failure, although there was no effect on the degree of proteinuria. The short follow-up period of patients and the worse than expected outcome of the control group have raised criticism of the study. Subsequent controlled studies have shown no benefit from the use of corticosteroids on MN. The two largest randomized controlled trials, one by the British Medical Research Trial and the second by the Toronto Glomerulonephritis Study Group, found no significant benefit of corticosteroid treatment alone in either induction of remission or preservation of renal function. Therefore, the evidence to date does not support the widespread use of oral corticosteroids as a single agent for the treatment of MN.

2. Cytotoxic agents combined with corticosteroids—In

patients with a moderate risk of progression, a significant benefit has been described when a cytotoxic agent alternating monthly with corticosteroids has been used. A number of randomized trials suggest that 6 months of this regimen (cyclophosphamide or chlorambucil as the cytotoxic agent) is four to five times more likely to induce a CR of the NS, and halt disease progression, compared to no therapy or corticosteroids alone. The largest studies with the longest observation time come from Ponticelli's group in Italy. The first study compared the effects of combined methylprednisolone (MTP) 1 g intravenously on the first 3 days of month 1, 3, and 5 followed by 27 days of oral methylprednisolone (0.4 mg/kg/day) or prednisone (0.5 mg/kg/day) alternating in months 2, 4, and 6 with chlorambucil at 0.2 mg/kg/day, versus conservative treatment in 62 patients with MN and nephrotic range proteinuria. The 32 patients who received the alkylating agent were followed for a mean of 31.4 ± 18.2 months. CR was achieved in 50% and PR in 31% of the cases. Among the controls, CR was achieved in 7% and PR in 23% of the patients. The regimen was remarkably safe with only four of the treated patients stopping therapy. After up to 10 years of follow-up, patients treated with combination therapy had a 92% probability of renal survival compared with 60% in the control group and only 8% of treated patients versus 40% of untreated ones had reached ESRD. In addition, the slope of the reciprocal of serum creatinine remained significantly slower in the treated group than in the untreated controls for up to 90 months. In terms of proteinuria, only 42% of the treated group, versus 78% of the placebo group, spent time in a nephrotic state over the 10-year follow-up. Women and patients with mild glomerular lesions (stage I and II) were more likely to enter remission after combined therapy in this study, and no patients had significantly impaired renal function at entry.

A second study compared 6 months of alternating monthly pulses of MTP (1 g), oral steroids, and chlorambucil as described above versus MTP pulses and steroids (0.4 mg/kg every other day) alone found that at 3 years, 66% of the patients given steroids and chlorambucil versus 42% of the patients given steroids alone were in remission, the difference being significant. At 4 years, however, this difference was no longer statistically significant, although a seemingly large 20% difference favoring the combined treatment still persisted. Combined therapy was also associated with a trend toward better preservation of renal function, as assessed by serum creatinine, although again the difference was not statistically significant.

In a third study from the same group, patients were enrolled in a 6-month study comparing MTP/prednisone alternating with chlorambucil (same doses as the prior studies)

to MTP alternating with oral cyclophosphamide (2.5 mg/kg/day). Among 87 nephrotic patients followed for at least 1 year, 82% of patients assigned to MTP and chlorambucil had complete or partial remission of the NS versus 93% of patients assigned to MTP and cyclophosphamide ($p = 0.116$, NS). The use of cyclophosphamide was associated with fewer side effects, but renal function was equally preserved in both groups for up to 3 years. However, a relapse rate in both treated groups of 25–30% was seen within 2 years. The incidence of CR 1 year following combined immunosuppressive treatment was approximately 28% in the first study, 20% in the second study, and 32% in the third study. In addition, these studies excluded all patients whose serum creatinine exceeded 1.7 mg/dL at entry.

More recently, in an uncontrolled trial, 39 patients with severe NS (proteinuria 8.9 ± 3.6 g/24 hours) and increased serum creatinine at entry (>1.5 mg/dL; creatinine clearance <60 mL/minute) were treated with chlorambucil (0.15 mg/kg/day) for 14 weeks plus oral prednisone 1 mg/kg tapered to 0.5 mg/kg/every other day over a 6-month period and were compared to a similarly affected historical control group from the 1970s. After 4 years of follow-up, there was a 90% probability of renal survival without dialysis in those who received treatment compared with only a 55% probability in those receiving conservative treatment. After 7 years, the renal survival was 90% and 20%, respectively.

These observations have been recently confirmed by Jha et al. who reported the 10-year follow-up of a randomized, controlled trial on 93 patients allocated to either conservative therapy or to receive a 6-month course of alternating prednisolone and cyclophosphamide. Proteinuria was 5.9 ± 2.2 and 6.1 ± 2.5 g/24 hour in the conservative and immunosuppressive therapy group, respectively. Renal function was well preserved with estimated GFR rates above 80 mL/minute in both groups. Of the 47 patients treated with immunosuppressive therapy, 34 achieved remission (15 C and 19 PR), compared with 16 (5 C, 11 PR) of 46 in the control group ($p < 0.0001$). The 10-year dialysis-free survival was 89 and 65% ($p = 0.016$), and the likelihood of survival without death, dialysis, and doubling of serum creatinine was 79% in the treated versus 44% ($p = 0.0006$) in the control group. The incidence of infections was similar in the two groups.

A recent meta-analysis of the available literature showed that the use of alkylating agents was associated with higher rates of remission (PR or CR), but there was no statistical difference when compared to placebo in ESRD or the death rate. Results of a meta-analysis need to be viewed with caution, since this technique is not a substitute for a well-designed randomized control trial of adequate size.

A number of uncontrolled studies have examined the effects of chlorambucil or cyclophosphamide on the outcome of MN in patients with advanced disease (serum creatinine >1.8 mg/dL). In one study eight patients with deteriorating renal function were treated with a modified Ponticelli's protocol using a lower chlorambucil dose (0.15 mg/kg/day) alternating monthly with cycles of prednisone. Proteinuria was reduced in all patients; creatinine clearance increased in six patients and the rate of renal function decline was reduced in the other two patients. However, adverse effects of chlorambucil were severe and patients with severe renal insufficiency (serum creatinine >3 mg/dL) had progressive deterioration in function.

Similarly, in another study 21 patients with heavy proteinuria and progressive renal failure (creatinine 2.0–5.4 mg/dL) were treated with alternating monthly cycles of prednisolone (125 mg on alternate days given in months 1, 3, and 5) and chlorambucil (10 mg/day in months 2, 4 and 6). In addition, nine patients received at least one course of three intravenous pulses of 1 g MTP at the start of the first cycle of treatment. After a mean period of follow-up of 39 months, three patients had died, six patients were on dialysis or had a serum creatinine ≥5.7 mg/dL, and one patient had progressive renal failure. Eleven patients had either stable or improved renal function, as judged by serum creatinine concentration. Treatment was associated with a high incidence of side effects, with significant complications related to drug therapy observed in >50% of subjects.

In an uncontrolled study, 32 high-risk patients were treated with monthly pulses of MTP (1 g intravenously on 3 consecutive days) followed by oral prednisone (0.5 mg/kg/day in months 1, 3, and 5) and chlorambucil (0.15 mg/kg/day in months 2, 4, and 6) ($n = 15$) or oral cyclophosphamide (1.5–2.0 mg/kg/day for 12 months) and steroids in a comparable dose ($n = 17$). All patients had evidence of deterioration of renal function prior to the start of therapy; serum creatinine was 2.5 ± 0.8 in the chlorambucil group and 3.0 ± 1.4 mg/dL in the cyclophosphamide group. Treatment resulted in rapid improvement in renal function in both groups (serum creatinine 1.9 ± 0.7 mg/dL in both groups at 6 months) but the improvement was short-lived in the chlorambucil group. At 6 months, there was a significant decrease in proteinuria in both groups, but again, the decrease was persistent only in the cyclophosphamide group (chlorambucil group 9.1 ± 2.6 g/day versus 6.8 ± 4.4 g/day and cyclophosphamide group 11.2 ± 5.3 g/day versus 2.0 ± 3.0 g/day at months 0 and 12, respectively). Overall, a partial remission of proteinuria was observed in five (33%) patients after chlorambucil treatment and in 15 (92%) patients after cyclophosphamide treatment ($p < 0.01$). Of these latter patients, six had complete remission, whereas none of the chlorambucil-treated patients did. Adverse effects were common and treatment had to be reduced, temporarily interrupted, or prematurely stopped in 6 of 17 cyclophosphamide-treated patients and in 11 of 15 chlorambucil-treated patients.

In contrast, in the only randomized study of patients at high risk of progression (mean creatinine 2.3–2.7 mg/day; proteinuria 11.1–12.5 g/day), 13 patients were assigned to monthly pulse cyclophosphamide combined with oral prednisone for 6 months and were compared to 13 patients treated with prednisone alone for the same period of time. At the

end of follow-up, there were no statistical differences regarding degree of proteinuria, frequency of remissions, or rate of decline of renal function between the steroid-alone and the combined-treatment group. Other small uncontrolled studies using cyclophosphamide alone have found similar results. These results clearly differ from those discussed above. One possible explanation is that daily cyclophosphamide is more effective than cyclophosphamide used in monthly intravenous pulses.

To address the long-term efficacy of cytotoxic therapy in these patients, 65 patients with MN and serum creatinine >1.5 mg/dL who were treated with oral cyclophosphamide (1.5–2.0 mg/kg/day for 12 months) and steroids (MTP pulses of 3 × 1 g intravenously at months 1, 3, and 5, and oral prednisone 0.5 mg/kg on alternate days for 6 months) were prospectively studied. Follow-up was 51 (5–132) months. Renal function improved or stabilized in all patients. Overall renal survival was 86% after 5 years and 74% after 7 years. A PR occurred in 56 patients followed by a CR in 17 patients. However, 11 patients had a relapse (28% relapse rate at 5 years), of whom 9 were retreated because of deteriorating renal function. Treatment-related complications occurred in two-thirds of patients, mainly consisting of bone marrow suppression and infections.

Thus, in a number of studies, both cyclophosphamide and chlorambucil in combination with corticosteroids appear to be effective in the treatment of patients with idiopathic MN and preserved renal function. This combination may also be effective in those with deteriorating renal function, but the supporting data are much less compelling, adverse effects are higher, and the likelihood of benefit is reduced in patients with severe renal failure (serum creatinine >3 mg/dL). The favorable effects are maintained well beyond the 1-year treatment period but relapse rates approached 35% at 2 years.

The adverse effects of cyclophosphamide when used long term are the major drawbacks to the universal application of this form of therapy. These include increased susceptibility to infections, anemia, thrombocytopenia, nausea, vomiting, sterility, and in the long-term secondary malignancy, in particular bladder cancer. In regard to chlorambucil, the major concern is the possibility of inducing acute leukemia or lymphoma. Even when chlorambucil was used in modified versions (lower doses) of the Italian regimen, the rate of adverse effects was high.

3. Cyclosporine—Early uncontrolled studies of cyclosporine suggested an initial benefit but a high relapse rate. In a recent single blind randomized controlled study, 51 patients with steroid-resistant MN were treated with low-dose prednisone plus cyclosporine A (CsA) compared to placebo plus prednisone. CsA was given at 3.5 mg/kg/day with a target whole-blood trough level of 125–225 ng/mL. All patients received prednisone at 0.15 mg/kg/day (up to a maximum of 15 mg/day). At the end of treatment at 26 weeks, 75% (21 of 28 patients) in the CsA group versus only 22% (5 of 23 patients) of controls had achieved a PR or CR (CR = 2 in the CsA group versus 1 in the placebo group). CsA was well tolerated, and no one had to discontinue treatment because of adverse effects. Relapses occurred in ~40% of patients within 1 year of discontinuation of CsA treatment, not dissimilar to what was found in controlled cytotoxic/corticosteroid regimens. There has been only one randomized controlled trial using CsA in patients with high-grade proteinuria and progressive renal failure, again conducted by the Toronto group. In this study, 64 patients were placed on a restricted protein diet (<0.9 g/kg) and followed for 12 months (phase 1). Seventeen patients with a loss in creatinine clearance of ≥8 mL/minute/year (but with creatinine clearance ≥30 mL/minute) and proteinuria ≥3.5 g/24 hours were randomly assigned to either CsA treatment (3.5 mg/kg/day; nine patients) or placebo (eight patients) for 12 months (phase 2). After 12 months, there was a significant reduction in proteinuria and in the rate of loss of renal function in the CsA group compared with the group that received placebo. In the CsA group, the slope of creatinine clearance was reduced from −2.4 to −0.7 mL/minute/month, whereas in the placebo group the change was insignificant, −2.2 to −2.1 mL/minute/month ($p < 0.02$). This improvement was sustained in ~50% of the patients for up to 2 years after CsA was stopped.

That prolonging the treatment results in a higher and more sustained rate of remission is supported by data from the German Cyclosporine in Nephrotic Syndrome Study Group. In this study, 41 high-risk patients with MN and proteinuria >3.5 g/24 hours (mean 10.9 ± 5.7 g/24 hours) were treated with CsA (average dose = 3.3 ± 1.1 mg/kg/day) for a median of 353 days (159–586 days). Approximately 65% of the patients also received ACEI plus corticosteroid treatment (~27.5 ± 21.2 mg/day). CR (proteinuria <0.5 g/24 hours) was achieved in 34% of the patients. The median treatment time to CR was 225 days (quartiles 120 days and 459 days). Taken together, these data would suggest that CsA will induce a remission (CR or PR) of the NS in 50–60% of patients. It is important to emphasize that although reduction of proteinuria usually occurs within a few weeks, the majority of CR occurred after more then 6 months of treatment. This would suggest that if urinary protein excretion is not significantly reduced within 3–4 months of initiating therapy it is unlikely that more prolonged therapy will result in a remission. This is an important observation and may explain why studies in which CsA was used for less then 6 months achieved low rates of CR whereas studies using CsA for up to 1 year, albeit uncontrolled, reported remission rates close to 80%. However, significant adverse effects including hypertension, gingival hyperplasia, gastrointestinal complaints, muscle cramps, and most important nephrotoxicity can accompany prolonged CsA treatment. The latter is dose/duration dependent as well as age dependent. Patients at particular risk are those with initial impaired renal function, especially if accompanied by chronic vascular plus or minus tubulointerstitial damage on renal biopsy. On the other hand, prolonged low-dose CsA

(~1.5 mg/kg/day) could be considered for long-term maintenance of patients with preserved renal function who achieve a CR or PR, but then relapse once CsA is discontinued, with little risk of nephrotoxicity.

4. Tacrolimus—Tacrolimus is a calcineurin inhibitor similar to CsA, but it is 50–100 times more potent as an immunosuppressive agent, on a molar basis, than CsA at suppressing lymphocyte proliferation *in vitro* and graft rejection *in vivo*. In animal models, pretreatment with tacrolimus prevented the development of experimental MN and significantly reduced urinary protein excretion in animals with established MN. The relevance of these data to human membranous nephropathy is unknown and data on the use of tacrolimus to treat human glomerulonephritis are limited. We have treated 10 patients with MN and proteinuria >5 g/24 hours with at least a 6-month course of tacrolimus monotherapy. Proteinuria decreased to subnephrotic levels in the majority of patients, but no patient achieved CR of the NS (unpublished observations).

A recent study by Praga et al. evaluated tacrolimus monotherapy in MN. In this study 25 patients with normal renal function (mean proteinuria ~8g/24h), received tacrolimus (TAC; 0.05 mg/kg/day) over 12 months with a 6-month taper, whereas 23 patients served as control. After 18 months, the probability of remission was 94% in the tacrolimus group but only 35% in the control group. Six patients in the control group and only one in the tacrolimus group reached the secondary end point of a 50% increase in their serum creatinine. Unfortunately, almost half of the patients relapsed after tacrolimus was withdrawn, and similar to patients treated with CsA, maintenance of remission may require prolonged use of tacrolimus in low doses.

5. Mycophenolate mofetil—Mycophenolate mofetil (MMF) has been used as an effective antirejection agent in solid organ transplants for >10 years. It is metabolized to mycophenolic acid, the active immunosuppressant compound, and selectively inhibits T- and B-lymphocyte proliferation through inhibition of *de novo* purine synthesis and inactivation of inosine monophosphate dehydrogenase. Mycophenolate mofetil directly suppresses the synthesis of antibodies by B cells and the generation of cytotoxic T cells, and decreases the expression of adhesion molecules on lymphocytes, thus impairing the ability of activated lymphocytes to bind to endothelial cells. The latter effect may reduce the influx of inflammatory cells into glomeruli after deposition of antibody. It does not share azathioprine's profile in regard to myelotoxicity, hepatotoxicity, and mutagenesis. Unlike cyclosporin A or tacrolimus, MMF is not nephrotoxic. Recognized side effects include nausea, vomiting, diarrhea, abdominal pain, anemia, and leukopenia. As with any immunosuppressive agent, patients on MMF are at risk of infections.

There has been a paucity of studies using MMF in MN. In a pilot study, 16 patients were treated with MMF, 1.5–2 g/day, for a mean of 8 months. These patients would be categorized as either medium or high risk for progression given the severity of their proteinuria and the fact that they had previously not responded to a variety of other immunosuppressive drugs. The results were modest: Six patients had a ≥50% reduction in their proteinuria, two had a minor reduction in proteinuria, four had no change, three were withdrawn because of significant adverse effects, and one stopped treatment on his own. There were no significant changes in mean serum creatinine, or serum albumin levels, over the course of the study. In patients who responded, the lowest degree of proteinuria was reached within 6 months, suggesting that patients who are likely to respond would do so in this time frame. This was a pilot study, and is somewhat difficult to interpret as negative or positive, given the setting of resistance to all other agents.

Similar results were reported in a retrospective analysis of 17 patients with MN (15 patients had nephrotic range proteinuria and 6 had renal insufficiency). Patients were either steroid dependent, steroid resistant, or steroid intolerant, with or without CsA, or had been resistant or had a suboptimal response to CsA, or had signs of progressive renal failure. Overall, there was a 61% reduction of proteinuria (7.8–2.3 g/24 hours; $p = 0.001$), with eight patients having a PR and two patients a CR. This group of MN patients was much more heterogeneous in terms of either a prior response to therapy or drug dependency before the initiation of MMF treatment.

More recently, Branten et al. reported on 32 patients with MN and renal insufficiency (serum creatinine >1.5 mg/dL) treated with MMF (1g twice daily) for 12 months and compared with results obtained on 32 patients from a historic control group treated for the same period of time with oral CYC (1.5 mg/kg/day). Both groups received high dose steroid treatment (MTP IV 1g × 3 on months 1, 3, and 5 followed by oral prednisone 0.5 mg/kg every other day for 6 months, with subsequent tapering). Overall, 21 MMF-treated patients developed PR of proteinuria; in 6 patients, proteinuria decreased by at least 50%, and no response was observed in five patients. Cumulative incidences of remission of proteinuria at 12 months were 66% in the MMF group versus 72% in the CYC group ($p = 0.3$). Side effects occurred at a similar rate between the two groups but relapses were much more common in the MMF treated group.

6. Rituximab—There is convincing evidence from both experimental and human studies that MN is mediated by the deposition of IgG antibodies in the subepithelial aspect of the GBM. Given the key role of IgG antibodies in MN, it is reasonable to postulate that suppression of antibody production by depleting B cells and/or plasma cells may improve or even resolve the glomerular pathology. Rituximab is a genetically engineered, chimeric, murine/human IgG$_1$κ monoclonal antibody against the CD20 antigen found on the surface of normal and malignant pre-B and mature B cells, but not expressed on hematopoietic stem cells, pro-B cells, normal plasma cells, or other normal tissues. The Food and Drug Administration approved it in 1997 for the treatment of relapsed or refractory low-grade or follicular, CD20$^+$, B cell non-Hodgkin's lymphoma. In a pilot study using rituximab in idiopathic MN, eight nephrotic patients with MN were prospectively treated with a 4 weekly course of Rituxan (375 mg/m^2) and followed for 1 year. All patients had complete depletion of circulating B cells lasting up to 1 year. Proteinuria significantly decreased from a mean ± SD of 8.6 ± 4.2 g at baseline to 4.3 ± 3.3 g (−51%, $p < 0.005$) at 3 months, 4.0 ± 3.1 g (−53%, $p < 0.005$) at 6 months, and to 3.0 ± 2.5 g (−66%, $p < 0.005$) at 12 months. At 12 months, proteinuria decreased to <0.5 g/24 hours in two patients and <3.5 g/24 hours in three other patients. Proteinuria decreased in the remaining patients by 74%, 44%, and 41%, respectively. Renal function remained stable in all patients. Adverse effects were reported as mild and included chills and fever in one patient and an anaphylactic reaction in another patient. This pilot study, although encouraging, needs to be confirmed by other studies before recommendations can be made regarding its use.

We recently conducted a prospective open-label pilot trial in 15 newly biopsied patients (<3 years) with IMN and proteinuria >4 g/24 hours despite ACEi/ARB use for >3 months and systolic BP <130 mm Hg. Thirteen males and 2 females, median age 47 (range 33–63), with a mean serum creatinine of 1.4 ± 0.5 mg/dL were treated with rituximab (1 g) on day 1 and 15. At six months, patients who remain with proteinuria >3 g/24 hours and in whom total CD19+ B cell count was >15 cells/μL received a second identical course of rituximab. All patients tolerated rituximab well, and achieved swift B lymphocyte depletion by day 28. Baseline proteinuria of 13.0 ± 5.7 g/24 hours (range 8.4–23.5) decreased to 9.1 ± 7.4 g, 9.3 ± 7.9 g, 7.2 ± 6.2 g and 6.0 ± 7.0 g/24 hours (range 0.2–20) at 3, 6, 9 and 12 months, respectively (mean ± SD). Fourteen patients completed a 12 months follow-up: complete remission (proteinuria <0.3 g/24 hours) was achieved in 2 patients, partial remission (<3 g/24 hours) in 6 patients, and 5 patients did not respond. Two patients progressed to ESRD. The mean drop in proteinuria from baseline to 12 months was 6.2 ± 5.1 g and was statistically significant ($p = 0.002$, paired t-test). Rituximab was well tolerated, and was effective in reducing proteinuria in patients with IMN. However, the responses varied widely among patients and further research is needed in order to identify a priori which patient is likely to benefit from rituximab treatment. A recent study has also shown that a single dose of rituximab is also effective in inducing remission in some patients. We are currently conducting a new study of 20 patients with MN being treated with rituximab (375 mg/m^2) weekly for 4 weeks where we have incorporated a number of mechanistic studies to see if we can predict response in these patients.

7. Eculizumab—The proinflammatory activities of the activated terminal complement components C5a and C5b-9 have been implicated in a wide range of inflammatory disease states including contributing to the glomerular injury in MN. Finding the C5b-9 membrane attack complex within the immune deposits and recognizing that experimental depletion of complement by cobra venom serum prevents subsequent proteinuria confirm the role of complement in the pathogenesis of MN. Eculizumab is a new, humanized anti-C5 monoclonal antibody designed to prevent the cleavage of C5 into its proinflammatory byproducts. In a recent randomized controlled trial (currently reported in abstract form only), 200 patients with MN were treated every 2 weeks with two different intravenous dose regimens and compared to a placebo group over a total of 16 weeks. Neither of the active drug regimens of eculizumab showed any significant effect on proteinuria or renal function when compared to placebo. It was later determined that adequate inhibition of C5 was seen in only a small percentage of patients, suggesting that the doses given were inadequate. More encouraging results were seen in a continuation of the original study in which eculizumab was used for up to 1 year, with a significant reduction in proteinuria in some patients (including two patients who went into complete remission). Whether complement inhibition with higher doses of eculizumab will prove to be more effective, as well as safe, in the treatment of MN remains a question for the future.

▶ Prognosis

Idiopathic MN is a glomerular disease usually of abrupt onset and is associated with the NS. Control of the NS, specifically a CR or PR, is clearly associated with prolonged renal survival and a slower rate of progression of renal disease. There are no standard or universal first-line specific therapeutic options for idiopathic MN. Supportive or conservative care should be given in all cases and should include the use of diuretics and antihypertensive (and potentially renal protective) agents such as ACEI and ARB therapy and lipid-lowering agents. In patients who are at low risk of progression, defined by normal renal function and proteinuria ≤4 g/day over a 6-month observation period, a conservative approach should suffice, given their excellent prognosis (<5% risk for progression over 5 years of observation). These patients need to be followed long term to ensure that there is no disease progression.

Patients at medium risk of progression, defined by normal renal function and persistent proteinuria between 4 and 8 g/day over a 6-month observation period despite maximum conservative treatment, or at high risk of progression, defined by deteriorating renal function and/or

by persistent high-grade proteinuria ≥8 g/day during the 6 months of observation, are candidates for immunosuppressive therapy. It is worth emphasizing that patients with persistent nephrotic range proteinuria exhibit marked abnormalities in their lipid profile and are at increased risk for CV complications. Proteinuria is a marker for predicting CV risk as demonstrated by data from the Framingham study showing that proteinuria predicts CV outcome. Data from recent studies (eg, LIFE and the AASK trials) show that CV risk increases with each increase in the level of proteinuria, making the link between chronic renal disease and cardiac disease so strong that few patients develop chronic kidney disease without clinically apparent or occult cardiac disease. The hypothesis that proteinuria is not only an indicator but is an inducer of kidney injury is supported by a number of studies showing that proteinuria plays a major role in the development of progressive tubular injury, interstitial fibrosis, and subsequent loss in GFR. There is overwhelming clinical evidence that higher sustained levels of proteinuria predict more rapid decline in renal function, more pronounced tubulointerstitial injury, and eventual kidney failure. Nephrotic patients are also at risk for thromboembolic events, with an incidence as high as 50% in patients with severe MN being reported. These events are associated with a mortality rate as high as 42% in high-risk patients.

These data emphasize that these life-defining events, in addition to the potential renal failure, are common in these patients. Therefore, even if the main benefit of immunosuppressive therapy is to speed up the induction of a remission that may have occurred spontaneously, it may still have value in the long term. A treatment algorithm that combines the predictive factors and best evidence for immunosuppressive therapy is presented in Figure 26–4. The recommendation to use cytotoxic/steroid or cyclosporine as the first line of therapy in the moderate or high-risk group is based on evidence from trials conducted in patients in these respective categories, but physicians must take into account individual patients and their wishes in order to decide which therapy should be initiated. These routines are not mutually exclusive and may follow sequentially (with a drug holiday) if the first one chosen does not succeed in reducing the proteinuria to the desired range and/or adverse side effects make completion of a course of therapy untenable. Patients who do not respond well or relapse after a first course of immunosuppression therapy may benefit from a second course of immunosuppression.

Preliminary evidence on the use of anti-CD20 antibodies suggests this is another agent that may be as effective, and safer, than our current regimens, but it needs to be assessed further before being widely recommended. Patients with severe renal insufficiency (serum creatinine ≥3 mg/dL) are less likely to benefit from immunosuppression therapy and the risk of treatment is significantly higher. These patients should be considered for conservative therapy only and plans should be made for transplantation in the future.

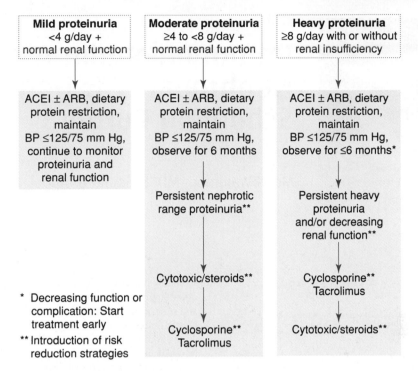

▲ **Figure 26–4.** MN treatment algorithm for membranous nephropathy.
ACEI, angiotensin-converting enzyme inhibitor; ARB, angiotensin receptor blocker; BP, blood pressure.

Autin HA, Illei GG: Membranous lupus nephritis. Lupus 2005;14:65.

Alexopoulos E et al: Induction and long-term treatment with cyclosporine in membranous nephropathy with the nephrotic syndrome. Nephrol Dial Transplant 2006;21:3127–3132.

Autin HA, Illei GG: Membranous lupus nephritis. Lupus 2005;14:65.

Branten AJ et al: Urinary excretion of beta2-microglobulin and IgG predict prognosis in idiopathic membranous nephropathy: a validation study. J Am Soc Nephrol 2005;16:169.

Branten AJ et al: Mycophenolate mofetil in idiopathic membranous nephropathy: a clinical trial with comparison to a historic control group treated with cyclophosphamide. Am J Kidney Dis 2007;50:248–256.

Cattran D: Management of membranous nephropathy: when and what for treatment. J Am Soc Nephrol 16: 2005;1188.

Cravedi P et al: Titrating rituximab to circulating B cells to optimize lymphocytolytic therapy in idiopathic membranous nephropathy. Clin J Am Soc Nephrol 2007;2(5):932–937

du Buf-Vereijken PW et al: Cytotoxic therapy for membranous nephropathy and renal insufficiency: improved renal survival but high relapse rate. Nephrol Dialysis Transplant 2004;19:1142.

du Buf-Vereijken PW, Wetzels JF: Efficacy of a second course of immunosuppressive therapy in patients with membranous nephropathy and persistent or relapsing disease activity. Nephrol Dialysis Transplant 2004;19:2036.

Fervenza FC et al: Rituximab treatment of idiopathic membranous nephropathy. Kidney Int 2008;73:117–125.

Glassock RJ: The treatment of idiopathic membranous nephropathy: a dilemma or a conundrum? Am J Kidney Dis 2004;44(3):562.

Jha V et al: A randomized, controlled trial of steroids and cyclophosphamide in adults with nephrotic syndrome caused by idiopathic membranous nephropathy. J Am Soc Nephrol 2007;18:1899–1904.

Perna A et al: Immunosuppressive treatment for idiopathic membranous nephropathy: a systematic review. Am J Kidney Dis 2004;44(3):385.

Praga M et al: Tacrolimus monotherapy in membranous nephropathy: a randomized controlled trial. Kidney Int 2007;71:924–930.

Troyanov S et al: Idiopathic membranous nephropathy: definition and relevance of a partial remission. Kidney Int 2004;66:1199.

Verhulst A et al: Inhibitors of HMG-CoA reductase reduce receptor-mediated endocytosis in human kidney proximal tubular cells. J Am Soc Nephrol 2004;15:2249.

Vidt DG et al: Rosuvastatin-induced arrest in progression of renal disease. Cardiology 2004;102:52.

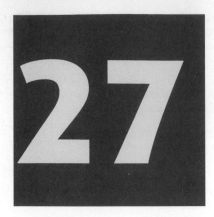

Immunoglobulin A Nephropathy & Henoch–Schönlein Purpura

Meryl Waldman, MD, & Gerald B. Appel, MD

IMMUNOGLOBULIN A NEPHROPATHY

ESSENTIALS OF DIAGNOSIS

► Immunoglobulin A nephropathy (IgAN) is the most frequent form of primary glomerulonephritis worldwide.

► Hematuria is typical. Younger patients often present with episodes of macroscopic hematuria coincident with mucosal infections or exercise. Adults often have asymptomatic hematuria and proteinuria.

► Abnormal glycosylation of immunoglobulin A (IgA) molecules is believed to be important in disease pathogenesis.

► The diagnosis is established by the presence of dominant or codominant IgA deposition by immunofluorescence microscopy typically in the mesangial region of the glomeruli.

► True IgA nephropathy is not just "benign recurrent hematuria." End-stage renal disease (ESRD) occurs in 15% of patients by 10 years and 20–40% by 20 years from onset.

General Considerations

IgAN is the most common form of primary glomerulonephritis worldwide. The prevalence of the disease shows geographic variations. In patients who undergo renal biopsy, IgAN accounts for approximately 30–40% of cases in Asia, 15–20% of cases in Europe, and 5–10% of cases in North America. These differences may be attributed to true differences in genetic susceptibility, or just as likely to differences in urinalysis screening practices, indications for renal biopsy, and possibly other factors. The disease is more common in whites, Asians, and American Indians and less common in blacks both in the United States and in Africa. It is most frequently diagnosed in young adults in the second and third decade of life and there is a male predominance.

Although numerous putative specific environmental or infectious agents have been suggested as the underlying stimulus for IgAN, none has been conclusively confirmed in the majority of patients. Familial clustering and a higher risk in identical twins suggest a role for genetic factors in susceptibility. A variety of genetic polymorphisms associated with susceptibility (and/or progression) in IgAN have been reported with conflicting results. Although IgAN is most commonly a primary (or idiopathic) renal disease, there are well-documented associations with a wide variety of conditions in individual patients (Table 27–1). In many of these conditions, IgA deposition in the glomerulus is not associated with inflammation and a progressive course, and thus, it may be clinically insignificant. This suggests that factors beyond the deposition of IgA or IgA-containing immune complexes must be involved in the pathogenesis of progressive disease in patients with idiopathic IgAN.

► Pathogenesis

The precise etiology of IgAN is unknown, but much evidence suggests that a basic abnormality in the IgA molecule itself plays a pivotal role in pathogenesis. Humans produce two isotype subclasses of IgA: IgA1 and IgA2. Plasma cells in the bone marrow, lymph nodes, and spleen mainly produce IgA1 (primarily monomeric), whereas both IgA1 and IgA2 are produced by the plasma cells in the respiratory and gastrointestinal tract (primarily polymeric). Analysis of kidney eluates from patients with IgAN reveals that the glomerular

Table 27–1. Diseases associated with immunoglobulin A (IgA) nephropathy.

Gastrointestinal	Chronic liver disease Celiac disease Inflammatory bowel disease
Infection	Human immunodeficiency virus Toxoplasmosis Leprosy *Yersinia enterocolitica* enteritis
Rheumatic	Ankylosing spondylitis Rheumatoid arthritis Reiter's syndrome Anterior uveitis
Pulmonary	Pulmonary hemosiderosis Interstitial pneumonitis
Malignancy	Lung adenocarcinoma Monoclonal IgA gammopathy Mycosis fungoides
Dermatologic	Dermatitis herpetiformis Psoriasis

deposits are almost exclusively polymeric IgA1. Furthermore, the hinge region of the IgA1 molecule in patients with IgAN is often abnormal with reduced galactose and/or sialic acid content. The mechanisms responsible for this underglycosylation are unclear, but reduced function of the enzyme responsible for performing this glycosylation may be involved. Nevertheless, the altered glycosylation pattern might favor self-aggregation of IgA1, formation of circulating IgA-containing immune complexes, defective clearance of abnormal IgA1 from the circulation, and increased binding of IgA1 to the extracellular matrix components in the kidney. Once deposited in the kidney, IgA1-containing immune complexes trigger cellular proliferation and enhance the production of proinflammatory cytokines, chemokines, and growth factors. Interleukin (IL)-6 may play a prominent role, but other factors including IL-1, platelet-derived growth factor, tumor necrosis factor, free oxygen radicals, and vascular cell adhesion molecule-1 have also been implicated as modulators of disease activity. Complement activation may be mediated by the alternative or lectin pathways since polymeric IgA1 and aberrantly glycosylated IgA1 are efficient at initiation.

▶ **Clinical Findings**

A. Symptoms and Signs

Patients with IgAN present in a variety of ways. Recurrent episodes of painless macroscopic hematuria (brown- or tea-colored urine) are more common in younger patients. These episodes often coincide with, or occur within, 1–2 days of an upper respiratory infection and are referred to as "synpharyngitic." Macroscopic hematuria may also be temporally related to other acute infections (gastroenteritis or urinary tract infection) and occasionally to strenuous exercise. Dull loin pain may accompany the hematuria, presumably due to renal capsular swelling.

In 30–40% of patients, IgAN is indolent with microscopic hematuria and proteinuria incidentally discovered on urinalysis. This asymptomatic presentation is more common in adults who are diagnosed with the urinary abnormalities at insurance physicals, pregnancy screening, and routine annual checkups. Other less common presentations include the nephrotic syndrome, acute renal failure (which may be the result of crescentic glomerulonephritis, renal tubular obstruction by red blood cells, or acute tubular necrosis), or chronic kidney disease representing long-standing disease that has gone undetected.

B. Laboratory Findings

There are no specific laboratory tests that distinguish IgAN from other glomerular diseases. The serum creatinine may be normal or elevated at presentation. Hematuria usually dominates the urinalysis. Proteinuria is often present, but the nephrotic syndrome is uncommon (~10–15% of patients). Urine microscopy typically reveals dysmorphic red blood cells and red blood cell casts indicating bleeding of glomerular origin. Complement levels are normal. Some, but not all IgAN patients have elevated levels of serum IgA (IgA1). Nevertheless, measurement of IgA levels has no diagnostic or prognostic value. Increased IgA levels alone are insufficient to cause disease. This conclusion is supported by observations that other diseases associated with increased serum IgA (ie, HIV, hepatobiliary disease, and IgA myeloma) infrequently result in IgAN.

A kidney biopsy is required for definitive diagnosis of IgAN. Immunofluorescence microscopy demonstrates the pathognomonic finding of dominant or codominant deposits of IgA in a diffuse granular pattern predominantly within the mesangium often with focal paramesangial and subendothelial extension (Figure 27–1). Other immunoglobulins and complement may be codeposited (with less intensity) including IgG, IgM, C3, and λ and κ light chains. Electron microscopy confirms the presence of electron-dense deposits in the mesangium. Light microscopic findings are variable and can reveal mesangial cell proliferation, mesangial expansion, focal or diffuse proliferative glomerulonephritis, crescentic glomerulonephritis, chronic sclerosing glomerulonephritis, and a membranoproliferative glomerulonephritis type I pattern. A subset of nephrotic patients with normal appearing glomeruli by light microscopy may have only prominent visceral epithelial cell foot process effacement on electron microscopy and appear indistinguishable from patients with minimal change disease.

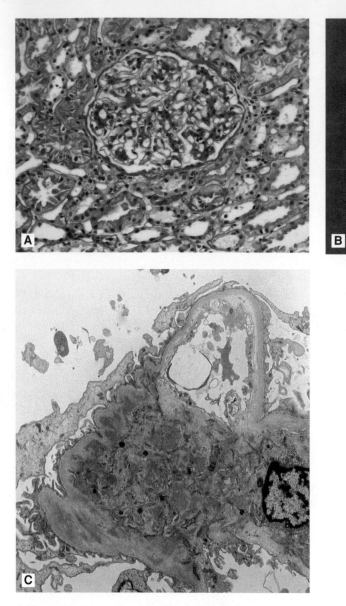

▲ **Figure 27–1.** Histology in IgA nephropathy. **A:** Light micrograph of mesangial glomerulonephritis typical of immunoglobulin A nephropathy. There are segmental areas of increased mesangial matrix and cellularity. **B:** Direct immunofluorescence microscopy demonstrating large, globular mesangial IgA deposits. **C:** Electron micrograph demonstrating electron-dense deposits in the mesangium.

Differential Diagnosis

Macroscopic hematuria due to IgAN is a much less common presentation in middle aged or elderly patients and thus its presence should raise suspicion of a nonglomerular etiology such as urinary tract malignancy or stones, and appropriate imaging should be performed to exclude these. Examination of the urine sediment is helpful in distinguishing glomerular from nonglomerular causes of hematuria. In children, postinfectious (streptococcal) glomerulonephritis may present with dark or smoky urine that may be confused with IgAN. However, the timing of the hematuria relative to the pharyngitis provides clues. Hematuria occurs consistently between 7 and 14 days after streptococcal infection as opposed to the synpharyngitic hematuria characteristic of IgAN. Episodic gross hematuria, often in association with upper respiratory infections, may also be seen in familial glomerular diseases such as thin basement membrane disease or Alport's syndrome.

Lupus nephritis is another glomerular disease associated with prominent mesangial IgA deposition. Lupus can be distinguished from IgA nephropathy by the more intense deposition of IgG compared to IgA, as well as the typical deposition of C1q, the characteristic "full house" immunofluorescent staining for IgA, IgG, IgM, C1q, and C3, and the serologic and clinical signs of lupus.

Treatment

A diagnosis of IgAN does not necessarily warrant immunosuppressive therapy since many patients will have a good outcome without treatment. The decision to treat depends on identification of those patients likely to progress based on adverse prognostic features. Patients with mild proteinuria (<500 mg/day), normal renal function, and normal blood pressure may be treated conservatively with close monitoring (every 6 months). Patients with normal renal function (creatinine <1.5 mg/dL) and greater degrees of proteinuria (500–1000 mg/day) may or may not benefit from other therapies. All certainly need optimal blood pressure control (goal <130/80). Many believe that use of angiotensin-converting enzyme inhibitors (ACEI) and angiotensin receptor blockers (ARBs) alone or in combination should be used to optimize blood pressure and decrease proteinuria in most patients with IgAN.

Because of the observed association of upper respiratory tract infections and macroscopic hematuria in IgAN, tonsillectomy has been proposed as a means of preventing progression of the disease. The results are at best conflicting with a lack of compelling evidence demonstrating long-term preservation of renal function. Nevertheless, in patients with recurrent episodes of severe tonsillitis associated with gross hematuria, tonsillectomy is reasonable.

The use of fish oils rich in omega-3 fatty acids, eicosapentaenoic acid (EPA), and docosahexaenoic acid (DHA) in large doses (12 g/day) may be beneficial. They may provide anti-inflammatory effects and retard renal injury by decreasing platelet aggregation and by competing with arachidonic acid to produce biologically less inflammatory prostaglandins and leukotrienes. Clinical trials with fish oils in IgAN have led to conflicting results. Some randomized controlled trials have shown significant preservation of renal function over time compared to placebo-treated patients, while others have failed to show a benefit. Given the potential efficacy and lack of toxicity, high doses of fish oil are often used in combination with ACEI/ARB therapy in patients with proteinuria (>1 g/day) and/or mildly impaired renal function. In some countries, combinations of dipyridamole and warfarin are used (with or without concomitant immunosuppressive agents) for their antiproliferative and antithrombotic effects. Dipyridamole has been shown to inhibit mesangial proliferation *in vitro*.

A trial of corticosteroids (6 months) may be warranted in IgAN patients with significant proteinuria (despite angiotensin inhibition) and normal renal function. In one randomized controlled trial, long-term follow-up of patients treated with 6 months of corticosteroids(1.0 g pulse of methylprednisolone at the beginning of months 1, 3, and 5 with continuous oral prednisone 0.5 mg/kg every other day) demonstrated improved renal survival and a decrease in proteinuria in treated patients compared to controls. However, patients with impaired renal function and more severe pathologic changes on renal biopsy appear to respond less favorably to steroids alone. Nevertheless, there are two forms of IgAN in which the use of prednisone is clearly indicated as initial treatment. Patients with the nephrotic syndrome and histologic findings characteristic of minimal change disease (minimal glomerular changes on light microscopy and diffuse foot process fusion on electron microscopy) typically go into remission with corticosteroids. Additionally, patients with clinical or pathologic features of rapidly progressive glomerulonephritis (RPGN) may also benefit from steroid therapy in conjunction with other agents.

Cytotoxic agents [short-term cyclophosphamide followed by maintenance with prednisone plus either azathioprine or mycophenolate mofetil (MMF)] may be indicated for patients with progressive disease but with creatinine less than 3 mg/dL. Improvement with such regimens is less likely when the plasma creatinine is greater than 2.5–3 mg/dL, which is considered past the "point of no return."

MMF has been used in at least five trials some of which were double blind and randomized. The results are conflicting with either favorable outcomes with treatment or no benefit. This may depend upon the population studied.

For patients who progress to ESRD, renal transplantation is suitable therapy. Histologic evidence of IgA deposition is reported in 30–60% of allografts by 10 years and 5–10% of affected allografts are lost to progressive disease. Contemporary immunosuppression regimens, which include cyclosporine, tacrolimus, and MMF, have not altered the recurrence rate.

Prognosis

The course of IgAN is highly variable. Certain features may confer a poor renal prognosis including male gender, absence of gross hematuria, elevated serum creatinine at time of biopsy, and greater severity of hypertension and proteinuria (except when the proteinuria is associated with a minimal-change-like lesion). Likewise, elevations of serum creatinine and proteinuria at the point of 1-year post-renal biopsy are predictive of a poor outcome.

It has been estimated that ESRD occurs in 15% of cases at 10 years and 20–40% of cases at 20 years, although this likely reflects a selection bias with follow-up of patients with more severe disease. Many patients have a very slow progressive decline in renal function over 10–20 years.

Alexopoulos E: Treatment of primary IgA nephropathy. Kidney Int 2004;65:341.

Ballardie FW: IgA nephropathy treatment 25 years on: can we halt progression? The evidence base. Nephrol Dial Transplant 2004;19:1041.

Donadio JV, Grande JP: The role of fish oil/omega-3 fatty acids in the treatment of IgA nephropathy. Semin Nephrol 2004;24:225.

Julian BA, Novak J: IgA nephropathy: an update. Curr Opin Nephrol Hypertens 2004;13:171.

Maes BD et al: Mycophenolate mofetil in IgA nephropathy: results of a 3-year prospective placebo-controlled randomized study. Kidney Int 2004;65:1842.

Samuels JA et al: Immunosuppressive treatments for immunoglobulin A nephropathy: a meta-analysis of randomized controlled trials. Nephrology (Carlton) 2004;9:177.

Xie Y et al: Relationship between tonsils and IgA nephropathy as well as indications of tonsillectomy. Kidney Int 2004;65:1135.

HENOCH–SCHÖNLEIN PURPURA

 ESSENTIALS OF DIAGNOSIS

- ▶ Henoch–Schönlein purpura (HSP) is the multisystem form of primary IgA nephropathy.
- ▶ It is a form of leukocytoclastic vasculitis with IgA-dominant immune deposits affecting small vessels of the skin, joints, gastrointestinal system, and kidney.
- ▶ It is most common in children.
- ▶ The classic tetrad of signs and symptoms includes rash, arthralgias, abdominal pain, and renal disease.

General Considerations

Henoch-Schönlein purpura, as defined by the International Consensus Conference on Nomenclature of Systemic Vasculitides, is "a vasculitis with IgA dominant immune deposits affecting small vessels and typically involving the skin, gut and glomeruli and associated with arthralgias or arthritis." There is much evidence to suggest that HSP and IgAN represent a spectrum of clinical presentations of similar disorders with HSP being the systemic form of IgAN. Both HSP and IgAN can occur consecutively in the same patient and each has been described in identical twins. Both diseases bear similar immunologic abnormalities and renal histologic findings. Furthermore, a history of recent or simultaneous infection (upper respiratory, gastrointestinal, or urinary tract) is common in children with both HSP and IgAN.

HSP can occur at any age, but preferentially affects children between the ages of 5 and 15 years. It is the most common cause of acute systemic vasculitis in children, with an incidence estimated at 10–20 cases per 100,000 children per year. In adults, the annual incidence is much lower (1.3–1.4/100,000), with a mean age of presentation of about 50 years.

Renal involvement varies depending on the diagnostic criteria used and method of detection of renal disease. In children, nephritis (HSPN) is manifested in 20–40% of cases but occurs more frequently in adults (50–85%).

Pathogenesis

There are significant gaps in our understanding of the pathogenesis of HSP, although abnormalities in IgA play a central role. Increases in both serum polymeric IgA1 and IgA1-containing immune complexes are present. Deposition of IgA1-containing immune complexes is associated with a systemic small vessel vasculitis and capillary damage. Complement activation, platelet activation, and release of cytokines and growth factors may all contribute to the pathogenesis. Why this leads to systemic vasculitis and extrarenal manifestations in HSP and not in isolated IgAN is unknown. Diminished galactosylation of IgA1 appears to correlate with the presence of nephritis as patients with HSP, but without nephritis, have normal IgA1 glycosylation.

Numerous infectious agents (ie, varicella, HIV, parvovirus B19, hepatitis A and B, mycoplasma, group A streptococci, Epstein-Barr virus, and *Campylobacter* enteritis) as well as other factors (medications, vaccinations, insect bites) have been linked to the development of HSP, but a causative relationship is unproven. IgA ANCA has also been found in some patients with HSP, but its pathogenetic role and clinical significance are unclear.

Clinical Findings

A. Symptoms and Signs

The classical clinical presentation includes palpable purpura (present in most cases), polyarthralgias (75–80% of cases), and abdominal pain (50–75% of cases). Symptoms and signs can occur in any order and at any time over a course of several days to weeks, and reflect the systemic leukocytoclastic vasculitis. The skin lesions usually appear as crops of palpable purpura on the lower limbs and buttocks. Gastrointestinal involvement is characterized by colicky abdominal pain sometimes associated with gastrointestinal bleeding (melena, hematochezia, or occult). Joint involvement, consisting of arthralgias or frank arthritis, is typically limited to the knees and ankles, and does not lead to permanent deformity. Pulmonary, neurologic, genitourinary, and cardiac manifestations may also occur.

Renal manifestations may occur within days or up to several weeks after onset of the clinical presentation of HSP, but rarely precedes the other major components of the disease. Renal findings include hematuria (microscopic or gross), proteinuria, and abnormal renal function tests.

B. Laboratory Findings

Laboratory tests are nonspecific. Coagulation tests and platelet counts are normal despite the presence of dramatic purpuric lesions. Plasma creatinine may be normal or elevated. Serum complement levels are normal and cryoglobulins are absent. Serum IgA levels may be elevated, but measurement of IgA levels is not diagnostic and they do not correlate with disease severity. Urinalysis in affected individuals reveals blood and protein, which is often mild (<500 mg/day), but can be in the nephrotic range. The urine sediment typically has red cells and cellular casts consistent with nephritis.

Confirmation of the diagnosis requires the identification of tissue deposition of IgA in the skin or kidney. Renal biopsy, the more invasive of the two options, is generally reserved for those with an unclear diagnosis or with evidence of more severe renal involvement. Biopsy of skin lesions reveals leukocytoclastic vasculitis with vessel wall necrosis and perivascular accumulation of inflammatory cells, mostly polymorphonuclear leukocytes and mononuclear cells, surrounding the capillaries and postcapillary venules of the dermis. Immunofluorescence reveals the presence of IgA. In some cases, these findings can be seen in areas of skin that appear uninvolved.

In renal biopsies, histologic findings resemble those of IgAN. A mesangioproliferative glomerulonephritis is typical, although some will have a membranoproliferative pattern. Necrotizing glomerular lesions, diffuse endocapillary proliferation, crescents, and fibrin deposits are more frequent in HSPN than in IgAN. Immunofluorescence microscopy demonstrates the characteristic granular deposition of IgA in the mesangium indistinguishable from that seen in IgAN. On electron microscopy, electron-dense deposits are scattered throughout the mesangium. In some patients, prominent capillary wall deposits of IgA and occasionally subepithelial deposits are present.

▶ Differential Diagnosis

In children, the characteristic tetrad of rash, joint, gastrointestinal, and renal involvement usually makes the syndrome of HSP clearly identifiable. Clotting disorders, septic emboli, and infections (ie, meningococcemia, gonococcemia, rickettsial) may mimic the findings of HSP. Any of the four major symptoms or signs may be present before the other, which may lead to misdirected evaluations (ie, abdominal pains alone may be mistaken for cholecystitis, appendicitis, and bowel infarction).

The differential diagnosis is much broader in adults and it must be distinguished from other forms of vasculitis including pauci-immune small vessel vasculitis, polyarteritis nodosa, systemic lupus erythematosis (SLE), cryoglobulinemia, and hypersensitivity vasculitis. Clinical and histologic characteristics in combination with serologic testing for ANCA, anti-GBM, cryoglobulins, hepatitis B and C, antinuclear antibody (ANA), and complement levels narrow the diagnosis.

▶ Treatment

In patients with normal kidney function, treatment is generally supportive. There are limited data available that define the optimal treatment for patients with renal involvement. Most patients require no specific therapy, as spontaneous remission is common. However, in patients with rapidly progressive renal failure caused by crescentic nephritis, aggressive therapy using high-dose pulse methylprednisolone in combination with cyclophosphamide followed by oral prednisone to decrease the inflammatory process may be beneficial. Uncertainty remains as to the optimal duration of therapy. Other regimens used with variable results include azathioprine, dipyridamole, urokinase, immune globulin, and plasma exchange. There are anecdotal reports of abatement of persistent HSP (purpuric rash, hematuria, and proteinuria) with fish oil in combination with ACEI, as well as cyclosporine A/steroid combinations. Prospective randomized clinical trials are needed to truly evaluate the efficacy of any of these agents.

▶ Prognosis

In the majority of patients, HSP is a self-limiting illness characterized by spontaneous resolution of manifestations and a good prognosis. One-third to one-half of patients will have one or more recurrences of symptoms, usually within 6 weeks, but they may recur as late as 3–7 years later.

Transient hematuria and proteinuria typically resolve within several months. Spontaneous recovery may also occur in patients with severe renal involvement including acute renal failure and nephrotic-range proteinuria. The incidence of long-term renal impairment varies among the different series in the literature. In children, renal survival is generally over 95% at 15 years. The prognosis of HSPN in adults may be worse than that of children with up to 30% of adults showing chronic decline in glomerular filtration rate with progression to ESRD. Nephrotic syndrome, persistent proteinuria, elevated serum creatinine at onset, extensive crescents (>50%), and advanced tubulointerstitial disease on renal biopsy are associated with a worse renal prognosis.

Recurrent renal disease can occur in renal transplants. Histologic recurrences of HSPN may occur in up to 50% of renal transplants and are associated with clinical disease in 20% and graft loss in 9% of cases. Graft loss may be more likely in patients who had aggressive initial disease with rapid progression to ESRD, or who undergo transplant either with living related donors or while still clinically active.

Dixit M et al: Managing Henoch–Schönlein purpura in children with fish oil and ACE inhibitor therapy. Nephrology 2004;9;381.

Kawasaki Y et al: Efficacy of methylprednisolone and urokinase pulse therapy combined with or without cyclophosphamide in severe Henoch–Schönlein nephritis: a clinical and histopathological analysis. Nephrol Dial Transplant 2004;19:858.

Tarshish P et al: Henoch–Schönlein purpura nephritis: course of disease and efficacy of cyclophosphamide. Pediatr Nephrol 2004;19:51.

Membranoproliferative Glomerulonephritis

28

Howard Trachtman, MD

ESSENTIALS OF DIAGNOSIS

▶ Characterized by persistent hypocomplementemia.

▶ Disease is most often primary or idiopathic.

▶ Fifty percent of patients progress to end-stage renal disease over 10–15 years.

▶ Prednisone is effective in pediatric patients but there is no proven treatment in adults.

▶ Disease recurs posttransplantation in approximately 25% of patients.

▶ General Considerations

Membranoproliferative glomerulonephritis (MPGN) is the classic renal nomenclature monstrosity that spreads fear among house officers and practitioners. This disease was first described by Rene Habib in 1961 and was linked to decreased serum complement levels in 1965. Since then it has been a recognized cause of serious glomerular disease in pediatric and adult patients throughout the world and represents an important cause of end-stage renal disease. It is defined by a characteristic histopathologic appearance that consists of a lobulated shape to the glomerular tuft, glomerular hypercellularity, thickening of the capillary wall, and splitting of the glomerular basement membrane with a double contour ("tram tracking"). On ultrastructural examination of renal tissue, there are electron-dense deposits in the capillary wall and the distinctive localization of the deposits results in classification of MPGN into type I (subendothelial and mesangial), type II (intramembranous dense deposits), and type III (subendothelial, mesangial, and subepithelial).

▶ Pathogenesis

The general mechanism of disease for the development of MPGN is dysregulated complement protein activation. Under normal circumstances complement activity, composed of various chemotactic factors and the membrane attack complex, is triggered either through the classical or alternative pathways. The third component of the cascade, C3, occupies a pivotal position in both pathways and is essential to the effector functions of the system. Therefore, a number of regulatory proteins are synthesized to modulate C3 convertase (C3bBb) activity and to prevent the deleterious consequences of uninterrupted complement activation. These include factors H and I, membrane cofactor protein (MCP), and decay accelerating factor.

MPGN is classified into primary and secondary forms. The pathogenesis of MPGN is linked to the underlying etiology of the glomerulopathy (Table 28–1). In the primary forms of MPGN, the mechanism of disease centers around abnormal activation of the complement cascade. In-depth studies of all components of the complement cascade suggest that there are three distinct patterns of complement activation in the three types of MPGN. Thus, in type I disease, the process is initiated by immune complex deposition within the glomerulus and involvement of the classical pathway. The source of the immune complexes is unknown in the idiopathic form of the disease. These patients have low levels of C3, C4, C6, C7, and/or C9. MPGN type I is sometimes associated with the presence of a circulating immunoglobulin (Ig)G or IgM autoantibody that stabilizes the C3 convertase (eg, C3 nephritic factor), thus engendering low C3 levels. A C4 nephritic factor has also been described. In the type II variant, the continuous overactivity of the complement cascade involves an amplification loop in the alternative pathway, characterized mainly by markedly depressed C3 levels. Abnormal complement activation in MPGN can also occur as a consequence of genetic mutations that result in reduced levels of endogenous inhibitors of the process, such as factor H, or because of the presence of C3 nephritic factor, the latter occurring in the majority of patients with MPGN type II (also called dense deposit disease). Animal models in mice and pigs demonstrate the

Table 28–1. Etiology of membranoproliferative glomerulonephritis.

Primary disease
    Type I
    Type II, dense deposit disease
        C3 nephritic factor
    Type III

Genetic forms
    Factor H defects
    C4 deficiency

Secondary
    Infections
        Lyme disease
        Hepatitis B
        Hepatitis C
        Bacterial endocarditis
        Hantavirus
        Malaria
        Schistosomiasis
    Chronic liver disease
    Collagen vascular disease
        Systemic lupus erythematosis
        Sjögren's syndrome
    Other autoimmune disease
        Thyroiditis/type 1 diabetes mellitus
    Malignancy
        Chronic lymphocytic leukemia
        Non-Hodgkin's lymphoma
    Medications
        Granulocyte colony-stimulating factor
        Interferon-α therapy

importance of factor H in regulating complement activation and the occurrence of MPGN when circulating levels of this protein are reduced. It is worth noting that unlike hemolytic uremic syndrome, which can develop in patients who have heterozygous genetic defects in factor H, MPGN occurs only in patients who carry homozygous mutations. Other genetic causes of MPGN include isolated C4 deficiency. Finally, the pathogenesis of MPGN type III appears to have features in common with type I disease as well as evidence of activation of the terminal complement pathway with low C3, C5, and properdin levels. In adults, the type III form frequently occurs in association with systemic infection, inflammation, or neoplasm. The presence of MGPN type III in adults should stimulate a search for an underlying systemic process causing it.

Secondary forms of MPGN can occur as a result of various infections including hepatitis B and C, bacterial endocarditis, mixed cryoglobulinemia, malignancies, collagen vascular disease, and chronic liver disease (including specific entities such as α_1-antitrypsin deficiency). Indeed, most cases of MPGN, particularly in adults, are attributable

to hepatitis C. The genetic forms of MPGN are rarely seen in adults. There are other entities that occur in rare association with MPGN such as Lyme disease and autoimmune thyroiditis. Moreover, the use of some newer medications has been linked to the occurrence of MPGN type I such as granulocyte colony-stimulating factor. Under these various circumstances, it is presumed that there is immune complex-mediated activation of the complement cascade. In animal models of cryoglobulinemia, overexpression of the membrane complement inhibitor, complement receptor 1-related gene/protein y (Crry), does not prevent the development of MPGN.

▶ **Prevention**

MPGN is either idiopathic or secondary to an underlying condition. The former category of diseases cannot be prevented. Secondary causes can be avoided by minimizing exposure to the etiologic agent or by primary prevention of the underlying disease.

▶ **Clinical Findings**

A. Symptoms and Signs

The incidence of MPGN is low and accounts for 5–30% of patients with new-onset nephrotic syndrome. It is lower in adults than in children. Several reports suggest that the incidence of MPGN has been declining over the past 10–20 years. Further epidemiologic studies are needed to clarify this issue. The disease is generally sporadic and familial cases are rare. Overall, the disease is equally prevalent in male and female patients but appears to be more common in white compared to black patients.

MPGN can present in a variety of fashions ranging from asymptomatic hematuria to a severe acute glomerulonephritis. In children, MPGN most often presents either as idiopathic nephrotic syndrome or an acute glomerulonephritis that closely resembles acute postinfectious nephritis. It accounts for 5–10% of pediatric cases of new-onset nephrotic syndrome. The profile of MPGN is distinct from minimal change disease and focal segmental glomerulonephritis, which occur more frequently in younger boys, because it is more common in female patients over 8 years of age. The clinical suspicion of MPGN in a child with acute nephritis rises when the C3 levels fail to normalize during the standard 8–12 week observation period or the C4 level is decreased at the onset of disease because it is only rarely decreased in acute postinfectious glomerulonephritis. Cases such as these account for nearly 30% of all instances of MPGN and may have concomitant reduction in the glomerular filtration rate (GFR). Hypertension is present in 50–80% of cases of MPGN and can be severe. Because of concern that corticosteroid therapy may exacerbate the elevation in blood pressure and trigger malignant hypertension, it is advisable to rule out MPGN in a high-risk patient such as an older female child before initiation of daily treatment with steroids, in cases where steroids might otherwise be indicated.

Occasional patients with persistent glomerular hematuria lasting longer than 6 months and hypocomplementemia with MPGN detected on renal biopsy have been reported. Reports from Japan confirm early detection of MPGN in pediatric patients following findings of hematuria and/or proteinuria on routine annual screening urinalyses. Although this testing enables detection of disease prior to the onset of significant hypertension, proteinuria, and/or azotemia, the cost effectiveness of this kind of program requires confirmation in other patient populations. In fact, there are even cases of typical MPGN in children being diagnosed because of persistent hypocomplementemia in the complete absence of any urinary findings. In patients with asymptomatic urinary abnormalities, type III MPGN is more likely to be detected than type I or II disease.

In adult patients, the clinical presentation may be the consequence solely of the renal involvement with edema, hypertension, or gross hematuria. However, in those patients with secondary disease the symptoms and signs usually reflect the underlying cause. Thus, patients with cryoglobulinemia may have weakness, arthralgias involving the knees, hips, and shoulders, and palpable vasculitic lesions on the buttocks and lower extremities. These symptoms may fluctuate over time. The distribution of the purpura is reminiscent of Henoch–Schönlein purpura. Those patients with disease secondary to infection, malignancy, or collagen vascular disease will have manifestations associated with the underlying disease. Interestingly, MPGN may be the first manifestation of hepatitis C infection because affected patients often have no clinical evidence of hepatic disease.

B. Laboratory Findings

MPGN is characterized by hypocomplementemia, namely reduced C3 and CH_{50} levels, which is confirmed in 80–90% of patients. In patients with type I MPGN, approximately 40% of those with a low C3 level will also have a low serum C4 level. This is less common in patients with type II or III MPGN. Although the different patterns of circulating complement component levels described above (see Pathogenesis) are useful in discriminating the types of MPGN, this testing is generally not performed in clinical chemistry laboratories and is available only in select research facilities. C3 nephritic factor activity is more common in type II disease, namely 60–70% of patients, compared to 20–25% of patients with type I or III disease. Interestingly, this autoantibody is also detectable in up to 50% of patients with secondary forms of MPGN. It is uncertain whether the presence of C3 nephritic factor indicates an increased risk of progression to end-stage renal disease. C3 nephritic factor can be measured in a hemolytic or a solid phase assay. In adults with cryoglobulinemia, testing should be performed for hepatitis

B and C infection. Hepatitis serology should also be evaluated in pediatric patients with MPGN even in the absence of mixed cryoglobulinemia. Other laboratory abnormalities will be present depending upon the underlying disease.

C. Pathology

The characteristic pathology in MPGN is diffuse mesangial and endothelial cell proliferation, thickening of the capillary wall, and splitting of the glomerular basement membrane (Figure 28–1). Depending upon the severity of the disease, crescent formation may be noted in a substantial percentage of glomeruli. The hypercellularity is enhanced by leukocyte and monocyte infiltration of the glomerular tuft. Special stains such as silver methenamine may be required to visualize the splitting and broadening of the glomerular basement membrane and the trichrome stain to facilitate localization of deposits (Figure 28–2). This is important in classifying the three types of primary MPGN—type I with subendothelial and mesangial, type II with intramembranous, and type III with subendothelial, mesangial, and subepithelial deposits. The trichrome stain is also useful in assessing fibrosis. Special stains such as thioflavin T have been advocated to detect intramembranous dense deposits, especially in cases with focal distribution of the material. The extent of the basement membrane broadening, thought by some to be due to mesangial interposition into the basement membrane, may be a marker of disease severity, with those patients with diffuse changes having a more guarded prognosis compared to those with focal abnormalities. Thus, in type I MPGN focal changes may represent an early manifestation of the disease

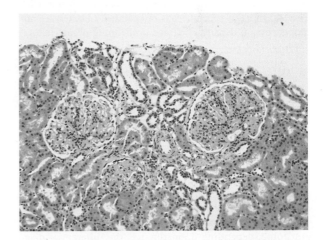

▲ **Figure 28–1.** Light micrograph of a hematoxylin and eosin-stained renal section illustrating the lobular appearance of the glomerulus, diffuse hypercellularity, and thickening of the capillary wall in a patient with membranoproliferative glomerulonephritis.

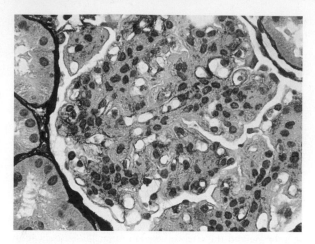

▲ **Figure 28–2.** Light micrograph of a silver-stained renal section illustrating classic splitting of the glomerular basement membrane and mesangial cell interposition (indicated by red arrows) in a patient with membranoproliferative glomerulonephritis.

and explain the more favorable outcome in response to treatment. The histopathologic appearance of cryoglobulinemic MPGN, which is the most common secondary variant in children, closely resembles type I disease.

Immunofluorescence staining is usually positive for C3, IgG, and IgM in a capillary wall and mesangial distribution. Classical complement cascade components are seen in type I but not type II and III MPGN. Electron microscopy confirms the precise location of the deposits, namely subendothelial, mesangial, intramembranous, or subepithelial. The deposits can be numerous or sparse in number, are homogeneous in density, and have no defining ultrastructural appearance.

▶ Differential Diagnosis

Other entities that need to be considered in a patient who is being evaluated for MPGN depend upon the specific clinical circumstances. Patients with urinary findings alone may have a mild postinfectious nephritis, hereditary nephritis, or immunoglobulin A (IgA) nephropathy. In those with an overt nephritic syndrome, possibilities include postinfectious nephritis, lupus nephritis, Henoch–Schönlein purpura nephritis, and vasculitis. The likelihood of the last two diseases is increased in patients with a rash, arthralgias, or fever. In those patients who present with the nephrotic syndrome, depending upon the age, the differential diagnosis includes minimal change nephrotic syndrome, focal segmental glomerulosclerosis, and membranous nephropathy. Paraproteinemias (light chain nephropathy), thrombotic microangiopathies, and fibrillary glomerulonephritis

can cause a histologic picture that resembles MPGN. Other than systemic lupus erythematosis (SLE) nephritis and atheroembolic renal disease, what distinguishes MPGN from all other diagnostic considerations is persistent hypocomplementemia.

▶ Complications

Patients with MPGN can develop sequelae related to the renal manifestations of the disease or the underlying illness. Thus, patients with acute nephritis may experience severe hypertension or congestive heart failure. Those patients with nephrotic syndrome may develop local infections, peritonitis, or thromboembolic events.

Patients with type II disease, which is more common in children than in adults, manifest partial lipodystrophy in nearly 25% of cases. This is characterized by a gradual loss of subcutaneous fat tissue in the face and upper body regions. *In vitro* studies demonstrate that addition of C3 nephritic factor to murine adipocytes results in cell lysis via a process that requires the presence of factor D and divalent cations. These findings may explain the linkage between MPGN and lipodystrophy. Leptin treatment of lipodystrophy in patients with MPGN for 4–36 months normalizes hyperfiltration and reduces proteinuria. The long-term consequences of this therapy on the progression of the renal disease have not been studied. Finally, there may be other associated findings in patients with MPGN such as mild visual fields and color defects. Retinal angiography demonstrates the presence of choroidal neovascularization.

Patients with MPGN in association with cryoglobulinemia may have ulcerative skin lesions, Raynaud's phenomenon, peripheral neuropathy, hepatomegaly, and signs of cirrhosis.

▶ Treatment

A. Pediatric Patients

Children with primary forms of MPGN who are clinically well and free of any symptoms, and who have only minor urinary abnormalities, generally do not require aggressive therapy. These patients may be treated with antihypertensive agents, specifically angiotensin-converting enzyme inhibitor or angiotensin receptor blocker, to reduce proteinuria and prevent progressive renal damage. However, after identification of the disease in 1965 and clarification of the ominous prognosis in the majority of patients, efforts were initiated to implement therapy to retard progression of MPGN. Initial studies performed by Clark West and colleagues at Cincinnati Children's Hospital indicated that prolonged alternate daily therapy with oral steroids favorably impacted on the disease course. The experience in 45 patients treated at that center was summarized in 1986. These patients were given prednisone 60 mg/m^2 or 2–2.5 mg/kg every other day for an average period of 6.5 years with an improved outcome compared to historic controls or patients treated at other centers. Hematuria resolved in 80%, renal function remained normal or improved in 73%, and 62% of those with nephrotic syndrome had normalization of serum albumin concentration. Hypocomplementemia resolves within 4–12 months of initiation of therapy in most patients. However, it may persist in some patients and does not necessarily indicate deteriorating renal histopathology. Repeat biopsies performed after 2 years of therapy indicated an increase in open capillary loops and a reduction in mesangial matrix expansion. However, it is important to note that there was an increase in glomerulosclerosis despite clinical improvement. This may reflect irreversible damage to nephrons prior to initiation of therapy. The efficacy of therapy was greater in patients who began treatment within 1 year of disease onset. In Japan where school urinary screening programs facilitate early detection of MPGN, treatment with prolonged alternate day steroids (4–12 years) after prednisolone pulse or cyclophosphamide therapy achieved remission and resulted in normalization of the urinalysis and stabilization of GFR in 15 patients and mild proteinuria in 4 others who were followed for 10–24 years.

The open-label treatment findings of the Cincinnati group have been confirmed in a randomized clinical trial performed by the International Study of Kidney Diseases in Children. Eighty children with MPGN (42 type I, 14 type II, 17 type III, and 7 nontypable) were assigned to prednisone 40 mg/m^2 every other day or placebo for an average of 41 months. All patients had significant proteinuria and a GFR >70 mL/minute/1.73 m^2. Treatment failure, defined as a 30% increase in the baseline serum creatinine or >35 μ mol/L increment, occurred in 55% of placebo versus 40% of prednisone-treated patients. Life table analysis indicated 61% renal survival at 130 months in prednisone-treated patients versus 12% in placebo-treated patients ($p = 0.07$). The response was comparable in type I and III MPGN. Although the outcome was less clear in type II disease, a response to more prolonged alternate day steroids in this subtype has been documented.

Based on this experience, it is recommended that alternate steroid therapy be given to all pediatric patients for at least 2 years if the GFR is well preserved (>70 mL/minute/1.73 m^2). The beneficial impact of treatment in patients with more advanced disease has not been established. The dose should be approximately 40–60 mg/m^2 every other day. Some investigators have reported good outcomes in a small series of patients given lower steroid doses; however, the minimum effective dose has not been systematically assessed. The need for prolonged therapy should be guided by the clinical response (serum complement level, degree of hematuria, urinary protein excretion, and calculated GFR) and repeat renal histopathologic assessment (after 2 years of steroid treatment, later in a course of therapy, or if there is evidence of recurrent disease).

B. Adult Patients

1. Steroid therapy—There is widespread concern about the risks of prolonged steroid therapy in adults. Therefore, the current evidence-based medicine recommendation is to prescribe steroids only for adults with nephrotic syndrome or impaired kidney function. Treatment is maintained for 6 months. The therapy may be extended until remission is achieved using the lowest possible dose of steroids. Patients with asymptomatic urinary findings and patients who fail to respond to steroids should be treated conservatively. Angiotensin-converting enzyme inhibitors have been demonstrated to be effective in reducing proteinuria in patients with MPGN.

2. Antiplatelet and anticoagulant therapy—It has been suggested that administration of the antiplatelet drug dipyridamole slowed deterioration in kidney function in patients with MPGN. However, a follow-up study failed to demonstrate efficacy of a combination of dipyridamole, cyclophosphamide, and warfarin. In a meta-analysis of five studies of antiplatelet therapy, no beneficial effect was discernible if the timing of the onset of treatment relative to the time of disease onset was accounted for. Thus, based on currently available evidence, these treatments are not recommended.

3. Cryoglobulinemic MPGN secondary to hepatitis C—In patients with hepatitis C infection and MPGN, interferon-α therapy for 6–12 months can achieve remission in 60% of patients. However, most will relapse within 3–6 months. Use of pegylated interferon and the addition of ribavirin to the regimen may improve the response. Current practice is to administer the combination of antiviral agents for 6 months and then switch to low dose every other day steroids. Removal of cryoglobulins with cryofiltration is an experimental modality that may work by removing cryoglobulins from the circulation. Dosing regimens for both pegylated interferon and ribavirin are controversial in patients with diminished renal function. Serious side effects have been observed in patients treated with these agents whose renal function is impaired.

4. Other therapies—There have been isolated case reports claiming that plasmapheresis is a useful therapy in patients with severe idiopathic MPGN and acute renal failure or rapidly deteriorating disease. However, the response was not uniform. Moreover, this treatment modality is invasive and costly. Therefore, it should not be utilized routinely as a first-line treatment. Mycophenolate mofetil has been tried in patients with cryoglobulinemic MPGN related to hepatitis B infection. Although treatment resulted in reduced proteinuria, viral replication was induced by the drug. Therefore, caution is advisable when considering this immunosuppressive agent for the treatment of MPGN. Plasmapheresis may be useful short term during the acute phase of treatment in patients with serious vasculitic flares from hepatitis C-associated cryoglobulinemia, although activation of the hepatitis is a concern.

▶ Prognosis

A. Pediatric Patients

In general, the long-term outlook for untreated patients with MPGN is guarded. Although occasional children and adolescents have been described who achieve a spontaneous remission, nearly 50% of patients progress to end-stage renal disease over 10–15 years. An elevated serum creatinine concentration at the time of diagnosis, nephrotic-range proteinuria, severe hypertension, crescents in >50% of glomeruli, diffuse interstitial fibrosis and tubular atrophy, and a reduced calculated GFR after 1 year of treatment are indicators of a poor outcome. The prognosis is worse in patients with primary versus secondary forms of MPGN. In addition, type II MPGN may have a more ominous long-term outlook compared to type I and III disease.

Recent reports confirm the poor prognosis of MPGN in pediatric patients. For example, in a series of 53 children, ranging in age from 13 months to 15 years, who were treated at two English centers over a 20-year period from January 1980 to December 1999, the mean renal survival time was 12.2 years. Interestingly, the histologic subtype, level of proteinuria below the nephrotic range, and specific therapy had no impact on the long-term outcome. However, the favorable experience in Japan, where MPGN is diagnosed as a result of school urinary screening programs, suggests that the prognosis may be improved following early detection and prompt implementation of corticosteroid therapy.

B. Adult Patients

Although there is an unstated concern that adults with MPGN do worse than children and adolescents, in general, the outcome of MPGN is comparable in adult versus pediatric patients. Thus, 50% of patients progress to end-stage renal disease within 5 years of the diagnostic renal biopsy and this percentage rises to 64% after 10 years of follow-up. The features associated with a poor prognosis are similar to those noted in pediatric patients, namely nephrotic syndrome at onset, more extensive tubulointerstitial lesions and interstitial fibrosis, and a reduced GFR. This is a compelling argument in favor of optimal control of blood pressure, preferably with an angiotensin-converting enzyme inhibitor or angiotensin receptor blocker. Treatment for hepatitis C with antivirals before renal involvement occurs may alter the incidence and natural history of secondary MPGN as treatment becomes more commonly implemented.

C. Recurrence Posttransplantation

One of the more discouraging features about primary MPGN is that the disease recurs in 20–30% of patients who receive a kidney transplant. The risk approaches 90% in those with type II disease. Time after transplant, HLA B8DR3, and a living related donor may be risk factors for recurrent MPGN. Hepatitis C MPGN can also recur in transplants or develop *de novo*. It is important to distinguish recurrent MPGN from allograft nephropathy, which can have a similar histopathologic appearance. The presence of immune deposits points toward recurrent disease. Nearly 40% of patients with recurrent MPGN will experience irreversible loss of graft function. This compounds the problem immeasurably because the likelihood of recurrent MPGN increases with each subsequent transplant procedure. There is no therapy to reduce this risk and patients should be managed on a case by case basis.

Appel GB et al: Membranoproliferative glomerulonephritis type II (dense deposit disease: an update. J Am Soc Nephrol 2005;16:1392.

Cansick JC et al: Prognosis, treatment and outcome of childhood mesangiocapillary (membranoproliferative) glomerulonephritis. Nephrol Dial Transplant 2004;19:2769.

Pickering MC et al: Uncontrolled C3 activation causes membranoproliferative glomerulonephritis in mice deficient in complement factor H. Nature Genet 2002;31:424.

Yanagihara T et al: Long-term follow-up of diffuse proliferative membranoproliferative glomerulonephritis type 1. Pediatr Nephrol 2005;20:585.

WEB SITE

The Web site www.medicine.uiowa.edu/kidneeds/ is organized by Dr. Richard Smith at the University of Iowa and deals with MPGN type II. It is highly recommended by C. Fred Strife, MD, at the University of Cincinnati Children's Hospital.

Goodpasture's Syndrome/ Anti-Glomerular Basement Membrane Disease

29

Sian Finlay, MD, & Andrew J. Rees, MD

ESSENTIALS OF DIAGNOSIS

▶ Rapidly deteriorating renal function, with or without hemoptysis and pulmonary shadowing on chest radiograph.

▶ Hematuria and proteinuria on urine dipstick and erythrocyte casts and/or dysmorphic erythrocytes on urine microscopy.

▶ Circulating antibodies directed against the glomerular basement membrane (GBM).

▶ Renal biopsy showing focal necrotizing glomerulonephritis with linear deposition of immunoglobulin.

General Considerations

Anti-glomerular basement membrane disease is a rare but well-characterized cause of glomerulonephritis, with an incidence of 1 case per million per year in white populations. All ages can be affected, but the peak incidence is in the third decade in young men and in the sixth and seventh decades in either sex. Lung hemorrhage occurs more often in younger patients, and isolated glomerulonephritis is more common in older patients. The disease is defined by the presence of pathogenic anti-GBM antibodies directed against the NC1 domain of the α_3 chain of type IV collagen [α_3(IV)NC1], a component of selected basement membranes including those of glomeruli and pulmonary alveoli. These cause focal necrotizing glomerulonephritis and result in widespread crescent formation on renal biopsy; clinically, the result is rapidly progressive glomerulonephritis. When this occurs in association with pulmonary hemorrhage, the condition is known as Goodpasture's syndrome.

The disease occurs in genetically susceptible individuals exposed to an environmental trigger. The HLA type strongly influences susceptibility; HLA types DR15 and DR4 predispose to disease, while HLA DR7 and DR1 are protective.

Environmental factors are involved in both triggering the disease and influencing its clinical presentation. Several reports describe clusters of cases, suggesting that an infective or other exogenous agent is involved in the pathogenesis, but no specific cause has been identified. Cigarette smoking has an important influence on the extent of lung injury, with pulmonary hemorrhage affecting almost all current smokers and being almost exclusively confined to this group. Lung hemorrhage following hydrocarbon exposure has also been described. In addition, genetic factors affect disease susceptibility.

Clinical Findings

A. Symptoms and Signs

Patients often have a history of malaise, arthralgia, and weight loss, but these features are generally far milder than in other causes of focal necrotizing glomerulonephritis, such as antineutrophilic cytoplasmic antibody (ANCA)-associated systemic vasculitis. Anemia is common, and may be symptomatic even in patients with minimal hemoptysis. The principal clinical symptoms relate either to pulmonary hemorrhage or to the development of renal failure. The severity of pulmonary hemorrhage varies and can range from minor hemoptysis to life-threatening hemorrhage with respiratory failure. Typically, hemoptysis is intermittent at the outset and can occur spontaneously or can be precipitated by intercurrent infections or fluid overload. There is a poor correlation between the severity of hemoptysis and the quantity of pulmonary blood loss, with other clinical signs being variable. These include inspiratory crackles and bronchial breathing, with patients often tachypnoeic and cyanosed. Historically hemoptysis has been the most common presenting feature, but its incidence is decreasing with the reduced prevalence of cigarette smoking. It now occurs in about 50% of cases. Even in those with life-threatening pulmonary hemorrhage, the lungs of patients who survive the acute illness recover completely and have no residual pulmonary symptoms of radiologic abnormalities. Histologically they are left with little residual lung pathology or fibrosis.

Renal disease can occur either alone or in association with pulmonary hemorrhage. Mild renal impairment may improve spontaneously, but once significant renal injury has occurred, improvement is rare and deterioration may be extremely rapid. Evolution from normal renal function to established renal failure is less than 12 hours in some patients. Microscopic hematuria is an early sign of renal pathology, and dysmorphic red cells and red cell casts are seen in the urine as the disease progresses. Proteinuria is present, but is usually modest (<3 g/L). Some patients present with macroscopic hematuria and severe loin pain, which are often features of very severe disease. Oliguria is a poor prognostic sign.

Without treatment anti-GBM disease almost always progresses to renal failure, but anti-GBM antibody synthesis is transient, often lasting for less than 2 months. Patients are treated with cytotoxic drugs and plasma exchange. Recurrence of anti-GBM disease is rare, but has been reported, sometimes precipitated by infection or exposure to a toxic agent. The outcome in these cases is generally better than with the original presentation, since the diagnosis is often made more quickly. The disease almost invariably recurs in renal allografts performed when circulating anti-GBM antibodies are still present, but transplantation is safe once they are no longer detectable. Exceptionally, however, renal transplantation can reinitiate anti-GBM antibody production, but this probably occurs in less than 1% of cases. Accordingly, transplantation is normally deferred for at least 6 months after the disappearance of circulating anti-GBM antibodies, and transplanted patients should be monitored closely for changes in urinary sediment or antibody titers.

B. Laboratory Findings

The diagnosis of Goodpasture's disease is dependent on the detection of anti-GBM antibodies either in the circulation or at renal biopsy. These antibodies are usually detected using an enzyme-linked immunosorbent assay (ELISA), and equivocal results can be confirmed by Western blotting. There is a clear correlation between the titer of anti-GBM antibodies and the severity of renal injury, but the pattern of lung disease is independent of antibody titer.

Other laboratory findings are nonspecific. Anemia is common, and is often microcytic and hypochromic. As in other types of rapidly progressive glomerulonephritis, there may be evidence of microangiopathy on the blood film, but this is mild. Abnormalities of the urinary sediment are an early sign of renal pathology, and are often followed by increases in serum urea nitrogen and creatinine as renal failure develops.

C. Imaging Studies

Chest radiographs can be normal or show alveolar shadowing in those with pulmonary hemorrhage. Typically this spares the bases and upper lung fields, but distinguishing

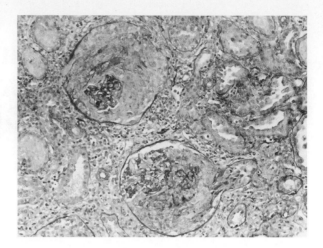

▲ **Figure 29–1.** Renal biopsy from a patient with Goodpasture's syndrome showing two glomeruli with segmental necrosis, leakage of blood into Bowman's space, and crescent formation. Renal tubules contain red cell casts and there is periglomerular and interstitial inflammation. Stained with acid fuchsin orange G-stain (AFOG).

pulmonary hemorrhage from infection or edema can be impossible. However, hemorrhage itself is not associated with curly B-lines and is not limited by fissures. Typically the radiologic changes appear and resolve more quickly than is the case for infection (Figure 29–1).

There are no specific morphologic abnormalities on any type of renal imaging and the appearance cannot be distinguished from other types of acute renal failure.

D. Special Tests

A renal biopsy is essential in the diagnosis and management of suspected anti-GBM disease (Figure 29–2). The early histologic changes include very minor mesangial expansion and hypercellularity and are followed by the development of a focal and segmental glomerulonephritis, often with marked neutrophil infiltration. This progresses to a focal necrotizing glomerulonephritis with rupture of glomerular capillaries and leakage of blood into Bowman's space. This initiates the formation of cellular crescents, composed of parietal epithelial cells and macrophages. There is some experimental evidence that crescents may also be comprised of visceral epithelial cells. Are we certain that is not the case in Goodpasture's disease? Characteristically all the crescents are at the same stage of evolution, a feature that reflects the explosive nature of the disease and distinguishes it from other forms of focal necrotizing and crescentic glomerulonephritis. Linear binding of antibody to GBM is found in all patients, regardless of the severity of the renal pathology. The antibody is

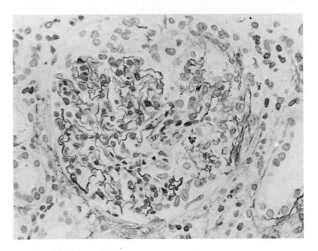

▲ **Figure 29–2.** Glomeruli from a patient with Goodpasture's disease showing linear deposition of IgG along the glomerular basement membrane detected by the immunoperoxidase method.

almost always immunoglobulin (Ig) G, but in one-third of cases IgA or IgM is also detected; exceptionally, reports describe deposition of IgA or IgM alone. Linear C3 is seen in 60–70% of patients, and its presence does not influence the severity of the renal injury.

▶ Differential Diagnosis

Goodpasture's disease must be distinguished from other causes of combined acute renal and respiratory failure, the most important of which are listed in Table 29–1. The detection of anti-GBM antibodies makes Goodpasture's disease

Table 29–1. Differential diagnosis of acute renal and respiratory failure.

Anti-glomerular basement membrane disease
Pulmonary edema secondary to acute renal failure of any etiology
Severe cardiac failure with renal hypoperfusion and pulmonary edema
Severe pneumonia (especially *Legionella*) associated with acute tubular necrosis
Systemic vasculitis—Wegener's granulomatosis, microscopic polyarteritis, systemic lupus erythematosis, Churg-Strauss syndrome
Other vasculitidies—rheumatoid vasculitis, Behçet's disease, cryoglobulinemia
Renal vein thrombosis with pulmonary emboli
Paraquat poisoning
Thrombotic microangiopathy (haemolytic uremic syndrome) with acute lung syndrome

very likely, but it is increasingly recognized that these antibodies are also found in a small proportion of patients with ANCA-associated focal necrotizing glomerulonephritis. The ANCA specificity in most of these patients is for myeloperoxidase, and their titer of anti-GBM antibodies is usually lower and more easily suppressed than in those patients with anti-GBM antibodies alone. Renal function in this group of patients may be recoverable even if they have severe renal failure at presentation.

▶ Treatment

The prognosis for Goodpasture's disease was very poor before the development of modern treatment regimens, with almost all patients dying of renal failure or pulmonary hemorrhage. The recognition that anti-GBM antibodies were pathogenic gave rise to the current treatment strategy, which is comprised of plasma exchange combined with immunosuppressive drugs. As more effective treatments were developed, it became apparent that the severity of the disease at presentation was a major determinant of the eventual outcome, especially with regard to recovery of renal function. Patients with microscopic hematuria and normal serum creatinine values often underwent spontaneous remission but remained at risk of developing devastating renal injury as long as anti-GBM antibodies remained in the circulation. In contrast, patients presenting with oligoanuric or dialysis-dependent renal failure almost never regain renal function.

Most centers now use protocols combining cyclophosphamide, prednisolone, and plasma exchange. A typical regimen is given in Table 29–2. However, the rarity of the condition makes it difficult to perform properly empowered randomized controlled clinical trials. The only controlled trial of treatment in Goodpasture's disease demonstrated a better outcome with plasma exchange than with immunosuppression and steroids alone, but used a less intensive plasma exchange regimen and lower doses of cyclophosphamide than those in common use. A study done at Walter Reed failed to demonstrate a significantly better outcome in the plasma exchange group. Nevertheless, the uniformly better results

Table 29–2. Protocol for treatment of acute Goodpasture's syndrome.

Prednisolone 1 mg/kg/day orally for 1 week; then reduce at weekly intervals to 45, 30, 25, 20, 15, 10, and 5 mg
Cyclophosphamide 3 mg/kg/day, rounded down to the nearest 50 mg (2 mg/kg in patients over 55 years)
Daily exchange of 4 L of plasma for 5% human albumin for 14 days or until the circulating antibody is suppressed; in the presence of pulmonary hemorrhage, or when there is concern about bleeding, 300–400 mL of fresh frozen plasma should be given at the end of each treatment

in series of patients treated with plasma exchange combined with alkylating agents such as cyclophosphamide provide strong evidence for their effectiveness.

Pulmonary hemorrhage is usually controlled within 24–48 hours, and moderately impaired renal function can be recovered in most patients (80% of patients with a creatinine <600 μmol/L show response to therapy). Advanced renal failure, in contrast, cannot usually be reversed by any current treatment, despite control of anti-GBM antibody levels. Consequently, the risk of treating patients with a serum creatinine over 600 μmol/L and no history of pulmonary hemorrhage probably outweighs the benefits and such patients are usually left untreated.

There are, however, a number of anecdotal reports of patients who recovered renal function despite having dialysis-dependent renal failure at presentation. These patients tend to have a short history of rapidly declining renal function and a renal biopsy showing either unexpectedly mild or very recent changes with fewer crescents than anticipated. Aggressive treatment should therefore be considered despite advanced renal failure in patients such as these, and a renal biopsy plays a key role in the evaluation. The need for early renal transplantation in cases in which regular dialysis would be particularly difficult provides another reason for aggressive treatment despite renal failure; plasma exchange regimens shorten anti-GBM antibody synthesis by up to a year.

Patients being treated by immunosuppressive drugs and plasma exchange need very careful monitoring, especially in the presence of severe renal failure. The $D_{L_{CO}}$, a measure of the diffusing capacity of the lung, is markedly elevated in pulmonary hemorrhage, and can be used in diagnosis. Minor reductions in $D_{L_{CO}}$ may occur long after resolution of the disease. Albumin solutions used as replacement fluid for plasma exchange have a high sodium concentration. Consequently plasma exchange is associated with sodium loading and can result in fluid accumulation and pulmonary edema. Accordingly, patients must be monitored carefully for fluid overload. Use of immunosuppressive drugs should also be monitored equally assiduously. Careful monitoring of the complete blood count is essential, and cyclophosphamide should be discontinued if the white cell count falls below 3.5×10^9/L. Progress can also be assessed by measuring serum creatinine, hemoglobin, and anti-GBM antibody titer, as well as by serial chest radiographs and $D_{L_{CO}}$ estimation. Recent studies have documented 1-year patient survival rates of 79–93%.

▶ Prognosis

Alport's syndrome is an inherited glomerular disease caused by mutations of the genes that encode the α_3, α_4, and α_5 chains of collagen, which together form the collagen network in glomerular capillaries. Consequently the GBM lacks these collagen chains. The disease usually progresses to end-stage renal failure and after renal transplantation, patients with Alport's syndrome are at risk of developing antibodies directed against the normal α chains in the renal allograft. The transient appearance of low titers of anti-GBM antibodies is quite common, and a small number of patients (3–5%) develop a focal necrotizing glomerulonephritis with crescents in the renal allograft. The clinical cause and morphologic appearances are indistinguishable from anti-GBM disease in native kidneys. Treatment is similarly identical, but the outcome is poor. Recurrence in subsequent grafts is the norm and usually occurs within days. Importantly, the anti-GBM antibodies are directed against the mutated α chain, most commonly the α_5 chain. Consequently most transplanted patients with Alport's syndrome have anti-α_5 antibodies rather than anti-α_3 antibodies, and these are detected poorly in standard anti-GBM ELISA assays. Loss of renal allografts due to *de novo* Goodpasture's syndrome in patients with Alport's syndrome is nevertheless uncommon. Recurrence of Goodpasture's syndrome is uncommon if the allograft is placed after anti-GBM titers are no longer present.

Browne G et al: Retransplantation in Alport post-transplant anti-GBM disease. Kidney Int 2004;65:675.

Levy JB et al: Long-term outcome of anti-glomerular basement membrane antibody disease treated with plasma exchange and immunosuppression. Ann Intern Med 2001;134:1033.

Postinfectious Glomerulonephritis

30

Bernardo Rodriguez-Iturbe, MD, & Sergio Mezzano, MD

This chapter deals with nephritis associated with bacterial infections. A variety of bacterial infections are associated with renal disease, among which are *Streptococcus* (group A and C), *Staphylococcus* (*aureus* and *epidermidis*), *Salmonella* (*typhi* and *paratyphi*), *Treponema pallidum*, and *Brucella abortus sui*. We will limit our considerations to three specific disease entities: Poststreptococcal glomerulonephritis, glomerulonephritis associated with infective endocarditis, and glomerulonephritis associated with infected atrioventricular shunts.

POSTSTREPTOCOCCAL GLOMERULONEPHRITIS

 ESSENTIALS OF DIAGNOSIS

▶ Acute nephritic syndrome (hematuria, edema, hypertension, ± oliguria), occasionally nephrotic syndrome, and rarely rapidly progressive azotemia.

▶ No evidence of systemic disease.

▶ Recent streptococcal infection (serology or culture).

▶ Reduced serum complement (CH_{50} and $C3$).

▶ General Considerations

The incidence of acute poststreptococcal glomerulonephritis (APSGN) has decreased dramatically in most industrialized countries. The association with alcoholism in adult patients has been noticed in central Europe. Nevertheless, in other countries, such as Singapore, Trinidad, and Venezuela, a poststreptococcal etiology is the causative factor in more than 70% of the children admitted to the hospital with glomerulonephritis. The reason for these geographic variations

in epidemiology may be the accessibility to early medical care and antibiotic treatment resulting from improvements in living standards. In addition, a lack of hygiene and sanitation prevalent in underdeveloped countries may predispose to a Th1 type of response (characteristic of APSGN) in contrast to the Th2 response that tends to favor minimal change disease in the industrialized countries with higher standards of hygiene. APSGN presents as sporadic cases, clusters of cases, or epidemics that follow streptococcal infections of the throat or the skin. The original epidemics were all due to group A streptococci, but the most recent large epidemic was due to the consumption of unpasteurized milk and cheese from cows with mastitis caused by *Streptococcus zooepidemicus*.

Streptococci of M types 47, 49, 55, and 57 are frequently the etiologic agents of pyodermitis-associated nephritis while types 1, 2, 4, and 12 correspond to upper respiratory streptococcal infections causing nephritis. There is a wide variability in the incidence of nephritis following a nephritogenic streptococcal infection, but the incidence among siblings is close to 40%, which indicates a familial predisposition to the disease; however, a genetic marker of susceptibility for APSGN has not been found.

APSGN is an immune complex-mediated disease. Humoral and cellular immune mechanisms are involved. Immune complexes formed in the circulation or *in situ* induce the local activation of the complement (preferentially by an alternative pathway) and coagulation systems (platelet consumption and activation) and the recruitment of inflammatory cells. Infiltration of helper T lymphocytes is an early feature and increased levels of interleukin (IL)-6, tumor necrosis factor (TNF)-α, and platelet-derived growth factor (PDGF) have been demonstrated. In addition, there is evidence of autoimmune reactivity attributed in part to neuraminidase-induced desialization of normal components.

Antineutrophil cytoplasmic antibody (ANCA), cryglobulins, serum rheumatoid factor titers, C3eNef, and anti-immunoglobulin (Ig) G renal deposits have all been demonstrated. These manifestations of autoimmune reactivity have undefined clinical significance except for the demonstration of ANCA that is more frequent in cases of greater severity.

The nature of the nephritogenic streptococcal antigen is still controversial. At present, streptococcal plasmin receptor [nephritis-associated plasmin receptor (NAPlr) or glyceraldehyde-3-phosphate dehydrogenase (GAPDH)] and streptococcal cationic exotoxin B and zymogen precursor (SPE B) are actively being investigated. Serum antibody response to these antigens has been found in 70–90% of the patients and both GAPDH and SPE B have been detected in renal biopsies obtained early in the course of the disease. Multicentric studies show that the antizymogen antibody titer is the best marker of nephritogenic streptococcal infection. Recently, evidence of colocalization of NAPlr and glomerular plasmin-like activity has been found, suggesting that the ability to bind to plasmin plays a critical pathogenetic role in APSGN.

APSGN induces long-term protective immunity as demonstrated by the fact that repeated attacks of the disease are extremely rare.

▶ Clinical Findings

APSGN is usually, but not exclusively, a disease of children and adolescents: The highest incidence occurs in patients between the ages of 4 and 15 years. Less than 5% of the patients are younger than 2 years and about 10% in most large series are older than 40 years.

A. Symptoms and Signs

The diagnosis of APSGN requires the demonstration of antecedent streptococcal infection in a patient who presents with acute glomerulonephritis. Nephritis may follow 7–15 days after streptococcal tonsillitis and 4–6 weeks after impetigo. It is not unusual for the active pyodermitis to have subsided at the time of APSGN but telltale skin scars and decoloration are present. Impetigo frequently complicates scabies and a clue to this association may be obtained by examination of the siblings of the patient.

The acute nephritic syndrome, characterized by edema, gross or microscopic hematuria, hypertension, and frequently oliguria, is the usual clinical presentation of APSGN and renal histology shows acute endocapillary glomerulonephritis with mesangial and capillary granular immune deposition. Hematuria, gross or microscopic, is almost universally present. The edema occurs in 80–90% of the patients, is usually the primary complaint, and varies in severity from swollen eyelids to anasarca, but in contrast with nephrotic syndrome, ascites is rarely present. Hypertension is found in 80% of the patients. The severity of hypertension is correlated with the degree of fluid retention and the volume-sensing hormonal systems reflect primary sodium retention with expansion of extracellular fluid volume: Suppressed renin–angiotensin–aldosterone system and stimulated secretion of atrial natriuretic peptide. The clinical manifestations of acute nephritic syndrome usually last less than 2 weeks.

Less than 4% of the children with APSGN have massive proteinuria and these patients usually have thick, garland-like immune deposits and large numbers of prominent "humps" as revealed by electron microscopy. Occasionally, a patient develops rapidly progressive azotemia and crescentic glomerulonephritis.

Asymptomatic cases, manifested by microscopic hematuria, reduction of the complement levels, and sometimes hypertension after a recent streptococcal infection, are in prospective studies four or five times more frequently than clinically apparent disease.

The clinical manifestations of APSGN in children are different from those in adult patients, who frequently have a more protracted course, higher incidence of complications, and a consistently poorer prognosis.

B. Laboratory Findings

The positivity of cultures in cases of APSGN has significant variability: 10–70% of the cases during epidemics and about 25% in sporadic cases. Most frequently, the poststreptococcal etiology is established by increasing titers of antistreptolysin O (ASO)(reported in 33–80% of the cases of APSGN that follow throat infections), anti-DNase B (increased in 73% of the postimpetigo cases), and the streptozyme test that measures antibodies to four antigens: DNase B, ASO, hyaluronidase, and streptokinase (positive in about 80% of the cases). Anti-NAPlr, anti-SPE B, and antizymogen (SPE B precursor) antibody titers are more sensitive (positive in close to 90% of the APSGN patients), but their determination is not generally available.

The complement system is preferentially, but not exclusively, activated by the alternative pathway. C4 levels are usually normal and CH_{50} and C3 are depressed in more than 90% of the cases and return to normal in less than 1 month. A normal serum complement in the acute phase as well as hypocomplementemia lasting longer than 1 month should raise the suspicion of a diagnosis different than APSGN. Serum IgG and IgM are usually elevated and IgA is normal. Cryoglobulins are present in one-third of the patients.

The urine sediment shows red blood cell casts and dismorphic erythrocytes, characteristic of glomerular hematuria. The fractional excretion of sodium is frequently less than 0.5 and increases with the reestablishment of diuresis.

C. Special Tests

Renal biopsy is not indicated in APSGN unless there are characteristics that make the diagnosis doubtful or have prognostic significance and therapeutic implications (see Differential Diagnosis below).

Differential Diagnosis

The initial approach to the patient with acute nephritic syndrome should indicate if a systemic disease is associated with the acute glomerulonephritis or if the clinical picture results from a primary renal disease. The lack of fever, gastrointestinal and pulmonary manifestations, arthralgias, or vasculitis skin lesions suggests primary renal disease. The serum complement levels are helpful as a first-line laboratory test because fewer than 10% of the patients with APSGN have a normal serum complement and such a findings should raise the possibility of other diseases such as IgA nephropathy, vasculitis, hemolytic uremic syndrome, or anti-glomerular basement membrane disease. In addition, the serum complement returns to normal levels in less than a month in APSGN and a persistently low C3 should make the clinician consider membranoproliferative glomerulonephritis (types 1 or 2) or lupus erythematosus.

Complications

Most children with APSGN have an uncomplicated clinical course. Pulmonary edema and hyperkalemia may sometimes be present if there is severe oliguria and fluids are not restricted. In contrast to the benign clinical picture in children, 40% of elderly patients with APSGN present with congestive heart failure. Massive proteinuria and azotemia, rare in children, may occur in as many as 20% and 80%, respectively, of the adults with the disease.

Rarely, APSGN is complicated by hypertensive encephalopathy or a rapidly progressive course characteristic of crescentic glomerulonephritis.

Treatment

Management of APSGN includes the treatment of the streptococcal infection and the treatment of the acute nephritic syndrome and its complications. Streptococcal infection should be treated with penicillin (a single dose of 1.2 million units of benzathine penicillin or 200,000 units of oral penicillin every 6 hours for 7–10 days) or if the patient is allergic, erythromycin (250 mg orally every 6 hours for 7–10 days). In small children these doses should be reduced by 50%.

The management of acute nephritic syndrome requires hospital admission in the adult or elderly patient and in most children with APSGN. Some children without severe edema or hypertension and normal serum creatinine may be followed at home if close contact is maintained, particularly in the first few days when the clinical picture may worsen.

All patients should have restricted sodium and fluid intake and most will benefit from the administration of loop diuretics in the first 24–48 hours of the disease. Hypertension usually subsides after diuresis is established. Oral nifedipine is generally sufficient to control hypertension. Nitroprusside may be required in very rare cases with hypertensive encephalopathy.

Pulmonary edema is treated with loop diuretics and oxygen; digitalis is contraindicated because it is ineffective and intoxication is frequent. Hyperkalemia and uremia may require dialysis.

Prognosis

The prognosis of the acute phase is excellent in children but in elderly patients the mortality in some series is as high as 20% because of the frequency of cardiovascular complications. Mild proteinuria and hematuria may persist for several months after the acute attack.

The long-term prognosis of APSGN has been debated for some time. Approximately 50% of the biopsies obtained up to 15 years after the acute attack show variable degrees of interstitial infiltration and glomerular sclerosis and the incidence of renal function abnormalities in the reported studies has significant variability. For instance, most studies indicate that proteinuria is found in 4–13% of patients, but the range extends from 1.4% to 46%. Similarly, the reported frequency of hypertension ranges from that found in the general population to as much as 46% of the patients. These discrepancies result, at least in part, from studying populations of different ethnic background, different age groups, and sporadic or epidemic cases. Nevertheless, the incidence of end-stage renal disease from the collected studies with 15 years of follow-up is less than 1%, and there is general agreement that the long-term prognosis is worse in adult patients and patients who develop massive proteinuria. A particularly bad prognosis has been reported in elderly alcoholic patients and in patients who develop proteinuria in the nephrotic range. A disturbingly high incidence of impaired renal function has been reported in a recent outbreak of APSGN occurring as a result of the ingestion of cheese contaminated with *S zooepidemicus*. In this study, which included mostly adult patients, 30% of the patients had impaired renal function 2 years after the acute attack.

Johnson RJ et al: Hypothesis: dysregulation of immunologic balance resulting from hygiene and socioeconomic factors may influence the epidemiology and cause of glomerulonephritis worldwide. Am J Kidney Dis 2003;42:575. [PMID: 12955687]

Oda T et al: Glomerular plasmin-like activity in relation to nephritis-associated plasmin receptor in acute poststreptococcal glomerulonephritis. J Am Soc Nephrol 2005;16:247. [PMID: 15574512]

Rodriguez-Iturbe B: Nephritis-associated streptococcal antigens: where are we now? J Am Soc Nephrol 2004;15:1961. [PMID: 15213287]

Yoshizawa N et al: Nephritis-associated plasmin receptor and acute poststreptococcal glomerulonephritis: characterization of the antigen and associated immune response. J Am Soc Nephrol 2004;15:1785. [PMID: 15213266]

GLOMERULONEPHRITIS ASSOCIATED WITH INFECTIVE ENDOCARDITIS

ESSENTIALS OF DIAGNOSIS

► Urinary abnormalities (hematuria and albuminuria), with or without elevated serum creatinine, nephrotic-range proteinuria, and occasionally rapidly progressive renal failure.

► Evidence of endocarditis (echocardiogram or physical examination).

► Positive blood cultures or serologic evidence of infection.

General Considerations

In the United States, 10,000 to 15,000 cases of infective endocarditis (IE) are diagnosed every year and a recent survey in France found an incidence of 31 cases per million population. Male:female ratios range from 2:1 to 9:1 and the disease is increasingly frequent in elderly individuals and in patients with no underlying heart disease. Intravenous drug usage, prosthetic heart valves, and structural heart disease are risk factors. Nosocomial endocarditis complicating bacteremia induced by invasive procedures or prosthetic devices may presently account for almost 10% of the cases of IE in some areas. Other less common predisposing conditions are HIV infection, immunosuppressed patients, hemodialysis arteriovenous fistulas, central venous catheters, and ulcerative colitis (*Streptococcus bovis* endocarditis).

The natural history of endocarditis-associated glomerulonephritis has been significantly altered with the changing epidemiology of IE and with the use of antibiotics. The average age of patients with endocarditis has increased to a current median age of 54 years. This change can be attributed to the decreasing prevalence of rheumatic heart disease, the increasing prevalence of underlying degenerative heart disease, and the increment of procedures and practices predisposing older patients to bacteremia. *Streptococcus viridans* was the most common organism in the preantibiotic era and glomerulonephritis occurred in 50–80% of cases. With the use of prophylactic antibiotics in patients with valvular heart disease and the mounting frequency of intravenous drug abuse, *S aureus* has replaced *S viridans* as the leading cause of infective endocarditis. The incidence of glomerulonephritis associated with *S aureus* endocarditis ranges from 22% to 78%, with the higher figure consisting predominantly of intravenous drug users. Renal complications of IE include infarcts, abscesses, and glomerulonephritis (all of which may coexist). In a recent survey of 62 out of 354 patients with IE in whom renal tissue was available for study, localized infarcts were reported in 31%, half of which were septic; focal or diffuse glomerulonephritis was found in 26%, of which many cases had vascular inflammation; interstitial nephritis, mostly attributable to antibiotics, was found in 10%, and cortical necrosis was found in 10% of the cases, all of them necropsy findings.

Pathogenesis

Focal and segmental proliferative glomerulonephritis, often with focal crescents, is the most typical finding on light microscopy. Some patients may exhibit a more diffuse proliferative endocapillary lesion with or without crescents. Immunofluorescence microscopy reveals granular capillary and mesangial deposits of IgG, IgM, and C3 and electron microscopy shows electron-dense deposits in mesangial, subendothelial, and occasionally in subepithelial localization. In subacute endocarditis, focal segmental proliferative lesions with fibrinoid necrosis or capillary thrombosis may be present. Tubulointerstitial cellular infiltration and variable degrees of atrophy and fibrosis may be found. The renal biopsy is important to clarify diagnosis or for prognosis.

The diffuse deposition of immunoglobulin, the depression of complement, and electron-dense deposits support an immune complex mechanism for the production of this form of glomerulonephritis. Further support for this pathogenesis is offered by the demonstration of specific antibody in kidney eluates and detection of bacterial antigen in the deposits. Both *S aureus* and hemolytic *Streptococcus* antigens have been identified. In addition, *S aureus* expresses "superantigens" that can also activate T cells directly.

Clinical Findings

The clinical presentation of infective endocarditis may vary from an indolent illness with few systemic manifestations, readily responsive to antibiotic therapy, to a fulminating septicemia with life-threatening destruction of heart valves and systemic embolization. The varied features of endocarditis relate in large measure to the different infecting organisms. S *viridans* is the prototype of bacteria that originate in the oral flora, infect previously abnormal heart valves, and may cause minimal symptoms despite progressive valvular damage. S *aureus*, in contrast, can invade previously normal valves and destroy them rapidly.

A. Symptoms and Signs

The diagnosis of endocarditis is usually suggested by the presentation of multiple clinical findings. A previous history of endocarditis is obtained in 2–9% of the patients. Peripheral signs of vascular and/or immunologic origin are seen with variable frequency: Petechiae in 20–40% of the patients, splinter hemorrhages (linear, red–brown streaks in nail beds) in 15%, Osler's nodes (painful nodules on the pads of digits) in 10–25%, Janeway lesions (painless dark spots on the palms or soles) in <10%, and Roth spots (pale areas surrounded by hemorrhage on funduscopic examination) in <5%.

The clinical renal manifestations usually consist of microscopic hematuria and mild proteinuria, with or without azotemia. One-third of patients with IE develop azotemia and the risk increases with age, previous history of hypertension, thrombocytopenia, and prosthetic valve infection. A rapidly progressive clinical course, if present, is associated with crescentic glomerulonephritis. Nephrotic syndrome is unusual, except in cases due to infected atrioventricular shunts.

B. Laboratory Findings

The positive yield of blood cultures depends on the number of cultures taken from separate venipuncture sites (three cultures give 98%), the amount of blood (>5 mL of blood gives 92%), and the organism involved. The probability of endocarditis in patients with *S aureus* bacteremia is particularly high and in bacteremia with *Enterococcus fecalis* is higher than with other enterococcal species. Other laboratory tests that are frequently positive in endocarditis are an elevated erythrocyte sedimentation rate, a normocytic normochromic anemia, and, especially in staphylococcal endocarditis, an elevated white cell count.

Decreased C3 and C4 levels, consistent with activation of the classical complement pathway, are found in 60–90% of patients with glomerulonephritis. The degree of complement activation correlates with the severity of renal impairment and the complement levels normalize with successful therapy of the infection. High titers of rheumatoid factor, circulating immune complexes, and mixed cryoglobulins may be present in up to 50% of patients with subacute IE, particularly if it is associated with glomerulonephritis. Positive cytoplasmic (C)-ANCA has been reported occasionally.

▶ Treatment

A. Antibiotic Prophylaxis

Despite the lack of definite proof of the benefits of prophylactic antibiotic therapy, the guidelines of the American Heart Association consider the use of antibiotic prophylaxis, recognizing that individual judgment must be exercised concerning its use. Most experts would prescribe antibiotic prophylaxis in patients with prosthetic heart valves, in patients with a previous history of IE, and in patients with congenital heart disease. Circumstances in which the risk of bacteremia is significant include invasive dental, oral, or upper respiratory procedures and, less frequently, invasive genitourinary procedures. In oral or upper respiratory procedures, amoxicillin (2 g orally, or 50 mg/kg in children), or in patients allergic to penicillin clindamycin (600 mg) or cephalexin (2 g), may be given 1 hour prior to the procedure. In high risk patients scheduled for genitourinary procedures, a combination of gentamycin (1.5 mg/kg) and amoxicillin (1 g) may be used.

B. Antibiotic Treatment

A number of different regimens have been advocated for the treatment of IE depending of the causative organisms. The common characteristic of all therapies is the need to give antibiotic treatment for 4–6 weeks, which, when the antibiotic is appropriate, usually results in complete eradication of endocarditis with correction of serologic abnormalities. The preferred antiobiotic selection is beyond the scope of the present work and requires determining bacterial resistance, but, in general, *S viridans, bovis,* and other streptococcal species may be reliably treated with penicillin (12–18 million units daily) or ceftriaxone (2 g daily) in allergic patients. Enterococci may be more successfully treated with a combination of antibiotics: Penicillin or vancomycin (if there is a high level of penicillin resistance) in association with gentamycin. Native valve endocarditis due to *S aureus* is best treated with nefcillin or oxacillin (2 g intravenously every 4 hours) with perhaps the addition of gentamycin in the first few days of therapy. Standard treatment for methicillin-resistant staphylococci is vancomycin.

Abnormal renal findings in patients with glomerulonephritis, among them microscopic hematuria, proteinuria, and elevation of serum creatinine, may persist for months after eradication of the infection. Normalization of C3 during the therapy correlates with a good outcome. Plasmapheresis and short-term courses of high dose steroids have been advocated in severe cases of crescentic nephritis.

▶ Prognosis

The prognosis of infective endocarditis depends on the severity and extent of the valvular damage and the infecting organism. The immediate prognosis of glomerulonephritis is in general good and is related to the prompt eradication of the infection. Patients with a rapidly progressive course and severe crescentic glomerulonephritis have the worst prognosis. Scarce information is available concerning the long-term prognosis of IE-related glomerulonephritis.

Couzi L et al: An unusual endocarditis-induced crescentic glomerulonephritis treated by plasmapheresis. Clin Nephrol 2004;62:461. [PMID: 15630906]

Hoen B et al: Association pour l'Etude et la Prevention de l'Endocardite Infectieuse (AEPEI) Study Group. Changing profile of infective endocarditis: results of a 1-year survey in France. JAMA 2002;288:75. [PMID: 12090865]

Koya D et al: Successful recovery of infective endocarditis-induced rapidly progressive glomerulonephritis by steroid therapy combined with antibiotics: a case report. BMC Nephrol 2004;21:18. [PMID: 15610562]

SHUNT NEPHRITIS

ESSENTIALS OF DIAGNOSIS

▶ Microscopic hematuria and proteinuria, frequently in the nephrotic range, occasionally elevated serum creatinine, and hypertension.

▶ Ventriculovascular shunt implanted for treatment of hydrocephalus.

▶ Prolonged fever or signs of chronic infection.

▶ General Considerations

Shunt nephritis refers to an immune complex-mediated glomerulonephritis that develops as a complication of chronically infected ventriculoatrial or ventriculojugular shunts inserted for the treatment of hydrocephalus. The renal outcome of shunt nephritis is good if early diagnosis and treatment are provided. Ventriculovascular (VV) shunts may become infected in about 30% of cases. Glomerulonephritis may develop in 0.7–2% of the infected VV shunts in an interval of time ranging from 2 months to many years after insertion. The infective organisms are usually *S epidermidis* and *S aureus* and less frequently *Propionibacterium acne,* *Pseudomonas,* and *Serratia* spp. In contrast to VV shunts, ventriculoperitoneal shunts are rarely complicated with glomerulonephritis. Due to the wide clinical spectrum of this disorder, as well as the indolent courses of shunt infections, the diagnosis is often delayed.

▶ Pathogenesis

The glomeruli typically exhibit a membranoproliferative glomerulonephritis type I, but a mesangial proliferative pattern may occasionally be present. By immunofluorescence, diffuse granular deposits of IgG, IgM, and C3 are demonstrated. Electron-dense mesangial and subendothelial deposits are found by electron microscopy. The pathogenesis of these lesions involves the deposition of bacterial immune complexes and activation of both the classic and alternative complement pathways.

▶ Clinical Findings

A. Symptoms and Signs

As a rule, patients present with signs of infection. The clinical course consists of recurrent fever, weight loss, paleness, arthralgias, and frequently hepatosplenomegaly, in association with evidence of increased intracranial pressure. The renal manifestations include hematuria (microscopic or gross), proteinuria (nephrotic syndrome in 30% of patients), renal insufficiency, and hypertension.

B. Laboratory Findings

Laboratory abnormalities include anemia, usually normochromic normocytic unless iron deficiency is also present, and elevated sedimentation rate and C-reactive protein levels. Elevated titers of rheumatoid factor, cryoglobulinemia, hypocomplementemia ($C3$, $C4$, and CH_{50}), and the presence of circulating immune complexes have all been demonstrated. Positive titers of ANCA specific for proteinase 3 have recently been reported in these patients.

▶ Treatment

Antibiotic therapy and prompt removal of the infected catheter usually lead to remission of the glomerulonephritis. However, cases of progressive chronic renal failure have been reported. Delay in the diagnosis and in the removal of the shunt worsens the prognosis of the renal lesion.

Iwata Y et al: Shunt nephritis with positive titers of ANCA specific for proteinase 3. Am J Kidney Dis 2004;43:e1-6. [PMID: 15112193]

Vasculitides

31

Patrick H. Nachman, MD, & Cynthia J. Denu-Ciocca, MD

ESSENTIALS OF DIAGNOSIS

▶ Vasculitides affecting the kidneys are typically associated with hematuria and proteinuria, frequently presenting as a rapidly progressive glomerulonephritis.

▶ Glomerular injury occurs in the setting of the small vessel vasculitides, associated with antineutrophil cytoplasmic autoantibodies (ANCA), antiglomerular basement membrane antibodies (anti-GBM), or the presence of immune complex formation such as with Henoch-Schönlein purpura (HSP), cryoglobulinemic vasculitis, and systemic lupus erythematosus (SLE).

▶ They may affect the kidneys alone, but are more frequently part of a multiorgan disease that may affect the skin, upper and lower respiratory tracts, and the musculoskeletal, gastrointestinal, and nervous systems.

▶ General Considerations

The classification of vasculitides is based on the predilection for injury of the different vascular beds (Table 31–1). The following sections provide an overview of the various groups of vasculitides. The remainder of this chapter will focus on the clinical aspects of small vessel vasculitis (SVV) because of their association with glomerulonephritis.

A. Large Vessel Vasculitis: Takayasu's Arteritis and Giant Cell Arteritis

Large vessel vasculitis affects the aorta and its major branches. During the acute phase of disease, large vessel vasculitis is characterized pathologically by chronic granulomatous inflammation that often contains giant cells in the inflammatory infiltrates. The chronic phase is characterized by extensive vascular sclerosis with little or no active inflammation. Inflammatory and sclerotic thickening of the aorta and the arteries causes narrowing of lumina, which in turn causes ischemia and the resultant clinical manifestations. Involvement of the renal artery may cause renovascular hypertension.

The two major large vessel vasculitides are Takayasu's arteritis and giant cell arteritis. Takayasu's arteritis most often involves the aorta and its major branches, although the pulmonary arteries may be affected. Takayasu's arteritis is most common in Asia, and rarely occurs in patients older than 40 years. Clinically, it often presents with diminished pulses, vascular bruits, claudication, and renovascular hypertension.

Giant cell arteritis rarely occurs in patients younger than 50 years and is most common in patients of northern European ethnicity. Like Takayasu's arteritis, giant cell arteritis affects the aorta and its major branches; however, it has a much greater predilection for the extracranial branches of the carotid artery. Frequent clinical manifestations include headache, jaw claudication, blindness, deafness, tongue dysfunction, extremity claudication, and reduced peripheral pulses. Pathologic involvement of the renal artery is common in giant cell arteritis, but symptomatic renovascular hypertension is rare. Polymyalgia rheumatica occurs in 40–60% of patients with giant cell arteritis. The presence of polymyalgia rheumatica may be useful for diagnosis, but symptoms may occur before, simultaneously, or after the onset of giant cell arteritis.

B. Medium-Sized Vessel Vasculitis: Polyarteritis Nodosa and Kawasaki's Disease

The medium-sized vessel vasculitides have a predilection for arteries that lead to major viscera and their initial branches. In the kidneys, the major targets are the interlobar and arcuate arteries, with less frequent involvement of the main renal artery and interlobular arteries. The two major medium-sized vessel vasculitides are polyarteritis

Table 31–1. Names and definitions of vasculitis adopted by the Chapel Hill Consensus Conference on the nomenclature of systemic vasculitis.

Large vessel vasculitis[1]	
Giant cell arteritis	Granulomatous arteritis of the aorta and its major branches, with a predilection for the extracranial branches of the carotid artery. Often involves the *temporal artery*. Usually occurs in patients older than 50 years and often is associated with *polymyalgia rheumatica*.
Takayasu's arteritis	Granulomatous inflammation of the aorta and its major branches. Usually occurs in patients younger than 50 years.
Medium-sized vessel vasculitis[1]	
Polyarteritis nodosa	Necrotizing inflammation of medium-sized or small arteries without glomerulonephritis or vasculitis in arterioles, capillaries, or venules.
Kawasaki's disease	Arteritis involving large, medium-sized, and small arteries, and associated with mucocutaneous lymph node syndrome. *Coronary arteries are often involved.* Aorta and veins may be involved. Usually occurs in children.
Small vessel vasculitis[1]	
Wegener's granulomatosis[2]	Granulomatous inflammation involving the respiratory tract, and necrotizing vasculitis affecting small to medium-sized vessels, eg, capillaries, venules, arterioles, and arteries. Necrotizing glomerulonephritis is common.
Churg–Strauss syndrome[2]	Eosinophil-rich and granulomatous inflammation involving the respiratory tract and necrotizing vasculitis affecting small to medium-sized vessels, and associated with asthma and blood eosinophilia.
Microscopic polyangiitis[2]	Necrotizing vasculitis with few or no immune deposits affecting small vessels, eg, capillaries, venules, or arterioles. Necrotizing arteritis involving small and medium-sized arteries may be present. Necrotizing glomerulonephritis is very common. Pulmonary capillaritis often occurs.
Henoch–Schönlein purpura	Vasculitis with IgA-dominant immune deposits affecting small vessels, eg, capillaries, venules, or arterioles. Typically involves skin, gut, and glomeruli and is associated with *arthralgias or arthritis*.
Cryoglobulinemic vasculitis	Vasculitis with cryoglobulin immune deposits affecting small vessels, eg, capillaries, venules, or arterioles, and associated with cryoglobulins in serum. *Skin and glomeruli are often involved.*
Cutaneous leukocytoclastic angiitis	Isolated cutaneous leukocytoclastic angiitis without systemic vasculitis or glomerulonephritis.

[1]"Large artery" refers to the aorta and the largest branches directed toward major body regions (eg, to the extremities and the head and neck); "medium-sized artery" refers to the main visceral arteries (eg, renal, hepatic, coronary, and mesenteric arteries); and "small artery" refers to the distal arterial radicals that connect with arterioles. Note large and medium-sized vessel vasculitides do not involve vessels other than arteries.

[2]Strongly associated with ANCA.

Reproduced with permission from Jennette JC et al: Nomenclature of systemic vasculitides. Proposal of an international consensus conference. Arthritis Rheum 1994;37(2):187.

nodosa (PAN) and Kawasaki's disease. Pathologically, both are characterized in the acute phase by necrotizing arteritis with transmural inflammation that can lead to the formation of pseudoaneurysms. In only a few days, the lesions evolve from an acute neutrophil-rich inflammation to a "chronic" inflammation with predominantly mononuclear leukocytes. Secondary complications of the arteritis include thrombosis, infarction, and hemorrhage. Sites of thrombosis and necrosis develop progressive scarring. Although medium-sized vessel vasculitides do not cause glomerulonephritis by definition, they can cause hematuria, proteinuria (usually less than 2 g/24 hours), and renal insufficiency as a result

of renal infarction. Pseudoaneurysms near the renal surface may rupture and cause severe, even fatal, retroperitoneal, and intraperitoneal hemorrhage.

Although the diagnostic term "polyarteritis nodosa" previously included all patients with any pattern of necrotizing arteritis, the new classification distinguishes it from vasculitides that predominantly affect small arterioles, capillaries, and venules [such as Wegener's granulomatosis, Churg–Strauss syndrome, and microscopic polyangiitis (MPA)]. By this approach, the presence of glomerulonephritis or pulmonary alveolar capillaritis with pulmonary hemorrhage rules out a diagnosis of polyarteritis nodosa and indicates the presence

Table 31-2. Clinical differences between polyarteritis nodosa and microscopic polyangiitis.

Clinical feature	Polyarteritis nodosa	Microscopic polyangiitis
Rapidly progressive nephritis	No	Very common
Pulmonary hemorrhage	No	Yes
Peripheral neuropathy	Yes	Yes
Microaneurysms by angiography	Yes	Rare
Renovascular hypertension	Occasional	No
Positive hepatitis B serology	Uncommon	No
Positive antineutrophil cytoplasmic antibodies serology results	Rare	Frequent
Relapses	Rare	Frequent

Reproduced with permission from Guillevin L et al: Antineutrophil cytoplasmic antibodies, abnormal angiograms and pathological findings in polyarteritis nodosa and Churg–Strauss syndrome: indications for the classification of vasculitides of the polyarteritis nodosa group. Br J Rheumatol 1996;35:958.

of some type of SVV. Testing for ANCA is typically negative in PAN as opposed to patients with small vessel vasculitides, MPA, Wegener's granulomatosis, or Churg–Strauss syndrome. Table 31–2 compares some of the features of polyarteritis nodosa and MPA.

The necrotizing arteritis of Kawasaki's disease is pathologically indistinguishable from polyarteritis nodosa. Kawasaki's disease is an acute febrile illness of childhood that is characterized by the mucocutaneous lymph node syndrome, which includes nonsuppurative lymphadenopathy, polymorphous erythematosus rash, erythema of the oropharyngeal mucosa, erythema of the palms and soles, conjunctivitis, and indurative edema and desquamation of the extremities. A major cause for morbidity and mortality in patients with Kawasaki's disease is the development of a necrotizing arteritis with a predilection for coronary arteries. Symptomatic renal involvement is rare in Kawasaki's disease.

Because Kawasaki's disease and polyarteritis nodosa are treated differently, differentiation between the two arteritides is very important. The presence or absence of the mucocutaneous lymph node syndrome is an effective diagnostic discriminator. Kawasaki's disease usually is treated with aspirin and intravenous γ-globulin therapy. One of the main goals of treatment of Kawasaki's disease is to reduce the incidence of coronary arteritis. Timely treatment with intravenous immunoglobulin (IVIG) and aspirin has been shown to reduce the incidence of cardiac lesions from 20–40% to <5%. Aspirin alone has not been shown to reduce

cardiac sequelae but combined therapy with IVIG appears to have an additive anti-inflammatory effect. If the patient fails initial treatment, repeated doses of IVIG, pulse methylprednisolone, cyclophosphamide, methotrexate, cyclosporin, and plasmapheresis have been utilized. Recently data suggest that infliximab may be an alternative therapy for patients with refractory disease.

Idiopathic polyarteritis nodosa is usually treated with high-dose corticosteroids and cyclophosphamide. This form of therapy has been shown to be beneficial, especially in those who have adverse prognostic factors. The optimal length of treatment is unknown, but a recent study has suggested that 6 months of therapy may be less effective than 12 months. For patients with hepatitis B virus-associated PAN, therapy with antiviral agents improves outcomes.

C. Small Vessel Vasculitis: Microscopic Polyangiitis, Wegener's Granulomatosis, and Churg–Strauss Syndrome

Small vessel vasculitides are characterized by necrotizing inflammation primarily targeting venules and capillaries, although arteries, arterioles, and veins may be affected. Unlike vasculitides of larger vascular beds, small vessel vasculitides frequently cause glomerulonephritis (Table 31–1).

The two major categories of SVV include the "pauci-immune small vessel vasculitides" and the "immune complex-mediated small vessel vasculitides" (Table 31–3). Immune complex-mediated vasculitides, such as HSP,

Table 31-3. Small vessel vasculitides.

Pauci-immune small vessel vasculitis (usually ANCA[1] positive)
Microscopic polyangiitis
Wegener's granulomatosis
Churg-Strauss syndrome
Drug-induced ANCA vasculitis
Immune complex small vessel vasculitis
Henoch–Schönlein purpura
Cryoglobulinemic vasculitis
Lupus vasculitis
Rheumatoid vasculitis
Goodpasture's syndrome
Serum sickness vasculitis
Hypocomplementemic urticarial vasculitis
Drug-induced immune complex vasculitis
Infection-induced immune complex vasculitis
Behçet's disease
Paraneoplastic small vessel vasculitis
Lymphoproliferative neoplasm-induced vasculitis
Carcinoma-induced vasculitis
Myeloproliferative neoplasm-induced vasculitis
Inflammatory bowel disease vasculitis

[1]ANCA, antineutrophil cytoplasmic autoantibodies.

Table 31–4. Comparison of approximate frequency of manifestations of microscopic polyangiitis with other forms of small vessel vasculitis.

	Pauci-immune		Immune complex		
	Microscopic polyangiitis (%)	Wegener's granulomatosis (%)	Churg–Strauss syndrome (%)	Henoch–Schönlein (%)	Cryoglobulinemic vasculitis (%)
Cutaneous	40	40	60	90	90
Renal	90	80	45	50	55
Pulmonary	50	90	70	<5	<5
Ear, nose, and throat	35	90	50	<5	<5
Musculoskeletal	60	60	50	75	70
Neurologic	30	50	70	10	40
Gastrointestinal	50	50	50	60	30

Adapted with permission from Jennette JC, Falk RJ: Small vessel vasculitis. N Engl J Med 1997;337:1512.

cryoglobulinemic vasculitis, lupus vasculitis, and anti-GBM vasculitis, have extensive localization of immunoglobulin and complement in vessel walls as a consequence of deposition of circulating immune complexes or *in situ* immune complex formation between circulating antibodies and planted or constitutive antigens. The pauci-immune necrotizing small vessel vasculitides have little or no vascular wall localization of immunoglobulins, and often present with a necrotizing and crescentic glomerulonephritis, either alone or as a component of a systemic disease. Pauci-immune crescentic glomerulonephritis is the most common type of crescentic glomerulonephritis (Table 31–4).

The three major systemic pauci-immune small vessel vasculitides are MPA, Wegener's granulomatosis, and Churg–Strauss syndrome. MPA is a necrotizing angiitis involving capillaries, venules, and arterioles of one or more organs either simultaneously or at different times, including the kidneys, lungs, skin, spleen, liver, heart, and muscle. Wegener's granulomatosis is characterized by necrotizing granulomatous inflammation found in the upper or lower respiratory tract and may occur without overt vasculitis. The Churg–Strauss syndrome is defined by the presence of eosinophil-rich granulomatous inflammation and vasculitis in patients with a history of eosinophilia and asthma. The necrotizing glomerulonephritis and vasculitis found in Wegener's granulomatosis and Churg–Strauss syndrome can be pathologically identical to that found in microscopic polyangiitis. It is characterized by segmental fibrinoid necrosis, crescent formation, and the absence of immune reactants.

ANCA SVV is more common in whites than in African-Americans, with a ratio of 7–8:1. Females and males are equally affected, and while patients are typically 55 years or older, patients of any age may have this disease.

Burns JC et al: Infliximab treatment for refractory Kawasaki syndrome. J Pediatr 2005;146:662.

Cantini F et al: Are polymyalgia rheumatica and giant cell arteritis the same disease? Semin Arthritis Rheum 2004;33:294.

Guillevin L et al: Treatment of polyarteritis nodosa and microscopic polyangiitis with poor prognosis factors: a prospective trial comparing glucocorticoids and six or twelve cyclophosphamide pulses in sixty-five patients. Arthritis Rheum 2003;49:93.

Guillevin L et al: Short-term corticosteroids then lamivudine and plasma exchanges to treat hepatitis B virus-related polyarteritis nodosa. Arthritis Rheum 2004;51:482.

Royle J et al: The diagnosis and management of Kawasaki disease. J Paediatr Child Health 2005;41:87.

▶ Pathogenesis

Conceptually, vasculitides may be organized on the basis of three different mechanisms of injury: (1) Immune complex-mediated vasculitis, (2) direct antibody-mediated attack, or (3) pauci-immune necrotizing vasculitides. Immune complex-mediated vasculitis includes HSP, cryoglobulinemic vasculitis, rheumatoid vasculitis, and lupus vasculitis. Direct antibody attack-mediated diseases include anti-GBM-mediated glomerulonephritis and Goodpasture's syndrome, and Kawasaki's disease mediated by antiendothelial cell antibodies. The pauci-immune small vessel vasculitides associated with ANCA will be the focus of this chapter as HSP, cryoglobulinemic vasculitis, lupus nephritis, and anti-GBM disease are described in detail in other chapters.

▶ Clinical Findings

A. Symptoms and Signs

Renal disease is manifested by hematuria with dysmorphic red blood cells and red blood cells casts. Proteinuria is usually moderate (2–3 g/day) but may be as much as 20 g/day. ANCA-associated glomerulonephritis frequently presents as a rapidly progressive glomerulonephritis, although the syndromes of asymptomatic hematuria with minimal amounts of proteinuria or acute nephritis are common as well.

At least 50% of patients with ANCA necrotizing glomerulonephritis have pulmonary disease spanning the spectrum from severe life-threatening pulmonary hemorrhage to fleeting alveolar infiltrates. Massive pulmonary hemorrhage affects about 10% of patients with ANCA glomerulonephritis, and is associated with an elevated risk of death.

In the evaluation of pulmonary disease in the setting of a glomerulonephritis, it is imperative to exclude the possibility of an infectious etiology, especially when pulmonary infiltrates with or without hemoptysis develop in the setting of prior or ongoing immunosuppressive treatment. Recurrent vasculitis must be differentiated from infection, with special attention to *Pneumocystis carinii, Mycobacterium tuberculosis,* or fungal pathogens. Bronchoscopy and bronchial alveolar lavage help differentiate infection from alveolar hemorrhage. Similarly, infections of the upper respiratory tract mimic vasculitic lesions in the nose, sinus, and ear. Fiberoptic transillumination of the upper airways with biopsy may allow differentiation of vascular inflammation from infection.

Common dermal vasculitic findings are palpable purpura (usually in the lower extremities), petechia, ulcers, nodules, urticaria, ecchymoses, and bullae. The neurologic manifestations of ANCA SVV are typically peripheral neuropathies (mononeuritis multiplex), while central nervous system involvement, specifically granulomatosis meningeal inflammation, occurs uncommonly. Several other organ systems may be involved. Gastrointestinal disease, which affects one-third of patients with ANCA SVV, may present with vasculitic ulcers of the small and large intestine resulting in bleeding or perforation. Iritis, uveitis, and episcleritis result in red, painful eyes. These lesions are frequently present in a "subclinical" fashion and require slitlamp ophthalmologic evaluation. Almost all patients have a prodrome of a "flu-like illness" with malaise, myalgias, and arthralgias. A migratory pattern of arthropathy is a typical presentation.

B. Laboratory Findings

Testing for ANCA is useful in diagnosing pauci-immune small vessel vasculitis or renal-limited pauci-immune crescentic glomerulonephritis. ANCA reacts with constituents of neutrophils and monocytes. By indirect immunofluorescence microscopy (IIFM) on alcohol-fixed neutrophils, two patterns of staining can be distinguished:

A cytoplasmic pattern (C-ANCA) and a perinuclear pattern (P-ANCA). The majority of C-ANCAs react with the lysosomal enzyme proteinase 3 (PR3-ANCA). In necrotizing SVV, P-ANCA reacts with myeloperoxidase (MPO-ANCA). Wegener's granulomatosis is usually associated with circulating PR3-ANCA, but as many as 20% of patients may have MPO-ANCA. Conversely, PR3-ANCA can be found in patients with microscopic polyangiitis and necrotizing glomerulonephritis without evidence of Wegener's granulomatosis. MPO-ANCA is more commonly found in patients with microscopic polyangiitis and those with necrotizing and crescentic glomerulonephritis without evidence of extrarenal SVV. MPO-ANCA is the most common ANCA subtype in Churg–Strauss syndrome. Thus, despite a predominance of antigenic specificity for each of the diseases, neither ANCA subtype differentiates between the three phenotypes of necrotizing vasculitis. While the majority of antibodies associated with a P-ANCA immunofluorescent pattern are antibodies to myeloperoxidase, a number of other antigens have rarely been associated with the P-ANCA pattern. These include antibodies to hyaluronidase, high mobility groups 1 and 2 (associated with gastrointestinal immune disorders), lactoferrin, cathepsin G, enolase, lysozyme, and azurocidin. Occasionally, an antinuclear antibody (ANA) pattern of immunofluorescence may be mistaken for a P-ANCA pattern.

C. Special Tests

1. Relationship of serial ANCA titers and disease activity—Despite numerous retrospective and a few prospective studies, it is still unknown how best to use serial ANCA testing in the management of patients with ANCA vasculitis and glomerulonephritis. In reality, the simple question of whether serial ANCA testing can be used to foresee and prevent the occurrence of relapse corresponds to a more complex problem as ANCA testing represents several tests, ANCA vasculitis represents several diseases, and the risk of relapse is not uniform among all patients with ANCA vasculitis. For serial ANCA testing to be clinically useful in the management of patients, ANCA titers must correlate with disease activity, a relapse must predictably follow a rise in ANCA titer within a reasonable time frame, and an effective, safe, and acceptable therapy must be available to abrogate the relapse. None of these requirements is fully met in ANCA vasculitis.

While ANCA titers have been shown to correlate with disease activity in cohort studies of patients with ANCA vasculitis, this correlation can be very poor for some individual patients. Clinical remission occurs in the setting of a persistently elevated ANCA titer, and conversely, clinical relapses occur in the setting of a persistently negative or low ANCA titer. Furthermore, what constitutes a clinically significant change in ANCA titer has been defined differently in various studies and remains to be determined for each of the various ANCA tests.

Notwithstanding these caveats, most of the available data specifically address the study of C-ANCA or PR3-ANCA in patients with Wegener's granulomatosis, whereas the data for P-ANCA, MPO-ANCA, and patients with microscopic polyangiitis or glomerulonephritis alone are much more limited. The reported rates of relapses following a rise in titer vary from 23% to 82% for C-ANCA determined by IIFM, and from 59% to 100% for PR3- or MPO-ANCA as determined by enzyme-linked immunosorbent assay (ELISA). The time between a rise in ANCA titer and the occurrence of relapse varies significantly. In a study of 85 patients with PR3-ANCA-positive Wegener's granulomatosis, ~50% of relapses occurred within 6 months after the rise in titer, while some relapses occurred more than 18 months later.

An important concern was recently raised pertaining to patients who maintain a persistently elevated ANCA titer despite a successful induction therapy. Based on relatively small numbers of patients, two retrospective studies suggest that patients with persistently elevated ANCA titers are more likely to suffer a relapse than patients with negative or declining titers. The question of whether to institute immunosuppressive therapy at the time of a rise in ANCA titer has been addressed in only one randomized, prospective study. In this study of patients with Wegener's granulomatosis, of nine patients preemptively treated with cyclophosphamide for 9 months after a ≥4-fold increase in titer none suffered a relapse [versus 6 of 11 (55%) nontreated patients]. Some relapses occurred more than a year after the rise in titer. Although preemptively treated patients received less immunosuppressive drugs by the end of the study, it employed a medication that is associated with a high risk for serious short- and long-term adverse effects.

In summary, although a rise in PR3-ANCA titer appears to presage a subsequent relapse, there is a relative paucity of data regarding microscopic polyangiitis, P-ANCA, and MPO-ANCA and the best way to define a rise in ANCA titer. Considering that the time to relapse can be very long, and that the risk/benefit of preemptive, prolonged immunosuppression is not established, it is fair to state that the use of preemptive immunosuppression is not justified. The decision to initiate a second course of treatment should rather be based on the constellation of findings on clinical course, physical examination, and serologies rather than ANCA titers alone.

2. Role of the kidney biopsy—Whether a renal biopsy is essential for the management of ANCA glomerulonephritis rests on the accuracy of the ANCA methodology, the risks associated with therapy, and the "pretest probability" based on the features of the patient's clinical syndrome. Based on a study of 1000 patients with proliferative and/or necrotizing glomerulonephritis, the sensitivity of ANCA for pauci-immune glomerulonephritis was only 80% with a specificity of 89%, corresponding to a positive predictive value of 86%, a false-positive rate of 14%, and a false-negative rate of 16%.

These results preclude the use of ANCA testing alone as the determinant for treatment. Conversely, if the pretest probability of ANCA vasculitis is high based on the presence of characteristic clinical findings, a positive ANCA test may be sufficient to establish a diagnosis of pauci-immune necrotizing glomerulonephritis. In the setting of a rapidly progressive glomerulonephritis, or a pulmonary-renal vasculitic syndrome, initiation of treatment with pulse methylprednisolone should not be delayed until a biopsy result is obtained, as prompt initiation of treatment is an essential determinant of outcome.

Han WK et al: Serial ANCA titers: useful tool for prevention of relapses in ANCA-associated vasculitis. Kidney Int 2003; 63:1079.

Langford CA: Antineutrophil cytoplasmic antibodies should not be used to guide treatment in Wegener's granulomatosis. Clin Exp Rheumatol 2004;22:S3-S6.34.

Slot MC et al: Positive classic antineutrophil cytoplasmic antibody (C-ANCA) titer at switch to azathioprine therapy associated with relapse in proteinase 3-related vasculitis. Arthritis Rheum 2004;51:269.

▶ Differential Diagnosis

The clinical differential diagnosis of ANCA-associated pauci-immune SVV also includes direct antibody attack-mediated and immune complex mediated SVV. Despite a great deal of overlap in organ system involvement among different types of small vessel vasculitides, certain clinical serologic and histologic features—described in Tables 31–4 and 31–5—differentiate among MPA, Wegener's granulomatosis, Churg–Strauss syndrome, cryoglobulinemic vasculitis, and HSP. Testing for ANCA, anti-GBM, cryoglobulins, hepatitis C or B, ANA, and complement component levels helps focus the differential diagnosis. Direct immunofluorescence microscopy of vessels in biopsy specimens, such as glomerular capillaries or dermal venules, demonstrates immunoglobulin (Ig) A-dominant vascular immunoglobulin deposits in HSP, IgG and IgM deposits in cryoglobulinemic vasculitis, and little or no immunoglobulin in pauci-immune SVV.

The differential diagnosis of pauci-immune necrotizing glomerulonephritis includes lupus nephritis, anti-GBM disease, and other aggressive forms of glomerulonephritis. Patients with thrombotic microangiopathies may present a picture that mimics necrotizing glomerulonephritis. However, these patients do not have MPO- or PR3-ANCA and have features typical of a microangiopathic hemolytic disease. About 20% of patients with anti-GBM disease may concomitantly express ANCA.

▶ Complications

The very nature of systemic SVV exposes patients to a number of potential complications related to irreversible end-organ damage as a result of the disease itself or its therapy. In fact, as many as 85–90% of patients with Wegener's

Table 31–5. Differentiation among various small vessel vasculitides.

	Immune complex mediated		Pauci-immune		
	Henoch-Schönlein purpura	Cryoglobulinemic vasculitis	Microscopic polyangiitis	Wegener's granulomatosis	Churg-Strauss syndrome
Small vessel vasculitis signs and symptoms[1]	+	+	+	+	+
IgA-dominant immune deposits	+	−	−	−	−
Cryoglobulins in blood and vessels	−	+	−	−	−
ANCA in blood	−	−	+	+	+
Necrotizing granulomas	−	−	−	+	+
Asthma and eosinophilia	−	−	−	−	−

[1]All of these small vessel vasculitides can manifest any or all of the shared features of small vessel vasculitides, such as purpura, nephritis, abdominal pain, peripheral neuropathy, myalgias, and arthralgias. Each is distinguished by the presence and just as importantly the absence of certain specific features.

ANCA, antineutrophil cytoplasmic autoantibodies.

Reproduced with permission from Jennette JC, Falk R: Small vessel vasculitis. N Engl J Med 1997;337:1512.

granulomatosis suffer some permanent end-organ damage that adversely affect their quality of life, such as end-stage renal disease (ESRD), chronic pulmonary dysfunction, hearing loss, destructive sinus disease, proptosis, motor or sensory neurologic deficits, and blindness.

ANCA vasculitis can also present with acute life-threatening manifestations. Diffuse pulmonary hemorrhage presents with gross hemoptysis and respiratory failure requiring mechanical ventilation. Without the use of plasmapheresis in addition to corticosteroids and cyclophosphamide, diffuse pulmonary hemorrhage is associated with a 50% mortality rate.

Patients with Wegener's granulomatosis may present with acute critical subglottic stenosis associated with stridor, and respiratory failure, which may require emergency tracheostomy. Unfortunately, surgical interventions on the trachea in patients with active Wegener's granulomatosis frequently leads to a chronic course characterized by poor healing and scarring, requiring repeat interventions. For this reason, early detection of subglottic involvement and the prompt institution of intralesional as well as systemic corticosteroids and immunosuppressant therapy are essential to avoid surgery or tracheostomy.

End-stage kidney disease (ESKD) may be the result of the acute injury or from progressive chronic scarring. In a cohort of 350 patients with ANCA vasculitis, 22% of patients presented with, or reached ESKD within 2 months of presentation. In addition, 10% of patients who responded to initial therapy later progressed to ESKD in a median of 106 months without clinical evidence of disease relapse.

Perhaps less recognized is the increased risk of venous thrombotic disease among patients with Wegener's granulomatosis. This was illustrated in a recent large clinical trial that detected an incidence of venous thrombosis of 7 per 100 patient-years, with 75% of the events occurring at the time of, or shortly preceding clinically active vasculitis.

The complications met during the course of vasculitis are often iatrogenic. Common to all forms of immunosuppression is the risk of serious infections including bacterial, viral, and fungal opportunistic organisms. The risk of serious infection is compounded by treatment-related neutropenia, which may occur in up to 55% of patients treated with cyclophosphamide or azathioprine. In that respect, the risk of neutropenia and associated infections is substantially lower with the use of monthly pulse cyclophosphamide than the daily oral regime.

Treatment with cyclophosphamide is also associated with long-term risks of gonadal failure and infertility in both men and women, and malignancies, especially cutaneous, hematologic, and urothelial cancers. These risks are commensurate with the cumulative dose of cyclophosphamide and other cytotoxic or antimetabolites received during the course of treatment. Use of glucocorticoids is also associated with multiple short- and long-term complications including diabetes mellitus, osteoporosis, avascular necrosis of bone, myopathy, and cataracts.

It would be useful to describe concomitant assessments and/or prophylactic medications that may be prescribed to minimize complications. For instance, at our institution we are using Bactrim (either SS once/day or DS 3/week) for *Pneumocystis* prophylaxis, and inconsistently use Mycelex to prevent thrush. We assess the patient for old tuberculosis (we have an immigrant population in which this problem is not uncommon) and we respond accordingly to a positive purified protein derivative (PPD) depending on prior treatment history. I do not know if there are standards for care here, but some attempt to address this issue would be practical and very helpful.

Similarly, on the osteoporosis side, we will use calcium carbonate 1 g/day and vitamin D along with Fosamax for patients with creatinine clearance (Ccr)>50. Again, there may not be evidence-based data, but if any of these things are actually done, it would be useful to begin a non-evidence-based discussion of these issues.

Etanercept plus standard therapy for Wegener's granulomatosis. N Engl J Med 2005;352:351.

Gluth MB et al: Subglottic stenosis associated with Wegener's granulomatosis. Laryngoscope 2003;113:1304.

Hoffman GS et al: Treatment of subglottic stenosis, due to Wegener's granulomatosis, with intralesional corticosteroids and dilation. J Rheumatol 2003;30:1017.

Jayne D et al: A randomized trial of maintenance therapy for vasculitis associated with antineutrophil cytoplasmic autoantibodies. N Engl J Med 2003;349:36.

Klemmer PJ et al: Plasmapheresis therapy for diffuse alveolar hemorrhage in patients with small-vessel vasculitis. Am J Kidney Dis 2003;42:1149.

Knight A et al: Urinary bladder cancer in Wegener's granulomatosis: risks and relation to cyclophosphamide. Ann Rheum Dis 2004;63:1307.

Merkel PA et al: Brief communication: high incidence of venous thrombotic events among patients with Wegener granulomatosis: the Wegener's Clinical Occurrence of Thrombosis (WeCLOT) Study. Ann Intern Med 2005;142:620.

Seo P et al: Damage caused by Wegener's granulomatosis and its treatment: prospective data from the Wegener's Granulomatosis Etanercept Trial (WGET). Arthritis Rheum 2005;52:2168.

▶ Treatment

A. Induction Therapy

The cornerstone of ANCA vasculitis treatment is based on a combination of corticosteroids and cyclophosphamide according to various regimens described in the literature. Since renal prognosis appears to be determined by early treatment, we typically initiate induction therapy with three daily pulses of methylprednisolone (7 mg/kg/day) followed by daily oral prednisone. Prednisone is started at a dose of 1 mg/kg for the first month, and tapered progressively over 3–4 months. Cyclophosphamide is administered either by monthly intravenous pulses (0.5–1 g/m^2) or orally (1–2 mg/kg/day). All forms of cyclophosphamide dosage should be titrated to keep the nadir leukocyte count >3000 cells/mm^3. When compared to treatment with corticosteroids alone, the use of cyclophosphamide is associated with a 5-fold decrease in the risk of death and a 3-fold decrease in the risk of relapse. Patients treated with either intravenous or oral cyclophosphamide have a long-term remission rate of between 60% and 85%.

Determining the optimum mode (oral versus intravenous) and duration of treatment with cyclophosphamide depends on several factors and considerations. The short- and long-term complications associated with the use of cyclophosphamide are commensurate with the cumulative dose received. In general, the intravenous regimen allows for a two to three times smaller total dose of cyclophosphamide than the oral regimen. In prospective and retrospective analyses, intravenous therapy was associated with a significant decrease in the rate of clinically significant neutropenia and other complications. In a meta-analysis of three randomized controlled trials comparing pulse versus oral continuous cyclophosphamide, intravenous cyclophosphamide resulted in a statistically higher rate of remission (odds ratio for failure to achieve remission 0.29; 95% CI 0.12–0.73) and lower rates of leukopenia (odds ratio 0.36; 95% CI 0.17–0.78) and infections (odds ratio 0.45; 95% CI 0.23–0.89). The final outcomes of patients (death or ESKD) were no different in the two groups despite a (statistically not significant) lower rate of relapse in the oral cyclophosphamide group.

The optimum length of therapy with cyclophosphamide has not been determined and is the subject of ongoing controversy. In patients achieving complete remission within 6 months of therapy, treatment can be stopped with the institution of close patient follow-up. In those individuals with persistently active disease at 6 months, it is reasonable to continue cyclophosphamide therapy for a full 12 months. An alternative regimen consists of switching cyclophosphamide to oral azathioprine at the end of 3 months if the patient is in remission. Azathioprine is then continued for 18 months. This regime offers the advantage of a limited use of cyclophosphamide and results in rates of remission and relapse similar to the cyclophosphamide-only-based therapies.

Patients presenting with pulmonary hemorrhage also benefit from the institution of plasmapheresis in a regimen similar to that used for patients with Goodpasture's disease. Although no controlled data are available, early and aggressive institution of plasmapheresis has substantially diminished the mortality rate associated with massive pulmonary hemorrhage. Plasmapheresis is typically performed daily until the pulmonary hemorrhage ceases and then every other day for a total of seven to ten treatments. The addition of plasma exchange to cyclophosphamide and corticosteroids also improves the chances of recovery of renal function of patients with severe renal dysfunction (serum creatinine >5.6 mg/dL) or needing dialysis at presentation. For patients without profound renal failure or with pulmonary hemorrhage, controlled and observational trials have not demonstrated a beneficial role to the addition of plasmapheresis to cyclophosphamide and corticosteroids.

B. Adjunctive, Alternative, and Maintenance Treatment Strategies

Several other therapies have been evaluated for a potential role in the management of patients with ANCA vasculitis. Considering the generally excellent response rates to treatment with cyclophosphamide and glucocorticoids, the goals of these therapies can conceptually be delineated in the broad categories of adjunctive therapy for patients at risk for treatment resistance; alternatives to the repeat use of cyclophosphamide; or as maintenance therapy aimed at preventing relapses. With a few notable exceptions, the data available in support of these treatments are limited to open-label, uncontrolled studies that are often limited in size. No agent has as yet been established as a clear alternative to cyclophosphamide for the induction therapy of patients with organ- or life-threatening disease. The following sections review the data regarding alternative, adjunctive, or maintenance therapies for ANCA vasculitis.

1. Trimethoprim-sulfamethoxazole—Trimethoprim-sulfamethoxazole is suggested as the initial treatment of selected patients with Wegener's granulomatosis limited to the upper respiratory tract, reserving corticosteroid therapy for patients who fail antibiotic therapy. In assessing the role of trimethoprim-sulfamethoxazole in the prevention of relapse in patients who were already treated with cyclophosphamide and/or prednisone, a prospective placebo-controlled trial with trimethoprim-sulfamethoxazole was performed in 81 patients with Wegener's granulomatosis. The number of relapses was significantly reduced in the groups assigned to trimethoprim-sulfamethoxazole, although the benefit was limited to relapse involving the upper respiratory tract, not the lower respiratory tract or the kidney. In contrast, "maintenance" therapy with trimethoprim-sulfamethoxazole (after cyclophosphamide treatment) has been associated with an increased rate of relapse when compared to no maintenance treatment (42% versus 29%, respectively).

Similarly, in a randomized trial of 65 patients with Wegener's granulomatosis comparing methotrexate and trimethoprim-sulfamethoxazole, methotrexate therapy was more effective in maintaining remission than trimethoprim-sulfamethoxazole used alone or in combination with prednisone. Thus, the use of trimethoprim-sulfamethoxazole in patients with Wegener's granulomatosis remains a matter of controversy, and its beneficial effects seem to be limited to the respiratory tract.

2. Methotrexate—The use of methotrexate (MTX) has been studied almost exclusively in patients with Wegener's granulomatosis, and primarily in patients with "limited," mild disease, and with little or no renal involvement. MTX has been evaluated as an alternative to cyclophosphamide for the induction of remission in an open-label, uncontrolled trial that revealed a response rate of 76% and a remission rate of 69%. The value of weekly MTX as an induction agent was compared to daily oral cyclophosphamide in a randomized controlled trial in 100 patients with "early" ANCA vasculitis who did not have organ- or life-threatening manifestations or significant renal involvement (patients with creatinine >150 μmol/L, urinary red cell casts, or proteinuria >1.0 g/day were excluded). Although the remission rate at 6 months was not statistically different between the two groups [MTX (89.8%) versus cyclophosphamide (93.5%) ($p = 0.041$)], remission was delayed among MTX-treated patients with more extensive disease or pulmonary involvement. MTX treatment was associated with a significantly higher rate of relapse than cyclophosphamide (69.5% versus 46.5%) and 45% of the relapses occurred while the patients were still receiving MTX.

Whether MTX is effective in preventing relapses after induction therapy with cyclophosphamide has also been evaluated in open-label, uncontrolled studies. These studies revealed relapse rates of 37–52% with 61–72% of relapses associated with glomerulonephritis and 69% of relapses involving the upper respiratory tract. In the absence of proper control groups, it is not possible to assess whether maintenance therapy with MTX reduces the rate or severity of relapses.

In summary, MTX appears to be an option in the treatment of patients with mild ANCA vasculitis and normal or near normal renal function. The data regarding its value for maintenance therapy are currently less convincing. The dose of MTX should be decreased by 50% in patients with renal insufficiency and its use is contraindicated if the Ccr is <10 mL/minute. Trimethoprim-sulfamethoxazole for prophylaxis against *Pneumocystis carinii* pneumonia cannot be used concomitantly with MTX.

3. Azathioprine—The role of azathioprine in the management of patients with ANCA vasculitis was examined for the maintenance of remission as an alternative to a prolonged course of cyclophosphamide. In a large multicenter European trial, 144 patients with ANCA vasculitis who attained remission with oral cyclophosphamide and prednisolone were randomized to either a continued course of oral cyclophosphamide for a total of 1 year or switched to oral azathioprine. All patients were switched to oral azathioprine after 12 months. At the end of 12 months of follow-up, the risk of relapse was not significantly different between the two groups (13.7% versus 15.5%, $p = 0.65$) nor was there a significant difference in the risk of adverse events.

In the past few years a number of new immunomodulatory agents, targeting T cells, B cells, or both, and a number of proinflammatory pathways have been introduced. Several of these agents have been evaluated in a limited way as adjunctive or maintenance therapy of ANCA vasculitis. These include the inhibitors of lymphocyte proliferation mycophenolate mofetil and leflunomide, the lymphocyte-depleting humanized anti-CD52 antibody alemtuzumab, the

B cell-depleting chimeric antibody rituximab, and blockers of the tumor necrosis factor (TNF)-α pathway infliximab and etanercept. All but etanercept were evaluated only as part of small open-label, uncontrolled studies. The possible role of etanercept for the maintenance of remission was evaluated in a randomized, placebo-controlled trial of 180 patients in the Wegener's Granulomatosis Etanercept Trial (WGET). In addition to etanercept or placebo, patients received standard therapy with glucocorticoids plus cyclophosphamide or MTX. After 3–6 months of cyclophosphamide, patients in remission discontinued cyclophosphamide and were treated with etanercept and either MTX or azathioprine (depending on their degree of renal insufficiency). Over a mean follow-up of 27 months, 72% of patients attained a sustained remission, but only 50% of patients remained in remission for the remainder of the trial. There were no significant differences between the etanercept and control groups in the rates of sustained remission (69.7% versus 75.3%, $p = 0.39$), in the relative risk of disease flares per 100 person-years of follow-up (0.89, $p = 0.54$), or in the severity of relapses. During the study, 56.2% of patients in the etanercept group and 57.1% of those in the control group had at least one severe or life-threatening adverse event or died ($p = 0.90$). It was concluded that etanercept was not effective for the maintenance of remission in patients with Wegener's granulomatosis.

C. Transplantation

Recurrence of ANCA vasculitis after renal transplantation occurs in about 20% of patients. Time to recurrence varies widely, from a few days to several years posttransplantation. Patients with Wegener's granulomatosis appear more likely to relapse than patients with microscopic polyangiitis or necrotizing crescentic glomerulonephritis alone, whereas the presence of circulating ANCA at the time of transplant does not seem to increase the risk of recurrence after transplantation. If the patient is clinically in remission, it is probably not necessary to delay transplantation until a negative ANCA serology is attained. We believe that transplantation should be delayed in patients with active disease. In the majority of reported cases, recurrent disease after transplantation responded well to treatment with cyclophosphamide and pulse corticosteroids.

D. Supportive Therapy

As corticosteroids and cyclophosphamide remain the cornerstone of therapy of ANCA SVV, special effort must be exercised to minimize the short- and long-term complications of treatment. Whenever corticosteroids are used, the development of osteoporosis can be minimized with the early institution of calcium and vitamin D supplementation, and in patients with established osteoporosis, calcitonin or bisphosphonates (if not contraindicated by azotemia or esophagitis). Rigorous control of blood pressure with sodium restriction and antihypertensive therapy is essential to minimize

the additive effect of hypertension in loss of renal function following active nephritis. Hormonal manipulation during cytotoxic therapy may allow the preservation of gonadal function. The prevention of cyclophosphamide-induced infertility was reported with the use of testosterone in men and leuprolide in women.

Booth A et al: Prospective study of TNFalpha blockade with infliximab in anti-neutrophil cytoplasmic antibody-associated systemic vasculitis. J Am Soc Nephrol 2004;15:717.

de Groot K et al: Randomized trial of cyclophosphamide versus methotrexate for induction of remission in early systemic antineutrophil cytoplasmic antibody-associated vasculitis. Arthritis Rheum 2005;52:2461.

Eriksson P: Nine patients with anti-neutrophil cytoplasmic antibody-positive vasculitis successfully treated with rituximab. J Intern Med 2005;257:540.

Keogh KA et al: Induction of remission by B lymphocyte depletion in eleven patients with refractory antineutrophil cytoplasmic antibody-associated vasculitis. Arthritis Rheum 2005;52:262.

Langford CA et al: Mycophenolate mofetil for remission maintenance in the treatment of Wegener's granulomatosis. Arthritis Rheum 2004;51:278.

Metzler C et al: Maintenance of remission with leflunomide in Wegener's granulomatosis. Rheumatology (Oxford) 2004;43:315.

Nzeusseu TA et al: Oral pamidronate prevents high-dose glucocorticoid-induced lumbar spine bone loss in premenopausal connective tissue disease (mainly lupus) patients. Lupus 2005;14:517.

Specks U: Methotrexate for Wegener's granulomatosis: what is the evidence? Arthritis Rheum 2005;52:2237.

▶ Prognosis

Untreated, systemic vasculitis is associated with an 80% 1-year mortality. The introduction of steroids, azathioprine, and cyclophosphamide led to a marked improvement in survival to 84% and 76% at 1 and 5 years, respectively. Predictors of death include increasing age and creatinine at presentation, disease extent and severity at diagnosis, pulmonary hemorrhage, and treatment-related infection.

A. Response to Treatment

The terms "remission" and "relapse" are defined in Table 31–6. Treatment with cyclophosphamide is beneficial over the use of corticosteroids alone for achieving a remission as well as for patient survival. Patients treated with either intravenous or oral cyclophosphamide have a long-term remission rate of between 70% and 92%. Based on a large observational cohort of 350 patients with ANCA vasculitis, female gender, black race, and potentially older age were associated with a higher likelihood of treatment resistance. Whether socioeconomic factors and access to health care account for these differences in response to treatment is unknown. Patients with PR3-ANCA may have a better chance of remission than patients with MPO-ANCA.

Table 31–6. Criteria for treatment response.

Remission: Stabilization or improvement of the renal function (as measured by serum creatinine), resolution of hematuria, and resolution of extrarenal manifestations of systemic vasculitis. Persistence of proteinuria was not considered indicative of persistence of disease activity.

Remission on therapy: The achievement of remission while still receiving immunosuppressive medication or corticosteroids given at a dose greater than 7.5 mg/day of prednisone or its equivalent.

Treatment resistance: (1) Progressive decline in renal function with the persistence of an active urine sediment, or (2) persistence or new appearance of any extrarenal manifestation of vasculitis despite immunosuppressive therapy.

Relapse: Occurrence of at least one of the following: (1) rapid rise in serum creatinine accompanied by an active urine sediment; (2) a renal biopsy demonstrating active necrosis or crescent formation; (3) hemoptysis, pulmonary hemorrhage, or new or expanding nodules without evidence for infection; (4) active vasculitis of the respiratory or gastrointestinal tracts as demonstrated by endoscopy with biopsy; (5) iritis or uveitis; (6) new mononeuritis multiplex; (7) necrotizing vasculitis identified by biopsy in any tissue.

Adapted with permission from Nachman PH et al: Treatment response and relapse in antineutrophil cytoplasmic autoantibody-associated microscopic polyangiitis and glomerulonephritis. J Am Soc Nephrol 1996;7:33.

B. Relapse

The risk of relapse after an initial response to treatment is of the order of 40%, but reports vary between 11% and 57%. The risk of relapse is not uniform among all patients with ANCA vasculitis. An increased risk of relapse has been associated with a diagnosis of Wegener's granulomatosis (as opposed to MPA). Based on a multivariate analysis of 258 patients, the presence of PR3-ANCA and lung and upper respiratory tract involvement were independent risk factors for relapse. Among patients presenting with none of the three risk factors, 26% relapsed in a median of 62 months (median among those who relapsed was 20 months). In contrast, 47% of the patients presenting with a single risk factor experienced a relapse in a median of 39 months (corresponding to a 2-fold increased risk for relapse; 95% CI: 1.1, 3.9, $p = 0.038$). Among patients presenting with all three risk factors, 73% relapsed in a median of 17 months (median time to relapse among those who relapsed was 15 months), corresponding to a 3.7 times increased risk of relapse (95% CI: 1.4, 9.7, $p = 0.007$) compared to those with no risk factor.

Relapse typically occurs in the same organ system initially affected by the disease, although new organ system involvement occurs as well. Relapses in the kidney are heralded by the recurrence of microscopic hematuria, red blood cell casts, and worsening renal function. Fluctuations in the amount of proteinuria are not good indicators of active disease, and are related to glomerulosclerosis. Fortunately, a similar rate of response is achieved in the treatment of relapse and initial disease. Full-blown vasculitic relapse should be treated with a repeat course of prednisone and cyclophosphamide. In general, these patients require maintenance on long-term immunosuppression with azathioprine, MTX, mycophenolate mofetil, or cyclophosphamide. How to best treat milder relapses is a matter of substantial investigation. In an effort to limit the exposure of relapsing patients to repetitive cycles of cytotoxic drugs and their associated risks, alternative or adjunctive, less toxic therapies are being evaluated.

C. Prognostic Factors

Several studies have examined the question of prognostic factors in ANCA SVV. In our experience, the presence of pulmonary hemorrhage was the most important determinant of patient survival, whereas other pulmonary findings (eg, infiltrates, nodules, or cavities) did not increase the risk of death.

The risk of ESRD is largely determined by the degree of renal dysfunction at the time of diagnosis. Serum creatinine is the single most important prognostic marker for long-term renal outcome as exemplified by a 1.24-fold increased risk for ESRD for each 1 mg/dL increase in serum creatinine at baseline. Nevertheless, there is no threshold of renal dysfunction below which treatment is futile, as remission occurs in 57% of individuals with an estimated GFR <10 mL/minute. Histopathologic measures of chronic renal scarring (glomerulosclerosis, interstitial fibrosis, and tubular atrophy) have consistently been associated with poor renal outcomes. The impact of renal damage as a predictor of resistance emphasizes the importance of early diagnosis and prompt institution of therapy.

Booth AD et al: Outcome of ANCA-associated renal vasculitis: a 5-year retrospective study. Am J Kidney Dis 2003;41:776.

Booth AD et al: Renal vasculitis—an update in 2004. Nephrol Dial Transplant 2004;19:1964.

Sanders JS et al: Risk factors for relapse in anti-neutrophil cytoplasmic antibody (ANCA)-associated vasculitis: tools for treatment decisions? Clin Exp Rheumatol 2004;22:S94.

as from side effects of treatment. While clinicians treating patients with LN have traditionally focused on therapeutic interventions to reduce the risks of renal failure, there is emerging appreciation that treatment may be required to interdict the cardiovascular and thromboembolic complications engendered by protracted nephrotic syndrome. Indeed, evidence of the benefit of achieving even partial remission of proteinuria (to the subnephrotic level) has a salutary effect on patient and renal survival. Beyond standard immunosuppressive therapies, the full armamentarium of renal protection strategies, particularly angiotensin antagonists and lipid-lowering statin drugs, is warranted in management of LN.

▶ Treatment

Optimal care of patients with LN usually requires integrated expertise of nephrologists and rheumatologists. Most SLE patients will require some dosage of corticosteroids, antimalarials, and nonsteroidal anti-inflammatory drugs for control of their commonly debilitating extrarenal disease, which are best evaluated and managed by rheumatologists. Conversely, delineation of the more arcane aspects of renal disease and integration of the results of renal biopsy are best evaluated

and managed by nephrologists. Conjointly staffed clinics offer the best environment for effective communication and comprehensive care of patients with SLE and LN.

Immunosuppressive drug options for management of patients with LN are summarized in Table 32–2. Evidence-based clinical recommendations derived from completed controlled clinical trials are limited and consensus in developing clinical practice guidelines has not been achieved. Results of ongoing multicentered clinical trials are expected to help prioritize the current therapeutic options for treatment of the various forms of LN within the next few years.

A. Corticosteroids

Patients with new onset Class III, IV, or V LN warrant a limited therapeutic trial of high-dose corticosteroids. Patients failing to achieve full remission of nephritis within 6–8 weeks should be treated with adjunctive cytotoxic drug therapy (cyclophosphamide or mycophenolate mofetil) as described below. Based on current evidence, those patients with substantial fibrinoid necrosis or cellular crescents on renal biopsy should be directly initiated on therapy with combined pulse methylprednisolone and pulse cyclophosphamide for a period of 6 or more months.

Table 32–2. Immunosuppressive drug options and guidelines for administration in lupus nephritis.

Corticosteroids

Prednisone: Start with 1 mg/kg/day for approximately 6–8 weeks; taper to approximately 0.25 mg/kg/day over the next 6–8 weeks; strive for low-dose alternate-day maintenance therapy; patients with membranous lupus nephritis are often initiated on treatment with comparable doses of alternate-day prednisone.

Pulse methylprednisolone: Start with three daily intravenous pulses, 1 g each; continue with single monthly pulses for 6 or more months in patients with severe lupus nephritis (usually in conjunction with pulse cyclophosphamide).

Cyclophosphamide

Pulse cyclophosphamide: If the estimated glomerular filtration rate (GFR) is >30 mL/minute, start single monthly doses of 0.75 g/m^2 body surface area (BSA) administered intravenously over 1 hour; if the GFR is <30 mL/minute, the starting dose is 0.5 g/m^2 BSA; adjust the subsequent doses to a maximum of 1.0 g/m^2 BSA according to the white blood cell (WBC) nadir count (should not be <1500) at days 10 and 14 after treatment. All cyclophosphamide pulse treatments should include bladder protection by administration of oral or intravenous mesna, forced fluids to achieve a diuresis of >150 mL/hour, and frequent voiding for 24 hours; consider preemptive antiemetic treatment with dexamethasone 10 mg single dose plus ondansetron or granisetron prior to cyclophosphamide infusions; pulse regimens usually continue monthly for 6 months with conversion to quarterly pulse cyclophosphamide or to alternative maintenance therapies with mycophenolate or azathioprine.

Daily oral cyclophosphamide: Start with 2 mg/kg/day (as single morning dose); taper the dose as necessary to keep WBC >4000; the duration of therapy is usually <3 months; after 3 months, consider a transition to maintenance therapy with azathioprine or mycophenolate (cost of cyclophosphamide at a dose of 150 mg/day: approximately $10.74/day).

Azathioprine

Start at 2 mg/kg/day as maintenance therapy (cost of azathioprine at a dose of 150 mg/day: approximately $2.79/day).

Mycophenolate mofetil

Start at 0.5 g twice daily, escalating weekly to a target of 1.0 g three times daily according to gastrointestinal tolerance (cost of mycophenolate mofetil at a dose of 3 g/day: approximately $33.60/day).

Cyclosporine

Start at 5 mg/kg/day adjusting the dose downward according to side effects, particularly azotemia and hyperkalemia (cost of cyclosporine A at a dose of 350 mg/day: approximately $17.50/day).

B. Cyclophosphamide

Results of early treatment of murine LN and meta-analyses of human trials indicate that cyclophosphamide is among the most effective immunosuppressive drugs for LN. Side effects of daily cyclophosphamide are formidable, particularly beyond 3 months, and for this reason, prescription of daily therapy has become limited. The therapeutic index of cyclophosphamide is improved by administration of intermittent pulse therapy, which has become widely accepted as the standard approach to administration of cyclophosphamide therapy.

The emergence of pulse cyclophosphamide as the therapeutic standard for proliferative LN arose from observations in several long-term clinical trials reported from the National Institutes of Health. The composite of evidence indicated that pulse cyclophosphamide achieved the most sustained rates of renal remission, the lowest rates of cumulative damage on renal biopsy, and ultimately the lowest rate of progression to end-stage renal failure. The substantive risk of gonadal toxicity incurred with extended courses of pulse cyclophosphamide has been the major impetus to continue the search for alternative therapies in LN.

C. Mycophenolate Mofetil

Mycophenolic acid was initially tested and shortly abandoned for treatment of rheumatic diseases in the 1960s. It was reformulated and initially compared to azathioprine in renal allograft recipients. Mycophenolate was licensed on the basis of its advantage over azathioprine in achieving a reduced frequency of acute rejection episodes. Doubts have been raised about the cost effectiveness of mycophenolate because of its high cost and its lack of proven benefit in extending allograft survival.

Several uncontrolled trials of mycophenolate in LN suggested that this therapy may be useful in patients failing to achieve satisfactory responses to cyclophosphamide. Since 2000, two controlled trials comparing induction therapy with mycophenolate mofetil versus cyclophosphamide (Chan study: Daily cyclophosphamide and Ginzler study: Monthly pulse therapy) indicated comparable rates of renal remission and short-term renal survival but fewer side effects in patients treated with 1–3 g/day of mycophenolate mofetil. A controlled trial led by Contreras comparing maintenance therapies with cyclophosphamide, azathioprine, and mycophenolate mofetil indicated that the best patient and renal outcomes were achieved with mycophenolate.

Because historical studies have shown that several treatments, including azathioprine, cyclophosphamide, a combination of azathioprine and cyclophosphamide, and even prednisone alone, achieve comparable short- and intermediate-term renal survival rates, many have argued that the definitive choice among the newer immunosuppressive drugs must await ascertainment of long-term renal outcomes after 5 or more years of observation.

D. Azathioprine

Azathioprine is a relatively weak immunosuppressive drug in studies of both murine and human LN. It has mostly been relegated to use as a steroid-sparing agent and as a less costly and well-tolerated maintenance after cyclophosphamide or mycophenolate induction therapies.

E. Experimental Therapies

Several studies involving novel therapeutic agents for LN are underway. The agents being evaluated in these studies are summarized in Table 32–3. The Web site www.clinicaltrials.gov is a potentially useful resource in searching for studies that may be recruiting patients, along with information about eligibility and exclusion criteria.

F. Membranous Lupus Nephritis With Stable Renal Function

Patients with membranous LN with normal renal function and subnephrotic proteinuria may not warrant aggressive immunosuppressive therapy and may be adequately managed with angiotensin antagonists and statins as needed for hyperlipidemia. Those with high-grade nephrotic-range proteinuria, particularly if protracted and unimproved by angiotensin antagonists, should be treated with similar but less intense regimens of corticosteroids plus cyclophosphamide or mycophenolate. If renal function is well preserved, cyclosporine is also an effective alternative in patients with membranous LN. The optimal duration of treatment is undefined, but relapse of proteinuria is particularly likely after cessation of cyclosporine. This has prompted a very protracted slow tapering of cyclosporine before discontinuation (unless there is clinical suspicion or pathologic evidence of significant cyclosporine nephrotoxicity).

Table 32–3. Experimental therapies for systemic lupus erythematosis and lupus nephritis.

Chemical agents
  Tacrolimus, Prograf
  Sirolimus, Rapamune

Monoclonal antibodies (targets)
  Rituximab, Rituxan (CD20, B cells)
  Epratuzumab (CD22, B cells)
  MEDI-545 (interferon-α)
  Belimumab, LymphoStat (BLyS cytokine)
  Tocilizumab, Actemra (interleukin-6 receptor)
  Infliximab, Remicade (tumor necrosis factor)

Costimulation inhibitors
  CTLA4-Ig, Abatacept, Belatacept (CD80/86)

Tolerogens
  Abetimus, LJP-394 (anti-DNA)

Autologous stem cell transplants

Prognosis

The prognosis of Class III and IV proliferative LN has improved from a 5-year renal survival of <20% during the period 1960–1980 to >80% during the period 1980–2000. This improvement in prognosis has been ascribed mostly to increasing use of cyclophosphamide. While preliminary data based on achievement of renal remission suggest that mycophenolate may have comparable benefits, it remains to be established if mycophenolate will achieve comparable long-term renal survival.

In patients progressing to end-stage renal disease due to LN, there is considerable controversy about the prevalence of active SLE during maintenance dialysis and the risk of recurrent LN in renal allografts. In general, patients should be clinically and serologically inactive for approximately 1 year before renal transplantation. Recent reports suggest that recurrence of low-grade LN is common, but fortunately clinically significant nephritis and allograft loss are rare.

Chan TM et al: Long-term outcome of patients with diffuse proliferative lupus nephritis treated with prednisolone and oral cyclophosphamide followed by azathioprine. Lupus 2005; 14:265.

Contreras G et al: Sequential therapies for proliferative lupus nephritis. N Engl J Med 2004;350:971.

Ginzler EM et al: Mycophenolate mofetil or intravenous cyclophosphamide for lupus nephritis. N Engl J Med 2005;353:2219.

Plasma Cell Dyscrasias

Richard J. Glassock, MD, & Arthur H. Cohen, MD

The kidneys may be affected in a variety of ways in the plasma cell dyscrasias; all of the important lesions result from the accumulation/deposition of the paraprotein in some or all of the renal components (Table 33–1). The different abnormalities are determined by properties of the paraprotein rather than the patient response. The kidneys may be the only organ affected [the lesion known as Bence Jones (myeloma) cast nephropathy] or may be part of systemic processes (amyloidosis, monoclonal immunoglobulin deposition disease). A diagnosis of a plasma cell dyscrasia is not always known prior to the discovery of abnormal kidney function. The renal biopsy, performed to identify the responsible lesion, is not infrequently the initial indication of a plasma cell dyscrasia. Although multiple myeloma (MM) may be diagnosed, it is important to appreciate that some of the disorders discussed here may be associated with either a monoclonal gammopathy of uncertain significance (MGUS) or only a minor increase in bone marrow plasma cells. The clinical manifestations depend on the type of renal involvement, the renal tissue component affected, and whether only one or more of the lesions are present. The definition of the specific lesion is dependent on the tissue pathologic features, for the clinical and laboratory findings often do not readily allow for a specific diagnosis.

Durie BG, Kyle RA, Belch A, Bensinger W, et al: Myeloma management guidelines: a consensus report from the Scientific Advisors of the International Myeloma Foundation. Hematol J 2003;4:379. [PMID: 14671610]

Herrera GA, Joseph L, Gu X, Hough A, Barlogie B: Renal pathologic spectrum in an autopsy series of patients with plasma cell dyscrasia. Arch Pathol Lab Med 2004;128:875. [PMID: 9740176]

AMYLOIDOSIS

 ESSENTIALS OF DIAGNOSIS

► Heavy proteinuria.
► Renal insufficiency.

► Monoclonal free light chains (LCs) in serum or urine.
► Renal biopsy disclosing characteristic extracellular deposits.

General Considerations

A contemporary classification of systemic amyloidosis (AL), based on the nature of the amyloid protein that is deposited in tissue, is given in Table 33–2. Amyloidosis is a disorder of abnormal protein folding in which normally soluble proteins are deposited in tissues as fibrillar structures that disrupt organ function and produce disease. The proteins are folded into a β-pleated sheet form that results in a high affinity for Congo red and several other metachromatic dyes. Only one variety of amyloidosis is also a paraprotein, namely AL amyloidosis, in which the fibrils are composed of one or the other of the immunoglobulin LCs. Although this discussion will focus on only this form of systemic amyloidosis, it should be recalled that amyloid may also occur in a localized form. Identification of the precise biochemical nature of the amyloid fibril requires the examination of a tissue specimen with a combination of immunofluorescence or immunoperoxidase and often biochemical tests. Genetic testing may also be needed in the case of the hereditary amyloidoses.

Amyloidosis is an uncommon disease affecting about 12 patients per million population per year, with about 15% representing hereditary forms and the remaining consisting of acquired, nongenetic forms. Any race, sex, or ethnicity can be affected.

Pathogenesis

AL amyloid fibrils are derived from the N-terminal region (variable domain) of monoclonal immunoglobulin LCs, more commonly λ than κ. The AL amyloid fibrils can deposit in almost any tissue except the brain. Certain LCs are more "amyloidogenic" than others. Furthermore, differences in the variable region of the LC (λ) may determine the sites of

Table 33–1. Selected renal disorders in plasma cell dyscrasias.

I. Monoclonal immunoglobulin deposition diseases	Typical paraprotein
A. Amyloid	λ
B. Light chain deposition disease	κ light chain
C. Heavy chain deposition disease	IgG heavy chain
D. Light and heavy chain deposition disease	IgG heavy chain or κ light chain or λ light chain
E. Glomerulonephritis with organized Monoclonal immunoglobulin deposits (Immunotactoid glomerulopathy [GOMIDD])	IgG, IgA, or IgM cryoglobulinemia
F. Monoclonal Cryoglobulinemia	
II. Bence Jones (myeloma) cast nephropathy	

Table 33–2. Classification and nomenclature for the systemic amyloidoses.

Amyloid protein	Precursor	Syndrome
AL	Ig light chain	"Primary" amyloid Multiple myeloma
AH	Ig heavy chain	"Primary" amyloid Multiple myeloma
AA	Serum amyloid A	"Secondary" amyloid
ATTR	Transthyretin	Hereditary, autosomal dominant (AD)
AApoI	Apolipoprotein AI	Hereditary, AD
AApoII	Apolipoprotein AII	Hereditary, AD
AGel	Gelsolin	Hereditary, AD
AFib	Fibrinogen α chain	Hereditary, AD
ACys	Cystatin C	Hereditary, AD
Aβ₂M	β₂-Microglobulin	Dialysis amyloid

Modified with permission from Editorial: Amyloid fibril protein nomenclature–2002. Amyloid 2002;9:197.

amyloid deposition. VλVI results in dominant renal involvement while others (VλII or III) are more likely to have dominant cardiac or other organ involvement. AL amyloidosis is also known as primary amyloidosis, largely a holdover from the older literature. A truncated monoclonal heavy chain may rarely cause amyloid (known as AH amyloid).

The fibrils in AL amyloidosis are composed of fragments of the variable portion of monoclonal LCs (λ more frequently than κ). In AA amyloidosis the fibrils are composed of the serum Amyloid A protein. In hereditary Amyloidosis the fibrils are composed of the mutant protein (e.g., Fibrinogen alpha chain). These can be differentiated by appropriate immunohistological studies of biopsy tissue (see below). As monoclonal LCs may deposit in tissue and result in another disease (see monoclonal immunoglobulin deposition disease), it is clear that an additional factor is necessary to form the characteristic morphologic features of amyloid. It is likely that the LCs need to be phagocytized by macrophages where the LCs are metabolized to preamyloid fragments that are secreted and precipitate in the tissues. In the kidneys, the major site of accumulation is the glomeruli, with arterioles, arteries, interstitium, and tubular basement membranes involved to somewhat lesser degrees.

▶ Clinical Findings

A. Symptoms and Signs

Almost any B cell dyscrasia can be associated with AL amyloidosis, which develops in about 10–15% of cases of MM. Most cases of AL amyloidosis are not associated with MM, but rather develop in association with MGUS or as a "primary" disorder. A monoclonal paraprotein of free LCs can be detected in the serum or urine of the majority of patients. Because older patients may not infrequently (5–10%) have an MGUS, it is necessary to be cautious not to overinterpret the significance of a small paraprotein "spike" in a serum protein electrophoresis.

Bone marrow aspirates or biopsies may reveal frank MM, but frequently do not. The disorder develops equally in men and women, but is quite uncommon in individuals <40 years of age. The clinical manifestations, which depend on the site or sites of amyloid deposition, can be quite varied. Cardiac [heart failure due to restrictive cardiomyopathy, atrioventricular (AV) nodal disease, or "pseudoinfarct" or low-voltage patterns on EKG], renal (nephrotic syndrome, symptomatic proteinuria, renal failure), tongue (macroglossia), gastrointestinal (malabsorption, motility disorders), peripheral nerve [sensory ("stocking and glove") and motor neuropathies, carpal tunnel syndrome], autonomic nerves (orthostatic hypotension, impotence, gastroparesis), skin (papules, nodules, purpura, ecchymoses with minimal trauma), joints (polyarthritis of the shoulder girdle), and coagulation (Factor IX and X deficiency with bleeding) are among the most common. Macroglossia is almost pathognomonic of AL amyloidosis. Patients presenting with unexplained proteinuria (including nephrotic syndrome), nonischemic cardiac failure, peripheral neuropathy, or hepatomegaly after age 40 years should always be suspected of having AL amyloidosis. Hypertension and hematuria are said to be uncommon in renal amyloidosis, but severe hypertension may be present when renal failure ensues, and normomorphic hematuria due to bladder involvement with amyloid may occur. Renal involvement is principally heralded by proteinuria, which sometimes can be massive (>20 g/day) and lead to problems of protein malnutrition, severe edema, and volume depletion.

The diagnosis of AL amyloidosis can be suspected on the basis of history and physical examination, but the diagnosis requires tissue confirmation. Biopsies of kidney (when proteinuria is present), abdominal fat pad aspiration, or rectal mucosal biopsies are preferred. Biopsy of an enlarged and firm liver in AL amyloidosis should be avoided because of the risk of bleeding. No such excessive bleeding risk appears to occur with a renal biopsy, unless the patient has a severe Factor IX or X deficiency.

Nonhistologic studies may be helpful but are not diagnostic. Cardiac ultrasound may reveal "sparkling" echogenicity and impaired contractility or relaxation of the ventricles in cardiac amyloidosis. Abdominal ultrasound studies often reveal normal sized or enlarged echogenic kidneys. Renal vein thrombosis may be detected by computed tomography (CT) or magnetic resonance imaging (MRI) in patients with the nephrotic syndrome.

Since serum amyloid P (SAP) component is universally present in amyloid (AL as well as other types), radioisotope-labeled SAP (^{125}I) has been used to detect amyloid deposits and to quantitate their changes or resolution with treatment; however, this test has very limited availability. Highly sensitive and specific assays for circulating free LCs have also been developed and should be used for both diagnosis and follow-up of patients with AL amyloidosis to assess the "burden" of LCs.

B. Pathological Findings

The light microscopic features of amyloid are characterized by the infiltration of extracellular sites by pale-staining acellular amorphous material that is Congo red positive and displays apple green birefringence when viewed with polarized optics (Figure 33–1). By electron microscopy, amyloid is composed of fibrils that are nonbranching, usually randomly arranged, of indefinite length, and approximately 10 nm in thickness. By immunofluorescence (IF), AL amyloid most commonly stains for the λ LC (approximately 75%) and less frequently for the κ LC; the pattern is of continuous amorphous or smudgy positivity. While these IF findings are generally the experience of many laboratories, a recent report has indicated that IF has a low degree of sensitivity for detecting a monoclonal LC.

The glomeruli are almost always involved. The amyloid deposits in mesangial regions, infiltrating and replacing mesangial matrix and compressing and displacing cells, and sometimes results in a nodular appearance; it also infiltrates and replaces capillary basement membranes.

▶ Differential Diagnosis

Once a tissue diagnosis of amyloidosis is established, there is no differential diagnosis of the type of kidney disease. However, the precursor protein needs to be established. Once an abnormal LC (or heavy chain) is documented in the tissue deposits and/or in serum, urine, or in bone marrow or other plasma cells, there are no further diagnostic considerations.

▶ Treatment

Treatment of AL amyloidosis is generally quite disappointing, but the outlook may be improving. In addition to supportive and symptomatic therapy, an attempt should be made to reduce the amount of amyloidogenic LC being produced. Oral melphalan (0.15 mg/kg/day for 7 days) and prednisone oral melphalan (20 mg three times per day for the same 7 days), repeated every 6 weeks depending on leukocyte counts, can slow the progression of the disease with a median survival of over 7 years in "responders" (reduced proteinuria, decreased amyloid "burden" in organs, and reduced circulating LC or monoclonal protein, if present).

All long-term survivors of AL amyloidosis have shown some objective response to chemotherapy, but unfortunately the majority of patients do not respond to melphalan-prednisone therapy. α-Tocopherol and interferon do not appear to be effective. High-dose dexamethasone plus interferon may yield some responses. 4'-Iodo-4'-deoxydoxorubicin has been effective in small studies, but the improvement in visceral amyloid deposits (VAD) has not been impressive. VAD regimens (previously described) have also been used in patients with AL amyloidosis (with and without MM) with benefits that seem to exceed those of the "standard" melphalan-prednisone therapy, at least in some studies. Thalidomide and its congeners, which are being evaluated for efficacy and safety in the treatment of MM, might also be effective in AL amyloidosis.

The most encouraging results have been seen with high-dose intravenous melphalan therapy followed by autologous bone marrow or peripheral stem cell transplantation; this may now be the treatment of choice for younger patients with limited organ system involvement, especially without cardiac involvement. However, recent controlled trials seem to

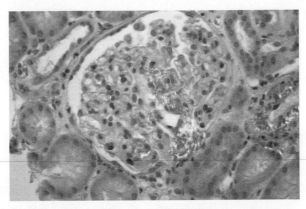

▲ **Figure 33–1.** Congo red stain with polarized optics; amyloid is in several segments in the glomerulus and in the wall of the arteriole.

indicate that the advantage of high-dose melphalan-prednisone plus autologous bone marrow transplantation therapy over high-dose melphalan-prednisone therapy alone for Systemic AL Amyloidosis is not as great as it was believed. Melpalan-prednisone plus autologous stem cell transplantation was not superior to high-dose melphalan-prednisone alone in this pivotal advanced study of advanced AL Amyloidosis. Stem cell transplants are very risky, with fatal outcomes common in patients with multisystem involvement and those with cardiac disease. Fractional survival for patients with two or fewer systems involved is about 75% at 5 years and is 25% or less at 2 years in those with cardiac involvement or more than two systems involved. Unfortunately, at present, the eligibility criteria for transplantation are such that only a minority of patients actually receive transplants. The best results are in patients with renal involvement as the sole or major manifestation of amyloidosis. Response duration and survival posttransplantation are superior to melphalan-prednisone treatment. A retrospective survey of over 700 patients with AL amyloidosis deemed "eligible" for high-dose intravenous melphalan and autologous stem cell transplantation revealed that only 44% actually received transplants and the median survival was 4.6 years; a complete hematologic response (disappearance of any evidence of a plasma cell dyscrasia) was achieved in 40% of patients. Mortality in the first 100 days was about 13% and was highest in those with cardiac involvement. The overall quality of life was greatly improved in those who achieved a complete hematologic and biochemical remission. Cardiac and/or renal allotransplantation has been performed, with anecdotal reports of prolonged survival. In the absence of specific therapy for the production of LC, recurrence of disease in the allograft can be anticipated.

General supportive therapy includes diuretics (for edema of nephrotic syndrome). Antihypertensive (angiotensin II inhibitors) agents should be used with great caution. Analgesics may be needed for neuropathic pain. Postural hypotension may limit the use of agents for hypertension present in the supine position. Midoridine and antigravity stocking may be of some benefit for severe postural hypotension. Cardiac glycosides (digoxin) and calcium channel antagonists are contraindicated, as they may worsen the cardiac manifestations.

Prognosis

The prognosis of AL amyloidosis, either in association with MM or as a "primary" disease, is poor, especially in the presence of clinically overt renal and/or cardiac involvement. In patients with renal involvement, the median time from diagnosis to end-stage renal disease (ESRD) is about 1 year and survival after dialysis is commenced is short, usually also less than 1 year. With current management, the principal cause of death is cardiac. In patients with restrictive myocardial disease (as determined by Doppler echocardiography), the 1-year survival is <50%. A low κ/λ ratio in bone marrow plasma cells may indicate a poor prognosis.

Novak L et al: AL-amyloidosis is underdiagnosed in renal biopsies. Nephrol Dial Transplant 2004;19:3050. [PMID: 15507480]

Jaccard A. Moreau P, Leblond V, et al. High-dose melphalan versus melphalan plus dexamethasone for AL amyloidosis. N Engl J Med 2007; 357 (11): 1083–1093.

MONOCLONAL IMMUNOGLOBULIN DEPOSITION DISEASE

 ESSENTIALS OF DIAGNOSIS

▶ Heavy proteinuria.

▶ Renal insufficiency.

▶ Hypertension.

▶ Monoclonal immunoglobulin (LC, heavy chain, both) in serum and/or urine.

▶ Renal biopsy with characteristic findings including extracellular deposition of paraprotein in in the basement membranes of glomeruli and tubules.

General Considerations

It is well recognized that several portions of the immunoglobulin molecule can deposit in the kidneys and elsewhere (largely in basement membranes) and result in homogeneous or microgranular "deposits" by electron microscopy. Initially considered the result of deposition of an abnormal κ LC resulting in what was initially termed LC deposit disease (LCDD), this systemic disorder has been expanded to include λ LC, heavy chain deposition (HCDD), and intact monoclonal immunoglobulin deposition (LHCDD). While many of these patients have multiple myeloma, monoclonal immunoglobulin deposition disease (MIDD) can develop in the absence of overt MM. POEMS, or the Crow-Fukase syndrome or Tatasuke syndrome, is an unusual variant that can be associated with a peripheral neuropathy, organomegaly, endocrinopathy, monoclonal gammopathy, and skin changes. Sclerotic bone lesions or Casteleman's disease commonly coexists. Papilledema, effusions, ascites, and thrombocytosis may appear.

Pathogenesis

In MIDD, most information about pathogenesis concerns LC deposit disease because it has been studied longer and is more common than heavy chain or LC and heavy chain deposit diseases. This discussion on pathogenesis will be related largely to LCDD. In a conceptual sense, this disorder is similar to amyloid in that it represents the systemic deposition of a paraprotein, with important pathologic and clinical manifestations in the kidneys. However, the LCs do not have the biochemical characteristics to change to a β pleated sheet configuration, form fibrils, and bind to Congo red stain. In contrast to amyloid, κ rather than λ is the predominant monoclonal protein and the tissue deposits are granular, not fibrillar. The factors that favor LC structure at deposition are not well understood; these may include degradation by macrophages, intrinsic properties of the intact LC, etc. Some MIDDs are associated with organized (fibrillar, crystalline or micro-tubular) deposits by electron microscopy. These include immunotactoid glomerulopathy, crystal cryoglobulinemia, and various forms of monoclonal cryoglobulinemia.

▶ Clinical Findings

A. Symptoms and Signs

MIDD represents a broad spectrum of clinical presentations and findings. LCDD is the most common form, representing about two-thirds of all cases. HCDD and LHCDD have about equal frequency and together represent about one-third of the cases. Intact IgG deposition is least common. LCDD is frequently (about 50%) accompanied by myeloma cast nephropathy (MCN). In HCDD the deposits are most often composed of γ chain while in LHCDD the deposits are composed of either IgGκ or IgGλ. In the uncommon intact monoclonal IgG DD, the deposits are composed of IgG subclass 1, 2, or 3 and the κ/λ ratio is about 1:1.

All subcategories of MIDD have a similar presentation; however, severe dialysis-requiring renal failure, including acute renal failure (ARF), is more common in LCDD complicated by myeloma cast nephropathy. Nephrotic-range proteinuria and an impaired glomerular filtration rate (GFR) are very frequently observed in MIDD without myeloma cast nephropathy, but heavy glomerular proteinuria is infrequent in LCDD associated with myeloma cast nephropathy. At the time of diagnosis, over 95% of patients have a serum creatinine over 1.2 mg/dL. Hypertension is very common, but somewhat less frequent in patients with LHCDD. The gender ratio is about 1:1. Most patients are over 50 years of age at the time of diagnosis. Patients with HCDD and deposition of the intact monoclonal IgG molecule may often have a "false-positive" antibody test for hepatitis C viral infection and hypocomplementemia (C3, C4, or C' H50). Liver function tests are normal in this circumstance. Serum or urinary protein electrophoresis for monoclonal proteins may be positive, more commonly in LHCDD and in HCDD (70–80%) than in LCDD (about 25%). A minority of patients will fulfill diagnostic criteria for multiple myeloma. A diagnosis of MM is more common in LCDD, almost always when myeloma cast nephropathy is also present. Some patients (60–70%) with HCDD or LHCDD will have an MGUS and others (10%) will have no identifiable B cell neoplasia. Hypogammaglobulinemia is common. The MIDD associated with cryoglobulinemia may have many systemic manifestations including hypocomplementemia, palpable purpura with cutaneous leukocytoclastic vasculitis, skin necrosis and alveolar hemorrhage. Immunotactoid glomerulopathy commonly presents as a renal-limited disease with hematuria and the nephrotic syndrome.

B. Pathological Findings

The hallmark of diagnosis is the documentation, by immunofluorescence, of only the abnormal LC (or light and/or heavy) chain in all basement membranes and other extracellular matrix in a continuous pattern. The κ LC is considerably more common than the λ LC in producing this disease (Figure 33–2A). The constant region of the immunoglobulin is typically deposited, resulting in strongly positive immunofluorescence for the monoclonal LC. In the kidneys, the tubular basement membranes, glomeruli, arterioles, and arteries are affected pathologically and clinically. This results in variable light and electron microscopic appearances. Some reports

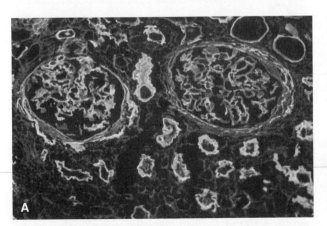 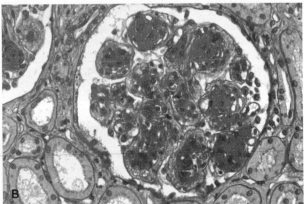

▲ **Figure 33–2. *A:*** Immunofluorescence with anti-κ antibody disclosing linear binding to basement membranes of glomerular capillaries and tubules. ***B:*** Glomerulus with nodular architecture (periodic acid–Schiff).

have indicated that the tubular basement membranes are more frequently affected than those in the glomeruli. However, the glomeruli are the major sites of clinical importance. The morphologic appearance of the glomeruli is typically considered to be of a nodular "glomerulosclerosis" with great similarity to the diabetic lesion (Figure 33–2B). However, there is considerable variation in appearance, especially in relation to the coexistence of Bence Jones cast nephropathy. Thus, glomeruli may have a normal appearance, may display mild or greater widening of the mesangium with or without increased cellularity, may have a membranoproliferative glomerulonephritis pattern of injury, and may have crescents or may have segmental sclerosis; consequently, the morphology of glomeruli is not an important diagnostic consideration. Glomeruli may be normal or near normal when the cast nephropathy coexists. By electron microscopy, there are continuous electron-dense coarsely granular deposits in capillary basement membranes and in mesangial matrix in glomeruli. This feature tends to be absent unless the nodular morphology is present. The tubular basement membranes are often thick and refractile by light microscopy and have ultrastructural findings similar to those in the glomeruli. Once again, the electron-dense "deposits" are not universally present. The MIDD with organized deposis uniformly have structural lesions by electron microscopy that differ from those described above. These are often referred to as non-Randall-type deposits, as the amorphous or granular deposits associated with the Light chain deposition diseases are referred to as Randall-type deposits.

Differential Diagnosis

This is very limited; the diagnosis is established by renal biopsy and, given the diagnostic immunofluorescence and electron microscopic findings, the differential diagnosis is quite limited.

Treatment

With such a poor prognosis, aggressive treatment measures have been employed in most cases. If MM is diagnosed, therapy with intermittent melphalan plus steroids or a vincristine–adramycin–dexamethasone (VAD) regimen is indicated. Similar regimens have also been employed in patients without overt MM. While some may respond to these therapies, it is difficult to determine in advance which patients will benefit. Those with ESRD clearly respond poorly or have complications to these regimens. Plasma exchange has been tried in some patients, mostly in those with protein electrophoreses showing a large amount of circulating paraprotein. Bortezomib (Velcade) is gaining favor over melphalan-prednisone regimens for treatment of overt Multiple Myeloma in patients who are ineligible for high-dose Melphalan regimens.

Younger patients without ESRD or major comorbidities who have MM may also become candidates for bone marrow or autologous peripheral stem cell transplantation. The treatment of choice for POEMS is also high-dose chemotherapy with autologous peripheral stem cell transplantation. Intravenous IgG and plasmapheresis are not effective therapies for POEMS. MIDD has a propensity to recur in renal transplants usually within 3 years following transplantation. Measures to control the synthesis of the monoclonal proteins (high-dose chemotherapy) should precede transplantation in all cases; careful monitoring of LC or heavy chain production (serum levels) should be regularly conducted posttransplantation.

Prognosis

The outcome is poor in most cases, with death or ESRD in the majority of patients. The mean time to ESRD is <6 months in LCDD and myeloma cast nephropathy and is somewhat longer in MIDD without myeloma cast nephropathy. Renal survival in pure MIDD has been estimated to be about 50% at 2 years, whereas it is only about 10% or less in MIDD with myeloma cast nephropathy (LCDD). Patient survival has been estimated to be about 75% at 2 years in pure MIDD, but is only 40% or less at 2 years for MIDD with myeloma cast nephropathy.

Leung N et al: Long-term outcome of renal transplantation in light-chain deposition disease. Am J Kidney Dis 2004;43:147. [PMID: 14712438]

Pozzi C et al: Light chain deposition disease with renal involvement: clinical characteristics and prognostic factors. Am J Kidney Dis 2003;42:1154. [PMID: 14655186]

BENCE JONES (MYELOMA) CAST NEPHROPATHY

 ESSENTIALS OF DIAGNOSIS

► Acute or less commonly chronic renal failure.

► Monoclonal LC in serum and/or urine.

► Renal biopsy with characteristic tubular casts with fracture lines or fragmentation surrounded by multinucleated foreign body giant cells and composed of the abnormal LC.

► Multiple myeloma.

General Considerations

Myeloma cast nephropathy had been considered synonymous with renal involvement in multiple myeloma and was formerly known as "myeloma kidney." However, with the definition of other lesions, including MIDD, it has become necessary to indicate the specific abnormality, as therapies and prognoses are different as indicated in the previous discussions. Thus, "myeloma kidney" is no longer a useful term. Bence Jones cast nephropathy may be the initial manifestation of multiple myeloma as ARF is often the presenting feature of this lesion.

Pathogenesis

Cast nephropathy results from the filtration of free monoclonal LCs by the glomeruli and their precipitation with Tamm–Horsfall protein in the distal nephron. It should be pointed out that while the distal nephron is a favored site of cast formation, the LCs may precipitate in any segment of the nephron, including the urinary spaces of glomeruli, presumably in the absence of Tamm–Horsfall protein. The monoclonal LCs are tubulotoxic, resulting in acute tubular necrosis. With subsequent destruction of the tubular walls in association with cast formation, an inflammatory process in the form of a foreign body reaction ensues and the casts are surrounded by multinucleated giant cells (Figure 33–3). The casts may be fragmented, crystal-containing, and have a brightly stained appearance; by immunofluorescence, the casts are composed of a single LC, the Bence Jones protein. It is this constellation of tissue findings that is almost pathognomonic of multiple myeloma and allows the pathologist to be the first to diagnose this marrow disorder by examining a renal biopsy performed in the work-up of ARF. As the casts are large, intranephron obstruction contributes to renal functional impairment.

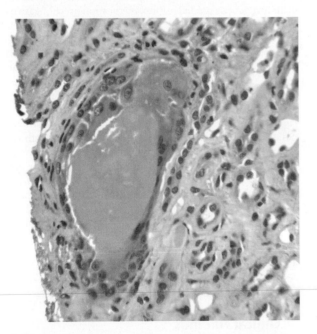

▲ **Figure 33–3.** Large tubular cast partially surrounded by multinucleated giant cells (hematoxylin and eosin).

Clinical Findings

Myeloma cast nephropathy is characterized by renal failure, including ARF, and high levels of urinary excretion of monoclonal LCs. It may represent the first manifestation of multiple myeloma and unless it is considered in the clinical differential diagnosis and unless a search for a paraprotein is not done, it is the renal pathologist who is responsible for establishing the diagnosis.

In the patients with ARF, a bland urine sediment, and negative or trace-positive dipstick for protein, urine protein should be evaluated by sulfosalicylic acid (SSA). The dipstick primarily detects albumin, not LCs; SSA detects nonalbumin proteins. Cast nephropathy without coexisting amyloid or MIDD is not associated with glomerular proteinuria (albumin).

Differential Diagnosis

Although Bence Jones cast nephropathy, as defined above, is pathognomonic of multiple myeloma, similar pathologic features have been described in B cell lymphoma and Waldenström's macroglobulinemia, both reflecting excretion of monoclonal LCs. Similar light microscopic cast morphology has been observed in some patients with pancreatic acinar cell carcinoma and renal transplants treated with tacrolimus and rapamycin; however, monoclonal LCs are not a component of casts in these settings.

Treatment

Myeloma cast nephropathy may respond to fluid volume expansion and increased water intake and a forced diureses (loop acting diuretics). Hypercalcemia (in MM), exposure to radiocontrast agents, nonsteroidal anti-inflammatory drugs (NSAIDs), diuretic-induced volume depletion, and hyperuricemia may all aggravate or precipitate an episode of MCN. It may also respond to loop-acting diuretics and to measures designed to decrease the production rate of LCs. Plasma exchange to reduce the levels of free LCs in the circulation in connection with an episode of ARF has been used to treat MCN, but the results are inconsistent and this procedure cannot be routinely recommended unless a hyperviscosity syndrome can be well documented.

Korbet SM, Schwartz MM: Multiple myeloma. J Am Soc Nephrol 2006;17:2533. [PMID: 16885408]

Lee CK et al: Dialysis-dependent renal failure in patients with myeloma can be reversed by high-dose myeloablative therapy and autotransplant. Bone Marrow Transplant 2004;33:823. [P MID: 14767499]

San Miguel JF, Schlag R, Khuageva NK, et al. Bortezomib plus melphalan and prednisone for initial treatment of multiple myeloma. N Engl J Med 2008;359 (9): 906–917.

Thrombotic Microangiopathies

Cynthia C. Nast, MD, & Sharon G. Adler, MD

The thrombotic microangiopathies (TMAs) are classified together due to their overlapping clinical and morphologic findings. Their major clinical manifestations include hemolytic anemia, microvascular thrombosis, and thrombocytopenia. Most TMAs have renal involvement with similar morphologic changes in the kidney reflecting the vasculopathy these lesions share. There are a number of underlying etiologic factors inducing TMA including systemic diseases, infection, and medications, which are summarized in Table 34–1.

TMAs originally were separated into the distinct disease entities of hemolytic uremic syndrome (HUS), thrombotic thrombocytopenic purpura (TTP), and scleroderma renal crisis according to their clinical features. In fact, HUS and TTP were suggested to be varying manifestations of a single disease. However, as the underlying pathogenetic factors are being elucidated, it is clear that the TMAs are distinct entities with specific etiologies and associated laboratory and clinical findings.

HEMOLYTIC UREMIC SYNDROME

ESSENTIALS OF DIAGNOSIS

▶ Microangiopathic hemolytic anemia.
▶ Thrombocytopenia.
▶ Renal involvement.

▷ General Considerations

Historically, HUS and TTP were considered to be variable expressions of the same disease process. With the identification of etiologic roles for factor H in HUS and for ADAMTS 13 in TTP, these are now thought to be distinct disorders with overlapping clinical features. HUS may present in a diarrheal (D+) or a nondiarrheal (D−) form. Most cases of D+ occur in summer and autumn, and result from Shiga-like toxin producing bacteria, primarily *Escherichia coli* O157:H7, although other organisms may be involved. Transmission has occurred via undercooked ground beef, contaminated water, and unpasteurized milk or apple cider, and epidemics may ensue. The Shiga-like toxin binds to colonic epithelium inducing inflammation and tissue injury thereby allowing the toxin to enter the circulation. The toxin then binds to vascular and renal tubular epithelial cell receptors resulting in endothelial injury, inflammation, thrombosis, and renal failure.

The D− form of HUS is less well understood. It is associated with a number of underlying clinical predisposing factors including genetic predisposition, medication use, nongastrointestinal infections, pregnancy, neoplasms, collagen-vascular diseases, systemic vasculitis, and bone marrow transplantation. Deficiency of prostacyclin PGI$_2$ has been implicated in some cases of D− HUS, while other cases likely result from an abnormality of the coagulation cascade or the endothelial cell membrane creating a prothrombotic milieu. A more common atypical subset of HUS is characterized by complement dysregulation due to factor H or membrane cofactor abnormalities. Factor H regulates the alternative complement pathway and membrane cofactor is a transmembrane complement regulatory protein. Mutations leading to deficiency or loss of activity of these regulatory elements allow activation of complement with deposition on and injury to glomerular and vascular endothelial cells and platelet aggregation resulting in thrombosis. Factor H deficiency is inherited in an autosomal recessive manner and is associated with low C3 levels and earlier disease onset. Factor H functional abnormalities are inherited in an autosomal dominant mode and these patients have normal serum complement levels, a later disease onset, and often other initiating events or stimuli.

▷ Clinical Findings
A. Symptoms and Signs

HUS classically presents as a triad consisting of microangiopathic hemolytic anemia, thrombocytopenia, and renal

Table 34–1. Etiologies of thrombotic microangiopathies.

Systemic disorders
Thrombotic thrombocytopenic purpura
Hemolytic uremic syndrome
Antiphospholipid syndrome
Systemic lupus erythematosus
Neoplasms
Malignant hypertension

Infections
Enteric pathogens
Escherichia coli 0157:H7
Shigella spp.
Salmonella spp.
Campylobacter jejuni
Yersinia
HIV
Streptococcus pneumonia
Mycoplasma pneumoniae
Legionella pneumophilia
Coxsackie A and B virus

Medications
Calcineurin inhibitors
Mitomycin C
Gemcitabine
Bleomycin
Cisplatinum
Cytosine arabinoside
Daunorubicin
Vincristine
Ticlopidine
Clopidogrel
Quinine

Miscellaneous
Vaccinations
Bone marrow transplantation
Pregnancy

D+ HUS is associated with infection, and the offending organism such as *E coli* 0157:H7, *Salmonella*, or *Shigella* may be identifiable in stool culture. Leukocytosis and fluid and electrolyte disturbances may be found.

Renal biopsy findings are identical in the D+ and D± forms, as they are in all TMAs and are characterized by the accumulation of fibrin in the lumina and walls of arteries, arterioles, and glomerular capillaries (Figure 34–1). By light microscopy, fibrin and platelet thrombi are present in variable numbers of glomerular capillaries. Glomeruli may appear ischemic with wrinkled and partially collapsed capillaries or develop a lobular appearance with capillary wall double contours. Fibrin is in the walls and/or lumina of arterioles and, to a lesser extent, arteries, which also show muscular hypertrophy and mucoid intimal thickening, and endothelial cell swelling resulting in luminal narrowing. This may have a concentric or "onion skin" appearance. Immunofluorescence discloses fibrin in vascular walls and lumina, and glomerular capillaries without immune complexes. On ultrastructural examination, glomerular capillary walls have wide subendothelial zones containing flocculent electron-lucent and electron-dense material representing altered fibrin, which may contain trapped erythrocytes. Often there is a new layer of basement membrane material beneath the widened subendothelial zones accounting for the double contour appearance of capillaries. There are no electron-dense (immune complex) deposits. It has been suggested that patients with HUS may have more fibrin and erythrocytes with fewer platelets within intrarenal thrombi compared with TTP, and that HUS is more likely to have renal cortical necrosis than other TMAs. However, there are no definitive distinguishing features among any of the TMAs on renal biopsy.

▶ Differential Diagnosis

The presence of thrombocytopenia, microangiopathic hemolytic anemia, and renal disease suggests the presence of a thrombotic microangiopathy. The renal biopsy most often cannot distinguish among the underlying causes. Therefore, the history, physical examination, and laboratory evaluation are important in distinguishing one form from another. HUS generally is associated with more severe renal involvement than TTP. The latter is sometimes also accompanied by the other features of the clinical pentad, including fever and central nervous system involvement. The finding of typical infectious agents on stool culture or a suspicious history in the D+ form indicates the likely diagnosis of HUS. Some laboratories are now performing clinical testing for ADAMTS13 (von Willebrand cleaving factor), which is currently the only definitive way to distinguish these syndromes. Markedly elevated blood pressure in the absence of other signs or symptoms of systemic disease suggests the presence of malignant hypertension. Systemic manifestations and/or laboratory findings of systemic lupus erythematosus (SLE) or scleroderma would implicate those

disease. The signs and symptoms overlap those of TTP, but in HUS there is a predominance of renal and hematologic features. D+ HUS is associated with watery to hemorrhagic diarrhea, and epidemics associated with ingestion of undercooked hamburger or unpasteurized milk or cider occur sporadically. The other systemic manifestations of the diarrheal and nondiarrheal forms are similar and include fever, severe hypertension, pulmonary edema, cerebral edema and seizures, congestive heart failure, and cardiac arrhythmias.

B. Laboratory Findings

The classical features are microangiopathic hemolytic anemia and renal dysfunction, frequently presenting as acute renal failure in adults, and less commonly in children.

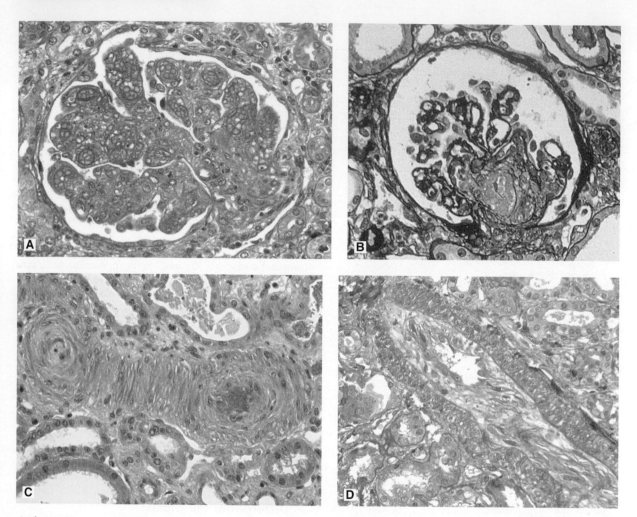

▲ **Figure 34–1.** Renal findings in thrombotic microangiopathy. **A:** Glomerulus with a lobular configuration, mesangiolysis, and thrombosed capillary lumina (×400). **B:** *Thrombosis of intraglomerular arteriole. The glomerulus is ischemic with wrinkled and partially collapsed capillary walls (×400).* **C:** Arteriole showing muscular hypertrophy with an "onion skin" appearance, absent lumen, and focal thrombosis (×200). **D:** *Artery with mucoid intimal thickening and swollen endothelial cells (×200). (continued).*

as the underlying cause, since most often, the TMA is not the initial presentation of these disorders. A history of fetal wastage and/or arterial or venous thrombosis may suggest underlying antiphospholipid syndrome. A history of particular medication ingestion or a viral or bacterial infection prodrome also may be helpful in implicating those as causative. All TMAs are in the differential diagnosis whenever thrombocytopenia, microangiopathic hemolytic anemia, and renal clinical or biopsy features are present. These include HUS, TTP, scleroderma renal crisis, and antiphospholipid syndrome, regardless of the etiology; malignant

hypertension may have a similar presentation and appearance on renal biopsy.

▶ **Treatment**

Therapy for HUS is primarily supportive only. Factor H replacement using fresh frozen plasma infusion has not been effective even in patients from families with documented factor H deficiency. However, recombinant Factor H currently is being developed as a potential therapy in this setting. Antibiotics, antiplatelet agents, anticoagulants, fibrinolytics, intravenous immunoglobulin, plasma infusion, plasmapheresis,

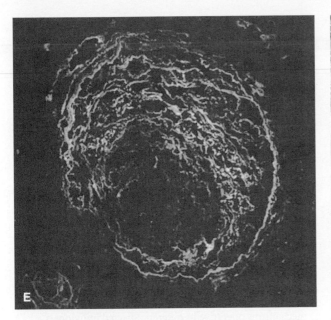
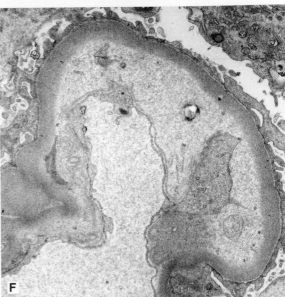

▲ **Figure 34–1. (*continued*) E:** Immunofluorescence of an artery demonstrating fibrin throughout the thickened vascular intima. ***F:*** *Electron micrograph of a glomerular capillary wall showing a markedly expanded subendothelial zone containing flocculent granular material (altered fibrin) with narrowing of the lumen.*

and prostacyclin infusion have not been proven efficacious in treating HUS.

Hosler GA et al: Thrombotic thrombocytopenic purpura and he-molytic uremic syndrome are distinct pathologic entities. Arch Pathol Lab Med 2003;127:834. [PMID: 12823037]

Siegler R et al: Hemolytic uremic syndrome; pathogenesis, treat-ment, and outcome. Curr Opin Pediatr 2005;17:200. [PMID: 15800412]

Tarr PI et al: Shiga-toxin-producing Escherichia coli and hae-molytic uraemic syndrome. Lancet 2005;365:1073. [PMID: 15781103]

THROMBOTIC THROMBOCYTOPENIC PURPURA

 ESSENTIALS OF DIAGNOSIS

▶ Microangiopathic hemolytic anemia.

▶ Thrombocytopenia.

▶ Fever.

▶ Central nervous system disorder, including mental sta-tus changes, seizures, focal neurologic abnormalities.

▶ Renal involvement.

▶ General Considerations

TTP previously was considered to be pathogenetically linked to HUS with a somewhat different clinical presen tation. However, the identification of an abnormal plasma protein in TTP has led to the understanding that TTP and HUS are pathogenetically distinct entities. Endothelial cells produce large multimers of von Willebrand factor (vWF) that normally are cleaved by a circulating zinc metallopro-tease termed ADAMTS13 (a disintegrin and metalloprote-ase with eight thrombospondin-1-like domains). In TTP, ADAMTS13 is reduced in amount or function, allowing persistence of many unusually large vWF multimers; iden-tification of these multimers is diagnostic for TTP. These multimers bind to extracellular matrix and platelets, induc-ing platelet aggregation and activation, thrombosis, and thrombocytopenia with organ ischemia. During times of remission, vWF multimers undergo normal cleaving. In the familial and chronic relapsing forms of TTP, gene muta-tions reduce functional ADAMTS13 to account for less than 5% observed in healthy individuals. The acquired form is due to the presence of an autoantibody interfering with the function of the cleaving protein and may be triggered by certain medications, of which quinine, mitomycin-C, cyclophilin inhibitors, and ticlopidine are the most com-mon. The acquired forms of TTP also may complicate collagen-vascular disorders such as scleroderma and SLE. Neoplasms and infections (most notably HIV) have been associated with TTP.

Clinical Findings

A. Symptoms and Signs

The classic pentad of TTP consists of fever, microangiopathic hemolytic anemia, TTP, renal disease, and central nervous system symptoms ranging from lethargy, somnolence, and confusion to focal neurologic signs, seizures, and/or coma. The neurologic symptoms often dominate the overall clinical picture. Renal signs and symptoms are common but often mild. It has been estimated that renal involvement is present in as many as 88% of patients

B. Laboratory Findings

The hemolytic anemia is characterized by many circulating fragmented erythrocytes in the form of schistocytes and helmet cells, which are thought to be produced by shear stress injury as blood flows through vessels narrowed by platelet thrombi. High lactate dehydrogenase (LDH) levels correlate with the severity of the disease. Renal manifestations include microscopic hematuria, rarely gross hematuria, mild to moderate proteinuria, and azotemia with up to 10% of patients having acute renal failure. Renal biopsy may show thrombi with a higher number of platelets and fewer erythrocytes or fibrin.

Treatment

Replacement of the missing cleaving protein activity through plasma or cryosupernatant (cryoprecipitate-poor plasma) infusion is the mainstay of therapy. Plasma exchange may provide additional benefit by removing circulating autoantibodies against ADAMTS13 in those with the acquired form of TTP, and by facilitating the infusion of large amounts of fresh frozen plasma (FFP)(average course of FFP is ~21 L). Steroids may be useful adjunctive therapy. Rituximab has been used with some success in a few refractory patients. Splenectomy and platelet inhibitors are occasionally used in patients refractory to standard therapy, but are not of proven value. Patients with renal failure may require supportive dialysis therapy. Aspirin and platelet transfusion are contraindicated. Response to therapy is best monitored by following serial serum LDH levels.

Haspel RL et al: The "cutting" edge: von Willebrand factor-cleaving protease activity in thrombotic microangiopathies. Transfus Apheresis Sci 2005;32:177. [PMID: 15784452]

Tsai H-M: Advances in the pathogenesis, diagnosis and treatment of thrombotic thrombocytopenic purpura. J Am Soc Nephrol 2003;14:1072. [PMID: 12660343]

SCLERODERMA RENAL CRISIS

 ESSENTIALS OF DIAGNOSIS

▶ Severe hypertension.
▶ Autoantibodies.

General Considerations

Scleroderma encompasses altered cell- and humoral-mediated immunity, abnormalities of the microvasculature, and aberrant production and accumulation of extracellular matrix resulting in vascular injury and fibrosis. The pathogenesis of scleroderma is not fully understood and incorporates complex genetic and environmental factors. Chemical, infectious, and physical agents all have been proposed as predisposing factors in the development of scleroderma, but the specific pathogenesis is unknown. It is possible that this heterogeneous disorder may have varying inciting events and mechanisms operative in different affected individuals.

Not until 1952 was renal disease recognized as a major cause of morbidity and mortality in systemic sclerosis. Scleroderma renal crisis likely is initiated by endothelial injury leading to vascular dysfunction. The endothelial damage may be prompted by effects of antiendothelial antibodies inducing upregulation of growth factors and cytokines, decreases in intrinsic complement regulatory proteins, cell-mediated immunity, and/or proteolytic activities in serum. This endothelial injury results in increased vascular permeability with intimal edema, myointimal proliferation, and increased extracellular matrix production, platelet aggregation and adhesion, and fibrin deposition. The consequent vascular luminal narrowing and reduced renal perfusion trigger increased renin production, thereby exacerbating hypertension. In the setting of scleroderma, fibroblasts express increased levels of tumor growth factor (TGF)-β receptors and become persistently activated by small amounts of TGF-β, overproducing extracellular matrix components. It is unclear whether this is an abnormal response to injury or a dysregulation of the relevant gene expression. When immune activation occurs due to one or more inciting events, fibroblasts produce excessive amounts of extracellular matrix material that accumulates in the target organs. Irrespective of the upstream pathogenetic mechanisms involved, fibroblast stimulation appears to be a final pathway in the sclerosis associated with scleroderma.

Numerous autoantibodies are associated with scleroderma, and there appears to be some specificity linked to the pattern of clinical disease presentation. Patients who develop scleroderma renal crisis often produce anti-RNA polymerase III and anti-Th/To RNP antibodies. These phenotype-specific antibodies may merely be markers of disease, or may have a pathogenetic role. The abnormal immune response may influence the onset or progression of scleroderma via several mechanisms. Autoantibodies may be directly pathogenic; between 25% and 85% of patients with scleroderma have antiendothelial cell antibodies, which could induce injury resulting in vascular damage as previously described. Antibody binding can change the sites of antigen proteolysis and/or promote the uptake of complexed proteins; this can spread the immune response to different antigenic components (epitope spreading) thereby enhancing the immune reaction. Involved organs often display T cell and macrophage infiltrates, possibly in response to environmental stimuli, with subsequent cytokine and growth factor release. In addition, altered B cells may upregulate complement receptor signaling further inducing target cell injury and augmenting T cell effector responses. These immune reactions may incite endothelial and fibroblast responses, leading to the vasculopathy and fibrosis of scleroderma. There is no firm evidence that cold temperatures, cardiac dysfunction, pregnancy, or specific drugs such as nonsteroidal anti-inflammatory drugs (NSAIDs) or calcium channel blockers induce this process, although high steroid doses over time have been linked to renal crisis.

▶ Clinical Findings

A. Symptoms and Signs

Classical scleroderma renal crisis occurs in approximately 10% of all patients with scleroderma, and is defined by the presence of new-onset often severe hypertension and/or rapidly progressive acute renal failure in this setting. However, this varies depending on the form of scleroderma. Patients with CREST (calcinosis, Raynaud's phenomenon, esophagitis, sclerodactyly, telangiectasias) syndrome and limited or localized systemic sclerosis are much less likely to develop renal crisis (~1%), although occasionally renal crisis may occur in those with minimal symptoms of scleroderma. In contrast, those with diffuse systemic sclerosis have the largest risk, with up to 25% of patients developing this complication. Renal crisis is more likely to develop in those with diffuse disease, rapid skin thickening on the trunk or proximal limbs, fatigue, weight loss, and polyarthritis; carpal tunnel syndrome; onset of scleroderma within the prior 5 years, especially the prior 1 year; antitopoisomerase III (Scl-70) as opposed to anticentromere antibodies; African-American ethnicity; male gender; edema; and tendon friction rubs.

Marked blood pressure elevation is the most common presenting manifestation, occurring in 90% of patients. Hypertension is severe with 30% having diastolic blood pressure in excess of 120 mm Hg, and may emerge abruptly; there are cases in which blood pressure was normal within days of an acute presentation. The hypertension may be manifest as a significant increase in blood pressure for that individual within the normal range, in the minority of patients with normal blood pressures. Extrarenal manifestations

occasionally precede the onset of renal crisis, and include pericardial effusions, congestive heart failure, and ventricular arrhythmias. Seizures rarely occur in those with renal crisis. Up to 50–60% of patients with systemic sclerosis who do not have renal crisis may have mild hypertension and up to 80% have abnormal morphologic findings in the kidney on renal biopsy.

B. Laboratory Findings

Plasma renin levels are invariably high in renal crisis, but whether this is the cause of the hypertension and renal ischemia or a reflection of it is unclear. The presence of microangiopathic hemolytic anemia and thrombocytopenia is a clinical clue to the presence of scleroderma renal crisis; the anemia is found in 43% of patients with renal crisis and thrombocytopenia occurs, but rarely is less than 50,000/mm^3. However, scleroderma, hemolytic anemia, thrombocytopenia, and acute renal failure occasionally may arise in the absence of severe hypertension, suggesting that thrombotic microangiopathy may occur in scleroderma via a mechanism independent of and/or in addition to malignant hypertension. Other laboratory features on presentation include nonnephrotic proteinuria, dysmorphic usually microscopic hematuria, and an elevated serum creatinine. These are not specific as microscopic hematuria, proteinuria, and diminished glomerular filtration rate (GFR) frequently accompany accelerated or malignant hypertension at presentation, and may occur in up to 50–60% of patients without renal crisis.

▶ Treatment

The standard treatment for patients with renal crisis is angiotensin-converting enzyme (ACE) inhibition, which has dramatically reduced the mortality associated with this disease. The mechanism of action of these agents likely is multifactorial as they are effective in patients with and without hypertension. When ACE inhibitors alone cannot adequately control hypertension, other antihypertensive agents should be prescribed to achieve a goal blood pressure of 125/75 mm Hg. It is recommended that ACE inhibitor therapy be continued in the setting of scleroderma renal crisis regardless of concerns that it may diminish renal perfusion pressure and exacerbate renal functional decline. Up to 50% of the patients who require dialysis during the course of renal crisis will become dialysis independent by 2 years after the initiation of therapy; therefore, ACE inhibition should be continued even if the patient requires dialysis. Anecdotal case reports suggest that combining ACE inhibition with angiotensin receptor blockers may worsen the renal outcome.

Denton CP et al: Scleroderma-clinical and pathological advances. Best Pract Res Clin Rheumatol 2004;18:271. [PMID: 15158741]

Rhew EY et al: Scleroderma renal crisis: new insights and developments. Curr Rheumatol Rep 2004;6:129. [PMID: 15016343]

ANTIPHOSPHOLIPID SYNDROME

ESSENTIALS OF DIAGNOSIS

▶ Thrombosis.

▶ Recurrent spontaneous abortions.

▶ Antiphospholipid, anticardiolipin, or anti-β_2 glycoprotein I antibodies.

▶ General Considerations

The antiphospholipid syndrome is an autoimmune disorder characterized by recurrent venous, arterial, or microvascular thrombosis or recurrent pregnancy loss. These events are induced by the actions of a family of autoantibodies with broad reactivity to phospholipid epitopes and/or to the phospholipid binding protein β_2-glycoprotein I. The syndrome may be present as a primary disorder or as a secondary disorder, the latter usually in association with SLE. The majority of the autoimmune anticardiolipin antibodies are directed against the phospholipid-binding protein rather than the phospholipid itself, and requires the binding protein to produce the effects.

Numerous mechanisms have been proposed to account for the hypercoagulable state. Antiphospholipid antibodies may interfere with the function of phospholipid-binding proteins involved in the regulation of coagulation. Candidates for such interference include β_2-glycoprotein I, prothrombin, protein C, and tissue factor. It has been postulated that through binding to cell receptors there is activation of endothelial cells with conversion from an anticoagulant to procoagulant phenotype with upregulation of adhesion molecules, the elaboration of cytokines, and alterations in the balance of prostacyclin and thromboxane. Antiphospholipid antibodies also bind to platelets via the apoER2' receptor. Oxidant-mediated endothelial injury may play a role, with autoantibodies to oxidized LDL occurring along with anticardiolipin antibodies. In fact, some anticardiolipin antibodies cross-react with oxidized LDL. Additionally, associated antibodies against tissue plasminogen activator with resulting reduced fibrinolysis may contribute to the clinical manifestations.

▶ Clinical Findings

A. Symptoms and Signs

A diagnostic classification of antiphospholipid syndrome was adopted in 1999 and requires at least one laboratory and one clinical manifestation (Table 34–2). The clinical criteria include a vascular occlusion involving veins, arteries, or capillaries in any organ or pregnancy complications including at least three miscarriages before the tenth gestational week, loss

Table 34–2. Criteria for definite antiphospholipid syndrome diagnosis.[1]

Clinical criteria
1. Thrombosis   Arterial, venous, or microvascular

2. Pregnancy loss
    Three or more consecutive miscarriages (<10 weeks gestational age)
    One or more fetal demise (>10 weeks gestational age)
    One or more premature births (34 weeks gestational age) due to preeclampsia, eclampsia, placental insufficiency

Laboratory criteria

1. Anticardiolipin antibody
    Moderate or high titer
    IgG and/or IgM

2. Lupus anticoagulant   On at least two measurements, 6 or more weeks apart

[1]Diagnosis requires at least one clinical and one laboratory criteria to be met.

of a normal fetus after 10 weeks, or prematurity of a normal fetus (earlier than 34 weeks). The antiphospholipid syndrome may involve one or more organs including the central nervous system, kidney, endocrine, gastrointestinal tract, lungs, skin, and cerebrovascular and cardiovascular systems. Renal manifestations are protean, and include acute renal failure, progressive chronic kidney disease sometimes culminating in kidney failure, cortical necrosis, mild to malignant hypertension, thrombotic microangiopathy, and thrombosis of renal allografts. The syndrome may occur in a "catastrophic" form, defined by involvement of at least three organ systems simultaneously. The kidney is the most frequently affected organ in the catastrophic form involved in 78% of cases, characterized by hypertension, which is often malignant. Dialysis is required in 25% of those with renal involvement. Other end-organ involvement includes pulmonary (66%), central nervous system such as cerebrovascular accidents (56%), cardiac including premature myocardial infarction (50%), and dermatologic (50%). Disseminated intravascular coagulation is uncommon.

B. Laboratory Findings

The diagnosis requires the presence of an antiphospholipid antibody, including immunoglobulin (Ig)G and/or IgM, anticardiolipin antibody, or lupus anticoagulant. Antibodies to phospholipid binding proteins frequently are present, but are not yet included in the diagnostic classification. Anticardiolipin antibodies are identified by immunoassays that measure pathologic reactivity to anionic phospholipids including the anticardiolipin antibody, antiphospholipid antibody, or false-positive VDRL test. Lupus anticoagulants are identified by abnormalities in coagulation assays including prolonged prothrombin time or partial thromboplastin time, particularly when the latter is not normalized when diluted with normal serum; abnormalities in the kaolin cephalin clotting time or the thromboplastin inhibition test; or abnormal Russel viper venom test. The anticardiolipin antibody or lupus anticoagulant must be detected twice at least 6 weeks apart according to the diagnostic criteria. Thrombocytopenia is frequent in antiphospholipid syndrome. Up to 5% of healthy individuals have circulating anticardiolipin antibodies, and it is unclear how many of these individuals eventually will develop antiphospholipid syndrome. It has been estimated that 12-30% of patients with SLE have anticardiolipin antibodies and 15–34% have evidence of a lupus anticoagulant. As many as 50–70% of these individuals may have an associated clinical event over the course of 20 years of follow-up.

▶ Treatment

The mainstay of therapy is anticoagulation, which is required long term. Warfarin therapy is recommended for the primary syndrome and for those with associated systemic lupus. A recently published study suggested there were low rates of recurrent thrombosis in patients in whom the international normalized ratio (INR) was kept in the range of 2–3, instead of the 3 previously recommended. Mortality for patients with the catastrophic syndrome is high, approaching 50%.

Patients should avoid prothrombotic drugs such as oral contraceptives, calcineurin inhibitors, hydralazine, procainamide, and chlorpromazine. Aspirin should be prescribed for women with prior pregnancy losses. Although not evidence based, the addition of steroids, plasmapheresis, and intravenous immunoglobulin has been implemented as salvage therapy in patients with severe and/or multiple organ involvement. The role of hydroxychloroquine and/or chloroquine to prevent thrombosis in patients with SLE is controversial.

de Groot PG et al: The antiphospholipid syndrome: clinical characteristics, laboratory features and pathogenesis. Curr Opin Infect Dis 2005;18:205. [PMID: 15864096]

Mackworth-Young CG: Antiphospholipid syndrome: multiple mechanisms. Clin Exp Immunol 2004;136:393. [PMID: 15147339]

Glomerular Disorders due to Infections

Jeremy S. Leventhal, MD, Michael J. Ross, MD,
Kar Neng Lai, MBBS, MD, Sydney Tang, MD, PhD

HIV-ASSOCIATED NEPHROPATHY

Jeremy S. Leventhal, MD, & Michael J. Ross, MD

ESSENTIALS OF DIAGNOSIS

► HIV-associated nephropathy (HIVAN) is a distinct and separate pathology with a unique combination of collapsing focal segmental glomerulosclerosis (FSGS), tubuloreticular inclusion bodies, microcystic dilation of renal tubules, and interstitial inflammation found in HIV-infected individuals.

► While HIVAN should be suspected in any HIV-infected person of African descent with proteinuria and decreased glomerular filtration rate (GFR), definitive diagnosis can be made only by renal biopsy.

► At-risk HIV-positive patients should be tested for proteinuria or decreased GFR to allow earlier detection of HIVAN.

► HIVAN is caused by expression of HIV-1 genes in renal epithelial cells.

► Highly active antiretroviral therapy (HAART) is the primary mode of treatment to retard progression of glomerular filtration decline and proteinuria.

► The diagnosis of HIVAN is an indication to begin HAART regardless of CD4 or viral counts.

► Angiotensin-converting enzyme (ACE) inhibitors and steroids may be of benefit in selected patients.

► General Considerations

At the onset of the HIV epidemic, little was known concerning the ability of the virus to cause organ-specific pathology.

By 1984, it became apparent that there was a renal syndrome associated with HIV infection that was characterized by severe proteinuria and rapidly progressive renal failure. Proteinuria was frequently severe with levels of protein excretion as high as 10 g daily. Patients were often asymptomatic until features of renal failure became manifest. As opposed to similar glomerulopathies, the nephropathy associated with HIV infection did not often result in severe hypertension or edema. On ultrasound imaging of the kidneys, nephromegaly was a common finding with increased kidney weight seen on autopsy. Renal biopsy of these patients revealed the presence of focal glomerulosclerosis, tubular microcystic dilation, and tubulointerstitial inflammation and fibrosis.

Now widely accepted to be a distinct renal disease, HIVAN does not affect all populations equally. In the United States, HIVAN is the third leading cause of end-stage renal disease (ESRD) in African-Americans between the ages of 25 and 64 years. International studies evaluating HIV-infected patients with proteinuria corroborate the U.S. data. Two studies in Thailand and Italy did not detect any cases of HIVAN among HIV-infected patients who underwent renal biopsy to evaluate the cause of proteinuria. Neither of these studies included any patients of African descent. A South African study, however, evaluated 30 patients with proteinuria and 7 patients with microalbuminuria. Renal biopsies revealed that 83% of the patients had pathology consistent with HIVAN, including six out of the seven patients with microalbuminuria. Moreover, ESRD due to HIVAN is 12.2 times more likely to occur in African-Americans than in whites and has the strongest racial predisposition of any form of acquired renal disease leading to ESRD.

Prior to the availability of HAART, the clinical course of HIVAN was characterized by a rapid decline of renal function resulting in the need for renal replacement therapy within weeks to months after diagnosis. The prognosis of these patients was dismal, approximately 1 year once on dialysis. However, since HAART became widely available, the outcome of HIV-infected patients has improved significantly.

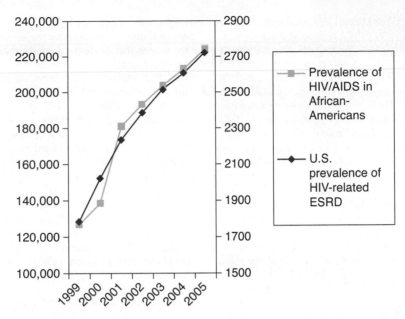

▲ **Figure 35–1.** The prevalence of patients with end-stage renal disease due to AIDS nephropathy in the United States continues to increase in parallel with the prevalence of HIV/AIDS in African-Americans, the group at highest risk of developing HIV-associated nephropathy (HIVAN). (Data adapted from the U.S. Renal Data System, USRDS 2007 Annual Data Report: *Atlas of Chronic Kidney Disease and End-Stage Renal Disease in the United States*. National Institutes of Health, National Institute of Diabetes and Digestive and Kidney Diseases, Bethesda, MD, 2007 and from the Centers for Disease Control and Prevention: *HIV/AIDS Surveillance Report, 2005*. Vol. 17, Rev ed. Atlanta, GA. Department of Health and Human Services, Centers for Disease Control and Prevention, 2007. Also available at http://www.cdc.gov/hiv/topics/surveillance/resources/reports/.

Note: The data here have been supplied by the USRDS. The interpretation and reporting of these data are the responsibility of the author(s) and in no way should be seen as an official policy or interpretation of the U.S. Government.

Similarly, the prognosis of HIV-infected patients with ESRD has improved. After the introduction of HAART in 1995, the mortality rate fell from about 72% to 24% for patients with both HIV and ESRD. Unfortunately, despite the improvements in the efficacy of medical treatment, the prevalence of ESRD in persons living with HIV/AIDS has continued to increase. This increase is closely paralleled by the increased prevalence of HIV/AIDS in African-Americans, the group at highest risk of developing HIVAN (Figure 35–1).

Patients with biopsy-proven HIVAN most often present with obvious signs of renal involvement. Severe proteinuria and impaired GFR are common indications for biopsy in patients with renal disease. However, even the presence of microalbuminuria may herald the presence of HIVAN. In recent years, as HAART has become widely used, the classic clinical presentation of HIVAN has become less common. However, the incidence of ESRD due to HIVAN has not changed appreciably in the past 10 years. While there are no large recent biopsy series of patients with renal disease while on HAART, it is likely that HAART usage has transformed HIVAN from a rapidly progressive disease with

severe proteinuria into an indolent disease with lower levels of proteinuria.

Acute kidney injury (AKI) and chronic kidney disease (CKD) are common problems in patients living with HIV/AIDS. Both outpatient and inpatient populations have been observed to have increased rates of AKI that are correlated with higher viral loads and lower CD4 counts; the most important predisposing factor to AKI is the presence of CKD. Interestingly, black race is not associated with increased risk for AKI in patients with HIV/AIDS, suggesting that HIVAN is not the underlying cause of CKD in most cases of AKI in HIV-infected patients. Analysis of over 2 million patients in the Veterans Administration (VA) database for a median time period of 3.7 years yielded a risk of ESRD for black individuals with HIV nearly 10 times that of white individuals with HIV. The most common cause of ESRD in blacks in this study was AIDS nephropathy, the diagnosis that is used by the U.S. Renal Data Service (USRDS) as a surrogate for HIVAN. Strikingly, HIV infection did not increase the risk of ESRD in white patients but did confer an increased risk of ESRD in black patients that was similar to diabetes. A similar study of

VA patients with stage III or higher CKD again found a similar risk for ESRD and rate of GFR decline in black patients with HIV as compared to their counterparts with diabetes.

While ESRD is clearly an important problem in patients with HIV/AIDS, the incidence and prevalence figures from the USRDS do not account for persons living with CKD who have not yet reached ESRD. Previous studies have shown that the prevalence of HIVAN in African-Americans with HIV/AIDS is approximately 4–12%, a figure that has not changed appreciably during the past decade. Extrapolating this prevalence to the 224,815 African-Americans known to be living with HIV/AIDS living in the United States, we predict that there are currently 8992–26,977 African-Americans living with HIVAN in the United States. Moreover, 24.7 million of the 39.5 million people living with HIV/AIDS worldwide reside in Sub-Saharan Africa. Recent evidence suggests that the burden of HIV-related renal disease in Africans is similar to that reported in African-Americans. Applying the same prevalence figure leads us to predict that 0.98–3.0 million people currently have HIVAN in Africa. Since most Africans with HIV/AIDS currently receive little or no treatment for their illness, it is likely that many die of opportunistic infections before renal disease becomes clinically apparent. As the health care delivery to Africans with HIV/AIDS improves, particularly with expanding access to antiretroviral therapy (ART), increased survival of patients can be expected. Almost certainly, HIVAN will emerge as a major complication of HIV-1 infection and will become an increasing cause of morbidity and mortality in Africa.

Centers for Disease Control and Prevention: HIV/AIDS Surveillance Report, 2005, Vol. 17, Rev ed. Atlanta, GA. Department of Health and Human Services, Centers for Disease Control and Prevention, 2007. Also available at http://www.cdc.gov/hiv/topics/surveillance/resources/reports/.

Choi A et al: Racial differences in end-stage renal disease rates in HIV infection versus diabetes. J Am Soc Nephrol 2007;18:2968.

Ross MJ et al: HIV-1 infection initiates an inflammatory cascade in human renal tubular epithelial cells. J Acquir Immune Defic Syndr 2006;42(1):1.

UNAIDS, 2006, UNAIDS/WHO AIDS Epidemic Update: December 2006.

U.S. Renal Data System, USRDS 2007 Annual Data Report: Atlas of Chronic Kidney Disease and End-Stage Renal Disease in the United States. National Institutes of Health, National Institute of Diabetes and Digestive and Kidney Diseases, Bethesda, MD, 2007.

Wyatt CM et al: Chronic kidney disease in HIV infection: an urban epidemic. AIDS. 2007;21(15):2101.

▶ Pathogenesis

A. Mouse Models

The mechanisms through which infection with HIV-1 results in the HIVAN phenotype are not completely known. How-

ever, much research has been done to elucidate important aspects of disease pathogenesis mainly through the use of animal models that develop a phenotype analogous to HIVAN.

Initially, controversy existed as to whether HIVAN resulted from viral infection of the renal parenchyma or from the cytokine milieu created by infection and activation of lymphocytes throughout the body. An HIV-transgenic mouse model was created in which the mice express an HIV-1 provirus under control of the endogenous HIV viral promoter with deletions in the *gag* and *pol* genes, rendering the virus noninfectious. A subsequent experiment performed with this transgenic mouse involved reciprocal transplantation with a mouse not possessing the HIV transgene. Wild-type mice receiving a kidney with an HIV transgene developed proteinuria, glomerular, and tubular changes similar to HIVAN. HIV-transgenic mice, receiving a wild-type kidney, did not develop the diseased status. These data suggest that expression of HIV gene products within the kidney is necessary for the development of HIVAN.

B. Molecular Basis of Pathogenesis

The HIV-1 genome is a 9 kb RNA that encodes nine genes, including three structural genes (*env, gag,* and *pol*) two regulatory genes (*tat* and *rev*), and four accessory genes (*vif, vpr, vpu,* and *nef*) (Figure 35–2). After processing, these nine genes yield 15 respective proteins, each of which plays a role in the life cycle of the virus. Of the 15 proteins, not all have been shown to be

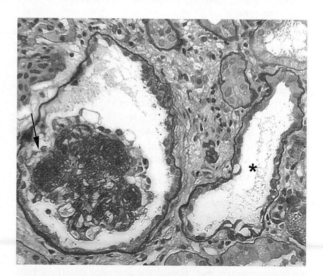

▲ **Figure 35–2.** Typical histopathologic findings in HIV-associated nephropathy (HIVAN). Periodic acid–Schiff staining demonstrates focal glomerulosclerosis with collapse of the glomerular tuft and overlying podocyte proliferation (arrow), microcystic tubular dilation (asterisk), interstitial inflammation, and interstitial fibrosis (×200).

involved in the pathogenesis of HIVAN (Figure 35–3). The *gag* and *pol* genes (accounting for seven HIV proteins after proteolytic cleavage), for example, are not functional in the Tg26 mouse model of HIVAN, suggesting that their presence is not necessary for the development of disease. Further research has indicated two genes whose function is most important for the development of the HIVAN phenotype: *nef* and *vpr*.

1. Nef gene—Several studies have attempted to determine the HIV-1 genes that are responsible for inducing HIVAN. *In vitro* studies have demonstrated that the *nef* gene is necessary and sufficient to induce the podocyte proliferation and dedifferentiation that are characteristic of HIVAN. Several transgenic murine models have also been developed to further delineate which viral genes are pathogenic to the kidney. HIV-transgenic mice that lack *gag*, *pol*, and *nef* develop FSGS. However, the breeding of these mice with *nef*-transgenic mice worsened the renal phenotype as compared to *nef*-mutant mice, suggesting that *nef* has deleterious effects in the kidney when other HIV gene(s) are present. In addition, transgenic mice expressing *nef* selectively in expression podocytes expression have increased podocyte proliferation and dedifferentiation, which are characteristic of HIVAN. However, these mice do not develop proteinuria or histologic glomerular disease, providing further evidence that while podocyte expression of *nef* is an important component of HIVAN pathogenesis, other HIV genes are necessary to induce the full phenotype.

2. Vpr gene—*Vpr* has been demonstrated to have a number of pathogenic effects upon infected cells. These include induction of cell cycle arrest in the G_2 phase, nuclear import of the HIV preintegration complex, transactivation of the viral long terminal repeat (LTR) promoter, and apoptosis. The ability of *vpr* to induce apoptosis has been linked to its ability to increase mitochondrial permeability. *In vitro*

studies have demonstrated the rapid release of apoptogenic proteins (cytochrome-*c* and apoptosis-inducing factor) from mitochondria when exposed to a carboxy-terminal construct of *vpr*. Vpr also promotes apoptosis by selectively increasing expression of proapoptotic molecules including caspase-9. Studies using a series of transgenic mice expressing HIV genes demonstrated that deletion of *vpr* eliminated the renal disease phenotype, further supporting the critical role of *vpr* in HIVAN pathogenesis.

3. Other HIV genes—Though several published *in vitro* studies have suggested that expression of HIV-1 genes other than *nef* and *vpr* may affect renal cells, *in vivo* animal studies have not supported a role for these genes in HIVAN pathogenesis. Several transgenic lines were created, each expressing one HIV gene (*vif*, *vpr*, *vpu*, *nef*, *rev*, *tat*) except for *gag* and *pol*, under the control of the podocyte-specific *Nphs1* promoter. Expression of the HIV transgene in the kidney was confirmed by real time polymerase chain reaction (PCR). No mouse expressing the transgenic product of *rev*, *tat*, *vif*, or *vpu* developed proteinuria or histologic glomerular lesions. Supporting the findings of previous studies, only transgenic mice expressing *nef* and/or *vpr* developed proteinuria and glomerular abnormalities, including FSGS. Furthermore, double-transgenic mice with kidney-specific expression of both *vpr* and *nef* developed proteinuria 1 week, as compared to 4 weeks, in mice transgenic for *vpr* or *nef* alone. *Nef–vpr* transgenic mice also developed markedly worsened renal function as compared to *vpr* transgenic and *nef* single transgenic mice by 4 weeks.

Taken together, the preponderance of published studies support the role of HIV-1 *vpr* and *nef* as the most important viral genes in the pathogenesis of HIVAN. While expression of either gene in the kidney can reproduce stereotypical

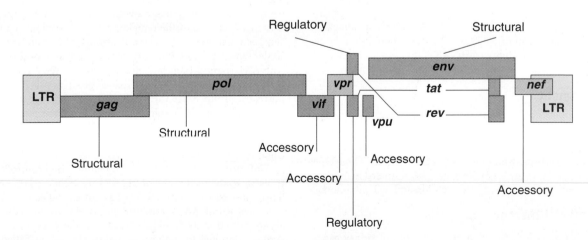

▲ **Figure 35–3.** A schematic representation of the HIV genome flanked by its long terminal repeat promoter regions. Genes nonessential to HIVAN pathogenesis in animal models are shown as dark gray.

features of HIVAN histology, coexpression results in the most severe phenotype, indicating an additive or synergistic effect of these genes.

Zuo Y et al: HIV-1 genes vpr and nef synergistically damage podocytes, leading to glomerulosclerosis. J Am Soc Nephrol 2006;17:2832.

▶ Clinical Findings

The most common pathologic finding in HIVAN biopsy specimens is focal glomerulosclerosis (FGS). This FSGS is often associated with retraction of the glomerular capillary walls resulting in narrowing of the lumen and wrinkling of the glomerular basement membrane causing the glomerulus to appear collapsed and is therefore described as "collapsing focal glomerulosclerosis."

The visceral epithelial cells of the glomerulus, known as podocytes, undergo characteristic phenotypic changes in HIVAN. Podocytes are usually terminally differentiated, quiescent cells, however, in HIVAN, they often become hypertrophic and proliferate. Prominent tubulointerstitial disease is present, the severity of which may exceed the glomerular pathology. Interstitial infiltrates are pleomorphic and may consist of lymphocytes, plasma cells, and macrophages. The tubular abnormalities include flattening and atrophy of tubular epithelial cells and dilation of the tubular lumen, which can be filled with proteinaceous casts. This "microcystic" dilation of the tubules is characteristic of HIVAN and can take place among multiple segments of the nephron.

On electron microscopy, several findings characterize the HIVAN lesion. There is almost complete effacement of podocyte foot processes and the visceral epithelial cytoplasm can have large, electron-dense resorption droplets. The endothelium has large tubuloreticular inclusions located within the cisternae of the endoplasmic reticulum or the Golgi bodies. This can also be seen in patients with lupus nephritis. However, is often not present in patients with the idiopathic collapsing variant of FSGS and therefore should alert the clinician to the possibility of HIVAN if the patient is HIV positive or if the HIV status of the patient is unknown.

Treatment

Strategies for the prevention and/or treatment of HIVAN have never been evaluated in prospective randomized controlled studies and most studies on the treatment of HIVAN have been retrospective and/or lack proper controls. Three types of medical therapy for HIVAN have been studied in humans: Antiretroviral therapy, corticosteroids, and ACE inhibitors.

A. HAART Therapy

Studies demonstrating that HIV infection of kidney parenchymal cells is necessary for the development of HIVAN support the hypothesis that antiretroviral medications should be beneficial for treating and/or preventing HIVAN. Early papers on the use of antiretroviral therapies were mainly case reports involving zidovudine. The first of multiple reports of HIVAN regression in response to zidovudine therapy was published in 1989. A retrospective study from France of patients with biopsy-proven HIVAN found that past use of antiretroviral therapy was associated with a relative risk of 1.9 for progression to ESRD. It was not clear whether use of antiretroviral medications worsened the outcome or if patients who progressed while on therapy were a treatment-resistant group and therefore at higher risk of worsening renal function.

Two of the largest studies looking at the effect of antiretroviral therapy in patients with HIVAN were both retrospective. The first study, published in 2004, assessed 3976 patients in a Baltimore AIDS clinic. Over the 12-year course of the study, HIVAN was diagnosed by biopsy or a conservative clinical protocol in 94 of the patients. Patients with HIVAN were evaluated in groups based on their treatment. The incidence of HIVAN was found to be 26.4, 14.4, and 6.8 per 100 patient-years in groups receiving no treatment, treatment with nucleoside analog only, or treatment with HAART, respectively. In addition, the study demonstrated a significant decrease in the incidence of HIVAN in the years 1998–2001 as compared to 1995–1997. The use of HAART appeared to be superior to nucleoside analog treatment alone, and appeared to account for the decreased incidence of HIVAN diagnosis. The decreasing incidence of HIVAN in this study contrasts with the relatively unchanged incidence of ESRD due to HIVAN over the past decade. This may reflect a change in the HIVAN phenotype in patients treated with HAART resulting in a more indolent disease that is less likely to be evaluated by diagnostic renal biopsy.

The second study, published in 2006, involved a cohort of 263 consecutive HIV-infected patients referred to the renal clinic at Johns Hopkins University. Of the 263 patients, 53 had biopsy-documented HIVAN. Seventeen were excluded because they required dialysis within a month of diagnosis. The characteristics of the remaining 36 were evaluated and compared with regard to their outcomes. Multivariate analysis demonstrated a significantly lower progression of disease with ART (hazard ratio of 0.30). The median renal survival was found to be 552 days in the treated group and 117 in the untreated group. Since this study included patients treated with nucleoside analog solo therapy (prior to the availability of HAART) and those treated with HAART, these results may underestimate the effect of modern ART upon renal outcomes.

Unfortunately, there have been no randomized controlled trials to evaluate the use of HAART in treating HIVAN. Since most patients with HIVAN have other indications for treatment with HAART, randomized placebo-controlled trials are not ethically feasible. Fortunately, the published literature continues to support the use of HAART in patients with HIVAN. As a result, the Infectious Diseases Society of America guidelines now state that a diagnosis of HIVAN is a strong indication for initiating HAART regardless of viral load or CD4 count.

The effect of stopping ART in patients previously diagnosed with HIVAN has not been studied. However, a case report of a woman who developed recurrent HIVAN after stopping HAART suggests that cessation of treatment may not be safe once a diagnosis of HIVAN is made and if antiretroviral medications must be withheld, patients should be monitored for worsening renal function or proteinuria.

Decades have passed since zidovudine was the sole antiretroviral available to treat chronic HIV infection. Available antiretroviral medications are increasingly diverse in their mechanisms of action and include nucleoside and nonnucleoside reverse transcriptase inhibitors, protease inhibitors, integrase inhibitors, and viral entry inhibitors. The ability to control viral replication and enact immune reconstitution therefore continues to improve. Hopefully, these advances in the treatment of HIV/AIDS will eventually translate into a decrease in the morbidity and mortality from HIV-mediated renal disease in these patients.

B. Angiotensin-Converting Enzyme Inhibitors and Receptor Blockers

Blockade of the renin–angiotensin system (RAS) has been shown to attenuate proteinuria in various glomerular diseases. There are also data from studies in HIV-transgenic models of HIVAN that suggest that RAS blockade using ACE inhibitors or angiotensin receptor blockers can decrease proteinuria and improve histologic and functional renal outcomes.

ACE inhibitors have been evaluated in several small studies. Initially, case reports in the early 1990s supported a beneficial role of ACE inhibitors in decreasing proteinuria and preserving renal function in HIVAN, but conclusions regarding the effect of these medications were made difficult by the concomitant use of ART. In 1996, a retrospective case–control study found that use of captopril was associated with slower progression to ESRD.

In 1997, the course of 20 patients with biopsy-proven HIVAN was documented. Seven of the 11 patients with non-nephrotic-range proteinuria and five of the nine patients with nephrotic-range proteinuria were treated with 10 mg of fosinopril daily. In the patients with initial nonnephrotic-range proteinuria, the mean serum creatinine went from 1.3 mg/dL and 1.0 mg/dL to 1.5 mg/dL and 4.9 mg/dL in the treated and untreated groups, respectively. Similarly, in the group with nephrotic-range proteinuria, the mean serum creatinine went from 1.7 mg/dL and 1.9 mg/dL to 2.0 mg/dL and 9.2 mg/dL in the treated and untreated groups. Proteinuria followed a similar trend. Diminished proteinuria was observed in the treated patients and proteinuria progressively worsened in the untreated patients. A subsequent study from the same group also suggested a beneficial effect of ACE inhibition upon renal outcomes; however, a confounding role for concomitant ART could not be ruled out.

Taken together, the strong evidence in the literature on the protective effect of RAS blockade in a variety of proteinuric renal diseases and the suggestive retrospective studies discussed above support a role for these medications in slowing the decline in renal function and in decreasing the rates of proteinuria in patients with HIVAN.

C. Prednisone

Tubulointerstitial inflammation is one of the most prominent histopathologic findings in HIVAN and the inflammatory response of renal parenchymal cells to HIV infection is an important component of HIVAN pathogenesis. It is therefore plausible that anti-inflammatory agents may be useful in the treatment of HIVAN. However, since patients with HIV/AIDS already have suppressed immune systems, use of immunosuppressive medications may expose these patients to excess risk of infection and/or malignancy.

In the early 1990s, case reports demonstrated improvements in proteinuria and renal function in patients with HIVAN who were treated with steroids for other indications. In 1996, a prospective case series of 20 consecutive patients with mostly biopsy-proven HIVAN (17 of 20) who were treated with oral prednisone was documented. Patients were treated with 60 mg/day for varying periods of time followed by a tapering course. Seventeen of the patients experienced a decrease in their serum creatinines from an average of 8.1 mg/dL to 3.0 mg/dL. Five patients who had an increase in their creatinine after cessation of treatment were then retreated. These patients again responded to the prednisone with subsequent decreases in serum creatinine measurements. There was, however, no control group in this study and six patients developed serious opportunistic infections while being treated with prednisone. Several other retrospective studies have also found a striking association between steroid treatment and improved renal outcomes in patients with HIVAN.

A beneficial effect of steroid treatment upon tubulointerstitial inflammation is suggested by a case report of a patient with biopsy-proven HIVAN who was rebiopsied when his creatinine began to increase as steroids were being weaned. The repeat biopsy revealed marked reductions in interstitial lymphocytes and macrophages after the steroid treatment, suggesting that prednisone reduced the interstitial inflammation in this patient.

Since there are still no prospective controlled studies demonstrating a benefit of corticosteroids in patients with HIVAN, we believe that they should be considered for use only as a short-term adjuvant while antiretroviral medications and ACE inhibitors are being titrated or in cases in which antiretroviral therapy and angiotensin blockade have failed.

Atta M et al: Antiretroviral therapy in the treatment of HIV-associated nephropathy. Nephrol Dialysis Transplant 2006;21:2809.

Bartlett JG, Lane HC: Guidelines for the use of antiretroviral agents in HIV-infected adults and adolescents. Department of

Health and Human Services, December 2007, page 64. Accessed 1/14/2008.

Ideura H et al: Angiotensin II provokes podocyte injury in murine model of HIV-associated nephropathy. Am J Physiol Renal Physiol 2007;293:F1214.

http://aidsinfo.nih.gov/contentfiles/AdultandAdolescentGL.pdf.

Ross MJ et al: HIV-1 infection initiates an inflammatory cascade in human renal tubular epithelial cells. J Acquir Immune Defic Syndr 2006;42(1):1.

Scialla J et al: Relapse of HIV-associated nephropathy after discontinuing highly active antiretroviral therapy. AIDS 2007;21(2):263.

▼ HEPATITIS-ASSOCIATED GLOMERULONEPHITS

Kar Neng Lai, MBBS, MD, Sydney Tang, MD, PhD

HEPATITIS C VIRUS-ASSOCIATED RENAL DISEASES

ESSENTIALS OF DIAGNOSIS

▶ The presence of circulating hepatitis C viral RNA and antibody.

▶ Type I membranoproliferative glomerulonephritis.

▶ Circulating type II mixed cryoglobulins [polyclonal immunoglobulin (Ig)G and monoclonal IgMκ rheumatoid factor].

▶ Strong association with hepatitis C virus (HCV) infection chronicity.

▶ Very low serum C4, C1q, and CH50, but normal C3 levels.

▶ General Considerations

A. Historic Perspective

The clinical manifestations associated with "mixed" cryoglobulinemia were first described in 1966. They included a constellation of clinical features that consisted of the triad of palpable purpura, arthralgias, and weakness plus variable degrees of glomerulonephritis, lymphadenopathy, and hepatosplenomegaly in some patients. Cryoglobulinemia in these patients had a "mixed" composition of IgG and IgM rheumatoid factor (RF). The cause of this disease was unknown in those days, and its association with hepatitis C virus (HCV) infection became increasingly apparent only after its discovery in 1989. It is now apparent that the classic clinical triad occurs in a minority of patients and that the main characteristic of the disease is the markedly heterogeneous manifestations of a systemic vasculitis, with purpuric skin lesions that show leukocytoclastic vasculitis on biopsy being an almost constant and predominant feature.

B. Hepatitis C Virus Virology

HCV is a small RNA virus that is included in the Flaviviridae family and has recently been classified as the sole member of the genus *Hepacivirus*. HCV is a small double-shelled virus consisting of a lipid envelope (E) with virally encoded glycoproteins (E1 and E2) and an inner nucleocapsid (core) that contains a positive-sense single-stranded RNA genome of 9500 nucleotides. It has well-defined structural (core, E1, and E2) as well as several nonstructural (from NS2 to NS5) proteins. The nonstructural proteins encode several proteases, a virus-specific helicase, and an RNA-dependent RNA polymerase responsible for replication of the genome. The evolution of HCV has been characterized by the emergence of six major genotypes based on sequence homology, and more than 50 subtypes.

C. Epidemiology

To date, around 170–200 million individuals worldwide are estimated by the World Health Organization to have chronic HCV infection. Although HCV infection appears to be primarily a disease that is almost exclusively confined to the liver, a wide variety of extrahepatic disease manifestations have been reported to be associated with HCV infection. The prevalence of extrahepatic diseases is not known with certainty, but it suggests that HCV is involved in nonhepatic pathologic processes.

Two immunologic features of HCV may predispose patients to manifestations of extrahepatic disease. First, HCV is known to evade immune elimination and lead to chronic infection and accumulation of circulating immune complexes. Membranoproliferative glomerulonephritis (MPGN) associated with HCV infection may be the result of this phenomenon. The second feature is that HCV stimulates production of monoclonal rheumatoid factors (mRF). This feature causes type II cryoglobulinemia that is responsible for most of the symptomatic cryoglobulinemic vasculitis. Although this manifestation occurs relatively infrequently, as do all the extrahepatic disease manifestations, it is an important extrahepatic involvement of chronic HCV infection responsible for much of the increased morbidity and mortality accompanying the disease.

The prevalence of mixed cryoglobulinemia increases with the duration of the hepatitis. Patients with chronic hepatitis C who have mixed cryoglobulinemia have an apparent duration of disease that is almost twice as long as those without cryoglobulinemia. A high prevalence of mixed cryoglobulinemia (35–90%) has been reported for patients with HCV infection. However, the prevalence of mixed cryoglobulinemia has not been assessed in populations of unselected HCV-infected patients. Hence, reports of high prevalence of mixed cryoglobulinemia may be influenced by selection bias, eg, studies on cirrhotic patients with long-standing HCV infection from gastroenterology centers. Frank symptomatic cryoglobulinemia occurs in 1% or less of patients and is usually associated with high levels of RF and cryoglobulins. Testing unselected patients with cryoglobulinemia has shown that up to 90% have anti-HCV antibody. Type I MPGN has long been regarded as idiopathic, but a considerable proportion of patients has concomitant chronic infection with HCV. The exact proportion of patients with type I MPGN who are anti-HCV-antibody positive is unknown.

The most frequent form of renal involvement in HCV infection is MPGN, described mainly in the United States and Japan. The real prevalence of MPGN without detectable cryoglobulinemia is difficult to assess. Such cases might represent a subclinical form of cryoglobulinemia because of failure to detect circulating cryoglobulins by standard laboratory techniques or inadequate methods. In addition, the production of IgM antibodies with anti-IgG activity might induce immune complexes without cryoprecipitable properties. Finally, these patients may develop detectable circulating cryoglobulinemia only later in the course of the disease.

▶ Pathogenesis

Cryoglobulinemia is defined as the presence in serum of immunoglobulins that precipitate at reduced temperatures (Figure 35–4). Therefore, blood samples obtained from patients for detection of cryoglobulins must be stored and transported at 37°C.

Cryoglobulins were classified based on their Ig composition, and three types were defined. Type I consists of a single monoclonal Ig without antibody activity, and can be found in patients with multiple myeloma, Waldenström's macroglobulinemia, or idiopathic monoclonal gammopathy. Types II and III, or mixed cryoglobulins, consist of polyclonal IgG and monoclonal IgMκ (type II) or polyclonal IgM (type III) with RF activity (Table 35–1). When no definite disease association is found, the condition is referred to as essential mixed cryoglobulinemia. The observation that up to 90% of unselected patients with cryoglobulinemia have anti-HCV antibody indicates that the disease is not genuinely "essential," but more likely is related to HCV infection. Hence, the term "essential" may be a misnomer and can no longer be used for the majority of cases, where cryoglobulins consist of complexes of RF, IgG, anti-HCV antibody, and HCV virions. The pathogenesis of cryoglobulinemia due to HCV infection is not well understood, but it appears to be related to excessive proliferation of B cells as a result of the chronic antigenic stimulation of HCV infection.

▶ Clinical Findings

A. Symptoms and Signs

1. Hepatitis C virus-related cryoglobulinemia—Full-blown symptomatic cryoglobulinemia occurs infrequently,

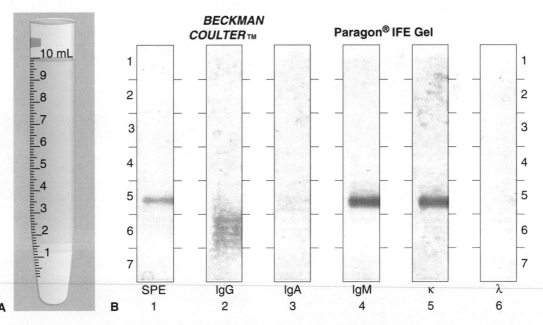

▲ **Figure 35–4. A:** Whitish cryoprecipitates forming in Wintrobe's tube after standing at 4°C for 72 hours followed by centrifugation at 400 × g for 10 minutes. The cryocrit is approximately 30%. **B:** Immunofixation of the washed, dissolved cryoprecipitate typed a monoclonal IgMκ with polyclonal IgG. By definition, these are type II cryoglobulins. (Courtesy of Dr Janette S.Y. Kwok, Department of Pathology, Queen Mary Hospital, Hong Kong, China.)

Table 35–1. Classification of cryoglobulins.

Type	Immunoglobulin composition	RF activity	Most common disease association	Other disease associations
I	Single monoclonal IgG, IgA, or IgM	No	Multiple myeloma	Waldenström's macroglobulinemia Idiopathic monoclonal gammopathy Chronic lymphocytic leukemia
II[1]	Polyclonal IgG and monoclonal IgM	Yes	HCV infection	Chronic lymphocytic leukemia Lymphoproliferative disease Essential[2]
III[1]	Polyclonal IgG and polyclonal IgM	Yes	Connective tissue disease, particularly RA	Lymphoproliferative disease Chronic liver disease Essential[3]

[1]Also known as mixed cryoglobulinemia due to the presence of more than one Ig type.
[2]When no definite disease association is found, these are known as essential mixed cryoglobulinemias.
RF, rheumatoid factor; RA, rheumatoid arthritis; Ig, immunoglobulin; HCV, hepatitis C virus.

and the typical symptoms are fatigue and palpable purpura, which histologically consists of a leukocytoclastic vasculitis (with complexes of anti-HCV antibody and HCV in injured tissue). These lesions are usually found on the lower limbs (Figure 35–5), although they can occur anywhere, and represent small vessel vasculitis. A smaller proportion of patients has fever, arthritis, Raynaud's phenomenon, and neuropathy. Peripheral neuropathy is usually characterized by paresthesias and variable degrees of motor deficits. Abdominal pain arises from mesenteric vasculitis, and may mimic an acute abdomen during disease flare. Hepatosplenomegaly is due to chronic liver disease as a result of HCV. Cryoglobulinemia is more common in women than men and typically occurs after a prolonged period, often years or decades, of HCV infection. Although the course of illness tends to wax and wane, occasionally the systemic illness can be severe or even fulminant. For instance, nodular pulmonary infiltrates from deposition of cryoglobulins leading to respiratory failure (Figure 35–6) and non-

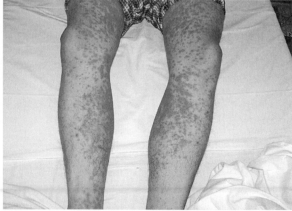

▲ **Figure 35–5.** Palpable purpuric skin lesions in the lower limbs of a patient with cryoglobulinemia. Such lesions are characteristic of any causes of small vessel vasculitis, but not pathognomonic of the rashes in cryoglobulinemia. (Courtesy of Dr. Chi-keung Yeung, Department of Medicine, Queen Mary Hospital, Hong Kong, China.)

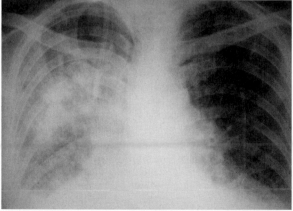

▲ **Figure 35–6.** Nodular pulmonary infiltrates in a patient with cryoglobulinemia. Note also a right internal jugular venous catheter *in situ* for plasmapheresis and hemodialysis.

Hodgkin's B cell and splenic lymphomas have been reported to arise in the setting of cryoglobulinemia. In addition, cryoglobulinemia has also been anecdotally reported in association with adenocarcinoma of the liver and stomach in Chinese.

2. Cryoglobulinemic glomerulonephritis—The principal renal manifestation of HCV infection is MPGN type I, usually in the context of cryoglobulinemia. Type II MPGN (eg, dense deposit disease) has not been described in association with HCV infection. From studies in Italy, the United States, and Japan, MPGN associated with type II cryoglobulinemia is the predominant type of glomerulonephritis clinically associated with HCV infection. The prevalence of MPGN in HCV type II cryoglobulinemia is approximately 30%. On the other hand, the prevalence of anti-HCV antibody among patients with MPGN is much lower in Chinese people. MPGN is also occasionally observed in patients with hepatitis C in the absence of cryoglobulinemia.

Renal disease is rare in children and the typical age of disease onset is in the fifth or sixth decade of life after long-standing infection, often in association with mild subclinical liver disease. Clinically, patients may have other symptoms of cryoglobulinemia, such as palpable purpura and arthralgias. Renal manifestations include nephrotic (20%) or nonnephrotic proteinuria and microscopic hematuria. Acute nephritic syndrome is the presenting feature in about 25% of cases. Progression to uremia is associated with male gender and old age. Renal insufficiency, frequently mild, occurs in about 50% of patients. Over 80% of patients have refractory hypertension upon presentation, which may be responsible for a considerable number of cardiovascular deaths.

The natural history of HCV-related cryoglobulinemia remains poorly defined. The clinical course can vary dramatically. The renal disease tends to have an indolent course and does not progress to uremia despite the persistence of urine abnormalities in the majority of patients. Around 15% of patients eventually require dialysis according to an Italian series.

B. Laboratory Findings

Laboratory testing coupled with renal biopsy establishes the diagnosis of HCV-related MPGN. Most patients will have anti-HCV antibody, as well as HCV RNA, in serum. Serum transaminase levels are elevated in 70% of patients. Cryoglobulins are detected in 50–70% of patients. Serum electrophoresis and immunofixation reveal type II mixed cryoglobulins (Figure 35–4B), in which the monoclonal rheumatoid factor, almost invariably an IgMκ, is a distinguishing feature of cryoglobulinemic glomerulonephritis. Their amount, usually measured as a cryocrit, varies from one patient to another, and varies from time to time in a given patient (ranging between 2% and 70%). Urine κ light chains are also commonly present. The serum complement

pattern, which does not change much with clinical activity, is also discriminative. Characteristically, the early complement components (C4 and C1q) and CH50 are at very low, or even undetectable, levels, while the C3 level tends to remain normal or only slightly depressed.

Renal histologic evaluation typically shows evidence of immune complex deposition in glomeruli and changes of MPGN. MPGN refers to a pattern of glomerular injury characterized by diffuse mesangial proliferation and thickening of the capillary wall, hence the synonym of mesangiocapillary glomerulonephritis (Table 35–2). In cryoglobulinemic MPGN, light microscopy reveals an increased number of mesangial cells, expansion of the mesangial matrix, and diffuse accentuation of glomerular tufts, which gives a lobular appearance to the glomeruli (Figure 35–7A). Glomerular capillary walls appear thickened because of the interposition

Table 35–2. Comparison of glomerulonephritis related to chronic hepatitis virus infection.

	HBV Membranous/ mesangiocapillary GN	HCV mesangiocapillary GN
Route of infection	Vertical or horizontal in children, intravenous or sexual in adult	Intravenous
Occurrence	Children and adult	Adult (fifth and sixth decade)
Male:female	3:1	2:3
History of liver disease	Absent in endemic areas	Yes
Abnormal liver function	Occasional	Yes
Renal presentation	Nephrotic syndrome/ proteinuria	Microscopic hematuria/ proteinuria, nephrotic syndrome <20%
Hypertension	25–40%	80%
Renal insufficiency	Occasional, 29% in 5 years	15% in 10 years
10-year probability of survival without dialysis	75–90%	49% mainly due to extrarenal complications
Extrarenal complications	Uncommon	40%—CVA, hematologic malignancy, infection, liver failure

HBV, hepatitis B virus; HCV, hepatitis C virus; GN, glomerulonephropathy; CVA, cerebrovascular accident.

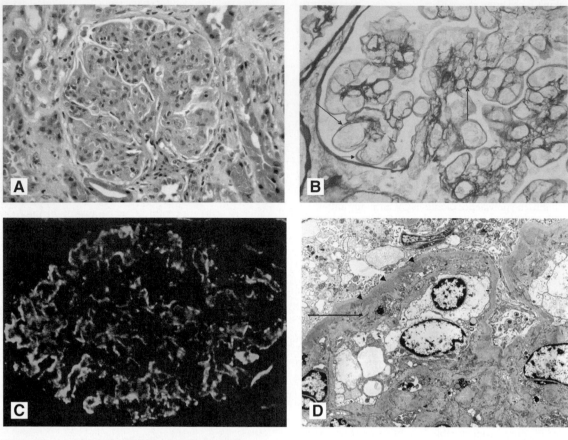

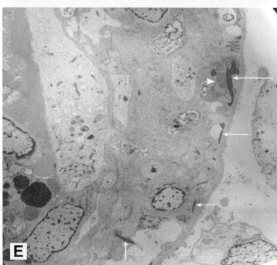

▲ **Figure 35–7.** Pathology of membranoproliferative glomerulonephritis type I associated with cryoglobulinemia. **A:** Glomerulus exhibits a diffuse increase in mesangial cellularity and matrix with accentuation of lobulation of tuft architecture, obliteration of capillary lumens, and leukocytic infiltrate (×200, H&E). **B:** Periodic acid–Schiff and methenamine silver staining reveal prominent double contours or tram-tracking (arrows) of the glomerular basement membrane (×400). **C:** Immunofluorescence reveals granular deposits of C3 (shown here) and IgG in the mesangium and in peripheral capillary loops (×200). **D:** Electron microscopy shows markedly increased glomerular cellularity and subendothelial deposits (arrowheads), indicative of cryoglobulin deposition. The thickened glomerular basement also incorporates cell processes (arrow), indicative of mesangial interpositioning (×10,500). **E:** Several tactoids are also seen. These are highly electron-dense deposits (arrows) that are most likely crystalline immune complexes as they are surrounded by accompanying nonstructured, less electron-dense materials (arrowhead) (×7800). (Courtesy of Dr. Kwok-wah Chan, Department of Pathology, Queen Mary Hospital, Hong Kong, China.)

of the mesangial matrix between the glomerular basement membrane (GBM) and the endothelium. Staining of the GBM with periodic acid–Schiff or silver stain shows splitting ("double contour") or "tram-tracking" due to insertion of the mesangial matrix (Figure 35–7B). Immunofluorescence reveals granular deposits of C3 and IgG in the mesangium and in peripheral capillary loops (Figure 35–7C). A similar morphologic appearance may be seen with infective endocarditis and infected ventriculoatrial shunts (shunt nephritis). In addition, glomerular capillaries may have marked inflammatory cell infiltrates with both mononuclear cells and polymorphonuclear leukocytes (Figure 35–7A), a distinguishing feature from noncryoglobulinemic MPGN. Intracapillary globular accumulations of eosinophilic material representing precipitated immune complexes or cryoglobulins may also be present. Viral HCV-containing antigens had previously been detected in glomerular structures using a three-stage indirect immunohistochemical monoclonal antibody technique but this has not been confirmed by subsequent studies. Electron microscopy shows subendothelial deposits (Figure 35–7D) that may have a tactoid pattern, size, and distribution (Figure 35–7E), suggestive of cryoglobulin deposition. These tend to be of 15–30 μm in size, distinguishing them from the smaller fibrillary deposits (12–25 μm). The presence of immunotactoid glomerulonephritis in a viral disease confirms the association of immunotactoid glomerulonephritis with a systemic disorder, while fibrillary glomerulonephritis is more frequently a "primary" condition. Fibrillogenesis may be favored by circulating paraproteins interacting with matrix proteins in the glomerulus, such as fibronectin. The animal model of membranoproliferative glomerulonephritis derived from induction of mixed cryoglobulinemia strongly suggests a pathogenetic role of cryoglobulins rather than a direct etiologic role of HCV infection. Of interest, however, and again in animal models, both rheumatoid factor and cryoglobulinemic properties may be necessary for the development of skin vasculitis, but cryoglobulin activity alone is sufficient to induce glomerular lesions.

Other forms of glomerular injury have been associated with HCV infection in individual case reports and small series, including membranous glomerulonephritis, IgA nephropathy, focal and segmental glomerulosclerosis, fibrillary glomerulonephritis, immunotactoid glomerulopathy, rapidly progressive glomerulonephritis, exudative–proliferative glomerulonephritis, and lupus nephritis. Membranous nephropathy in HCV carriers is characterized by the absence of cryoglobulins and male predominance.

▶ Treatment

In general, therapy can be directed at two levels: (1) Removal of cryoglobulins by plasmapheresis and (2) inhibition of their synthesis through either attenuation of the immune responses (using corticosteroid or cytotoxic agents) or suppression of viral replication (using interferon and ribavirin).

Before the association between HCV and cryoglobulinemic MPGN was unraveled, corticosteroid and cyclophosphamide were the mainstay of treatment. High-dose pulse methylprednisolone (1 g/day for 3 consecutive days), followed by oral steroids, was used to control the systemic illness. Plasmapheresis may be applied to remove circulating cryoglobulins, thus preventing their deposition in glomeruli and blood vessel walls. Cyclophosphamide ameliorates the vasculitic injury and inhibits the production of monoclonal rheumatoid factors by B-lymphocytes.

Our current understanding of the association between mixed cryoglobulinemia and HCV infection has resulted in a more rational approach to the treatment of this condition. Controlled trials have shown that antiviral therapy with interferon-α is associated with improvements in systemic symptoms of immune complex disease. However, relapse after therapy occurs in a large proportion of patients, particularly with interferon monotherapy given for short durations. Combination therapy with interferon-α2b plus ribavirin represented an important milestone in the treatment of chronic hepatitis C and acute hepatitis C after renal transplantation. Such cocktail therapy has also produced favorable results in mixed cryoglobulinemia, although nonresponses and relapses after initial improvements still occur. In some instances in which sustained viral eradication was unsuccessful, long-term maintenance interferon therapy has led to amelioration of disease. The introduction of pegylated forms of interferon (peginterferon) in 2000 represented another breakthrough in the treatment of chronic hepatitis C. Pegylation refers to the covalent attachment of a large inert molecule of polyethylene glycol (PEG) to a protein to yield a molecule that retains biological activity, but has delayed absorption and clearance, allowing for weekly rather than daily or three times a week administration. Delayed clearance also led to greater, more potent, and longer lasting antiviral effects. Recent data on peginterferon and ribavirin combination therapy in treating HCV infection are encouraging. Furthermore, the higher treatment failure rate of HCV carriers with genotype 1 is recognized.

Despite reports that antiviral therapy can occasionally be associated with the worsening of renal disease or a variable response, there are increasing observational studies suggesting the effectiveness of peginterferon and ribavirin combination therapy in treating HCV-associated cryoglobulinemic membranoproliferative glomerulonephritis. One therapeutic drawback lies in the hemolytic effect that complicates ribavirin therapy, particularly in patients with functional renal impairment. This therapeutic difficulty has been overcome by adjusting the dose according to the glomerular filtration rate instead of body weight alone and utilizing recombinant erythropoietin to overcome anemia. It is necessary to follow ribavirin serum levels when using this approach. Posttreatment renal biopsy showed histologic improvement in two of the three patients who received combination therapy for 12 months. In another study in which the viral genotypes were documented, genotype 1 was again associated with a lower sustained virologic response rate even with combined interferon-α and ribavirin therapy. In severe acute flares of cryoglobulinemia with glomerulonephritis or vasculitis, an appropriate approach is to include corticosteroids and cyclophosphamide as needed to control severe cryoglobulinemic symptoms in addition to combination antiviral therapy. In the most severe cases, plasmapheresis (three to four times weekly exchanges of 3 L of plasma for 2–3 weeks) can be helpful. For refractory cases, monoclonal antibody against the B cell surface antigen CD20 (Rituximab) has been reported to be efficacious with a favorable side-effect profile.

Au WY et al: Life-threatening cryoglobulinemia in HCV-negative-Southern Chinese and a novel association with structural aorticabnormalities. Ann Hematol 2005;84:95.

Hadziyannis SJ et al: Peginterferon alpha2a and ribavirincombination therapy in chronic hepatitis C: a randomized study of treatment duration and ribavirin dose. Ann Intern Med 2004;140:346.

Roccatello D et al: Long-term effects of anti-CD20 monoclonalantibody treatment of cryoglobulinemic glomerulonephritis. Nephrol Dial Transplant 2004;19:3054.

Uchiyama-Tanaka Y et al: Membranous glomerulonephritisassociated with hepatitis C virus infection: case report and literature review. Clin Nephrol 2004;61:144.

HEPATITIS B VIRUS-ASSOCIATED RENAL DISEASES

 ESSENTIALS OF DIAGNOSIS

▶ Membranous nephropathy is the most frequent association.

▶ The presence of circulating hepatitis B virus (HBV) or DNA.

▶ The presence of HBV-specific antigen(s) or viral genome in the glomerulus.

▶ Serum C3 and C4 levels may be low in 20–50%.

▶ General Considerations

A. Historic Perspective

Following the landmark discovery in 1965 of the Australian antigen, subsequently renamed the hepatitis B surface antigen (HBsAg), the occurrence of membranous nephropathy (MN) due to glomerular deposition of Australian antigen-containing immune complexes was described in a 53-year-old man in 1971. Different histologic types of glomerular lesions have since been described in association with HBV carriage; however, the most striking is still MN.

B. Hepatitis B Virus Virology

HBV is a hepatotropic, double-stranded DNA virus belonging to the family Hepadnaviridae. HBV has a double-shelled virion 42–47 nm in diameter, a 27-nm internal core, an excess of incomplete 22-nm spheres, and a circular DNA, with a length varying between 3000 and 3300 base pairs. The DNA genome contains only four genes that encode viral proteins. These include the surface (S) gene, which encodes the three forms of HBsAg, the precore/core (PC/C) gene, which encodes the core protein and hepatitis B e antigen (HBeAg), the X gene, which encodes the X protein, and the polymerase (P) gene, which encodes the viral DNA polymerase. HBV is itself not cytopathic; hepatitis develops as a result of the host's immune reaction toward infected hepatocytes. HBV utilizes a replication strategy closely related to retroviruses, in that transcription of RNA into DNA is a critical step. Unlike retroviruses, HBV DNA is not integrated into host cell DNA during replication. After an HBV particle binds to and enters a hepatocyte, HBV DNA enters the cell nucleus and is converted into covalently closed circular DNA (cccDNA), which is highly stable acting as the intermediate template for transcription of RNA copies. This pregenomic mRNA is transported to the cytoplasm and has the dual functions of acting as a template for synthesis of new HBV DNA and carrying genetic information to direct the synthesis of viral proteins.

C. Epidemiology

An estimated 350–400 million people worldwide are now infected with HBV. The reported prevalence of HBV-associated nephropathy, particularly MN, closely parallels the geographic patterns of prevalence of HBV. HBV infection occurs throughout the world and is endemic in developing countries, such as Africa, Eastern Europe, the Middle East, Central Asia, China, Southeast Asia, the Pacific Islands, and the Amazon basin of South America (with prevalence rates up to 10% or higher).

In endemic areas, transmission is usually vertical from infected mother to child. Horizontal transmission occurs via direct contact with blood (as in blood transfusions) or mucous membranes (as in sexual contacts), or via the percutaneous route upon contact with blood or body fluids (as in illicit intravenous drug use and needle-sharing practices).

▶ Pathogenesis

The only definitive means to prove that a particular glomerulopathy is etiologically associated with HBV infection is to fulfill the following criteria:

1. The presence of circulating HBV antigen or DNA and HBV-specific antigen(s) or the viral genome in the glomerulus or viral particles identified on ultrastructural examination.

2. The absence of other causes of renal disease.

3. Regression of the pathologic lesion with viral eradication.

4. Reproducibility of the pathology in animal models infected with the virus.

Observations from chronic hepatitis virus infection in woodchucks revealed three types of glomerulonephritis, namely, membranous nephropathy with HBcAg deposits, mesangial proliferative glomerulonephritis with mesangial deposits of HBsAg, and mixed membranous and mesangial proliferative glomerulonephritis with capillary deposits of HBcAg and mesangial deposits of HBsAg. The natural animal model of woodchuck hepatitis reveals pathologic findings similar to those of humans. HBV-associated membranous nephropathy is particularly frequent in male children. Mesangial proliferative forms with IgA deposits appear to be more common in adults. In the woodchuck, the membranous pattern of injury appeared more frequently in the young, whereas the mesangial proliferative pattern of injury tended to appear in older animals. Nevertheless, in humans, it is difficult to rule out the chance occurrence of two common disorders (eg, HBV and IgA nephropathy) presenting in the older population in an endemic area as a cause of this association. The male/female ratio of affected woodchucks was significantly greater than that of the chronic carrier population. One major difference is that the HBeAg system has not been characterized in woodchucks. In clinical practice, regression of the pathology with viral eradication is not easily demonstrable because of ethical concerns involving repeat renal biopsies in human subjects after clinical remission. Hence the diagnosis of HBV-associated renal disease in reality relies heavily upon the demonstration of HBV-specific antigen(s) in the glomeruli.

▶ Clinical Findings

A. Symptoms and Signs

Pediatric and adult patients tend to have slightly different clinical manifestations of HBV-related MN. In children, there is a strong male preponderance, and the most frequent presentation is nephrotic syndrome together with microscopic hematuria and normal or mildly impaired renal function. Pediatric chronic HBV carriers often do not have overt liver disease, and transaminase levels are usually normal. In adults, proteinuria and the nephrotic syndrome are the most common manifestations, though male predominance is less obvious than that observed in children. In addition, adults are more likely than children to have hypertension, renal dysfunction, and clinical evidence of liver disease.

The prognosis of HBV-associated MN in children is favorable with stable renal function and high rates of spontaneous remission reported in several high prevalence areas, including Hong Kong, South Africa, and Turkey. On the other hand, adults with HBV-associated MN typically develop progressive disease. In Hong Kong, up to 29% of patients had progressive renal failure, and another 10% developed ESRD over 5 years. The prognosis is even worse in patients with nephrotic-range proteinuria and overt hepatitis at presentation, with over 50% of patients requiring renal replacement therapy over 3 years.

B. Laboratory Findings

Laboratory tests to be followed for diagnostic purposes and also to assess response to treatment include standard liver biochemistries (serum alanine aminotransferase, γ-glutamyltransferase, and bilirubin levels) and HBV serologies (HBsAg, HBeAg, anti-HBe, and anti-HBc antibodies). HBeAg is present in 80% of patients, who may also have high titers of anti-HBc. Subjects with biochemical hepatitis should also be tested for circulating HBV DNA levels and should undergo liver biopsy. In addition, α-fetoprotein assay could be an important adjunct. Serum C3 and C4 levels may be low in 20–50% of patients.

Light microscopic findings are similar to that of idiopathic MN, with some differentiating features. The characteristic glomerular lesion is a diffuse thickening of the glomerular capillary walls to form thick "membranes" (Figure 35–8A). It is now firmly established that this alteration is caused by immune complexes that accumulate subepithelially on the outer aspect of the GBM, which assumes a "membranous" morphology in a stepwise manner. Other pertinent light microscopic findings are reflected in the reactive structural changes of the GBM induced by immune complexes. Therefore special stains highlighting the GBM, such as methenamine silver and periodic acid–Schiff (PASM or silver stain) or trichrome stain, are more useful (Figure 35–8B). The earliest change on silver staining is a mottled appearance best seen on tangential sections and represents slight indentations of the GBM by immune complexes adhering to its surface. The most specific change of the GBM is the so-called "spike" formation (Figure 35–8C). These are projections of GBM material between immune complexes that lead to a saw tooth-like appearance of the GBM. This pattern is pathognomonic of full-blown membranous glomerulonephropathy. Disease progression results in a diffuse thickening of the GBM. The major constituents of the immune complexes are IgG together with C3. IgM, IgA, and C1q may be present. Ultrastructural findings typically consist of both subepithelial and occasional subendothelial deposits. The presence of subendothelial deposits, sometimes referred to as membranoproliferative glomerulonephritis type III changes, favors a secondary case of MN such as HBV associated rather than idiopathic. The presence of mesangial proliferation on light microscopy is helpful in distinguishing this form of secondary MN from idiopathic MN.

Apart from MN, other renal pathologies have also been associated with HBV infection. These include MPGN with or without cryoglobulinemia, mesangial proliferative glomerulonephritis, and IgA nephropathy. Polyarteritis nodosa has also been reported in some patients with HBV and may

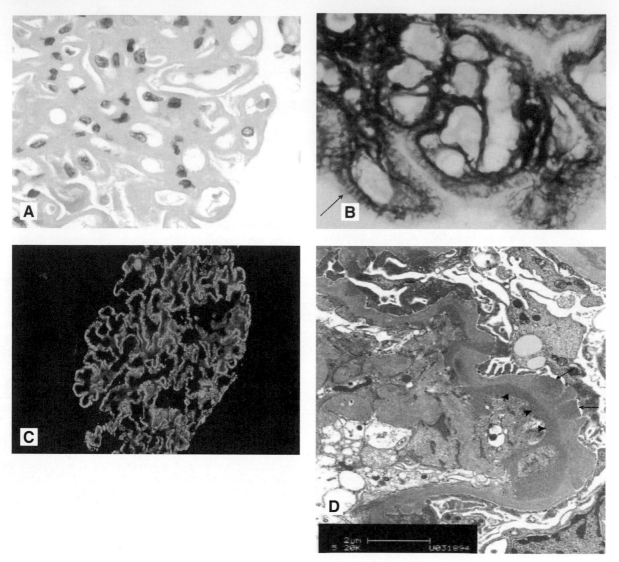

▲ **Figure 35–8.** Pathology of hepatitis B virus (HBV)-associated membranous nephropathy (MN). **A:** On light microscopy, the characteristic glomerular lesion is a diffuse thickening of glomerular capillary walls to form thick "membranes" (H&E, ×200). **B:** Periodic acid–Schiff and methenamine silver staining highlight the characteristic epimembranous "spike" formation (arrow), projections of glomerular basement membrane (GBM) material between immune complexes that lead to a saw tooth-like appearance of the GBM (×400). **C:** Immunofluorescence reveals granular deposits of IgG (shown here) together with C3. IgM, IgA, and C1q may be present. **D:** Ultrastructural findings typically consist of both subepithelial (arrows) and occasional subendothelial (arrowheads) deposits. The presence of subendothelial deposits, sometimes referred to as membranoproliferative glomerulonephritis (MPGN) type III changes (an amalgam of membranous and MPGN type I pathologies), favors a secondary case of MN, such as HBV-related rather than idiopathic. (Courtesy of Dr. Yun-hoi Lui and Dr. Chung-ying Leung, Department of Pathology, United Christian Hospital, Hong Kong, China.)

respond to corticosteroids and interferon-α therapy. Occasionally, overlapping of these pathologic forms leading to double glomerulopathies may be seen. For instance, MN and IgAN have been reported to coexist in an HBV carrier.

Regardless of the pathologic finding, it is important to localize HBV-specific antigens in the biopsy. To document an etiologic association between HBV and MN or other forms of glomerular lesion, the demonstration of HBV-specific antigens by immunofluorescence is indispensable. The three major antigens are HBsAg, HBeAg, and hepatitis B core antigen (HBcAg). Monoclonal antibodies recognize a single antigenic epitope and are in general less sensitive than polyclonal antibodies that bind to more than one epitope. Commercial polyclonal anti-HBc preparations cross-react with both anti-HBc and anti-HBe, as HBeAg is an integral component of HBcAg. HBsAg is characteristically localized in the mesangium while HBeAg is found in the capillary loop. Furthermore, HBV DNA and mRNA have been detected in the glomerulus and tubular epithelia by polymerase chain reaction and *in situ* hybridization with specific HBV RNA probes.

▶ **Treatment**

Unlike childhood disease in which there is a high rate of spontaneous remission, adults with HBV-associated MN typically develop progressive disease. Various strategies have been tried, although an ideal agent has yet to be found. Treatment for HBV-associated renal disease should ideally achieve the following objectives:

1. Amelioration of nephrotic syndrome and its complications, such as hyperlipidemia, edema, infection, and venous thrombosis.

2. Preservation of renal function.

3. Normalization of liver function and prevention of hepatic complications of HBV.

4. Permanent eradication of HBV.

In view of the immune complex nature of the disease, immunosuppressive therapy, similar to that applied in the idiopathic form of the disease, was once fashionable. Although it has previously been reported that corticosteroids achieve symptomatic relief in isolated cases, the contemporary view

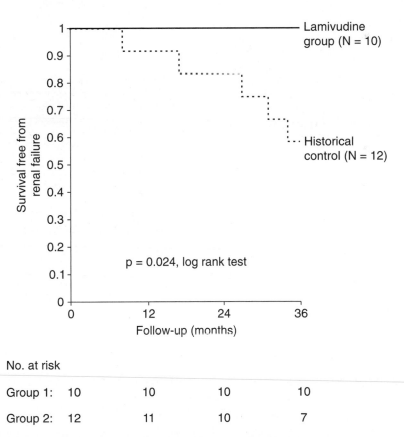

No. at risk				
Group 1:	10	10	10	10
Group 2:	12	11	10	7

▲ **Figure 35–9.** Renal survival in 10 patients who received lamivudine treatment for hepatitis B virus-associated membranous nephropathy (solid line) versus 12 matched patients from the prelamivudine era (dotted line).

is that steroids and cytotoxic agents may cause deleterious hepatic flares or even fatal decompensation by enhancing viral replication upon treatment withdrawal.

Another approach is treatment with an antiviral agent. Interferon-α is a naturally occurring cytokine produced by B-lymphocytes, null lymphocytes, and macrophages, and possesses antiviral, antiproliferative, and immunomodulatory effects. While reported to be useful in children, interferon-α has produced mixed results in adults with HBV-associated MN.

The introduction of the nucleoside analog lamivudine has revolutionized the treatment of chronic HBV infection. Lamivudine is the (−)-enantiomer of 3′-thiacytidine, and it inhibits DNA synthesis by terminating the nascent proviral DNA chain through interference with the reverse transcriptase activity of HBV. In children and adults with HBV-associated MN, lamivudine has been anecdotally reported to induce remission of nephrotic syndrome and suppress viral replication. In our analysis of 10 adult nephrotic patients with HBV-related MN who received lamivudine treatment versus 12 matched historic control subjects who presented in the prelamivudine era, lamivudine treatment significantly improved proteinuria, ALT levels, and renal outcome over a 3-year period (Figure 35–9). Randomized studies in a larger cohort of patients are needed. A potential limitation of prolonged treatment with lamivudine is the emergence of drug-resistant strains due to the induction and selection of HBV variants with mutations at the YMDD motif of DNA polymerase. One agent that might be considered in case of lamivudine resistance is adefovir dipivoxil, an acyclic nucleotide analogue that is effective against both lamivudine-resistant HBV mutants as well as wild-type HBV. However, this agent is potentially nephrotoxic and there are no clinical data on its efficacy in HBV-related MN that does not respond to lamivudine treatment. There are data to suggest that the recommended dose of 10 mg adefovir dipivoxil is associated with a lower risk of nephrotoxicity.

In the absence of an ideal agent for treatment of HBV-associated glomerulopathy, active immunization remains the most effective measure of immunoprophylaxis. Vaccination for all newborns in some endemic areas such as Hong Kong has dramatically reduced the incidence of chronic HBV infection and its associated complications in children and adolescents. In Taiwan, the introduction of active immunization to all newborns since 1984 has led to a dramatic (10-fold) decline in the incidence of neonatal HBV infection and its subsequent sequelae. In the United States, universal vaccination of infants began in 1991, and a 67% reduction in HBV infection was recorded 10 years later. In 2003, the World Health Organization recommended that all countries provide universal HBV immunization programs for infants and adolescents.

Janssen HL et al: Polyarteritis nodosa associated with hepatitis virus infection. The role of antiviral treatment and mutations in the hepatitis B virus genome. Eur J Gastroenterol Hepatol 2004;16(8):801.

Locarnini S: Molecular virology of hepatitis B virus. Semin Liver Dis 2004;24(Suppl 1):3.

Poland GA, Jacobson RM: Clinical practice: prevention of hepatitis B with the hepatitis B vaccine. N Engl J Med 2004;351:2832.

Yuen MF, Lai CL: Adefovir dipivoxil in chronic hepatitis B infection. Expert Opin Pharmacother 2004;5:2361.

Acute Tubulointerstitial Nephritis

36

Edgar V. Lerma, MD

ESSENTIALS OF DIAGNOSIS

► Acute onset of renal failure.

► Fever, skin rash, and peripheral eosinophilia in a minority of cases.

► Mild proteinuria, hematuria, and sterile pyuria; eosinophiluria detected by Hansel's or Wright's stain.

► Tubular dysfunction, manifested as glycosuria, aminoaciduria, potassium wasting, magnesium wasting.

TUBULOINTERSTITIAL DISEASES

► General Considerations

Disease processes involving the part of the renal parenchyma that consists of the tubules and interstitium are primarily referred to as tubulointerstitial diseases. Tubulointerstitial diseases can be classified as acute or chronic and can present either as primary or secondary (to a systemic disease) processes. Histopathologically, the presentation can vary from a subtle accumulation of lymphocytes, monocytes, or macrophages in the interstitium or tubular atrophy or dilation to extensive interstitial fibrosis, which may be accompanied by glomerulosclerosis.

There are several ways in which injury to the tubulointerstitium can occur, and these can involve either immune-mediated or non-immune-mediated (direct toxicity) mechanisms.

Although not commonly performed, a renal biopsy still provides the most definitive means of diagnosis. From a practical standpoint, however, the diagnosis is usually based upon a combination of epidemiologic, clinical, and laboratory findings.

As an example, a simple urinalysis provides a gamut of information on tubulointerstitial diseases. Examination of the urinary sediment for red blood cells (RBCs),

white blood cells (WBCs), and casts is particularly valuable. Dipstick analysis for protein is frequently positive, and when quantified, it is usually <2 g/day. Depending on which part of the tubules is injured, it is possible to observe glucosuria or aminoaciduria (proximal tubules), potassium or magnesium wasting (distal tubules), and salt wasting, as well as urinary concentrating defects or isosthenuria (medullary loop of Henle), manifested by polyuria. Normal anion gap metabolic acidosis is commonly observed, as in the various types of renal tubular acidoses.

Glomerular diseases are a distinct and separate pathologic entity, characterized by heavy or nephrotic-range proteinuria >3.5 g/day, RBC casts on urinalysis, as well as hypoalbuminemia. It is not uncommon, however, for both glomerular and tubulointerstitial disease to occur in a single patient.

Patients are often hypertensive at the time of presentation.

Acute tubulointerstitial nephritis (ATIN) usually presents as an acute rise in blood urea nitrogen (BUN) and creatinine values. The majority of affected patients typically present with nonspecific symptoms. The classic triad of fever, skin rash, and peripheral eosinophilia is seen in a minority of patients. Mild to moderate proteinuria, hematuria, and sterile pyuria are seen in the majority of cases. The occurrence of nephrotic-range proteinuria usually suggests concomitant glomerular disease. It must be noted that eosinophiluria is not specific for ATIN, as has also been demonstrated in other disease processes such as rapidly progressive glomerulonephritis and acute prostatitis as well as atheroembolic renal disease.

Under the microscope, the eosinophilic granules are more clearly demonstrated when Hansel's stain is used, although, in some cases, Wright's stain would suffice. Renal tubular acidosis features, such as glucosuria, aminoaciduria, as well as phosphaturia, indicate tubular injury.

Although the diagnosis of ATIN is usually suspected based on clinical grounds, the definitive diagnosis is established primarily by histopathologic features.

▶ Pathogenesis

The causes of ATIN are conveniently classified into three general categories: Drug-induced ATIN, infection-associated ATIN, and systemic disorders, with immune-mediated mechanisms.

The patient's history is crucial in determining the exact cause of ATIN because the majority of cases have been causally related to medication use, with approximately one-third of such cases being secondary to antibiotic usage.

There are four different mechanisms by which a drug can induce ATIN (Figure 36–1).

A. Antibiotic-Induced Acute Tubulointerstitial Nephritis

The prototype agent for antibiotic-induced ATIN is methicillin. Because of this it is rarely if ever used in clinical practice today. In fact, it is no longer available in the United States. The list of medications causing ATIN continues to grow (Table 36–1).

All β-lactam antibiotics (penicillins and cephalosporins) have been associated with ATIN. It can occur from as much as 10–20 days after the first exposure to the culprit drug to as little as 2–3 days after reexposure to a drug to which an individual has previously been sensitized. Frequently, ATIN presents as an acute oliguric renal failure.

ATIN has also been noted to occur secondary to drugs that are taken discontinuously, with the classic example being interrupted therapy with rifampin for tuberculosis. Interestingly, case reports of rifampin-induced ATIN have demonstrated the occurrence of circulating antirifampin antibodies and immunoglobulin G (IgG) deposits along the tubular basement membrane as well as casts containing immunoglobulin light chains in tubular lumens similar to that seen in patients with myeloma.

Recently, even the use of proton pump inhibitors has been associated with ATIN.

Note, however, that the development of drug-induced ATIN is not dose dependent.

B. Nonsteroidal Anti-inflammatory Drug-Induced Acute Tubulointerstitial Nephritis

Nonsteroidal anti-inflammatory drugs (NSAIDs) produce ATIN with several unique features. It usually occurs after several weeks to months of exposure to the culprit NSAID. In contrast to other causes of ATIN that typically present with

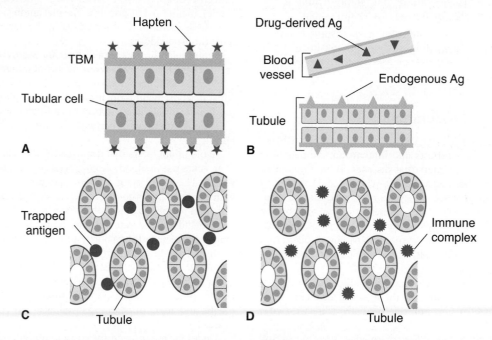

▲ **Figure 36–1.** Mechanisms whereby a drug (or one of its metabolites) can induce acute interstitial nephritis (AIN). **A:** The drug can bind to a normal component of the tubular basement membrane (TBM) and act as a hapten. **B:** The drug can mimic an antigen normally present within the TBM or the interstitium and induce an immune response that will also be directed against this antigen. **C:** The drug can bind to the TBM or deposit within the interstitium and act as a planted ("trapped") antigen. **D:** The drug can elicit the production of antibodies and become deposited in the interstitium as circulating immune complexes. (Adapted with permission from Rossert J: Kidney International 2001;60:804.)

Table 36–1. Drugs causing acute tubulointerstitial nephritis (ATIN).

Antimicrobial agents	Ketoprofen
Acyclovir	Mefenamic acid
Ampicillin[1,2]	Meloxicam
Amoxicillin	Mesalazine (5-ASA)
Aztreonam	*Naproxen*
Carbenicillin	*Phenylbutazone*
Cefaclor	*Piroxicam*
Cefamandole	Sulfasalazine
Cefazolin	Sulindac
Cephalexin	*Tolmetin*
Cephalothin	**Anticonvulsants**
Cefoxitin	Carbamazepine
Cefotaxime	Diazepam
Cidofovir	Phenobarbital
Ciprofloxacin	*Phenytoin*[2]
Cloxacillin	Valproate sodium
Colistin	**Diuretics**
Cotrimoxazole[2]	Chlorthalidone
Erythromycin	Ethacrynic acid
Ethambutol	*Furosemide*[2]
Foscarnet	Hydrochlorothiazide[2]
Gentamicin	Indapamide
Indinavir	Triamterene[2]
Interferon	**Others**
Isoniazid	
Lincomycin	*Allopurinol*[2]
Methicillin[2]	α-Methyldopa
Mezlocillin	Azathioprine
Minocycline	Bethanidineb
Nafcillin	Bismuth salts
Nitrofurantoin[2]	Captopril[2]
Norfloxacin	Chlorpropamide[2]
Oxacillin[2]	Cyclosporine
Penicillin G[2]	*Cimetidine*
Piperacillin	Clofibrate
Polymyxin acid[2]	Clozapine
Quinine	D-Penicillamine
Rifampicin[2]	Fenofibrate[2]
Sulfonamides	Gold salts
Teicoplanin	Griseofulvin
Tetracycline	Interferon
Vancomycin	Interleukin-2
NSAIDs including salicylates	*Omeprazole*
Alclofenac	*Phenindione*[2]
Azapropazone	Phenothiazine
Aspirin	Phenylpropanolamine
Diclofenac	Probenecid
Diflunisal[2]	Propranolol
Fenclofenac	Propylthiouracil
Fenoprofen	Ranitidine
Ibuprofen	Streptokinase
Indomethacin	Sulfinpyrazone
	Warfarin

[1]Drugs most commonly involved are shown in *italic* letters.
[2]Drugs that can induce granulomatous acute interstitial nephritis.

mild proteinuria, NSAID-induced ATIN is characterized by the occurrence of nephrotic syndrome (hypoalbuminemia, edema, and nephrotic-range proteinuria). Typically, affected patients tend to be elderly, perhaps because of an increased incidence of painful arthritic conditions. In patients subjected to renal biopsy, features of minimal change disease have been reported, especially in those with concomitant nephrotic-range proteinuria.

It must be emphasized, however, that in the workup of acute renal failure, NSAIDs can cause not only ATIN, but also hemodynamic perturbations of renal perfusion related to its vasoconstrictive properties, especially in the setting of volume depletion.

NSAID-induced ATIN is more likely to cause permanent renal injury as compared to other drugs causing ATIN.

C. Infection-Induced Acute Tubulointerstitial Nephritis

Infectious disease processes primarily involving the kidneys, such as acute pyelonephritis, have also been associated with ATIN. This topic is discussed in more detail in Chapters 37 and 38.

D. Other Causes of Acute Tubulointerstitial Nephritis

Recently, proton pump inhibitors have been implicated in the causation of ATIN. The timing from initiation of proton pump inhibitors to presentation with renal involvement varies, with an average of 9–10 weeks. Reexposure after discontinuation of the drug results in a faster onset of kidney damage. Renal biopsy typically shows the presence of an interstitial infiltrate with or without tubulitis. The presence of eosinophils in the tubulointerstitium is seen in the majority of cases. Glomeruli are typically spared (Figure 36–2).

Early recognition and prompt withdrawal of the offending proton pump inhibitor are crucial in portending a good prognosis. The majority of affected patients have partial or complete renal recovery.

▶ Clinical Findings

A. Symptoms and Signs

The main histopathologic feature of ATIN is diffuse or patchy infiltration of inflammatory cells within the renal interstitial space, accompanied by edema, with particular sparing of the glomeruli and blood vessels; this is accompanied by pathologic changes in the renal tubules. The interstitial infiltrate can be T lymphocytes and monocytes, eosinophils, plasma cells, or neutrophils. The particularly type of inflammatory cell involved depends on the particular culprit causing the reaction. This cellular infiltrate is eventually replaced by interstitial fibrosis (Figure 36–3).

In general, there is a poor correlation between clinical and laboratory findings and the underlying histopathology.

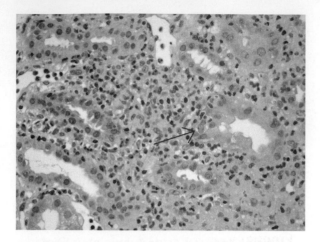

▲ **Figure 36–2.** Acute tubulointerstitial nephritis in a 39-year-old male with a history of intake of omeprazole who presented with acute renal failure and a serum creatinine of 5.9 mg/dL. There is interstitial edema, an inflammatory infiltrate composed of lymphocytes, macrophages, and numerous eosinophils. Tubulitis is also evident (arrow). Hematoxylin and eosin (×400). (Courtesy of Dr. Shane Meehan, Department of Pathology, University of Chicago.)

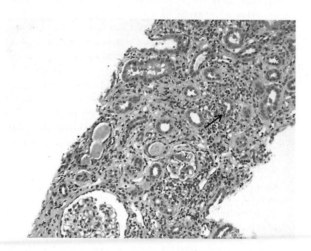

▲ **Figure 36–3.** Acute and chronic tubulointerstitial nephritis in a 14-year-old female with a serum creatinine of 2.0 mg/dL and a history of exposure to amoxicillin. The interstitium has mononuclear inflammatory cell infiltrates and increased pink matrix material indicative of collagen deposition. The tubules are shrunken and focal tubulitis is evident (arrow). Hematoxylin and eosin (×200). (Courtesy of Dr. Shane Meehan, Department of Pathology, University of Chicago.)

In NSAID-induced ATIN the typical glomerular lesion is that of minimal change disease with normal findings on light microscopy and a demonstration of foot process effacement on electron microscopy. Membranous nephropathy has also been associated with NSAID use in some published reports.

Histopathologic findings considered markers of poor prognosis include interstitial granulomas, interstitial fibrosis, and tubular atrophy.

Patients with ATIN usually present with generalized nonspecific symptoms consistent with acute renal failure, such as oliguria, generalized malaise, nausea and vomiting, or decreased appetite. Typically, the diagnosis is initially suspected in a patient presenting with asymptomatic or symptomatic elevation of BUN and serum creatinine (azotemia) values in the setting of recent infection or usage of medications, in particular antibiotics.

Those with drug-induced ATIN can present with an allergic type reaction that consists of the triad of erythematous rash, fever, and peripheral eosinophilia. Recent studies, however, have demonstrated the occurrence of such a triad of symptoms in only a minority of cases.

B. Laboratory Findings

Aside from the usual elevation in BUN and serum creatinine, urinalysis shows a predominance of WBCs, some RBCs, and WBC casts. The presence of RBC casts point to underlying glomerular disease, which may be primary or may occur concomitantly.

Eosinophiluria is usually shown with a Hansel's stain, which demonstrates the eosinophilic granules more clearly, in contrast to that of a simple Wright's stain. Defined as the presence of >−1% eosinophils (out of WBCs) in the urine, it is no longer considered specific for ATIN as it has been described in cases of acute cystitis or prostatitis, acute pyelonephritis, as well as postinfectious or rapidly progressive glomerulonephritis, and even renal atheroembolic disease. It has also been seen during transplant rejection. In a recent review of four large series, the estimated sensitivity of eosinophiluria was 67% with a specificity of 83%. Current data suggest that the presence or absence of eosinophiluria neither confirms nor excludes the diagnosis of ATIN, respectively.

Mild proteinuria, usually <1 g/day, is a common occurrence in ATIN. Nephrotic-range proteinuria, >3 g/day, has been described in those using NSAIDs for a chronic period of time or those with biopsy-proven minimal change disease.

C. Special Tests

Renal ultrasound shows nonspecific findings, such as normal to slightly enlarged kidney sizes, with a mild degree of increased echogenicity in ATIN. There are, however, no specific sonographic features that would reliably distinguish ATIN from other causes of acute renal failure.

Gallium scanning plays an important role in distinguishing ATIN from acute tubular necrosis (ATN). A positive result is usually indicated by showing diffuse, intense uptake bilaterally, consistent with the interstitial inflammatory infiltrate. In one small series, patients with ATIN were shown to have positive gallium scans; this is in contrast to those with ATN who have negative gallium scans. Such utility is limited, however, by its lack of specificity and increased occurrence of false-positive results, especially in those with iron overload or advanced liver disease. Gallium has some structural similarity to the ferric iron and can bind to transferrin and ferritin.

▶ Differential Diagnosis

Although the history and clinical features are truly suggestive of ATIN, the definitive diagnosis can be arrived at only by performing a renal biopsy and demonstrating the histopathologic features discussed above.

In most cases, however, when ATIN is highly suspected, the offending agent is immediately removed or discontinued. If renal function subsequently shows an improving trend in the following days to a week, then no further evaluation or therapy is rendered. A renal biopsy is definitely indicated if there is no evidence of recovery or resolution after discontinuation of the offending agent, if the patient has rapidly progressed to overt renal failure, or if there is significant uncertainty concerning the actual diagnosis.

For those patients highly suspected of having ATIN who may have a contraindication for renal biopsy, a trial of steroids, eg, prednisone 1 mg/kg/day, may be considered. Those who respond to this form of treatment usually improve within 1–2 weeks of initiation of steroid therapy and return to baseline renal function (Figure 36–4).

▶ Treatment

The mainstay of treatment in ATIN is primarily supportive therapy. Once a presumptive diagnosis of ATIN is made, the first step in management is immediate discontinuation of the offending agent or treatment of the underlying infection. The diagnosis should be made promptly as ATIN is usually easily reversible in the earlier stages. However, it may take several days to weeks to see an improvement in renal function (based on serum creatinine) and for it to return to baseline levels.

Pharmacologic therapy should be considered considered in those patients in whom drug discontinuation does not result in any evidence of improvement in renal function, such as declining serum creatinine.

In 40% of cases there is a persistent elevation in serum creatinine despite earlier removal of the culprit agent. In those patients who do not show any significant improvement in renal function within 10–15 days after the withdrawal of the suspected agent, the accepted treatment is pulse methylprednisolone followed by oral prednisone, tapered over 4–8 weeks, although this has not always been effective. At present, there is no definitive evidence that corticosteroid therapy offers any benefit to those with NSAID-induced ATIN. One study, however, suggested that a course of prednisone be tried in

those with renal failure that is still persistent 1–2 weeks after the discontinuation of the culprit NSAID.

Recently, Gonzalez, et al reported that "early" initiation of steroid treatment improved the recovery of renal function in patients with drug-induced acute interstitial nephritis. An earlier onset of use of corticosteroids after discontinuing the offending drug (13 versus 34 days) was associated with a better recovery of renal function. In their study, the etiology of the drug-induced ATIN (antibiotic versus NSAID) did not appear to influence the eventual outcome.

Recently, mycophenolate mofetil has been used in the treatment of those patients with ATIN who have been steroid resistant or intolerant. This would include patients with obesity, diabetes, or other conditions that make steroids not an ideal agent.

▶ Prognosis

The majority of patients with ATIN will have either partial or complete recovery of renal function depending on the underlying cause. If recovery of renal function is not achieved after 3 weeks, it is unlikely that there will be any recovery. This is considered to be another negative prognosticator.

NEPHROPATHIA EPIDEMICA

Nephropathia epidemica is characterized by an acute onset of fever accompanied by abdominal or loin pain, myalgias and arthralgia, and acute myopia with conjunctival injection. Urinalysis reveals proteinuria, microscopic hematuria, and leukocyturia. Transient nonselective glomerular-type proteinuria has been described, implicating a transient lesion involving the glomerular filtration barrier. Such an increase in glomerular permeability may be attributed to an immunologic response to the viral infection. Antibodies against hantavirus have been demonstrated in affected patients.

Histopathologically, findings consistent with ATIN are seen; some reports have also described concurrent slight glomerular mesangial changes.

Thrombocytopenia is also common. The etiologic agent is believed to be the Puumala hantavirus of the Bunyavirus family that is carried by rodents.

Although spontaneous renal recovery is the rule, some reports suggest that a previous infection with hantavirus may be a risk factor for the development of hypertension.

IDIOPATHIC ACUTE INTERSTITIAL NEPHRITIS

There is a subset of patients whose renal biopsies clearly show evidence of AIN, but no medication or infection could be identified as the culprit. These patients are labeled as having idiopathic AIN. Although the pathogenesis remains unclear, some cases may demonstrate evidence of an immune-mediated mechanism, ie, circulating antibodies against the tubular basement membrane or linear immunofluorescence along the tubular basement membrane.

Similarly, these patients clinically present with acute renal failure or tubular function abnormalities.

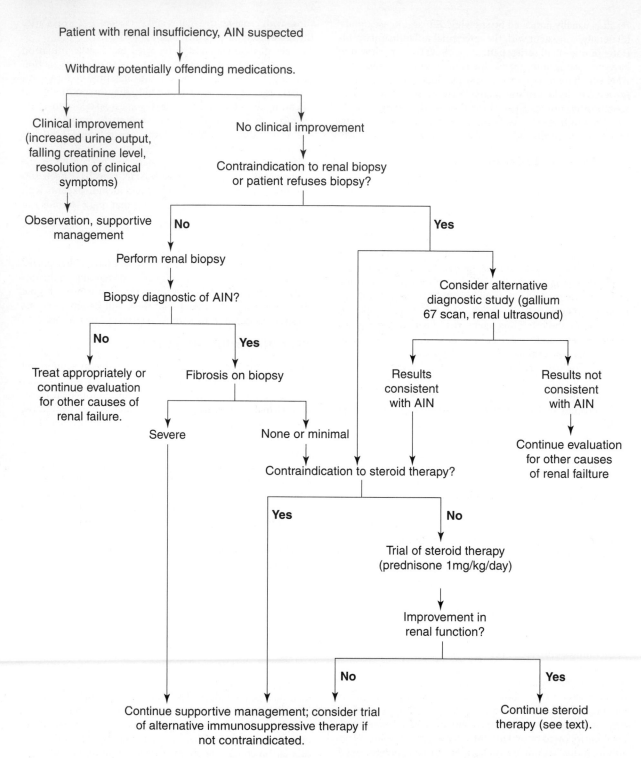

▲ **Figure 36–4.** Algorithm for the diagnosis and treatment of acute tubulointerstitial nephritis. AIN, acute interstitial nephritis.

Appel GB, Bhat P: Nephrology VIII. Tubulointerstitial diseases. In: *ACP Medicine*. Dale DC (editor). WebMD, Inc., 2006.

Baker RJ, Pusey CD: The changing profile of acute tubulointerstitial nephritis. Nephrol Dial Transplant 2004;19:8.

Brewster UC, Perazella MA: Acute kidney injury following proton pump inhibitor therapy. Kidney Int 2007;71:589.

Clarkson MR et al: Acute interstitial nephritis: clinical features and response to corticosteroid therapy. Nephrol Dial Transplant 2004;19:2778.

González E et al: Early steroid treatment improves the recovery of renal function in patients with drug-induced acute interstitial nephritis. Kidney Int 2008;73:940–946.

Kodner CM, Kudrimoti A: Diagnosis and management of acute interstitial nephritis. Am Fam Phys 2003;67(12):2527–2534.

Kshirsagar AV: The significance of urine eosinophils. In: *UpToDate 15.3*. Rose BD (editor). UpToDate 2008, Waltham, MA.

Kshirsagar AV, Falk RJ: Treatment of acute interstitial nephritis. In: *UpToDate 15.3*. Rose BD (editor). UpToDate 2008, Waltham, MA.

Miettinen MH et al: Ten-year prognosis of Puumala hantavirus-induced acute interstitial nephritis. Kidney Int 2006;69(11):2043.

Preddie DC et al: Mycophenolate mofetil for the treatment of interstitial nephritis. Clin J Am Soc Nephrol 2006;1:718.

Rose B: NSAIDs: acute renal failure and nephritic syndrome. In: *UpToDate 15.3*. Rose BD (editor). UpToDate 2008, Waltham, MA.

Rose BD, Appel GB: Clinical manifestations and diagnosis of acute interstitial nephritis. In: *UpToDate 15.3*. Rose BD (editor). UpToDate 2008, Waltham, MA.

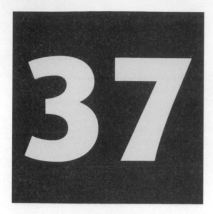

Chronic Tubulointerstitial Nephritis

Edgar V. Lerma, MD

Chronic interstitial nephritis (CIN) is by definition tubulointerstitial nephritis that has failed to resolve on its own or has been resistant to whatever treatment was rendered after several months or years. However, it can also arise *de novo* as a consequence of chronic, low-grade, or injurious exposures of the tubulointerstitium to the culprit agent, ie, medication, physical factor, infectious agents, etc. Such exposures may be intermittent or persistent. Histopathologically, it is characterized by the presence of interstitial chronic inflammation, interstitial fibrosis, and tubular atrophy (Figure 37–1).

Depending on the culprit agent, the disease may have a particular predilection for either the proximal tubules, the distal tubules, or both. The functional abnormalities usually depend on the tubular site of involvement, ie, distal tubule dysfunction may be characterized by acidosis and hyperkalemia, as seen in obstructive uropathies, whereas injury involving the renal medulla is characterized by an impaired ability to concentrate urine as seen in sickle cell nephropathy (Table 37–1).

As CIN progresses, there may be concomitant glomerular abnormalities, probably secondary to maladaptive alterations in the glomeruli or a result of the tubulointerstitial processes. At that time, patients may present with nephrotic-range proteinuria, which can cloud the primary underlying disease process.

The various causes of CIN can be classified into several categories (Table 37–2).

PRIMARY OR IDIOPATHIC

EPSTEIN–BARR VIRUS

The localization of Epstein–Barr virus (EBV) DNA in the proximal tubule cells in patients with CIN of unknown etiology has suggested a causative role for the Epstein–Barr virus. However, further studies need to be done to demonstrate if a true cause and effect of EBV renal scarring actually exists.

BK VIRUS NEPHROPATHY

In immunosuppressed individuals, such as transplant recipients, BK polyoma virus infection has been shown to cause interstitial nephritis. The virus has been demonstrated in the transitional cells in the urine (so-called 'decoy cells') via urine microscopy, but correlation with renal allograft function status and histologic evidence of renal involvement is very poor. Accurate diagnosis of BK polyomavirus infection requires a very high index of suspicion. Electron microscopy is very sensitive in depicting the presence of BK virions, but the finding of viral particles is not by itself diagnostic. An increase in CD20 and a decrease in cytotoxic T cells in allografts is characteristic of polyoma virus infection.

Clinically, it is difficult to distinguish interstitial nephritis versus acute cellular rejection.

Management of patients with polyoma virus nephropathy is difficult since there is no specific antiviral therapy available at this time. Aside from reducing immunosuppressive therapy, other novel treatments include IVIg and Cidofovir. The latter is also nephrotoxic, and has been described to cause acute interstitial nephritis.

SECONDARY

INFECTIONS

ACUTE PYELONEPHRITIS

Acute pyelonephritis (discussed in more detail in Chapter 38) is classified under the category of complicated urinary tract infections. Patients clinically present with a combination of symptoms that includes fever and chills, dysuria, urgency, and increased frequency. They commonly complain of flank discomfort with a physical correlate of costovertebral angle tenderness. Urine microscopy usually reveals an active urinary sediment consisting of leukocytes and leukocyte casts, and even red blood cells (RBCs) on occasion.

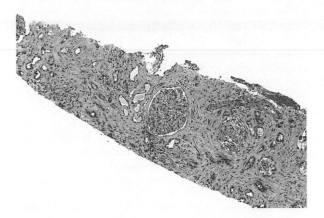

▲ **Figure 37–1.** Chronic tubulointerstitial nephritis with interstitial fibrosis, fibroblasts, and scattered mononuclear inflammatory cells. There is extensive tubular atrophy and loss. Glomeruli are spared. Hematoxylin and eosin (×200). (Courtesy of Dr. Shane Meehan, Department of Pathology, University of Chicago.)

Histopathologically, there is infiltration of polymorphonuclear cells and lymphocytes and edema grossly distorting the normal tubulointerstitial architecture.

The majority of cases respond to appropriate antibiotic therapy targeting the causative organism, which is most commonly a gram-negative *Escherichia coli*. In those who do not respond to antimicrobial therapy readily, or who develop recurrent infections, there may be renal scarring and possible progression to chronic pyelonephritis.

CHRONIC PYELONEPHRITIS

Chronic bacterial infections of the urinary tract are among the most common causes of chronic tubulointerstitial nephritis (CTIN). The majority of these cases are associated with vesicoureteral reflux (VUR), hence the term "reflux nephropathy" (discussed in more detail in Chapter 39). However, for those not associated with VUR, the disease is termed "chronic pyelonephritis."

Clinically, patients with chronic pyelonephritis present with fever and chills, dysuria, vague flank or back pain, as well as hypertension. Some patients may present with tubular abnormalities such as impaired urinary concentrating ability, hyperkalemia, and salt wasting, all of which reflect distal tubular dysfunction. Chronic or repeated urinary tract infections are predisposing risk factors.

Examination of the urine often reveals an active urinary sediment consisting of leukocytes and leukocyte casts. Grossly, the kidneys appear contracted.

Histopathologically, the findings are similar to other forms of CTIN, with tubular atrophy and interstitial fibrosis.

Table 37–1. Clinical features of chronic tubulointerstitial nephritis.

Electrolyte and acid–base disorders

Proximal RTA or Fanconi syndrome
  Myeloma
  Dent disease
  Cystinosis
  Sjögren's syndrome

Distal RTA
  Bacterial pyelonephritis
  Reflux nephropathy
  Lithium
  Lead
  Myeloma
  Light chain disease
  Lupus nephritis
  Hypercalcemia

Hyperkalemia (Type 4) RTA
  Reflux nephropathy
  Lead
  Lupus nephritis
  Sickle cell nephropathy

Sodium wasting

Clinical syndromes

Kidney stones
  Hypercalcemia
  Hyperoxaluria
  Uric acid nephropathy
  Dent disease
  Sarcoidosis

Nephrogenic diabetes insipidus
  Lithium
  Cisplatin
  Hypokalemia
  Hypercalcemia
  Dent disease

ARF
  Pyelonephritis
  Analgesic nephropathy
  Lithium
  Calcineurin inhibitors
  Cisplatin
  Myeloma
  Lymphoma
  Lupus nephritis
  Hypercalcemia
  Uric acid nephropathy
  Radiation nephritis

Papillary necrosis
  Acute pyelonephritis
  Analgesic nephropathy
  Sickle cell nephropathy

RTA, Renal tubular acidosis; ART, acute renal failure.

Table 37–2. Causes of chronic tubulointerstitial nephritis.[1]

Primary or idiopathic
Epstein–Barr virus

Secondary
Infections
Polyoma virus
Pyelonephritis (acute and chronic)
Drugs
Analgesic abuse nephropathy
Lithium-induced renal disease
Acyclic nucleoside inhibitors (Chapters 14 and 35)
Calcineurin inhibitors
Aristolochic acid/Chinese herb nephropathy
Chemotherapeutic agents: Cisplatin, ifosfamide, carmustine
Heavy metals
Lead nephropathy
Cadmium
Hematologic diseases (Chapter 33)
Multiple myeloma
Lymphoproliferative disorders
Light chain disease
Sickle cell nephropathy (Chapter 49)
Obstructive uropathy (Chapter 16)
Reflux nephropathy (Chapter 39)
Immune-mediated diseases
Sarcoidosis
Primary Sjögren's syndrome
Tubulointerstitial nephritis with uveitis (TINU)
Idiopathic hypocomplementemic
Interstitial nephritis
Metabolic disorders
Hyperoxaluria
Hyperuricemia/hyperuricosuria
Hypercalcemia/hypercalciuria (Chapters 6 and 40)
Hypokalemic nephropathy
Genetic disorders
Cystinosis (Chapter 40)
Dent disease
Miscellaneous
Endemic (Balkan) nephropathy
Radiation nephritis

[1]For those conditions not discussed in detail in this chapter, refer to the corresponding chapter(s) given in parentheses.

Lymphocytes and mononuclear cells predominate in the chronic inflammatory infiltrative population.

XANTHOGRANULOMATOUS PYELONEPHRITIS

Persistent chronic pyelonephritis can progress to a localized infection called "xanthogranulomatous pyelonephritis." Its exact pathogenesis is unknown. Typically, there is an underlying urinary tract obstruction, eg, nephrolithiasis, which is complicated by the infection, leading to ischemia and de-struction of renal parenchymal tissue, with granuloma formation subsequent to the accumulation of lipid deposits. These lipid deposits are actually lipid-laden macrophages, called "foam cells."

The symptoms are similar to those of chronic pyelonephritis, including hypertension. Characteristically, a distinct mass may be palpable over the affected "nonfunctioning" kidney. Urine cultures are usually positive for *E coli* and other gram-negative bacilli or *Staphylococcus aureus*.

Computed tomography (CT), the imaging modality of choice, demonstrates that the kidney is significantly enlarged. Other findings include the predisposing renal calculus as well as low-density masses or xanthomatous tissues. Neoplastic renal disease must be excluded among the differentials.

On intravenous pyelography (IVP) the involved kidney may contain a localized "abscess-looking" area that may look like a complex cyst or tumor. This is usually distinguished by either magnetic resonance imaging (MRI) or CT.

Current treatment recommendations consist of appropriate coverage with broad-spectrum intravenous antibiotics combined with total or partial nephrectomy.

MEDICATION-RELATED CHRONIC INTERSTITIAL NEPHRITIS

ANALGESIC ABUSE NEPHROPATHY

 ESSENTIALS OF DIAGNOSIS

▶ The most common cause of CIN.

▶ Long-term ingestion of phenacetin, acetaminophen, aspirin, and caffeine or combinations of such.

▶ Most common in women in their 60s or 70s with a history of chronic low back pain, chronic or recurrent headaches, and chronic joint pains.

▶ Hypertension is common.

▶ Imaging studies: Papillary necrosis on IVP, papillary calcifications and bumpy renal contours on CT scan, and small echogenic appearing kidneys on ultrasonography.

▶ General Considerations

Analgesic abuse nephropathy (AAN) is the most common cause of CTIN. There has been a positive correlation between the incidence of renal disease secondary to analgesic nephropathy and the daily consumption of analgesics, in particular phenacetin and other analgesic mixtures.

In the past, it was believed that only phenacetin-containing analgesics were responsible for the disease, but it has been reported on numerous occasions that all analgesics, including acetaminophen, and aspirin can actually cause the same disease process.

Nonsteroidal anti-inflammatory drugs (NSAIDs) are another common cause of CIN. This is discussed in detail in Chapter 15.

Pathogenesis

The main site of renal injury in analgesic nephropathy is the renal medulla (area of the medullary loops of Henle, the vasa recta, and collecting ducts), primarily because of its inherent low oxygen tension. This is also the region in which toxic metabolites of various analgesic compounds build up as a result of the countercurrent mechanism. As the vasoconstrictive effects on the renal medulla predominate, ischemic injury continues, leading to cortical atrophy and eventual interstitial changes.

Clinical Findings

AAN is most commonly seen in females in their 60s or 70s who have chronic pain syndromes, eg, headaches, joint pains or back pains. Ingestion of 1 g of analgesic preparations daily for more than 2 years is considered the minimum dosage and time required to produce clinical analgesic nephropathy. Peptic ulcer disease and gastrointestinal symptoms are a common occurrence.

Renal dysfunction is manifested by isosthenuria (impaired urinary concentration) as well as impaired sodium conservation that may predispose to intravascular volume depletion. Renal tubular acidification defects are also seen. Urinalysis may show evidence of sterile pyuria, urinary tract infection, microscopic or macroscopic hematuria, and mild proteinuria.

Occasionally, patients can present with flank pain or gross hematuria associated with papillary necrosis. Such papillae can slough off and cause obstructive manifestations. These are usually demonstrated on IVP or ultrasonography. Papillary calcification and characteristic "bumpy" renal contours are usually demonstrated on CT. In some instances, the kidneys can appear bilaterally atrophic or asymmetric in size.

Patients with analgesic nephropathy are also at increased risk for transitional cell carcinoma of the uroepithelium.

The oxidative effects of phenacetin are believed to be responsible for the increased formation of atherogenic low-density lipoprotein (LDL), thereby predisposing patients to an increased risk of premature atherosclerosis with attendant cardiovascular morbidity and mortality.

Treatment

Management is primarily supportive, including discontinuation of the culprit analgesic agent. Even after cessation of the analgesic, close monitoring, especially for the development of new symptoms such as gross hematuria, is recommended due to increased risk of uroepithelial tumors.

LITHIUM-INDUCED RENAL DISEASE

ESSENTIALS OF DIAGNOSIS

▶ CIN is the most common pathologic finding in those with chronic lithium nephropathy.

▶ Polydipsia and polyuria are presenting symptoms of nephrogenic diabetes insipidus (NDI).

▶ Incomplete distal renal tubular acidosis (RTA) in up to 50% of patients.

▶ Pathology: Cystic dilation of the distal tubules leads to the formation of "microcysts."

▶ Increased incidence of uroepithelial tumors.

General Considerations

Lithium has been commonly used in patients treated for bipolar disorders. Chronic lithium ingestion is a known cause of NDI. Lithium enters the collecting tubule cells via the sodium channels; by inhibiting adenylate cyclase and subsequent cyclic AMP (cAMP) production it interferes with the ability of antidiuretic hormone (ADH) to increase water reabsorption. Likewise, it decreases the expression of the water channels (aquaporin 2) in the collecting tubules. A positive correlation has been described between the length of duration of treatment (average 6.5–10 years) with lithium and such impairment of urinary concentrating ability manifested by polyuria (and polydipsia). An incomplete distal (type 1) RTA, secondary to lithium-induced decreased H ATPase pump activity in the distal tubule, has been described.

Lithium has also been associated with hypercalcemia. It has been suggested that it induces morphologic changes in the parathyroid glands, resulting in increased parathyroid volume and parathyroid hormone secretion (hyperparathyroidism), which consequently promote bone resorption and subsequent release of calcium into the bloodstream, leading to hypercalcemia.

Clinical Findings

Pathologically, lithium-induced nephropathy is characterized by the formation of "microcysts" (cortical and medullary tubular cysts) in the distal convoluted tubules and collecting ducts (Figure 37–2). Such distal tubular involvement clinically correlates with NDI, manifested by polyuria and polydipsia.

Typically, renal dysfunction secondary to chronic lithium use is mild to moderate. However, patients with serum creatinine levels greater than 2.5 mg/dL at the time of presen-

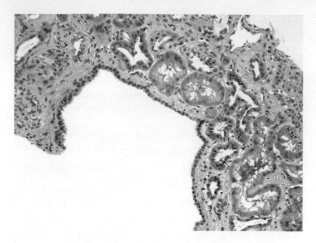

▲ **Figure 37–2.** Lithium nephrotoxicity with a collecting duct microcyst and interstitial fibrosis in a kidney biopsy from a 62-year-old male with chronic renal failure and a 15 year history of lithium intake. Hematoxylin and eosin (×200). (Courtesy of Dr. Shane Meehan, Department of Pathology, University of Chicago.)

tation progress to end-stage renal disease (ESRD) even after cessation of lithium. However, in patients with less severe renal dysfunction, such discontinuation of lithium usually leads to stabilization of kidney function.

Amiloride, a potassium-sparing diuretic, has been shown to reduce polyuria and to block lithium uptake in the sodium channels of the collecting duct. In contrast, although thiazide diuretics can reduce lithium-induced polyuria, they can also cause intravascular volume depletion, which can lead to increased sodium and lithium reabsorption in the proximal tubule, thereby aggravating acute lithium toxicity.

▶ **Treatment**

For those patients on chronic maintenance therapy with lithium, a regular follow-up of serum creatinine, estimated glomerular filtration rate (GFR), and 24-hour urine volume is recommended. Elevations in creatinine should lead to either appropriate dose reduction or complete withdrawal of the drug.

The average latent period between initiation of lithium therapy and onset of ESRD was 20 years.

CALCINEURIN INHIBITOR INDUCED

 ESSENTIALS OF DIAGNOSIS

▶ Commonly seen in recipients of solid organ (kidney, pancreas, heart) transplants, with histopathologic features similar to those seen in chronic rejection.

▶ Electrolyte abnormalities are common, in particular hyperkalemia and hypomagnesemia.

▶ Pathology: "Striped" pattern of patchy interstitial fibrosis and tubular atrophy.

▶ **General Considerations**

Cyclosporine and tacrolimus, which belong to a class of immunosuppressive agents primarily called calcineurin inhibitors, are commonly used in solid organ transplantation. Cyclosporine has also been commonly used in the treatment of various autoimmune diseases. These agents also cause acute and chronic renal failure. The pathogenesis can be attributed to the drugs' predominantly vasoconstrictive effect on the afferent arteriole, thereby causing glomerular ischemia.

▶ **Clinical Findings**

Pathologically, the tubulointerstitial damage occurs in a band-like pattern, referred to as "striped interstitial fibrosis," involving the cortex and medulla. Tubular injury secondary to calcineurin inhibitors can lead to hyperkalemia and a non-anion gap metabolic acidosis. Other electrolyte abnormalities include hypomagnesemia, hypophosphatemia, and hyperuricemia.

▶ **Treatment**

Treatment of renal dysfunction requires a significant reduction in the dose of the offending agent, which often translates to an improvement in GFR. Mycophenolate mofetil and rapamycin are alternative immunosuppressive agents commonly used in transplant recipients.

Interestingly, calcineurin inhibitor-induced nephropathy is rare in bone marrow transplant recipients due to the shorter duration and lower doses of the usual treatment regimens.

ARISTOLOCHIC ACID NEPHROPATHY OR CHINESE HERB NEPHROPATHY

 ESSENTIALS OF DIAGNOSIS

▶ Aristolochic acid nephropathy is commonly seen among users of Chinese herbal medications for weight reduction.

▶ Nephrotoxicity is usually attributed to "aristolochic acid."

▶ Pathology: Hypocellular interstitial fibrosis with marked tubular atrophy.

▶ Increased incidence of uroepithelial tumors.

General Considerations

Typical changes of CIN have been described in mostly middle-aged women in Belgium who were using Chinese herb pills as part of a weight losing diet regimen in 1992. The culprit active ingredient was discovered to be aristolochic acid, which was not only nephrotoxic, but carcinogenic as well.

Clinical Findings

Interestingly, affected patients have normal blood pressure readings. There is a positive correlation between the total dose of aristolochic acid and the decline in GFR.

Treatment

If untreated, patients usually rapidly progress to ESRD. Histopathologically, a hypocellular interstitial fibrosis with marked tubular atrophy is seen. A short course of oral steroids has been shown to slow progression of renal failure.

CHEMOTHERAPY INDUCED

Changes in CIN have been associated with chemotherapeutic agents, especially those with predominant renal routes of excretion. Cisplatin-induced CIN appears to be mediated by increased production of tumor necrosis factor (TNF)-α. Pentoxyphyllin (a known TNF-α inhibitor) has been shown to prevent such cisplatin-induced injury. Damage to the tubulointerstitial areas leads to salt wasting, which may be complicated by orthostatic hypotension, as well as hypomagnesemia and hypocalcemia. Other CIN lesion-producing chemotherapeutic agents include ifosfamide and carmustine. Findings of interstitial fibrosis and chronic inflammatory changes are quite common.

Treatment entails discontinuing the culprit agent and avoiding coadministration of other agents with potential nephrotoxicities.

ACUTE PHOSPHATE NEPHROPATHY

Acute phosphate nephropathy is a newly described entity commonly seen in patients after exposure to oral sodium phosphate solutions (OSPS) used as bowel cleansers in preparation for colonoscopy. This is characterized by low-grade proteinuria as well as hyperphosphatemia. Histopathologically, there is evidence of acute and chronic tubular injury with interstitial edema, accompanied by tubular atrophy and interstitial fibrosis. The distinctive feature of this entity is the presence of abundant calcium phosphate deposits in the distal tubules and collecting ducts. The following factors predispose patients to acute renal failure: Volume depletion, advanced age, hypertension, concurrent treatment with angiotensin-converting enzyme inhibitors (ACEIs) or angiotensin receptor blockers (ARBs), diuretics and NSAIDs, baseline creatinine elevation, or inappropriate use of OSPS in those with underlying chronic kidney disease (CKD).

Preventive measures include adequate hydration and possibly withholding ACEIs, ARBs, diuretics, and NSAIDs on the day prior to and on the day of colonoscopy. OSPS should be used cautiously in elderly individuals.

HEAVY METALS

CADMIUM

Years of prolonged environmental or occupational exposure to cadmium also leads to CIN and eventual progression to renal failure. Proximal tubular dysfunction, presenting as Fanconi syndrome, characterized by glucosuria, aminoaciduria, and tubular proteinuria, is common.

Increased urinary cadmium excretion is characteristic. At present, treatment for cadmium nephrotoxicity is primarily supportive.

LEAD

Similar to cadmium, the proximal tubule cells tend to be the site of accumulation for lead, thereby leading to a Fanconi type picture. CIN secondary to lead exposure for several years is characterized histopathologically by progressive tubular atrophy and widespread fibrosis, which clinically translate into a significant decline in GFR. There seems to be an inverse relationship between the serum lead measurement and renal function as estimated by GFR. Hypertension is also quite common.

Lead nephropathy also reduces urinary excretion of uric acid, thereby leading to hyperuricemia and gout. In contrast, acute exposure to high levels of lead is usually characterized by acute onset of abdominal discomfort and encephalopathic manifestations as well as anemia.

The diagnosis of lead nephropathy is established by increased urinary excretion of chelated lead, that is, after administration of ethylenediamine tetraacetic acid (EDTA). Cumulative body stores of lead are estimated by the EDTA mobilization test or by x-ray fluorescence, which determines bone lead content. In the EDTA mobilization test, 2 g of EDTA is administered either by the intravenous or intramuscular route, with subsequent measurement of 24-hour urine lead excretion. Urinary lead >0.6 g/day is considered abnormal. One major limitation of the EDTA mobilization test is that it cannot mobilize lead deposits in bone. Reduced levels of erythrocyte aminolevulinate dehydrase (ALAD) compared to levels of ALAD "restored" by the addition of dithiothreitol may be even more efficient in detecting increased body lead burden in patients with chronic renal failure.

Note that serum levels of lead, although elevated during acute exposure, are not very helpful in the chronically exposed. The explanation for this is that during acute exposure, lead is concentrated in the RBCs, which later die, hence extracting lead into the bones and other tissues. Renal biopsy shows nonspecific findings seen in CIN. The treatment of

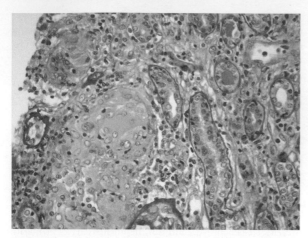

▲ **Figure 37–3.** Noncaseating granulomatous inflammation in a patient with sarcoidosis. Periodic acid–Schiff (×400). (Courtesy of Dr. Shane Meehan, Department of Pathology, University of Chicago.)

choice is EDTA chelation therapy or oral succimer, which has been shown to slow the progression of CKD.

IMMUNE MEDIATED

SARCOIDOSIS

Renal involvement in sarcoidosis can occur in a variety of ways. Most commonly, patients have hypercalcemia secondary to increased production of 1,25-dihydroxyvitamin D_3 by the activated macrophages in the characteristic granulomatous tissues. Such hypercalcemia can lead to other renal manifestations such as nephrogenic diabetes insipidus, hypercalciuria-related nephrolithiasis, and, in some cases, renal failure.

Sarcoidosis can also present as a form of interstitial nephritis with associated "noncaseating granulomas" (Figure 37–3).

Typical tubular manifestations include mild proteinuria, sterile pyuria, and impaired ability to concentrate urine.

Treatment is with corticosteroids 1 mg/kg/day, which has been reported to lead to improved renal function. More commonly, however, because the renal involvement is long standing, recovery is usually incomplete, even in those treated with steroids.

SJÖGREN'S SYNDROME

Sjögren's syndrome-associated CIN characteristically presents as type 1 RTA, with hypokalemia and a normal anion gap metabolic acidosis. Although the mechanism for this is incompletely understood, it is believed to be related to autoantibodies against carbonic anhydrase II. Treatment with high-dose corticosteroids has resulted in a dramatic improvement in renal function.

TUBULOINTERSTITIAL NEPHRITIS WITH UVEITIS SYNDROME

ESSENTIALS OF DIAGNOSIS

▶ Presents as acute renal failure.
▶ Commonly affects young adult females and adolescents.
▶ Accompanying "uveitis" develops in relation to underlying interstitial nephritis.
▶ Pathology: Predominance of CD4 and CD8 T lymphocytes in renal biopsy.

▶ General Considerations

Tubulointerstitial nephritis with uveitis (TINU) was first described in 1975. It is usually seen in adolescents and young adults, with a female preponderance and no particular racial predilection.

▶ Pathogenesis

The exact pathogenesis remains unclear, but the predominance of T lymphocytes in the tissues and possible association with *Chlamydia* and Epstein–Barr virus suggest that delayed type hypersensitivity and suppressed cell-mediated immunity may play major roles.

▶ Clinical Findings

Clinically, patients present with nonspecific signs and symptoms, ie, fever, generalized malaise, anemia, and asthenia. Typically, uveitis of the anterior chamber is seen bilaterally, presenting as redness and pain over the eyes. Occasionally, patients complain of accompanying blurring of vision and photophobia. Uveitis can occur as quickly as 2 months prior to, simultaneously with, or up to 14 months after the onset of interstitial nephritis, presenting as acute renal failure.

Renal manifestations include both proximal and distal tubular dysfunction, ie, tubular proteinuria. Increased urine β_2-microglobulin (a marker of tubulointerstitial disease) has been noted. Ultrasonography may reveal enlarged swollen kidneys.

▶ Differential Diagnosis

A definitive diagnosis is established by demonstrating typical findings of interstitial nephritis, ie, tubulointerstitial edema with infiltration of lymphocytes, plasma cells, and histiocytes. A predominance of CD4 and CD8 T lymphocytes, monocytes, and macrophages has been described. Eosinophils and noncaseating granulomas may also be seen.

The above findings combined with the temporal relation to the concomitant uveitis make the diagnosis likely.

Other common causes of tubulointerstitial disease process with uveitis include sarcoidosis and Sjögren's syndrome.

▶ Treatment

Renal disease frequently resolves spontaneously over the course of 12 months without steroid therapy. However, for those with moderately advanced chronic kidney disease, prednisone 1 mg/kg/day (usually 40–60 mg orally daily) can be given for 3–6 months depending on the response, and then tapered subsequently. Note that this steroid regimen is somewhat similar to that given for patients with persistent ATIN, except that the duration of therapy is slightly more prolonged because of more frequent relapses noted with TINU. While the renal manifestations may resolve spontaneously and respond well to a course of systemic steroids, the uveitis often has a chronic or relapsing course that may require more aggressive therapy. For uveitis, topical or systemic corticosteroids have been used.

▶ Prognosis

As in other chronic tubulointerstitial diseases, there is a positive correlation between prognosis and the degree of interstitial fibrosis.

IDIOPATHIC HYPOCOMPLEMENTEMIC INTERSTITIAL NEPHRITIS

This disease is usually seen in older men, and as the name implies, is characterized by decreased levels of C3 and C4 (hypocomplementemia) in the absence of evidence of systemic lupus erythematosus (SLE) or Sjögren's syndrome. Histopathology reveals extensive tubulointerstitial infiltration with lymphocytes as well as Ig and complement deposits; these suggest local immune complex formation as the pathogenetic mechanism. Treatment consists of glucocorticoids and cyclophosphamide.

METABOLIC

HYPEROXALURIA

Oxalate is normally excreted via renal means. However, when combined with calcium, it becomes highly insoluble. The calcium oxalate product can cause nephrolithiasis and CTIN. The diagnosis is established by demonstrating birefringent positive crystals (using polarized light microscopy) not only in the interstitial spaces but also in the tubular lumens, with surrounding inflammation and interstitial fibrosis.

Commonly seen in those with autosomal recessive, primary hyperoxalurias, affected individuals may present with gross hematuria and renal colic secondary to oxalate stones. The majority of patients progress to ESRD by the second decade of life. The recommended treatment for those with recurrent nephrolithiasis and/or ESRD is combined liver and kidney transplantation.

Ingestion of ethylene glycol (antifreeze) and inhalation of methoxyflurane (an anesthetic agent commonly used in the past) are other sources of oxalate. They both cause severe renal failure and residual tubulointerstitial damage in those who recover.

Interestingly, ingestion of a sour "star fruit," which is noted for its very high oxalate content, is another cause of acute interstitial oxalate deposition leading to interstitial nephritis and eventual renal failure.

In enteric hyperoxaluria, because of chronic diarrhea, less calcium is available in the intestines to bind oxalate. Because of this, much of the unbound oxalate is reabsorbed and excreted in the urinary tract, thereby increasing urinary oxalate levels. In addition to severe hyperoxaluria, patients may also have secondary hypocalciuria and hypocitraturia. This is commonly seen in those who have undergone extensive small bowel resections or jejunoileal bypass procedures.

Individuals who consume excessive amounts of ascorbic acid can also develop oxalate stones and CIN, as ascorbic acid is metabolized to glyoxylate and oxalate.

HYPERURICEMIA/HYPERURICOSURIA

In tumor lysis syndrome (discussed in more detail in Chapter 13) there is massive release of uric acid, thereby accounting for the occurrence of hyperuricemia and hyperuricosuria. Histopathologically, urine uric acid and crystals deposit in the interstitium, leading to tubular atrophy, a predominance of interstitial inflammatory infiltrates, and eventual fibrosis.

HYPERCALCEMIA/HYPERCALCIURIA

Hypercalcemia and hypercalciuria are discussed in more detail in Chapters 6 and 40.

CHRONIC HYPOKALEMIA

In patients with eating disorders who abuse laxatives and diuretics, chronically low levels of potassium have been described. Chronic hypokalemia has had histopathologic correlates consisting of proximal tubular cell vacuolization, dilated intercellular spaces, and medullary cysts; these clinically correlate with an impaired ability to concentrate urine (nephrogenic diabetes insipidus), conserve salt, and hypertension. It remains unclear, however, how often CIN occurs secondary to chronic hypokalemia.

MISCELLANEOUS

ENDEMIC (BALKAN) NEPHROPATHY

As the name implies, endemic (Balkan) nephropathy (EN) is particularly endemic in the so-called Balkan states, or the former Yugoslavia, Bulgaria, and Romania. No specific etiologic cause has yet been identified, but due to its "specific" geographic distribution, environmental factors have long been suspect. Genetic and immune-related factors have also been identified.

Balkan nephropathy is a slow, yet progressive form of CTIN that eventually leads to ESRD.

Dietary consumption of aristolochic acid (see the discussion above on Chinese Herb Nephropathy) has been linked to this disease and its attendant risk of transitional cell cancer.

Clinically, a characteristic early feature is normochromic normocytic anemia, the degree of which is significantly disproportionate to the stage of CKD. Urinalysis usually shows mild proteinuria (increased urine β_2-microglobulin has been noted) with few RBCs and WBCs. Patients tend to be normotensive in the earlier stages of the disease with eventual progression to hypertension in more advanced stages. Grossly, the kidneys may appear symmetrically reduced in size.

An important complication of this disease is the development of uroepithelial carcinoma involving the urinary bladder or one or both ureters and renal pelvis.

Treatment is primarily supportive.

RADIATION NEPHRITIS

Radiation nephritis is classified into two categories, based on the onset of symptom presentation: Acute radiation nephritis and chronic radiation nephritis.

Acute radiation nephritis usually presents after 6–12 months of exposure to radiation. Patients usually have edema, hypertension (occasionally accelerated hypertension), as well as marked proteinuria. Normochromic normocytic anemia secondary to intravascular hemolysis (microangiopathic hemolytic anemia) accompanying acute renal failure is common.

Chronic radiation nephritis, however, which usually presents after more than 18 months of radiation exposure, is also characterized by proteinuria, hypertension, and progression of CKD toward ESRD.

Although the exact pathogenesis remains elusive, it is believed that exposure of the kidneys to >1500–2500 rads leads to endothelial cell injury and eventual swelling, which leads to vascular occlusion, congestion, and chronic ischemic

injury. Radiation can also cause direct injury to the tubular epithelial cells. Furthermore, patients receiving radiation therapy for some underlying malignancy also receive concomitant chemotherapy. The latter may potentiate the toxic effects of radiation to the kidneys.

Histopathologically, aside from the common findings of tubular atrophy and interstitial fibrosis, there is characteristic thickening of the capillary walls, which may also demonstrate "splitting." Interposition of deposits between the split layers of the GBM is noticeably similar to that seen in hemolytic uremic syndrome (HUS) and thrombotic thrombocytopenic purpura (TTP), thereby supporting the postulated role of endothelial cell injury, leading to intravascular congestion and chronic ischemic injury, as alluded to earlier.

In bone marrow transplant recipients treated with radiotherapy followed by chemotherapy, ie, cyclosporine, pathologic findings similar to those found in thrombotic microangiopathies are similarly found, as opposed to when only chemotherapy is used.

Prevention is the only way to approach radiation nephritis. Proper shielding of the kidneys, especially in those with underlying CKD should be emphasized. Fractionizing the total irradiation dose into several small doses over several days may also have some merit. Likewise, minimizing the total irradiation dose is also suggested.

For those with radiation nephritis who develop hypertension, an ACE inhibitor is the recommended antihypertensive agent.

Appel GB, Bhat P: Tubulointerstitial diseases. In: *ACP Medicine.* American College of Physicians, 2007.

Braden GL et al: Core curriculum in nephrology: tubulointerstitial diseases. Am J Kidney Dis 2005;46(3):560.

Grollman AP et al: Aristolochic acid and the etiology of Balkan (endemic) nephropathy. Proc Natl Acad Sci USA 2007;104(29):12129.

Markowitz GS et al: Acute phosphate nephropathy following oral sodium phosphate bowel purgative: an underrecognized cause of chronic renal failure. J Am Soc Nephrol 2005;16:3389.

Walker R: Chronic interstitial nephritis. In: *Comprehensive Clinical Nephrology.* Johnson RJ, Feehally J (editors). Elsevier, 2005.

Urinary Tract Infection

Kamaljit Singh, MD, Sampath Kumar, MD, Ronald Villareal, MD, & Edgar V. Lerma, MD

Urinary tract infections (UTIs) result in 3.6 million office visits each year and greater than 100,000 hospital admissions in the United States annually. They may be confined to the lower urinary tract resulting in *cystitis* or involve the upper urinary tract and cause *pyelonephritis*. This is an important distinction as *pyelonephritis* may result in renal parenchymal damage, urosepsis, and death. Enteric or coliform bacteria are responsible for most UTIs with *Escherichia coli* being the most commonly identified organism. UTIs are further divided into (1) *uncomplicated UTIs*, where there is no structural or anatomic abnormalities of the urinary tract, and (2) *complicated UTIs*, where they may be either structural or anatomic abnormalities of the urinary tract or functional predispositions to infection. In addition, microorganisms in patients with complicated UTIs are frequently multidrug resistant.

Because of certain unique characteristics of affected individuals, UTIs can also be classified according to the population affected, eg, in young women, in young men, during pregnancy, in diabetic patients, etc.

Ascending infection from the urethra is the most common route of infection. The periurethral epithelium is normally colonized by enteric bacterial flora that invade the bladder. This probably accounts for the markedly greater frequency of infections in females, in whom the urethra is short and is in close proximity to the vulvar and perianal areas, thereby increasing the likelihood of contamination. While the majority of UTIs are due to *E coli*, only a few serogroups of *E coli* (O1, O2, O4, O6, O7, O8, O75, O150, and O18ab) can actually cause infections. An important virulence factor of these uropathogens is the presence of adherence factors, such as Type I fimbriae, or P fimbriae which allow binding of the organism to uroepithelial cells. Bacteria rapidly multiply in the bladder and may travel up the ureters to the renal pelvis and parenchyma, thereby causing pyelonephritis.

Hematogenous spread to the renal parenchyma and/or bladder is less common, but should be considered in infections due to *Staphylococcus aureus*.

Multiple risk factors are described for UTIs (summarized in Table 38–1), but the most important ones for acute cystitis in young women are recent or frequent sexual activity and a history of previous episodes of cystitis.

The majority of UTIs are caused by gram-negative enteric bacilli. *E coli* is the most commonly identified etiology in cases of uncomplicated cystitis and pyelonephritis. In a study of community acquired UTIs in the United States, *E coli* was recovered from 72% of outpatient urine samples from women aged 15–50 years and from 53% of samples from women above 50 years of age. *Klebsiella pneumoniae*, *Enterococcus* spp., and *Proteus mirabilis* were the next most commonly isolated organisms and were also noted to be more common in elderly women. *Staphylococcus saprophyticus* is common in younger, more sexually active women, reportedly accounting for 5–15% of episodes of acute cystitis, but recent studies have shown lower rates of isolation of 0.2–2%.

In recurrent UTIs or complicated UTIs, the relative frequency of infections caused by organisms other than *E coli*, such as, *Pseudomonas aeruginosa*, *Proteus* spp., *Klebsiella* spp., *Enterobacter* spp., enterococci, and staphylococci increases greatly. Previously less encountered organisms are becoming increasingly recognized as important nosocomial pathogens, and these include *Corynebacterium urealyticum*, *Candida* spp., and *Acinetobacter baumanii*, especially in patients with indwelling catheters who are receiving long-term antibiotic therapy. *S aureus* may be isolated from patients with indwelling urinary catheters, but invasion of the kidney via the hematogenous route should be suspected in noncatheterized patients, especially if intrarenal or perinephric abscesses are found. Fastidious organisms that have been isolated from the urine in women include *Gardnerella vaginalis*, *Ureaplasma urealyticum*, and *Mycoplasma hominis*; however, their pathogenic role remains unclear. *Mycobacterium tuberculosis* is an important cause of chronic UTIs in developing countries.

Table 38–1. Risk factors for urinary tract infections.

Female sex

Previous urinary tract infection

Sexual intercourse

Lack of circumcision (children and young adults)

Vesicoureteric reflux

Urologic instrumentation or surgery

Urethral catheterization

Urinary tract obstruction, including calculi, prostatic hypertrophy

Neurogenic bladder

Polycystic kidney disease

Renal transplantation

Lack of urination after intercourse

Spermicide use

Diaphragm use

Pregnancy

Lower socioeconomic group

Diabetes

Sickle cell trait in pregnancy

Human immunodeficiency virus with high viral load

Neurologic disease, eg, spinal cord injury

Older age

Estrogen deficiency (loss of vaginal lactobacilli)

Bladder prolapse

ACUTE UNCOMPLICATED CYSTITIS

 ESSENTIALS OF DIAGNOSIS

▶ Triad of dysuria, frequency, and urgency.

▶ Suprapubic or low back pain.

▶ Afebrile.

▶ Positive urinalysis.

General Considerations

Acute cystitis is an infection of the bladder. It is the classic example of an uncomplicated UTI and it commonly affects women in the reproductive age group. It is estimated that approximately 50–60% of adult women will have an episode of cystitis at some point during their lifetime. Infection is most commonly due to gram-negative enteric bacteria. Viral cystitis due to adenovirus can be seen in children, and together with BK virus may cause hemorrhagic cystitis in immunosuppressed adults.

Risk factors for cystitis include increased frequency of sexual intercourse, recent use of a diaphragm with a spermicidal agent (for contraception), delayed postcoital micturition, and a history of a recent UTI.

▶ Clinical Findings

A. Symptoms and Signs

The symptoms of uncomplicated lower UTI or cystitis are classically manifested by the triad of dysuria, frequency of urination with small amounts of cloudy urine, and urgency. Occasionally patients complain of grossly bloody urine, particularly at the end of micturition, and suprapubic or pelvic pain. Fever is usually absent in infection confined to the lower urinary tract. Physical examination is generally unremarkable, but a pelvic examination is indicated if the patient reports any symptoms of urethritis or vaginitis, eg, vaginal irritation or discharge.

B. Laboratory Findings

The diagnosis of lower UTIs is often based on the patient's history alone. The probability of cystitis in a woman who presents in the outpatient setting with dysuria and frequency of urination without any vaginal discharge is about 96%.

Urine microscopy demonstrating the presence of pyuria (defined as greater than five white blood cells per high powered field) in a clean-catch urine specimen has a high sensitivity for infection (95%) but a relatively low specificity (71%). The presence of visible bacteria on microscopy is more specific (85–95%).

Urine dipstick testing has gained increased popularity because it is fast and convenient, especially in the outpatient setting. The presence of either nitrite or leukocyte esterase is considered a positive result (a sensitivity of 75% and a specificity of 82%).

Urine culture is usually performed on a clean-catch midstream urine sample. The traditional criterion of 100,000 bacteria or colony-forming units (cfu/mL) has a high specificity, but the sensitivity is only 50%. In young women with symptoms of dysuria and frequency, lowering the threshold to 1000 cfu/mL raises the sensitivity with minimal reduction in specificity.

C. Special Tests

Testing is generally not necessary in healthy, nonpregnant women with a strongly positive history of acute uncomplicated cystitis and presumptive therapy can be initiated. The

Table 38–2. Oral regimens for acute uncomplicated cystitis.

Antimicrobial agent	Dosage	Duration (days)	U.S. Food and Drug Administration pregnancy category	Adverse effects
Trimethoprim-sulfamethoxazole (DS 160/800 mg)	One tablet q12h	3	C	Anorexia, nausea, vomiting, rash, blood dyscrasias, Stevens–Johnson syndrome
Trimethoprim	100 mg q12h	3	C	Diarrhea, rash, blood dyscrasias, hypersensitivity, taste changes
Ciprofloxacin	250 mg q12h	3	C	Headache, dizziness, nausea, diarrhea, psychosis, tendon rupture
Levofloxacin	250 mg q24h	3	C	As for ciprofloxacin
Gatifloxacin	400 mg q12h	3	C	As for ciprofloxacin
Nitrofurantoin monohydrate macrocrystals	100 mg q12h	7	B	Anorexia, nausea, vomiting, headache, hemolytic anemia, pulmonary hypersensitivity
Amoxicillin-clavulanate	500/125 mg q12h	7	B	Nausea, diarrhea, rash, blood dyscrasia
Cephalexin	250 mg q8h	7	B	Nausea, diarrhea, rash, blood dyscrasia

causative organisms and their antimicrobial susceptibility profiles are predictable in this group of patients. In women with neither a strongly positive nor negative history of UTIs, appropriate testing should be performed. Usually, a urinalysis with urine microscopy, Gram's staining, and rapid leukocyte esterase (LE) testing by dipstick is considered appropriate testing. A positive dipstick finding will result in a high post-test probability of cystitis and empiric therapy can be prescribed without the need for a urine culture. In those women with a negative urine dipstick result, a urine culture should be performed as there may still be an approximately 20% posttest probability of a UTI.

▶ Differential Diagnosis

Because patients with cervicitis or vaginitis may also complain of dysuria or urinary frequency, it is important to differentiate urethritis caused by *Neisseria gonorrhea* or *Chlamydia trachomatis* from vaginitis due to *Candida* or *Trichomonas* spp. The concurrent presence of copious vaginal discharge and irritation may point more toward urethritis or vaginitis. Occasionally, symptoms due to genital herpes simplex virus infection may also mimic symptoms of cystitis. It is therefore important to elicit a sexual history from the patient including a history of new sexual partners in the past few weeks, the presence of urethral symptoms in the sexual partner, and the presence of vaginal irritation or discharge.

▶ Treatment

A 3-day course of trimethoprim-sulfamethoxazole (TMP/SMX) remains a suitable first-line antibiotic for the majority

of uncomplicated UTIs in young healthy, nonpregnant women between 15 and 50 years old, an age group in which the rates for resistance to TMP/SMX are the lowest (Table 38–2). The Infectious Disease Society of America guidelines recommend the use of TMP/SMX only in areas in which *E coli* resistance rates are <20% and hence the decision to use TMP/SMX must be guided by local antibiotic resistance. Of note, at least 50% of women infected with a resistant organism are successfully treated with TMP/SMX and clinical cure rates of approximately 85% can be expected even when the resistance rates approach 30%. A 3-day course of a fluroquinolone, eg, levofloxacin, ciprofloxacin, or gatifloxacin, is a reasonable alternative in patients with TMP/SMX intolerance or risk factors for TMP/SMX resistance such as prior recent use of TMP/SMX, a UTI in the past 6 months, older age, and recurrent UTIs. A 7-day course of a B-lactam antibiotic, eg, amoxicillin-clavulanate or nitrofurantoin, and oral cephalosporins are other potential alternatives. Infection with *S saprophyticus* should be treated with a 7-day course of antibiotics. Cystitis typically responds rapidly to antibiotic therapy. However, in situations in which a 3-day regimen fails (either due to persistence of symptoms or relapse within 4 weeks after treatment completion) urine cultures (to look for the presence of resistant bacteria) and imaging studies should be performed to rule out complicated infection. A 14-day antibiotic regimen is recommended in these situations.

Approximately 20–30% of women who have been treated for acute uncomplicated cystitis will have a recurrent episode. It can be either from relapse or reinfection. Relapse is caused by an organism that has previously been sequestered either in the kidney or bladder epithelium. Reinfection, on the other hand, which is the more common cause of recurrent UTIs, is caused by an organism that is reintroduced from the fecal reservoir. The longer it takes for recurrent UTIs to occur, from the time of the previous UTI, the less likely it is going to be. Risk factors that have been identified include increased frequency of sexual intercourse, use of a spermicide, a new sexual partner, a history of the first UTI occurring before 15 years of age (regardless of the cause), as well as a maternal history of UTIs.

Continuous or postcoital prophylaxis can be used effectively to treat women who have recurrent UTIs. Continuous prophylaxis is an option for women with frequent recurrent infections, eg, at least two symptomatic infections during a 6-month period or three or more infections in 1 year. Continuous prophylaxis with daily or three times weekly administration of TMP/SMX (80/400 mg), TMP alone (100 mg), or nitrofurantoin (50 mg) diminishes recurrences by 95%. Continuous prophylaxis is usually prescribed initially for 6 months to 1 year. Postcoital prophylaxis is an alternative for women who report a strong association between intercourse. The same prophylactic antibiotic regimens taken after sexual intercourse have been shown to prevent episodes of symptomatic infection. Women who prefer not to take continuous prophylaxis or who are not sexually active can self treat with a short course of a fluoroquinolone or TMP/SMX.

ACUTE PYELONEPHRITIS

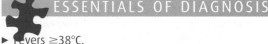

ESSENTIALS OF DIAGNOSIS

▶ Fevers ≥38°C.

▶ Chills.

▶ Flank pain or costovertebral angle tenderness.

▶ Positive urine culture.

▶ General Considerations

Pyelonephritis is an infection that involves the upper urinary tract, more specifically the kidney and the renal pelvis. Most episodes are generally considered to be uncomplicated. The microbiology of pyelonephritis is similar to cystitis with a predominance of enteric gram-negative bacteria including *E coli*, *K pneumoniae*, and *Proteus* spp. Among gram-positive organisms, *Enterococcus* spp. are the most commonly isolated.

▶ Clinical Findings

A. Symptoms and Signs

Acute uncomplicated pyelonephritis is often suggested by fever (≥38°C with or without chills) and flank or back pain. Associated symptoms including those of cystitis and nausea

and vomiting, which may be prominent. In elderly patients, symptoms of upper tract infection are often atypical and may suggest diagnoses other than a UTI, eg, abdominal pain, change in mental status. Physical examination is significant for fever and tachycardia. There may be costovertebral angle tenderness on palpation. Sepsis parameters, eg, hypotension, may be present in severely ill patients.

The diagnosis of acute pyelonephritis should be made on clinical grounds, based on the presence of characteristic signs and symptoms, together with concurrent laboratory evidence of a UTI, as previously discussed.

B. Laboratory Findings

Leukocytosis with a left-shift (predominance of bands) on a complete blood count or leukopenia in the setting of severe urosepsis may be present. A gram stain performed on the unspun urine specimen is useful for guiding immediate empiric antibiotic selection. Pretreatment urine culture and antimicrobial susceptibility testing of uropathogens should be performed routinely in women with acute pyelonephritis. Peripheral blood cultures may be positive and are indicated in women with moderate to severe pyelonephritis and in all hospitalized patients. Histopathologically, findings consistent with interstitial nephritis are seen such as patchy edema and the predominance of polymorphonuclear cells and lymphocytes invading the tubulointerstitium.

▶ Differential Diagnosis

Occasionally patients may report pain with radiation into the groin suggesting the presence of a renal calculus or pain from the kidney that is referred to or near the epigastrium or lower quadrants suggesting gallbladder disease, pancreatitis, or appendicitis. Elderly patients may report symptoms of frequency and incontinence that may be unrelated, eg, due to diverticulitis. In addition, symptoms of UTI are often difficult to elicit in older adults because of underlying dementia or use of indwelling urinary catheters. It is worth noting that patients with UTIs in the presence of an indwelling urinary catheter usually have no lower tract symptoms, but fever and bacteriuria may be present. A diagnosis of urosepsis may be made erroneously in the absence of urinary symptoms because of the presence of bacteriuria, which is common in this population.

▶ Treatment

Healthy, nonpregnant women who present with acute uncomplicated pyelonephritis can be managed in the outpatient setting if they do not have signs of systemic toxicity and are able to take oral antibiotics. For such patients, a 14-day course of a fluoroquinolone is recommended. However, women with mild symptoms can be treated with a 7-day course of an oral fluoroquinolone. Patients who are unable to maintain oral hydration or take medications, who are poorly compliant or have uncertain social situations, or who have complicated infection or signs of systemic toxicity should be admitted for parenteral antibiotics initially. Intravenous fluoroquinolones or a broad-spectrum cephalosporin with or without an aminoglycoside, ertapenem, or piperacillin-tazobactam provide adequate coverage against likely pathogens. For suspected infections due to *P aeruginosa*, an antipseudomonal antibiotic such as ceftazidime, cefepime, imipenem-cilastin, or meropenem with or without an aminoglycoside should be considered. Antibiotics can be adjusted once the infecting microorganism is identified and susceptibilities are known. Fourteen days of antibiotic therapy is usually needed. Patients who are initially on intravenous antibiotics can be switched to oral antimicrobials after clinical improvement (Table 38–3).

▶ Prognosis

Patients with acute uncomplicated pyelonephritis usually respond to antibiotic therapy within 48–72 hours. Patients who fail to respond during this time period, or whose conditions worsen with appropriate antibiotic therapy, should be reevaluated, with repeat urine and blood cultures, to determine if there is an emergence of resistance or an alternate etiologic organism. Evaluation of the upper urinary tract with imaging studies such as an ultrasound or computed tomography (CT) may be necessary. CT is the preferred imaging study because of its higher sensitivity (as compared to ultrasonography) in detecting anatomic and structural abnormalities of the urinary tract. These abnormalities may include perinephric and intrarenal abscesses as well as emphysematous pyelonephritis, all of which may necessitate urologic evaluation.

A. Complicated Urinary Tract Infection

A complicated UTI is defined as an infection in a patient with a structural or functional abnormality that would reduce the efficacy of antimicrobial therapy. Children and men with UTIs as well as nosocomial or nursing home-acquired infections and infections in a kidney allograft should be considered complicated. These patients are at increased risk for bacteremia and sepsis, perinephric and intrarenal abscess formations, and emphysematous pyelonephritis.

Note that by definition, the presence of a resistant organism does not necessarily mean that the UTI is "complicated." This is because even with a resistant organism, the duration and prognosis of the illness should remain unaltered for as long as appropriate antibiotic therapy is administered. Similarly, male gender or the elderly status of an individual does not necessarily signify a "complicated" UTI.

Nosocomial UTIs are frequently caused by multidrug-resistant organisms and hence it is important to obtain culture data before starting specific antimicrobial therapy. Empiric therapy for patients with mild to moderate illnesses may include a fluoroquinolone. For severe illness, a parenteral antibiotic should be used, at least initially (see Table 38–3). Patients can be switched to oral antimicrobials after clinical improvement. At least 10–14 days of therapy is usually needed.

B. Urinary Tract Infections in Men

In the past, UTIs in men were considered "complicated." Recent publications, however, showed that men with symptoms of a UTI, in the absence of structural or anatomic abnormalities of the urinary tract, can be classified as having an "uncomplicated" UTI, and would be appropriate

Table 38–3. Parenteral regimens for acute uncomplicated pyelonephritis.[1]

Antimicrobial agent	Dosage	U.S. Food and Drug Administration pregnancy category	Adverse effects
Levofloxacin	500 mg q24h	C	Headache, dizziness, nausea, diarrhea, psychosis, tendon rupture
Ciprofloxacin	400 mg q12h	C	As for levofloxacin
Ceftriaxone	1 g q24h	B	Nausea, diarrhea, rash, blood dyscrasia
Ceftazidime	1–2 g q8h	B	As for ceftriaxone
Cefepime	1–2 g q12h	B	As for ceftriaxone
Pieracillin-Tazobactam	3.375 g q6h	B	As for ceftriaxone
Ertapenem	1 g q24h	C	As for ceftriaxone
Imipenem	500 mg q6h	B	As for ceftriaxone
Meropenem	1 g q8h	B	As for ceftriaxone
Gentamicin	3–5 mg/kg/24 hours	D	Ototoxicity, dizziness, nephrotoxicity

[1]Switch to oral regimen to complete 14 days therapy.

candidates for shorter antibiotic courses as compared to those for complicated UTI.

Risk factors for UTIs in men include anal intercourse, lack of circumcision, and having a sexual partner with *E coli* vaginal colonization.

For treatment, a 7-day regimen of TMP/SMX, trimethoprim, or a fluoroquinolone should be used. A pretreatment urine culture should be collected prior to starting treatment and symptoms and signs of prostatitis should be elicited.

C. Catheter-Associated Urinary Tract Infection

Catheter-associated UTI (CAUTI) is the most common cause of nosocomial infections in the United States and is also considered the most common source of gram-negative septicemia in hospitals. This, however, affects not only hospitalized patients but also nursing home residents as well as those living in extended care facilities. Advanced age, an increasing degree of underlying illness, and the duration of catheterization are risk factors specific for UTIs in patients with an indwelling catheter. Such catheters are used frequently in a myriad of clinical settings, such as patients with dementia, spinal cord injuries, developmental abnormalities, and other physical or neurologic disabilities who are residing in nursing homes and chronic long-term care facilities.

The majority of patients with a catheter-associated UTI tend to be asymptomatic and, therefore, should not receive antimicrobial therapy. Approximately 10–25% of those patients, however, develop signs and symptoms of infection, and those are the ones who would require antibiotic coverage.

Pyuria is more common in patients with indwelling bladder catheters, and can be seen whether the affected patient has or does not have symptoms, making it clinically insignificant; it should not be used to guide the decision to initiate antibiotic therapy.

Symptomatic (manifested as fever or hypothermia, hypotension, hypoglycemia, or hyperglycemia or altered level of consciousness) patients should be treated with antimicrobial agents as recommended for treatment of complicated UTIs.

An indwelling bladder catheter is a common means of introducing infection inside the urinary tract. Therefore, prevention is the key. Catheter placements should be avoided unless absolutely necessary and prompt removal should be undertaken as soon as possible. Screening the urine 48 hours after removing a catheter is highly recommended. Catheters should be replaced when infected. All catheter-related infections are classified under "complicated" UTIs. Every attempt should be made to reevaluate the real need for a urinary catheter.

D. Candiduria or Funguria

The appearance of *Candida* in the urine is an increasingly common complication of indwelling catheters, particularly for patients in ICU settings, on broad spectrum antibiotics, or those with underlying diabetes. For most patients, isolation of *Candida* spp. in the urine represents colonization only. Risk factors for candiduria include use of a chronic indwelling urinary catheter, antibiotic usage, and older age.

In asymptomatic patients, removal of the urinary catheter results in eradication of infection in as many as 40% of patients. Recently published Infectious Disease Society of America guidelines on treatment of candidiasis caution against treatment of patients with asymptomatic candiduria. Antibiotic treatment should be reserved for patients with symptoms (fever with or without symptoms of cystitis) and should consist of oral fluconazole 200 mg/day for 7–14 days coupled with removal of the urinary catheter where possible. In patients who are severely ill with pyelonephritis and fungemia, systemic treatment with fluconazole 6 mg/kg/day or amphotericin B 0.6 mg/kg/day is an option. Less nephrotoxic liposomal formulations of amphotericin B are reserved for those with renal insufficiency.

E. Asymptomatic Bacteriuria

As the name implies, asymptomatic bacteriuria is a significant bacteriuria, ≥100,000 cfu/mL on two successive urine cultures in asymptomatic women or from a single culture in asymptomatic men or from a catheterized urine specimen. Asymptomatic bacteriuria is common in older women and men and is found in approximately 25–50% of ambulatory elderly women and 15–40% of men in long-term care facilities. It is because of this high prevalence in the elderly that it is not possible to diagnose a UTI on the basis of a positive urine culture alone. Although symptomatic infection develops in a few of these patients, such complications are rare and do not appear to justify either screening or the routine use of antibiotics for treatment or prevention. Treatment of asymptomatic bacteriuria is recommended in only three settings: In pregnant women, prior to urologic surgery (involving mucosal disruption), and after renal transplantation. Treatment of asymptomatic bacteriuria in those with neutropenia or immunosuppressed individuals, such as recipients of solid organ or bone marrow transplants (except kidney transplants), is not currently recommended as supporting clinical evidence is still lacking. In diabetic women, large studies have shown that there was no difference in the time period to the first symptomatic UTI between treated and untreated patients with asymptomatic bacteriuria.

F. Urinary Tract Infection during Pregnancy

The prevalence of urinary tract infections during pregnancy is 4–7%. Early screening and treatment of asymptomatic bacteriuria during pregnancy result in better outcomes when compared to no treatment or placebo. It has been well established that there is a direct relationship between a symptomatic UTI and premature delivery and the risk of complication is greater with pyelonephritis then with cystitis.

Neither acute uncomplicated cystitis nor asymptomatic bacteriuria has been demonstrated to be more common in pregnant women as compared to nonpregnant women, but studies have shown that the predilection for progression to pyelonephritis is significantly accelerated in the pregnant populace. This is probably related to anatomic or structural, as well as functional changes that occur in the urinary tract of pregnant women. This threat to both mother and fetus makes the prompt diagnosis and treatment of UTIs particularly important.

Recommendations for prenatal follow-up include screening for asymptomatic bacteriuria at week 16 of gestation.

Pregnant women with significant bacteriuria or symptomatic cystitis should therefore receive 7 days of antibacterial therapy. The isolated organisms are similar to those in nonpregnant women, with *E coli* being the most common, followed by *S saprophyticus*, group B *Streptococcus*, *Klebsiella* spp., and other enteric gram-negative bacilli. Therapeutic options include amoxicillin-clavulanate, nitrofurantoin, an oral cephalosporin, or fosfomycin as a single dose. Pyelonephritis with pregnancy should be treated with a parenteral antibiotic until the patient is afebrile for 24 hours, followed by a 10–14 day course of treatment. Asymptomatic bacteriuria in pregnancy should always be treated as 30–40% of the patients will develop a symptomatic UTI and pyelonephritis. Pregnant woman with recurrent UTIs should have postcoital prophylaxis with a cephalosporin or nitrofurantoin. Sulfonamides should be avoided in the first and third trimesters of pregnancy. Quinolones should also be avoided during pregnancy.

G. Urinary Tract Infections in Diabetic Patients

The incidence of acute uncomplicated cystitis and asymptomatic bacteriuria is increased in diabetic women as compared to nondiabetic women. In hospitalized patients, the incidence of pyelonephritis in diabetic patients is also higher, and this has been attributed to poor bladder function, eg, neurogenic bladder secondary to autonomic neuropathy, and bladder catheterization.

In addition, diabetic patients are also predisposed to emphysematous pyelonephritis. This is a fulminant, necrotizing infection involving the renal parenchyma and perirenal tissue, caused by gas-forming organisms such as *E coli*, *K pneumoniae*, *P aeruginosa*, and *P mirabilis*. The usual pathology is that of papillary necrosis causing obstruction. Diabetes is present in more then 90% of patients who may have some degree of urinary tract obstruction.

Diagnosis is established by demonstrating the presence of gas in the urinary tract combined with UTI. CT is the imaging modality of choice, as the accurate localization of gas correlates with the prognosis.

Emphysematous pyelonephritis can be divided into four prognostic categories depending on the location of gas in the urinary tract.

1. Gas in the collecting system only.
2. Gas in the renal parenchyma without extrarenal extension.
3. Perinephric extension of gas.
4. Bilateral emphysematous pyelonephritis.

The third and fourth categories will require surgical intervention, eg, possible nephrectomy combined with appropriate antibiotic therapy. They are also associated with a high mortality rate. Percutaneous drainage and relief of urinary tract obstruction combined with appropriate antibiotic coverage should suffice in the first two categories.

Medical therapy alone carries a mortality rate of 60–80%.

PROSTATITIS

The term prostatitis refers to a number of different conditions, both infectious and noninfectious. Prostatitis occurs in approximately 2–10% of men during their lifetime. The microbiology of prostatitis includes gram-negative bacilli: *E coli*, *Proteus* spp., *Klebsiella* spp., *P aeruginosa*, and, rarely, enterococci and *S aureus*. It is believed to be secondary to the reflux of infected urine from the urethra into the prostatic ducts. Prostatic calculi may serve as a nidus for the infecting organism and may also contribute to antibiotic resistance.

A classification scheme was introduced by the National Institutes of Health to distinguish various syndromes of prostatitis based on the presence or absence of pyuria and culture-proven infection. This classification scheme divides prostatitis into four categories:

1. Acute bacterial prostatitis: Symptoms and signs of prostatitis usually with positive urinary tract cultures.

2. Chronic bacterial prostatitis: Chronic or recurrent bacterial infection of the prostate or urinary tract.

3. Chronic pelvic pain syndrome or chronic nonbacterial prostatitis: Pelvic discomfort greater than 3 months with or without pyuria and negative prostate or urinary tract cultures.

4. Asymptomatic inflammatory prostatitis: The presence of pyuria in prostatic secretions or tissue with an absence of clinical symptoms.

ACUTE BACTERIAL PROSTATITIS

 ESSENTIALS OF DIAGNOSIS

▶ Fevers ≥38°C.
▶ Perineal pain.
▶ Tender prostate.
▶ Positive urine culture.

▶ General Considerations

Acute bacterial prostatitis is the result of ascending infection from the urethra. Patients often have concurrent UTIs. Most cases are due to enteric gram-negative bacteria including *E coli*, *K pneumoniae*, and *Proteus* spp.

▶ Clinical Findings

A. Symptoms and Signs

Patients commonly present with fever ($\geq 38°C$ with or without chills), perineal discomfort, and urinary complaints, eg, dysuria, frequency, or urinary retention. Patients may also complain of pelvic or lower back pain. The physical examination is significant for an exquisitely tender and edematous prostate. In patients suspected of having acute prostates, massage of the prostate is absolutely contraindicated, as it may serve as a means to precipitate bacteremia. Sepsis with positive blood cultures may be present in severely ill patients.

B. Laboratory Findings

Leukocytosis with a left shift may be seen on complete blood count. Urinalysis is abnormal with pyuria and urine cultures are usually positive. Peripheral blood cultures may also be positive.

▶ Differential Diagnosis

In patients with prominent urinary complaints and bacteriuria, the diagnosis of prostatitis may be confused with pyelonephritis. It is also important to differentiate patients with urethritis or epididymoorchitis caused by *N gonorrhea* or *C trachomatis*. A sexual history should be elicited including a history of urethral discharge.

▶ Treatment

Antibiotic selection should be guided by results of urine cultures and susceptibility results. Appropriate empiric antibiot-ics include a fluoroquinolone (eg, ciprofloxacin 500 mg every 12 hours or levofloxacin 500 mg once daily) or TMP/SMX (one double-strength tablet every 12 hours). A total of 4–6 weeks of antibiotic therapy should be administered to prevent the development of chronic bacterial prostatitis. Patients who are too ill for oral therapy or are septic on presentation should be hospitalized for initial parenteral treatment (intravenous quinolones with or without an aminoglycoside). Urethral catheterization is contraindicated in patients who develop urinary outflow obstruction and a percutaneous suprapubic cystostomy should be performed. Antibiotics can be switched to oral antimicrobials after clinical improvement to complete 4–6 weeks of therapy. Repeat urine cultures should be performed to ensure eradication of infection.

Patients with acute bacterial prostatitis usually respond to antibiotic therapy within 72 hours. Patients who fail to respond should have a urologic consultation and transrectal ultrasound (TRUS) or CT to rule out prostatic abscesses. Prostatic abscesses usually require surgical drainage for cure.

Kravchick S et al: Acute prostatitis in middle-aged men: a prospective study. BJU Int 2004;93:93.

Nicolle LE et al: Infectious Diseases Society of America Guidelines for the Diagnosis and Treatment of Asymptomatic Bacteriuria in Adults. Clin Infect Dis 2005;40:643.

Pappas PG et al: Guidelines for treatment of candidiasis. Clin Infect Dis 2004;38:161.

Scholes D et al: Risk factors associated with acute pyelonephritis in healthy women. Ann Intern Med 2005;142(1):20.

Wilson ML, Gaido L: Laboratory diagnosis of urinary tract infections in adult patients. Clin Infect Dis 2004;38:1150.

Zhanel GG et al: Antibiotic resistance in outpatient urinary isolates: final results from the North American Urinary Tract Infection Collaborative Alliance (NAUTICA). Int J Antimicrob Agents 2005;26:380.

Reflux Nephropathy

Hiep T. Nguyen, MD, & Emil A. Tanagho, MD

ESSENTIALS OF DIAGNOSIS

▶ Renal scarring associated with intrarenal reflux of infected urine (ie, acquired reflux-associated nephropathy).

▶ Congenital nephropathy associated with vesicoureteral reflux (VUR) but in the absence of infection.

▶ Nephropathy associated with VUR and impairment of urinary flow (ie, secondary VUR).

▶ General Considerations

A. Demographics

1. Acquired reflux nephropathy—It is estimated that the general incidence of primary VUR in the population is 0.4–1.8%. In children who present with a febrile urinary tract infection (UTI), the incidence of VUR increases significantly to 12–50%. Approximately 30–60% of children with VUR will have established renal scars at the time of diagnosis. Moreover, 12% of children with VUR and normal kidneys will develop scarring, irrespective of medical or surgical management. In young children, acquired reflux nephropathy is more common in girls than boys, with a ratio of 4 to 1, similar to the sex prevalence in patients with VUR detected after evaluation for a UTI. In older children, the incidence of reflux nephropathy is equivalent among the sexes, but males appear to be more severely affected. In adults, bilateral nephropathy is more common in men than in women.

2. Congenital reflux nephropathy—With the advent of routine prenatal ultrasonography, many children with VUR are detected prior the development of a UTI. It is estimated that the incidence of VUR in patients with prenatally diagnosed hydronephrosis is approximately 15–20%. In contrast to the sex prevalence of VUR diagnosed following a UTI, VUR detected during evaluation for prenatal hydronephrosis is more common in boys than in girls. It is estimated that

30–50% of these children will have renal abnormalities such as decrease in size, dysmorphic features, or imaging findings similar to renal scarring. The degree of renal abnormalities correlates with the increasing severity of the reflux.

B. Overall Incidence of Renal Abnormalities

Whether VUR is diagnosed following a UTI or in the evaluation for prenatal hydronephrosis, renal abnormalities/scarring are common at the time of diagnosis. Reflux nephropathy was found to be present in 27% of patients with VUR at the time of presentation. Of children less than 1 year of age, 20% had diffuse abnormalities while 5% had focal abnormalities. In children 1–5 years of age, the same percentage of patients had diffuse abnormalities but 16% had focal abnormalities. Similarly, in children older than 5 years of age, the number of patients with diffuse renal abnormalities was constant at 18% but 20% had focal abnormalities. Dysmorphic kidneys were more commonly seen in children younger than 1 year of age at the time of evaluation, while focal scarring was more commonly seen in older children. In children younger than 1 year of age the male to female ratio with reflux nephropathy was 1.6:1. In contrast, the ratio of male to female changed to 1:4 in older children.

The risk of scarring is greatest in children younger than 1 year of age; reflux nephropathy occurs uncommonly after 5 years of age. It has been observed that new scars developed in 24% of children younger than 2 years of age but in only 10% of children between 2 and 4 years of age and 5% of children older than 5 years of age. These findings suggest the susceptibility of the developing kidney to damage from reflux of infected urine.

▶ Pathogenesis

A. Acquired Reflux Nephropathy

1. Intrarenal reflux—Acquired renal scarring results from an episode or repeated episodes of acute pyelonephritis caused by infected urine in the presence of VUR. Intrarenal reflux allows a retrograde flow of urine into the collecting ducts and into the renal periphery (Figure 39–1). It allows direct transmission of bladder pressures to the renal pelvis, exposing the renal tubules to abnormal pressures. In addition, it exposes the renal parenchyma to urine that is in the bladder, which may have some toxic effects on the kidney cells. More importantly, intrarenal reflux provides a means for urinary pathogens to access renal parenchyma.

Renal scarring is more likely to occur in the polar regions of the kidney; this is related to the variation in renal papillary morphology. During renal development, different papillary types are formed. Compound papillae arise when two or more individual papillae are joined. This type of papillae is usually found in the renal poles, while simple papillae are more often seen in the other segments of the kidneys. The tips of the papillae project into the renal pelvis and provide a valvular action against the retrograde flow of urine into the collecting tubules. However, the tips of compound papillae are often flattened (Figure 39–2). In animal studies, intrarenal reflux occurs only through the round or gaping ducts of Bellini that open on the flattened (concave) tips of the compound papillae. In contrast, simple papillae tend to have

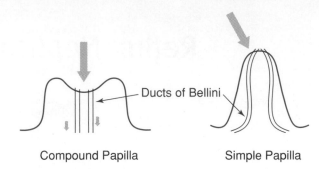

▲ Figure 39–2. The flat surface of the compound papillae allows pathogens to directly enter the renal parenchyma. In contrast, the convex surface of the simple papillae provides a valvular mechanism against the efflux of urine into the ducts of Bellini.

convex surfaces with a slit-like ductal opening and, thus, do not permit reflux. These papillary configurations and their predisposition for intrarenal reflux have also been observed in children with VUR. Renal scarring occurs only in area with intrarenal reflux. Moreover, physical distortion such as from hydronephrosis, high-pressure voiding, or adjacent renal scarring could convert nonrefluxing to refluxing papillae.

2. The role of infection—Renal scarring appears to occur more often when both VUR and infection are present. In a pig model, it has been observed that renal scarring does not occur when VUR is created on one side. However, when a bacterial infection is introduced into the bladder, renal scarring develops only on the side with VUR, while the nonrefluxing renal unit remains normal. This process begins with small discrete abscesses developing in individual tubules, which later coalesce into a confluent mass. Acutely, the interstitium is infiltrated with inflammatory cells, inducing tubular destruction and a variable amount of interstitial fibrosis. Within 2 weeks, the active interstitial inflammatory cell infiltration becomes patchier in distribution, with lymphoid follicles becoming more prominent and irreversible scarring being established. By 3 weeks, scar contraction occurs. These histopathologic findings are identical to those found in children with reflux nephropathy. Furthermore, treatment with antibiotics during the first week after infection appears to limit inflammation, and consequently, scar formation. Only fine linear scars extending through the cortex and small dimpling of the renal surface are evident if appropriate antibiotic therapy is instituted during the early inflammatory phase.

Bacterial virulence also plays an essential role in the development of renal scarring. Bacteria express factors that facilitate adhesion to the uroepithelium and increase the propensity for renal injury. Pyelonephritogenic strains of *Escherichia coli* commonly have fimbriae that fail to react with mannose on the host cell surface and express P blood group

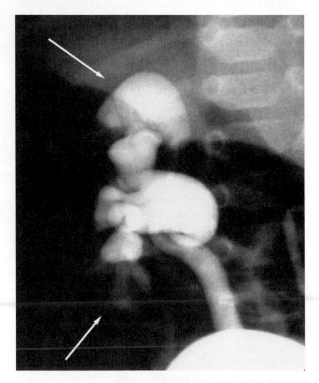

▲ Figure 39–1. Intrarenal reflux (arrows) occurring in the renal poles allows bacteria direct access into the renal parenchyma.

ligands on their fimbriae. Other virulence factors such as hemolysin and K-antigen augment the host inflammatory response and the degree of tissue destruction. Bacteria that express several virulence factors can cause acute pyelonephritis in the absence of VUR. However, in the presence of VUR, less virulent bacteria cause similar episodes of pyelonephritis. It is presumed that VUR compromises host defense mechanisms such as the antegrade flow of urine from the kidneys and the normal configuration of the papillae, which then allow the bacteria to have direct assess into the renal tubules.

3. The mechanism of renal damage from infection—

Infection activates a cascade of mediators, which leads to renal epithelial cells damage. In animal models, bacterial infection that reaches the kidney rapidly induces the activation of complement, granulocytic aggregation, and capillary obstruction. Phagocytosis of the bacterial endotoxins causes the release of proteolytic enzymes from granulocytes, inducing cell injury and death. More importantly, ischemia and reperfusion injury induce further renal damage through the release of superoxide and other free-oxygen radicals, which in turn destroy the lipid cell membranes. The ischemia results from a focal decrease in renal blood flow, due in part to a transient elevation in renal vein renin during the early inflammatory phase of pyelonephritis, compression of the vasa recta and peritubular capillaries by edema, and obstruction of the renal microvasculature by platelets and granulocyte aggregations. Free-oxygen radicals are also produced by the respiratory burst from neutrophilic leukocytes engaging in bacterial phagocytosis and by the metabolism of products produced by the anaerobic metabolism of adenosine triphosphate. The effects of ischemia and reperfusion injury on the renal epithelial cells could be limited by modulating the formation of free-oxygen radicals through the administration of exogenous superoxide dismutase, complement depletion, or pretreatment with allopurinol. Currently, the efficacy of these methods in modulating renal injury induced by pyelonephritis in humans remains unknown.

4. Acquired renal scarring in the absence of infection—

Renal scarring can also occur in the absence of infection. It is believed that the reflux sterile urine can induce an inflammatory response in the renal parenchyma that leads to scarring. From radiographic observations, it is noted that VUR not only goes into the collecting ducts (ie, pyelotubular) but also extends into the interstitium (ie, pyelointerstitial, either via the collecting ducts themselves or through a direct break into the epithelial lining of the collecting system. It is known that when it escapes outside the epithelium-lined surface, sterile urine can produce a severe inflammatory reaction, leading to a fibrotic response and subsequent scarring. This process of renal damage might be slower compared to that induced by the backflow of infected urine, but nevertheless, can cause the same extensive damage. Histologic evidence concerning the effects of sterile refluxed urine on the renal parenchyma has been seen from pathologic specimens from children and adults with severe renal scarring and VUR without any documented urinary tract infection.

B. Congenital Reflux Nephropathy

Reflux nephropathy does occur in children with VUR prior to the development of febrile UTIs and this process may occur during renal development. The pathogenesis of congenital reflux nephropathy is not well understood. Two theories have been proposed to explain the pathogenesis of renal damage in the presence of VUR but in the absence of infection: (1) Abnormal bladder dynamics/the water-hammer effect and (2) abnormal ureteric bud-metanephric mesenchyme interaction.

1. Abnormal bladder dynamics and the water-hammer effect—

In the pig, lamb, dog, and primate model, sterile reflux alone does not cause renal scarring. However, renal abnormalities such as dysplasia and hypoplasia are seen when VUR occurs concordantly with extreme hydrodynamic conditions such as those associated with urinary obstruction. Similarly, this is observed clinically in children with secondary VUR from posterior urethral valves, urethral strictures, or neurogenic bladder.

In the fetal sheep, occlusion of the urachus results in hydroureteronephrosis, cortical thinning, and medullary loss in males but not the females. These features are more pronounced after VUR is experimentally created *in utero*. After birth, the male sheep with VUR created during fetal development had persistent bladder instabilities and acquired renal scarring in the absence of UTIs. These findings in the animal model provide a plausible explanation for why high-grade VUR and associated renal abnormalities are more commonly seen in male infants. In support of these findings, it is observed in the pig model that with increased bladder pressure due to obstruction, the nonrefluxing simple papillae start to show gaping ductal openings and free intrarenal reflux.

How then does pyelotubular backflow of sterile urine induce renal injury? Renal injury may result from the direct transmission of high bladder pressure to the renal epithelial cells by VUR, inducing direct cellular insult or indirectly through the compression of the peritubular arteries with resultant ischemia. Alternatively, the efflux sterile urine into the developing renal parenchyma may provide a noxious stimulus that interferes with normal tubular development. Currently, there is no direct evidence to support either of these theories.

2. Abnormal ureteric bud-metanephric mesenchyme interaction—

An alternative explanation for the pathogenesis of congenital reflux nephropathy is based upon the interaction between the ureteric bud and the metanephric mesenchyme. This interaction determines not only renal development but also the configuration of the ureterovesical junction (Figure 39–3). A ureteric bud that is positioned closer to the urogenital sinus predisposes to primary reflux,

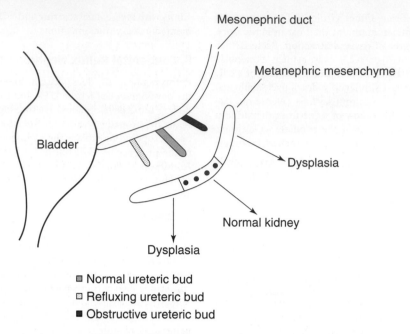

▲ **Figure 39–3.** Interaction between the ureteric bud and metanephric mesenchyme determines not only the type of renal development but also the configuration of the ureterovesical junction (reflux, normal, or obstructive). When the ureteric bud arises from a position much lower on the mesonephric duct than normal, its contact with the periphery of the metanephric mesenchyme leads to development of a dysplastic renal unit with a reflux ureter.

while those positioned inferiorly are often more obstructed. The metanephric mesenchyme is a long ridge of tissue, and only its center is likely to be capable of developing into normal renal tissue. If the ureteral bud arises in the proper position on the mesonephric duct, it will make contact with the metanephric mesenchyme in the center and a normal kidney will develop. The rest of the ridge will atrophy. However, if the bud develops too high or too low on the duct, it will make contact with the ridge's periphery, which is not capable of normal renal development. With closer contact to the center of the ridge, fewer dysplastic changes are seen in the affected renal unit. This explains why partial dysplasia of the kidney usually involves the upper or lower pole and why, in duplication, the chances of associated dysplasia are high. The same is true in refluxing ureters. Minimal reflux results from a ureteral bud that arises slightly lower than the normal takeoff point. Since it contacts the metanephric mesenchyme close to the center, renal development is in most cases normal. However, severe reflux results from a ureteral bud that arises very low on the mesonephric duct. Due to its abnormal contact with the ridge, dysplasia ensues. This results in the pathologic findings associated with congenital reflux nephropathy.

It should be noted that clinically, sterile VUR does not seem to affect renal growth or glomerular function. In

minipigs, sterile VUR does not affect renal growth or the glomerular filtration rate (GFR) even in the presence of elevated bladder pressure. However, sterile VUR has been shown to affect the renal concentrating ability by disrupting the countercurrent mechanisms in the loop of Henle. In addition, it has been demonstrated that sterile VUR can also modulate regional renal blood flow, especially during voiding.

▶ Prevention

The only reliable method of preventing reflux nephropathy is through the proper identification of patients at risk. Factors that are important in the development of renal scarring include young age, the severity of VUR, bladder dynamics, the character of UTIs, and the number of pyelonephritic episodes. Early identification of those at risk allows for early aggressive treatment of UTIs, minimization of intravesical pressure, and education of parents, physicians, and patients. It is not known if aggressive treatment of VUR reduces the risk of renal scarring. In a recent meta-analysis of randomized controlled trials for antibiotics and surgery for treatment of VUR, it was observed that combined treatment resulted in a 60% reduction in febrile UTIs by 5 years but without a concomitant significant reduction in the risk of new or progressive renal damage. Nevertheless, new scars are likely to develop with breakthrough UTIs without appropriate treatment for VUR whether it be medical or surgical.

▶ Clinical Findings

A. Symptoms and Signs

1. Acquired reflux nephropathy—In patients with reflux nephropathy associated with VUR and UTI, the kidneys are characteristically small with an irregular surface and areas of depression. The renal parenchyma is reduced in thickness with a net reduction in the ratio of cortical to medullary thickness. Coarse segmental scars are often seen overlying dilated calices and involving both the renal cortex and medulla. Wedges of fibrous tissue (scars) are sharply demarcated from surrounding tissue. There is hypertrophy of the unaffected area, leading to the lobular appearance of the renal outline. These changes are often seen in and are more prominent in the renal poles.

On microscopic examination, a variable amount of chronic inflammatory cell infiltration (primarily of lymphocytes and plasma cells) and occasional lymphoid follicles can be seen in the affected renal segments. There is generalized tubular atrophy and loss. Of the remnant tubules, the tubular basement membrane is markedly thickened. Nonfunctioning of tubules leads to an accumulation of an eosinophilic material within the lumen (termed thyroid tubules). Due to the loss of renal tubules, the glomeruli are crowded together in all stages of injuries, from periglomerular sclerosis to hyaline bodies (Figure 39–4). There is often marked interstitial fibrosis. The renal blood vessels show a reduced ratio of lumen to wall thickness. In more advanced cases, intimal hyperplasia and replacement of medial muscle by fibrosis are seen. Interestingly, these changes in association with acquired reflux nephropathy are very similar to those of obstructive nephropathy, suggesting that the mechanisms of injury may be similar.

2. Congenital reflux nephropathy—Renal changes may also occur in patients with VUR prior to the development of UTIs. These changes presumably evolve on a congenital basis. On pathologic evaluation, these kidneys often show evidence of renal hypoplasia or dysplasia. The affected kidneys appear small and smooth. On microscopic examination, primitive ducts lined by columnar epithelium and surrounded by mantles of mesenchymal cells are seen throughout the renal parenchyma (Figure 39–5). Less often, only focal or segmental dysplasia is evident, resembling in appearance the segmental scarring seen in the acquired (UTI associated) form of reflux nephropathy. In addition to dysplasia, hypoplasia characterized by a reduction in nephron number can also be seen in the affected kidneys. Both dysplasia and hypoplasia lead to global renal atrophy and potential impaired renal growth.

B. Imaging Studies

1. Intravenous urography—Identification of renal abnormalities is essential for the diagnosis of reflux nephropathy. In the past, renal scars have been detected by intravenous urography (IVU). Established scars are visualized from the appearance of caliceal deformity or clubbing with corresponding areas of focal parenchymal thinning contrasting with hypertrophy in unaffected areas. A variable degree of scarring may be visualized with IVU, from solitary polar defects to global defects as manifested by small, shrunken kidneys with little or no function. It is important to recognize

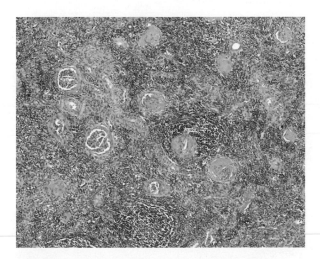

▲ **Figure 39–4.** With acquired reflux nephropathy, varying degrees of glomerular injury are observed in a region of scarring. Note the interstitium is primarily replaced by chronic inflammatory cell infiltrate.

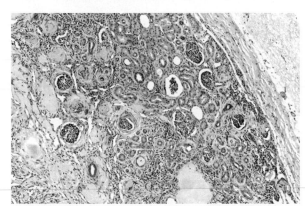

▲ **Figure 39–5.** With congenital reflux nephropathy, dysplasia characterized by primitive ducts surrounded by mesenchymal cells can be seen throughout the renal parenchyma.

that scarring detected on IVU may not be evident for some time after the causative pyelonephritic episode.

2. Nuclear renal scan—Renal imaging with technetium-99m dimercaptosuccinic acid (⁹⁹ᵐTc-DMSA) recently replaced IVU as the more common and reliable method of detecting and assessing renal scars. In contrast to IVU, which provides only structural information, a DMSA scan is able to provide functional assessment. Its other advantages include reduced radiation exposure, avoiding the risk of contrast-induced reactions, and improved visualization of the kidney by negating the issue of an overlying bowel overshadowing the renal morphology during evaluation with IVU. A DMSA scan is highly sensitive for detecting renal injury associated with acute pyelonephritis and more established scars. In addition, it can provide a quantitative assessment of the relative contribution of each kidney to global renal function.

⁹⁹ᵐTc-DMSA binds to functioning renal tubular cells; consequently, nonfunctioning or poorly functioning renal parenchyma is represented as photon absent or deficient areas. In human and animal models, transient injury from acute pyelonephritis correlates with focal abnormalities with an intact renal outline on DMSA image. In contrast, established scars are seen as focal abnormalities with a disrupted outline (Figure 39–6). More generalized or diffuse abnormalities with poor ⁹⁹ᵐTc-DMSA uptake or small kidneys are more commonly seen in patients with congenital reflux nephropathy (Figure 39–7). However, focal abnormalities on DMSA scan similar to those seen in patients with acquired reflux nephropathy can also be seen in patients with congenital reflux nephropathy.

▶ Complications

A. Hypertension

1. Incidence—Patients with renal scars are at risk for developing hypertension. Approximately 5–27% of children with renal scars and approximately 38–50% of adults with reflux nephropathy develop hypertension. There is a continued risk of hypertension in patients with reflux nephropathy irrespective of age. In some adults with renal scarring, hypertension has been detected as long as 27 years after VUR was diagnosed. Along with proteinuria, the development of hypertension is a common feature of progressive deterioration in renal function in patients with reflux nephropathy. In children with reflux nephropathy, focal segmental glomerulosclerosis (FSGS) has been consistently observed in the affected renal units.

Several mechanisms for hypertension-induced renal dysfunction in patients with reflux nephropathy have been suggested including immunologic injury, macromolecular trapping and mesangial dysfunction, and glomerular hyperfiltration. Of these, glomerular hyperfiltration resulting from

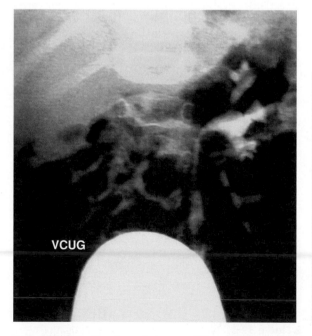

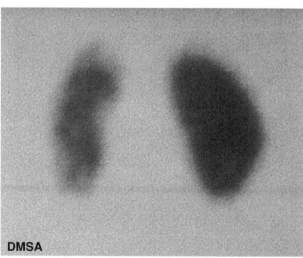

▲ **Figure 39–6.** Focal renal abnormalities with a disrupted renal outline and decreased renal function are seen in the left kidney of a girl with left vesicoureteral reflux and recurrent urinary tract infections. VCUG, vesicoureterogram.

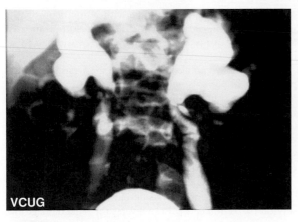
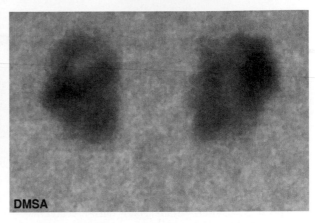

▲ Figure 39–7. Diffuse renal abnormalities are seen in both kidneys of a newborn with bilateral high-grade vesicoureteral reflux diagnosed following evaluation for prenatal hydronephrosis, prior to the development of urinary tract infections. Note the dysmorphic calyces seen on the vesicoureterogram that are usually associated with congenital reflux nephropathy.
DMSA, dimercaptosuccinic acid.

altered intrarenal and glomerular hemodynamics mediated through the renin-angiotensin system appears to be the most important. Cortical scarring with the destruction of nephrons may subject the remaining nephrons to compensatory hypertrophy and hyperfiltration, leading to FSGS and subsequent renal dysfunction.

2. Risk factors—There are several risk factors for the development of hypertension in patients with reflux nephropathy, including age, gender, degree of reflux and renal scarring, and pregnancy. The risk of hypertension appears to be greatest during adolescence and adulthood. As indicated previously, the prevalence of hypertension in adults with renal scarring is much higher than that in children. However, it should be noted that in adults, hypertension is associated with proteinuria and renal dysfunction; thus, it is difficult to determine if the hypertension in adults with renal scarring results primarily from reflux nephropathy or is secondary to the renal dysfunction. Gender also appears to be a risk factor for the development of hypertension. Males with reflux nephropathy proportionally appear to have a higher incidence of hypertension than their female counterparts. In addition, the degree of reflux and renal scarring also positively correlates with the development of hypertension. Patients with severe bilateral VUR or bilateral renal scarring are more likely to develop hypertension compared to those with unilateral VUR or renal scarring.

In women with reflux nephropathy, there is an increased risk of hypertension during pregnancy when it may present as a first manifestation of clinically latent reflux nephropathy. The development of hypertension during pregnancy is highest in women with bilateral renal scarring and has significant associated maternal complications such as urine infection, proteinuria, edema, hematuria, or renal stones. In addition,

if during pregnancy the hypertension is associated with some reduction in renal function, women with reflux nephropathy are at higher risk of developing further deterioration in renal function. Moreover, hypertension poses a significant risk to the fetus; if maternal hypertension is present at the time of conception, the risk of fetal death is increased 4- to 5-fold.

3. Mechanisms—There are several potential mechanisms in the pathogenesis of hypertension in patients with reflux nephropathy. Renal scarring results in focal, segmental ischemia, which in turn can activate the renin-angiotensin system and induce hypertension. Increased peripheral plasma renin activity (PRA), which manifests as either absolute abnormal levels or levels that fail to decrease normally with chronologic age, is frequently found in patients with reflux nephropathy and hypertension. However, there is no direct correlation between PRA and blood pressure, and PRA offers no predictive values in identifying patients who may later develop hypertension. Another potential mechanism for hypertension in patients with reflux nephropathy is abnormal sodium transport. In children and adolescents with reflux nephropathy, there is a reduction in the activity of the sodium-potassium ATPase-dependent pump, which can lead to sodium retention and, consequently, hypertension. Finally, other factors that may also contribute to the pathogenesis of hypertension in patients with reflux nephropathy include hypervolemia associated with renal impairment, accumulating nitric oxide synthase inhibitors, and a genetically determined predisposition to develop essential hypertension.

B. Renal Impairment

The estimated risk of end-stage renal disease (ESRD) in patients with reflux nephropathy is less than 1%. However, approximately 5–12% of patients with ESRD have reflux nephropathy. Recently, it was reported that in Italy, the leading cause of chronic renal failure was renal hypoplasia/dysplasia associated with urinary tract malformations, with the most common being associated with VUR. It was noted that there was a steep decline in renal function during puberty and early postpuberty. Genetic markers such as HLA subtypes have been found in patients with reflux nephropathy and renal dysfunction and suggest a genetic susceptibility to renal damage.

Lesser degrees of renal dysfunction can also be seen with reflux nephropathy, which may progress with time. In a long-term study following 294 patients with reflux nephropathy into adulthood, only 2% had renal insufficiency at presentation, but in follow-up 24% had a mild to moderate degree of renal dysfunction. Other parameters of renal function may also be affected including defects in concentrating abilities, which may resolve following cessation of VUR.

▶ **Treatment**

The management of renal failure in patients with reflux nephropathy is similar to that of other causes. Aggressive treatment of hypertension, prevention of breakthrough UTIs, and the use of angiotensin-converting enzyme (ACE) inhibitors can decrease the rate of renal deterioration and preserve renal function.

The management of hypertension is essential for preventing progression to ESRD. Treatment with ACE inhibitors is effective in treating the hypertension and in having positive effects on cardiac and renal function. Treatment of patients with severe renal scarring and microalbuminuria with ACE inhibitors decreases proteinuria, maintains the GFR and serum creatinine, and slows the progression of renal damage. Since early treatment of hypertension may slow the progression of renal injury, it may also be appropriate to consider ACE inhibitor therapy in children with reflux nephropathy who have proteinuria and a rise in blood pressure compared to previous measurements, who are not considered to be hypertensive.

Nephrectomy can also be useful in the treatment of hypertension in patients with reflux nephropathy and hypertension if the source of the hypertension can be lateralized. However, in some cases the differential renal vein renin activity might not localize the increased renin release to the scarred kidney. In addition, the removal of a scarred kidney with a presumed normal contralateral kidney does not always cure the hypertension.

It is generally agreed that once proteinuria, hypertension, or renal dysfunction has developed, it is unlikely that surgical correction of VUR can reverse the renal damage and the sequelae of reflux nephropathy. However, there are diverse opinions as to whether antireflux surgery done early in the disease process could prevent these complications. Surgical correction of VUR does seem to reduce the incidence of UTIs but does not seem to affect the incidence of hypertension or other complications. When compared to medical management with antibiotic prophylaxis, there is no difference in the development or progression of renal scars. Proponents of early antireflux surgery suggest that if surgery is to be beneficial it must be undertaken very early in life, when the growing kidney is most sensitive to injury.

Ardissino G et al: Epidemiology of chronic renal failure in children: data from the Italian Kidney project. Pediatrics 2003;111:e382.

Phan V et al: Vesicoureteral reflux in infants with isolated antenatal hydronephrosis. Pediatr Nephrol 2003;18:1224.

Wheeler D et al: Antibiotics and surgery for vesicoureteric reflux: a meta-analysis of randomised controlled trials. Arch Dis Child 2003;88:688.

Nephrolithiasis

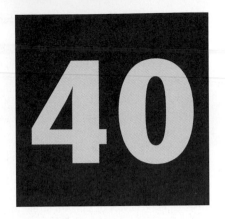

Elaine M. Worcester, MD, & Fredric L. Coe, MD

ESSENTIALS OF DIAGNOSIS

▶ Definitive diagnosis is via passage or removal of stone material; material passed should be retrieved and analyzed to determine composition.

▶ Diagnosis is also made by radiologic visualization of stones; composition may be inferred from Hounsfield units, but only analysis is definitive.

▶ Typical history of renal colic is suggestive but not diagnostic in the absence of one of the above.

▶ Underlying causes of stone formation can usually be determined by an organized evaluation of urine and serum chemistries.

General Considerations

Stones affect males about twice as often as females; the lifetime prevalence of stones in males is 12% and in females 6%, and appears to be increasing in the United States. Calcium oxalate and calcium phosphate stones account for about 80% of all stones passed, uric acid and struvite about 5–10% each, and cystine about 2%. Recurrence rates of common calcium oxalate stones are about 50% at 5–10 years; recurrence of cystine, uric acid, or struvite stones is higher, without treatment. Stones smaller than 5 mm in diameter are usually able to pass spontaneously; stones above that size are less likely to do so, and will often require urologic procedures for removal, such as extracorporeal shock wave lithotripsy (ESWL), or cystoscopic removal.

Stamatelou KK et al: Time trends in reported pevalence of kidney stones in the United States: 1976–1994. Kid Int 2003;63:1817.

Pathogenesis

The final common pathway to stone formation for any stone type is supersaturation of the urine with respect to the components making up the stone. Supersaturation means that the ambient concentrations of the stone materials (for example, calcium oxalate) exceed their solubility, and are therefore high enough to permit crystals to form and grow. Moderate levels of supersaturation, particularly with respect to calcium oxalate, may be tolerated because of the presence of substances that retard crystal formation and growth; inhibitors include glycoproteins, such as inter-α-trypsin inhibitor and osteopontin, glycosaminoglycans, and small molecules such as citrate. Stone formers may lack adequate levels of inhibitors; alternatively, persistently high levels of supersaturation may overwhelm such protection. Supersaturation may result from increased excretion of poorly soluble substances such as calcium, oxalate, or cystine, in addition to other confounding factors, for example, from low urine volume that raises the concentrations of such substances, or in some cases from persistently low or high urine pH, which decreases the solubility of uric acid or calcium phosphate, respectively. The type of stone formed correlates with the supersaturations found in the urine. In general, the urine of stone formers is more supersaturated with stone minerals than is the urine of non-stone formers, and prevention is aimed at lowering supersaturation for the relevant stone components.

Both heredity and environmental factors play a role in stone formation. Cystinuria is an example of a monogenic disorder resulting in stone formation, in which an abnormal dibasic amino acid transporter in the proximal tubule results in stone formation because of decreased renal reabsorption of cystine. There are a few examples of calcium oxalate stone formation, such as primary hyperoxaluria, or Dent's disease, in which monogenic disorders are causal, but most stone formers do not have identifiable disorders of this kind. That heredity still plays a role in many cases is evidenced by the increased risk of stone formation in men with a family history of stones, and increased concordance for stones in monozygotic compared with dizygotic twins, indicating a genetic component to stone formation. This is likely a polygenic disorder, with a large role played by environmental factors in its expression, such as diet and obesity.

Goldfarb DS et al: A twin study of genetic and dietary influences on nephrolithiasis: a report from the Vietnam Era Twin (VET) Registry. Kidney Int 2005;67(3):1053.

Taylor EN et al: Obesity, weight gain, and the risk of kidney stones. JAMA 2005;293(4):455.

▶ Risk Factors

Certain groups are at increased risk for stone formation, such as patients with bowel resections, gout, obesity, and first-degree relatives of calcium stone formers. Maintaining adequate urine volume is probably protective. Certain dietary factors are known to play a role in increasing risk of idiopathic stone formation, including diets high in animal protein, salt, and sucrose, which may all increase urinary calcium excretion; conversely, calcium restriction has been found to be of no help, and in fact decreased dietary calcium intake also appears to be a risk factor for incident stone formation. The reason may be that low calcium intake leads to an increase in absorption of oxalate from the diet, and therefore higher urinary oxalate excretion. In patients with neurogenic bladder, avoidance of chronic instrumentation seems to be helpful in prevention of bacterial colonization and resultant formation of struvite stones.

▶ Prevention

People who have formed one or more stones should be evaluated as detailed below to determine the factors leading to stone formation, so that measures can be taken to prevent future stones. Prevention is usually based on measures that lower urine supersaturation with respect to the mineral that formed the patient's stones. Institution of effective preventive measures can significantly decrease the number of stone recurrences and the need for surgical treatment of stones.

von Unruh GE et al: Dependence of oxalate absorption on the daily calcium intake. J Am Soc Nephrol 2004;15:1567.

▶ Clinical Findings

A. Symptoms and Signs

Pain of stone passage begins suddenly, and mounts to a plateau of severity over perhaps 30 minutes to 2 hours. The pain is not improved or worsened by posture or movement, although patients usually move about to distract themselves. Flank location is not too helpful, but initial flank location with subsequent downward migration anteroinferiorly is very suggestive of a moving stone. Other suggestive patterns are persistent urinary frequency without evident infection, from a stone at the ureterovesical junction. Most

characteristic of colic is its mysterious disappearance without residual effects; no pain in clinical medicine of such severity disappears completely over minutes. Hematuria with suggestive pain increases diagnostic likelihood. No pain closely matches or resembles the pain associated with severe renal colic. Its character is indescribable, even by writers and poets. Rarely, stones may present with painless hematuria, or with renal insufficiency caused by obstruction.

B. Laboratory Findings

1. Stone analysis—Any objects said to have been passed should be analyzed via infrared spectroscopy or x-ray diffraction to determine if they are indeed one of the recognized human stone types—usually calcium oxalate, calcium phosphate, uric acid, cystine, or struvite, rarely ammonium acid urate or a drug stone. Artifacts can be presented to feign disease. Given a proven stone type, or one suggested by radiography, treatment can be focused on preventing formation of that particular material. Because stone type can change with time and treatment, all stones should be analyzed.

2. Urinalysis—Urinalysis may reveal some diagnostic information. Crystalluria is frequent, and may be due to uric acid, calcium phosphate, or calcium oxalate; the latter occurs as the monohydrate—dumbbell-shaped and small, or the dihydrate—double pyramids. Crystals form in urine of normal people, although less copiously; however, persistent crystalluria in the urine of a stone former predicts recurrence. Struvite crystals look like coffin lids and are not found without urinary infection with bacteria that can hydrolyze urea to ammonia, so they are of importance. Likewise, the finding of cystine crystals in the urine is diagnostic of cystinuria. Hematuria, pyuria, and proteinuria are all clinically important, but not specific to stone formers. Urine pH and specific gravity may provide clues to causes of stone recurrence or compliance with therapy.

3. Routine blood chemistry—High serum calcium, even if only slight, suggests hyperparathyroidism, sarcoidosis, hyperthyroidism, or possible lithium use, and is very important. Benign familial hypocalciuric hypercalcemia is important because it requires no treatment and does not usually progress to renal failure.

4. Twenty-four-hour urines—Analysis of two or three 24-hour urines is indicated for diagnosis of factors contributing to stone formation in all but single calcium stone formers with normal blood chemistry, in whom conservative therapy with fluids is justified. In recurrent calcium stone formers the most common abnormality found is elevated excretion of calcium with normal blood calcium, so-called idiopathic hypercalciuria. Other abnormalities may also be contributory, including elevated excretion of oxalate, decreased citrate excretion, and persistent low volume. These factors all serve to raise the level of urinary supersaturation (SS) with respect to the stone salt.

Treatment with diet and medication is aimed at normalization of specific abnormalities to prevent stone recurrence, and will be described below. Urine testing is available from many commercial sources and always includes the analytes shown in Table 40–1, which permits calculation of excretion rates as well as of SS for uric acid (UA), calcium oxalate (CaOx), and calcium phosphate (CaP), the three main kinds of stones. A qualitative test for cystine, to detect unsuspected cystinuria, is often done on the initial urine as well. A single urine can suffice, but because of high variability day to day among patients it is more prudent to obtain two to avoid missing abnormalities and gauge average trends. Normal ranges for urine excretion of the relevant substances are suggested in Table 40–1, but it should be remembered that these merely inform us of values that are generally outside the range found in non-stone formers. In truth, there is a great deal of overlap between the two groups, and each of these values should be thought of as continuous risk factors. Risk of incident kidney stones increases progressively as the urine calcium concentration rises, for example. Likewise, stone risk drops as urine volume increases.

C. Imaging Studies

Radiographic confirmation of stones is best done via noncontrast computed tomography (CT). Stone type can be suggested by the Hounsfield number—radiographic density—of the stone; low numbers suggest uric acid or cystine; higher numbers suggest calcium phosphate or calcium oxalate stones. Struvite stones have a laminar rugged appearance, and are often full casts of the renal pelvis and calyces, the so-called stag horn conformation.

D. Special Examinations

Patients should be instructed to list the dates of all stone occurrences, procedures, and complications of stones before their visit, saving time; old records are best obtained as well, for confirmation. Points of history related to stone causes (Table 40–2) are best taken at the initial visit. Family history matters in that some stones— struvite, those due to primary hyperparathyroidism—are not familial, while others have a genetic component.

Daudon M et al: Serial crystalluria determination and the risk of recurrence in calcium stone formers. Kidney Int 2005;67(5):1934.

Table 40–1. Twenty-four-hour urine stone chemistries.

Analyte	Units	Normal Values (non-stone formers)
Volume	L/day	>1.5
pH		5.8–6.2
Calcium	mg/day	<250 (women), <300 (men), <4 mg/kg or <140 mg/g creatinine (both sexes)
Oxalate	mg/day	30–50
Citrate	mg/day	>550 (women), >450 (men)
Uric acid	mg/day	<750 (women), <800 (men)
Phosphate	mg/day	500–1500
Magnesium	mg/day	50–150
Sulfate	mmol/day	20–80
Ammonia	mmol/day	15–60
Sodium	mmol/day	50–150
Potassium	mmol/day	20–100
Creatinine	mg/day	15–19 mg/kg (women), 20–24 mg/kg (men)
SS CaOx		6–10
SS CaP		0.5–2
SS uric acid		0–1

SS, supersaturations; CaOx, calcium oxalate; CaP, calcium phosphate.

Table 40–2. Clinical findings.

History specific to stone evaluation
Dates of stones and their related procedures
Stone analyses performed in the past
Potential stone causes
   Dehydration—occupation, travel, sports
   Calcium supplements
   Lithium—for mood disorders, usually
   Hyperthyroidism
   Sarcoidosis
   Chronic urinary infections
   Bowel disease; especially bowel surgery
   Urinary obstruction, congenital anomalies
   Immobilization for a significant period
   Glucocorticoid use for a significant period

Physical findings specific to stone disease
Ocular changes of Wilson's disease
   Hyperthyroidism; eye changes, goiter
   Hepatosplenomegaly—sarcoid suggested
   Evidence of past surgeries
   Large bladder after voiding

▶ Differential Diagnosis

Very few things are confused with renal stone passage. Flank pain and hematuria may be caused by papillary necrosis, renal emboli, or renal tumors, and frequency and hematuria may be confused with urinary tract infection, which can coexist with stone passage in some cases. The pain of gallbladder disease or diverticulitis may transiently mimic that of stone passage, but the diagnosis is seldom in doubt for long.

Diagnosis of the causes of stone formation is detailed below, and relies on the results of stone analysis and serum and blood chemistries. Certain systemic illnesses can include kidney stones as one of their manifestations; Table 40–3 presents some patterns of serum and urine findings that may suggest one of these. Most idiopathic stone formers have relatively normal serum chemistries, and no other systemic manifestations.

▶ Complications

Acute episodes of stone passage may lead to obstruction, and then require urologic intervention such as ESWL or ureteroscopy. Urinary tract infection may complicate instrumentation and lead to complicated infection in the setting of obstruction. A history of stones is associated with decreased renal function, and an increased risk of hypertension, and may in rare instances contribute to development of end-stage renal failure.

Table 40–3. Patterns of laboratory abnormalities found in some systemic disorders associated with stones or nephrocalcinosis.[1]

Serum	Urine	Significance
TB:High Ca	High Ca	Primary HPT
High Ca	Nl/low Ca	FHH: Loss of function CaR
Low Ca	Nl/high Ca	ADH: Gain of function CaR
Low Mg	High Ca	FHHN
Low K, high HCO$_3$	High Ca	Bartter syndrome, Types 1 or 2
Low K, low HCO$_3$	High Ca, pH >6	Distal RTA
Low K	Low K	Diuretics, vomiting

Ca, calcium; Mg, magnesium; K, potassium; Nl, normal; HPT, hyperparathyroidism; FHH, familial hypocalciuric hypercalcemia; CaR, calcium receptor; ADH, autosomal dominant hypocalcemia; FHHN, familial hypomagnesemia with hypercalciuria and nephrocalcinosis; RTA, renal tubular acidosis.

Gillen DL et al: Decreased renal function among adults with a history of nephrolithiasis: a study of NHANES III. Kidney Int 2005;67(2):685.

▶ Treatment

A. Struvite Stones

These stones are produced by urinary tract infection with urease-producing bacteria, and cannot be treated without a combined medical—surgical approach. Usually they are too large (>2 cm) for ESWL and must be removed via percutaneous lithotomy or, in some instances, ureteroscopic laser lithotripsy. The surgery must create a stone-free kidney in that infected fragments can readily reform a large new stone. Antibiotics are useful in the immediate perioperative and postoperative periods, but chronic use has no basis. Acetohydroxamic acid (AHA) inhibits bacterial urease and can prevent growth and formation of struvite stones, but significant side effects, such as headache and thrombotic events, make it less useful. The usual organisms that cause struvite stones are *Proteus, Klebsiella, Pseudomonas,* and *Enterobacter* spp., often highly resistant to antibiotics. Repeated treatments for urinary infection and prior urologic procedures can lead to their colonization of the urinary tract. Loss of renal function can occur because of persistent obstruction and infection. Struvite stone formers may have passed prior stones due to other causes, such as cystinuria, low urine pH with uric acid stones, or calcium stones from any one of their causes. Therefore, they should be evaluated fully, in the sequence below, to find preventable causes of stone recurrence.

B. Cystine Stones

Only autosomally recessive inherited abnormalities of the dibasic amino acid transporter found in the proximal tubule of the kidney cause these stones. Two types of cystinuria have been identified clinically. Recent genetic studies have linked Type A (or Type I) to a defect in rBAT, the heavy unit of the heteromeric amino acid transporter; Type B (type non-I) is linked to abnormalities of b$^{0,+}$AT, the light subunit of the transporter. The clinical presentations of these two groups are the same. Cystinuria is detected via stone analysis and spot urine cystine screening tests. If the latter is positive a 24-hour urine must be collected for creatinine and cystine to confirm either the heterozygote—usually non-stone-forming- or homozygous-stone-forming—state. Urine cystine levels above 300 mg daily are almost always the latter. Treatment is with urine volumes above 3 L daily, up to 5 L depending on the urine cystine excretion. As a general rule, 300 mg/L can be dissolved and it is preferable to achieve about a 2-fold more urine volume than is necessary, ie, 2 L for 300 mg/day of cystine and 4 L for 600 mg of cystine daily. Cystine dissolves more readily in urine of pH >7; potassium citrate, 20–30 mEq twice daily, is a reasonable starting dose; follow-up urine testing is needed to be sure of pH and volume. Serum potassium must be tested, ideally at 1 week of treatment, to be sure hyperkalemia has not occurred. Any elevation of serum creatinine requires special caution in the use of potassium alkali.

Because urine pH is increased by treatment, and because cystinuric patients may harbor abnormalities that foster calcium stones and can be worsened by high urine pH, all patients must be studied fully with 24-hour urine testing for stone risk factors. If they are present, follow-up testing must include risk factors and an assessment of their changes with treatment to prevent overgrowth of calcium salts on cystine stones (eggshell stones). Cystine stones are difficult to fracture with ESWL so other modalities are usually preferred.

When fluid and alkalinization alone are unsuccessful in preventing recurrence, chelating agents may be used. These drugs form a mixed thiol-cysteine disulfide that is more soluble than cystine. D-Penicillamine has been used in the past, but because of side effects, it has largely been supplanted by α-mercaptopropionylglycine (tiopronin), which appears to be somewhat better tolerated. The usual dose is 100 mg tablets, three to six daily in divided doses, which may be increased up to 1200 mg/day; side effects include loss of taste—remedied in part by supplemental zinc—and occasionally serious reactions including fever, proteinuria and serum sickness syndromes. Captopril also binds cysteine, but fall in blood pressure and allergic reactions limit its use, and its efficacy is controversial.

C. Uric Acid Stones

In all cases, these stones occur because of low (<5.6) 24-hour urine pH; low urine volume may be a contributing factor in some cases, such as patients with chronic diarrhea. High urine uric acid excretion is almost never of importance. Any uric acid in stones is sufficient grounds to perform 24-hour urine stone risk testing, which will reveal not only urine pH but other possible abnormalities that might cause conversion to calcium stones when pH is raised in treatment.

Treatment of uric acid stones consists of raising urine pH to 6, avoiding very high pH values (>6.5) that can promote calcium phosphate stones. Potassium citrate 10–30 mEq twice daily is a reasonable starting dose. Follow-up at 6 weeks can be used to gauge the need for adjusting the dose. Allopurinol is specifically not indicated for uric acid stones, as it is not sufficient or necessary.

Uric acid stone formers are often obese or diabetic, conditions that lower urine pH via insulin resistance. Stone management in obese persons, and preservation of renal tissue in patients with diabetes make stone prevention especially important in this population. Even one uric acid stone is sufficient for complete evaluation and treatment. Given the wide range of urine pH and given that response to treatment cannot be predicted, there is no basis for empirical treatment with an arbitrary dose of alkali without urine testing. As well, in patients with diabetes, and those with other disorders of potassium handling, follow-up must include serum potassium. Our practice is to check this at 1 week if baseline potassium is even high normal, or serum creatinine is above normal, or if drugs that reduce renal potassium excretion are being used. We also check serum potassium any time urine retesting is performed.

Ammonium acid urate stones are different in cause. This salt precipitates at a higher pH (about 5.7) when urine ammonia is high. In humans, the cause is almost always chronic diarrhea, organic or from laxative abuse, with hypokalemia, which stimulates ammonia production. Treatment requires correction of the underlying intestinal problem.

D. Calcium Stones

1. Single stones

—Unlike the situation for struvite, cystine, or uric acid stones, where even one stone requires specific treatment, patients who have formed only one calcium stone have two practical and medically sound options. In patients who avoid dehydration and maintain a reasonable urine volume of 2 L or so daily, only one-third will experience stone recurrence within 5 years. Massive hydration, with urine flows near 3 L, and sustained, will lower that rate to about 10%, an impressive reduction. Patients who are well educated about stone disease play a major role in their own treatment, as they often decide which conservative medical measure they will use. We have known some patients who are content with the odds, while others, perhaps more squeamish, prefer more active protection. A very high intake of fluids is reasonable for them. If they desire more, they can be managed as if they had multiple stones. In labeling someone a single stone former, we include radiography; single means only one stone, clinically and by x-ray.

2. Multiple stones

A. THE MOST ABUNDANT STONE FORMERS—Struvite, cystine, and uric acid stone formers together scarcely match even a fraction of those with multiple calcium stones. In clinical practice well over half, even two-thirds of cases will be calcium stones. Even so, we would not enlarge our comments except that causes of calcium stones are most diverse, and treatments vary. Evaluation is similar to that for all stone formers, except that at least two complete stone risk urines (Table 40–1) are advisable to detect the cause of stones and guide treatment (Table 40–4). In all multiple calcium stone formers, the highest urine volume achievable for a given patient is the proper clinical goal. We will not repeat this clinical maxim, but always practice it.

(1) Idiopathic hypercalciuria (IH)—High urine calcium (>250 or 300 mg/day, women and men, or >4 mg/kg/day, either sex), normal serum calcium, and exclusion of hyperparathyroidism, hyperthyroidism, vitamin D excess, calcium supplement excess, rapidly progressive bone disease, malignancy, sarcoidosis, and immobilization make the diagnosis. Almost all stone formers with hypercalciuria have IH. The

Table 40–4. Causes of calcium stones.[1]

Idiopathic hypercalciuria	Hypercalciuria + normocalcemia + clinical exclusions
Primary HPT	Hypercalciuria + hypercalcemia + clinical exclusions
Hypocitraturia	Low urine citrate
Hyperuricosuria	High urine uric acid
RTA	Low serum HCO_3, urine pH >6.5, low serum K
Dietary hyperoxaluria	High urine oxalate
Enteric hyperoxaluria	High urine oxalate + small bowel malabsorption
Primary hyperoxaluria	High urine oxalate + clinical exclusions
Colon resection, ileostomy	Clinical setting
Habit, environment	Clinical setting

[1]HPT, hyperparathyroidism; RTA, renal tubular acidosis.

etiology is not yet understood, but the familial nature of the disorder points to a genetic predisposition. Patients have increased calcium absorption from food, and increased loss of calcium in the urine. Although protocols to divide patients into "absorptive" and "renal leak" subtypes have been proposed, in practice, the two groups are not clearly differentiated. In addition, recent studies document the occurrence of bone mineral loss and increased fractures in patients with kidney stones, and this suggests some risk of bone mineral loss in all hypercalciuric patients. Thus, low calcium diet is seldom used in the treatment of hypercalciuria, as it may worsen bone mineral loss; in addition, it has not been found to be effective.

Treatment of IH is aimed at lowering urine calcium loss, and thereby decreasing urine supersaturation. Three treatment trials document the efficacy of thiazide diuretics to reduce urine calcium excretion and reduce stone recurrence. Trial drugs have included chlorthalidone 25–50 mg daily, hydrochlorothiazide, 25 mg twice daily, and indapamide 2.5 mg daily, and stone reductions have decreased, on average, from a 3 year recurrence rate of 50–70% to about 15–20%. Dietary factors are known to influence calcium excretion in IH. One study has documented excellent outcomes with a reduced sodium-reduced protein diet in males versus poorer outcomes from a low calcium diet.

Thiazide use is conventional; potassium wasting is minimized by lowering diet sodium intake. Replacement is best with potassium citrate if urine citrate is low, but a potassium chloride salt is preferable if urine pH is above 6.2 because the citrate can increase pH and promote conversion to phosphate

stone formation. Follow-up urine testing is recommended to be sure of a reduction of urine calcium, and to adjust diet sodium as needed. Serum potassium must be measured and hypokalemia treated. Amiloride 5 mg tablets, one or two daily, can be used if needed to reduce potassium losses. Potassium depletion can reduce urine citrate (see below) and this is corrected with potassium repletion.

(2) Primary hyperparathyroidism—Hypercalciuria with hypercalcemia suggests this disease. Reduced serum phosphate is supportive. Serum parathyroid hormone (PTH) should be measured, and the diagnosis requires the PTH be not reduced. A normal or high PTH with high serum calcium is sufficient for the diagnosis provided thiazide is excluded—which can raise serum calcium—and lithium use, which causes abnormal parathyroid regulation.

Similarly, hyperthyroidism also produces this result. Sarcoidosis, most malignant hypercalcemic states, and vitamin D excess all suppress serum PTH. The elevation of serum calcium can be modest (10.5 or less) so multiple blood samples are prudent given a scattering of borderline high results. This disease requires surgical treatment at the present time. The new calcimimetic agents are not as yet proven remedies, and are extremely expensive.

(3) Hypocitraturia—Low urine citrate (below 450 and 350 mg/day, women and men, respectively) is not uncommon and could promote calcium stones because citrate binds calcium ions and inhibits calcium salt crystallization. Three trials of potassium citrate have led to conflicting results. Two well done trials show positive results almost identical to those of thiazide for IH. The third showed no effect of citrate, mainly because recurrence in the placebo arm was as low as with thiazide or citrate. Sodium citrate salts have never been used in a trial and have the theoretical disadvantage of possibly increasing blood pressure and urine calcium. Typical products include many generic potassium citrate powders that must be dissolved in water as a beverage and used at 25–30 mEq twice daily. Only one proprietary pill form (Urocit K, Mission Pharmacal) exists, 10 mEq tablets, one or two to be taken two or three times daily. Follow-up urine testing is needed to confirm results. As with uric acid stone formers, serum potassium requires testing at appropriate intervals for safety. Potassium salts should be used with extreme care if renal function is reduced, or if drugs are being given that impair potassium excretion.

(4) Hyperuricosuria with calcium oxalate stones—Daily urine uric acid excretion above 750 or 800 mg in women and men, respectively, appears to promote CaOx stones, perhaps by fostering CaOx crystallization. In one trial allopurinol 200 mg daily reduced stone recurrence with the same efficiency as cited for thiazide and potassium citrate. Hyperuricosuria is a dietary phenomenon, related to high intakes of meat, and can be reduced by diet. No trials document benefits

of diet, and it can be hard to accomplish. If stones are a serious clinical problem allopurinol is a reasonable alternative.

(5) Distal renal tubular acidosis (RTA)—This is a rare condition of reduced renal ability to lower urine pH normally, which may be genetic or acquired. Acid excretion is reduced causing metabolic acidosis. Hypokalemia is usual, as is hypocitraturia. Urine calcium can be elevated because of the acidosis, and the high urine pH fosters calcium phosphate stones and nephrocalcinosis. Potassium citrate, 2–4 mEq/kg/day in divided doses, can correct the acidosis and hypokalemia and may reverse the hypercalciuria. If urine calcium remains high, thiazides can be used. Genetic RTA need not cause progressive renal disease if treated. Sjögren syndrome is a more common cause of RTA with stones, and is an immune disorder that can cause chronic renal failure. Other causes of RTA include any hyperglobulinemic state, including the rheumatoid and collagen vascular diseases.

(6) Dietary hyperoxaluria—In dietary hyperoxaluria oxalate is usually between 50 and 80 mg daily (normal oxalate <50 mg daily) and variable. Sources of preformed oxalate are of plant origin, and spinach, nuts, cocoa, and pepper excess are very common in practice. High protein intakes stimulate endogenous oxalate production. Perhaps the most common situation is a low calcium diet, which permits diet oxalate to be absorbed instead of precipitated in the gut lumen. Dietary management includes a normal calcium intake (800–1000 mg) from foods, not supplements, reduced protein intake, and avoidance of excessive high oxalate foods. No trials substantiate these measures, however.

(7) Enteric hyperoxaluria—Enteric hyperoxaluria is a syndrome of small bowel malabsorption from any cause, but usually from Crohn's disease, bowel resection, or intestinal bypass for obesity, and subsequent excessive colonic oxalate absorption. Urine oxalate levels can range from 50 to 150 mg daily, and the diagnosis is based on the clinical setting. In addition to avoidance of high oxalate foods and excessive protein intake, calcium carbonate supplements—500–1000 mg— can be used during each meal to precipitate diet oxalate. Reduced diet fat content can reduce binding of calcium by undigested fatty acids, and reduce urine oxalate. Cholestyramine 2–4 g with each meal will adsorb both fatty acids and oxalate and reduce urine oxalate. Potassium citrate will offset the enteric bicarbonate loss usually encountered, and raise urine pH and citrate levels. These measures can reduce stones in our experience, although no trials prove that assertion. Enteric hyperoxaluria can cause renal damage including end-stage renal disease, so treatment must be aggressive and persistent.

(8) Primary hyperoxaluria (PHO)—PHO Types I and II arise from genetic mutations of one of two genes that control oxalate production, mainly by the liver. The urine oxalate can range from 80 mg to 300 mg daily. Patients can present with stones beginning even in childhood, and renal failure is a common outcome because of damage from the high oxalate. A fraction of patients lower their urine oxalate in response to pyridoxine, in doses ranging from 10 mg to 300 mg daily; it is best to try this in all cases, beginning at the lowest doses and working up. Very high urine volume, and perhaps potassium citrate and neutral potassium phosphate (Neutraphos, 1–2 g daily in divided doses), may lower urine oxalate. However, in practice, no one should attempt to manage this condition without continued guidance from a stone referral center, which usually means patients must travel. Preemptive liver and kidney transplantation is the definitive treatment for Type I PHO as renal disease begins to progress, because systemic oxalosis can damage blood vessels, nerves, and the heart.

(9) Colon resection—Colon resection, often with ileostomy, causes diarrhea with resulting low urine volume, bicarbonate loss, and consequent low urine pH and citrate levels, and thereby leads to calcium oxalate and uric acid stones. Management is obvious: Fluids, sodium or potassium alkali replacement, and dietary measures to minimize the diarrhea. These goals are difficult to achieve in practice.

(10) Habit and environment—With or without a metabolic stone-forming abnormality, some people are predisposed to conditions of low fluid intake and/or dehydrating environments and tend to become stone formers. Simple habitual low urine volume is not rare and is difficult to treat. Dehydration at work arises from many causes, such as hot environments, frequent air flight, deliberate fluid restriction —in school teachers and surgeons, for example—and outdoor workers. Such people may change their habits briefly when their 24-hour urines are to be collected, so you do not know their true habits and they may not tell you unless you ask. Treatment is obvious but can be challenging.

(11) The problem of calcium phosphate stones—Calcium will crystallize with phosphate instead of oxalate when urine pH is persistently high, that is, above 6.3 on a 24-hour basis. Calcium monohydrogen phosphate (brushite) is one form, and such stones are associated with plugging of terminal collecting ducts with crystals and significant renal disease. Apatite is the other usual stone, and its renal pathology has not yet been determined. All stones should, therefore, be analyzed and if a calcium phosphate phase is predominant, or if any brushite is present, alkali supplements should be avoided; they will not be needed to raise urine pH as it is certainly already high. Hypocitraturia with alkaline urine pH poses a common and special problem, sometimes referred to as incomplete RTA in that blood is normal but low citrate with high urine pH suggests an acidification defect.

We have become skeptical of this formulation, and leery of alkali; if potassium citrate can raise urine citrate in such circumstances without an increase in urine pH, we use it. If not, we use fluids and other means.

Abate N et al: The metabolic syndrome and uric acid nephrolithiasis: novel features of renal manifestation of insulin resistance. Kidney Int 2004;65(2):386.

Evan AP et al: Crystal-associated nephropathy in patients with brushite nephrolithiasis. Kidney Int 2005;67:576.

Parks JH et al: Clinical implications of abundant calcium phosphate in routinely analyzed kidney stones. Kidney Int 2004;66(2):777.

▶ Prognosis

Recurrence of calcium stones can be decreased with treatment using a combination of medication and diet; without treatment, recurrence is likely, although it may be after a number of years. Cystine and uric acid stones, and stones associated with hyperoxaluria, are very prone to frequent recurrences without treatment. Although most calcium stones pass, some require surgical intervention. Repeated episodes of stone passage, and the attendant obstruction and procedures, may result in some loss of renal function. Whether prevention is able to preserve function has not been tested, but is possible. Preventive therapy can decrease the need for surgical procedures to remove stones.

Primary (Essential) Hypertension

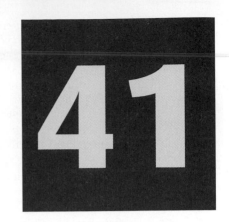

Peter D. Hart, MD, &
George L. Bakris, MD

ESSENTIALS OF DIAGNOSIS

▶ Primary hypertension in adults aged 18 years and older is defined as blood pressure of 140/90 mm Hg or more, based on an average of two or more properly measured seated blood pressure (BP) readings at each of two or more clinic visits.

▶ Normal BP is a systolic BP (SBP) <120 mm Hg and diastolic BP (DBP) <80 mm Hg.

▶ Prehypertension is defined as an SBP of 120–139 mm Hg or DBP of 80–89 mm Hg.

▶ Stage 1 hypertension is defined by an elevation in either SBP 140–159 mm Hg or diastolic BP of 90–99 mm Hg.

▶ Stage 2 hypertension is defined by an elevation in either SBP of ≥160 mm Hg or DBP of ≥100 mm Hg.

▶ The level of BP alone is inadequate for diagnosis and it should be interpreted in the context of the overall cardiovascular risk of the patient, which is most easily estimated by evaluating other concomitant disorders and target-organ damage (TOD).

▶ General Considerations

Hypertension affects more than 29% adult Americans and is the most common reason for office visits to physicians in the United States. The prevalence of hypertension is expected to increase largely due to the epidemic of obesity and the aging population in the United States. Indeed, data from the Framingham health study suggest that people with a normal BP (<120/80 mm Hg) at 55 years of age have a 90% lifetime risk of developing hypertension. Additionally, it is now well established that a linear relationship exists between BP and risk of cardiovascular events, thus the more elevated the BP the greater the likelihood

of myocardial infarction, congestive heart failure, kidney failure, or stroke.

Despite the increased prevalence of hypertension and its associated morbidity and mortality, current control rates are inadequate. Only 34% of people with hypertension have their BP controlled to a goal of BP < 140/90 mm Hg. Key factors for the inadequate BP control include failure of physicians to prescribe (1) lifestyle modifications, (2) adequate doses of antihypertensive medications, and (3) appropriate drug combinations and increased occurrence of pure systolic hypertension in the elderly, which is considerably more difficult to treat.

Risk Factors

The Joint National Committee (JNC) 7 recommends that specific public health interventions such as decreasing calories, saturated fat, and salt intake, especially in processed foods, and increasing physical activity be strongly encouraged at school and community levels. This strategy can achieve a downward shift in the distribution of a population's BP and thus potentially decrease the lifetime risk of morbidity and mortality from hypertension in an individual.

▶ Clinical Evaluation

A. Measurement of Blood Pressure

Accurate measurement and interpretation of BP is crucial for the diagnosis and treatment of hypertension. The recommendations outlined below will help standardize the technique and improve the accuracy of BP readings:

- Patients should abstain from drinking caffeine or alcohol-containing beverages or using tobacco within 30 minutes prior to a BP measurement.
- The cuff size appropriate for the patient's arm circumference should be used (the cuff bladder should encircle at least 80% of the arm).

- The cuff bladder should be centered over the brachial artery, with its lower edge within 2.5 cm of the antecubital fossa.

- Listen over the brachial artery using the bell of the stethoscope with minimal pressure exerted on the skin. Inflate the cuff 20 mm Hg higher than the pressure at which the palpable pulse at the radial artery disappears. Use a properly calibrated syphgmomanometer.

- The deflation rate of the column of mercury should be 2–3 mm Hg/second.

- Multiple measurements should be made on different occasions in the sitting position with the back supported for 5 minutes and the arm at heart level.

- At least two readings should be taken on each visit separated by as much time as possible.

- Attempt to avoid "terminal digit preference" (more than 20% of measurements ending with a specific even digit).

- Measure BP in both arms initially, and in the arm with the higher BP thereafter if the difference is greater than 10/5 mm Hg.

1. Home blood pressure measurements—Home BP measurements are indicated for (1) evaluating white-coat hypertension, (2) assessing TOD in response to antihypertensive drug therapy, and (3) improving patients' adherence to therapy. Home BP readings are typically lower (by an average of 12/7 mm Hg), and correlate better with a risk of future mortality, than office BP measurements. Persons with home BP readings of >135/85 mm Hg are generally considered to have hypertension.

2. Ambulatory blood pressure monitoring—Ambulatory BP readings provide BP data during daily activities and sleep and correlate better than home or office readings with TOD, left ventricular hypertrophy (LVH), and cardiovascular event rates. They are indicated for the evaluation of white-coat hypertension in the absence of TOD, episodic hypertension, apparent drug-resistant hypertension, drug-induced hypotensive symptoms, and autonomic dysfunction. As in home BP readings patients are considered to have hypertension if their mean BP during the day is >135/85 mm Hg or >125/75 mm Hg during sleep. Recent outcome studies have demonstrated increased cardiovascular risk associated with abnormal ambulatory blood pressure monitoring (ABPM) profiles (eg, "nondipping" of BP at night).

WHITE-COAT HYPERTENSION—Approximately 25% of those with hypertension have BP readings that are considerably higher in the doctor's office or hospital than those measured at home, at work, or by ABPM. This occurs more commonly among the elderly. The clinical consequences of this diagnosis are higher risk for cardiovascular events and related mortality as compared to normotensive, non-white-coat hypertension patients, but with a lower risk than those with

primary hypertension. Twenty-four hour ambulatory monitoring is needed along with a normal physical examination to confirm the diagnosis. It has been suggested that such stimuli raise BP only transiently and reversibly while others think that these patients will all eventually become sustained hypertensives. Currently, lifestyle modifications with frequent BP monitoring are recommended.

B. Laboratory Findings

Patients with essential hypertension should undergo a limited work-up because extensive laboratory testing may be unrewarding.

1. Cardiac tests—LVH is an objective measure of both the severity and duration of hypertension. It should be routinely evaluated in all patients with an electrocardiogram although an echocardiogram appears to be a better predictor of future cardiovascular events. Other initial laboratory tests include a 9–12 hour fasting lipid profile that includes high-density lipoprotein (HDL), low-density lipoprotein (LDL), and triglycerides, hematocrit, and routine blood chemistries including glucose.

2. Kidney function tests—Current recommendations for evaluation of kidney function include a serum blood urea nitrogen and creatinine, estimated glomerular filtration rate (GFR), electrolytes, and spot urinalysis to detect red blood cells, white blood cells, casts, or proteinuria. Optional tests include measurement of urine albumin excretion or albumin/creatinine ratio and microalbuminuria (protein excretion between 30 and 300 mg/day). Note: All patients with even trace positive protein on routine dipstick should have a spot urine albumin:creatinine checked.

C. Special Examinations

The initial clinic evaluation of a person with elevated BP readings should include the following objectives:

- Determine an accurate diagnosis of hypertension.
- Define the presence or absence of TOD related to hypertension (Table 41–1).
- Screen for other cardiovascular (CV) risk factors or comorbidity that often accompany hypertension (Table 41–1).
- Stratify the risk for cardiovascular disease.
- Assess the likelihood of secondary hypertension and initiate further diagnostic testing to confirm or exclude the diagnosis.
- Obtain data that may be helpful in the choice of therapy and prognosis.

The most important aspects of the history include the natural history of the hypertension, aggravating factors, the extent of TOD, and the presence of other risk factors. Clinical clues suggestive of the possible presence of secondary hypertension must be recognized. The main goals of the physical

Table 41–1. Cardiovascular risk factors and target-organ damage associated with hypertension.

Major risk factors
Hypertension
Cigarette smoking
Obesity (body mass index ≥30)
Physical inactivity
Dyslipidemia
Diabetes mellitus
Microalbuminuria or chronic kidney disease
Age (men >55 years or women >65 years)
Family history of premature cardiovascular disease (men >55 years or women >65 years)
Target-organ damage
Left ventricular hypertrophy
Angina pectoris or prior myocardial infarction
Prior coronary revascularization
Congestive heart failure
Chronic kidney disease
Stroke or transient ischemic attack
Peripheral artery disease
Retinopathy

examination are to evaluate for features of target-organ damage and for evidence of secondary hypertension. Keys areas include verification of the BP in the contralateral arm, fundoscopy, body mass index, waist circumference, auscultation for carotid, abdominal, and femoral bruits, and detection of lower extremity edema.

▶ Complications

Hypertension is associated with major cardiovascular risks such as premature cardiovascular disease, congestive heart failure, LVH, stroke, chronic kidney disease, and end-stage renal disease.

▶ Treatment

The primary goal of antihypertensive therapy is to reduce cardiovascular and renal morbidity and mortality using the least intrusive means possible. Indeed, in clinical trials adequate BP control has been associated with mean reductions of >50% in the incidence of congestive heart failure, >20% in myocardial infarction, and >35% in stroke. Thus, JNC 7 and other national guidelines recommend that all patients with hypertension should have their SBP lowered to below 140 mm Hg and DBP below 90 mm Hg. In patients with hypertension and diabetes or chronic kidney disease, the recommended BP goal is less than 130/80 mm Hg.

Appropriate lifestyle modifications are strongly recommended for all patients with either prehypertension or hypertension. Antihypertensive medications should be started if the BP is >140/90 mm Hg despite an adequate trial of nonpharmacologic treatment. The initiation of two drugs should be strongly considered in all patients with a baseline BP of more than 20/10 mm Hg above goal or stage 2 hypertension. This strategy will increase the likelihood of achieving goal BP within a reasonable time period but should be used cautiously in patients with diabetes and the elderly who are at a higher risk of developing orthostatic hypotension.

A. Life-Style Modification

JNC 7 recommends weight loss for overweight or obese patients with hypertension, limitation of dietary sodium intake to ≤100 mEq/L/day (ie, 2.4 g of sodium or 6 g of sodium chloride) as part of the Dietary Approaches to Stop Hypertension (DASH) eating plan, and moderate alcohol intake of no more than two drinks per day. Increased physical activity such as brisk walking for at least 30 minutes for about 5 days/week is also advised (Table 41–2). Additionally, smoking cessation is also recommended to improve cardiovascular health. The benefits of these interventions include lowering BP, enhancement of antihypertensive efficacy, and reduction of cardiovascular risks.

B. Pharmacologic Treatment

Recent clinical trials have convincingly shown that reduction of BP by most antihypertensive agents will reduce the cardiovascular and renal morbidity and mortality associated with hypertension. The JNC 7 recommends that low-dose thiazide-type diuretics (eg, 12.5–25 mg of chlorthalidone or hydrochlorothiazide) should be used as initial therapy for most patients with hypertension either alone in stage 1 hypertension or in combination with other agents such as angiotensin-converting enzyme (ACE) inhibitors, angiotensin receptor blockers (ARBs), calcium channel blockers (CCBs) or β-blockers in stage 2 hypertension. The thiazide-diuretic based regimen has been shown by recent clinical trials including Antihypertensive and Lipid-Lowering Treatment to Prevent Heart Attack Trial (ALLHAT) to prevent or reduce the cardiovascular complications of hypertension and is associated with a low rate of metabolic complications. Most patients will need two or more antihypertensive agents to achieve the recommended BP goal. If the low-dose thiazide monotherapy is inadequate to achieve the BP goal an ACE inhibitor or ARB should be added. This combination is synergistic and effective in lowering BP, especially among African-Americans and the elderly. Other antihypertensive agents can be added sequentially or substituted at monthly intervals until the BP goal is reached (Figure 41–1). After the BP goal has been achieved and remains stable, patients can be followed up at 3- to 6-month intervals.

Table 41-2. Lifestyle modifications to manage essential hypertension.[1]

Modification	Recommendation	Approximate Reduction in Systolic Blood Pressure[2]
Weight reduction	Maintain normal body weight (body mass index 18.5–24.9 kg/m^2)	5–20 mm Hg/10 kg
Adopt DASH eating plan	Consume a diet rich in fruits, vegetables, and low-fat dairy products with a reduced content of saturated and total fat	8–14 mm Hg
Dietary sodium reduction	Reduce dietary sodium intake to no more than 100 mmol/day (2.4 g sodium or 6 g sodium chloride)	2–8 mm Hg
Physical activity	Engage in regular aerobic physical activity such as brisk walking (at least 30 minutes/day, most days of the week)	4–9 mm Hg
Moderation of alcohol consumption	Limit consumption to no more than two drinks (eg, 24 oz beer, 10 oz wine, or 3 oz 80-proof whiskey) per day in most men and to no more than one drink per day in women and in lighter-weight persons	2–4 mm Hg

[1]For overall cardiovascular risk reduction, stop smoking.
[2]The effects of implementing these modifications are dose and time dependent and could be greater for some individuals.
DASH, Dietary Approaches to Stop Hypertension.

C. Treatment of Specific Clinical Conditions

The general recommendations for initial therapy should be adapted for particular clinical conditions in which specific antihypertensive agents have been shown to be beneficial by outcome data from clinical trials, what JNC 7 refers to as compelling indications. These include the demonstration that renin–angiotensin–aldosterone blockers such as ACE inhibitors or ARBs improve outcome in high-risk settings such as patients with diabetes mellitus, congestive heart failure, myocardial infarction, stroke, chronic kidney disease, or albuminuria and that β-blockers improve survival in patients with systolic heart failure and prior myocardial infarction.

1. Diabetes and hypertension—The combination of hypertension and diabetes significantly increases the risk of cardiovascular events and end-stage renal disease than either risk factor alone. Recent clinical outcome trials and guidelines have solidified the role of renal angiotensin aldosterone antagonists such as ACE inhibitors and ARBs in delaying the progression of diabetic nephropathy and reducing cardiovascular events and they are indicated as agents of first choice in all patients with diabetes. Additionally, based on the ALLHAT Trial, thiazide diuretics must be included as part of the drug therapy for most patients with diabetes. Combinations of two or more antihypertensive drugs are

usually needed to achieve the recommended goal BP of less than 130/80 mm Hg. If the BP goal is not achieved other drugs such as CCBs and vasodilating β-blockers are added until goal BP is attained.

2. Congestive heart failure (CHF)—Hypertension is a major risk factor for the subsequent development of both systolic and diastolic heart failure. For many patients, LVH is an important intermediate step, resulting in "hypertensive heart disease" with impaired LV filling and increased ventricular stiffness. The BP goal for most patients with CHF is less than 140/90 mm Hg. Asymptomatic patients with "reduced LV function" [left ventricular ejection fraction (LVEF) <40%] improve both their BP and long-term prognosis with an ACEI and β-blocker while patients with symptomatic systolic heart failure will require additional agents such as ARBs, aldosterone antagonists, and loop diuretics. Treatment of hypertension in CHF patients with preserved LV function has not been as well studied. In general, β-blockers or non-dihydropyridine (DHP)-CCBs are recommended to increase diastolic filling time and decrease heart rate, but there are currently no randomized clinical trials with outcome data to demonstrate their long-term efficacy.

3. Coronary artery disease (CAD)—The coexistence of CAD and hypertension is an indication for therapy with multiple antihypertensive drugs to achieve a goal BP of less

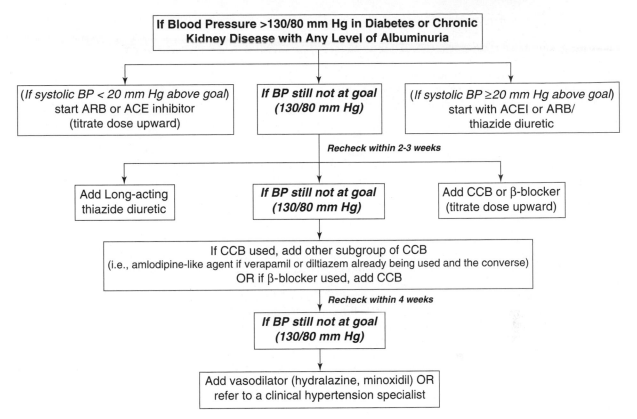

▲ Figure 41–1. Algorithm for the management of essential hypertension in kidney disease. BP, blood pressure; ACE, angiotensin-converting enzyme; ACEI, ACE inhibitors; ARB, angiotensin receptor blockers; CCB, calcium channel blockers.

than 140/90 mm Hg. In patients with hypertension and stable angina, β-blockers are strongly recommended but long-acting CCBs are suitable and effective alternatives based on the results of recent outcome trials such as the International Verapamil/Trandolapril Study in which more than 22,000 patients with hypertension and coronary disease were randomized to either atenolol or verapamil. Patients with acute coronary syndromes or post-myocardial infarction should be initially treated with ACE inhibitors, β-blockers, and aldosterone antagonists. Additional recommendations include intensive treatment of dyslipidemia (to achieve or exceed an LDL-cholesterol target of <100 mg/dL) and anti-platelet therapy with aspirin or dypyridamole.

4. Left ventricular hypertrophy (LVH)—LVH is a well-recognized independent risk factor for cardiovascular events and premature death. It is common in the elderly and is often associated with diastolic dysfunction. Intensive BP management with agents that induce regression of LVH and reduce BP to a goal of less than 140/90 mm Hg is recommended. Recent clinical trials indicate that ARBs are very effective agents for the reduction of LVH but other interventions

such as weight loss, exercise, and sodium restriction are also effective.

5. Stroke—In acute ischemic stroke, the optimal level of BP is controversial. Acute lowering of the BP may lead to a reduction in blood flow to "watershed" areas of the brain with worsening of the neurologic function. In this setting, control of BP to intermediate levels of 160/100 mm Hg is appropriate. In stable patients, ACE inhibitors and thiazide diuretics are recommended to lower BP to a goal of less than 140/90 mm Hg and reduce recurrence of stroke.

6. Chronic kidney disease (CKD)—A majority of patients with CKD have hypertension and the therapeutic goals are to slow the progression of renal disease and to prevent cardiovascular disease. Optimal BP control to a goal of less than 130/80 mm Hg is strongly recommended. ACE inhibitors and ARBs are recommended for initial therapy because they have been shown to retard the progression of both diabetic and nondiabetic renal disease. An increase of the serum creatinine level by as much as 35% over baseline after initiation of these drugs should not lead to discontinuation because of the long-term benefits of these agents. For increases of serum creatinine larger than 35%, an assessment for concomitant nonsteroidal anti-inflammatory drug (NSAID) use, volume depletion, and/or renovascular hypertension is appropriate. Most patients will require three or more BP drugs to achieve the goal BP and loop diuretics are usually added when the estimated GFR is less than 30 mL/minute/1.73 m^2.

7. Albuminuria/proteinuria—In all patients with hypertension, albuminuria or proteinuria is an established risk marker for progression of renal disease and has also emerged as an independent marker of cardiovascular risk. Recent pharmacologic interventions with agents that lower BP and reduce albuminuria have resulted in a significant delay and even an arrest in the progression of microalbuminuria to CKD. Moreover, a reduction in proteinuria of more than 50% from baseline following 6 months of treatment reduces the risk of end-stage renal disease by 72% at 5 years. Recent outcome clinical trial data and current guidelines recommend that patients with hypertension with albuminuria should be started on agents that block the renin–angiotensin–aldosterone system, such as ACE inhibitors or ARBs. It has also been shown that maximal dose combinations of ACE inhibitors and ARBs agents further reduce albuminuria by an additional 30–35% over either agent alone, which correlates with slower kidney disease progression independent of BP. Nondihydropyridine CCBs such as verapamil or diltiazem also reduce proteinuria in patients with hypertension with proteinuric kidney disease, and have additive effects when combined with ACE inhibitors.

ALLHAT Officers and Coordinators for the ALLHAT Collaborative Research Group. Major outcomes in high-risk hypertensive patients randomized to angiotensin-converting enzyme inhibitor or calcium channel blocker vs. diuretic: The Antihypertensive and Lipid Lowering Treatment to Prevent Heart Attack Trial (ALLHAT). JAMA 2002; 288:2981.

Bakris GL et al: Differential effects of calcium antagonist subclasses on markers of nephropathy progression. Kidney Int 2004;65(6):1991.

Chobanian AV et al: The Seventh Report of the Joint National Committee on the Detection, Evaluation, and Treatment of High Blood Pressure (JNC 7). JAMA 2003;289:2560.

Clement DL et al: Prognostic value of ambulatory blood pressure recordings in patients with treated hypertension. N Engl J Med 2003;348:2407.

Ibsen H et al: Reduction in albuminuria translates to reduction in cardiovascular events in hypertensive patients: losartan intervention for endpoint reduction in hypertension study. Hypertension 2005;45:198.

Nakao N et al: Combination treatment of angiotensin-II receptor blocker and angiotensin-converting enzyme inhibitor in non-diabetic renal disease (COOPERATE): a randomized controlled trial. Lancet 2003;361:117.

Pepine CJ et al: A calcium antagonist vs. a non-calcium antagonist hypertension treatment strategy for patients with coronary artery disease. The International Verapamil-Trandolapril Study (INVEST): a randomized controlled trial. JAMA 2003;290:2805.

Pitt B et al: Eplerenone, a selective aldosterone blocker, in patients with left ventricular dysfunction after myocardial infarction. N Engl J Med 2003;348:1309.

Secondary Hypertension

William J. Elliott, MD, PhD, Priya Kalahasti, MD,
Sey M. Lau, MD, Joseph V. Nally, Jr., MD, &
Celso E. Gomez-Sanchez, MD

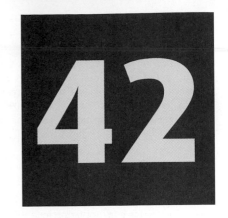

▼ GENERAL APPROACHES

William J. Elliott, MD, PhD

ESSENTIALS OF DIAGNOSIS

► Abrupt onset of hypertension.

► Blood pressure ≥160/100 mm Hg.

► Considerable target-organ damage.

► Positive result of a highly specific diagnostic test.

► Adequate response to therapy for the specific type of secondary hypertension.

More than 95% of Americans with hypertension have no specific cause for their elevated blood pressure (BP). It is important, however, to consider the possibility that newly diagnosed hypertension has a specific cause, for three reasons. First, BP control is often difficult to achieve in people with secondary causes of hypertension; diagnosing it early is likely to get BP to goal more quickly. Second, and particularly important in younger people, diagnosing and treating secondary hypertension will reduce the future burden of treatment (both expenditures for pills and follow-up and adverse effects of therapy) and improve the quality of life. For some secondary causes, specific and potentially curative therapy is available. Lastly, routine consideration of secondary causes when the diagnosis of hypertension is first made will ensure that at least once during the person's lifetime the possibility of secondary hypertension will be entertained. The risks and benefits of further testing can therefore be critically evaluated.

Patients with an identifiable secondary cause of hypertension typically present with a relatively abrupt onset of symptoms (BP ≥160/100 mm Hg) and with considerable target-organ damage. They typically do not respond as well to lowering BP and to antihypertensive drug therapy as do patients with primary hypertension. The BP-lowering response to specific antihypertensive drugs may offer important clues to the presence and type of secondary hypertension; for example, patients with early renovascular hypertension often have an impressive BP-lowering response to an angiotensin-converting enzyme (ACE) inhibitor and those with bilateral adrenal hyperplasia as a cause of primary aldosteronism respond well to spironolactone, but not vice versa. The most common forms of secondary hypertension and useful tests for each will be discussed individually. The choice of tests and the order in which they are obtained depend not only on the pretest probability of the disease, but also on safety, availability, local expertise with the test, and its cost.

▼ RENOVASCULAR HYPERTENSION

Priya Kalahasti, MD, Sey M. Lau, MD, & Joseph V. Nally, Jr., MD

ESSENTIALS OF DIAGNOSIS

► Renovascular hypertension (RVHT) is the most common cause of secondary hypertension in the United States.

► RVHT is an elevation of blood pressure (BP) due to activation of the renin–angiotensin system in the setting of renal artery occlusive disease.

► The diagnosis of RVHT can be made only if BP improves following intervention, thereby making RVHT a retrospective diagnosis.

► The presence of anatomic renal artery stenosis (RAS) is not synonymous with RVHT.

► Progressive and occlusive renovascular disease may lead to impaired kidney function, termed "ischemic nephropathy."

▶ General Considerations

A. Clinical Clues

Recognition of important clinical clues for RVHT is paramount in the clinical diagnosis of this condition. RVHT probably occurs in less than 1% of unscreened patients with mild hypertension. By comparison, 10–30% of white patients with severe or refractory hypertension may have renal artery disease. Pertinent clinical clues for RVHT are summarized in Table 42–1.

B. Epidemiology

Essential or primary hypertension is the most common form of Hypertension, occurring in >90% of the more than 50 million Americans with elevated BP (Table 42–2). Of the 5–10% of hypertensive patients with secondary hypertension, RVHT accounts for 0.2–3%. However, at autopsy the prevalence of anatomic RAS attributable to atherosclerosis (ASO) in the elderly is quite common. Clinically, RAS may coexist in 20–25% of patients undergoing cardiac catheterization for coronary artery disease (CAD). Similarly, approximately 6% of patients with end-stage renal disease (ESRD) have a concomitant diagnosis of RAS. However, it is unclear whether the occlusive RAS was etiologic in the development of end-stage kidney failure.

C. Etiology

The etiology of RAS is usually attributable to ASO or fibromuscular disease (FMD). As can be seen in Table 42–2, ASO accounts for over 70% of RAS. It is generally seen in an older hypertensive population with concomitant diffuse ASO in other vascular beds (eg, coronary, carotids, and peripheral circulation). The RAS lesion due to ASO occurs at the ostium or in the proximal 2 cm of the renal artery. In contrast, FMD accounts for 20–25% of RAS and is typically seen in younger female hypertensive patients. Table 42–3 lists other less common causes of RAS.

Table 42–1. Clinical clues to renovascular hypertension.

Severe or refractory hypertension
Age of onset younger than 30 years or older than 55 years
Abrupt acceleration of stable hypertension
Severe hypertension in the setting of generalized atherosclerosis
Systolic-diastolic bruit in the epigastrium
Flash pulmonary edema
Unexplained azotemia
ACE inhibitor- or ARB-induced renal dysfunction

ACE, angiotensin-converting enzyme; ARB, angiotensin receptor blocker.

Table 42–2. Classification of hypertension.

Classification	Prevalence (%)
Essential (primary) hypertension	90 to 95
Secondary hypertension	5 to 10
Renal	2.6 to 6.0
Renovascular hypertension	0.2 to 3.0
Endocrine (primary aldosteronis, pheochromocytoma, thyroid disease, etc.)	1 to 2

▶ Pathogenesis

The pathophysiology of renovascular hypertension is best explained by the sentinel animal experiments by Goldblatt. These animal models consist of occluding one or both renal arteries with constricting clips. The two-kidney one-clip (2K-1C) model represents unilateral RAS whereas the two-kidney two-clip (2K-2C) model represents bilateral RAS. Unilateral stenosis in a solitary functioning kidney, such as in renal transplant patients, is represented by the one-kidney one-clip (1K-1C) model. Both the 2K-2C and 1K-1C models share similar features.

The mechanism of development of hypertension is mediated via the renin–angiotensin–aldosterone system (RAAS) with salt and water retention. In unilateral RAS (2K-1C model), renal perfusion pressure is decreased in the kidney distal to the stenosis, which leads to increased renin production, which in turn forms angiotensin II (AT II). AT II causes vasoconstriction directly and also stimulates aldosterone production, which causes salt and water

Table 42–3. Etiology of renovascular hypertension.

Cause	Prevalence (%)	Clues/characteristics
Atherosclerosis (ASO)	70	Older patients (>55 years of age)
		Concomitant diffuse ASO in other vascular beds
		Ostial or proximal (2 cm) renal artery lesions
Fibromuscular dysplasia (FMD)	20	Younger women
		Unclear etiology
Others		Extrinsic compression by tumor
		Retroperitoneal mass
		Arterial dissection
		Vasculitis
		Aneurysm

retention. The normal contralateral kidney undergoes a pressure natriuresis, which maintains volume status. Due to the constantly elevated levels of renin in the 2K-1C model, this form of RAS is referred to as renin-mediated hypertension.

On the other hand, in the 2K-2C or 1K-1C models representing bilateral RAS or RAS to a solitary kidney, there is an initial increase in renin, which in turn causes an increase in AT II and aldosterone. As in the model described, resultant salt and water retention occurs, but the absence of a normal contralateral kidney prevents pressure natriuresis. Suppression of renin occurs due to volume expansion attributed to the increases in salt and water retention. This form of hypertension is considered volume mediated, whereas the 2K-1C model of unilateral RAS is renin mediated.

A. What Is Significant Stenosis?

Stenosis that causes hemodynamic changes with a reduction in renal perfusion pressure is called critical stenosis. In Goldblatt's experimental models, 80–85% renal artery constriction induces significant hemodynamic changes. In humans, a >75% degree of RAS is thought to cause critical hemodynamic changes. Clinically, this is of importance as modest RAS may be present in many older patients, but may not be sufficient to produce hemodynamically significant lesions.

B. Stages of Experimental Renovascular Hypertension

1. Phase 1: Acute phase—There is an immediate rise in BP as a result of increased levels of renin. This initial rise in BP, whether in the 2K-1C or in the 1K-1C model, is renin–angiotensin mediated. Removal of the stenosis reverses the hypertension.

2. Phase 2: Transition phase—This phase lasts for few days to many weeks in the experimental model. Salt and water retention occur, along with a subsequent fall in plasma renin. Nevertheless, in this phase, removal of the stenosis may reverse the hypertension.

3. Phase 3: Chronic phase—Over time, vascular changes and renal parenchymal disease may develop due to the hemodynamic and nonhemodynamic effects of AT II. The importance of this phase is that removal of the stenotic lesion fails to correct the hypertension. In this phase, blockade of RAAS may not decrease the BP.

▶ Clinical Findings

The two major goals of the evaluation of the hypertensive patient are to recognize clinical clues for secondary forms of hypertension and to identify evidence of target-organ damage (TOD) from the hypertension. The clinical clues suggestive of RVHT are listed in Table 42–1

A. Symptoms and Signs

RVHT should be suspected in patients presenting with severe, sudden-onset hypertension prior to 30 years of age or after 55 years of age. For reasons that are not well understood, RVHT is relatively less common in African-Americans in whom severe hypertension is most frequently essential. Because fibromuscular dysplasia occurs in younger patients (mainly women), those presenting with hypertension before 30 years of age should be suspected of having RVHT. However, RVHT due to ASO is likely to present in older patients with significant hypertension in the setting of generalized ASO in other vascular beds. Malignant hypertension with neurologic symptoms and advanced fundoscopic changes with papilledema should raise the possibility of RVHT. Similarly, severe or refractory hypertension defined as hypertension requiring three or more drugs as well as severe hypertension with heart failure/ flash pulmonary edema may also be one of the presenting features of RVHT. Importantly, this sudden onset of worsening azotemia after the institution of an angiotensin-converting enzyme (ACE) inhibitor or AT II receptor blockers (ARB) should suggest RVHT, especially bilateral RAS or RAS with a solitary functioning kidney. In such patients, with all of their functioning kidney mass distal to a critical RAS, maintenance of the glomerular filtration rate (GFR) is dependent upon efferent arteriolar vasoconstriction mediated by AT II. Once this preservation of function is lost after administration of an ACE or ARB, a decline in renal function is seen.

The presence of severe stage II hypertension (greater than 160–100 mm Hg) may be a critical clue to the presence of RVHT. The presence of an abdominal bruit in the setting of increased BP is also a strong clinical clue to RAS. The bruit is systolic–diastolic in nature and is located near the epigastrium. This is seen more commonly in fibromuscular dysplasia and, in fact, correlates with surgical outcomes. The absence of such a bruit does not exclude RAS. The presence of stage III or IV hypertensive retinopathy on fundus examination is highly suggestive of RVHT. Evidence of diffuse ASO in the peripheral vascular, coronary, and cerebral vascular beds may be suggestive of RVHT due to ASO renal artery disease in the older hypertensive population.

By definition RVHT requires an elevation of BP due to the activation of the renin–angiotensin system in the setting of renal artery occlusive disease. The diagnosis of RVHT can be made only if BP improves after a correction of RAS, thereby making RVHT a retrospective diagnosis. The primary goal in screening for RVHT is to identify a subset of patients who may have a reversible hemodynamic cause of their hypertension and/or renal dysfunction. Table 42–4 summarizes the specificity and sensitivity of these diagnostic modalities

B. Laboratory Findings

1. Electrolytes—Hypokalemia may be a surrogate marker of hemodynamically significant renal artery occlusive disease

Table 42–4. Specificity and sensitivity.

Test	Sensitivity (%)	Specificity (%)
Plasma renin activity (PRA)	50–80	84
Functional studies		
Captopril PRA	74	89
Captopril scintigraphy/ renography	85–90	93–98
Anatomic studies		
Duplex ultrasound scanning	90	90–95
Spiral (helical) computed tomography scanning	98	94
Magnetic resonance Angiography	90–100	76–94

Modified with permission from Nally JV et al: Advances in non-invasive screening for renovascular disease. Cleve Clin J Med 1994;61:328.

secondary to stimulation of the renin–angiotensin system with secondary hyperaldosteronism. The hyperaldosteronism results in urinary sodium retention and kaliuresis, which may be responsible for the development of hypokalemia.

2. Renal function—RVHT may be seen in patients with or without renal dysfunction. RVHT and possible ischemic nephropathy may be suspected in patients with unexplained azotemia occurring in the setting of generalized ASO and asymmetric kidney sizes (possibly due to the occlusive RAS). As noted previously, azotemia following the administration of an ACE inhibitor or ARB is a strong clinical clue suggestive of hemodynamically significant renal artery disease.

3. Plasma renin activity and direct renin—Historically, plasma renin activity (PRA) was measured to evaluate patients with RVHT. PRA was determined indirectly by measurement of AT I because the amount of AT I produced from angiotensinogen is proportional to the renin enzyme concentration. This reaction is dependent on the amount of angiotensinogen present and can underestimate the renin concentration in patients with severe heart or liver failure who have markedly low levels of angiotensinogen. Direct renin measurements are now determined by specific monoclonal antibodies to renin. Direct renin assays are now available clinically and may offer clinical advantages in terms of accuracy and more rapid reporting of results (a prior PRA level of 1 ng/mL/hour converts to a direct renin level of 8.4 mU/L).

Unfortunately, PRA has been an insensitive method of screening with elevated levels present in only 50–80% of patients with RVHT. Moreover, up to 15% of patients with essential hypertension have elevated PRA levels, making PRA a nonspecific determinant of RVHT. Although infrequently used in usual medical practices today due to its low sensitivity and specificity, a very low PRA (if plasma renin activity is very low, <1 ng/mL/hour, in the absence of drugs known to suppress renin) can strongly argue against RVHT as the cause of elevated BP. Captopril-stimulated PRA testing may be preferable to PRA determination alone in the evaluation of the patient with RVHT.

C. Imaging Studies

1. Renal scintigraphy/renography—Commonly used radionuclide agents include technetium-99m diethylenetri-aminepentaacetic acid (DTPA), which is used as a marker of GFR because it is exclusively excreted by glomerular filtration, and technetium-99m-labeled mercaptoacetyltriglycine (MAG3), which is used to approximate the renal plasma flow rate and, in contrast to DTPA, is excreted both by glomerular filtration and tubular secretion.

2. Captopril scintigraphy/renography—Since the ischemic kidney is dependent upon the effects of AT II to induce efferent artery vasoconstriction to maintain the GFR, the introduction of captopril is expected to lower the GFR of the affected kidney distal to the stenosis. The results after captopril are demonstrated by a decreased uptake of DTPA (decreased GFR) with little change in MAG3 uptake (preserved renal plasma flow rate), but a delayed excretion phase of MAG3 compared to renal scans without captopril provocation (Figure 42–1). Limitations of this technique for screening include decreased sensitivity in patients with renal dysfunction. A positive finding provides clear evidence that the occlusive disease is hemodynamically significant and that intervention is likely to improve BP control.

3. Atherosclerotic renal artery stenosis—Atherosclerotic lesions are ostial or proximal within the first 2 cm of the renal artery, and typically do not occur in the distal portion of the renal arteries.

4. Fibromuscular disease—Medial fibroplasia will appear as a "string of beads"(the beads are of larger caliber than the artery), and is often located at the mid to distal portion of the renal artery.

5. Renal angiography/arteriography—The gold standard in detecting renal artery occlusive disease remains renal angiography/arteriography because it provides maximum information about the vascular architecture as well as an opportunity for intervention if hemodynamically significant lesions are found. With the advent of digital subtraction angiography, less contrast media can be given to obtain images, thus decreasing the risk of developing contrast-induced

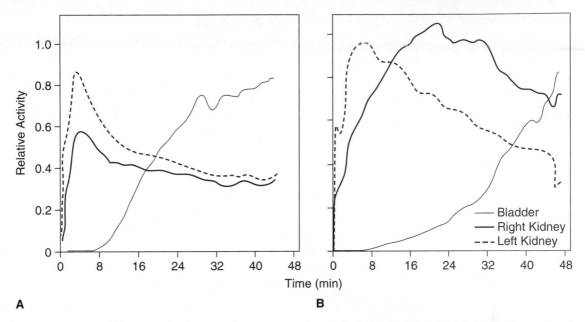

A   **B**

▲ **Figure 42–1.** Captopril scintigraphy/renography. A Tc-DTPA time–activity curve at baseline **(A)** and after captopril **(B)** in a patient with stenosis of the right renal artery. The diagnosis of renal artery stenosis is based on asymmetry of renal size and function, as well as a delayed time to maximal activity (>11 minutes), significant asymmetry of the peak activity of each kidney, marked cortical retention of the radionuclide, and marked reduction in calculated glomerular filtration rate of the ipsilateral kidney. (Adapted with permission from Nally JV et al: Advances in noninvasive screening for renovascular hypertension disease. Cleve Clin J Med1994;61:328.)

nephropathy. Techniques developed to avoid the use of contrast media include carbon dioxide (CO_2) angiography, which lowers the risk of renal toxicity, but also lowers the resolution of the image. Other complications that can result from invasive renal angiography include renal artery dissection and generation of atheroemboli.

6. Magnetic resonance angiography—A noninvasive method of defining the renal artery vasculature includes magnetic resonance angiography (MRA), which modifies the magnetic resonance imaging (MRI) to examine patterns of blood flow. In renal vascular disease, there is reduced blood flow distal to a stenotic lesion that causes a loss of MRA signaling. Unfortunately, loss of MRA signaling is also commonly encountered in distal vessels of normal patients thereby exaggerating the amount of narrowing found, especially in the distal half of the artery. Gadolinium MRA has been shown to significantly improve the images of the distal arteries and accessory renal arteries. Although gadolinium-enhanced MRA has previously been suggested to be an alternative non-nephrotoxic method in defining the renal artery vasculature, its use should be avoided in those with renal dysfunction due to the well-described association between gadolinium and the development of nephrogenic fibrosing dermopathy (NFD) and systemic fibrosis (NSF). Contraindications to the use of MRA include patients with claustrophobia and those with

metallic implants/foreign bodies. MRA may not be as useful in detecting FMD as compared to renal angiography due to the increased spatial resolution of MRA (1 mm versus 200 νm).

7. Spiral (helical) computed tomography scanning—High quality images, as well as three-dimensional images, of the renal arteries can be obtained using this technique. By using a continuously rotating tube and an advancing table, images can be obtained in less than 1 minute, thereby significantly reducing motion artifact. Unfortunately, as with conventional renal angiography, contrast media must be administered and therefore the concerns for nephrotoxicity exist.

8. Duplex ultrasound scanning—Over the years, the non-invasive renal ultrasound has replaced intravenous pyelography (IVP) as the preferred method of obtaining information regarding the assessment of kidney size. Direct visualization of the renal arteries can be obtained (by B-mode imaging) and measurement of hemodynamic factors can be achieved by pulse Doppler ultrasound. Duplex ultrasound scanning is generally reported as lesions causing 0–59% stenosis and those causing 60–99% stenosis. Areas that are 0–59% stenosed are unlikely to cause lesions that are hemodynamically significant, whereas lesions that are 60–99% stenosed indicate a further need for investigation. A drawback to duplex ultrasound scanning is that the procedure is operator dependent due to its high technical demands.

9. Renal resistive indices—Renal resistive indices are also provided by duplex ultrasound. RI approximates the amount of renal arterial impedance. In patients with RAS, an increase in renal resistive index >80% is associated with poorer post-revascularization outcome as well as an increased risk of progressive renal dysfunction.

D. Special Tests

1. Captopril-stimulated plasma renin activity test—By comparing PRA at baseline and at 1 hour after an oral dose of 25–50 mg of captopril (a short-acting ACE inhibitor), the predictive value of PRA may be increased and used to discriminate essential hypertension from RVHT. Studies have shown larger elevations in PRA and greater reductions in BP after captopril in patients with RVHT compared to those with essential hypertension (see Table 42–5). Major limitations to the widespread use of this screening method include decreased reliability of the test in patients with renal dysfunction, inability to determine unilateral versus bilateral disease, nonstandardized assay methodology of PRA between institutions, and improper patient preparation prior to testing. Ideally patients should ingest dietary salt *ad libitum* and hold antihypertensive medications for 2 weeks (especially ACE inhibitors, diuretics, and β-blocking agents) prior to the captopril PRA testing.

2. Differential renal vein renin determinations—Historically used to assess the functional significance of renal vascular stenosis, the determination of the renal vein renin ratio has fallen out of favor because of the invasive nature of the procedure, the associated technical difficulties, the inability to detect bilateral stenosis, and the high false-negative rate. The procedure is done by obtaining blood samples from each of the renal veins and the inferior vena cava (below the level of the renal artery). Lateralization of the renal vein renin ratio predicts substantial improvement in BP control after surgical intervention. Renal vein renin ratios are considered to be lateralized when the ratio is greater than 1.5 (ipsilateral to contralateral kidney).

Table 42–5. Renin criteria for captopril test that distinguish patients with renovascular hypertension from those with essential hypertension.

Stimulated plasma renin activity of 12 ng/mL or more
Absolute increase in PRA of 10 ng/mL/hour or more
Percent increase in PRA
Increase in PRA of 150% if baseline PRA >3 ng/mL/hour
Increase in PRA of 400% if baseline PRA <3 ng/mL/hour

Reproduced with permission from Pohl MA: Renovascular hypertension and ischemic nephropathy. In: *Atlas of Diseases of the Kidney.* Schrier RW, Ed. Blackwell Science/Current Medicine Inc., 1998, p. 3.11 (http://www.kidneyatlas.org/book3/adk3-03.QXD.pdf).

▶ Treatment

The goals of therapy are optimal control of hypertension and preservation of renal function, which can be achieved either through medical therapy, percutaneous renal angioplasty (PTRA) with or without stenting, or renovascular bypass surgery. The optimal treatment of patients with RVHT remains an elusive goal because there are no randomized controlled trials comparing medical versus surgical versus renal angioplasty versus renal stents on BP control and/or the preservation of kidney function.

A. Medical Therapy

Medical therapy is often required either for short-term management prior to an intervention or for long-term management of unstable patients or those whose BP is easily controlled with preserved GFR. Long-term medical therapy is often recommended for patients who are not optimal surgical candidates, patients with multiple comorbidities, and those with technically difficult revascularization. The medical management of RVHT is similar to that of primary hypertension, yet three important distinctions exist: (1) Hypertension may be more difficult to control and often requires multiple medications from different classes, (2) vigilant attention must be given to preserving kidney function, and (3) coexistent atherosclerotic cardiac and carotid disease are more prevalent and may require specific intervention. The response to a specific drug may be variable and highly individualized. All patients with RVHT may not readily respond to antihypertensive therapy. Historically, early studies in the 1960s did not show much success when a thiazide diuretic and hydralazine were employed. Later, with the advent of β-blockers and agents that interrupt the renin–angiotensin system, major improvements in medical therapy were seen.

1. Angiotensin–converting enzyme inhibitors and angiotensin II receptor blockers—In patients with unilateral RAS, ACE inhibitors are the preferred agent of choice. To achieve optimal control of hypertension, these agents are often combined with other antihypertensive agents, especially diuretics. Optimal control may be achieved in up to 96% of patients with an ACE inhibitor. The initial review of captopril therapy in 269 patients showed successful short-term control of BP in 74%. In a comparison study of Enalapril and a diuretic with standard triple drug therapy, control was seen in 96% of patients on an ACE inhibitor versus 62% on triple drug therapy. In unilateral RAS, the fall in GFR in the stenotic kidney due to AT II inhibition by an ACE inhibitor is not reflected, as the total GFR does not fall due to compensation of filtration in the contralateral kidney. In bilateral RAS, the GFR is maintained by AT II. Inhibition of AT II by an ACE inhibitor can cause hemodynamic changes causing a further reduction in GFR. A loss in the autoregulatory mechanism of efferent arteriolar constriction occurs in patients who are on an ACE inhibitor. This effect is also potentiated by volume contraction induced by a diuretic. Thus, in patients with bilateral RAS, a combination of an ACE inhibitor and diuretic should be used with caution. Despite the reduction of the potent vasoconstrictor AT II, medical control of hypertension is often difficult to achieve with these agents, especially if the hypertension has been present for over 3–5 years. Underlying severe ASO and/or the presence of chronic kidney disease (CKD) makes the hypertension difficult to manage.

2. Calcium channel blockers—Calcium channel blockers (CCBs) are effective in lowering the BP in patients with RVHT. They also maintain renal blood flow through vasodilation in the afferent arteriole. The benefit of using CCBs in RVHT is they have a more favorable effect on renal function compared to an ACE inhibitor. They can be used safely in patients with bilateral RAS without concern for a significant decline in the GFR. In one study, nifedipine produced a smaller reduction in GFR as compared to captopril. All three categories of CCBs, the dihydropyridines (nifedipine, felodipine, amlodipine), benzothiazipines (diltiazem), and phenylalkylamines (verapamil), have been used as antihypertensive medications for patients with or without RAS.

B. Surgical Therapy

1. Percutaneous renal artery intervention—Selected patients with RAS may benefit from percutaneous revascularization. Revascularization is often recommended when control of hypertension becomes difficult despite multiple antihypertensive medications. Patients with long-standing renal parenchymal disease may not benefit from PTRA. Nevertheless, a recent pronounced decline in GFR before PTRA may predict a favorable outcome. Renal angiography with and without renal artery stenting has become the major form of renal revascularization. The technical success rate is high, yet long-term studies reporting BP control or preservation of kidney function are either inconclusive or in progress. Recommendations vary as to whether the RAS is due to FMD or to ASO.

2. Percutaneous renal artery intervention for fibromuscular dysplasia—PTRA is the initial choice in younger patients with fibromuscular disease. Correction is indicated to control hypertension and to prevent progressive renal disease. Results for percutaneous intervention in the majority of patients with FMD have been very good and comparable to surgical therapy. Indication for surgical intervention in these patients is due to branch renal artery involvement, which makes PTRA technically difficult. As many as 30% of FMD patients may have branch renal artery disease requiring surgical intervention.

3. Atherosclerotic renal artery stenosis—There have been three randomized controlled trials comparing the merits of medical therapy versus percutaneous revascularization in terms of BP control and/or renal function in RAS

attributable to atherosclerosis (ASO-RAS). Fifty-five hypertensive patients with sustained hypertension attributed to RAS with a minimum diastolic BP of 95 mm Hg on at least two antihypertensive drugs were randomized to either medical therapy or PTRA without stenting. In patients with bilateral RAS randomized to angioplasty, a significant fall in BP was observed at the latest follow-up (3–54 months). There was no clinically or statistically significant difference noted in either the medical or the angioplasty arm in patients with unilateral stenosis. No significant renal outcomes were noted in either unilateral or bilateral stenosis.

The largest randomized controlled trial of PTRA without stenting was conducted by the Dutch Renal Artery Stenosis Intervention Cooperative Study Group. They randomized 106 patients with ASO-RAS to medical therapy or PTRA. At the end of 12 months, there were no significant differences between the two groups in BP, renal function, and antihypertensive drug therapy. They concluded that angioplasty has little advantage over medical therapy. The limitation of the study was the high crossover rate from medical therapy to intervention and lack of stent use. Currently, studies examining medical therapy versus renal artery angioplasty with stenting are ongoing.

4. Renal artery bypass surgery—Earlier reports had suggested a survival benefit for RAS patients who underwent renal artery bypass surgery versus medical therapy. However, these observations came from nonrandomized studies in which there was an inherent bias for healthier patients to undergo surgery. To date, there is a single randomized trial comparing medical therapy and renovascular surgery in patients with high-grade bilateral RAS or RAS to a solitary kidney. The primary endpoints were doubling of serum creatinine, uncontrolled hypertension, renal failure, or death. There were no significant differences between the medical and surgical groups in this randomized, controlled study. Given the lack of a clear mandate in the treatment of patients with hemodynamically significant renovascular disease, recent guidelines by the National Kidney Foundation suggest referral of such patients to an expert in the field of hypertension and kidney disease for specific medical and/or interventive therapy tailored to that individual. Currently, percutaneous angiography with stent placement is increasingly being used in the treatment of ASO-RAS. Although this form of intervention is more likely to maintain artery patency when clinically successful, there is a lack of clinical evidence from long-term trials that stenting has demonstrable benefits on BP control, preservation of kidney function, or patient morbidity and mortality from cardiovascular events. At present, three trials are ongoing in the United States and abroad comparing medical therapy to renal angioplasty with stenting in patients with ASO-RAS. Definitive recommendations regarding the management of RVHT awaits the conclusions of these important trials.

Izzo JL, Black HR, Eds. *Hypertension Primer*, 3rd ed. American Heart Association, 2003.

▼ ENDOCRINE HYPERTENSION

Celso E. Gomez-Sanchez, MD

Several endocrine organs produce hormones that participate in the control of blood pressure (BP) by the regulation of salt and water homeostasis or vascular tone. The mechanisms of hypertension vary according to the hormonal disorder and may be direct, eg, neralocorticoid hypertension and pheochromocytoma or indirect, as in hyperparathyroidism or acromegaly.

The adrenal gland produces mineralocorticoids, glucocorticoids, and androgens. Aldosterone, the most important mineralocorticoid, is secreted by the zona glomerulosa of the adrenal cortex and is regulated primarily by angiotensin II (AT II) and potassium. Aldosterone activates mineralocorticoid receptors in transporting epithelia resulting in the expression of multiple factors that mediate an increase in sodium and water reabsorption and potassium and hydrogen ion excretion. The specificity of the mineralocorticoid receptor for the natural and far more abundant glucocorticoid cortisol is similar to that of aldosterone. The specificity of the receptor for aldosterone in target epithelia is exerted by the coexpression of the enzyme 11β-hydroxysteroid dehydrogenase type 2 with the mineralocorticoid receptor. This enzyme inactivates cortisol and prevents its activation of mineralocorticoid receptors expressed in the same cell, leaving mineralocorticoid functions under the control of the less abundant steroid. Inhibition of 11β-hydroxysteroid dehydrogenase type 2 allows cortisol to bind the mineralocorticoid receptor and produce an apparent mineralocorticoid hypertension identical to that of aldosterone excess, but aldosterone is suppressed, as is its major secretagogue, AT II. Thus mineralocorticoid hypertension is defined by the excessive activation of the receptor, not the identity of the steroid, and is classified as low renin, high aldosterone hypertension and low renin, low aldosterone hypertension (Table 42–6).

PRIMARY ALDOSTERONISM

ESSENTIALS OF DIAGNOSIS

▶ Hypertension, frequently refractory to usual medical therapy.

▶ Hypokalemia, unprovoked or easily provoked, although a normal potassium level is frequently found.

▶ Screen by measuring serum aldosterone and plasma renin activity.

▶ Tentative diagnosis: Serum aldosterone/plasma renin activity ratio greater than 30 and a serum aldosterone greater than 15 ng/dL.

▶ Confirmation of the diagnosis by finding an elevation in the production of aldosterone during the ingestion of a high sodium diet (>200 mEq/day) for 3 days with a urinary excretion rate of aldosterone greater than 12 μg/day, lack of suppression of serum aldosterone to below 7.5 ng/dL after a 2-L saline infusion over 4 hours, or lack of suppression of serum aldosterone below 5 ng/dL after 3 days of a high sodium diet and oral fludrocortisone acetate 0.1 mg every 6 hours.

▶ General Considerations

Primary aldosteronism was originally described by Conn in the 1950s. For many years it was believed to be relatively rare, affecting 0.1–0.5% of hypertensive patients. Advances in the screening procedure for primary aldosterone dramatically increased the identification of patients with primary aldosteronism resulting in a prevalence rate of 6–10% among patients with essential hypertension and the realization that primary aldosteronism is the most common form of secondary hypertension. The incidence is higher in the most severe cases of hypertension. The concept that primary aldosteronism was a benign disorder has been disproved and it is now clear that the incidence of left ventricular hypertrophy and cerebrovascular events is greater in primary aldosteronism than in matched patients with essential hypertension.

▶ Clinical Findings

A. Symptoms and Signs

The most common findings in primary aldosteronism are moderate to severe hypertension and hypokalemia. Patients with primary aldosterone are frequently refractory to

Table 42–6. Causes of mineralocorticoid hypertension.

Increased mineralocorticoid secretion
Primary aldosteronism
Aldosterone-producing adenoma (APA)
Idiopathic hyperaldosteronism
Glucocorticoid-remediable aldosteronism (GRA)
Adrenocortical carcinoma
Congenital adrenal hyperplasia
11β-Hydroxylase deficiency
17β-Hydroxylase deficiency
Increased mineralocorticoid action
Apparent mineralocorticoid excess (AME)
Congenital
Licorice ingestion
Ectopic corticotropin production
Activating mutation of the mineralocorticoid receptor
Increased sodium transport in renal epithelia
Liddle syndrome
Pseudohypoaldosteronism type II or Gordon syndrome

antihypertensive medications requiring several drugs to attain control. The incidence of primary aldosteronism increases to up to 20% in patients referred for refractory hypertension. When symptoms are present, they are the result of potassium depletion and include neuromuscular symptoms (weakness, paralysis, cramps, or tetany), fatigue, and polyuria (due to hypokalemia-induced renal concentrating defect). Potassium depletion can impair insulin secretion and cause glucose intolerance or diabetes. Edema is seldom seen in primary aldosteronism. End-stage organ damage occurs more frequently, with left ventricular hypertrophy being more pronounced than in matched patients with essential hypertension. Structural damage to the renal, cerebral, and retinal vasculature is also more common. Proteinuria occurs in about 50% of patients with primary aldosteronism and renal failure in about 15% of patients. Removal of an aldosterone-producing adenoma results in improvement in left ventricular hypertrophy even if the BP remains elevated.

Primary aldosteronism has several etiologies, the most important ones being aldosterone-producing adenoma (40–70%) and idiopathic hyperaldosteronism or bilateral hyperplasia (30–60%). Other less common causes include unilateral hyperplasia, adrenocortical carcinoma, and glucocorticoid-suppressible aldosteronism, probably accounting for 1–4% of patients. The differentiation between an aldosterone-producing adenoma and idiopathic hyperaldosteronism is crucial because an adenoma is a surgically correctable disease while idiopathic hyperaldosteronism is treated medically.

B. Laboratory Findings

Hypokalemia is frequently found in patients with primary aldosteronism provided that sampling is collected without the use of a tourniquet or fist clenching. It is an infrequent finding due to the common practice of using a tourniquet and fist clenching for blood collection. The incidence of potassium <3.5 in patients with primary aldosteronism from samples collected using a tourniquet and fist clenching is approximately 10%, while samples obtained from the same patients collected without the tourniquet gave an incidence of 69%.

Screening for primary aldosteronism is done by the measurement of serum aldosterone (ng/dL) and plasma renin activity (PRA) (ng/mL/hour) and the expression of the results as the ratio. The blood sampling is taken in the sitting position. Patients should preferably be off antihypertensive drugs for at least a week, but since this is often difficult to do, it can be done while patients are on most drugs including angiotensin-converting enzyme (ACE) inhibitors, AT II receptor blockers, α-blockers, calcium channel blockers, and less desirably on thiazide diuretics and sodium channel inhibitors. Mineralocorticoid receptor blockers (spironolactone or eplerenone) should be discontinued for at least 3 weeks. β-Blockers also interfere because they lower renin and spuriously alter the ratio. A ratio greater than 30 is highly suspicious if the absolute level of serum aldosterone is greater than 15 ng/dL. Patients with a high aldosterone/PRA ratio, but levels of serum aldosterone less than 9 ng/dL, are almost never found to have primary aldosteronism.

In recent times, the measurement of PRA is being superseded by the immunologic measurement of active renin. To calculate the ratio, active renin may be estimated by dividing the PRA by 8. Aldosterone measurements should be measured after correction of the hypokalemia.

C. Imaging Studies

High-resolution computed tomography (CT) scan or magnetic resonance imaging (MRI) usually can detect adrenal masses greater than 0.5 cm in diameter. As many adenomas are smaller than 0.5 cm and are not detected, the error in properly diagnosing a unilateral aldosterone-producing adenoma can be as high as 50%. Patients with idiopathic hyperaldosteronism frequently have bilateral macronodules and/or micronodules that can be uneven in size and might appear to be a unilateral adenoma. The diagnosis of a unilateral adenoma with sufficient confidence for surgical correction requires the use of a bilateral adrenal catheterization with measurements of aldosterone and cortisol from both adrenal veins and inferior vena cava. The results are expressed as an aldosterone/cortisol ratio; a ratio of aldosterone/cortisol from one side versus the opposite side that is greater than 4 establishes a diagnosis of a unilateral adrenal adenoma. The catheterization of the right adrenal vein requires considerable experience. Failure to do an adrenal vein catheterization results in a surgical error of around 25–30%. In patients below the age of 40 years, the presence of an adrenal mass by CT scan >1 cm with an attenuation less than −10 Hausfield units considerably improves the likelihood of a proper identification of an aldosterone-producing adenoma. Above this age the greater incidence of nonfunctional adrenal incidentalomas decreases the reliability.

D. Special Tests

Three tests have been employed for confirmation of the diagnosis. The most common is the measurement of the excretion of urinary aldosterone on the third day of a 200 mEq/day sodium diet. An excretion level above 12 μg aldosterone per day is diagnostic. A second test is the measurement of serum aldosterone at the end of the infusion of 2 L of 0.9% sodium chloride over 4 hours. A value below 7.5 ng/dL (or 5 ng/dL depending on the measuring technique) is normal. Finally, less commonly used is the measurement of serum aldosterone after 3 days of a high sodium diet plus the administration of fludrocortisone 0.1 mg four times a day. A value less than 5 ng/dL is normal.

In recent years, identification of glucocorticoid-suppressible aldosteronism has become more common. This disorder is characterized by an uneven crossover recombination between the promoter region and the first two to four exons of the *CYP11B1* gene (11β-hydroxylase) and the last five to seven exons of the *CYP11B2* gene (aldosterone synthase) resulting in gene duplication. This gene is expressed in the zona fasciculata of the adrenal, is regulated by adrenocorticotropic hormone (ACTH), and synthesizes aldosterone. A genetic test is available for the diagnosis. Patients with a familial history of hypertension, especially those diagnosed with hypertension at a young age or those with a family history of early cerebrovascular events, should be screened.

▶ Treatment

The treatment of an aldosterone-producing adenoma is surgical excision using a laparoscopic technique if possible. Patients with idiopathic hyperaldosteronism should be treated medically with a mineralocorticoid receptor antagonist. Two agents are available. Spironolactone is administered at doses of 25–200 mg/day. Patients are started with 25 mg/day and increased to response (up to 300 mg/day). Spironolactone has multiple side effects. It is also an androgen receptor antagonist and progesterone receptor agonist that produces a high incidence of impotence and gynecomastia in men and menstrual irregularities and breast tenderness due to progestational effects in women. A recent new spironolactone derivative, eplerenone, has been introduced that has significantly fewer side effects. It is administered at doses of 50–250 mg/day in divided doses. In patients who do not tolerate these drugs, a thiazide diuretic combined with a sodium channel antagonist, amiloride, can also be used, but supplemental potassium is frequently required. Patients frequently require further antihypertensive drugs. Patients with an aldosterone-producing adenoma who are not surgical candidates can also be treated medically.

11β-HYDROXYLASE DEFICIENCY

ESSENTIALS OF DIAGNOSIS

▶ The second most common cause of congenital adrenal hyperplasia in some areas of the world.
▶ Autosomal recessive disorder.
▶ Low renin, low aldosterone hypertension.
▶ Hyperandrogenism.
▶ Elevated secretion and levels of 11-deoxycortisol and deoxycorticosterone and decreased secretion of cortisol and aldosterone.

▶ General Considerations

11β-Hydroxylase deficiency is a rare autosomal recessive disorder of the *CYP11B1* gene and the second most common cause of congenital adrenal hyperplasia in some areas of the world. The defect results in a decrease in the synthesis of cortisol with an increase in the secretion of precursors, including 11-deoxycortisol and deoxycorticosterone, which have mineralocorticoid activity. The shunting of precursors to the androgen pathway results in androgenization. Patients usually present in early life with hypertension and frequently hypokalemia. The diagnosis is established by demonstrating elevated concentrations of deoxycorticosterone and 11-deoxycortisol.

▶ Clinical Findings

The diagnosis is more easily suspected in young girls, as they present with virilization and hypertension. In boys and men, the diagnosis is suspected in young patients with low renin hypertension and sometimes pseudoprecocious puberty. The diagnosis is established by demonstrating low renin, aldosterone, and cortisol levels and high levels of deoxycorticosterone.

▶ Treatment

Treatment involves replacement of the cortisol deficit with hydrocortisone and the addition of mineralocorticoid receptor antagonists such as spironolactone or eplerenone.

17α-HYDROXYLASE DEFICIENCY

ESSENTIALS OF DIAGNOSIS

▶ Low renin, low aldosterone hypertension.
▶ Rare genetic disorder, autosomal recessive.
▶ Female phenotype in male patients.
▶ Sexual infantilism in female patients.
▶ Elevated secretion of deoxycorticosterone and corticosterone.
▶ No production of cortisol.

▶ General Considerations

17α-Hydroxylase deficiency is a rare genetic autosomal recessive disorder of the *CYP17* gene resulting in the lack of formation of any 17-hydroxylated steroids including cortisol and androgens and excessive production of the 17-deoxysteroids corticosterone and deoxycorticosterone. The presentation is that of patients with low renin, low aldosterone hypertension with sexual infantilism with undervirilization in males and failure of spontaneous pubertal development in females. The diagnosis is established by the demonstration of high levels of corticosterone and deoxycorticosterone and the absence of 17β-hydroxylated steroids.

Treatment

Treatment involves replacement with hydrocortisone and the use of mineralocorticoid receptor antagonists. The deficit of estrogens is usually treated with oral contraceptives. Males usually are raised as girls due to the lack of development of male genitalia.

APPARENT MINERALOCORTICOID EXCESS

 ESSENTIALS OF DIAGNOSIS

▶ Low renin, low aldosterone hypertension.

▶ Severe hypertension in very young patients.

▶ Acquired as the result of overconsumption of licorice or its derivatives.

▶ Abnormal ratio of the excretion of urinary free cortisol to urinary free cortisone or the ratio of the metabolites of cortisol and cortisone: Tetrahydrocortisol + allotetrahydrocortisol to tetrahydrocortisone.

General Considerations

Apparent mineralocorticoid excess (AME) was originally described as a potentially fatal disorder involving juvenile low-renin, low-aldosterone hypertension, hypokalemic alkalosis, low birth weight, failure to thrive, and, frequently, nephrocalcinosis. It is caused by a deficiency of the enzyme 11β-hydroxysteroid dehydrogenase 2. It is an autosomal recessive syndrome. Adult patients with the syndrome have also been found. However, in adults the acquired form due to the ingestion of licorice in the form of candy or its derivative carbenoxolone, used in some places for the treatment of duodenal ulcers, is more common. Acquired AME is not as common in the United States as in Europe, because licorice candy in the United States is generally made with artificial flavoring rather than the extract of the root of the true licorice, *Glycyrrhiza glabra,* containing the active compound glycyrrhizic acid. Chewing tobacco in the United States, however, is often flavored with real licorice. The mineralocorticoid receptor has affinity for the abundant glucocorticoid cortisol equal to that for aldosterone and cortisol normally circulates at 100–1000 times the concentrations of aldosterone. Specificity of the mineralocorticoid receptor in renal transporting epithelia is due to the coexpression of the enzyme 11β-hydroxysteroid dehydrogenase 2, which metabolizes cortisol to inactive cortisone. A deficiency of the enzyme results in occupancy of the receptors by cortisol and enhanced mineralocorticoid effect.

In ectopic corticotropin-secreting tumors producing Cushing syndrome, the massive increase in the production of cortisol saturates the 11β-hydroxysteroid dehydrogenase 2 and allows cortisol to activate the mineralocorticoid receptor.

Clinical Findings

A. Symptoms and Signs

The diagnosis is suspected in patients with low renin, low aldosterone hypertension with hypokalemic alkalosis. In infants it should be suspected when severe hypertension and hypokalemia and a history of low birth weight and failure to thrive are present. Nephrocalcinosis is a frequent finding. The syndrome is autosomal recessive and should be suspected in patients with a strong history of cosanguinity. In adult patients a history of ingestion of licorice candy, usually of European origin, or use of licorice-flavored chewing tobacco in large quantities is an important clue. Patients present with hypertension with hypokalemia and a frequent history of changes in mood and irritability. Withdrawal of licorice results in resolution of the syndrome.

Patients with Cushing syndrome due to ectopic corticotropin production most often present after the diagnosis of a cancer and experience profound weakness, hypertension, and hypokalemia. Patients at this stage of the natural history of their cancer are frequently not diagnosed with Cushing syndrome because ectopic ACTH production is a late event and the classical phenotypic manifestations are absent. Other forms of Cushing syndrome can also present with this form of hypertension and hypokalemia, and these findings correlate with the severity of the abnormality in cortisol production.

B. Laboratory Findings

The diagnosis is determined by the measurement of the excretion of urinary free cortisol to urinary free cortisone, whereas the ratio is less than 1 in normal individuals and is clearly increased in patients with AME syndrome. The ratio of the metabolites of cortisol and cortisone, tetrahydrocortisol + allotetrahydrocortisol to tetrahydrocortisone, is also measured in patients with AME. The ratio is around 1 in normal individuals and is usually higher than 2 in patients with AME. In these patients the total cortisol production is lower than normal, but the blood concentrations are normal. This is reflected by total cortisol metabolite excretion in the urine.

Treatment

Patients with congenital AME are treated with mineralocorticoid receptor antagonists (spironolactone or eplerenone).

Some patients benefit from treatment with dexamethasone, which does not have mineralocorticoid properties. Acquired forms are treated by withdrawal of the offending licorice or carbenoxolone. Ectopic corticotropin production is treated by management of the cancer, if possible.

Prognosis

The prognosis in patients with congenital AME depends on the adherence to therapy, but is relative poor, with significant morbidity and mortality at a young age. Patients with licorice-induced hypertension have a good prognosis if the licorice intake is eliminated. Patients with ectopic corticotropin production have a poor prognosis as the presentation of the syndrome usually occurs late in the history of the cancer.

LIDDLE SYNDROME

 ESSENTIALS OF DIAGNOSIS

▶ Autosomal dominant disease.

▶ Hypertension and hypokalemia.

▶ Hyporeninemic hypoaldosteronism.

▶ Lack of response to mineralocorticoid receptor antagonists.

▶ Good response to epithelial sodium channel blockers.

▶ Clinical Findings

Liddle described a family of patients that presented with severe hypertension, hypokalemia, low PRA, and low plasma aldosterone concentrations. He demonstrated that adrenal steroids were not involved and there was no response to the administration of mineralocorticoid receptor antagonists, but there was to sodium channel blockers. It was later that the genetic defect was demonstrated to be mutations affecting the C-terminal portion of the β or γ subunit of the sodium channel. Renal transplantation improves the syndrome.

▶ Treatment

Patients are treated with sodium channel antagonists, primarily amiloride, at doses between 5 and 15 mg twice a day.

PSEUDOHYPOALDOSTERONISM TYPE II OR GORDON SYNDROME

 ESSENTIALS OF DIAGNOSIS

▶ Hypertension.

▶ Hyperkalemia.

▶ Metabolic acidosis.

▶ Normal renal function.

▶ Defects in the WNK1 or the WNK4 (without lysine kinases).

▶ Clinical Findings

Pseudohypoaldosteronism type 2 is a familial autosomal dominant disease in which patients present with a history of hypertension, hyperkalemia, metabolic acidosis, and normal renal function. Patients have low-renin, low-aldosterone hypertension. The hypertension and hypokalemia respond to thiazide therapy. The various families with the syndrome show linkages to chromosomes 1, 17, and 12. The ones linked to chromosome 12 have been associated with an intronic defect in the gene for WNK1. The deletion results in overexpression of the WNK1, which inhibits the action of the WNK4 in sodium and potassium transport. The one linked to chromosome 17 involves mutations in the WNK4 resulting in an increased activity of the sodium chloride cotransporter (thiazide-sensitive cotransporter) and in potassium and chloride transport. The gene defect in syndromes associated with chromosome 1 remains unknown.

▶ Treatment

Patients respond to the administration of thiazide diuretics.

PHEOCHROMOCYTOMA

 ESSENTIALS OF DIAGNOSIS

▶ Pheochromocytomas are tumors of neuroectodermal origin arising from chromaffin cells.

▶ Paroxysmal hypertension occurring in 30–50% of patients.

▶ Sustained hypertension in at least 50% of the patients.

▶ Classic triad of severe headaches, palpitations, and diaphoresis.

▶ Approximately 90% are benign and 10% are malignant.

▶ Approximately 15% are bilateral.

▶ Most are sporadic, but at least 10% are familial.

▶ Approximately 25% of patients with sporadic pheochromocytoma have a germ line mutation suggesting that they are founders.

▶ Biochemical diagnosis. Measurement of urinary or plasma free metanephrines is more sensitive, and should precede localization efforts.

▶ General Considerations

Catecholamine-producing tumors are neoplasias of chromaffin cells that most often originate in the adrenal medulla (pheochromocytoma), but may also originate extraadrenally, in the paraganglia (paragangliomas). They are an uncommon cause of hypertension with a prevalence of less than 0.1% among hypertensive patients, although around 0.5% of patients with hypertension are screened for a pheochromocytoma in the United States. The diagnosis of a pheochromocytoma is important because it is a curable form of hypertension that is highly lethal if undiagnosed. Pheochromocytomas are components of the multiple endocrine neoplasia (MEN) syndromes type 2a and 2b. They are also present in a significant proportion of patients with von Hippel disease where the incidence varies according to the family and can be as high as 50% of affected individuals. Neurofibromatosis type 1 is also associated with an incidence of pheochromocytomas of around 1–5%. Mutations of the succinate dehydrogenase subunits B, C, and D are associated with extra adrenal paragangliomas. Germ line mutations in sporadic pheochromocytomas are present in about 24% of patients. Since there is no family history of pheochromocytomas in these patients, it might represent a founder effect.

▶ Clinical Findings

A. Symptoms and Signs

Elevation of BP is the most common manifestation of a pheochromocytoma. Sustained elevation of BP is present in above 50% of the patients and intermittent hypertension in about a third, while normal BP or postural hypotension is present in about 20% of patients. The most dramatic presentation of a pheochromocytoma is an acute episode of severe hypertension, severe headache, palpitations, tachycardia, and diaphoresis. Arrhythmias are frequent, as is the presentation with chest pain. Catecholamines can cause coronary vasospasm and acute myocarditis with electrocardiographic and enzymatic changes that may be diagnosed as an acute myocardial infarction. Dilated cardiomyopathy with low cardiac output, pulmonary edema, and occasional hypotension is common. Shock unresponsive to norepinephrine occurring after a hypertensive crisis can also be a presentation that can easily be missed. Cerebrovascular accidents occur due to the profound vasoconstriction of the cerebrovascular arteries or emboli from a catecholaminergic-dilated cardiomyopathy. Certain drugs such as tricyclic antidepressants, antidopaminergics (metoclopramide), naloxone, and β-blockers (when not preceded by α-adrenergic blockade) can precipitate an acute hypertensive crisis in a patient with a pheochromocytoma. Children with pheochromocytoma usually have sustained hypertension with nausea, headaches, and sweating. Lactic acidosis in the absence of shock should be an indication for considering the diagnosis of a pheochromocytoma.

B. Special Tests

The diagnosis is established by the demonstration of increased catecholamines and their metabolites. Measurement of vanillylmandelic acid (VMA) is very insensitive and is represented more in large tumors. Currently there are two different approaches toward the diagnosis of a pheochromocytoma; one involves the measurement of plasma free metanephrines and catecholamines (to a lesser extent) and the other involves the measurement of urinary fractionated metanephrines. The NIH group has proposed the use of plasma metanephrines as the most sensitive way of diagnosing a pheochromocytoma; the sensitivity of the test is very high while the specificity of the diagnosis is around 85%. The Mayo Clinic has proposed that the measurement of urinary fractionated metanephrines and catecholamines has a lower sensitivity (90%) but a higher specificity (98%).

In some cases in which the degree of suspicion is high, but the plasma or urinary measurements are equivocal, the clonidine suppression test is useful. The test consists of administering clonidine 0.3 mg orally with plasma catecholamines and free metanephrines collected 3 hours later while patients are supine. A decrease of less than 40% for plasma metanephrines and less than 50% for plasma catecholamines is positive for a pheochromocytoma. Once a pheochromocytoma has been diagnosed biochemically, localization is usually accomplished using CT scanning or MRI with T_2-weighted images. For those that cannot be located using these techniques, radionuclide imaging with $[^{131}I]$MIBG can be done. In some cases positron emission tomography (PET) scanning can also be useful using $[6\text{-}^{18}F]$ fluorodopamine or $[^{18}F]$ fluorodeoxyglucose.

▶ Differential Diagnosis

Multiple disorders can mimic symptoms of a pheochromocytoma and some are associated with increased catecholamine secretion. Clonidine or alcohol withdrawal, cerebrovascular events, subarachnoid hemorrhages, migraines, and intracranial lesions may mimic a pheochromocytoma. Drugs such as ephedrine, cocaine, phencyclidine, and LSD can also produce a similar episodic syndrome. Panic attacks, hypoglycemic episodes, or just severe hypertension with a hyperdynamic circulation might resemble episodes of pheochromocytoma.

▶ Complications

Undiagnosed pheochromocytoma is associated with a high incidence of sudden death, cerebrovascular events, and dilated cardiomyopathy.

▶ Treatment

The treatment of pheochromocytomas is primarily surgical if the tumors are located. Patients are pretreated with an α-blocker such as phenoxybenzamine and/or an $α_1$-blocker (prazosin, doxazosin, or terazosin) and a β-blocker (after the administration of an α-blocker). A combined β-blocker and α-blocker (labetalol) is particularly useful. Surveillance after an isolated pheochromocytoma has been removed should continue because a significant proportion involve germ line mutations and can recur in the other adrenal or ganglia.

▶ Prognosis

Undiagnosed and untreated pheochromocytoma patients experience a high incidence of sudden death and cardiovascular and cerebrovascular events. A hypertensive crisis frequently occurs during routine procedures. Patients who are properly treated with α- and β-blockers and surgery have a good prognosis, but there is a 10–15% incidence of recurrence. The course of malignant pheochromocytomas is highly variable; some behave aggressively while others have an indolent course.

Calhoun DA et al: Aldosterone excretion among subjects with resistant hypertension and symptoms of sleep apnea. Chest 2004;125:112.

Funder, JW, Carey, RM, Fardella, C, Gomez-Sanchez, CE, Mantero, F, Stowasser, M, Young, WF, Jr., and Montori, VM Case detection, diagnosis, and treatment of patients with primary aldosteronism: an endocrine society clinical practice guideline. J Clin Endocrinol Metab 2008; 93:3266.

Kahle KT et al: Regulation of diverse ion transport pathways by WNK4 kinase: a novel molecular switch. Trends Endocrinol Metab 2005;16:98.

Mulatero P et al: Increased diagnosis of primary aldosteronism, including surgically correctable forms, in centers from five continents. J Clin Endocrinol Metab 2004;89:1045.

New MI et al: Monogenic low renin hypertension. Trends Endocrinol Metab 2005;16:92.

Pacak K et al: Biochemical diagnosis, localization and management of pheochromocytoma: focus on multiple endocrine neoplasia type 2 in relation to other hereditary syndromes and sporadic forms of the tumour. J Intern Med 2005;257:60.

Rossi G et al: Aldosterone as a cardiovascular risk factor. Trends Endocrinol Metab 2005;16:104.

Unger N et al: Comparison of active renin concentration and plasma renin activity for the diagnosis of primary hyperaldosteronism in patients with an adrenal mass. Eur J Endocrinol 2004;150:517.

Yang CL et al: Mechanisms of WNK1 and WNK4 interaction in the regulation of thiazide-sensitive NaCl cotransport. J Clin Invest 2005;115:1379.

▼ COARCTATION OF THE AORTA

William J. Elliott, MD, PhD

ESSENTIALS OF DIAGNOSIS

▶ Unexpected differences in BPs in the extremities (eg, right > left arm, arms > legs).

▶ Imaging study (typically echocardiogram) of the aorta demonstrating the site of coarctation.

▶ General Considerations

Most aortic coarctations occur between the ligamentum arteriosum and the left subclavian artery. In children, coarctation occurs commonly in conjunction with other congenital abnormalities. Coarctation is more common in males (66–75%). Differences in BP may clue the location of the coarctation: If it is proximal to the left subclavian artery, systolic BP is typically higher in the right arm than the left arm. More commonly, the coarct is more distal, and the systolic BP in the right leg is lower than that in the right arm.

▶ Clinical Findings

A. Symptoms and Signs

Although children with coarctation sometimes note dyspnea, fatigue, headache, cold feet, and even claudication (especially with vigorous exercise), most adults are asymptomatic. The traditional characteristic physical sign is a diminished or delayed left radial or right femoral pulse, in comparison to the right radial pulse. A loud systolic murmur, often with a thrill and occasionally heard in the back, may be accompanied by other murmurs, depending on the presence or absence of other cardiac abnormalities (eg, bicuspid aortic valve, present in 50–80% of children). "Notching" (typically of the inferior posterior aspects) of the ribs (third through eighth) is characteristic, and the number and location of notched ribs may provide information as to the location of the coarctation.

B. Special Tests

An echocardiogram is typically recommended as the first test, since it can identify about 95% of coarctations through the first 8 cm of the descending aorta (which probably covers 99% of cases). Computed tomography (CT) and magnetic resonance imaging (MRI) have also been used successfully. Angiography is sometimes not required if the other images are acceptable to a vascular surgeon.

▶ Differential Diagnosis

The differential diagnosis includes Takyusu's arteritis and Moyamoya disease (both of which can affect a major artery in one arm, which is more common than both legs and not an arm).

▶ Treatment

A systolic pressure gradient across the coarct of more than 20 mm Hg generally requires intervention. A variety of surgical approaches have been successful, depending on the location of the coarctation. Postoperative elevation in systolic BP is a predictor of long-term adverse outcomes (including death). Balloon dilatation with or without endovascular stenting is more popular now, but few long-term results have been reported. This is especially important in still-growing children, in whom repeat aortoplasty has been successful up to 3 years after the initial stent placement. Aortoplasty has also been successfully used after an initial surgical repair. Hypertension recurs in about 25–33% of patients with repaired coarctation in long-term follow-up; exercise-induced hypertension is even more common (25–56%).

Prognosis

The mean age at death for untreated coarctation is about 34 years. The degree of BP lowering after a corrective procedure in patients who present with aortic coarctation in adulthood is controversial. Two of three studies indicated that most patients have a lower BP about 3 months after the operation than before it, but after 5 years about a third were hypertensive. Older age was generally associated with a higher risk for postprocedure hypertension.

Prisant LM et al: Coarctation of the aorta: a secondary cause of hypertension. J Clin Hypertens 2004;6:347. [PMID: 15187499]

▼ SLEEP APNEA

William J. Elliott, MD, PhD

ESSENTIALS OF DIAGNOSIS

- ▶ Elevated BP that is lowered after a formal diagnosis and effective treatment for sleep apnea.
- ▶ A formal polysomnographic sleep study that demonstrates an apnea–hypopnea index [Total number of apneic episodes (greater than 10 seconds) + number of hypopneic episodes (reduction in airway pressure by ≥30% and drop in oxygen saturation by ≥4%)/(number of hours of sleep)] > 5.

General Considerations

There are no reliable estimates of the incidence or prevalence of hypertension due to sleep apnea. Sleep apnea itself is thought to affect 17–26% of men and 9–28% of women older than 20 years of age, and is more common among African-Americans than whites. It is much more frequently found in overweight and obese individuals (mean body mass index ~35 kg/m^2) with a mean age of about 60 years. In several epidemiologic studies, sleep apnea has been a significant independent risk factor for the development of hypertension, but these results are confounded by close correlations of both hypertension and sleep apnea with age, gender, body mass index, alcohol intake, and smoking. In one study, sleep apnea was the cause of resistant hypertension in 83% of investigated cases.

Pathogenesis

The mechanisms responsible for the increased prevalence of hypertension in patients with sleep apnea have not yet been elucidated. Sleep apnea increases sympathetic activity and catecholamine levels, which can secondarily affect many mechanisms that lead to elevated BP. Sleep apnea is also associated with increased C-reactive protein, endothelial dysfunction, elevated leptin levels, and weight gain, all of which are characteristics of hypertension.

Clinical Findings

A. Symptoms and Signs

The typical patient with sleep apnea has daytime sleepiness and drowsiness (typically while driving), poor sleep quality (typically described as "restless sleep"), morning headache and sore throat, and excessive fatigue. The bed partner will usually report loud snoring and irregular breathing, and an astute observer may note cessation of breathing, gasping, and choking sounds during the night.

B. Special Tests

The Berlin Questionnaire is a validated screening tool for sleep apnea that has 86% sensitivity, 77% specificity, and 89% predictive value after evaluation in 744 primary care patients subsequently formally evaluated with polysomnography. Those who score highly are typically asked to undergo formal multichannel polysomnography to verify the diagnosis.

Treatment

Traditionally, three options are offered to treat sleep apnea: Weight loss (successful in a minority of cases in the long term), laryngeal surgery (if excessive pharyngeal tissue is sufficient to cause airway obstruction), and continuous positive airway pressure (CPAP) during sleep, usually delivered with a mask connected to a pressurized air-delivery system. For patients who tolerate sleeping with the apparatus in place, reductions in BP are typically seen within 4 weeks. As with most long-term therapies, adherence to an initially successful intervention wanes over time.

Recently, several uncontrolled cohort studies have reported that spironolactone is useful in the treatment of hypertension in patients with sleep apnea. A comparative trial of CPAP and spironolactone has not yet been done.

Prognosis

There are no long-term studies of CPAP or other therapies directed to improving sleep apnea that report results of BP lowering. Laryngeal surgery in appropriately selected patients improves short-term BP control. Long-term weight loss and CPAP are recommended on the basis of short-term improvements in BP.

Goodfriend TL et al: Resistant hypertension, obesity, sleep apnea and aldosterone: theory and therapy. Hypertension 2004;43:518. [PMID: 14732721]

Wolk R et al: Obesity, sleep apnea and hypertension. Hypertension 2003;42:1067. [PMID: 14610096]

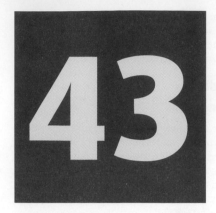

Hypertension in High-Risk Populations

David Martins, MD, Keith Norris, MD,
Tiina Podymow, MD,
& Phyllis August, MD, MPH

▼ HYPERTENSION IN AFRICAN-AMERICANS

David Martins, MD, & Keith Norris, MD

▶ General Considerations

Hypertension is a persistent and frequently progressive elevation in blood pressure. The level of systolic and/or diastolic blood pressure at which the elevation assumes the diagnosis of hypertension depends on the presence or absence of coexisting comorbidities. The current classification of blood pressure and the level of blood pressure that defines hypertension for the major comorbid conditions as recommended in the seventh report of the Joint National Committee on Prevention, Detection, Evaluation, and Treatment of high blood pressure are shown in Table 43–1. The prevalence of hypertension varies with age and sex. It is estimated that 23% of adult Americans between the ages of 20 and 74 years have hypertension. About 75% of women aged 75 years and over have hypertension and about 64% of men aged 75 years and over have hypertension. At all ages and in both sexes African-Americans have the highest prevalence of hypertension in the United States. In African-Americans hypertension tends to develop at an earlier age and tends to be more severe than in other races. Some patients with systemic hypertension will have a specific identifiable cause for the elevated systemic blood pressure. The estimated proportion of the cases of secondary hypertension among patients with systemic hypertension ranges from about 5% to 10% and has not been shown to exhibit racial predilection. Patients with secondary hypertension usually exhibit suggestive constellations of signs and/or symptoms on initial evaluation and should undergo further evaluation for specific causes of hypertension regardless of their race and/or ethnicity.

Hypertension is one of the major risk factors for cardiovascular disease. Uncontrolled hypertension leads to specific target organ damage that contributes to overall cardiovascular morbidity and mortality. African-Americans exhibit a greater increase in target organ damage than other racial and ethnic groups. In fact, the heart disease mortality rate is 50% higher, the stroke mortality rate is 80% higher, and the incidence of hypertension-related end-stage renal disease (ESRD) is 6-fold higher in African-Americans than in whites. It is apparent that hypertension along with its cardiovascular morbidity and mortality is an even greater challenge for the African-American community than it is for the rest of the nation. Many of the factors responsible for the disparities in the incidence, prevalence, detection, treatment, and control of hypertension have been well described and can be useful in the design and development of programs and policies targeted to the diagnosis and control of hypertension within the population.

▶ Pathogenesis

Blood pressure is a continuous variable determined by multiple factors and demonstrates a fairly normal distribution within the population. Some of the factors that determine blood pressure level are genetic and may account for about 30–50% of the blood pressure variation in the general population. The development of essential or idiopathic hypertension, however, is believed to require a genetic predisposition and an environmental precipitation in most instances. The search for specific genes responsible for hypertension has resulted in the discovery of some rare monogenetic causes of both high and low blood pressure. While several physiologic characteristics such as low renin levels, lower bioavailability of nitric oxide, increased salt sensitivity, and increased aldosterone levels are more prevalent in African-Americans, specific genetic underpinnings have yet to be identified. In spite of popular expectation there is still no identified genetic basis for the excess prevalence of hypertension in the African-American community. However, several lifestyle and environmental risk factors for hypertension have been identified with important differences among racial and ethnic groups.

Table 43–1. Classification of blood pressure for adults.

Blood pressure category	Blood pressure reading, mm Hg	
	Systolic	Diastolic
Normal range	<120	and <80
Prehypertension	120–139	or 80–90
Hypertension		
Stage 1	140–159	or 90–99
Stage 2	≥160	or ≥100

Data from the Seventh Report of the Joint National Committee on Prevention, Detection, Evaluation, and Treatment of High Blood Pressure: JNC VII.

Excess body fat, particularly in the upper body, is an important risk factor for hypertension. Whether expressed as overweight or obesity, excess body fat is more common among African-Americans, Hispanics, and several other ethnic minorities. Dietary salt intake in the form of sodium chloride has been associated with the level of blood pressure and the rise in blood pressure with age. As a group, African-Americans have higher salt intake and greater sensitivity to changes in blood pressure in response to dietary salt intake. In contrast a low potassium intake has been associated with hypertension and there is evidence that high dietary potassium, particularly in the form of fresh fruits and vegetables, may offer protection from hypertension and perhaps reduce the need for antihypertensive drug therapy. The diets of many African-Americans are generally low in fruits and vegetables and the average dietary potassium intake among African-Americans is less than that of other major racial and ethnic groups in the United States.

Physical inactivity is a risk factor for hypertension and cardiovascular mortality. Optimum physical activity requires 20–60 minutes of rhythmic and aerobic large-muscle activity such as walking, running, and cycling 3–5 days a week for blood pressure control and cardiorespiratory fitness. Physical activity is suboptimal in over 60% of the U.S. adults, about 25% of whome are totally inactive. Physical inactivity is more common among older adults, women, less affluent people, and Hispanic and African-American adults.

The intake of three or more standard drinks of alcohol per day, where a standard drink is defined as 14 g of ethanol and is contained in 1.5 oz of distilled spirit, a 5-oz glass of table wine, or a 12-oz glass of beer, has been associated with serious adverse psychosocial and health consequences including hypertension. It is estimated that about 60% of Americans ages 18 years and over ingest alcohol and about 30% have five or more standard drinks on the same occasion at least once in that year. Many of these Americans are African-Americans.

The low educational status and high unemployment rate prevalent among minority populations in the United States predispose many minority communities, including African-American, to adverse political and socioeconomic conditions that contribute to environmental and psychosocial stress as well as reduced access to quality health care. Acute stress can transiently raise blood pressure, while chronic stress has been associated with sustained hypertension. The job-strain model of psychosocial conflict, designed to assess the impact of occupational stress on the health of the worker, characterizes jobs into high and low strain jobs. Workers with high decision latitudes exhibit little or no distress because they have more flexibility in deciding how best to meet their work-related demands, while those in occupations that combine high demands with low decision latitudes exhibit high stress levels and its attendant cardiovascular morbidity. African-Americans are more likely to be employed in these positions. Indeed, men employed in these typically blue-collar jobs have a 3-fold increase in hypertension and those who remain in these jobs for 3 or more years have a reported blood pressure that is 11/7 mm Hg higher than men in low strain jobs.

While genetic and biological differences may influence the distribution of blood pressure levels within a population, the prevailing body of evidence seems to suggest that lifestyle and socioeconomic disparities have a greater influence on the expression of hypertension and the disproportionate burden of hypertension and cardiovascular disease in African-Americans. This suggests that it is not genetics alone but the gene–environment interaction that is responsible for the higher prevalence of hypertension among African-Americans. Further evidence supporting the unique role of environment is the fact that the excess risk for hypertension in African-Americans is more strongly linked to being born and living in the United States than with African ancestry.

Racial and/or ethnic differences in combined cardiovascular endpoints assume less significance in hypertensive-treated patients after an adjustment for differences in socioeconomic and demographic factors. The treatment and control of hypertension for optimal outcomes require an appropriate sensitivity to and an understanding of the unique sociocultural aspects of race/ethnicity to maximize effective access to care, adherence to treatment, and scheduled follow-ups. Such approaches will ultimately assist in overcoming many of the barriers to the control of hypertension and will lead to improved cardiovascular outcomes for all Americans.

▶ Treatment Strategies

A. Hypertension

Severe hypertension and suboptimal blood pressure control rates perpetuate the disproportionate burden of cardiovascular disease (CVD) and premature death among African-Americans. Biobehavioral and socioeconomic factors frequently cited as plausible explanations for the lack of awareness and treatment of high blood pressure among African-Americans may not fully explain the failure to achieve recommended blood pressure goals. Several large-scale multicenter studies with substantial enrollment of African-American patients have demonstrated that blood pressure can be treated to goal levels, although more aggressive therapy may be needed. African-Americans seem to have a slightly greater blood pressure response to diuretics and calcium channel blockers than do other ethnic groups and less response to angiotensin-converting enzyme inhibitors (ACEIs) and β-blockers. Nevertheless, these differences do not seem to translate into different clinical outcomes based on class of antihypertensive therapy as long as target blood pressure levels are achieved. Thus, the search for cardiovascular risk factors and target organ damage, both of which are more prevalent among hypertensive African-Americans, and the selection of the appropriate therapeutic agent by compelling indication based on the coexisting comorbidities should supersede the search for specific agents for blood pressure control among African-Americans.

B. Cardiovascular and Related Complications of Hypertension

Hypertension is not only a major risk factor for CVD, but often occurs with one or more cardiovascular risk factors such as obesity, diabetes, and/or dyslipidemia in a syndrome known as the metabolic syndrome. A race-specific role for emerging cardiovascular risk factors such as aldosterone and inflammatory mediators has yet to be determined. The clinical and laboratory search for cardiovascular risk factors and target-organ damage is particularly important for African-American hypertensive patients. The awareness and identification of specific end-organ damage and coexisting cardiovascular risk factors should help prioritize nonpharmacologic recommendations, the selection of compelling evidenced-based medical treatment, and the establishment of appropriate target goals.

C. Left Ventricular Hypertrophy

Left ventricular hypertrophy is a common complication of hypertension and an independent predictor of increased mortality among hypertensive patients. It is more common among female and African-American patients with hypertension and may account for some of the ethnic and gender differences in cardiovascular mortality rates.

The treatment and control of hypertension by β-blockade and renin–angiotensin inhibition have been associated with regression of left ventricular hypertrophy. The blood pressure reduction and left ventricular mass regression associated with both of these treatments in most studies were similar in African-American and other racial and ethnic participants. A diminished response among African-Americans treated with angiotensin receptor blocker (ARB) therapy in one study

may have been related to fewer African-Americans achieving target blood pressure goals, but a differential outcome based on race cannot be excluded.

D. Congestive Heart Failure

Congestive heart failure (CHF) in blacks is characterized by a higher frequency of hypertension as the etiology, a worse prognosis, and perhaps less of a response to evidenced-based CHF medical therapy in comparison to their white counterparts. There is abundant evidence that β-blockade and renin–angiotensin inhibition are beneficial for improving both mortality and hospitalization outcomes among patients with CHF, and overall these treatment strategies when adjusted for other covariates appear similar for both African-American and other racial/ethnic patients. While there are reports of higher readmission rates for African-American patients receiving these treatments, posthospitalization mortality data suggest that when quality care is provided, the apparent racial disparities in CHF outcomes dissipate. The treatment of CHF patients should therefore encompass class-specific therapy (eg, ACEI, ARB, β-blocker) in combination with diuretics as indicated for the general population regardless of race or ethnicity. The addition of aldosterone blockade has also led to improved CHF outcomes, although there are no data on racial differences. However, isosorbide dinitrate and hydralazine have been shown to reduce CHF mortality by 43% compared to placebo for African-Americans.

E. Stroke

African-American patients with hypertension exhibit the highest stroke rates of any racial or ethnic group. The recent decline in stroke mortality observed in other racial and ethnic groups is attenuated for African-American patients with hypertension. Blood pressure control and antiplatelet therapy remain the principal strategies for reducing stroke events among patients with hypertension. The degree of protection conferred by blood pressure control may vary for different classes of antihypertensive medications. A relative-risk reduction in stroke as high as 40% has been reported for African-Americans with diuretic therapy compared to therapy with ACEIs. Diuretics and calcium channel blockers (CCBs) have emerged as the preferred antihypertensive treatment for reducing stroke events for all hypertensive patients, including African-Americans. There are no reported racial and/or ethnic differences in the prevention of recurrent stroke and myocardial infarction with ticlopidine and aspirin. Aspirin is more cost effective and should therefore be the preferred agent for antiplatelet therapy. Ticlopidine should be reserved for patients with aspirin intolerance and allergy.

F. Chronic Kidney Disease

ESRD secondary to hypertension is six times more common in African-Americans than in the general population. The use of ACEIs in comparison to β-blockers and dihydropyridine CCBs was associated with a reduction in adverse clinical outcomes (doubling of creatinine, ESRD, or death) for African-American patients with hypertensive nephrosclerosis. Thus, the existing body of evidence suggests that optimal clinical outcomes are achieved when inhibition of the renin–angiotensin system is used as initial antihypertensive therapy with diuretics in African-Americans with hypertensive nephrosclerosis. Diabetes is the leading cause of ESRD for all racial and ethnic groups and over 90% of patients with diabetic nephropathy have hypertension. Multiple studies support the use of ACEIs and ARBs as the mainstay of therapy. The inclusion of nearly 15% African-American participants in two of the pivotal prospective randomized trial studies, suggests that the positive outcomes extend to blacks as well as nonblacks. Thus, interruption of the renin–angiotensin system has emerged as the initial recommended therapy in combination with diuretics for treating hypertensive and diabetic nephropathy, and usually represents the minimum treatment regimen needed to achieve the more aggressive recommended treatment goal of 130/80 mm Hg for patients with chronic kidney disease.

G. Therapeutic Lifestyle Changes

Therapeutic lifestyle changes are equally effective across racial and ethnic groups and sometimes even more effective among African-American patients. These changes are particularly important for African-American patients with hypertension because many of the major risk factors for hypertension in these patients are behavioral and modifiable. The identification and communication of risk-attributable behaviors (such as dietary indiscretion, physical inactivity, excessive alcohol intake, and smoking), particularly within the context of the established burden of cardiovascular disease, should engage and encourage the patient to be proactive in the implementation of therapeutic lifestyle changes.

Practical suggestions for the effective implementation of therapeutic lifestyle changes are listed in Table 43–2. Many of the barriers to successful implementation of therapeutic lifestyle changes among African-Americans are listed in Table 43–3. The recommendations for therapeutic lifestyle changes, such as weight control, dietary salt reduction, regular physical activity, and adherence to clinic visits and a medication regimen, should be provided in specific detail with a practical design, making it possible to break through some of these common barriers and achieve successful implementation. This may frequently necessitate the inclusion of additional healthcare professionals (eg, dietitian, pharmacist, social worker) and/or family members in the dialogue.

Table 43–2. Therapeutic lifestyle changes.

Medical target	Practical plan to achieve goal
Weight loss	Lose weight gradually by making permanent changes in daily diet for the entire family Initiate 800–1500 kcal/day diet and set a reasonable weight loss goal (1–2 lb/week for the first 3–6 months)
Dietary goals	
Low fat Low sodium High potassium Adequate calcium	Eat more broiled and steamed foods Eat more grains, fresh fruits, and vegetables Eat fewer fats and use healthier fats, such as olive oil Eat fewer processed foods, fast foods, and fried foods Read labels and pay attention to the sodium, potassium, and fat content of foods Do not add salt when cooking; instead use vinegar, lemon juice, or sodium substitutes such as potassium instead of standard table salt for seasoning Do not season foods with smoked meats, such as bacon and ham hocks If lactose intolerant, try lactose-free milk or yogurt, or drink calcium-fortified juices or soy milk
	No more than two beers, one glass of wine, or one shot of hard liquor per day (even less for women)
Physical fitness	Increase physical activity as part of the daily routine: eg, if currently sedentary, get off the bus six blocks from home or walk in the evening with your spouse, a friend, or a group Gradually increase the time spent at an enjoyable physical activity to 30–45 minutes 3–5 days/week
Adapt a low stress lifestyle	Teach coping skills for specific stressors in the work and/or home environment Meditation, relaxation, yoga, biofeedback, others
Additional considerations	Maintain a smoke-free environment and limit alcohol intake

Modified with permission from Martins D, Norris K: Hypertension treatment in African Americans: physiology is less important than sociology. Cleve Clin J Med 2004;71(9):735.

Table 43–3. Barriers to therapeutic lifestyle changes and adherence in African-Americans.

Overweight/obese (body mass index >25/30 kg/m^2)	Cultural concern that a thin body habitus is associated with poor health
High dietary intake of sodium and fat	Cultural food preparation and conditioned tasting likely were initiated or exacerbated during slavery when high salt and fat content were needed for preservation and/or palatability of suboptimal food sources (Salt sensitivity is more common in African-Americans than in whites; if BP is not controlled, check 24-hour urinary sodium excretion to assess dietary adherence)
Low dietary calcium intake	Low milk and dairy intake due to high prevalence of lactose intolerance
Inactivity for women	Cultural emphasis on hair styling and relatively high cost of hair maintenance contribute to avoidance of routine exercise with increased heart rate and sweating
Low adherence to prescribed treatment plan	Assess for medication side effects (particularly impotence among males and increased angioedema among African-Americans taking ACEI) High rate of poverty, low rates of insurance (check prescription plan) and/or ability to pay for prescribed medications (adjust therapy as needed) Assess biobehavioral barriers and family support structure Recognize distrust of the medical establishment
Missed office appointments	Transportation difficulties: Many patients may not have a car and many cities have poor mass transportation systems Competing priorities such as child/grandchild care and elder care (often related to extended family home structure; child care and elder care facilities are often geographically disconnected from health centers) Limited ability to leave work to attend health care appointments in many job settings

BP, blood pressure; ACEI, angiotensin-converting enzyme inhibitor.
Modified with permission from Martins D, Norris K: Hypertension treatment in African Americans: physiology is less important than sociology. Cleve Clin J Med 2004;71(9):735.

▶ Prognosis

The mainstay of hypertensive therapy for African-Americans remains diuretics and therapeutic lifestyle changes. The selection of supplemental antihypertensive agents should be tailored to the presence of coexisting risk factors, comorbid medical conditions, and/or the presence of hypertension-related target organ damage. Many of these patients will need two to four antihypertensive agents to achieve target blood pressure goals. The preference for agents that block the renin–angiotensin system as supplemental antihypertensive agents among patients with CHF, diabetes, and kidney disease cannot be overemphasized. It is, however, pertinent to note that the use of some of these agents among African-Americans is associated with a slightly higher rate of side effects, such as angioedema with ACEIs. Thus, strategies for the treatment of hypertension should be driven by the prevalence of coexisting cardiovascular risk factors and an understanding of sociocultural influences that impact access to care and adherence to evidenced-based treatment rather than minor differences in blood pressure response by racial and ethnic categories. Such approaches will ultimately reduce the disproportionate impact of hypertension and CVD within the African-American community.

Grim CE et al: Hyperaldosteronism and hypertension: ethnic differences. Hypertension 2005;45(4):766.

Heart Disease and Stroke Statistical Update: *2004 Update.* American Heart Association, 2004.

Julius S et al: Cardiovascular risk reduction in hypertensive black patients with left ventricular hypertrophy: the LIFE study. J Am Coll Cardiol 2004;43(6):1047.

Martins D, Norris K: Hypertension treatment in African Americans: physiology is less important than sociology. Cleve Clin J Med 2004;71(9):735.

Martins D, Norris K: Hypertension in African Americans. In: *Handbook of Black American Health, ed 2: Policies and Issues Behind Disparities in Health.* Livingston I (editor). The Greenwood Publishing Group, 2004.

Norris KC, Francis CK: Gender and ethnic differences and considerations in cardiovascular risk assessment and prevention in African Americans. In: *Practical Strategies in Preventing Heart Disease.* Wong N, Gardin JM, Black HR (editors). McGraw-Hill, 2004.

Taylor AL et al: African-American Heart Failure Trial Investigators. Combination of isosorbide dinitrate and hydralazine in blacks with heart failure. N Engl J Med 2004;351(20):2049. Erratum in N Engl J Med 2005;352(12):1276.

▼ HYPERTENSION IN THE ELDERLY

▶ General Considerations

In the past few years there has been a major paradigm shift in thinking about hypertension, with systolic blood pressure (BP) now accepted as the primary clinical concern in adults. Systolic hypertension is generated principally by functional and structural changes in the aorta and large arteries and can be viewed as a condition that differs distinctly from diastolic hypertension. Isolated systolic hypertension is considerably more difficult to treat than diastolic hypertension and expert clinical judgment is often required in establishing acceptable BP targets and in choosing optimal drug therapy.

Age-related BP patterns in industrialized societies are complex (Figure 43–1): Systolic BP increases linearly with age, while diastolic BP increases until about age 50 years and then declines. Mean arterial pressure (MAP) thus increases until about age 50 years and then plateaus, whereas pulse pressure (PP) is constant until age 50 years and then increases. In adults, systolic hypertension is thus the predominant form of the condition. Contrary to popular belief, systolic hypertension is not just "burned out" diastolic hypertension. Rather, it can arise *de novo* at any age, either preceding or without the presence of diastolic hypertension. Aging is not inexorably associated with systolic hypertension: In primitive or cloistered societies there is no relationship between age and BP.

Aging and hypertension dramatically increase the risk for cardiovascular disease (CVD). Overall, each 20 mm Hg increase in systolic BP (or 10 mm Hg increase in diastolic BP) at least doubles the risk of cardiovascular disease or stroke over the range of 115/75 to 185/115 mm Hg. The risk associated with systolic BP is robust and log-linear irrespective of age, while the relationship between diastolic BP and risk is weaker and more complex; the risk for CVD is proportional to diastolic BP until about age 50 years, after which *decreased* diastolic BP and "wide pulse pressure hypertension" are the major markers of increased risk for CVD.

The value of therapy in isolated systolic hypertension has been clearly established for thiazide-based therapy in the Systolic Hypertension in the Elderly Program (SHEP) and for calcium antagonist-based therapy in the Systolic Hypertension in Europe (Syst-EUR) study. In both of these studies, individuals over age 60 years with stage 2 isolated systolic hypertension (pretreatment systolic BP values >160 mm Hg with diastolic BP values <90 mm Hg) experienced a relative reduction in stroke by about one-third when active therapy was compared to placebo. The net differences in systolic BP between the active and control arms in SHEP and Syst-EUR were about 10–12 mm Hg. To date, no study has been completed that demonstrates an outcome benefit of treating stage 1 systolic hypertension (140–159 mm Hg), but it has recently been found that treating prehypertension (systolic BP 120–139 mm Hg) for 2 years with an angiotensin blocker reduces the subsequent incidence of hypertension for at least 2 years after cessation of therapy.

▶ Pathogenesis

The predominant clinical form of hypertension in middle-aged and elderly individuals is isolated systolic hypertension (ISH); combined systolic–diastolic hypertension (SDH) is much less common and isolated diastolic hypertension (IDH) is increasingly rare (Figure 43–2). These clinical subtypes are related to the underlying hemodynamic abnormalities, which are quite heterogeneous from a pathophysiologic perspective. In the past, the pathogenesis of hypertension was oversimplified as a syndrome of arteriolar vasoconstriction and vascular smooth muscle hypertrophy leading to high systemic vascular resistance (SVR) with normal cardiac output.

In reality, hypertension is a collection of hemodynamic anomalies that includes various proportions of (1) increased impedance in large arteries (generating systolic or wide pulse pressure hypertension), (2) decreased luminal diameter of distal arterioles (generating diastolic or mean arterial hypertension), (3) inappropriately high cardiac output, and

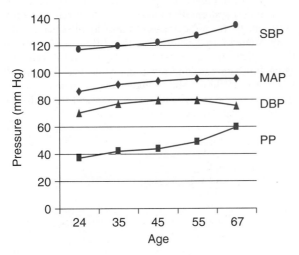

▲ **Figure 43–1.** Age and blood pressure trends. In the third National Health and Nutrition Examination Survey (NHANES III) of the U.S. population, systolic blood pressure (SBP) increased with age, diastolic blood pressure (DBP) increased until about age 50 years and then declined, mean arterial pressure (MAP) reached a plateau at about age 50 years, and pulse pressure (PP) continued to increase with age especially in later years. Data shown are for white males; trends are similar for all races and both genders. (Adapted with permission from Burt VL et al: Prevalence of hypertension in the US population: results from the Third National Health and Nutrition Examination Survey, 1988–1991. Hypertension 1995;25:305.)

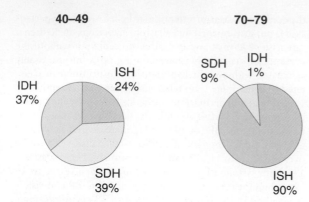

▲ Figure 43–2. Age and prevalence of systolic and diastolic hypertension. Isolated systolic hypertension (ISH) is much more common in older individuals (age 70–79 years) than in younger individuals (age 40–49 years). Combined systolic-diastolic hypertension (SDH) also diminishes with age. Isolated diastolic hypertension (IDH) almost disappears in older individuals. [Adapted with permission from Franklin SS et al: Predominance of isolated systolic hypertension among middle-aged and elderly US hypertensives: analysis based on National Health and Nutrition Examination Survey (NHANES)III. Hypertension 2001;37:869.]

(4) increased blood pressure reactivity to environmental stimuli, most commonly recognized as the "white-coat syndrome." In contrast to IDH, the characteristic sign of increased SVR, ISH is associated with significant increases in aortic impedance and sometimes with increased stroke vol-

ume, with only minimal to moderate increases in SVR (Figure 43–3). In some cases, especially in women and smaller people, increased aortic impedance can be caused by a relatively small aortic diameter with normal aortic wall elastic properties, whereas in older people the aortic wall is stiffer because of thickening and a reduced elastin:collagen ratio. In either case, the widened pulse pressure is the result of the net imbalance between pressure and flow during peak systole. Isolated increases in cardiac output are rare, but in many cases stroke volume is higher than would have been expected given the elevated systemic BP. Understanding which of these anomalies is present is important because each requires different treatment strategies for optimum results.

Increases in large and small arterial impedances usually have opposing effects on diastolic BP. Increased distal impedance (ie, SVR) usually exacerbates systolic hypertension (Figure 43–2) because diastolic BP is the basis of any accompanying systolic elevation in BP. In contrast, increased aortic impedance tends to lower diastolic BP because stiffer central arteries have reduced capacitance function and less elastic recoil. Thus, of each stroke volume less is stored by the aorta during systole and less is available to be delivered by elastic recoil during diastole to sustain distal flow and pressure.

Arm cuff systolic BP values are not fully representative of systolic BP (or pulse pressure) values in other parts of the body. Altered transmission of systolic BP from the heart to the periphery is causally related to changes in BP seen with aging and hypertension. In young people, peak systolic BP in the arm is almost always higher than that measured at the aortic root due to the impedance gradient caused by the progressive taper of peripheral conduit arteries. Yet older or

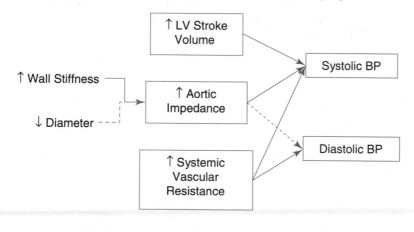

▲ Figure 43–3. Pathogenesis of systolic and diastolic blood pressure (BP) elevations. Increased systemic vascular resistance (SVR) causes parallel elevations in systolic and diastolic BP. Increased left ventricular (LV) stroke volume causes elevated systolic BP. The determinant of wide pulse pressure is increased aortic impedance due to either a smaller aortic diameter or increased effective wall stiffness. Increased aortic impedance simultaneously increases systolic and decreases diastolic BP, thus widening pulse pressure.

hypertensive individuals often have equal aortic and brachial systolic BP values due to the added dimension of enhanced pressure wave reflection. In these individuals, the increased magnitude of the reflected pressure wave in late systole causes late systolic pressure augmentation (where there is summation of the forward and reflected pressure waves). This added systolic BP burden increases cardiac loading and promotes left ventricular hypertrophy.

▶ Treatment

A. Blood Pressure Measurement Issues

For the majority of older patients, the accuracy of brachial cuff BP values is no worse than that of younger people. Peak brachial systolic BP is principally determined by the interaction of the heart and large arteries in early systole (at about 80–90 milliseconds after ventricular contraction begins). Arm cuff BP readings are generally not affected by reflected waves because the primary reflected wave appears much later in systole (about 140 milliseconds), after peak systolic flow has begun to decline rapidly. Pseudohypertension (spuriously high systolic BP readings due to abnormally stiff calcified peripheral arteries) has been reported, but this phenomenon is quite rare in usual medical practice. In fact, older individuals with hypertension often have normal or *increased* peripheral arterial compliance values.

B. Goal Pressures

Despite the continuous relationship between risk and BP, current guidelines have maintained rigid cutoff values for therapy at 140/90 mm Hg in patients without complications or 130/80 mm Hg in patients with diabetes or chronic kidney disease. The value of intensive lowering of BP to values substantially below 140/90 mm Hg has not been tested and some experts still question whether there is a clinically relevant "J-curve" that limits the degree of safe lowering of BP; overall, however, most experts believe that "lower is better." In all cases, sound clinician judgment is needed to individualize therapy.

One useful rule to establish a BP goal in an individual with wide pulse pressure is to calculate the estimated mean arterial pressure (MAP = diastolic + 1/3 pulse pressure) and compare this value to a theoretical threshold value of 100 mm Hg (equivalent to a BP of 140/80 or 130/85 mm Hg). Using this method, if BP is lowered from 170/70 (MAP = 103) mm Hg to 150/70 (MAP = 97) mm Hg, the risk for cardiovascular disease can be reduced hypothetically by as much as 50%. In some cases it may be necessary to proceed more slowly, having established an intermediate level of BP control during an initial stabilization period with systolic BP values <160 mm Hg.

C. Nonpharmacologic Therapy

Controversy still abounds regarding the utility of hygienic measures in older individuals and no clinical study has demonstrated unequivocal outcome benefits of lifestyle modification in older individuals or in ISH. Nevertheless, current guidelines recommend that all individuals with hypertension be instructed in lifestyle modifications that lower BP. Weight loss is probably most important, but sustained weight loss is not usually achieved without some form of increased physical activity. Smoking cessation, moderation of alcohol intake, salt restriction, and increased dietary potassium intake are also recommended.

D. Drug Choices

In general, any drug that lowers BP satisfactorily and does not cause untoward side effects is an appropriate antihypertensive agent for a patient of any age. Choosing among individual drug classes is less important for BP control than it is for the treatment of concomitant conditions or hypertensive complications present in that patient. Yet certain trends have emerged suggesting that each class of antihypertensive drugs has a slightly different profile of optimal outcome benefits.

The most consistently effective and reliable drugs for elderly patients are thiazide diuretics and calcium antagonists, which have been shown to cause effective reduction of BP, stroke, and cardiovascular disease. Yet these same drugs do not appear to protect against chronic kidney disease. Thiazides are safe and effective in modest doses (up to 25 mg hydrochlorothiazide daily). Angiotensin-converting enzyme (ACE) inhibitors or angiotensin blockers are recommended as first-line therapy for individuals with diabetes or chronic kidney disease. These agents have also achieved outcome benefits in ischemic heart disease and heart failure. ACE inhibitors have an inconsistent record in preventing primary or secondary strokes, but angiotensin blockers have demonstrated stroke protection. The reason for the apparent outcome differences between ACE inhibitors and angiotensin blockers is unclear, but inadequate ACE inhibitor dosing has plagued clinical trials with these agents. The least attractive antihypertensives are β-blockers, which are less effective than the other major classes in lowering peripheral and central systolic BP, in protecting the kidney, or in preventing strokes and cardiovascular disease. For these reasons, β-blockers are not ideal choices unless overt ischemic heart disease or heart failure is present.

Ultimately, combination drug therapy is almost unavoidable because the majority of individuals at any age require more than one drug to achieve and sustain a meaningful reduction in BP. The most effective two-drug regimens combine a thiazide diuretic or calcium antagonist with an ACE inhibitor or an angiotensin blocker. Optimal three-drug regimens in the elderly often combine a thiazide diuretic, calcium antagonist, and either an ACE inhibitor or an angiotensin blocker.

E. Barriers to Blood Pressure Control in the Elderly

In general, elderly individuals are more receptive to treatment than their younger counterparts. Nevertheless, there are several specific biological barriers to effective therapy.

1. Central arterial stiffness—With the exception of β-blockers, standard antihypertensive drugs (thiazides, calcium antagonists, ACE inhibitors, and angiotensin blockers) work by directly or indirectly causing arteriolar (and to a lesser degree venous) relaxation. Unfortunately, currently available agents do relatively little to reverse the aortic stiffness that causes isolated systolic hypertension. For this reason, idealized BP targets cannot always be attained in older individuals with longstanding systolic hypertension and very wide pulse pressure. Because the diastolic BP value is relatively fixed in most individuals with wide pulse pressures, the effects of antihypertensive drugs (except β-blockers) are seen mainly in the form of decreases in systolic BP; in the majority of patients, systolic BP can be brought down to levels below 160 mm Hg. Even if ideal goals are not achieved in these patients, substantial benefit can be derived because of the log-linear association between risk and systolic BP.

2. Orthostatic hypotension—Many elderly individuals have impaired postural adaptation reflexes and thus can exhibit clinically significant orthostatic decreases (>20 mm Hg systolic or 10 mm Hg diastolic) in blood pressure. Cardiovascular disease risk is elevated by over 64% in such individuals compared to age-matched controls. Thus, it would be desirable to treat such patients aggressively. Unfortunately, the presence of orthostatic hypotension usually limits aggressive therapy in these individuals due to symptoms such as dizziness and weakness, along with an increased risk of falling. Although there are no formal studies testing individual drug classes in individuals with orthostatic hypotension, it is wise to avoid drugs that can affect postural adaptation, including potent venodilators such as α-blockers, α-β-blockers, organic nitrates, and phosphodiesterase inhibitors. It is also wise to avoid loop diuretics and high doses of thiazide diuretics, which exacerbate orthostatic hypotension by reducing venous return and cardiac filling.

3. Increased blood pressure variability—Because of the low blood flow during diastole in individuals with wide pulse pressure, diastolic BP is relatively fixed. The wide range of variability in BP seen in this group thus occurs mainly in systolic BP, which responds to ambient physiologic stress levels. Regardless of whether the stimulus tends to increase cardiac stroke volume (eg, aerobic exercise) or arteriolar constriction (eg, isotonic exercise), the systolic BP responds. Furthermore, elderly individuals with stiff carotid arteries have reduced baroreflex sensitivity and thus cannot maintain buffered control of sympathetic nervous outflow. The result is often a marked increase in systolic BP variability that is often seen in the form of increased home-office BP differences (including white-coat hypertension). Therapy in these individuals is often difficult and confusing because home BP monitoring may reveal normal BP readings, whereas office values may be very high. In such patients it is important to note that standard antihypertensive drugs have minimal effects on these acute stress-induced changes in BP. Thus, attempts to treat

high "office" pressures can be met with episodes of symptomatic hypotension at home. In most instances, the clinician should carefully assess whether target organ damage (TOD) is present (especially left ventricular hypertrophy or signs of chronic kidney disease). In patients without significant TOD, therapy can be less aggressive. In patients with TOD, every attempt should be made to lower BP with agents appropriate for that individual.

Franklin SS et al: Predictors of new-onset diastolic and systolic hypertension: the Framingham Heart Study. Circulation 2005;111:1121.

Izzo JL Jr: Arterial stiffness and the systolic hypertension syndrome. Curr Opin Cardiol 2004;19:341.

Julius S et al: Trial of Preventing Hypertension Study I. Feasibility of treating prehypertension with an angiotensin-receptor blocker. N Engl J Med 2006;354:1685.

McEniery CM et al: Increased stroke volume and aortic stiffness contribute to isolated systolic hypertension in young adults. Hypertension 2005;46:221.

Williams B et al: Differential impact of blood pressure-lowering drugs on central aortic pressure and clinical outcomes: principal results of the Conduit Artery Function Evaluation (CAFE) study. Circulation 2006;113:1213.

Zhang H et al: Blood pressure lowering for primary and secondary prevention of stroke. Hypertension 2006;48:187.

▼ HYPERTENSION IN PREGNANCY

Tiina Podymow, MD, & Phyllis August, MD, MPH

▶ General Considerations

Hypertension is the most common medical disorder of pregnancy and complicates a reported 6–10% of pregnancies. Of four million women giving birth in the United States each year, an estimated 240,000 are affected by hypertension. Hypertension and preeclampsia can cause serious maternal and fetal problems and account for ~15% of maternal deaths in the United States. Worldwide, preeclampsia causes at least 63,000 maternal deaths yearly.

There are four major hypertensive disorders in pregnancy: (1) Chronic hypertension, (2) preeclampsia, which is pregnancy-induced hypertension associated with proteinuria, (3) preeclampsia superimposed on chronic hypertension, and (4) gestational hypertension. All four types may lead to maternal and perinatal complications, although preeclampsia with severe hypertension is associated with the highest maternal and fetal risks. The diagnosis essentially depends on the gestational age at presentation of hypertension and the presence or absence of proteinuria (Figure 43–4).

A. Chronic Hypertension

Chronic hypertension is blood pressure (BP) >140/90 mm Hg that either predates pregnancy or presents earlier than

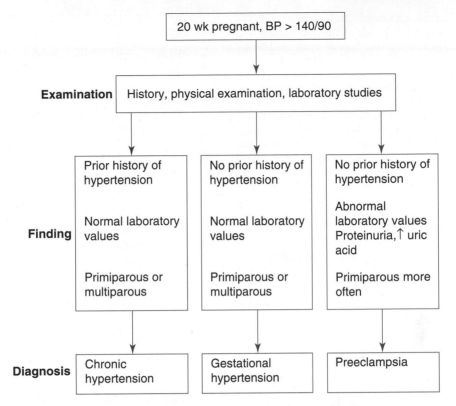

▲ **Figure 43–4.** Algorithm for diagnostic evaluation of pregnant women with hypertension. BP, blood pressure.

20 weeks of pregnancy. It is not associated with proteinuria and complicates approximately 3% of pregnancies.

B. Preeclampsia–Eclampsia

Preeclampsia, a pregnancy-specific syndrome that develops in the latter half of pregnancy (after 20 weeks) in 5–6% of all pregnant women, and is characterized by increased BP (>140/90 mm Hg) and new onset proteinuria (>0.3 g daily) in a woman who had normal BP before 20 weeks. Eclampsia is the occurrence of seizures that cannot be attributed to other causes and complicates approximately 3% of preeclamptic women.

A severe variant of preeclampsia that features hemolysis, elevated liver enzymes, and low platelets (the HELLP syndrome) occurs in 1 in 1000 pregnancies.

C. Preeclampsia Superimposed on Chronic Hypertension

Women with chronic hypertension are at increased risk for the development of superimposed preeclampsia, which complicates 25% of chronic hypertensive pregnancies (versus 5% of nonhypertensive pregnancies). The diagnosis of superimposed preeclampsia is made if proteinuria develops for the first time after 20 weeks in association with an (even higher) increase in BP. In women with both hypertension and proteinuria before 20 weeks of gestation (for example, patients with diabetic nephropathy and proteinuria), superimposed preeclampsia is diagnosed (1) when there is a sudden increase in proteinuria or a sudden increase in BP in the latter half of pregnancy in a woman whose hypertension had previously been well controlled or (2) as part of the HELLP syndrome when there is new onset thrombocytopenia with hemolysis and elevated levels of alanine aminotransferase or aspartate aminotransferase.

D. Gestational Hypertension

Gestational hypertension, seen in 6% of pregnancies, develops in the latter half of pregnancy and is not associated with features of preeclampsia (eg, proteinuria). Some women may ultimately develop signs of preeclampsia, so the final diagnosis can only be made postpartum.

▶ Clinical Findings

A. Maternal Risks

Women with chronic hypertension in pregnancy may develop superimposed preeclampsia; morbidity and mortality rates (both maternal and fetal) are greater in these women than in women with other forms of hypertension in pregnancy. The risk of abruptio placenta is increased 3-fold in women with chronic hypertension. Other risks include accelerated hypertension and cerebrovascular catastrophe; if preeclampsia is superimposed, risks are even worse for accelerated hypertension and fatal intracerebral hemorrhage, which account for 15% of maternal deaths.

Women with secondary hypertension due to renal disease or collagen vascular disease may experience irreversible deterioration in renal function or multiorgan system morbidity regardless of the development of superimposed preeclampsia. If significant azotemia is present (creatinine >1.9 mg/dL, 168 μmol/L), the maternal and fetal outcomes are poor, with worsening azotemia, proteinuria, and hypertension in the mother and growth restriction in the fetus. Finally, pregnancies in women with uncomplicated chronic hypertension are usually successful, but such women are more likely to undergo cesarean delivery and be hospitalized for high BP.

B. Fetal Risks

Perinatal death is higher in pregnancies of women with chronic hypertension than in normotensive women, and superimposed preeclampsia is associated with an even greater risk. Maternal chronic hypertension is a risk factor for intrauterine growth restriction (IUGR, defined as birth weight <10th percentile), which is seen in 5–13% of cases. With superimposed preeclampsia IUGR is seen in 35% of cases and delivery resulting in prematurity occurs in up to 54% of cases; fetal death is the outcome in <1%. Thus, chronic hypertension is associated with increased risk of perinatal death, IUGR, and premature delivery, which are considerably magnified in the presence of superimposed preeclampsia.

▶ Differential Diagnosis

The prevalence of hypertension in premenopausal women is close to 25% and increases with age. Approximately 2–5% of pregnancies are complicated by chronic hypertension. Preexisting hypertension may be more common, particularly in industrialized urban areas where women often postpone child bearing to later years.

If hypertension was clearly documented before conception, the diagnosis of chronic hypertension in pregnancy is straightforward (Figure 43–4). Chronic hypertension is also the most likely diagnosis when hypertension (and no proteinuria) is present before 20 weeks of gestation. In normotensive patients, BP falls in early pregnancy. Systolic pressure changes little, whereas diastolic pressure falls by ~10 mm Hg within 13–20 weeks, with a nadir at 24 weeks, and then rises again to prepregnancy levels in the third trimester (weeks 28–40) (Figure 43–5). This physiologic fall may be even more exaggerated in women with chronic hypertension, and difficulties in diagnosis arise when pregnant women with undiagnosed chronic hypertension are seen for the first time in the second trimester, during the time of the physiologic decrease in BP. In

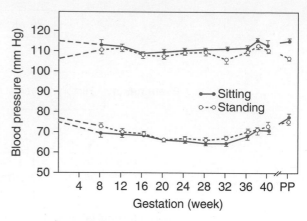

▲ **Figure 43–5.** Blood pressure during normal gestation. The decrease in blood pressure is apparent by the end of the first trimester of pregnancy and often approaches prepregnancy levels at term.

this circumstance, women may appear normotensive (when it is really the physiologic decrease in BP); later they are inaccurately diagnosed with gestational hypertension or preeclampsia when BP rises to prepregnancy levels in the third trimester. In such cases the diagnosis of preeclampsia is ruled out by the absence of proteinuria (greater than "trace" on dipstick is abnormal) and the absence of other classic laboratory abnormalities of preeclampsia or HELLP syndrome such as uric acid greater than 5.5 mg/dL (325 μmol/L), elevated liver function tests, and decreased platelets.

White-coat hypertension (elevated office BP with normal BP outside the medical setting) may be seen in up to 29% of women without preexisting hypertension. A noninvasive 24-hour blood pressure monitor can distinguish white-coat hypertension from true hypertension in the pregnant patient. White-coat hypertension does not appear to predispose paatients to preeclampsia.

Women who present with hypertension before gestational week 20 likely have chronic hypertension. Young women may have secondary hypertension (eg, renal disease, renovascular hypertension, primary aldosteronism, Cushing's syndrome, pheochromocytoma). When secondary hypertension is suspected, noninvasive evaluation may be appropriate (Figure 43–6). For example, if proteinuria is documented in early pregnancy, noninvasive evaluation for renal disease is indicated. This might include 24-hour urinary protein excretion, creatinine clearance, renal ultrasound, and serologic testing to rule out systemic lupus erythematosus if there are suggestive symptoms. Another form of secondary hypertension that should be considered is pheochromocytoma, which although rare is associated with a high rate of morbidity and mortality during pregnancy. This entity should be considered in women with severe hypertension, especially when associated with symptoms such as headache, palpitations, pallor, and

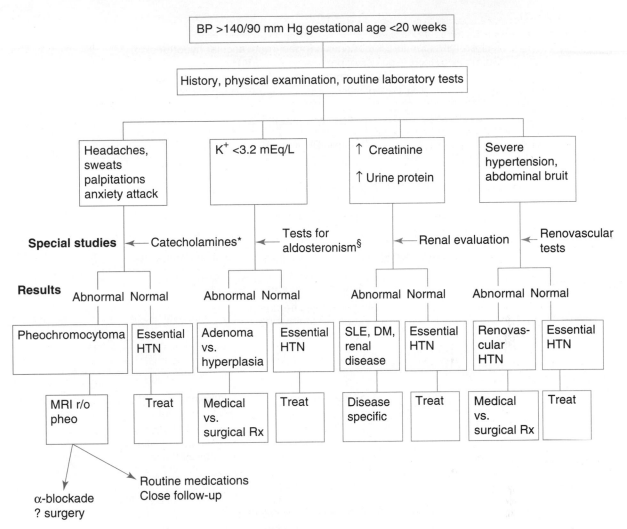

▲ **Figure 43–6.** Algorithm for the diagnosis and treatment of secondary hypertension in pregnancy. *Serum and urine. §Renin, urine aldosterone, and urine potassium; difficult to interpret in pregnancy. Renal evaluation: serologic evaluation, 24-hour urine, and renal ultrasound. Renovascular tests: renin (normally elevated in pregnancy), Doppler ultrasound of renal arteries, magnetic resonance imaging. BP, blood pressure; DM, diabetes mellitus; HTN, hypertension; Rx, treatment; pheo, pheochromocytoma; SLE, systemic lupus erythematosus.

sweats. Significant hypokalemia (potassium <3.2 mEq/L) may be a sign of primary aldosteronism.

Baseline laboratory tests including uric acid, platelets, liver function tests, urea, creatinine, and 24-hour urine for protein should be performed in women with early pregnancy hypertension, as this is helpful in determining the clinical significance of later increases in BP accompanied by abnormal laboratory tests.

Distinguishing between chronic hypertension (that is first noted in pregnancy) and gestational hypertension is not possible until after delivery. In some instances, women with undocumented hypertension before pregnancy will have normal BP throughout their entire pregnancy, only to return to prepregnancy hypertensive levels in the postpartum period; this accounts for the mysterious cases of isolated postpartum hypertension.

▶ **Treatment**

A. Preconception

Management of the pregnant woman with chronic hypertension begins before conception to establish the diagnosis and to rule out forms of secondary hypertension such as renal disease and renovascular hypertension (Figure 43–7).

Preconception
Screen for secondary hypertension (pheo, renovascular hypertension) Counseling: Increased risk of preeclampsia (25%) Lifestyle adjustments: Increase rest, decrease excercise Adjust medications: Discontinue ACE inhibitors

First trimester		
Diastolic BP, mm Hg		
<90	90–100	≥100
Consider careful decrease in BP medication	Adjust medications: Stop ACE and angiotensin II β blockers Decrease diuretic dose	Increase medication
Baseline evaluation for secondary hypertension if clinically suspected		

Second trimester		
Nonpharmacologic treatment ❑ Home BP monitoring ❑ Adequate rest		
Diastolic BP, mm Hg		
<90	90–100	≥100
Consider careful decrease in BP medication	Continue treatment	Indicates significant hypertension: Consider stopping work; close surveillance for preeclampsia

Third trimester
Increased surveillance for preeclampsia Check BP every 2 weeks

▲ **Figure 43–7.** Treatment algorithm of chronic hypertension. pheo, pheochromocytoma; ACE, angiotensin-converting enzyme; BP, blood pressure.

Patients who have had hypertension for longer than 5 years, older women, and women with chronic illnesses such as diabetes may be evaluated for target organ damage such as left ventricular hypertrophy, fundoscopic changes, azotemia, and cardiac disease. Ideally, medications should be adjusted before pregnancy, and medications with deleterious fetal effects, such as angiotensin-converting enzyme inhibitors (ACEIs) and angiotensin II receptor blockers (ARBs), can be assessed. Preconception is also the time to discuss the risks posed by pregnancy. Women should be informed of the likelihood of a favorable outcome if they have chronic hypertension, but should be apprised of the risks of superimposed preeclampsia

and fetal complications. Patient education regarding these issues helps to increase compliance and may improve outcome, and frequent visits will increase the likelihood of detecting preeclampsia and other complications before they become life threatening.

B. Postconception

1. Nonpharmacologic management—Treatment of hypertension in the gravid patient represents a departure from guidelines for treatment of nonpregnant hypertensive women. Patients are not advised to exercise vigorously as the concern is that women with chronic hypertension are at risk for preeclampsia, a condition characterized by decreased uteroplacental blood flow that vigorous exercise may further compromise. Of note, women who work outside the home had both higher blood pressure and an increased risk of preeclampsia in one study. Decreased work hours and more rest may theoretically increase placental blood flow and decrease BP.

Excessive weight loss during pregnancy is not advisable, even in obese women. Salt restriction is an important component of the management of many nonpregnant hypertensive individuals, but extremely low sodium intake (<2 g sodium) is not advisable during pregnancy. Calcium supplementation in excess of the recommended dietary allowance has not been shown to reduce the incidence of superimposed preeclampsia; however, in the developing world, in women with low dietary intake, calcium supplementation may prevent preeclampsia.

2. Pharmacologic management—In nonpregnant adults, control of BP can decrease the long-term incidence of cardiovascular disease and mortality. During the 9 months of pregnancy, however, untreated mild to moderate hypertension is unlikely to lead to adverse maternal outcomes. An important issue for women with chronic hypertension is the prevention of preeclampsia; however, there is little evidence that the treatment of mild to moderate hypertension in pregnancy reduces the incidence of superimposed preeclampsia.

The appropriate level of BP in a pregnant woman with hypertension is consensus rather than evidence based. International guidelines vary concerning both the thresholds for starting treatment and the targeted BP goals. Recommendations here are in accord with those of the National High Blood Pressure Education Programs' (NHBEP) working Group Report on High Blood Pressure in pregnancy. When maternal BP reaches levels $\geq150/90$–95 mm Hg, treatment should be instituted to avoid hypertensive vascular damage, with BP generally targeted to 140/90 mm Hg.

As BP normally drops in the first two trimesters of pregnancy, including women with chronic hypertension, clinicians can consider discontinuing antihypertensive drugs and monitoring. Therapy can then be initiated at a BP of $\geq150/90$ mm Hg for otherwise healthy pregnant women with mild to moderate hypertension, regardless of type. A wide variety of reasonable agents are available for use (Table 43–4). The Food and Drug Administration classification of drugs in pregnancy designates most antihypertensive medications as category C, indicating that the drug should be given only if potential benefits justify potential risks to the fetus. This category cannot be interpreted as no risk, and is so broad that it is not clinically useful. The most recent evidence assessing the risks and benefits of drugs useful in treating hypertension in pregnancy will be reviewed. These medications have the longest history of safe use in pregnancy; however, they are rarely used in the nonpregnant population due to side effects or inconvenient dosing.

3. Central adrenergic agonists

A. METHYLDOPA—Methyldopa remains the drug of first choice for treatment of hypertension in pregnancy; it has not been found to be teratogenic after a 40-year history of use. In treated patients it has been found to be useful in decreasing the occurrence of severe hypertension and hospital admissions compared with untreated patients. Birth weight and development in the first year as well as development to the age of 7 years were similar in children exposed to methyldopa compared to children in the placebo group. Methyldopa is metabolized to α-methylnorepinephrine and replaces norepinephrine to decrease sympathetic tone centrally. The adverse effects are due to its action at the brainstem and include decreased mental alertness, impaired sleep, and decreased salivation leading to xerostomia. It can cause elevated liver enzymes in 5% of patients, with hepatitis or hepatic necrosis rarely reported. It has been associated with Coombs' positivity without (except rarely) hemolytic anemia as well as a positive antinuclear antibody (ANA).

B. CLONIDINE—Clonidine is another α_2-adrenergic agonist comparable to methyldopa, although it is not used in preference to methyldopa given the proven safety of the latter. There is a greater potential for rebound hypertension when this drug is abruptly discontinued, and its use is reserved for individuals who cannot tolerate the other medications.

C. β-ADRENOCEPTOR BLOCKERS—β-Adrenoceptor blockers have been studied extensively in pregnancy and none has been associated with teratogenicity. Individual agents are not distinguishable with the exception of atenolol, which has been associated with decreased fetal weight compared to placebo. Oral and parenteral β-blockade have been associated with neonatal bradycardia, which was not clinically significant for the most part.

Maternal outcomes have been found to improve with the use of β-blockers, which control maternal BP and decrease both the incidence of severe hypertension and the rate of admission to hospital prior to delivery. They have been compared and found to be equivalent to methyldopa in 15 trials. Adverse effects due to β-blockade include fatigue, lethargy, exercise intolerance, sleep disturbance, and bronchoconstriction in patients with asthma.

Labetalol, a nonselective β-blocker with vascular α_1-receptor blocking capabilities, has gained wide acceptance for use in pregnancy. When administered orally in patients with chronic hypertension, it is as safe and effective as methyldopa. Parenterally it is used to treat severe hypertension, and when compared to hydralazine has been associated with a lower incidence of maternal hypotension and other side effects.

D. CALCIUM CHANNEL BLOCKERS—Calcium channel blockers have been used to treat chronic hypertension, mild preeclampsia, and urgent hypertension in preeclampsia. Orally administered nifedipine and verapamil do not appear to

Table 43–4. Drugs for chronic hypertension in pregnancy.[1,2]

Drug (FDA risk[3])	Dose	Concerns or comments
Preferred agent Methyldopa (B)	0.5–3.0 g/day in two or three divided doses	Drug of choice according to the NHBEP working group; safety after the first trimester is well documented, including 7-year follow-up of offspring
Second-line agents[4] Labetolol (C)	200–1200 mg/day in two or three divided doses	May be associated with fetal growth restriction and neonatal bradycardia
Nifedipine (C)	30–90 mg/day of a slow-release preparation	May inhibit labor and have a synergistic interaction with magnesium sulfate
Hydralazine (C)	50–300 mg/day in two to four divided doses	Few controlled trials; long experience with a few adverse events documented; useful only in combination with sympatholytic agents; may cause neonatal thrombocytopenia
β-Receptor blockers (C)	Depends on the specific agent	May cause fetal bradycardia and decrease uteroplacental blood flow, which may be less for agents with partial agonist activity; may impair fetal response to hypoxic stress; risk of growth restriction when started in the first or second trimester (atenolol)
Hydrochlorothiazide (C)	25 mg/day	The majority of controlled studies are in normotensive pregnant women rather than in hypertensive patients; can cause volume depletion and electrolyte disorders; may be useful in combination with methyldopa and vasodilators to mitigate compensatory fluid retention
Contraindicated ACE inhibitors and AT1 receptor antagonists (D[5])	—	Leads to fetal loss in animals; human use in the second and third trimester is associated with fetopathy, oligohydramnios, growth restriction, and neonatal anuric renal failure, which may be fatal

[1]No antihypertensive has been proven safe for use during the first trimester.
[2]Drug therapy is indicated for uncomplicated chronic hypertension when diastolic BP >100 mm Hg (Korotkoff V). Treatment at lower levels may be indicated for patients with diabetes mellitus, renal disease, or target organ damage.
[3]U.S. Food and Drug Administration classification.
[4]Some agents are omitted (eg, clonidine, α-blockers) due to limited data on their use for chronic hypertension in pregnancy.
[5]Authors would classify in category X during the second and third trimesters.
FDA, Food and Drug Administration; NHBEP, National High Blood Pressure Education Programs; ACE, angiotensin-converting enzyme.

pose teratogenic risk to fetuses exposed in the first trimester. Maternal side effects of the calcium channel blockers include palpitations, peripheral edema, headaches, and facial flushing. Most investigators have focused on the use of nifedipine, although there are reports on nicardipine, isradipine, felodipine, and verapamil as well; amlodipine is still unstudied in pregnancy.

A concern with the use of calcium antagonists for control of BP in preeclampsia is the concomitant use of magnesium sulfate to prevent seizures; drug interactions with nifedipine and magnesium sulfate have been reported to cause neuromuscular blockade, myocardial depression, or circulatory collapse, although in practice these medications are commonly used together and the actual risk appears to be low.

(E) DIURETICS—Although diuretics are widely used in the treatment of nonpregnant hypertensive patients,

obstetricians are reluctant to use diuretics because of a concern that they will interfere with the physiologic volume expansion of normal pregnancy. However, in a meta-analysis of trials involving >7000 subjects diuretics appeared to prevent preeclampsia. While volume contraction might be expected to limit fetal growth, data have not supported this concern. Of note, mild volume contraction with diuretic therapy may lead to hyperuricemia, and in so doing may invalidate serum uric acid levels as a laboratory marker in the diagnosis of superimposed preeclampsia.

Diuretics are commonly prescribed in essential hypertension prior to conception and, given their apparent safety, the NHBEP Working Group on High Blood Pressure in Pregnancy concluded that they may be continued through gestation or used in combination with other agents, especially for women deemed likely to have salt-sensitive hypertension. Hydrochlorothiazide may be continued; utilization of low doses, no more than 25 mg daily, can minimize the side effects of impaired glucose tolerance and hypokalemia. Spironolactone is not recommended due to theoretic antiandrogen effects during fetal development.

F. DIRECT VASODILATORS—Hydralazine is effective orally, intramuscularly, or intravenously; parenteral administration is useful for rapid control of severe hypertension. Adverse effects, mostly due to excessive vasodilation or sympathetic activation, include headache, nausea, flushing, or palpitations. In rare cases, chronic use can lead to a pyridoxine-responsive polyneuropathy or to a drug-induced lupus syndrome.

Hydralazine has been used in all trimesters of pregnancy and is not associated with teratogenicity. It has been widely used for chronic hypertension in the second and third trimesters, but use has been supplanted by agents with more favorable side effect profiles. For acute severe hypertension later in pregnancy, intravenous hydralazine has been associated with more maternal and perinatal adverse effects than intravenous labetalol or oral nifedipine, such as maternal hypotension, oliguria, cesarean sections, placental abruptions, and APGAR scores <7. Furthermore, the common side effects such as headache, nausea, and vomiting mimic the symptoms of deteriorating preeclampsia. A recent meta-analysis of the use of intravenous hydralazine for severe hypertension in pregnancy does not support its use first line, and suggests that parenteral labetalol or oral nifedipine may be preferable.

Nitroprusside is seldom used in pregnancy; it is used only as a last resort in cases of life-threatening hypertension with heart failure. Adverse effects include excessive vasodilation and syncope in the mother and a risk of cyanide toxicity in the fetus.

Isosorbide dinitrate has been investigated in a small study of gestational hypertensive and preeclamptic patients. It was found to lower BP but not cerebral perfusion, thus decreasing the risk for ischemia and infarction when BP is lowered.

G. SEROTONIN₂ RECEPTOR BLOCKERS—Ketanserin is a selective S_2 receptor-blocking drug that appears to be safe and useful in the treatment of chronic hypertension in pregnancy, preeclampsia, and HELLP syndrome. Ketanserin is used in Australia and South Africa, but has not been approved by the Food and Drug Administration for use in the United States.

H. ANGIOTENSIN-CONVERTING ENZYME INHIBITORS AND ANGIOTENSIN RECEPTOR ANTAGONISTS—ACEIs and angiotensin receptor agents are contraindicated in pregnancy due to toxicity associated with reduced perfusion of the fetal kidneys; their use is associated with a fetopathy similar to that observed in Potter's syndrome, ie, bilateral renal agenesis, oligohydramnios due to fetal oliguria, calvarial hypoplasia, pulmonary hypoplasia, intrauterine growth retardation, and neonatal anuric renal failure leading to death. Use of ARBs in pregnancy has also caused fetal demise amid the same pathogenic features.

The available evidence on first trimester exposure to ACEIs is not consistent with high teratogenic risk, although a small risk cannot be ruled out. Most cases of malformations have been associated with second or third trimester use. As such, inadvertent first trimester drug exposure is not considered to be an indication for elective termination of the pregnancy. Of note, many women at risk for hypertension during pregnancy, particularly those with underlying diabetes mellitus, may benefit from use of ACEIs prior to conception. Since all cases of ACEI-associated fetopathy or renal failure occurred with drug use in the latter two trimesters, it seems reasonable to use these drugs when appropriate and to counsel women to switch to alternate agents either while attempting to conceive or as soon as the pregnancy is diagnosed.

C. Preeclampsia

1. Clinical features and diagnosis—Preeclampsia is the development of hypertension in association with new-onset proteinuria (>0.3 g daily), edema, and hyperuricemia after 20 weeks of gestation. Edema alone has been abandoned as a marker of preeclampsia because it is present in too many normal pregnant women to be a specific indicator of disease. Mild preeclampsia can be distinguished from severe preeclampsia: features of severe preeclampsia include severe hypertension (systolic pressure greater than 160/110 mm Hg on two occasions), eclampsia (seizures), pulmonary edema, cortical blindness, proteinuria >5 g/24 hours, renal failure or oliguria (<500 mL/24 hours), hepatocellular injury (serum transaminase levels ≥2 × normal), thrombocytopenia (<100,000 platelets/mm³), coagulopathy, or HELLP syndrome.

Important findings on physical examination in addition to elevated BP include hyperreflexia, generalized edema, and vasospasm on fundoscopic examination.

It is important to determine which women are at increased risk for preeclampsia, because such individuals need to be followed more closely during pregnancy. Those at increased risk for preeclampsia include women with chronic hypertension, women who had early (before 34 weeks of gestation) or severe preeclampsia in a previous pregnancy, and women with diabetes, collagen vascular disease, renovascular disease, renal parenchymal disease, or a multifetal pregnancy, or women who were the product of a pregnancy complicated by preeclampsia (Table 43–5). Such women should have a baseline laboratory evaluation performed early in gestation. Recommended tests that are helpful to compare and to discriminate preeclampsia from chronic or transient hypertension later in pregnancy include hematocrit, hemoglobin, platelet count, serum creatinine, uric acid, alanine aminotransferase, and aspartate aminotransferase. If qualitative dipstick proteinuria is documented, a 24-hour urine collection should be performed for the determination of protein and creatinine clearance. There is an extensive literature reporting the ability of various clinical signs or laboratory tests to predict, early in

Table 43–5. Risk factors for preeclampsia.

Risk factors

Nulliparity

Multiple gestation [relative risk (RR) 2.93]

Family history of preeclampsia (mother or sister) (RR 2.9)

History of preeclampsia before 34 weeks in a previous pregnancy (40% recurrence)

History of HELLP syndrome (50% risk of preeclampsia in subsequent pregnancy)

Obesity body mass index ≥35 (odds ratio for preeclampsia 4.5)

Hydatidiform mole

Age ≥40 years

Underlying medical conditions

    Preexisting hypertension (odds ratio 3.8)

    Preexisting renal disease

    Preexisting diabetes (RR 3.56)

    Presence of antiphospholipid antibodies (R.R 9.72)

What to do after the risk assessment

Offer women referral before 20 weeks to a specialist in the medical complications of pregnancy (internist, nephrologist, hematologist, or endocrinologist as appropriate) for input to their antenatal care plan if they have one of the following (grade D evidence):

    Previous preeclampsia

    Multiple pregnancy

    Underlying medical conditions

        Preexisting hypertension or booking diastolic blood pressure ≥90 mm Hg

        Preexisting renal disease or booking proteinuria (positive on more than one occasion or ≥300 mg/24 hours)

        Preexisting diabetes

        Presence of antiphospholipid antibodies

HELLP, hemolysis, elevated liver enzyme, and low platelets.

pregnancy, which patients will later develop preeclampsia. While many of these tests reflect important pathophysiologic features of preeclampsia, none is considered sensitive or specific enough to use at this time.

2. Prevention—Strategies to prevent preeclampsia, including sodium restriction, diuretics, high protein diets, low dose aspirin, calcium supplementation, fish oil, magnesium, antioxidants, and antihypertensive medication, have been largely ineffective. Baby aspirin is a relatively benign drug that is still used in select cases, although in large meta analyses its utility appears uncertain.

3. Pathophysiology—The pathophysiology of preeclampsia can be divided into two stages: Alterations in placental perfusion and the maternal syndrome. Abnormalities begin in the vascular supply of the developing placenta, leading to placental ischemia and production of vasculogenic substances, which upon reaching the maternal circulation produce the maternal clinical syndrome. There is evidence for the importance of the placenta in the pathogenesis of preeclampsia, which can develop without a fetus in the case of molar pregnancies (a rapidly growing placenta with trophoblastic tissue) and in multiple gestations (increased placental mass).

There is an increased incidence of preeclampsia in women with medical conditions associated with microvascular disease such as hypertension, diabetes, and collagen vascular disease, as the impaired placental perfusion leading to ischemia may be the common starting point of this disease.

Impaired placental perfusion appears to cause the release of "factors" into the maternal circulation. Angiogenic proteins such as placental growth factor (PlGF) and vascular endothelial growth factor (VEGF), which are both required for normal angiogenesis and endothelial function in pregnancy, are reduced in women with preeclampsia. Recent studies report elevated maternal serum levels of a protein that appears to scavenge these factors and induce endothelial dysfunction: sFlt-1, a soluble fms-like tyrosine kinase. This molecule functions to neutralize VEGF and PlGF. In experimental studies, increased serum levels of sFlt-1 and reduced levels of PlGF have been found to predict the development of preeclampsia in humans. The mechanism for the upregulation of sFlt-1 and whether normalization of VEGF and PlGF levels might halt progression of preeclampsia are yet unknown.

4. Blood pressure—High BP in preeclampsia is due mainly to a reversal of the vasodilation of normal pregnancy, replaced by a marked increase in peripheral vascular resistance. Preeclamptic patients do not develop overt hypertension until late gestation (after week 20, and usually not until the third trimester-weeks 28–40), but vasoconstrictor influences may be present much earlier. For instance, longitudinal and epidemiologic surveys show that women destined to develop preeclampsia have slightly higher "normal" blood pressure (eg, diastolic levels >70 mm Hg) as early as the second trimester.

BP in preeclampsia is characteristically labile, and there is a reversal of the normal circadian rhythm, with BP levels often being higher at night. These changes should be kept in mind when evaluating a woman with preeclampsia, because two observers may obtain different readings, reflecting lability and not measurement error. In addition, increases in peripheral vascular resistance and BP that characterize preeclampsia have been found to be mediated by an increase in sympathetic vasoconstrictor activity, which reverts to normal after delivery. These observations lend mechanistic support to the use of methyldopa and labetalol.

5. Treatment—Most cases of preeclampsia present close to term. They are managed by obstetricians with an approach that includes bed rest, consideration of the use of antihypertensive medications, and delivery of the fetus, followed by seizure prophylaxis with magnesium sulfate. Although there are no proven strategies for the prevention of preeclampsia, early diagnosis is important to avoid severe complications. When early signs of preeclampsia are detected, hospitalization should be strongly considered to permit close monitoring of the patient. If preeclampsia is diagnosed early, bed rest and close monitoring of maternal and fetal conditions may enable prolongation of pregnancy and improve maternal and fetal outcomes.

Lowering BP does not cure preeclampsia but may prolong the pregnancy, because uncontrolled hypertension is frequently an indication for delivery. In a woman with preeclampsia it prevents the maternal cerebrovascular and cardiovascular complications that result from elevated BP. There is a consensus that severe hypertension, defined as >160/110 mm Hg, requires treatment because these women are at increased risk of intracerebral hemorrhage and because lowering BP leads to a decrease in maternal death. Women with hypertensive encephalopathy, hemorrhage, or eclampsia (seizures) require treatment with parenteral agents to lower mean arterial pressure (two-thirds diastolic + one-third systolic BP) by 25% over minutes to hours, and then to further lower BP to ≤160/100 mm Hg over subsequent hours. In women with preeclampsia, treatment of acute severe hypertension should be initiated at lower doses, as these patients may be intravascularly volume depleted and are at increased risk for hypotension. The parenteral medications used to treat acute hypertension in women with preeclampsia are listed in Table 43–6. If delivery is not anticipated immediately (within 24–48 hours) antihypertensive therapy should be considered when diastolic BP reaches 100 mm Hg; in this instance, oral agents are appropriate.

Maternal factors that may signal the time for delivery in preeclampsia include gestational age over 38 weeks, platelet count $<100 \times 10^3$, progressive deterioration in liver and renal function, suspected abruptio placenta, and uncontrolled severe hypertension despite medication. Fetal factors include fetal growth restriction, nonreassuring fetal testing results, and oligohydramnios.

Renal function is usually well preserved, and because relative oliguria is often a manifestation of renal vasoconstriction rather than impaired glomerular filtration rate it is not advisable to "push fluids" in such circumstances to increase urine output. Aggressive hydration of women with preeclampsia may result in acute pulmonary edema, a rare manifestation that may develop when abundant intravenous fluids are administered or on the backdrop of preexisting coronary disease. Decreased urinary output will usually resolve within 24 hours of delivery and will not be associated with acute tubular necrosis.

Some, although not all women develop considerable peripheral edema in association with preeclampsia. The mechanisms are likely a combination of hypoalbuminemia, increased renal sodium reabsorption, and local tissue factors such as increased capillary permeability. Despite the presence of edema, plasma volume is reduced in most cases, presumably as a consequence of vasoconstriction as opposed to underfilling of the arterial circulation. In view of the reduced plasma volume, there is a reluctance to administer diuretic

Table 43–6. Drugs for urgent control of severe hypertension in pregnancy.[1]

Drug (FDA risk[2])	Dose and route	Concerns or comments[3]
Labetolol (C)	20 mg intravenously, then 20–80 mg every 20–30 minutes, up to a maximum of 300 mg; or constant infusion of 1–2 mg/minute	Experience in pregnancy less than with hydralazine. Probably less risk of tachycardia and arrhythmia than with other vasodilators
Hydralazine (C)	5 mg, intravenously or intramuscularly, then 5–10 mg every 20–40 minutes, or a constant infusion of 0.5–10 mg/hour	Drug of choice according to NHBEP working group; long experience of safety and efficacy
Nifedipine (C)	Tablets recommended only: 10–30 mg orally; repeat in 45 minutes if needed	Reports of synergistic interaction with magnesium sulfate
Relatively contraindicated: Nitroprusside (C[4])	Constant infusion of 0.5–10 μg/kg/minute	Possible cyanide toxicity; agent of last resort.

[1]Indicated for acute elevation of diastolic blood pressure >105 mm Hg; the goal is a gradual reduction to 90–100 mm Hg.
[2]U.S. Food and Drug Administration classification; C indicates either that studies in animals have revealed adverse effects on the fetus (teratogenic, embryocidal, or other) and/or there are no controlled studies in women, or studies in women and animals are not available. Drugs should be given only if the potential benefits justify the potential risk to the fetus.
[3]Adverse effects for all agents, except as noted, may include headache flushing, nausea, and tachycardia (primarily due to precipitous hypotension and reflex sympathetic activation). NHBEP, National High Blood Pressure Education Programs.
[4]We would classify this in category D: There is positive evidence of human fetal risk, but the benefits of use in pregnant women may be acceptable despite the risk (eg, if the drug is needed in a life-threatening situation or for a serious disease for which safer drugs cannot be used or are ineffective).

therapy to women with preeclampsia, even when edema is present, because diuretics may further reduce plasma volume and potentially compromise uteroplacental perfusion. However, in the postpartum period, edema may become considerably worse due to administration of intravenous fluids during surgery. Moreover, hypertension may be worse in the first postpartum week, and tends to reach its maximum by the fifth postpartum day. Thus, on occasion, it may be necessary to administer small doses of diuretics when edema becomes marked and causes discomfort, particularly when BP is elevated.

Seizures are generally preceded with complaints of headache. The contribution of uncontrolled hypertension to the eclamptic seizure has been disputed. Some have argued that eclampsia is a manifestation of hypertensive encephalopathy, while others cite data indicating that many women who seize have BP levels that are only mildly elevated. However, uncontrolled hypertension may lower the seizure threshold, and although the treatment of hypertension does not necessarily prevent eclamptic seizures, BP levels should be maintained in a "safe" range of 130–150/80–100 mm Hg. Most of the cases of intracerebral hemorrhage and death due to eclampsia have occurred in women with preexisting hypertension and uncontrolled BP. Antihypertensive therapy should be combined with intravenous magnesium sulfate in the postpartum period, because it is the anticonvulsant of choice to prevent eclamptic seizures. Reversible posterior leukencephalopathy (transient cortical blindness) resolves with BP management as above.

The liver may be involved in severe cases of preeclampsia, usually in association with hemolysis and thrombocytopenia (the HELLP syndrome). The HELLP syndrome is associated with a poor prognosis and is usually an indication for urgent delivery. Women with liver involvement may develop epigastric or right upper quadrant pain resulting from hepatocellular necrosis, edema, and ischemia leading to stretching of the Glisson capsule. Periportal hemorrhagic necrosis in the periphery of the liver lobule results in elevations in liver enzymes. On rare occasions, there may be bleeding from these lesions, and hepatic rupture is a fatal complication of preeclampsia if not recognized early and treated aggressively with supportive therapy and surgery. The consultant should be familiar with these complications of preeclampsia and should recognize the potential severity of the development of epigastric, chest, or abdominal pain in a woman with preeclampsia.

6. Obstetric issues: Fetal monitoring and delivery—
Once preeclampsia is diagnosed, monitoring of the fetus is indicated to identify fetal distress, which, if present, would be an indication for urgent delivery. One of the most difficult management issues in preeclampsia is the timing of delivery in cases in which fetal maturity is questionable. Delivery is always appropriate therapy for the mother. However, delivery is not indicated for a preterm fetus with no evidence of fetal compromise in a woman with only mild preeclampsia. Important decisions are based on whether the fetus is more likely to survive without significant neonatal complications *in utero* or in the nursery and whether maternal safety will be jeopardized by the postponement of delivery.

Delivery is always indicated when preeclampsia develops at term and should be strongly considered in women who have severe preeclampsia beyond 32–34 weeks of gestation. In women with preeclampsia remote from term (23–32 weeks) prolongation of pregnancy is possible in only a select group of women with easily controlled hypertension, no evidence of fetal distress, and no indication of serious maternal disease (headache, abdominal pain, and signs of the HELLP syndrome).

▶ Prognosis

Hypertension frequently persists after delivery in women with antenatal hypertension or preeclampsia, and BP may be labile in the weeks postpartum. BP may increase even higher if patients are treated with nonsteroidal anti-inflammatory agents. The goals of treatment are to prevent severe hypertension (and its consequences of cerebral hemorrhage and eclampsia). Antihypertensive treatment given antenatally should be reordered postpartum and then discontinued in days to weeks after BP normalizes. If BP was normal prior to conception, then normalization is likely to return after 2–12 weeks. Hypertension that persists beyond that may represent previously undiagnosed chronic hypertension or secondary hypertension and should be evaluated and followed.

Evaluation should also be considered postpartum for patients who developed preeclampsia early (at less than 34 weeks of gestation), who had severe preeclampsia, who had a recurrence of this condition, or who continue to have persistent proteinuria. In these cases, renal disease, secondary hypertension, and thrombophilias (eg, factor V Leiden) may be evaluated.

Counseling for future pregnancies requires consideration of different recurrence rates for preeclampsia depending on the pathogenesis and population. The earlier in gestation, the higher the risk of recurrence; before week 30, recurrence may be as high as 40%. If preeclampsia has developed in a nulliparous woman close to term (ie, after 36 weeks), the risk of recurrence is thought to be 10%. Patients who had HELLP syndrome appear to have a high risk of subsequent obstetric complications, with preeclampsia occurring in 55%; however, the rate of recurrent HELLP appears to be low, only 6%.

Hypertensive diseases of pregnancy have been associated with the risk of hypertension and stroke later in life. In one study, gestational hypertension was associated with a relative risk (RR) of 3.72 for later hypertension, and preeclampsia with a RR of 3.98 for later hypertension and 3.59 for stroke. Preeclampsia is also a risk factor for coronary disease when studied retrospectively. These associations serve to increase awareness for the need to monitor patients for future hypertensive and cardiovascular disorders.

In general, antihypertensive drugs that are bound to plasma protein are not transferred to breast milk. Lipid-soluble drugs achieve concentrations higher than water-soluble drugs. Neonatal exposure to methyldopa, labetalol, captopril, and nifedipine via nursing is low, and these medications are considered safe in breastfeeding. Atenolol and metoprolol are concentrated in breast milk, possibly to levels that could affect the infant, and are not recommended. Finally, although the concentration of diuretics in breast milk is usually low, these agents may reduce milk production due to mild volume contraction and may interfere with the ability to successfully breast feed.

Levine RJ et al: Urinary placental growth factor and risk of pre-eclampsia. JAMA 2005;293(1):77.

Milne F et al: The pre-eclampsia community guideline (PRECOG): how to screen for and detect onset of pre-eclampsia in the community. BMJ 2005;330(7491):576.

Sibai BM: Diagnosis, controversies, and management of the syndrome of hemolysis, elevated liver enzymes, and low platelet count. Obstet Gynecol 2004;103(5 Pt 1):981.

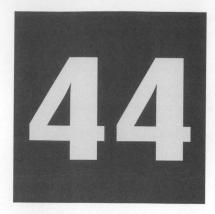

44

Refractory Hypertension

Luis M. Ruilope, MD, & Julian Segura, MD

ESSENTIALS OF DIAGNOSIS

▶ Blood pressure above the recommended values (140/90 mm Hg) despite the use of greater than or equal to 3–4 antihypertensive agents, each belonging to a different class.

▶ Insufficient treatment prescription and lack of adherence to prescribed drugs, dietary restrictions, and lifestyle recommendations are the most frequent causes.

▶ Associated with obesity, sleep apnea, diabetes, chronic kidney disease, advanced age, high dietary salt intake, and black race.

As the 21st century unfolds, hypertension remains a challenging medical problem. Hypertension continues to be a common reason for office, urgent care center, and emergency room visits. If not properly controlled, hypertension can lead to blindness, renal failure, heart disease, and stroke. In spite of the establishment of extensive health action programs, blood pressure (BP) values remain above the recommended objectives in the majority of patients with hypertension. Data from the National Health and Nutrition Examination Survey 1999–2000 showed that in only 34% of all persons with hypertension in the United States was blood pressure controlled to meet recommended values. Similar data come from different countries.

Common factors associated with the development of resistant hypertension include obesity, sleep apnea, diabetes, chronic kidney disease, advanced age, high dietary salt intake, and black race. Interfering substances such as nonsteroidal anti-inflammatory drugs and excessive alcohol consumption can worsen blood pressure control. However, an insufficient treatment prescription and the lack of adherence to the prescribed drug and lifestyle recommendations (eg, the moderation of alcohol consumption, the restriction of salt intake, the reduction of body weight) seem to be the most frequent causes of uncontrolled BP. Other causes of resistance to treatment include cases of spurious hypertension, such as isolated office (white-coat) hypertension, and failure to use large cuffs on large arms. Nevertheless, a significant number of patients adequately diagnosed and treated still have uncontrolled BP. The real prevalence of refractory hypertension is difficult to determine. Published studies describe a prevalence that oscillates between 3% and 30% in hypertension units. Further, the existence of different diagnostic and therapeutic strategies makes a comparison between different published studies difficult.

This review focuses on those causes of resistance to treatment that can be evaluated in the outpatient setting. These include a search for nonadherence, assessing the adequacy of the treatment regimen, and ruling out drug interactions and associated conditions. In the absence of the above factors, assessment for secondary causes of hypertension is appropriate. This careful stepwise evaluation is not only cost effective, but also capable of identifying the contributing factors in the vast majority of patients with apparently resistant hypertension.

▶ General Considerations

The recent joint directives of the European Society of Hypertension/European Society of Cardiology (ESH-ESC) define the treatment of refractory hypertension as a therapeutic plan that includes attention to lifestyle measures and the prescription of at least three drugs (including a diuretic); however, in adequate doses this has failed to lower systolic and diastolic BP sufficiently. Moreover, the VII Joint National Committee report further notes the exclusion of potential causes of secondary hypertension (including the use of agents that may increase BP), with special attention to the type of diuretic and the dose used in the case of renal insufficiency. Both directives agree on the need to refer the patient to a specialist because of frequently associated target-organ damage.

▶ Pathogenesis

Recent clinical trials indicate that resistant hypertension is common, affecting 20–30% of the different study populations.

Such clinical outcome studies provide good estimates of the true frequency of resistant hypertension because they employ an intensive treatment regimen mandating drug titrations if BP remained elevated, provide medications free of charge, and closely monitor adherence to the treatment regime with pill counts.

In the Antihypertensive and Lipid-Lowering Treatment to Prevent Heart Attack Trial (ALLHAT) more than 33,000 subjects aged 55 years or older with a history of hypertension and one other cardiovascular risk factor were randomized to receive chlorthalidone, amlodipine, or lisinopril. The dose of the randomized medication was titrated first; non-study-related antihypertensive medications were then added as long as BP remained above 140/90 mm Hg. After a 5-year follow-up, 34% of subjects had not achieved goal BP, and overall, 27% of subjects were receiving three or more medications.

In the Controlled ONset Verapamil INvestigation of Cardiovascular End Points trial (CONVINCE), more than 16,600 subjects were randomized to controlled-onset, extended-release verapamil or conventional anti-hypertensive therapy (atenolol or hydrochlorothiazide), with other medications added as necessary to reduce BP below 140/90 mm Hg. After a mean follow-up of 3 years, 33% of subjects had not achieved goal BP and 17–18% of subjects were receiving three or more antihypertensive medications. In studies of even more patients with complicated hypertension, control rates were even poorer.

In the Losartan Intervention For Endpoint Reduction in Hypertension (LIFE) study, which enrolled hypertensive patients with left ventricular hypertrophy, only 46–49% of subjects had a BP of <140/90 mm Hg after almost 5 years of intensive antihypertensive treatment.

▶ Clinical Findings

A. Symptoms and Signs

Table 44–1 lists factors that have been suggested to be causes for resistance; they are often displayed as associated factors in the same patient.

1. White-coat phenomena—Some studies suggest that white-coat or isolated clinic hypertension is as least as common in patients with resistant hypertension as the general population, with a prevalence ranging from 28% to 52%. The white-coat effect is defined as an increase in BP that occurs at the time of a clinical visit and dissipates soon after. It has been known for more than 50 years that BP recorded by a physician can be as much as 30 mm Hg higher than BP taken by the patient at home, using the same technique and in the same posture. Physicians also record higher pressures than nurses or technicians. The white-coat effect is usually defined as the difference between the clinic and daytime ambulatory pressure. The underlying mechanisms are not well understood, but may include anxiety, a hyperactive alerting response, or a conditioned response. The white-coat

Table 44–1. Causes of refractory hypertension.

Inadequate treatment
Noncompliance
Inadequate doses
Inappropriate combinations
Failure to modify lifestyle including obesity, alcohol abuse, tobacco
False refractivity
Isolated office (white-coat) hypertension
Pseudohypertension
Improper blood pressure measurement (one measurement, failure to use large cuff on long arms)
Other associated factors
Volume overload due to excessive sodium intake, inadequate diuretic therapy, and/or progressive renal insufficiency Sleep apnea
Drug-induced resistant hypertension
Nonsteroidal anti-inflammatory drugs (oral contraceptives, sympathicomimetic agents, corticosteroids, cocaine, cyclosporine, erythropoietin)
Secondary hypertension
Primary aldosteronism
Renal artery stenosis (fibromuscular dysplasia, atherosclerosis)
Renal parenchymal disease
Pheochromocytoma

effect is seen to a greater or lesser degree in most if not all hypertensive patients, but is much smaller or negative in normotensive subjects or those with masked hypertension. A closely linked but discrete entity is white-coat hypertension, which refers to a subset of patients who are hypertensive according to their clinic BP but normotensive at other times.

2. Secondary causes of arterial hypertension—The most common secondary causes of resistant hypertension are hyperaldosteronism, renal parenchymal disease, renal artery stenosis, and sleep apnea (Table 44–2). However, recent prospective studies indicate that hyperaldosteronism is the most common cause of secondary hypertension.

Table 44–2 lists the symptoms and signs frequently associated with secondary hypertension; these can guide us toward undertaking the necessary diagnostic tests in each case.

3. Hyperaldosteronism—Hyperaldosteronism is being increasingly recognized as a common underlying cause of hypertension. In an extensive evaluation that included more than 600 subjects with hypertension, Mosso et al reported that the prevalence of aldosteronism increases according to the severity of the hypertension. Applying the Joint National Committee on the Prevention, Detection, Evaluation, and Treatment of High Blood Pressure sixth report staging criteria to untreated subjects, primary aldosteronism was diagnosed

Table 44–2. Indicative symptoms and signs of secondary hypertension.

Primary aldosteronism

Muscle cramps, weakness

Most patients are normokalemic (some of them show hypokalemia) and clinically undistinguishable from essential hypertensives

More severe target-organ damage than other hypertensives

Elevated plasma aldosterone concentrations and increased ratio of aldosterone concentration to plasma renin activity

Renal parenchymal disease

Renal insufficiency indicated by an elevated serum creatinine and reduced creatinine clearance

Patients are often volume expanded and have increased sensitivity to salt

Renovascular disease

Fibromuscular dysplasia

It typically affects young women (15–50 years old)

Patients generally do not develop renal insufficiency

There is usually a good clinical response to interventions such as percutaneous renal artery angioplasty

Atherosclerosis

It generally occurs in patients over 50 years old and is more common in smokers and in patients with other atherosclerotic diseases

Duplex ultrasonography, gadolinium-enhanced magnetic resonance angioplasty, or computed tomography can provide effective screening of atherosclerotic renal disease

Sleep apnea

Repeated episodes of partial (hypopnea) or complete (apnea) cessation of breathing during sleep; such episodes may be of central origin, or due to mechanical obstruction of the airways, or to a combination of the two

The cardinal manifestations of the obstructive sleep apnea syndrome are snoring and daytime sleepiness

Patients are generally obese

Morning headaches

The gold standard for diagnosing sleep apnea is polysomnography

Pheochromocytoma

Sustained or episodic hypertension complicated by headache, palpitations, or diaphoresis

Great variability in blood pressure values

Other rare causes of secondary hypertension

Cushing syndrome

Coarctation of the aorta

Hypercalcemia

Carcinoid syndrome

Central nervous system tumors

Acromegaly

in 2% of subjects with stage 1 hypertension (140–159 mm Hg/90–99 mm Hg), 8% of subjects with stage 2 hypertension (160–179 mm Hg/100–109 mm Hg), and 13% of subjects with stage 3 hypertension (>180/110 mm Hg). This is just one of many reports that indicate a prevalence of hyperaldosteronism of 15–30% among general and selected hypertensive populations.

Primary aldosteronism (PA) is particularly common in subjects with resistant hypertension. In a prospective evaluation of African-American and white subjects with resistant hypertension, defined as uncontrolled hypertension despite use of three or more antihypertensive agents, the reported prevalence of aldosteronism was approximately 20%. These results are consistent with a study from separate investigators reporting a prevalence of aldosteronism of 17% among subjects referred to hypertension specialists for uncontrolled hypertension. Thus, PA should be excluded in all patients in whom secondary hypertension is suspected.

4. Sodium ingestion—volume overload—An increased salt sensitivity may be a cause of refractory hypertension. There is a subset of patients who are more likely to manifest increased salt sensitivity, including blacks, the elderly, and patients with underlying renal insufficiency. In any patient, excessive sodium intake can blunt the antihypertensive benefit of most agents. With the exception of calcium channel blockers (CCBs), antihypertensive drugs show greater effectiveness when the patient follows a low sodium diet. Also, treatment with vasodilators or adrenergic blockers can favor an expansion of volume and resistance to the treatment (pseudoresistance). When a volume overload is suspected, 24-hour measurement of sodium urinary excretion can be insufficient to determine sodium intake. The quantification of total plasmatic volume can provide reliable information about the degree of volume overload, and can serve as a guide at the time of prescribing a diuretic.

B. Special Tests and Examinations

The auscultatory method of BP measurement with a properly calibrated and validated instrument should be used. Patients should be seated and should relax for at least 5 minutes in a chair rather than on an examination table, with feet on the floor and arm supported at heart level. Measurement of BP in the standing position is indicated periodically, especially in those at risk for postural hypotension. An appropriate-sized cuff bladder (encircling at least 80% of the arm) should be used to ensure accuracy. At least two measurements should be made.

The readings should take place in a calm environment, after a rest time of 5–15 minutes, at least 30 minutes after the consumption of stimulants such as coffee or tobacco, since nicotine as much as caffeine can temporarily elevate BP readings. However, the possible alertness reaction that may take place during the consultation limits BP readings and contributes to an increase in the prevalence of uncontrolled hypertension. The use of a correct technique with several consecutive measurements (especially by nurse personnel) offers results comparable to ambulatory measurements and provides a better evaluation of hypertensive patients. When ambulatory BP monitoring (ABPM) is used, 20–50% of patients previously diagnosed with high BP display normal BP values. Noninvasive, 24-hour ABPM has evolved over the past 25 years from a novel research tool of limited clinical use to an important and useful modality for stratifying cardiovascular risk and guiding therapeutic decisions. Early clinical uses of ABPM mostly focused on identifying patients with white-coat hypertension; however, growing evidence now points to greater prognostic significance in determining risk for hypertensive end-organ damage compared with office BP measurements. Ambulatory measurement of BP using automated devices has demonstrated the benefit in treatment resistance and borderline hypertension, and is recommended by the Joint National Committee for the Prevention, Detection, Evaluation, and Treatment of High Blood Pressure in a number of clinical scenarios.

On the other hand, self-measurement of BP (SMBP) at the patient's home with the correct technique and a valid and properly calibrated digital device provides very useful information on BP values of everyday life. The potential advantages of having patients take their own BP are two-fold: The distortion produced by the white-coat effect is eliminated, and multiple readings can be taken over prolonged periods of time. SMBP plays an increasing role in the diagnosis of hypertension. It may be used as a first step in the evaluation of patients with suspected white-coat hypertension, as recommended in JNC 7. There is also evidence that SMBP can improve BP control.

Pseudohypertension is another factor that can lead to a false misdiagnosis of refractory hypertension when intra-arterial pressures are actually normal or below normal. It refers to the phenomenon whereby vascular stiffening results in falsely high auscultatory BP measurements. Some studies suggest that pseudohypertension may be common among the elderly, but definitive evaluation is lacking. Pseudohypertension might be suspected if some of the following occur:

1. Severe hypertension in the absence of demonstrable target-organ deterioration.

2. Symptoms of hypotension in patients with seemingly resistant hypertension.

3. Radiologic evidence of calcification of the brachial artery.

4. BP values more elevated in the brachial artery than in the legs.

5. Severe isolated systolic hypertension.

The Osler maneuver (the ability to palpate the brachial or radial artery despite ipsilateral occlusion of the artery by a BP cuff inflated to suprasystolic values) constitutes a simple screening test for pseudohypertension. Another of value when pseudohypertension is suspected is the use of ultrasonic or oscillometric measuring instruments since their readings correlate more closely with intra-arterial pressure values than those obtained by an indirect auscultatory sphygmomanometer.

Complications

A. Insufficient or Inadequate Treatment

When physicians fail to prescribe lifestyle modifications, adequate antihypertensive drug doses, or appropriate drug combinations, inadequate BP control may result. Most patients with hypertension will require two or more antihypertensive medications to achieve their BP goals. The addition of a second drug from a different class should be initiated when use of a single drug in adequate doses fails to achieve the BP goal. When BP is more than 20/10 mm Hg above goal, consideration should be given to initiating therapy with two drugs, either as separate prescriptions or in fixed-dose combinations. In a review of cases of refractory hypertension in a hypertension unit, an inadequate therapeutic regime was the most frequent (43%) cause of resistance. After the corresponding adjustment in these therapeutic regimes, especially after the use of diuretics, BP came under control. CCBs and α-adrenergic receptor blockers (α-blockers) promote sodium and fluid retention, which may favor an inadequate control of BP, mainly when they are not used in combination with a diuretic. The administration of a drug with an active effect not sufficiently prolonged can bring about insufficient BP control that appears to be resistant to treatment. Likewise, the use of an inadequate drug combination, either belonging to the same pharmacologic group, or with a similar mechanism of action, or with opposing effects, can have negative consequences for obtaining adequate BP control. However, the administration of an adequate drug combination, with synergistic effects, including the administration of fixed doses, can significantly improve the observed response rates over those achieved with the use of each drug by itself.

Figure 44–1 shows a model of synergistic combinations proposed in the last European directives that can be useful in testing the adjustment of the associations.

Table 44–3 gives several recommendations for optimal pharmacologic treatment.

B. Poor Patient Compliance

Poor patient compliance remains the most important reason for inadequate BP control. The lack of adherence to hypertensive treatment is one of the major determinants of the excess morbidity and mortality observed in hypertensive patients, and must be taken into account in all patients with refractory hypertension. Studies have demonstrated that in some patient groups at 1 year, fewer than 30% of patients are still taking their antihypertensive medication. There are

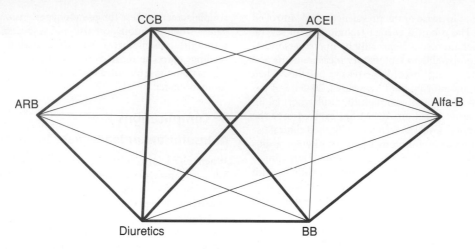

▲ **Figure 44–1.** Synergistic antihypertensive drug combinations. CCB, calcium channel blocker; ARB, angiotensin II receptor blocker; BB, β-blocker; Alfa-β, α-blocker. (Reproduced with permission from Guidelines Committee: 2003 European Society of Hypertension-European Society of Cardiology guidelines for the management of arterial hypertension. J Hypertens 2003;21:1011.)

multiple factors that influence patient compliance, including education, socioeconomic status, and drug costs. There have been numerous studies concerning the reasons for the lack of adherence to treatment and how to detect it. However,

Table 44–3. Measures to optimize blood pressure control.

Improve compliance to treatment
Simpler regimes
One daily dose
Make the patient aware of the importance of the treatment
Build trust by empathy
Use the most efficient drugs and those best tolerated by the patient
Titrate or combine medications, when necessary
Favor the use of a fixed combination rather than multiple tablets
Use fixed drug associations that permit neutralization of the side effects of each of the drugs alone
Visits not excessively spaced apart in time
Clarify the therapeutic objective
Simple, summarized, and easy to memorize directives
Assume that blood pressure depends on the individualized risk stratification of each patient
Importance of achieving both systolic and diastolic blood pressure
Optimize the pharmacologic treatment
Use drugs in the total recommended doses
Stimulate the use of fixed associations with synergistic or additive effects
Intensive therapy is directed toward control (associate the necessary number of drugs with a synergistic or additive action, whenever they are tolerated

direct questioning of the patient on the correct taking of the medication continues to be the most practical measure to confirm lack of adherence to treatment. In these cases, the taking of medication under the supervision of health personnel is usually accompanied by a noticeable reduction in BP, although this measurement is not regularly made. Also, the use of electronic devices to objectively monitor following of the therapeutic treatment has contributed to an awareness of standards of behavior of patients and restores more adequate measures of control. Additionally, the role of nurse personnel in support and education programs for hypertensive patients is of great importance.

The two main factors that have been shown to be most important in influencing patient compliance are the side effect profiles of the antihypertensive agents and the convenience of the dose schedule.

1. Adverse events—The side effects that are associated with antihypertensive agents, as well as those perceived by patients to be associated with antihypertensive agents, remain by far the most important cause of poor patient compliance. It is thus crucial and almost always possible to find drugs or drug combinations that can be well tolerated by individual patients, and a concerted effort should be made to find the right drugs. It should be kept in mind that almost all side effects associated with antihypertensive agents are dose related, and utilizing smaller doses will frequently alleviate the side effects.

2. Convenience—It has been clearly demonstrated that patients who need to take antihypertensive agents twice a day take their drugs less readily than those provided with only one daily dose. Thus, wherever possible, patients should be treated with once-a-day agents. In selecting once-a-day agents, it is important to use those with a true 24-hour effect. The risk of nonembolic strokes and of myocardial infarction peaks in the early morning and coincides with the rapid surge of BP. This occurs during arousal from sleep (typically between 6 AM and noon). Adequate BP control during this period seems to be associated with fewer cardiovascular events. Antihypertensive agents taken once daily in the morning that do not provide 24-hour efficacy may leave patients with no control at a time when they are at greatest risk of developing cardiovascular events. The duration of action of a particular antihypertensive drug can be assessed in the clinical setting by measuring BP at the trough of drug action (24–26 hours after dosing). Patients should omit taking their medication on the morning of the clinic visit so that BP is measured at trough. If BP is controlled, the agent is providing 24-hour coverage; if not, it should be replaced or two daily doses prescribed.

Table 44–3 summarizes some of the keys to improving adherence to treatment.

▶ Treatment

The best treatment for resistant hypertension is based on identification and reversal of contributing factors. Accordingly, it is mandatory to make a thorough search for noncompliance to treatment and to evaluate the adequacy of the treatment regimen, drug interactions, and associated conditions (Figure 44–2). Noninvasive, 24-hour ABPM may be an important and useful modality for identifying patients with white-coat hypertension. In the absence of the above factors, assessment for secondary causes of hypertension, in particular hyperaldosteronism, is appropriate.

Addition of low-dose spironolactone (12.5–50 mg) was associated with a mean decrease in BP of 21 ± 20 mm Hg/10 ± 14 mm Hg at 6 weeks and 25 ± 20 mm Hg/12 ± 12 mm Hg

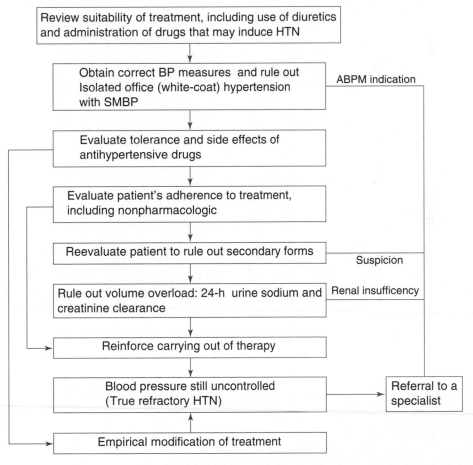

▲ **Figure 44–2.** Algorithm for the diagnostic and therapeutic management of a patient with refractory hypertension. SMBP, self-monitoring of blood pressure; ABPM, ambulatory blood pressure monitoring; HTN, hypertension.

at 6-month follow-up in subjects with resistant hypertension. The reduction in BP was similar to subjects with high urinary aldosterone excretion and normal or low aldosterone excretion. Also, spironolactone lowered BP equally in African-American and white subjects. These results demonstrate that an aldosterone antagonist can be effective in treating hypertension resistant to multidrug regimens that include a diuretic and an angiotensin-converting enzyme inhibitor or an angiotensin receptor blocker. Additional reduction in BP was also achieved in subjects without hyperaldosteronism. Benefits in such subjects may have been secondary to additional diuretic effects of the aldosterone antagonist or may reflect a broad role of aldosterone in causing resistant hypertension even in the absence of demonstrable hyperaldosteronism. Recent clinical trials document the efficacy of eplerenone, a selective aldosterone antagonist, in treating hypertension in subjects with primary hypertension. Eplerenone would likewise be effective as an additional therapy in subjects with resistant hypertension while avoiding the antiandrogenic and antiprogesteronic effects of spironolactone. Studies evaluating eplerenone specifically in this setting are warranted.

With an aging and increasingly obese population, the prevalence of resistant hypertension will undoubtedly increase. Even now, failure of multidrug regimens of three or more medications to control BP is common. Aldosterone antagonists can provide significant reductions in BP in these difficult-to-treat patients. Hyperkalemia or acute renal insufficiency occurs rarely, and should be monitored for, particularly in patients with chronic kidney disease and/or diabetes.

The general benefit of an aldosterone blockade in subjects with resistant hypertension suggests that aldosterone excess may be a more common cause of hypertension than previously thought. However, the aldosteronism that we are reporting as being so common is undoubtedly different from the classic syndrome of primary aldosteronism. The regulatory abnormalities, distinct from classic aldosteronism, resulting in such a high prevalence of aldosteronism are unknown. Recognition of such abnormalities may allow prevention and/or development of even more effective treatment strategies.

▶ Prognosis

Truly refractory hypertension, hypertension in which all known refractory causes can be excluded, could become a rarity. Nonetheless, from a practical point of view we offer a series of steps to detect, control, or diminish the conditioning factors, emphasizing the need to arrive at a correct diagnosis. For this diagnosis, the basic pillars are an adequate measuring of pressure, a guarantee of correct associations, an acceptable carrying out of the prescribed regime, and, lastly, ruling out secondary forms of hypertension. Arriving at this point, the intervention of a specialist can ensure the control of BP by means of the combined use of four or more antihypertensive agents.

Bansal N et al: Blood pressure control in the hypertension clinic. Am J Hypertens 2003;16:878.

Black HR et al: Principal results of the Controlled Onset Verapamil Investigation of Cardiovascular End Points (CONVINCE) Trial. JAMA 2003;289:2073.

Chobanian AV et al: The Seventh Report of the Joint National Committee on Prevention, Detection, Evaluation, and Treatment of High Blood Pressure: the JNC 7 report. JAMA 2003;289:2560.

Cushman WC et al: Success and predictors of blood pressure control in diverse North American settings: the Antihypertensive and Lipid-Lowering Treatment to Prevent Attack Trial (ALLHAT). J Clin Hypertens (Greenwich) 2002;4:393.

Guidelines Committee: 2003 European Society of Hypertension-European Society of Cardiology guidelines for the management of arterial hypertension. J Hypertens 2003;21:1011.

Llisterri Caro JL et al: Blood pressure control in Spanish hypertensive patients in Primary Health Care Centers. PRESCAP 2002 Study. Med Clin (Barc) 2004;122:165.

Mancia G et al: Blood pressure control according to new guidelines targets in low- to high-risk hypertensives managed in specialist practice. J Hypertens 2004;22:2387.

Mosso L et al: Primary aldosteronism and hypertensive disease. Hypertension 2003;42:161.

Nishizaka MK et al: Efficacy of low-dose spironolactone in subjects with resistant hypertension. Am J Hypertens 2003;16:925.

O'Brien E: European Society of Hypertension recommendations for conventional, ambulatory and home blood pressure measurement. J Hypertens 2003;21:821.

Pickering TG: Measurement of blood pressure in and out of the office. J Clin Hypertens 2005;7:123.

Pickering TG et al: Recommendations for blood pressure measurement in humans: An AHA Scientific Statement from the Council on High Blood Pressure Research Professional and Public Education Subcommittee. J Clin Hypertens 2005;7:102.

Primatesta P, Poulter NR: Hypertension management and control among English adults aged 65 years and older in 2000 and 2001. J Hypertens 2004;22(6):1093.

White WB et al: Effect of the selective aldosterone blocker eplerenone versus the calcium antagonist amlodipine in systolic hypertension. Hypertension 2003;41:1021.

Hypertensive Emergencies & Urgencies

William J. Elliott, MD, PhD

ESSENTIALS OF DIAGNOSIS

▶ Emergency: Very elevated blood pressure with acute, ongoing target-organ damage that should be lowered within minutes.

▶ Urgency: Very elevated blood pressure without acute, ongoing target-organ damage that should be lowered within hours (controversial).

General Considerations

Many patients present to emergency departments or physician offices with very elevated BPs, but few of these involve either hypertensive emergencies or urgencies. True hypertensive emergencies occur in only one to two people per 100,000 population per year in developed countries, but may be up to four times more common in developing nations, minority populations, economically challenged individuals, and those who are nonadherent to prescribed antihypertensive drugs. To triage such patients appropriately it is important to identify symptoms or signs indicating acute, ongoing target-organ damage. This can take several forms, but usually involves the central nervous system (including the optic fundi), cardiovascular system, kidneys, and/or uterus (see the first three columns of Table 45–1). Patients with acute, ongoing target-organ damage are at very high risk of cardiovascular events and generally should be treated within minutes in a heavily monitored setting with a short-acting intravenously delivered antihypertensive agent (typically sodium nitroprusside). Individuals who do not have acute, ongoing target-organ damage may be referred to a source of ongoing care for hypertension (if at low risk), or treated with orally administered antihypertensive agents (if at moderate risk) and the BP response observed.

Examples of hypertensive urgencies that would usually be treated in a hospital include patients with very elevated BPs in the perioperative period, organ transplant recipients (especially if the transplant was recent), and patients with severe burns. Most other hypertensive urgencies are treated in the outpatient department; whether such treatment is beneficial in the emergency department is controversial and depends on traditions local to the specific jurisdiction.

Pathogenesis

The key pathophysiologic feature in understanding hypertensive emergencies is that the normal blood pressure–blood flow curve in most vascular beds is shifted to the right in patients who develop hypertensive emergencies. Over time, their arteries adapt to the very high BPs in order to maintain organ perfusion, a process called "autoregulation." If the BP is lowered too quickly or if the BP is too low to maintain autoregulation, blood flow to important organs will be compromised and ischemia (to the brain, heart, or kidneys) may result.

Clinical Findings

See the first three columns of Table 45–1.

Differential Diagnosis

Neurologic subtypes of hypertensive emergencies are the most difficult to distinguish from each other. The distinction is very important, since drug therapy to lower BP is usually withheld in the setting of an ischemic stroke in evolution, whereas it is not only beneficial, but often diagnostic in hypertensive encephalopathy. The results of CT or MRI scans are often helpful.

Many other syndromes include acute, ongoing target-organ damage (eg, papilledema) that could be (but is not) directly related to hypertension (eg, hematuria from glomerulonephritis, acute elevation in serum creatinine from toxic nephropathy), but these generally lack the very elevated BP that is characteristic of the hypertensive emergency.

Table 45–1. Common hypertensive emergencies with signs/symptoms and other findings.

Type of emergency	Symptoms and signs	Other findings	Recommended drug	Blood pressure target
Neurologic emergencies				
Hypertensive encephalopathy (typically a diagnosis of exclusion)	Mental status changes, generally without focal neurologic signs; papilledema is common	No other findings to explain mental status changes	Nitroprusside[1]	25% reduction over 2–3 hours
Acute ischemic stroke	Focal neurologic signs, headache	CT or MRI may show infarcted or ischemic area	Nitroprusside[1] (controversial)	Blood pressure is generally not treated unless it is higher than 180–220/110–120 mm Hg
Intracranial hemorrhage	Headache, focal neurologic signs	CT or MRI typically shows hemorrhagic area	Nitroprusside[1] (controversial)	0–25% reduction over 6–12 hours (controversial)
Subarachnoid hemorrhage	Headache	Lumbar puncture shows xanthochromia and/or blood	Nimodipine	Up to 25% reduction in previously hypertensive patients, 130–160 mm Hg systolic for normotensive patients
Acute head injury/trauma	Headache, signs of external trauma	CT or MRI may show area of traumatized brain	Nitroprusside[1]	0–25% reduction over 2–3 hours (controversial)
Cardiovascular emergencies				
Acute myocardial infarction	Chest discomfort, dyspnea, anxiety	Electrocardiogram may show hyperacute T-wave elevation; troponin is typically elevated	Nitroglycerin	Cessation of ischemia (typically only a 5–10% decrease is required)
Acute left ventricular failure/ acute pulmonary edema	Dyspnea, pulmonary rales	Chest x-ray shows pulmonary vascular redistribution	Nitroprusside[1] or nitroglycerin	Improvement in failure (typically a 10–15% decrease)
Acute aortic dissection	"Tearing" chest pain, pulse deficit in legs	Widened mediastinum on chest x-ray, "intimal flap" on echocardiogram, CT, or MRI	β-Blocker + nitroprusside[1]	120 mm Hg systolic in 30 minutes (if possible)
Recent vascular surgery	Tense suture lines	None	Nitroprusside[1]	Typically ~160/100 mm Hg
Epistaxis unresponsive to packing	Uncontrolled blood from the nose (anteriorly or posteriorly)	None	Nitroprusside[1]	To control bleeding (typically only a 5–10% decrease is required)
Renal emergencies				
Acute deterioration in renal function	None that is characteristic of this condition	Significant elevation of serum creatinine relative to recent level	Fenoldopam	0–25% reduction in mean arterial pressure over 1–12 hours
Hematuria (typically gross)	Red or brown urine, flank pain	4+ blood on urinalysis	Fenoldopam	To reduce bleeding rate (typically a 0–10% reduction over 1–12 hours
Catecholamine-excess states				
Pheochromocytoma	Headache, sweating attacks, orthostatic hypotension	Elevated plasma metanephrines and urinary catecholamine metabolites; mass seen on CT or T_2-weighted images on MRI	Phentolamine	To control paroxysms and/or symptoms

Type of emergency	Symptoms and signs	Other findings	Recommended drug	Blood pressure target
Drug-related conditions (tyramine ingestion with monoamine oxidase inhibitor; withdrawal of antihypertensive drug; phencyclidine/cocaine use)	Headache, mental status change, tachycardia (often, but not always)	None characteristic of this condition	Phentolamine	Typically only one dose is necessary
Pregnancy-related conditions				
Eclampsia/preeclampsia	Seizure/headache, edema (no longer required for diagnosis)	Proteinuria (dipstick or 24-hour collection); occasionally thrombocytopenia, elevated AST or ALT	$MgSO_4$, methyldopa, hydralazine, labetalol, nifedipine	Typically <90 mm Hg diastolic, but often lower

[1]Some physicians prefer an intravenous infusion of either fenoldopam or nicardipine, neither of which has potentially toxic metabolites, over nitroprusside. Acute improvements in renal function occur during therapy with fenoldopam, but not with nitroprusside.
CT, computed tomography; MRI, magnetic resonance imaging; AST, aspartate aminotransferase; ALT, alanine aminotransferase.

▶ Complications

Because of the extreme BP level and the existence of acute, ongoing target-organ damage, patients with hypertensive emergencies are at very high short-term risk for cardiovascular and renal complications if left untreated. Treatment, however, can lead to an even greater risk if carried out improperly. The most feared complication of treatment for a hypertensive emergency is reduction of the BP too quickly or to a too low level for autoregulation to be maintained. This results in reduced blood flow to important organs and is ischemic in cardiac, neurologic, renal, or peripheral beds. The major reason for not using quick-acting oral hypotensive drugs is that they can precipitously lower BP and lead to major complications (myocardial infarction, stroke, acute renal failure).

Patients with hypertensive urgencies are at much lower cardiovascular risk than patients with hypertensive emergencies. There are currently no data to indicate that such patients benefit from acute treatment of their hypertension, but they certainly can be harmed if treatment is too aggressive (eg, oral nifedipine capsules).

▶ Treatment

Patients with hypertensive emergencies are best treated in a closely monitored environment (eg, intensive care unit) with a short-acting, quickly reversible intravenously administered drug (see the last two columns of Table 45–1). Sodium nitroprusside is the drug with the longest track record and is very inexpensive, but it carries the risk of cyanide and thiocyanate toxicity with prolonged use or at high doses. After the BP is maintained at the target range for several (typically 6–12) hours, oral therapy (typically with an intermediate-acting calcium antagonist) can be given, and the intravenously administered drug can be tapered and discontinued.

▶ Prognosis

Left untreated, patients with hypertensive emergencies have a dismal prognosis (typically a 5-month mean survival); in 1928 (when the term was introduced), "malignant hypertension" reflected a prognosis that was as poor as patients with cancer. Since the introduction of effective antihypertensive drug therapy, the prognosis depends more on the level of renal, cardiac, and neurologic function at presentation than on the initial level of BP. Sufficient kidney function sometimes returns to allow stopping of dialysis, if it is required acutely for a hypertensive emergency, particularly if the BP is well controlled during follow-up.

Elliott WJ: Management of hypertensive emergencies. Curr Hypertens Rep 2003;5:486. [PMID: 14594569]

Vaughan CJ et al: Hypertensive emergencies. Lancet 2000;356:411. [PMID: 10972386]

Cystic Diseases of the Kidney

Qi Qian, MD, & Vicente E. Torres, MD, PhD

Renal cystic disease comprises a wide range of disease entities. They can be classified as either (1) hereditary or acquired or (2) systemic or renal confined diseases that have the common feature of multiple renal cysts. Each disease entity differs in its presentation, prognosis, and management.

Renal cysts are smooth-walled, fluid-filled circular structures formed by focal outpouching of renal tubules. The pathogenesis of cyst formation has not been entirely elucidated. However, tremendous strides have been made in recent years. For autosomal dominant and autosomal recessive polycystic kidney diseases (ADPKD and ARPKD), a picture is starting to emerge. Defects in the primary ciliary sensing mechanisms, intracellular calcium regulation, and cellular cyclic AMP (cAMP) accumulation all seem to play a role in the altered cellular phenotype and functions.

Today, treatment includes risk modification, management of complications, and renal transplant or dialysis. There is no definitive therapy to eliminate or to retard cyst growth. A better understanding of its pathogenesis offers hope in the near future for correcting the underlying abnormalities in cystic pathways.

AUTOSOMAL DOMINANT POLYCYSTIC KIDNEY DISEASE

 ESSENTIALS OF DIAGNOSIS

► Two renal cysts unilaterally or bilaterally before age 30 years by renal ultrasound in patients with a family history of ADPKD.

► Two cysts in each kidney between the ages of 30 and 59 years by renal ultrasound in patients with a family history of ADPKD.

► Four or more cysts in each kidney after age ≥60 years by renal ultrasound in patients with a family history of ADPKD.

► General Considerations

ADPKD is the most common life-threatening monogenic disease. It occurs worldwide and in all races, affecting 1 in 400–1000 individuals. In the United States, approximately 500,000 people are affected and about 2000 begin hemodialysis each year.

ADPKD is an autosomal dominantly transmitted disease. It is composed of two types: ADPKD1, caused by mutations in the *PKD1* gene and responsible for 85% of the clinical cases of ADPKD, and ADPKD2, caused by mutations in the *PKD2* gene and accounting for approximately 15% of cases. A very small percentage of ADPKD patients, with a milder form of disease not linked to mutations in either *PKD1* or *PKD2*, might have mutation(s) in a yet to be identified third *PKD* gene.

In addition to its renal manifestations, ADPKD is a multisystemic disorder with prominent extrarenal cystic and noncystic manifestations including polycystic liver disease and cysts in diverse organ systems (pancreas, arachnoid membrane, pineal gland, and seminal vesicles), intracranial saccular aneurysms, thoracic aortic aneurysms and dissections, coronary artery aneurysms, mitral and/or tricuspid valve prolapse, aortic valve insufficiency, aortic root dilation, and possibly colonic diverticula.

The severity of cystic renal dysfunctions is highly heterogeneous with significant interfamilial and intrafamilial variations. In general, ADPKD1 is more severe and is marked by an early onset of end-stage renal failure (mean age of 54 years) versus that of ADPKD2 (mean age of 74 years). Compared to female patients male ADPKD2 patients tend to develop more extensive cystic renal dysfunction, although they have less cystic liver disease.

▶ Clinical Findings

A. Symptoms and Signs

1. Renal manifestations—With age, cystic renal enlargement occurs in all ADPKD patients. The severity of structural abnormality generally correlates with the renal manifestations including pain, hematuria, hypertension, and renal dysfunction. Massively enlarged kidneys can also cause compression of the neighboring organs and the inferior vena cava, leading to early satiety, dyspnea, and lower extremity edema.

A. Hypertension—Hypertension (HTN) occurs before the onset of renal failure in more than 80% of ADPKD patients. Although the prevalence increases with age, ADPKD is associated with an earlier onset and a significantly increased incidence of HTN compared to those in the general population.

The cause of HTN is multifactorial including activation of the intrarenal renin–angiotensin system, defects in nitric oxide endothelium-mediated vasorelaxation, elevated sympathetic activity, and possible defects in vascular smooth muscle cells directly associated with the *PKD* mutations.

Early onset and/or uncontrolled HTN are significant risk factors for faster renal disease progression and for mortality from cardiac complications such as left ventricular hypertrophy and coronary artery disease. Uncontrolled HTN can also worsen valvular heart disease and increase the risk of intracranial aneurysmal rupture and morbidity associated with rupture.

B. Pain—Episodes of acute flank pain are common. The potential etiologies are cyst hemorrhage, infection, stone, or, rarely, renal tumor. Massively enlarged kidneys can cause mechanical lower back pain. A small group of patients develops chronic flank pain without an identifiable etiology except for the enlarged kidneys. These patients are at risk for narcotic and/or analgesic dependence and medication-related complications.

C. Hematuria, cyst hemorrhage, and retroperitoneal hemorrhage—Gross hematuria may be the initial presenting symptom. It occurs in up to 42% of ADPKD patients and can result from cyst hemorrhage, stone, infection, or renal tumor.

Most cyst hemorrhages are self-limited and resolve within 2–7 days. First episodes occurring in patients older than 50 years or episodes persisting for more than a week should be investigated to rule out neoplasm.

Occasionally, hemorrhagic cysts can rupture into the retroperitoneum causing retroperitoneal bleeding. This can be severe and life threatening.

D. Urinary concentration defect—A urine concentration defect, often associated with mild polyuria, is the most common and earliest manifestation of ADPKD. It usually goes unnoticed and is well compensated by adequate fluid intake.

E. Nephrolithiasis—Nephrolithiasis occurs in approximately 20% of ADPKD patients and is five times more common than in the general population. The majority of stones are composed of uric acid and/or calcium oxalate. Uric acid stones occur more frequently in ADPKD than in non-ADPKD stone formers. Factors that may contribute to the lithogenicity are urinary stasis due to distorted renal architecture, hypocitraturia, and low urinary pH (promoting uric acid stone formation). The symptoms and signs of nephrolithiasis are similar to those of non-ADPKD stone patients.

F. Urinary tract or cyst infections—Whether urinary tract infections occur more frequently in ADPKD patients is unclear, but their risk of complicated infections is clearly increased. Infections include cystitis, pyelonephritis, renal cyst infection, and perinephric abscesses. They occur more frequently in females than in males. The main pathogens are *Escherichia coli*, *Klebsiella*, *Proteus*, and other Enterobacteriaceae. Symptoms and signs are urinary frequency and urgency for cystitis; fever, chills, nausea, vomiting, and flank pain for pyelonephritis, renal cyst infection, and perinephric abscesses.

G. Renal failure—ADPKD1 is associated with a 20-year earlier onset of end-stage renal failure compared to that of ADPKD2. Once the renal clearance starts to decline, it decreases linearly at a rate of approximately 5.0–6.4 mL/minute/year. Both genetic and environmental factors play a role in renal disease progression. Among patients with ADPKD1, the location of the *PKD1* mutation may influence renal outcome. The mutations located in the first half of the *PKD1* gene (5′region) were shown to be associated with a slightly earlier onset of renal failure compared to the mutations located in the second half of the gene (3′region).

Additional risk factors that portend a poor renal outcome include male gender, sickle cell trait, diagnosis of ADPKD before age 30 years, first episode of gross hematuria before age 30 years, hypertension before age 35 years, hyperlipidemia, low high-density lipoprotein (HDL), and cigarette smoking.

The symptoms and signs of renal failure in ADPKD, which begin to appear when the glomerular filtration rate is reduced to <30–40 mL/minute/1.73 m^2, mirror those of non-ADPKD chronic renal failure.

2. Extrarenal manifestations

A. Polycystic liver disease—Polycystic liver disease (PLD) is the most common extrarenal manifestation of ADPKD. Liver cysts originate from small clusters of intralobular bile ductules surrounded by fibrous tissue termed biliary microhamartomas and from peribiliary glands. The occurrence of PLD in ADPKD increases with age from 0% in ADPKD children to 20% in the third decade and over 75% in the seventh decade of life. Women, especially those with multiple pregnancies and/or on oral contraceptive or on estrogen replacement therapy, tend to have an earlier onset and worse PLD.

The majority of PLD patients are asymptomatic. When occurring, the symptoms usually result from either mass effect or cyst-related complications such as cyst hemorrhage, rupture, or infection. The liver synthetic functions are typically preserved because, despite even a significant degree of cystic liver involvement, the total amount of unaffected hepatic parenchyma is not reduced.

Symptoms associated with mass effect are dyspnea, orthopnea, early satiety, gastroesophageal reflux, mechanical back pain, uterine prolapse, rib fracture, and, in severe cases, failure to thrive. In rare cases, a massively enlarged cystic liver can cause obstructions to the hepatic venous outflow tract, portal vein and/or bile duct, or the inferior vena cava. These patients may develop portal hypertension, esophageal and/or gastric varices, ascites, and, rarely, obstructive jaundice.

Hepatic cyst hemorrhage and ruptures can present as acute abdominal pain, extrinsic bile duct compression, and liver enzyme elevation. Rarely, cysts can rupture into the peritoneum and cause acute ascites and life-threatening hemoperitoneum.

Patients with hepatic cyst infection may present with fever, chills, localized upper abdominal pain, leukocytosis, and elevation of alkaline phosphatase. Bacteremia is frequently present. The major pathogens are Enterobacteriaceae.

B. INTRACRANIAL ANEURYSMS AND OTHER VASCULAR MANIFESTATIONS—The incidence of intracranial aneurysms (ICAs) and ICA ruptures in ADPKD is increased by 5- to 10-fold compared to that in the general population. Family clustering is evident. Patients with a family history of ICA or subarachnoid hemorrhage (SAH, the consequence of ICA rupture) have an ICA occurrence of 21% versus 6% in those without such history.

The majority of ADPKD-associated ICAs are small (<7 mm in diameter) and are located in the anterior circulation (approximately 90%). Although compared to sporadic ones, ICAs in ADPKD have a younger mean age of aneurysmal rupture (39 versus 51 years).

The risk of ICA rupture (extrapolated from the International Study of Unruptured Intracranial Aneurysms) depends on the size and location of the ICAs and whether the patient has a prior episode(s) of SAH.

The yearly risk of rupture is less then 0.1% for the small sized (<7 mm in diameter) anterior circulation ICAs in patients without a prior SAH. The risk is higher for ICAs >7 mm in diameter or in the posterior circulation or in patients with a prior history of SAH.

Unruptured ICAs are generally asymptomatic. Rarely, patients can present with focal neurologic symptoms such as cranial nerve palsy or seizure due to local compression. Rupturing or ruptured ICAs typically present with prominent symptoms including episodes of sudden onset intense headache or headache with a quality different from that experienced before. The pain can radiate to the occipital and cervical region and may be accompanied by nuchal rigidity. Other associated symptoms are nausea, vomiting, photophobia, cranial nerve palsy, seizure, lethargy, and coma.

Other vascular manifestations more frequently seen (an approximately 10-fold increase) in ADPKD are thoracic aortic and cervicocephalic arterial dissections, intracranial arterial dolichoectasia, and coronary artery aneurysms. The symptoms and signs of these complications are similar to those seen in non-ADPKD patients.

C. VALVULAR HEART DISEASE—Valvular heart diseases occur more frequently in ADPKD patients than in their nonaffected family members or the general population. Of those, mitral valve prolapse is the most common and can be detected by echocardiography in up to 20% of ADPKD patients. Other more frequent valvular heart diseases include mitral insufficiency, tricuspid insufficiency, tricuspid prolapse, and aortic insufficiency often associated with aortic root dilation. Symptoms vary from asymptomatic or episodic palpitations to, in rare cases, congestive heart failure. When a cardiac murmur is heard, antibiotic prophylaxis against subacute bacterial endocarditis is indicated.

D. RENAL CELL CARCINOMA—Despite the frequent occurrence of hyperplasia and microscopic adenomas on renal pathology, the overall incidence of renal carcinoma in ADPKD is not increased. However, when occurring, the renal cancer tends to affect younger patients (mean age of 45 versus 55 years in the general population), be multifocal, and possess high-grade sarcomatoid features.

B. Laboratory Findings

1. Renal pathology—Grossly, numerous spherical cysts varying in size are obvious and are distributed evenly in both the cortex and medulla. The enlarged kidneys typically retain their reniform shape. However, renal tubular systems are distorted beyond recognition.

Microscopically, significant abnormalities are evident even in patients with mild renal insufficiency. These abnormalities include interstitial fibrosis frequently associated with inflammatory cell infiltration, tubular epithelial hyperplasia associated with flat nonpolypoid or polypoid hyperplasia and microscopic adenoma, and advanced sclerosis of preglomerular vessels including both afferent arterioles and interlobular arteries, which are more severe compared to those of non-ADPKD patients with the same degree of renal insufficiency.

2. Liver pathology—Grossly, the size of cysts varies from pinpoint to huge. The cysts tend to cluster and spare segments of the hepatic parenchyma free of disease.

Microscopically, cyst walls are thin and lined with a single layer of flattened or cuboidal cells of biliary origin. Biliary microhamartomas are often seen in association with cysts on serial sections. Cysts derived from peribiliary glands can cause extrinsic compression of bile ducts.

3. Urinary abnormalities—Urinary abnormalities include reduction in maximal urine concentration, hypocitraturia and low urine pH, microscopic or macroscopic hematuria, and mild to moderate proteinuria.

C. Imaging Studies

Although renal ultrasonography (US) is efficacious for polycystic kidney disease (PKD) screening, it provides limited anatomic definition. Magnetic resonance imaging (MRI) and contrast-enhanced computer tomography (CT) can accurately assess renal volume, cyst volume, and preserved renal parenchyma. CT without intravenous contrast is sensitive in detecting and localizing renal stones (including uric acid stones) and hemorrhages (Figure 46–1). Both CT and MRI detect renal neoplasms with similar sensitivity. MRI is often preferred because nephrotoxic intravenous contrast can be avoided.

To identify infected liver cysts, the combination of contrast-enhanced CT or MRI and nuclear scintigraphy may be helpful. CT or MRI might show thickened cyst walls, increased density of cyst contents, and air-fluid levels. Although limited by its imprecise anatomic definition, nuclear scintigraphy such as [111] In-labeled leukocyte scans can help to localize the infected cysts. A definitive diagnosis lies in a positive identification of microorganism in cyst fluid by aspiration.

An MR or CT angiogram is the test of choice for detecting ICAs. It has an estimated sensitivity of >90% in detecting aneurysms ≥3 mm in diameters. Thin cut, noncontrast CT is the initial test of choice for identifying SAH. Hemorrhage appears as areas of increased density. If the CT result is equivocal and clinical suspicion is high, lumbar puncture should be performed to establish the diagnosis.

▶ Differential Diagnosis

Renal cystic diseases can be a sequela of many systemic disease entities. This should be kept in mind especially when the patient's overall presentation is atypical for ADPKD. A correct diagnosis lies in a careful identification of extrarenal manifestations that are not typically associated with ADPKD.

ADPKD must be differentiated from ARPKD, ACKD, multiple simple cysts, glomerulocystic kidney disease, tuberous sclerosis complex, and von Hippel–Lindau disease. The features separating ADPKD from these conditions are outlined in Table 46–1.

▶ Treatment

Currently, no definitive treatment modality is available to halt cystic disease progression or to induce cyst regression. Risk factor modification, early detection and management of

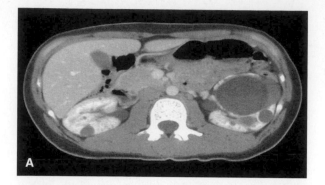

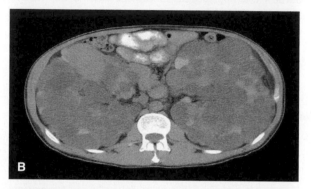

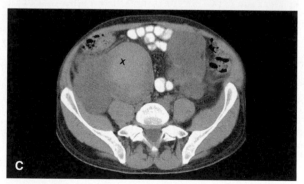

▲ **Figure 46–1.** Autosomal dominant polycystic kidney disease. **A:** Contrast-enhanced CT scan in a 26-year-old female with early stage polycystic kidney disease. Note a dominant left renal cyst. **B:** Noncontrast CT scan in a 42-year-old male with advanced cystic disease and bilateral renal enlargement. Note innumerable renal cysts, many of which are hyperdense (hemorrhagic or with high protein content). **C:** The lower pole of the right kidney from the same patient in **(B)** contains a large cyst with increased and heterogeneous densities representing clots (marked by 'X') and recent hemorrhage.

ADPKD complications, and avoidance of potentially nephrotoxic agents are the mainstays of management aiming to limit morbidity and premature death.

Table 46–1. Distinguishing features of autosomal dominant polycystic kidney disease.

Disease	Inheritance	Extrarenal characteristics	Renal manifestations
ADPKD	AD	Early adult onset of HTN; flank pain; gross hematuria; polycystic liver enlargement; SAH	Urine concentration defect; bilateral cystic renal enlargement; cysts arise from cortex and medullar; nephrolithiasis; renal failure with cystic disease progression
ARPKD	AR	Infantile "Potter's phenotype"; infantile HTN; portal hypertension: esophageal and gastric varices; hypersplenism	Large kidneys; bilateral fusiform collecting duct dilation; urine concentration defect; chronic renal failure
ACKD	Not inherited	Longstanding renal failure; risk of renal cancer	Normal sized or small kidneys; cysts arise from cortex; cyst wall calcification, papillary cystadenomas and renal cancer
Glomerulocystic kidney disease	AD (some)	Heterogeneous group of diseases	Cysts arise from the Bowman's capsules
Simple renal cysts	Not inherited	Associated with aging	Identified incidentally
Tuberous sclerosis complex (TSC)	AD	Prominent skin lesions; CNS: Giant cell astrocytomas and cortical tubers; cardiac rhabdomyomas; pulmonary lymphangioleiomyomatosis	Cysts; renal angiomyolipomas; renal carcinomas (rare)
von Hippel–Lindau disease (VHL)	AD	No skin lesion; retinal and CNS hemangioblastomas; pheochromocytomas; pancreatic cysts	Cysts; renal cell carcinomas (common)
Orofacial syndrome type 1	X-linked dominant	Cleft tongue and palate; broad nasal root; digital abnormalities	Cysts (may resemble ADPKD)
Medullary cystic disease	AD	Hyperuricemia	Adult onset of renal failure
Nephronophthisis	AR	Retinal degeneration (retinitis pigmentosa)	Childhood or adolescent onset of renal failure
Medullary spongy disease	Usually not familial		Papillary calcifications and renal stones; normal glomerular filtration rate

ADPKD, autosomal dominant polycystic kidney disease; ARPKD, autosomal recessive polycystic kidney disease; AD, autosomal dominant; AR, autosomal recessive; HTN, hypertension; SAH, subarachnoid hemorrhage; CNS, central nervous system.

A. Dietary Recommendations and Patient Education

In general, a diet of low sodium (<90 mEq/day), low cholesterol (<200 mg/day), high fiber, and 0.8 g/kg of ideal body weight/day protein is recommended. Avoiding or at least limiting caffeinated beverages to one to two servings per day is encouraged, because *in vitro* studies suggest that caffeine stimulates cAMP-mediated fluid secretion by the cyst-lining cells, which might promote cyst growth. Cessation of cigarette smoking should be stressed, because smoking is associated with a faster decline of renal function and an increased risk of ICA rupture.

Patients should be informed about and vigilant in monitoring the occurrence of ADPKD-associated manifestations because early detection and treatment can improve the overall disease outcome.

B. Hypertension

The best antihypertensive regimen for this patient population has not been clearly defined. In the majority of patients, angiotensin-converting enzyme inhibitors (ACEIs) and/or angiotensin receptor blockers (ARBs) are well tolerated and efficacious. If necessary, β- or combined α/β-blockers, a central α-adrenergic agonist, calcium channel blockers, or a low-dose thiazide diuretic (6.25–12.5 mg/day) may be added to optimize blood pressure control.

β-Blockers are indicated if patients have aortic root dilation or supraventricular tachycardia associated with mitral valve prolapse. High-dose diuretics should be avoided because they can reduce the renal blood flow and trigger acute gouty episodes.

C. Flank Pain

Nonopioid agents are preferred for pain. Narcotic analgesics are reserved for managing the acute and severe episodes of pain exacerbation. Care should be taken to identify the underlying etiology and treat the correctable causes such as infection, renal stone, or tumor. Long-term use of potentially nephrotoxic analgesics such as combination analgesics or nonsteroidal anti-inflammatory drugs should be avoided.

Clinically significant chronic pain may be treated with tricyclic antidepressants after the correctable causes are ruled out and/or treated. Splanchnic nerve blockade with local anesthetics or steroids may provide prolonged pain relief in some cases and can be an adjunctive therapy.

Cyst decompression should be considered when conservative measures fail. Cyst aspiration followed by sclerosis and surgical or laparoscopic cyst decompression are the effective options.

For patients with a few dominant cysts deemed to cause pain, cyst aspiration followed by alcohol sclerosis (under US or CT guidance) can be carried out by an interventional radiologist and be both diagnostic and therapeutic. Minor complications include microscopic hematuria, localized pain, and transient fever. Severe complications, occurring mainly after aspirating the centrally located cysts, are rare including pneumothorax, perirenal hematoma, arteriovenous fistula, urinoma, and infections.

For patients with a large number of cysts contributing to pain, laparoscopic or surgical cyst fenestration can be effective for 80–90% at 1 year postoperation. Sixty to 80% have sustained pain relief for 2 years or longer. Laparoscopic or retroperitoneoscopic procedures have a shorter and less complicated recovery compared to open surgery. A relative contraindication is prior abdominal surgery with possible adhesions.

Other modalities that have been tried are laparoscopic renal denervation combined with cyst fenestration, laparoscopic or retroperitoneal nephrectomy, and embolization of the renal artery for patients with end-stage renal failure.

D. Cyst Hemorrhage

The majority of cyst hemorrhages are self-limited and respond to conservative management including bed rest, analgesics, and adequate fluid intake to prevent obstructing urinary blood clots. Rarely, the bleeding may be severe with formation of subcapsular or retroperitoneal hematoma, a fall in hemoglobin concentration, and, in severe cases, hemodynamic instability. These patients should be hospitalized for investigation by CT or angiography, volume resuscitation with transfusion if necessary, and, for refractory bleedings, arterial embolization or surgery.

E. Urinary Tract and Renal Parenchymal/Cyst Infection

Prompt treatment of symptomatic urethritis or cystitis with an oral antimicrobial is crucial in preventing retrograde seeding to renal parenchyma and/or cysts. Highly lipophilic antimicrobials such as trimethoprim-sulfamethoxazole, fluoroquinolones, or, rarely, chloramphenicol are the agents of choice. If available, the results of blood and urine cultures should also guide the selection of antimicrobial. Acute episodes of parenchymal or cyst infection usually require initial parenteral therapy.

If cyst infection persists after 1–2 weeks of treatment, percutaneous or surgical drainage should be considered. If fever recurs after the discontinuation of antibiotics, reevaluation is necessary to rule out complications such as obstruction, perinephritic abscess, or stone. If no complication can be identified, a prolonged treatment (several months) may be necessary to eradicate the infection.

F. Nephrolithiasis

The principles of stone management for ADPKD patients are the same as for idiopathic stone patients. Potassium citrate is a well-suited treatment for three main causes of stones in ADPKD: uric acid lithiasis, hypocitraturic calcium oxalate lithiasis, and distal acidification defects. For acute stone attack, treatment includes parenteral fluid, analgesics, and, when indicated, lithotripsy or urologic procedures.

G. Renal Failure

1. Dialysis—ADPKD patients, in general, tolerate dialysis as well or better than patients with renal failure from other causes. This is possibly due to their higher production of endogenous erythropoietin and higher blood hemoglobin concentration. Rarely, hemodialysis can be complicated by episodes of intradialytic hypotension due to inferior vena cava compression caused by medially located right renal cysts or by hepatic cysts. This problem can be effectively managed by cyst aspiration or resection.

Peritoneal dialysis can also be safely carried out in ADPKD patients, although there is an increased risk of inguinal and umbilical hernias.

2. Transplantation—Transplantation is the treatment of choice for ADPKD end-stage renal failure. No difference is noted in posttransplant patient or graft survival between ADPKD and non-ADPKD patients. ADPKD-related complications such as mitral valve prolapse, aortic aneurysmal rupture, and hepatic or renal cyst infection are not adversely affected by renal transplant or posttransplant immune suppression.

Pretransplant cystic kidney nephrectomy is not routinely performed because native kidneys contribute to the maintenance of postoperative hemoglobin concentration and, in case of acute allograft failure, native kidneys may assist in fluid management. Pretransplant nephrectomy, however, is indicated if the patient has a history of cyst infection, frequent cyst hemorrhages, severe hypertension, or massive symptomatic renal enlargement.

H. Polycystic Liver Disease

The majority of PLD cases are asymptomatic and require no treatment. Estrogens, both oral contraceptives and estrogen replacement therapy, may contribute to cyst enlargement and should be discontinued if the risk of cyst growth outweighs the benefit of estrogen therapy.

When symptoms due to cyst compression occur, therapy is directed toward reducing cyst and hepatic volume. The options are (1) percutaneous cyst aspiration and sclerosis if a few dominant cysts give rise to symptoms, (2) laparoscopic fenestration for a limited number of large symptomatic cysts, (3) surgical partial hepatectomy and fenestration if symptoms are caused by a voluminous cystic liver for which percutaneous or laparoscopic treatment is not feasible, and rarely (4) liver transplantation if cystic involvement is extensive, refractory to other treatment, and not resectable.

When cyst infection is suspected, a percutaneous aspiration should be carried out to confirm the diagnosis. The combination of antibiotic therapy for at least 6 weeks and percutaneous cyst drainage is necessary to eradicate the infection. Trimethoprim-sulfamethoxazole and the fluoroquinolones have good cyst penetration and are effective against typical pathogens. The results of cyst-fluid culture should be used to guide the antimicrobial selection.

I. Intracranial Aneurysms

For ruptured or symptomatic ICAs, the therapy is surgical clipping of the ICA or, recently, endovascular coiling. Early recognition and urgent neurosurgical consultation are critical, because ICA rupture carries a high (50%) combined severe morbidity and mortality, and timely management can improve its outcome.

For asymptomatic ICAs, depending on the risk of rupture, the treatment options are observation with risk prevention and intervention including surgical clipping or endovascular coiling.

For anterior circulation ICAs under 7 mm in diameter in patients without a history of aneurysmal rupture, observation and follow-up (at 6 months initially and then yearly) with aggressive blood pressure control and smoking cessation are indicated. For the larger sized or posteriorly located ICAs and for ICAs in patients with a prior history of SAH, the choice of treatment depends on the patient's age, presence of comorbidities, local institutional experience, and expertise of care-providing physicians. The benefits of intervention should be weighed against the complications associated with intervention.

Presymptomatic ICA screening is usually not recommended for ADPKD patients without a family history of ICAs. It is indicated for patients with a family history of SAH, a high risk occupation such as pilots, or prior to major elective surgeries with anticipated hemodynamic instability. Screening should also be provided for patients with significant anxiety about ICAs.

Everson GT et al: Management of polycystic liver disease. Curr Gastroenterol Rep 2005;7(1):19. [PMID: 15701294]

Ong AC: Molecular pathogenesis of ADPKD; the polycystic complex gets complex. Kidney Int 2005;67:1234. [PMID: 15780076]

AUTOSOMAL RECESSIVE POLYCYSTIC KIDNEY DISEASE

 ESSENTIALS OF DIAGNOSIS

▶ Recessive pattern of transmission; parental consanguinity.

▶ Presentations for the neonatal period and infancy: Oligohydramnios, Potter's phenotype, pulmonary hypoplasia, and large echogenic kidneys with poor corticomedullary differentiation.

▶ Presentations for older children and adolescents: Portal fibrosis and increased hepatic echogenicity, hepatosplenomegaly, dilated intrahepatic ducts, and medullary sponge kidney (MSK) and renal cysts.

▶ General Considerations

ARPKD is a recessively inherited disease with an incidence of approximately 1 in 20,000 live births. It is caused by mutations of the *PKHD1* gene. It affects all racial and ethnic groups and is an important cause of neonatal and infantile morbidity and mortality.

In its severe form, enlarged ARPKD kidneys can be detected during the fetal or perinatal period. Twenty to 30% of these patients will not survive beyond infancy. For patients who survive the neonatal period, 20–45% will progress to end-stage renal failure by age 15–20 years.

In contrast to ADPKD, ARPKD has a more restricted pattern of presentation, with abnormalities confined mainly to the kidneys and biliary tract. The majority of patients present in infancy with prominent symptoms of respiratory distress due both to pulmonary hypoplasia (Potter's phenotype) from oligohydramnios and to a restricted diaphragmatic movement due to massively enlarged kidneys (Figure 46–2). Some patients have less prominent symptoms and present later in their childhood or adolescence with significant periportal fibrosis and portal hypertension, but less severe renal involvement.

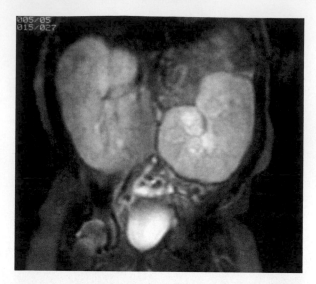

▲ **Figure 46–2.** Autosomal dominant polycystic kidney disease. Coronal T_2-weighted MRI of a 1-year-old ARPKD patient. The kidneys are massively enlarged with a lobular, reniform contour.

Prenatal diagnosis is made by ultrasound at ≥20 weeks of gestation. However, some ARPKD kidneys may not show sonographic abnormalities until the latter part of the third trimester. Thus, a normal renal ultrasound in the second or early third trimester cannot rule out ARPKD. Mutation analysis is now available.

▶ Clinical Findings

A. Symptoms and Signs

1. Neonatal and infancy—ARPKD infants can present with Potter's phenotype: Pulmonary hypoplasia leading to pulmonary insufficiency; specific facial characteristics including widely set eyes, a prominent inner canthus, a beaked nose, and large low-lying ears; and spine and limb contractures. Pulmonary insufficiency with respiratory distress is the major manifestation and the primary cause of morbidity and mortality in this group of patients. The kidneys are typically large and palpable. Renal function is impaired in the majority of these patients. Polyuria and renal tubular defects can be prominent. These defects can lead to dehydration, volume depletion, and metabolic acidosis, especially when patients are under concurrent stress conditions such as infection, poor oral intake, and/or diarrhea. Hypertension occurs in up to 80% of these patients and can be severe.

2. Childhood and adolescence—The main manifestations in this stage may be related to biliary dysgenesis caused by insufficient remodeling of the primitive intrahepatic biliary system (ductal plate), leading to congenital hepatic fibrosis

and intrahepatic bile duct dilation (Caroli's disease). The hepatocytes are unaffected. The clinical sequelae of portal hypertension include esophageal and/or gastric varices and variceal bleeding, and cytopenia due to hypersplenism. Renal disease may be mild. Papillary collecting duct ectasia and renal cysts may be incidentally detected. Chronic renal insufficiency may develop in some cases.

3. Cholangitis—Ascending cholangitis can occur at any age, especially in patients with significant intrahepatic bile duct dilation. Manifestations include fever, right upper quadrant abdominal pain, leukocytosis, liver enzyme elevation, and gram-negative bacterial sepsis.

4. End-stage renal failure—Growth failure, anemia, and osteodystrophy are presentations associated with end-stage renal failure.

B. Laboratory Findings

1. Renal pathology—Grossly, the kidneys from an infant or a young child are enlarged with a reniform configuration. Small cysts (1–2 mm) are visible on the renal capsular surface. Microscopically, collecting duct ectasia is prominent. The ectatic collecting ducts are fusiform, coursing radially through the cortex, and remain connected with the tubular system. The corticomedullary junction is not clearly demarcated.

With age, the overall size of the kidneys decreases. Macroscopic cysts develop and interstitial fibrosis becomes more prominent. The appearance of the kidneys at this stage may be difficult to distinguish from that of ADPKD.

2. Hepatic pathology and functional studies—Grossly, the liver size can be normal or enlarged. Microscopically, biliary dilation and portal fibrosis are present in all ARPKD patients to a varying degree. The fibrosis progresses with increasing age. Because hepatocytes are unaffected, the liver synthetic functions such as serum transaminase and albumin levels are typically maintained within normal limits.

C. Imaging Studies

Ultrasound is helpful in evaluating infants and children with suspected ARPKD. Bilateral symmetric renal enlargement with increased echogenicity and loss of corticomedullary differentiation is characteristic. Small tubular microcysts of 2–5 mm are common. With age, the kidneys will decrease in size and further increase in echogenicity. Macrocysts of >1 cm in diameter may become prominent. These features are ultrasonographically indistinguishable from those of ADPKD. US is also effective in assessing the degree of hepatobiliary involvement of ARPKD. With progression of periportal fibrosis, the hepatic echotexture becomes coarse and biliary dilation with thickened ductal walls can be prominent.

CTs of liver and kidneys are useful in defining the extent of hepatic and renal disease. However, their value is limited by the need for intravenous contrast, which could be detrimental to diseased kidneys. An MRI evaluation can be very helpful in these circumstances. MRI is excellent in evaluating the kidney size, cyst size, and number and extent of biliary abnormalities.

Differential Diagnosis

ARPKD should be differentiated from childhood-onset ADPKD, glomerulocystic kidney disease, and nephronophthisis. Table 46–1 lists specific features that might help to differentiate ARPKD from other cystic renal diseases. Additionally, a number of syndromic congenital disorders such as Meckel–Gruber syndrome, Bardet–Biedl syndrome, or asphyxiating thoracic dystrophy can present with the combination of renal abnormalities and hepatic fibrosis. However, these conditions can be easily differentiated because they are associated with other multiple congenital defects that are not found in ARPKD.

Treatment

A care team composed of intensivists, nephrologists, gastroenterologists, specialized nurses, dietitians, social workers, and sometimes psychiatrists is often needed to provide comprehensive care to neonates and children with ARPKD and to support their families, who can suffer from severe psychosocial stresses.

A. Pulmonary Hypoplasia

Aggressive respiratory support with whatever measures necessary is of paramount importance. Mechanical ventilation and/or nephrectomy (to make room for ventilation) might be required for severe, refractory cases.

B. Hypertension

ACEIs and ARBs are usually effective in treating the hypertension in these patients; α/β-blockers, calcium channel blockers, or diuretics can be added, depending on the clinical situation.

C. Polyuria due to Concentration Defect

Because of a urine concentration defect, these patients are susceptible to dehydration, especially during episodes of acute febrile illness. Special attention should be paid to this and maintenance fluids should be given to prevent its occurrence.

D. End-Stage Renal Failure

Both hemotoneal and peritoneal dialysis have been successfully performed for ARPKD patients with end-stage renal failure. A renal transplant is preferred to dialysis, because a successful transplant improves patient survival and prevents growth retardation and osteodystrophy. Nephrectomy may be indicated for massively enlarged kidneys to accommodate

the renal allograft. Splenectomy may be indicated in severe cases of hypersplenism with leukocytopenia and thrombocytopenia.

E. Complications of Hepatic Fibrosis and Portal Hypertension

Bacterial cholangitis should be promptly diagnosed and treated with appropriate antimicrobials. Periodic abdominal ultrasound and upper endoscopy may be necessary to assess the degree of hepatosplenomegaly and varices. Primary prevention of variceal bleeding with β-blockers or endoscopic variceal sclerosis or banding can be helpful in preventing acute bleeding episodes. Portosystemic shunting may also be helpful for selected cases. Liver transplant, including living-donor liver transplant, is indicated in patients with severe hepatic complications.

Bergmann C et al: PKHD1 mutations in autosomal recessive polycystic kidney disease (ARPKD).Hum Mutat 2004;23(5):453. [PMID: 15108277]

TUBEROUS SCLEROSIS COMPLEX

 ESSENTIALS OF DIAGNOSIS

- ▶ Multiple cortical tubers on MRI (>2 needed for diagnosis).
- ▶ Radial migrating lines on head MRI (>3 needed for diagnosis).
- ▶ Subependymal nodules or giant cell astrocytomas (>2 needed for diagnosis).
- ▶ Astrocytic retinal hamartomas (>2 needed for diagnosis).
- ▶ Facial angiofibromas or fibrous forehead plaques (>2 needed for diagnosis).
- ▶ Ungual fibroma (>2 needed for diagnosis).
- ▶ Cardiac rhabdomyomas (fetus, infant, or child).
- ▶ Multiple renal cysts and angiomyolipomas or renal cell carcinoma.
- ▶ See Table 46–2 for diagnostic criteria.

General Considerations

Tuberous sclerosis complex (TSC) is an autosomal dominantly inherited disease. It affects 1 in 6000 individuals. It can be caused by mutations in either *TSC1* (chromosomal 9) or *TSC2* (chromosomal 16) genes. *De novo* (newly occurred) *TSC* mutations, in which approximately two-thirds are *TSC2* mutations, account for two-thirds of all TSC cases. The *TSC2* gene is located immediately adjacent to *PKD1* (the gene responsible for ADPKD1) in a head-to-head configuration on chromosome 16p13.3. Some

Table 46–2. Features of tuberous sclerosis complex and diagnostic criteria.

Major features
Facial angiofibromas or forehead plaques
Nontraumatic ungual or periungual fibroma
Hypomelanotic macules (more than three)
Shagreen patch (connective tissue nevus)
Multiple retinal nodular hamartomas
Cortical tuber
Subependymal nodule
Subependymal giant cell astrocytoma
Cardiac rhabdomyoma, single or multiple
Lymphangiomyomatosis
Renal angiomyolipoma
Minor features
Multiple, randomly distributed pits in dental enamel
Hamartomatous rectal polyps
Bone cysts
Cerebral white matter radial migration lines
Gingival fibromas
Nonrenal hamartomas
Retinal achromic patch
"Confetti" skin lesions
Multiple renal cysts
Diagnostic criteria[1]
Definitive tuberous sclerosis complex (TSC): Either two major features or one major feature plus two minor features probable TSC: One major plus one minor feature possible TSC: Either one major feature or two or more minor features

[1]These diagnostic criteria were adopted at the Consensus Conference on TSC held in Annapolis, Maryland, on July 10, 1998, under the auspices of the National Tuberous Sclerosis Association.

Adapted with permission from *Tuberous Sclerosis Complex*, ed 3. Rodriguez Gomez M (editor). Oxford University Press, 1999.

deletional mutations can disrupt both the *TSC2* and *PKD1* genes causing a *TSC2–PKD1* contiguous gene syndrome: A TSC phenotype plus an early-onset, severe polycystic renal disease.

TSC genes are tumor suppressor genes. Their protein products, hamartin (*TSC1*) and tuberin (*TSC2*), form a complex that deactivates small G protein (Rheb) and mammalian target of rapamycin (mTOR)-mediated cell growth and cell cycle progression. Thus, the mutations of either the *TSC1* or *TSC2* gene will result in abnormal cell growth, proliferation, and the formation of hamartomas (angiomyolipomata) in multiple organ systems and renal neoplasms. Angiomyolipomata are benign tumors composed of a circumscribed group of dysplastic smooth muscle cells, fat, and blood vessels.

These cells have a poor structural organization and propensity to multiply. Additionally, TSC mutations can give rise to renal neoplasms including benign and malignant tumors.

The most frequently involved organs by angiomyolipomata in TSC are the skin, brain, retina, heart, kidney, and lung. Spinal cord lesions are rare; the peripheral nerves or the skeletal muscles are not known to be involved. Compared to *TSC1* mutations, *TSC2* mutations tend to have a more severe clinical phenotype. The leading cause of death in TSC is, overall, central nervous system (CNS) complications. However, in the adult TSC population, renal complications including uremia, retroperitoneal bleeding, and metastatic renal cancers are the leading cause of death.

Genetic testing is available from Athena Diagnostics, Inc. (Worcester, MA). However, a 20% false-negative rate limits its practical utility. The test is indicated when clinical diagnosis is unclear or when parents of an affected child are making decisions in family planning. Today, clinical criteria are still the quickest and the most accurate and inexpensive way to establish a diagnosis.

▶ Clinical Findings

A. Symptoms and Signs

The presentations of TSC are age dependent (Figure 46–3). Cortical tubers and intracardiac rhabdomyomas may occur at the perinatal period and can be detected by imaging studies such as CT or MRI. Intracardiac rhabdomyomas typically reach their maximal size at birth and regress in the postnatal years. They can cause cardiac outflow tract obstruction.

Other perinatal or neonatal manifestations include cutaneous hypomelanotic macules, facial angiofibromas (facial forehead plaques), arrhythmia due to Wolff–Parkinson–White (WPW) syndrome, and renal cysts.

Subependymal nodules occur in early childhood. They may reach their peak rate of growth at puberty and cease to grow by the end of the third decade of life. Subependymal nodules may evolve into subependymal giant cell astrocytomas.

Seizure, regression of social-adaptive behavior, and mental retardation usually associated with seizure activity in infancy can be evident during childhood.

Retinal hamartomas usually appear during early childhood. They have limited growth potential, frequently become calcified, and usually remain asymptomatic.

Facial angiofibromas (also called adenoma sebaceum), shagreen patches, and ungual fibromas develop during childhood and affect up to 80% of TSC patients. Minor features such as enamel pits, gingival fibromas, retinal achromic patches, confetti skin lesions, and hamartomatous rectal polyps can also be evident.

Pulmonary lymphangioleiomyomas (LAMs), which occur exclusively in women (up to 40%), can cause pneumothorax or chylothorax, hypoxia, and respiratory failure.

The renal manifestations of TSC include angiomyolipomata, epithelioid angiomyolipomata, cysts, epithelial cell

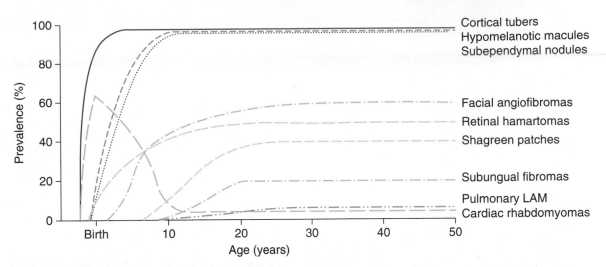

▲ Figure 46–3. Autosomal dominant polycystic kidney disease. Estimated age of development and age-adjusted prevalence of the main extrarenal manifestations of the tuberous sclerosis complex. LAM, lymphangioleiomyomatosis. (Reproduced with permission from Torres VE et al: Update on tuberous sclerosis complex. In: *Rare Kidney Diseases.* Schieppati A (editor). S. Karger AG, 2001.)

neoplasms, interstitial fibrosis associated with focal segmental glomerulosclerosis, and a variety of other lesions (see Table 46–3).

Angiomyolipomata are benign, slow growing, fat-containing tumors occurring multicentrically in both kidneys. They tend to be larger and more numerous in women. This female predilection might be related to the expression of estrogen and progesterone receptors on the tumor cells. The main clinical presentations include hemorrhage and abdominal or flank mass and tenderness. Hemorrhagic episodes present as sudden, painful, and sometimes life-threatening events. Angiomyolipomata can also cause hypertension, renal insufficiency, and fever of unknown origin. In general, tumors with diameters of greater than 4 cm are prone to become symptomatic.

Table 46–3. Renal manifestations of tubulosclerosis complex.

Angiomyolipomas
Cysts
Epithelioid angiomyolipomas
Renal cell carcinomas
Renal oncocytomas
Focal segmental glomerulosclerosis with interstitial fibrosis
Glomerular microhamartomas
Lymphangiomatous cysts
Rare associations (renal artery stenosis, ureteropelvic junction obstruction, nephrocalcinosis)

Epithelioid angiomyolipomata are a non-fat-containing variant of angiomyolipomata. They are composed of aberrant vascular smooth muscle cells bearing an epithelioid phenotype. Although these tumors are considered to have a malignant potential, their natural history and clinical presentation have not been clearly defined.

Epithelial neoplasms associated with TSC include benign papillary adenomas and oncocytomas and malignant clear cell, papillary or chromophobe carcinomas. The clinical presentations of these tumors are similar to those of sporadic renal tumors, except that TSC-associated tumors tend to be multicentric and bilateral. Rapid growth of tumors and lack of a fat component on surveillance imaging are indicative of malignancy.

Multiple renal cysts are another feature of TSC. The cysts, in general, are not numerous or overtly symptomatic. However, in a subset of TSC patients, the cystic renal involvement can be extensive, indistinguishable from that of ADPKD. The majority of these patients have a contiguous *TSC2–PKD1* gene syndrome. Complications associated with renal cysts are hemorrhage, hematuria, hypertension, and renal failure.

B. Laboratory Findings

1. Renal pathology—Angiomyolipomata (including their epithelioid variant), cysts, and benign or malignant neoplasms are the principal renal pathologic findings in TSC. They frequently coexist.

Angiomyolipomata are composed of proliferative mixtures of blood vessel, smooth muscle, and fatty tissues. At the early stage, they appear as multicentric, wedge-shaped cortical lesions with their bases facing the surface of the kidney. On enlarging, the tumors may penetrate into the renal parenchyma or extend to the perirenal fat becoming exophytic. Epithelioid angiomyolipomata are a variant of angiomyolipomata. They are composed of epithelioid vascular smooth muscle cells with irregular nuclei and higher mitotic activity. These tumors do not contain adipose tissues.

Renal cysts can originate from any section along the nephrons. They are composed of hypertrophic and hyperplastic epithelium. Cystic renal involvement can be extensive in patients with contiguous *TSC2–PKD1* gene syndrome.

Renal cancers in TSC tend to be multifocal and may possess aggressive sarcomatoid features.

Other pathologic changes that can be associated with TSC include interstitial fibrosis, focal segmental glomerulosclerosis, renal vascular dysplasia, and glomerular microhamartomas.

2. Urine study—Mild to moderate proteinuria may be present.

C. Imaging Studies

The imaging (US, CT, or MRI) appearance of renal cysts is indistinguishable from that of simple cysts or ADPKD cysts. The coexistence of angiomyolipomata distinguishes TSC from other renal cystic diseases.

The imaging diagnosis of angiomyolipomata requires the identification of fat in the tumor, which shows an increase in echogenicity on US, a low attenuation on CT, and high signal intensity on T_1-weighted MRI. Renal cancer should be suspected if a tumor shows no identifiable fatty tissue and when there is evidence of intratumoral calcification. Surgical exploration is usually indicated in these cases.

▶ Differential Diagnosis

TSC must be differentiated from ADPKD, ARPKD, ACKD, multiple simple cysts, glomerulocystic kidney disease, and von Hippel–Lindau disease. The features that can separate TSC from these conditions are listed in Table 46–1.

▶ Treatment

Depending on clinical scenarios, current treatment options for TSC renal manifestations include observation, arterial embolization, and partial or total nephrectomy.

For slowly growing angiomyolipomata of <4 cm in diameter, semiannual or annual observational follow-up may be sufficient. For larger (>4 cm) or rapidly growing angiomyolipomata, intervention may be considered to prevent acute hemorrhage. Renal-sparing tumor resection is the preferred approach. A decision for nephrectomy should be carefully balanced against the loss of renal function and the negative impact on the patient's long-term care. For highly vascular lesions or lesions that are deemed to have a high risk of intraoperative bleeding, arterial embolization to obliterate the regional blood supply should be considered. The embolization can be used alone or be followed by renal sparing tumor resection.

For episodes of acute hemorrhage due to angiomyolipomata or cysts, treatment options include supportive observation, arterial embolization, and, in refractory cases, partial or total nephrectomy.

Because the loss of inhibition to mTOR resulting from TSC mutations is the cause of tumor formation, rapamycin (an mTOR-inhibiting agent) becomes a potential pharmacologic treatment agent of choice to prevent tumor formation and growth. Its utility is being tested in human trials.

For TSC patients with uremia due to loss of renal function from multiple renal resections, replacement of renal tissue by tumors, or severe PKD, dialysis or renal transplant is indicated. Bilateral nephrectomy is usually indicated because of the risk of bleeding and renal cancer.

Inoki K et al: Dysregulation of the TSC-mTOR pathway in human disease. Nat Genet 2005;1:19. [PMID: 15624019]

Maria BL et al: Tuberous sclerosis complex: pathogenesis, diagnosis, strategies, therapies, and future research directions. J Child Neurol 2004;19:632. [PMID: 15563008]

Sancak O et el: Mutational analysis of the *TSC1* and *TSC2* genes in a diagnostic setting: genotype-phenotype correlations and comparison of diagnostic DNA techniques in tuberous sclerosis complex. Eur J Hum Genet 2005;13(6):731. [PMID: 15798777]

VON HIPPEL–LINDAU DISEASE

 ESSENTIALS OF DIAGNOSIS

▶ In patients with a family history of von Hippel–Lindau (VHL) disease:

  –Cerebellar hemangioblastomas.

  –Retinal hemangioblastomas.

  –Renal cysts and renal cell carcinoma.

  –Pheochromocytomas.

▶ In patients without a family history of this disease:

  –Retinal hemangioblastomas (≥ 2).

  –Cerebellar hemangioblastomas (≥ 2).

  –Single hemangioblastomas plus a visceral tumor.

▶ A diagnosis can be made with one of the above findings (the number needed for diagnosis is given in parentheses).

▶ General Considerations

VHL disease is an autosomal dominant neoplastic disease that affects approximately 1 in 35,000 individuals worldwide.

It occurs in all ethnic groups and is caused by mutations in the *VHL* gene located on chromosome 3p25.

VHL is a tumor suppressor gene. pVHL, the protein product of *VHL*, binds to a group of partner proteins (Elongin B, Elongin C, Cul2, and Rbx1) and forms a stable multiprotein complex. Depending on the level of cellular oxygenation, the pVHL complex regulates the degradation of an oxygen sensor protein named hypoxia-inducible factor (HIF). HIF induces the expression of hypoxia-inducible proteins, including angiogenic peptides [ie, vascular endothelial growth factor (VEGF)] and erythropoietin. Overproduction of these proteins is associated with tumor formation.

Under adequate tissue oxygenation, via ubiquitinating HIF, the pVHL complex promotes HIF degradation and thus suppresses the production of HIF-dependent protein. In VHL disease, mutant pVHL fails to degrade HIF, causing an overproduction of HIF-dependent proteins and tumorigenesis. Moreover, converging evidence indicates that the pVHL complex also possesses HIF-independent tumor suppressive functions. Taken together, mutations in the *VHL* gene invariably lead to tumor formation.

VHL disease, based on its clinical presentations, is divided into type 1 (low risk of pheochromocytoma) and type 2 (high risk of pheochromocytoma) diseases (see Table 46–4). These clinical phenotypes are correlated with the types of *VHL* mutations.

Type 1 VHL disease is marked by a frequent occurrence of hemangioblastoma, renal cell carcinoma, and a low occurrence of pheochromocytoma. This type of clinical presentation is associated primarily with the truncating *VHL* mutations (a part of pVHL is cut off). Type 2 VHL diseases, further classified into 2A, 2B, and 2C, are almost invariably associated with missense mutations (a change of a single amino acid within pVHL). In addition to its high risk of hemangioblastoma and pheochromocytoma, type 2A is characterized by a low risk of renal cell carcinoma, 2B by a high risk of renal cell carcinoma, and 2C by a sole occurrence of pheochromocytoma without significant risk of hemangioblastoma or renal cell carcinoma. Each subtype is associated with specific variants of missense mutations.

Table 46–4. Classification of von Hippel–Lindau disease.

Type 1	Hemangioblastoma
	Renal cell carcinoma
Type 2	Pheochromocytomas (common for type 2 von Hippel-Lindau disease)
	Plus 2A: Hemangioblastoma
	Renal cell carcinoma (low occurrence)
	2B: Hemangioblastoma
	Renal cell carcinoma (high occurrence)
	2C: Pheochromocytomas (only)

VHL patients typically develop tumors in their second to fourth decades of life. Renal cell cancer, with a lifetime occurrence of approximately 70% in this patient population, is the leading cause of death.

Genetic testing information can be found at http://www.vhl.org/dna/. Currently, diagnosis is established by the clinical presentations.

▶ **Clinical Findings**

A. Symptoms and Signs

Multiple retinal and CNS hemangioblastomas are the most common and earliest manifestations of VHL disease. If untreated, retinal hemangioblastomas can cause local hemorrhage, retinal detachment, and blindness. Because these retinal tumors are frequently located in the periphery of the retina, a careful ophthalmologic examination with pupillary dilation is indicated.

The cerebellum is the most frequent site for CNS hemangioblastomas, followed by the spinal cord and the brain stem. Although these tumors do not metastasize, their space-occupying growth at multiple locations can cause devastating neurologic defects.

Renal manifestations include renal cysts, hemangiomas, benign adenomas, and renal cell carcinomas.

Most VHL patients develop renal cysts. Although, in general, the cysts are not extensive or overtly symptomatic, a small fraction of VHL patients develops significant cystic renal disease sometimes indistinguishable from ADPKD. Complications include cyst hemorrhage, hematuria, hypertension, and renal dysfunction. Renal cysts in VHL are precursor lesions of renal cell carcinomas.

Renal hemangiomas and benign adenomas are mostly asymptomatic and are typically identified during evaluation for other clinical manifestations of VHL.

Renal carcinomas, mainly of the clear cell type, are often preceded by the growth of premalignant renal cysts. These cancers tend to be multifocal and bilateral and have a high rate of recurrence after resection(s).

Compared to the sporadic renal carcinomas, VHL-associated renal cancers have a younger age of onset (mean age of approximately 40 versus 59 years) and lack male predominance. Tumors that exceed 3 cm in diameter may invade renal veins and metastasize to distant organs including the adrenal gland, liver, lungs, CNS, and bone.

The clinical presentation of renal cancers in VHL disease is not different from that of sporadic ones. However, because of the high rate of cancer occurrence and risk of mortality, regular surveillance by imaging studies should be carried out.

Other less frequently involved organs are the adrenal gland (pheochromocytomas), pancreas (cysts, adenomas, and carcinomas), inner ear (endolymphatic sac tumor), epididymis (cysts and rare hemangiomas), and spleen (angiomas). Because pancreatic cysts are uncommon in the general population,

VHL should be considered in the differential diagnosis when a patient presents with multiple pancreatic cysts.

Pheochromocytomas in VHL disease have the same presentation as sporadic ones. Arteriography or surgery can trigger hypertensive crises in these patients. Thus, prior to undergoing these procedures, VHL patients should be screened to rule out pheochromocytomas.

B. Laboratory Findings

1. Pathology—The gross appearance of retinal and CNS tumors depends on their composition. Microscopically, these tumors are composed of vessels lined with endothelial cells, stromal cells, and pericytes.

The VHL kidney contains numerous macroscopic and microscopic tumor foci, each surrounded by a fibrous pseudocapsule. These carcinomas are composed of clear cells. Focal calcifications can be identified within these tumors.

2. Other laboratory abnormalities—Other laboratory abnormalities include erythrocytosis secondary to the production of erythropoietin by tumor cells and elevation of 24-hour urine metanephrine in patients with pheochromocytomas (type 2 VHL disease).

C. Imaging Studies

CT and MRI are the tests of choice for cerebellar hemangioblastomas. On CT, these tumors typically appear as round and hypodense cystic nodules, and are intensely enhanced by intravenous contrast administration. On MRI, the cystic part of the tumors are sharply demarcated and mural nodules can clearly be detected as high signal intensity on T_2-weighted images compared to that of the surrounding gray matter. The nodules typically enhance with gadolinium administration.

CT or MRI is also the test of choice for renal cancer screening and surveillance. The tumors are intensely enhanced by intravenous contrast and can be detected by either method.

▶ Differential Diagnosis

VHL disease must be differentiated from ADPKD, multiple simple cysts, and TSC. The features that can separate VHL disease from these conditions are listed in Table 46–1.

▶ Treatment

A. Central Nervous System and Retinal Hemangioblastomas

Surgical resection is usually indicated for cerebellar hemangioblastomas. Radiotherapy can be tried for symptomatic lesions that are not amenable to surgery. Posttreatment annual follow-up is necessary. Cryocoagulation or photocoagulation is the treatment of choice for retinal hemangioblastomas.

B. Renal Carcinomas

Tumors <3 cm in diameter have a low risk of metastases and are relatively slow growing. Semiannual or annual follow-up with serial imaging studies, CT or MRI, is recommended. For larger sized renal cell cancers (>3 cm in diameter), intervention is indicated because of the high risk of metastasis. Surgical tumor resection is the standard treatment. Renal-sparing tumor resections should always be tried when possible to preserve the patient's quality of life and prevent or delay the need for dialysis or transplantation. At the time of surgery, all accessible renal tumors and cysts should be removed. Because of predictable tumor recurrence, ongoing screening after initial resection and repeated resections are often necessary.

Image-guided percutaneous radiofrequency ablation or cryoablation can be a feasible alternative to surgery in certain cases, including preemptive treatment of small cancers and high operative risk conditions. These procedures are minimally invasive, associated with a very low rate of complication, and can be carried out repeatedly. The absolute contraindications include irreversible coagulopathy and active infection such as sepsis.

Humanized VEGF neutralizing antibody has been shown to delay the progression of metastatic renal cancers in a randomized phase II trial and is being tested in a phase III trial. If the results from this trial are confirmatory, humanized VEGF neutralizing antibody could be a valuable addition to the current repertoire of treatment modalities.

For patients with end-stage renal disease secondary to bilateral nephrectomy, dialysis or renal transplant (in the absence of a metastatic tumor) is indicated.

Hines-Peralta A et al: Review of radiofrequency ablation for renal cell carcinoma. Clin Cancer Res 2004;10(18Pt2):6328S. [PMID: 15448026]

Sufan RI et al: The role of von Hippel–Lindau tumor suppressor protein and hypoxia in renal clear cell carcinoma. Am J Physiol Renal Physiol 2004;287:F1. [PMID: 15180922]

NEPHRONOPHTHISIS & MEDULLARY CYSTIC DISEASE

 ESSENTIALS OF DIAGNOSIS

▶ Small kidneys with tubular atrophy and interstitial fibrosis.

▶ Renal cysts located in the corticomedullary junction.

▶ Chronic renal failure with minimal or low-grade proteinuria.

▶ General Considerations

Nephronophthisis and medullary cystic disease constitute a rare group of heterogeneously inherited cystic tubulointerstitial renal diseases. Although having nearly identical clinical and pathologic features, they are genetically separated entities. Nephronophthisis is autosomal recessive; five genes (*NPHP1*, *INVS*, *NPHP3*, *NPHP4*, and *NPHP5*) responsible for this disease have been identified. Medullary cystic disease is autosomal dominant; one gene (UMOD) and one 2.1-Mb gene locus (1q21) have been identified.

▶ Clinical Findings

A. Symptoms and Signs

The onset of both diseases is insidious. The earliest sign is polyuria accompanied by polydipsia due to urinary concentration defect. It precedes the decline of renal function. Hypertension can be absent at the early stages of renal dysfunction because of renal salt wasting. With a progressive decline in renal function, hypertension, anemia, and sequelae of uremia will ensue. Nephronophthisis has a childhood or adolescent onset of end-stage renal failure, whereas in medullary cystic disease real failure occurs in adulthood.

Nephronophthisis and medullary cystic disease have different extrarenal clinical manifestations (Table 46–1). Some patients with nephronophthisis develop retinitis pigmentosa (approximately 1 in 10 affected individuals) while a fraction of patients with medullary cystic disease develops hyperuricemia and gouty arthritis.

B. Laboratory Findings

1. Renal pathology—The kidneys are small. Cysts of variable size are located mostly at the corticomedullary junction. Microscopically, tubular atrophy, irregular thickening of the tubular basement membrane, and interstitial fibrosis are diffuse. The interstitial fibrosis is frequently associated with patchy infiltrations of inflammatory cells.

2. Urinary findings—Urinary findings include a reduction in maximal urine concentration, urine salt wasting, and bland urine sediment with a mild degree or absence of proteinuria.

C. Imaging Studies

Renal US shows normal to small-sized echogenic kidneys with a smooth contour. Small corticomedullary cysts may be seen. A CT scan or MRI shows bilaterally small kidneys. Renal cysts are confined to the medulla and corticomedullary junction.

▶ Treatment

No specific treatment is available for renal dysfunction. If present, water and electrolyte imbalance should be corrected. Hyperuricemia or gout associated with medullary cystic disease should be treated with allopurinol. For end-stage renal failure, renal transplant is preferred to chronic dialysis. No treatment is available for visual loss secondary to retinitis pigmentosa.

Bichet DG et al: The quest for the gene responsible for medullary cystic kidney disease type 1. Kidney Int 2004;66(2):864. [PMID: 15253745]

Hoefele J et al: Mutational analysis of the NPHP4 gene in 250 patients with nephronophthisis. Hum Mutat 2005;25(4):411. [PMID: 15776426]

Otto EA et al: Nephrocystin-5, a ciliary IQ domain protein, is mutated in Senior-Loken syndrome and interacts with RPGR and calmodulin. Nat Genet 2005;37(3):282. [PMID: 15723066]

MEDULLARY SPONGE DISEASE

ESSENTIALS OF DIAGNOSIS

▶ Precalyceal tubular ectasia with a pathognomonic "paint brush appearance" on excretory urogram.

▶ Usually without a positive family history and with normal renal clearance.

▶ General Considerations

Medullary sponge disease is a benign condition frequently identified incidentally during evaluation of renal colic. It may be associated with a variety of congenital abnormalities including congenital hemihypertrophy, Beckwith–Wiedemann syndrome, and Ehlers–Danlos syndrome. Although renal failure may occur due to recurrent stone-induced obstructive uropathy, the majority of patients maintain a normal glomerular filtration rate.

▶ Clinical Findings

A. Symptoms and Signs

Many patients are asymptomatic. Some can present with nephrolithiasis, recurrent urinary tract infections, and microhematuria. Stones are composed of calcium oxalate or calcium phosphate. The mechanisms underlying the lithogenicity in this disease have not been fully elucidated. Tubular dilation, urinary stasis, hypercalciuria, and hypocitraturia are thought to contribute to the stone formation.

B. Laboratory Findings

1. Renal pathology—Grossly, kidneys are of normal size. The main abnormality is a papillary deformity with calcifications. Microscopically, calcified ectatic or cystic dilations of the medullary collecting ducts are present.

2. Urinary abnormalities—Urinary abnormalities include microscopic hematuria, high urine pH, hypercalciuria, and hypocitraturia.

C. Imaging Studies

Excretory urography shows linear striated densities in one or more papillae resembling a "paint brush," which is pathognomonic of this disease.

Differential Diagnosis

Table 46–1 lists features that could separate medullary sponge disease from other renal cystic diseases.

Treatment

Treatment of nephrolithiasis is the same as for sporadic renal stone patients. Prolonged antimicrobial therapy may be required to treat the urinary tract infections.

Milliner DS et al: Urolithiasis. In: *Pediatric Nephrology*, ed 5. Avner ED, Harmon W, Niaudet P (editors). Lippincott, Williams & Wilkins, 2004, pp 1091–1112.

ACQUIRED CYSTIC KIDNEY DISEASE

ESSENTIALS OF DIAGNOSIS

▶ Four or more cysts in each kidney by ultrasonography or CT in patients with advanced chronic renal failure or in a uremic state.

▶ Absence of inherited cystic renal diseases.

General Considerations

Acquired cystic kidney disease (ACKD) is a condition in which a noncystic kidney develops cysts in the context of advanced chronic renal failure. Patients do not need to be on dialysis to have ACKD. The chronic uremic milieu is thought to promote the cystic transformation. The prevalence and severity of ACKD increase with the duration of end-stage renal failure. Ten to 20% of patients with renal failure have ACKD at the onset of dialysis; approximately 50% have ACKD after 5 years of dialysis and more than 90% have ACKD after 10 years of dialysis.

A major concern with ACKD is its association with renal cancer. Two to 7% of these patients will develop renal cancer, a marked increase (>100-fold) in prevalence compared to that of the general population. The mean duration of dialysis prior to the detection of cancers is about 8 years. The cancer in ACKD tends to be bilateral and multifocal and can be either clear cell or papillary carcinomas (1:1 occurrence ratio). In patients with a successful renal transplant, ACKD can regress. However, preexisting renal carcinomas in native kidneys can progress and become metastatic. This may be associated with posttransplant immune suppression. ACKD

and its associated risk of renal cancer can also occur in children with chronic renal failure.

Clinical Findings

A. Symptoms and Signs

The majority of ACKD patients are asymptomatic. Infrequently, patients can develop flank pain, hematuria, or perinephric hematoma due to cyst hemorrhage or renal cancer. Rarely, severe retroperitoneal hemorrhage can develop, requiring resuscitation and surgical or radiologic intervention. Symptoms and signs that might be paraneoplastic, such as fever, erythrocytosis, and hypercalcemia, should raise suspicion for renal cell cancer.

B. Laboratory Findings

Grossly, kidneys usually are small with cysts varying in size from pinpoint to a few centimeters. They are located mostly in the renal cortex. Microscopically, these cysts are lined with a single layer or multiple layers of renal epithelial cells. Some of these lining cells appear proliferative and dysplastic. Cyst walls are often calcified, and papillary cystadenomas can frequently be identified within these cysts. With time, renal enlargement may ensue.

C. Imaging Studies

To define the extent of AKCD, either renal ultrasound or CT is sufficient. To detect renal cancer, CT with intravenous contrast or MRI with gadolinium is necessary to demonstrate an enhancement.

Differential Diagnosis

ACKD should be differentiated from ADPKD, ARPKD, multiple simple cysts, glomerulocystic kidney disease, TSC, and VHL disease. The features that can separate ACKD from these conditions are listed in Table 46–1.

Treatment

Treatment is indicated when ACKD patients develop significant complications such as retroperitoneal hemorrhage, infection, and/or renal cancer (≥3 cm in diameter). Bilateral nephrectomy is usually indicated in these cases.

Although the rate of renal cancer is increased, routine screening for renal cancer is not indicated for all ACKD patients. This is mainly because a large number of renal failure patients have multiple comorbidities such as diabetes, hypertension, or atherosclerotic vascular diseases, which can limit their life expectancy to such an extent that they are more likely to succumb to diseases other than ACKD-associated renal cancer. However, for patients who have less comorbidity, have a good life expectancy, and have been on dialysis for at least 3 years, screening for renal cancer is indicated.

Ikeda R et al: Proliferative activity of renal cell carcinoma associated with acquired cystic disease of the kidney: comparison with typical renal cell carcinoma. Hum Pathol 2002;33(2):230. [PMID: 11957150]

SIMPLE RENAL CYSTS

ESSENTIALS OF DIAGNOSIS

▶ By renal US:

–Rare in individuals less than age 30 years.

–1.7% of individuals at age 30–49, 11.5% at age 50–70, and 22–30% at age greater than 70 years have at least one renal cyst.

▶ Conventional US underestimates the number of renal cysts compared to that of CT or MRI.

▶ General Considerations

Simple renal cysts originate from focal dilation of renal tubules and are common in the aging population. The number of individuals with renal cysts and the number and size of the cysts increase with age.

▶ Clinical Findings

A. Symptoms and Signs

In most cases, simple renal cysts are asymptomatic. They are typically identified incidentally on imaging studies of the abdomen. Occasionally, flank pain, cyst hemorrhage, hematuria, or, rarely, cyst infection can occur. Simple renal cysts have been reported to be associated with renin-mediated hypertension and erythropoietin-mediated erythrocytosis,

B. Laboratory Findings

Pathologically, simple renal cysts are more commonly located in the cortex with sizes varying from a few millimeters to over 20 cm. Microscopically, cysts are lined with a single flattened layer of cyst-lining epithelia. The surrounding renal parenchyma is usually normal.

C. Imaging Studies

Ultrasonographically, simple cysts present as round, smooth, and thin-walled cysts with sharply defined margins, without internal echoes. On CT, they are round, smooth, and homogeneous with a density near that of water and do not enhance with intravenous contrast administration. If a cyst has internal echoes on ultrasound or shows enhancement on CT with contrast, further diagnostic evaluation such as cyst aspiration and/or angiography should be considered.

▶ Differential Diagnosis

Multiple simple renal cysts should be differentiated from ADPKD, ARPKD, ACKD, glomerulocystic kidney disease, TSC, and VHL disease. The features that can separate multiple simple cysts from these conditions are listed in Table 46–1.

▶ Treatment

Treatment is needed only when complications such as pain, cyst hemorrhage, or cyst infection develop and is as discussed for patients with ADPKD.

Terada N et al: The natural history of simple renal cysts. J Urol 2002;167(1):21. [PMID: 11743266]

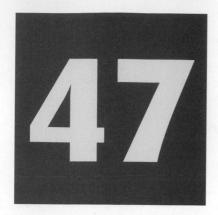

Familial Hematurias: Alport Syndrome & Thin Basement Membrane Nephropathy

Clifford E. Kashtan, MD

Hematuria is a relatively common abnormality. About 0.25% of school-age children have persistent microscopic hematuria. In adults the prevalence of hematuria increases with age and is greater in women. The causes and consequently the workup of hematuria vary with age. Glomerular disorders are responsible for most cases of pediatric hematuria, while urinary tract malignancy is an important cause of hematuria in individuals over 40 years of age.

Because thin basement membrane nephropathy (TBMN) typically has a benign course, it is likely that this condition is underdiagnosed, and that the true prevalence of familial hematuria is higher than we might think. TBMN and Alport syndrome account for a substantial fraction of children with isolated hematuria referred to pediatric nephrology clinics. TBMN was diagnosed in 40–70% of patients with asymptomatic microscopic hematuria and a negative urologic evaluation.

ALPORT SYNDROME

 ESSENTIALS OF DIAGNOSIS

▶ Microscopic hematuria.

▶ Abnormal tissue expression of type IV collagen α_3, α_4, and α_5 chains, or the presence of *COL4A3, COL4A4,* or *COL4A5* mutation(s).

▶ Characteristic thickening and lamellation of glomerular basement membranes (GBM).

▶ High-frequency sensorineural deafness.

▶ Anterior lenticonus or perimacular retinal flecks.

General Considerations

Alport syndrome is a progressive nephropathy caused by mutations in type IV collagen, the predominant collagenous constituent of basement membranes. These mutations result in critical defects in the structure and function of glomerular, cochlear, and ocular basement membranes.

Pathogenesis

The type IV collagen family consists of six proteins, designated α_1 (IV) – α_6 (IV), encoded by six distinct genes, *COL4A1–COL4A6*. These genes are organized in pairs on three chromosomes: *COL4A1–COL4A2*, chromosome 13; *COL4A3–COL4A4*, chromosome 2; and *COL4A5–COL4A6*, X chromosome. Within each pair the genes are oriented in a 5′–5′ fashion, separated by regulatory domains of varying length.

Type IV collagen α chains associate into trimers that in turn form supermolecular networks. Three trimers have been identified in mammalian basement membranes: $\alpha_1\alpha_1\alpha_2$, $\alpha_3\alpha_4\alpha_5$, and $\alpha_5\alpha_5\alpha_6$. The $\alpha_1\alpha_1\alpha_2$ trimer is found in all basement membranes, including glomerular mesangium, but it is a relatively minor component of mature GBM. The predominant type IV collagen species in GBM, and in the basement membrane of the organ of Corti and certain ocular basement membranes, is the $\alpha_3\alpha_4\alpha_5$ trimer. The $\alpha_3\alpha_4\alpha_5$ trimer is also present in Bowman's capsules (BC) and the basement membranes of distal (dTBM) and collecting (cTBM) tubules. The $\alpha_5\alpha_5\alpha_6$ trimer is expressed in BC, dTBM, and cTBM, but not in GBM. The $\alpha_5\alpha_5\alpha_6$ trimer is also highly expressed in epidermal basement membranes (EBM).

Alport syndrome arises from mutations in the *COL4A3, COL4A4,* and *COL4A5* genes. About 80% of individuals with Alport syndrome have the X-linked form of the disease (XLAS), due to mutations in *COL4A5*. Autosomal recessive Alport syndrome (ARAS) is caused by mutations in both alleles of *COL4A3* or *COL4A4*, and accounts for about 15% of people with the disease. Finally, about 5% of individuals with Alport syndrome have autosomal dominant disease (ADAS), resulting from a mutation in one allele of *COL4A3* or *COL4A4*. Heterozygous *COL4A3* or *COL4A4* mutations are an important cause of thin basement membrane nephropathy.

The usual result of COL4A5 mutations in males with XLAS is the complete disappearance of $\alpha_3\alpha_4\alpha_5$ and $\alpha_5\alpha_5\alpha_6$ trimers, and the supermolecular networks formed by these trimers, from all basement membranes. Heterozygous females with XLAS typically exhibit mosaic expression of these trimers in their basement membranes. In most patients with ARAS, $\alpha_3\alpha_4\alpha_5$ are absent from all basement membranes, but $\alpha_5\ \alpha_5\ \alpha_6$ trimers persist in BC, dTBM, cTBM, and EBM. These observations in human subjects have been confirmed in various animal models of XLAS and ARAS and have several implications that have received support from *in vitro* studies. First, the interactions among the six members of the type IV collagen family are specific and can produce only three trimers: $\alpha_1\alpha_1\alpha_2$, $\alpha_3\alpha_4\alpha_5$, and $\alpha_5\ \alpha_5\ \alpha_6$. Second, a mutation in a type IV collagen α chain disrupts the formation and deposition of all trimers in which that chain participates. Lastly, since disappearance of $\alpha_3(IV)$, $\alpha_4(IV)$, and $\alpha_5(IV)$ chains from basement membranes is specific for Alport syndrome, immunostaining for these chains in tissues is diagnostically useful.

▶ Clinical Findings

A. Symptoms and Signs

1. Renal—Hematuria is a constant feature of Alport syndrome, occurring in 100% of affected males and about 95% of affected females. It is often detectable in infancy, and episodic gross hematuria is common during childhood.

Overt proteinuria develops in all affected males, typically in late childhood or adolescence, and in many affected females. In affected females, proteinuria is a risk factor for the development of end-stage renal disease (ESRD).

2. Cochlear—Sensorineural hearing loss (SNHL) is detectable in 50% of males with XLAS by the age of 25 years and 90% by the age 40 of years, while the prevalence of SNHL in females is 10% before the age of 40 years and 20% by the age of 60 years. SNHL in Alport syndrome is never congenital, always bilateral, and invariably accompanied by renal symptoms.

In affected males SNHL is frequently detectable by audiometry in late childhood or early adolescence, and initially affects high-frequency tones (2000–8000 Hz). Over time the hearing deficit extends into conversational speech. Recent histologic studies of the Alport's cochlea suggest that SNHL may be due to a defective function of the basement membrane of the organ of Corti, leading to abnormal mechanical relationships between outer hair cells and the basilar membrane.

3. Ocular—Ocular defects occur in 15–30% of individuals with Alport syndrome. The pathognomonic ocular lesion of Alport syndrome is anterior lenticonus, in which the central region of the lens protrudes into the anterior chamber. Anterior lenticonus is associated with marked attenuation of the lens capsule, the basement membrane that surrounds the lens, and becomes apparent during adolescence and young adulthood. Other ocular changes associated with Alport syndrome include perimacular retinal flecks, corneal endothelial vesicles, and recurrent corneal erosions. These lesions may also arise from defective basement membranes: Bruch's membrane (perimacular flecks), Descemet's membrane (corneal endothelial vesicles), and corneal epithelial basement membrane (corneal erosions).

4. Leiomyomatosis—Coinheritance of XLAS and leiomyomatosis of the esophagus, tracheobronchial tree, and female external genitalia has been described in approximately 20 kindreds. In addition to symptoms of Alport syndrome, affected individuals may display dysphagia, postprandial vomiting, retrosternal or epigastric pain, recurrent bronchitis, dyspnea, cough, and stridor, typically beginning in late childhood.

B. Imaging Studies

Leiomyomatosis suspected by chest x-ray or barium swallow may be confirmed by computed tomography or magnetic resonance imaging.

▶ Differential Diagnosis

The cardinal symptom of Alport syndrome is persistent microscopic hematuria. In children the differential diagnosis of persistent microscopic hematuria includes Alport syndrome, TBMN, IgA nephropathy and other chronic forms of glomerulonephritis, and hypercalciuria. The clinical features of these conditions are compared in Table 47–1. The differential diagnosis in adults would include these conditions as well as urologic lesions, particularly in individuals over 40 years of age.

Kidney biopsy, supplemented by clinical and pedigree data, is still the key procedure for the differentiation of Alport syndrome from other glomerular causes of persistent microscopic hematuria. The presence on electron microscopy of diffuse thickening of the GBM with multilamellar splitting of the lamina densa is diagnostic of Alport syndrome. However, GBM thinning due to lamina densa attenuation is typical of both early Alport syndrome and TBMN, so that in some instances these conditions cannot be distinguished by routine renal biopsy evaluation.

Immunostaining for the α_3, α_4, and α_5 chains of type IV collagen is a very valuable tool for confirming a diagnosis of Alport syndrome and for distinguishing the X-linked and autosomal recessive forms of the disorder. These chains are entirely absent from renal basement membranes in about 80% of males with XLAS, while 60–70% of female heterozygotes with XLAS exhibit mosaic expression of these chains. In most patients with ARAS, the α_3 (IV) and

Table 47–1. Clinical features of common causes of persistent microscopic hematuria in childhood.

	Episodic gross hematuria	Family history often positive	Hearing deficit	Proteinuria	Hypertension	Hypercalciuria
Alport syndrome	Common	Hematuria, ESRD, Hearing loss	Common[1]	Common[1]	Common[1]	Rare
Thin basement membrane nephropathy	Common	Hematuria	Rare	Rare	Rare	Rare
IgA nephropathy	Common		Rare	Rare	Rare	Rare
Hypercalciuria	Rare	Urolithiasis	Rare	Rare	Rare	Always present

[1]After age 10 years in affected males.

α_4 (IV) chains are not expressed in renal basement membranes, while the α_5 (IV) chain is absent from the GBM but present in Bowman's capsule and distal and collecting TBM. The heterozygous mutations in *COL4A3* or *COL4A4* responsible for many cases of TBMN cause no discernible changes in the expression of $\alpha_3\alpha_4\alpha_5$ trimers in basement membranes.

XLAS can also be diagnosed by skin biopsy, since the α_5 (IV) chain is undetectable in EBMs of about 80% of XLAS males and is mosaically expressed in 60–70% of females with XLAS. In interpreting the results of type IV collagen immunostaining of skin and kidney it is important to remember that normal expression of the α_3(IV), α_4(IV), and α_5(IV) chains does not exclude a diagnosis of Alport syndrome. However, normal results of type IV collagen immunostaining can buttress a provisional diagnosis of TBMN in patients with attenuated GBM, normal hearing, and no family history of ESRD.

Complications

Common complications of Alport syndrome include hypertension, ESRD, and SNHL. Some patients with anterior lenticonus develop cataracts that require removal. Patients with XLAS and diffuse leiomyomatosis may need surgical treatment of esophageal and tracheobronchial smooth muscle tumors.

Treatment

To date there have been no controlled therapeutic trials in patients with Alport syndrome. In an uncontrolled study of a small number of males with XLAS, cyclosporine reduced proteinuria and appeared to stabilize renal function, but this observation has yet to be confirmed by other investigators. Studies of murine and canine models of Alport syndrome suggest that angiotensin blockade may retard progression to ESRD.

▶ Prognosis

Not surprisingly for an X-linked disorder, gender has a marked impact on the prognosis of XLAS. Fifty percent of males with XLAS reach ESRD by the age of 25 years, and close to 100% of XLAS males have reached ESRD by the age of 40 years. The nature of the underlying mutation in the *COL4A5* is an important determinant of the rate of progression to ESRD in XLAS males. While only about 12% of females with XLAS develop ESRD before the age of 40 years, the probability of ESRD increases to about 30% by the age of 60 years and 40% by the age of 80 years. Risk factors for ESRD in XLAS females include a history of gross hematuria, sensorineural deafness, proteinuria, and extensive GBM thickening and lamellation.

Patients with ARAS typically reach ESRD before the age of 40 years, regardless of gender. ADAS tends to advance less aggressively than XLAS or ARAS, with 50% of affected men reaching ESRD by the age of 50 years, compared to 25 years of age for males with XLAS.

Kashtan CE: Familial hematuria due to type IV collagen mutations: Alport syndrome and thin basement membrane nephropathy. Curr Opin Pediatr 2004;16:177. [PMID: 15021198]

Merchant SN et al: Temporal bone histopathology in Alport syndrome. Laryngoscope 2004;114:1609. [PMID: 15475791]

Rheault MN et al: Mouse model of X-linked Alport syndrome. J Am Soc Nephrol 2004;15:1466. [PMID: 15153557]

WEB SITES

A detailed review of the molecular pathogenesis and clinical features of Alport syndrome can be found on the GeneReviews website at http://www.genereviews.org/.

THIN BASEMENT MEMBRANE NEPHROPATHY

ESSENTIALS OF DIAGNOSIS

▶ Microscopic hematuria.

▶ Diffuse attenuation of GBM.

▶ Normal tissue expression of type IV collagen α_3, α_4, and α_5 chains.

▶ Absence of family history of renal failure.

General Considerations

TBMN is, like Alport syndrome, a heritable form of glomerular hematuria associated with genetic defects in type IV collagen. It is estimated that 40% of cases of TBMN arise from heterozygous mutations in *COL4A3* and *COL4A4*, the genes that code for the α_3 and α_4 chains of type IV collagen, respectively. The absence of genetic linkage to *COL4A3* or *COL4A4* in some TBMN families suggests the existence of additional TBMN loci.

Although TBMN and Alport syndrome may have similar clinical presentations and pathologic manifestations, especially in childhood, the two disorders differ in several key respects. Unlike those with Alport syndrome, individuals with TBMN rarely exhibit deafness, ocular abnormalities, proteinuria, hypertension, or renal insufficiency, and the family history is typically negative for relatives with kidney failure.

Pathogenesis

Heterozygous mutations in the *COL4A3* and *COL4A4* genes are associated with at least three possible phenotypes: no symptoms, isolated microscopic hematuria with thin GBM, and hematuria progressing to renal failure and typical histologic features of Alport syndrome (autosomal dominant Alport syndrome). To date it has not been possible to correlate a particular phenotype with the type and/or location of the heterozygous defect in the *COL4A3* or *COL4A4* gene. Most of the mutations identified thus far are single nucleotide substitutions, although frame-shifting and splicing mutations have also been described.

It is tempting to speculate that heterozygous mutations in *COL4A3* or *COL4A4* result in haploinsufficiency of the relevant type IV collagen chain [α_3(IV) or α_4(IV)] and diminished expression of the $\alpha_3\alpha_4\alpha_5$ type IV collagen network in GBM, leading to an attenuated, mechanically fragile GBM. Hematuria in these patients would arise from focal, transient ruptures in the weakened GBM. The presence of some quantity of the $\alpha_3\alpha_4\alpha_5$ network in the renal basement membranes of TBMN patients may prevent the secondary processes that lead to renal fibrosis in Alport's patients, whose renal basement membranes typically lack expression of the $\alpha_3\alpha_4\alpha_5$ network.

Clinical Findings

The typical patient with TBMN has isolated microscopic hematuria, which may be persistent or intermittent. Acute infections may be associated with transient gross hematuria.

Family history is frequently positive for hematuria but negative for renal failure, and pedigree analysis often indicates that the hematuria is transmitted as an autosomal dominant trait. When a patient with isolated microscopic hematuria has such a family history, the clinician can make a presumptive diagnosis of TBMN without requiring confirmation of GBM attenuation by renal biopsy.

Proteinuria and hypertension are rarely observed in patients with TBMN, but have been described in association with glomerulosclerosis. Some patients with presumed TBMN who develop proteinuria and/or hypertension have been misdiagnosed and actually have Alport syndrome or a chronic glomerulonephritis. Patients with microscopic hematuria who have proteinuria, hypertension, or a family history of renal failure are candidates for histologic diagnosis.

Differential Diagnosis

The differential diagnosis of microscopic hematuria includes Alport syndrome, TBMN, immunoglobulin A (IgA) nephropathy and other chronic forms of glomerulonephritis, hypercalciuria, and, in adults, urologic abnormalities. A diagnostic approach is described in the section on Alport syndrome.

Complications

TBMN is typically a benign condition. Individuals with hematuria due to TBMN have on occasion encountered problems obtaining health or life insurance.

Treatment

Most people with TBMN do not require any form of therapeutic intervention. Treatment, preferably with an agent that targets the renin–angiotensin axis, is indicated in the TBMN patient with proteinuria and/or hypertension.

Prognosis

Individuals with TBMN have an excellent prognosis. Because some people who carry a diagnosis of TBMN eventually develop proteinuria and/or hypertension, intermittent monitoring of urinalysis and blood pressure is recommended.

Hall CL et al: Clinical value of renal biopsy in patients with asymptomatic microscopic hematuria with and without low-grade proteinuria. Clin Nephrol 2004;62:267. [PMID: 15524056]

van Paassen P et al: Signs and symptoms of thin basement membrane nephropathy: a prospective regional study on primary glomerular disease—The Limburg Renal Registry. Kidney Int 2004;66:909.

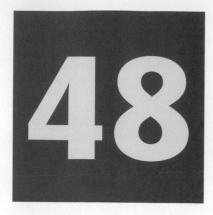

Fabry Disease

Robert J. Desnick, PhD, MD

ESSENTIALS OF DIAGNOSIS

► X-linked recessive lysosomal storage disease.

► Males.

–Deficient plasma and/or leukocyte α-galactosidase A (in classic phenotype <1% of normal mean activity; in later-onset variants >1% of normal mean activity).

–Certain α-galactosidase A gene mutations provide genotype/phenotype correlations.

–Accumulation of globotriaosylceramide (GL-3).

–Presence of angiokeratomas, acroparesthesias, hypohidrosis, corneal and lenticular changes, renal failure, cardiac disease, and cerbrovascular disease.

► Females.

–Due to random X-chromosome inactivation, commonly females may have plasma and leukocyte α-galactosidase A activity varying from severely deficient to normal.

–α-Galactosidase A mutation analysis required for definitive diagnosis.

–Females vary in clinical symptoms from asymptomatic to as severe as classically affected males. Symptoms may appear at later ages than in affected males.

► General Considerations

Fabry disease is an X-linked inborn error of glycosphingolipid catabolism caused by the deficient activity of the lysosomal enzyme, α-galactosidase A (α-Gal A). This enzymatic defect results in the progressive accumulation of GL-3 and related glycosphingolipids with terminal α-galactosyl moieties in the lysosomes of endothelial, epithelial, perithelial, and smooth muscle cells throughout the body. In classically affected males who have little, if any, α-Gal A activity, the glycosphingolipid deposition in the vascular endothelium is responsible for the major clinical manifestations of the disease, including angiokeratomas, acroparesthesias, and hypohidrosis. With advancing age, the progressive vascular glycosphingolipid accumulation leads to renal failure, cardiac and cerebrovascular disease, and early death. Based on the United States and European dialysis and transplantation registries, most classically affected males go into renal failure between the ages of 35 and 45 years. Prior to the advent of renal transplantation and dialysis, the average age of death for classically affected males in one series was 41 years. The incidence of classical Fabry disease is estimated to be ~1 in 40,000–60,000 males.

In addition to the classic Fabry disease phenotype, later-onset variants have been identified that do not include the classic manifestations of Fabry disease, the acroparesthesias, angiokeratoma, hypohidrosis, or corneal and lenticular lesions (Table 48–1). Cardiac variants who present in the fifth to eighth decades of life have left ventricular hypertrophy, mitral insufficiency and/or cardiomyopathy, and mild to moderate proteinuria with normal renal function for age. Residual α-Gal A activity and primarily cardiomyocyte glycosphingolipid deposition are present. Renal variants also lack the classic manifestations of Fabry disease but renal insufficiency develops. Screening of patients with end-stage renal disease (ESRD) of unknown causes has identified mutation-positive patients with Fabry disease. The incidence of the later-onset phenotypes has been estimated at 1 in 4000 males.

Because of random X-chromosome inactivation, heterozygous females may have clinical symptoms of Fabry disease that range from asymptomatic to as severe as in affected males. Heterozygous females are generally less severely affected than males and their symptoms may occur later in life than in affected males.

Enzyme replacement therapy for Fabry disease has recently become available and has been shown to be effective (see Treatment section).

Affected males with the classic and later-onset phenotypes can be reliably diagnosed by the demonstration of

Table 48–1. Fabry disease: major manifestations in classical and variant patients.

Manifestation	Classical Type	"Renal Variant"	"Cardiac Variant"
Age at onset	4–8 years	>25 years	>40 years
Average age at death	41 years	?	>60 years
Angiokeratoma	+ +	–	–
Acroparathesias	+ +	–	–
Hypohidrosis/anhidrosis	+ +	–	–
Corneal/lenticular opacities	+	–	–
Heart	Ischemia/LVH	LVH	LVH/myopathy
Brain	TIA/strokes	?	
Kidney	Renal failure	Renal failure	± Proteinuria
Residual α-Gal A activity	<1%	>1%	>1%

LVH, left ventricular hypertrophy; TIA, transient ischemic attack; +, present; –, absent.

deficient α-Gal A activity in plasma, isolated leukocytes, and/or cultured cells. Classically affected males have essentially no α-Gal A activity, while later-onset cardiac and renal variants exhibit residual activity (>1% of normal). Identification of a mutation in the patient's α-Gal A gene confirms the diagnosis of Fabry disease.

Heterozygous females have markedly variable α-Gal A activities because of random X-chromosomal inactivation and, therefore, measurement of plasma and/or leukocyte α-Gal A activity may be misleading. For example, some obligate heterozygotes (daughters of affected males) may have α-Gal A levels ranging from normal to very low activities similar to those of affected males. Many females (~90%) have the characteristic corneal dystrophy of Fabry disease. Accurate diagnosis of heterozygous females requires demonstration of the specific mutation in the α-Gal A gene. Such testing is recommended for all at-risk females.

▶ Pathogenesis

The pathogenesis of Fabry disease is directly related to the progressive accumulation of GL-3 and related glycosphingolipids in tissue lysosomes and body fluids. GL-3 is synthesized primarily in the liver and secreted into the plasma associated with low-density lipoprotein (LDL) particles. GL-3 is taken up by endothelial and other cells by the LDL receptor-mediated pathway. A significant amount of GL-3 is deposited in the lysosomes of the vascular endothelium and other cell types. In the kidney, the earliest lesions are due to the accumulation of glycosphingolipids in endothelial and epithelial cells of the glomerulus and of Bowman's space and in the epithelium of the loops of Henle and of distal tubules.

In later stages, and to a lesser extent, proximal tubules, interstitial histiocytes, and fibrocytes accumulate the glycosphingolipid. Lipid-laden distal tubular epithelial cells desquamate and may be detected in the urinary sediment. These cells have been shown to account for about 75% of the urinary cells shed by a classically affected hemizygote.

Concurrently, renal blood vessels are involved progressively and often extensively. An early finding is arterial fibrinoid deposits, which may result from the necrosis of severely involved muscular cells. Other histologic changes in the kidney are the sequelae of nonspecific ESRD with evidence of severe arteriolar sclerosis, glomerular atrophy and fibrosis, pseudotubular proliferation of residual glomerular epithelium, tubular atrophy, and diffuse interstitial fibrosis. Kidney size increases during the third decade of life, followed by a decrease in the fourth and fifth decades.

Histologic and ultrastructural studies of kidney tissue from a 75-year-old male with the later-onset cardiac variant of Fabry disease showed that lysosomal glycosphingolipid deposition was extensive in podocytes, rare in tubular epithelial cells, and absent in mesangial, interstitial, and vascular endothelial and smooth muscle cells.

▶ Clinical Findings

A. Symptoms and Signs

In classically affected males, Fabry disease typically begins in childhood with episodes of pain and discomfort in the hands and feet (acroparesthesias). The painful episodes may be brought on by exercise, fever, fatigue, stress, or change in weather conditions. In addition, young patients develop a dark red macular papular skin rash, called angiokeratoma, seen most densely from the umbilicus to the knees, a decreased ability to perspire, and characteristic corneal and lenticular changes observed on slitlamp microscopy that do not affect vision. Patients may have gastrointestinal problems including abdominal postprandial pain, diarrhea, vomiting, and nausea. Patients also experience heat or cold intolerance and exercise intolerance. Mild proteinuria, isothenuria, and urinary sediment abnormalities are early evidence of renal involvement.

The disease progresses very slowly and symptoms of kidney, heart, and/or neurologic involvement often do not occur until the ages of 30–45 years. In fact, many patients are first diagnosed when the accumulated storage material begins to affect kidney or heart function. Renal dysfunction leading to uremia with or without hypertension and progressing to ESRD may occur. Cardiovascular dysfunction may include myocardial infarction, cardiac hypertrophy, valvular abnormalities, and arrhythmias while cerebrovascular complications include risk of early stroke, hemiplegia, hemianesthesia, and transient ischemic attacks. Particularly in smokers, there may be pulmonary complications like airflow obstruction and dyspnea.

Patients die from complications of renal disease, cardiac involvement, and/or cerebrovascular disease. Some or all of the symptoms of Fabry disease may occur in heterozygous females but at a later age than in affected males.

B. Laboratory Findings

1. Biochemical testing

A. MALES—The most efficient and reliable method for the diagnosis of affected males is the determination of α-Gal A activity in plasma and/or isolated leukocytes. The test is a fluorometric assay and uses the substrate 4-methylumbeliferyl-β-D-galactopyranoside. Affected males with classic Fabry disease will have essentially no α-Gal A activity while those with later-onset cardiac and renal variants have some residual activity ($>$1% of mean normal).

B. HETEROZYGOUS FEMALES—Measurement of plasma and/or leukocyte α-Gal A activity is unreliable for heterozygote detection because of random X-chromosomal inactivation. Some heterozygous females may have normal α-Gal A enzyme levels while other heterozygous females may have very low to intermediate levels of enzymatic activity. α-Gal A mutation analysis is required for the definitive diagnosis of heterozygous females.

2. Molecular genetic testing—Mutation analysis by DNA sequencing of the α-Gal A gene is the most definitive way to confirm the diagnosis of Fabry disease in males and is required for females suspected of being heterozygotes. A mutation in the α-Gal A gene has been identified in $>$99% of affected males with decreased α-Gal A activity. To date, over 450 α-Gal A mutations have been described; most

mutations identified have been private, occurring only in single pedigrees.

3. Special tests—Males suspected of having Fabry disease and women suspected of being heterozygotes should have a slitlamp examination by a qualified ophthalmologist to detect the characteristic corneal and lenticular changes present in Fabry disease. The corneal opacities are found in classically affected males and most heterozygous females ($\sim$ 90%), and are typically absent in later-onset variants.

▶ Differential Diagnosis

The pain symptoms in Fabry disease are similar to those of other disorders, including rheumatoid arthritis, juvenile arthritis, rheumatic fever, erythromelalgia, lupus, "growing pains," petechiae, Raynaud's syndrome, fibromyalgia, and multiple sclerosis.

Differential diagnosis of the cutaneous lesions must exclude the angiokeratoma of Fordyce, angiokeratoma of Mibelli, and angiokeratoma circumscriptum, none of which has the typical histologic or ultrastructural pathology of the Fabry lesion. The angiokeratoma of Fordyce is similar in appearance to that of Fabry disease, but is limited to the scrotum, and usually appears after age 30 years. The angiokeratoma of Mibelli includes warty lesions on the extensor surfaces of extremities in young adults and is associated with chilblains. Angiokeratoma circumscriptum or naeviformus can occur anywhere on the body, is clinically and histologically similar to that of Fordyce, and is not associated with chilblains.

Angiokeratoma, reportedly similar to or indistinguishable from the clinical appearance and distribution of the cutaneous lesions in Fabry disease, has been described in patients with other lysosomal storage diseases, including fucosidosis, sialidosis (α-neuraminidase deficiency with or without β-galactosidase deficiency), adult-type β-galactosidase deficiency, aspartylglucosaminuria, adult-onset α-galactosidase B deficiency, β-mannosidase deficiency, and a recently reported lysosomal disorder that presents with mental retardation and some features of the mucopolysaccharidoses.

▶ Treatment

The first level of treatment for Fabry patients is preventive. The episodes of pain generally have precipitating causes such as stress, exposure to the sun or heat, changes in temperature, physical exertion, or fever and illness. Patients should make every effort to avoid these precipitating factors, if possible. Patients with frequent severe pain may benefit from medications such as diphenylhydantoin (Dilantin), carbamazapine (Tegretol), or gabapentin (Neurontin). These medications must be taken every day to prevent the onset of pain and to reduce the frequency and severity of painful attacks. Other preventive measures include avoidance of smoking and in those patients with mitral valve prolapse, taking prophylactic antibiotics when undergoing dental procedures or surgery. Regular visits to a physician who will monitor general health and, in particular, urinary albuminuria and protein is a vital part of preventive therapy. For kidney health, a low sodium low protein diet and presymptomatic treatment with angiotensin receptor blockers (ARBs) or angiotensin-converting enzyme (ACE) inhibitors should be considered. For those patients with severely compromised kidney function, dialysis and kidney transplantation are available. The success of kidney transplantation offers the ability to restore kidney function in Fabry patients and has improved the overall prognosis for this disease. The disease does not reoccur in the kidney.

Recently, enzyme replacement therapy for Fabry disease has become available in many countries. There are two preparations of recombinant human α-Gal A: Fabrazyme, manufactured by Genzyme Corporation, and Replagal, manufactured by TKT Inc; only Fabrazyme is approved by the Food and Drug Administration for use in the United States. Extensive preclinical, Phase 1/2, 3, and 4 clinical trials of Fabrazyme demonstrated that recombinant human α-Gal A is well tolerated and safe and demonstrated that the patients treated with Fabrazyme (1 mg/kg every 2 weeks) maintained GL-3 clearance from the vascular endothelium in the kidney, heart, and skin, the key sites of pathology in this disease. In addition, histologic examination of other renal, cardiac, and skin cell types revealed complete or partial clearance of accumulated GL-3. Plasma GL-3 was also cleared by Fabrazyme.

Patients on enzyme replacement therapy also reported improved quality of life including decreased pain and gastrointestinal problems, and increased sweating, heat tolerance, and energy. A randomized double-blind placebo-controlled Phase 4 study involving 82 Fabry patients with mild to moderate renal disease (serum creatinine >1.2, but <3.0 mg/dL) demonstrated that the patients who received 1 mg/kg of Fabrazyme every 2 weeks were 61% less likely to experience a clinically significant renal, cardiovascular, or cerebrovascular event after an adjustment for baseline proteinuria between the treated and placebo groups. The most pronounced benefit of Fabrazyme was seen when therapy was started in patients with milder renal disease, emphasizing the importance of early treatment.

A consensus report of physicians expert in Fabry disease recommended that all males with Fabry disease (including those with ESRD) and heterozygous females with substantial disease manifestations should be treated by enzyme replacement therapy as early as possible. Dialysis and transplanted patients with Fabry disease suffer from the nonrenal cardiac and cerebrovascular complications of the disease and, therefore, should be treated with enzyme replacement therapy. Recent studies have shown that Fabrazyme can be administered during hemodialysis as the enzyme is not filtered.

Banikazemi M et al: Agalsidase-beta therapy for advanced Fabry disease: A randomized trial. Ann Intern Med 2007;146:77.

Desnick RJ et al: α-Galactosidase A deficiency: Fabry disease. In *The Metabolic and Molecular Bases of Inherited Disease*, ed 8. Scriver CR et al (editors). McGraw-Hill, 2001, 3733.

Desnick RJ: Enzyme replacement therapy for Fabry disease: lessons from two α-galactosidase A orphan products and one FDA approval. Expert Opin Biol Ther 2004;4:1167.

Desnick RJ et al: Fabry disease, an under-recognized multisystemic disorder: expert recommendations for diagnosis, management, and enzyme replacement therapy. Ann Intern Med 2003;138:338.

Eng C et al: Safety and efficacy of recombinant human alpha-galactosidase A replacement in Fabry's disease. N Eng J Med 2001;345:9.

Germain DP et al: Sustained, long-term renal stabilization after 54 months of agalsidase beta therapy in patients with Fabry disease. J Am Soc Nephrol 2007;18:1547.

Kosch M et al: Enzyme replacement therapy administered during hemodialysis in patients with Fabry disease. Kidney Int 2004;66:1279.

MacDermot KD et al: Anderson-Fabry disease: clinical manifestations and impact of disease in a cohort of 60 obligate carrier females. J Med Genet 2001;38:769.

Meehan SM et al: Fabry disease: renal involvement limited to podocyte pathology and proteinuria in a septuagenarian cardiac variant. Pathologic and therapeutic implications. Am J Kidney Dis 2004;43:164.

Nakao S et al: Fabry disease: detection of undiagnosed hemodialysis patients and identification of a "renal variant" phenotype. Kidney Int 2003;64:801.

Shabbeer J et al: Fabry disease: 45 novel mutations in the α-galactosidase A gene causing the classical phenotype. Mol Genet Metab 2002;76:23.

Spada M et al: High incidence of later-onset Fabry disease revealed by newborn screening. Am J Hum Genet 2006;79:31.

Thadhani R et al: Patients with Fabry disease on dialysis in the United States. Kidney Int 2002;61:249.

Wilcox WR et al: Long-term safety and efficacy of enzyme replacement therapy for Fabry disease. Am J Hum Genet 2004;75:65.

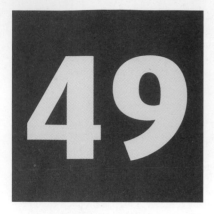

49

Sickle Cell Nephropathy

Jon I. Scheinman, MD

The major clinical consequences of sickle cell disease (SCD) are crises from vascular obstruction by sickled cells and anemia because of red blood cell (RBC) destruction. The obstruction can cause hematuria and renal papillary necrosis (RPN) with a defect in tubular function, especially in urinary concentration. The chronic consequences include sickle cell glomerulopathy, more indirectly related to sickling, and a specific form of renal malignancy.

▼ HEMATURIA & RENAL PAPILLARY NECROSIS

 ## ESSENTIALS OF DIAGNOSIS

▶ Acute gross hematuria or persistent microscopic hematuria.

▶ Without RBC casts or dysmorphic (other than sickle) RBCs.

▶ Ultrasound or helical computed tomography (CT) shows distinctive medullary abnormalities.

▶ General Considerations

Hematuria in SCD is a specialized form of the sickle crisis, the consequence of renal medullary sickling, vascular obstruction, and RBC extravasation. The low PaO_2, high osmolality, and acidic environment of the renal medulla lead to sickling.

▶ Pathogenesis

The renal pathology associated with isolated hematuria, shows relatively insignificant changes, primarily medullary congestion. The later RPN in SCD is a focal process, with some collecting ducts surviving within a diffuse area of fibrosis. The relevant medullary pathology in SCD is found in the region of the collecting ducts, the inner medulla, and the papilla. Within the medullary fibrosis the vasa rectae are destroyed, following initial dilation and engorgement. The RPN of SCD contrasts with the RPN observed in analgesic abuse, in which the vasa rectae typically are spared, and most lesions occur in peritubular capillaries. Because calyces are affected separately and sequentially in SCD, acute obstruction and renal failure are uncommon.

▶ Clinical Findings

A. Symptoms and Signs

Gross and often painless hematuria is dramatic and is usually unilateral (L>R) due to increased left renal vein pressure. Hematuria occurs at any age and is more often seen with a (higher gene frequency) sickle trait (HbAS).

RPN is usually discovered by radiologic investigation of patients with painless gross hematuria. However, hematuria is not invariably present in RPN, with no difference in the incidence between symptomatic (65%) and asymptomatic (62%) patients. RPN can be found even in young children.

Acute renal failure is not uncommon in SCD; it is seen most often with infections and evidence of rhabdomyolysis, and in patients with lower hemoglobin (Hb) (~6.4 versus 8.7 g/dL). Volume depletion is a common precipitating cause. It is likely that nonsteroidal anti-inflammatory agents are partly responsible for some episodes of acute renal failure, in view of the maintenance of the glomerular filtration rate (GFR) in SCD by prostaglandin mechanisms.

Rhabdomyolysis with acute renal failure and disseminated intravascular coagulation has been seen, albeit rarely, in those with sickle trait who undergo rigorous military training, and there is an apparently increased risk of sudden unexplained death in patients with sickle trait.

Priapism is a specialized vasoocclusion of the penis, which was found as often as 42% in one series. A painful, hot, tender erection, most often on waking, lasts up to 3 hours. This can be preceded by days or weeks of "stuttering."

B. Laboratory Findings

A drop in Hb is unusual in acute hematuria.

C. Imaging Studies

Increased echodensity of medullary pyramids on ultrasound is typical of SCD, and in the absence of hypercalciuria, medullary echodensity in a patient with hematuria should suggest a sickle hemoglobinopathy (Figure 49–1).

In one series, 39% of 189 patients had at least calyceal clubbing and 23% had definite RPN. Cortical scarring, as found in pyelonephritis, should not accompany the calyceal clubbing of SCD, but a history of infection appears more common in RPN in SCD. A "medullary" form of RPN is common, with an irregular medullary cavity, often with sinus tracts. Sonography can sometimes identify the early medullary form of papillary necrosis. Later, a distinctive "garland" shadowing pattern of calcification of the medullary pyramids can be present.

Unusually, pyelography has been done when SCD was not recognized. Helical CT can detect RPN earlier than sonography. Ultrasound reflectivity in young SCD patients (aged 10–20 years) has found diffuse or medullary echogenicity in a minority of patient, a finding that is not RPN.

▷ Differential Diagnosis

Sickle cell crises are painful episodes of vasoocclusion, often accompanied in the second or third day by fever without documented infection. The abdominal crisis is similar to a "surgical" abdomen but usually without rebound tenderness. In the presence of gross hematuria, the origin of the pain is often assumed to be the kidney, but careful palpation of the kidneys should be distinctive.

Continued or persistent gross hematuria likely represents a form of renal "sickle crisis" in a known HbSS or HbAS patient. Other treatable causes of hematuria, including the recently described distinctive renal medullary carcinoma in patients with sickle hemoglobin, must be excluded. Severe pain makes the diagnosis of renal sickle crisis less likely, whereas moderate discomfort often lateralizes the bleeding. Renal and bladder ultrasound can rule out bleeding from a stone or tumor and may aid in the diagnosis of RPN (see below).

▷ Treatment

1. In view of the benign pathology in SCD hematuria, conservative management is appropriate. Bed rest is often recommended to avoid dislodging hemostatic clots.

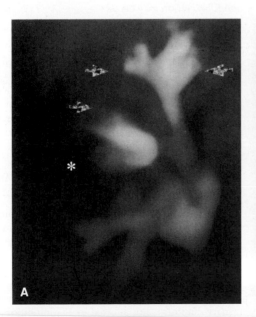 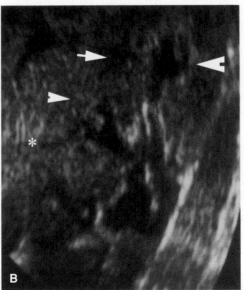

▲ **Figure 49–1.** ***A:*** Tomographic pyelography of an 18-year-old patient with abdominal pain and hematuria. Papillary necrosis is evident from blunted medullary cavities, especially the upper pole (closed arrows). The bases of the calyces are preserved. The middle pole calyx has a possible sinus tract (*). ***B:*** Ultrasonographic visualization of the same kidney. The middle pole exhibits deep extensions into the papilla, likely sinus tracts, typical of the "papillary" form of RPN. (Reproduced with permission from Scheinman JI: The kidney in sickle cell disease. In: *Primer on Kidney Diseases.* Greenberg A (editor). Academic Press, 1998.)

2. It is advisable to maintain high rates of urine flow by encouraging increased intake or infusion of hypotonic fluids(4 L/1.73 m^2 surface area per day) combined with administration of diuretics (a thiazide or a loop diuretic such as furosemide), which should help clear clots from the bladder. The resulting diuresis would reduce medullary osmolarity, which would help to alleviate sickling in the vasa rectae. Sodium-containing fluids may tend to increase sodium retention (see below).

3. Alkalinization of the urine by 8–12 g $NaHCO_3$ (per 1.73 m^2) per day may reduce sickling in a urine environment, but this may not be relevant to medullary sickling. The O_2 affinity of Hb is theoretically increased in a more alkaline environment.

4. After failure of treatment with fluid administration and alkalinization, ε-aminocaproic acid (EACA) can be tried to inhibit fibrinolysis, allowing clots to mediate hemostasis. The effective dosage in an adult is 8 g/day.

5. Arteriographic localization and local embolization of the involved renal segment may avoid nephrectomy, only rarely required for uncontrolled bleeding.

6. Newer surface-active polymers may abort sickle crises, and could possibly abort the acute hematuria of SCD.

7. General treatment strategies for SCD, by decreasing the proportion of rheologically abnormal cells, can reduce the risk of recurrence of cerebral vasculopathy and probably other complications. These include frequent transfusions and measures to increase fetal Hb including 5-azacitidine and hydroxyurea.

Ballas SK et al: Safety of purified poloxamer 188 in sickle cell disease: phase I study of a nonionic surfactant in the management of acute chest syndrome. Hemoglobin 2004;28:85.

Lang EK et al: Multiphasic helical CT diagnosis of early medullary and papillary necrosis. J Endourol 2004;18:49.

Rees DC et al: Guidelines for the management of the acute painful crisis in sickle cell disease. Br J Haematol 2003;120:744.

▼ TUBULAR DYSFUNCTION

ESSENTIALS OF DIAGNOSIS

▶ Concentrating defect—maximum 414 mOsm/kg after 8–10 hours of thirst, compared with 911 mOsm/kg in controls. This is reversible by transfusion in children. Urinary diluting capacity is normal.

▶ Incomplete *distal renal tubular acidosis* (RTA) (minimum urine pH 5.8 versus 5.1 in controls).

▶ Impaired K^+ secretion–an aldosterone resistance.

▶ Less creatinine (Cr) secretion.

▶ General Considerations

The tubular dysfunction of SCD manifests a defect in urine concentration, while dilution is maintained. Hydrogen ion and potassium secretion functions are only mildly affected, and proximal tubular mechanisms are exaggerated.

▶ Pathogenesis

Sickling and vascular congestion of the medulla, accompanying gross hematuria, with sluggish blood flow that fails to remove reabsorbed sodium, are probably responsible for reversible concentrating defects in younger children. Medullary fibrosis and permanent destruction of collecting ducts result in irreversible concentrating defects.

Generation of vasopressin is normal in SCD, and the concentrating defect is not responsive to vasopressin.

Since urinary dilution depends upon solute reabsorption in the cortical ascending loop of Henle, which is not involved in SCD patients, the urine diluting capacity is normal.

Since acid excretion depends upon a proton gradient most associated with the (nonaffected) cortical "intercalated" collecting duct cells, a severe acidification defect is unlikely. However, since juxtamedullary nephrons, which reabsorb HCO_3^-, are also severely involved in SCD, some defect in acid and K^+ excretion may occur.

A. Tubular Secretory Processes

Tubular secretory processes are spared in SCD, so there is a significant disparity between creatinine clearance (CCr) and inulin clearance (CIn), an expression of increased tubular secretion of Cr in SCD. The increased CCr normally produced by a Cr load is lost in SCD, showing loss of Cr secretory reserve. Uric acid secretion is increased and may be a functional adaptation to high uric acid generation.

B. Role of Prostaglandins in Sickle Cell Disease Tubular Dysfunction

Increased vasodilatory *prostaglandins* (PG) may help to explain SCD tubular dysfunction. PG inhibition by indomethacin usually decreases the fractional excretion of Na (FE_{Na}) minimally (by 16%). However, in SCD this decline in FE_{Na} is even more exaggerated (42%). PGs also appear to have a greater than normal effect on the delivery of sodium to the distal diluting segment. Whereas in normal conditions urinary dilution is not affected by PG inhibition, in SCD it decreases such urinary diluting capacity.

SCD patients fail to increase net acid excretion in response to indomethacin inhibition of PG synthesis because of decreased NH_4^+ excretion. It is likely that NH_4^+ excretion is normally maintained at maximum in SCD by endogenous PGs.

▶ Clinical Findings

A. Symptoms and Signs

The most common tubular abnormality in SCD is a *urinary concentrating defect*, which can even be measured in sickle trait. In children, the concentrating defect may be accompanied by enuresis and an increased risk of dehydration during water deprivation. The concentrating defect is unique to sickling hemoglobinopathies, as no concentrating defect have been described in other anemias. Urinary dilution remains normal.

B. Laboratory Findings

An incomplete distal RTA may complicate SCD, but is usually not a clinical problem. The minimum urine pH achieved in response to NH_4Cl loading is not as low as in controls (5.8 versus 5.1), but total NH_4 excretion is normal. Consequently, titratable acidity is reduced. With the tendency to decreased K^+ secretion, this resembles a type IV renal tubular acidosis, resulting from an aldosterone-independent end-organ failure secondary to medullary fibrosis.

While there is a shift of K^+ into cells that is protective against the large load of K^+ released from sickled cells, this shift is under β_2 stimulation, so that β-blockers or ACE inhibition may result in hyperkalemia.

Diuretic response is poor in SCD, because it depends on this increased distal sodium delivery. Proximal tubular phosphate reabsorption, which usually parallels sodium reabsorption, is also increased. This may also cause hyperphosphatemia, especially in the presence of an increased phosphate load generated by hemolysis.

▶ Treatment

Treatment of tubular disorders in SCD is usually unnecessary if renal function is normal. The risk of dehydration caused by decreased urinary concentrating ability requires earlier treatment of diarrhea or vomiting.

1. Avoid volume expansion as a treatment for sickle crises. Administration of large volumes of standard sodium-containing fluids to significantly anemic patients with increased sodium reabsorption may result in congestive heart failure.

2. The edema accompanying severe anemia may be difficult to treat because the response to diuretics is diminished.

3. K^+ may be elevated by hemolysis, especially if there is renal insufficiency. β-Blockers or angiotensin-converting enzyme (ACE) inhibition should be avoided as they may aggravate hyperkalemia.

Bayazit AK et al: Renal function in children with sickle cell anemia. Clin Nephrol 2002;57(2):127.

SICKLE CELL GLOMERULOPATHY & CHRONIC RENAL INSUFFICIENCY

ESSENTIALS OF DIAGNOSIS

▶ Proteinuria is the hallmark of chronic steroid-sensitive nephropathy (SSN). Of adults with SCD 15–40% are found to have abnormal proteinuria or nephrotic syndrome.

▶ Progression to kidney failure for nephrotic syndrome in SCD may be more rapid than in other causes of nephrotic syndrome.

▶ Hypertension is unusual in SCD (2–6%) compared to the published incidence for the black population in the United States of 28%, at all age ranges.

▶ General Considerations

Chronic renal failure (CRF) is a major organ failure in SCD, probably the consequence of the progression of focal segmental glomerulosclerosis (FSGS). Overall, 5–18% of SCD patients will develop CRF.

▶ Pathogenesis

Hyperfiltration is recognized in SCD by increased GFR, especially in children. An even greater increase in effective renal plasma flow (ERPF) (all plasma that goes through the filtering units) results in a lower than normal filtration fraction, the proportion of a substance flowing through the kidney that is filtered. Increased cortical blood flow itself could cause decreased tubular secretion by limiting diffusion from rapidly flowing plasma. Alternatively, a distinctive increased glomerular permeability (tested by dextrans) may exist in SCD nephropathy, not explained by purely hemodynamic changes. Proximal tubular "hyperfunction" in SCD may be a compensation for the distal tubular injury, mediated by the PG systems (see above). The net effect of PG inhibition is to reverse hyperfiltration. The dramatically increased ERPF and decreased filtration fraction of SCD are returned toward normal. If hyperfiltration is a necessary predecessor of glomerulopathy in SCD, then prostaglandins may explain the early development of FSGS.

Glomerulopathy in SCD has been attributed to immunopathogenic mechanisms, because of a reported membrano-proliferative glomerulonephritis (MPGN). However, most now agree that evidence of immune complex deposition is usually lacking in SCD patients with heavy proteinuria.

Possible mechanisms of the SCD nephropathy associated with FSGS include hyperfiltration and glomerular hypertrophy. Hyperfiltration, combined with direct endothelial damage by occlusion with sickled cells, might lead to endothelial hyperplasia and ultimately fibrosis. Any hypothesis should take into account that glomerular hypertrophy is always present in SCD, probably related to the anemia itself, but proteinuria is not invariable in SCD and appears to be unrelated to the number and severity of SCD crises or the presence of hematuria or demonstrated RPN.

Systemic hypertension is notably absent in these patients. The presence of hyperfiltration, glomerular hypertrophy, and FSGS does not imply that these findings are sequential or causative. A common stimulus may be operative, such as the growth-promoting hormones and inflammatory cytokines, to which the glomerulus may be sensitive. It is possible that FSGS is the consequence rather than the cause of interstitial fibrosis, which might obstruct the efferent glomerular capillaries, raising intraglomerular pressure and resulting in progressive (reactive) sclerosis.

The iron deposited as hemosiderin in tubular cells has been suspected of playing a role in the chronic nephropathy of SCD, but the mechanism is not clear. Experimentally, saturated iron complexes can induce a nephrotic syndrome in rabbits.

▶ Prevention

The prevention of sickle cell nephropathy (SCN), or preventing its progression, may involve measures to prevent both sickle crises and hyperfiltration (see below).

▶ Clinical Findings

A. Symptoms and Signs

The association of significant *proteinuria* with SCD was often recognized sporadically and usually described as a nephritic process.

The definition of SCN that is most accepted now is associated with nephrotic-range proteinuria. While long-term studies have not been done, it appears to have a more rapid course than other causes of nephrotic syndrome. Two-thirds of patients developed renal failure within 2 years. The onset of renal failure was heralded by increasingly inadequate erythropoiesis, and carried a survival time of 4 years.

B. Laboratory Findings

Hyperfiltration complicates the estimation of GFR, whose upper limits of the normal range are not certain even with the "gold standard" of inulin clearance. The reliability of the clearance methods that can substitute for inulin clearance have certainly not been validated in the elevated range. For most clinical purposes, an accurate measure of GFR is unnecessary. A decrease in GFR, particularly when accompanied by proteinuria, is ominous.

C. Imaging Studies

For clinical purposes, renal ultrasound should be adequate to estimate kidney size and to exclude the likelihood of renal medullary carcinoma (see Figure 49–1).

D. Special Tests

The usual glomerular finding in sickle cell nephropathy is FSGS, which is intimately associated with glomerular hypertrophy. Immunofluorescence is positive only for IgM, C3, and C1q irregularly in sclerotic segments. Electron microscopy confirms the absence of immune complex-type dense deposits. There was focal electron-lucent expansion of the subendothelial zone with occasional mesangial cell interposition. No new mesangial matrix material is observed to suggest MPGN.

▶ Differential Diagnosis

Proteinuria detected by dipstick in a patient with SCD should be quantified and renal function assessed. Diseases other than sickle cell glomerulopathy should be considered. If hematuria is present, RBC casts may point to pathology other than sickle cell glomerulopathy. Hypertension, hypocomplementemia, and antinuclear antibodies also suggest other diagnoses. Judging from the relatively uniform findings in our series, few other additional studies are indicated. Microalbuminuria has been found in SCD patients >9 years of age, and may predict those with future glomerulopathy.

▶ Treatment

- Slowing the progression of SCN to chronic renal insufficiency (CRI) in SCD involves modifications in physiology, which also affect growth factors.
- Efforts to reduce sickling crises are of unknown value.
- Renal transplantation for end-stage kidney failure can dramatically improve patient survival compared to dialysis.

The patients with proteinuria in our series were not those with either the most frequent sickle crises or the severest anemia. Nevertheless, some factors in the sickle cell condition must predispose to the nephropathy. Therefore, it is reasonable to attempt to minimize sickling and those factors known to promote FSGS in other primary diseases or in animal models, but it is unknown whether hemodynamic alterations can alter the progression of FSGS to CRI.

A. Protein Restriction

Because high protein intake accelerates the development of FSGS in uninephrectomized rats, without necessarily causing glomerular hyperperfusion, it is attractive to consider protein restriction in the management of SCD nephropathy, as is being tried in several forms of renal disease. In children, restriction of protein intake may carry unreasonable risks. Delayed growth and development are already particular risks in the patient with SCD. Therefore, we advise only the avoidance of an unusually high protein intake that is greater than the recommended dietary allowance.

B. Angiotensin-Converting Enzyme Inhibition

Glomerular hyperperfusion and proteinuria could be mediated through increased glomerular capillary pressure, reduction of which by ACE inhibition might protect the glomerulus from FSGS.

In our 2-week trial of enalapril therapy in 10 patients with mild SCD nephropathy, blood pressure, GFR (CIn), and ERPF (p-aminohippuric acid clearance) did not change significantly, whereas proteinuria diminished by 57%, rebounding after treatment withdrawal. A more recent 6-month controlled trial of enalapril in 22 SCD patients with microalbuminuria showed a significant decrease in the treatment group, while the control group increased. Whether long-term ACE inhibitor therapy has a salutary effect in preventing renal insufficiency is untested.

C. Other Treatments

Specific treatment of the patient with SCD and renal failure has been poorly explored, and the problems of CRI are only magnified by SCD. Patients with renal failure, even mild, can have symptomatic anemia requiring transfusion. In some patients, treatment with erythropoietin can variably restore hemoglobin concentrations to higher levels. A few patients have been treated with hydroxyurea plus erythropoietin with apparent benefit.

D. Dialysis and Transplantation

Renal transplantation is a better option than long-term dialysis for the SCD patient with CRI.

In our review of the U.S. Renal Data System files for 2000, we found 1656 SCD patients, 237 transplanted and 1419 not transplanted, who did not have causes of CRI other than likely SCN. While in the transplanted SCD patient survival was worse than that of all African-American patients without SCD, the lifetable projected survival times were still quite close, with approximately 50% survival at 15 years. Using an age-adjusted cohort of African-American patients as controls, the difference statistically disappeared. Comparing the nontransplanted SCD patients with the cohort of African-American patients, survival was quite different, but both were extremely poor: 14% for SCD patients and 25% for African-American patients at 10 years. A comparison of the 153 transplanted SCD patients with those who received no transplant showed a far better survival curve, 56% versus 14% at 10 years.

These results indicate that transplantation is a better option for the SCD patient with renal failure. However, results may be less satisfactory than for other African-American patients, and grafts have been lost due to demonstrable massive sickling events.

Bone marrow transplantation can cure SCD, and the possibility of its coupling with other transplants will undoubtedly be explored. Caution will be needed, in view of the possible increase in parvovirus, a common agent of aplastic crisis that might be especially dangerous in the transplant patient.

Animal experiments have shown the promise of genetic transduction of an antisickling hemoglobin to cure sickling in mice.

Datta V et al: Microalbuminuria as a predictor of early glomerular injury in children with sickle cell disease. Indian J Pediatr 2003;70:307.

Papassotiriou I et al: Increased erythropoietin level induced by hydroxyurea treatment of sickle cell patients. Hematol J 2000;1:295.

▼ RENAL MALIGNANCY

ESSENTIALS OF DIAGNOSIS

▶ Presents with gross hematuria and abdominal flank pain, less commonly with weight loss and a palpable mass.

▶ Its possibility requires that hematuria be investigated with some imaging modality, at least ultrasound.

▶ With survival of only 15 weeks from the time of surgery, and little evidence of response to different immunotherapies and chemotherapies, early diagnosis is the best therapeutic option.

▶ General Considerations

A distinctive renal medullary cell carcinoma in some patients with SCD is exceptionally aggressive. Its development is probably related to the other renal medullary pathology of SCD, RPN, and medullary fibrosis.

Saxena AK et al: Should early renal transplantation be deemed necessary among patients with end-stage sickle cell nephropathy who are receiving hemodialytic therapy? Transplantation 2004;77:955.

Scheinman JI: Sickle cell disease and the kidney. Semin Nephrol 2003;23:66.

Hemodialysis

Michael V. Rocco, MD, MSCE, &
Shahriar Moossavi, MD, PhD

▶ General Considerations

The major forces responsible for solute transport across the membrane are diffusion and convection. Diffusion is influenced by the concentration gradient of the solute, the solute characteristics (eg, molecular weight and charge), and the membrane characteristics (eg, pore size and number). Removal of solutes by diffusion is enhanced by a large concentration gradient, small solute size, and a membrane with a large surface area and many large pores. The concentration gradient is maximized by using countercurrent flow of blood and dialysate.

In convection, hydrostatic or osmotic pressure forces water across the membrane. The water transport facilitates the passage of solutes across the membrane. The term ultrafiltration describes the solute and fluid removal via convection.

In hemodialysis, the predominant mechanism for solute removal is through diffusion, with a smaller amount of solute clearance occurring by convection. Thus, hemodialysis is very effective in removing solutes of small-molecular-weight, but is relatively inefficient in removing solutes of larger sizes. In addition, hemodialysis is an inefficient means of removal of protein-bound substances. Only the free portion of these solutes can diffuse across the membrane and be removed. The removal rate of protein-bound compounds thus depends on the concentration of the unbound solute, the size of the protein, and the replacement rate of the unbound solute.

In hemofiltration, the predominant mechanism for solute removal is through convection; thus, this procedure has the ability to remove solutes of larger molecular size when coupled with a dialysis membrane with a large pore size.

▶ Treatment

A. Indications for Starting Chronic Dialysis Therapy

Patients should be considered for initiation of chronic hemodialysis therapy once the estimated glomerular filtration rate (GFR) is less than 15 mL/minute. In most patients, the four variables in the Modification of Diet in Renal Disease (MDRD) equation can be used to estimate the GFR. A 24-hour urine collection for creatinine and urea should be considered in those patients who have reduced muscle mass due to medical conditions such as amputations or limitation on mobility due to congestive heart failure, claudication, chronic lung disease requiring oxygen therapy, etc. There are no randomized trials that suggest an optimal time to initiate chronic dialysis therapy, so clinical judgment is important in making this decision in individual patients.

1. Earlier initiation of dialysis—There are specific indications for starting chronic hemodialysis therapy at a level above a GFR of 15 mL/minute. These conditions include intractable fluid overload not responsive to diuretics, hyperkalemia unresponsive to medical therapy, metabolic acidosis not fully corrected by medical therapy, malnutrition or weight loss not ascribed to other medical conditions, or decreasing functional status. It may also be desirable to start home dialysis therapies at a higher level of GFR to minimize training difficulties due to neurologic dysfunction at lower levels of GFR.

2. Later initiation of dialysis—Patients can be considered for a later initiation of dialysis if they are asymptomatic from a uremic standpoint, have adequate nutritional status, and do not have a decline in either dry weight or serum albumin levels. If renal replacement therapy is delayed, then the patient should be reassessed on a regular basis for a change in these parameters.

B. Apparatus

The major parts of the dialysis machine are the blood pump, dialyzer, dialysate pump, safety monitors, and alarms (Figure 50–1).

1. Dialyzer—The artificial kidney or dialyzer consists of the blood compartment, the dialysate compartment, and the

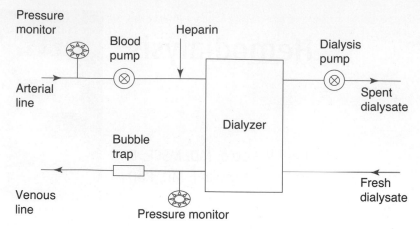

▲ **Figure 50–1.** Hemodialysis machine apparatus.

semipermeable membrane. The surface area of the dialyzer membrane can be increased by using either parallel plates or hollow fibers. Most dialyzers used in adults have a surface area between 1.5 and 2.1 m². Parallel plate dialyzers are rarely used today. Most dialysis membranes in use today are made from a variety of synthetic materials including polyamide, polymethylmethacrylate, acrylonitrile-sodium methallylsulfonate (AN-69), polyacrylonitrile, polycarbonate, and polysulfone. Cellulose membranes are being used with decreasing frequency in the United States.

The contact of blood with the membrane can result in activation of the complement system, with the release of bradykinin or cytokines. The biocompatibility of the dialysis membrane depends not only on the material used but also on the degree of blood contact with the dialysate. Unsubstituted cellulose membranes activate the complement system. To decrease complement activation, the hydroxyl groups of cellulose have been replaced with acetate or a synthetic material has been added to cellulose.

2. Membrane characteristics and solute clearance—A high efficiency membrane has the ability to remove small solutes well. The removal of small solutes is a function of the membrane surface area. High-efficiency membranes have a large surface area. The efficiency of a dialyzer is measured by the clearance of urea (MW 60) and is expressed as KoA_{urea}. Larger molecular-weight solutes are removed to a greater degree by membranes with larger membrane pores. These membranes are referred to as high-flux membranes. High-flux and many high-efficiency membranes also have the ability to achieve a high ultrafiltration rate. The water permeability of a membrane is specified by its ultrafiltration coefficient (K_{uf}).

The clearance of creatinine (MW 113) by a dialyzer is usually about 20% less than the dialyzer urea clearance, despite the minimal difference in molecular weight. The removal of

phosphorus (MW 31) by dialysis depends mostly on the time provided for dialysis per week, and also on the dialyzer efficiency and the predialysis phosphorus level. During dialysis, phosphorus is removed rapidly from plasma but not from the intracellular compartment. The slow equilibration between these compartments and bone is the major limiting factor of phosphorus removal.

Historically, middle molecule clearance was defined by the clearance of vitamin B_{12} (MW 1355). However, the clearance of vitamin B_{12} is low due to its high degree of protein binding. Thus, many high-flux dialyzers are now classified based on the clearance of molecules such as β_2-microglobulin (MW 11,800). With the introduction of high-flux dialyzers, the clearance of β_2-microglobulin has improved. Despite these improvements, the serum concentration of β_2-microglobulin remains markedly elevated in anuric hemodialysis patients using high-flux dialyzers. β_2-Microglobulin deposition is the cause of dialysis-associated amyloidosis.

3. Dialyzer reuse—Reuse of dialyzers is a common practice in outpatient dialysis units in the United States, but is less common in other countries. A method for the reuse process used in the United States has been written by the Association for the Advancement of Medical Instrumentation (AAMI). Each dialyzer should be labeled with the patient's identifying information. The total cell volume (TCV) should be measured prior to its first use. After the dialysis treatment, the membrane is rinsed with normal saline, pressure washed, and then cleansed with either bleach or a hydrogen peroxide mixture. Bleach can damage the membrane and increase protein loss with dialysis if it is used in inappropriately high concentrations. Once the membrane has been cleaned, its performance is evaluated by measuring the TCV. If the new value for TCV is >80% of the original TCV, it passes the performance test, and the membrane can be reused after disinfection and sterilization with a mixture of hydrogen peroxide, formaldehyde,

or glutaraldehyde. The polysulfone membranes can also be heat sterilized. The final step of the reuse process is the removal of the germicide. Residual germicide can cause a burning sensation, itching, or other allergic reactions. The reuse of dialyzers needs an informed consent. Patients with bacteremia or hepatitis B are excluded from dialyzer reuse. HIV and hepatitis C infection are not considered contraindications to reuse. In general, membrane biocompatibility improves with dialyzer reuse. Exposure of the membrane to blood can result in the protein coating of the membrane. This protein coating may decrease complement activation. Dialyzers can be reused dozens of times without a significant loss of efficacy. A decrease in the reuse number may suggest an increased rate of clotting of the hollow fibers and can often be improved by adjusting the anticoagulation prescription.

4. Dialysis machine—The blood pump moves the blood from the arterial line through the dialyzer back to the venous line. The speed of the blood pump can be adjusted to between 200 and 600 mL/minute. At any given time about 200–250 mL of blood is outside the patient. The dialysis pump sucks the dialysis fluid (dialysate) away from the dialyzer producing the transmembrane pressure. The transmembrane pressure can be adjusted to achieve the desired fluid removal. In modern dialysis machines, the transmembrane pressure is automatically adjusted by the dialysis machine based upon the amount of volume to be removed during the dialysis session and the type of ultrafiltration profiling chosen. The dialysate flow rate is usually between 500 and 800 mL/minute and is usually set between 100 and 200 mL/minute higher than the blood flow rate. The dialysate temperature can be adjusted. A lower temperature can cause peripheral vasoconstriction in the patient and thus improve hemodynamic stability.

The arterial and venous pressures are monitored during the dialysis treatment. The arterial pressure is measured before the blood pump to avoid excessive suction of blood and the venous pressure is measured before the blood returns to the access to avoid excessive resistance. A high venous pressure in the access is suggestive of an impairment to flow in the venous outflow tract that could be due to stenosis in the venous outflow of the access, clotting in the venous chamber of the catheter, stenosis in native vessels through which the access drains, or kinking of the blood lines. A high negative arterial pressure is indicative of immature access, stenosis or scarring in the accessed area, suctioning against the vessel wall, or the use of long or small gauge needles or catheters.

Other safety guards included on dialysis machines are the air trap to detect air embolism, the blood leak detector to detect blood in the dialysate compartment, and the measurement of dialysate conductivity to detect a malfunction in mixing the dialysis solution. If one of these safety guards is triggered, the machine will alarm and in some cases shut down. If a blood leak is detected, the dialyzer will be replaced and the patient will be administered antibiotics to treat any possible contamination of blood with the dialysis solution.

5. Dialysis solution—The major electrolyte components of the dialysis solution are sodium, potassium, calcium, magnesium, chloride, bicarbonate, and glucose (Table 50–1). In some dialysis machines, the sodium concentration can be changed during the same treatment (sodium modeling). The concentration of potassium and calcium can be varied to some extent based on the patient's blood chemistries. Calcium and magnesium can react with the bicarbonate in an alkaline environment and precipitate as carbonate salts. These components are stored separately and the final dialysis solution is prepared during the treatment by mixing a concentrated solution of these components with treated water.

6. Water treatment—Dialysis water is obtained by processing water from the municipal water supply (Figure 50–2). The water is processed using guidelines developed by the AAMI. With each dialysis treatment over 100 L of water is used to make the dialysis solution. Tap water is contaminated with organic and inorganic compounds, heavy metals and trace elements, bacteria, and endotoxins. In areas in which tap water is hard, a water softener can be used to facilitate calcium and magnesium removal. Organic contaminants such as chloroethylene, benzene, toluene, pesticides, herbicides, chloramine, chlorine, and other halogens are removed by a carbon filter. Chloramine is added by some municipal water agencies to help in the water cleaning process; this agent can cause hemolysis even at very low concentrations. Once the tap water is processed in these preliminary steps, the final processing for removal of contaminants occurs using either reverse osmosis (RO) or deionization. In RO, contaminants are removed by forcing water across a semipermeable membrane using high pressures. RO is very effective in removing bacteria, viruses, pyrogens, and heavy metals such as aluminum. Ultraviolet light can also damage and fragment bacteria. This bacterial debris, however, needs to be removed by the RO system. With deionization, the ionic contaminants are replaced by hydrogen or hydroxyl ions. In addition, various filters can be added to improve water quality. A 5-μm prefilter is used to remove large particles at the beginning of the water treatment system. Fine particles are removed

Table 50–1. Composition of dialysis solution.

Sodium	137 (135–148) mEq/L
Potassium	2.0 (0–3.0) mEq/L
Calcium	2.5 (0–3.5) mEq/L
Magnesium	0.75 mEq/L
Chloride	106 mEq/L
Bicarbonate	33 mEq/L
Acetate	4.0 mEq/L
Dextrose	200 mg/dL

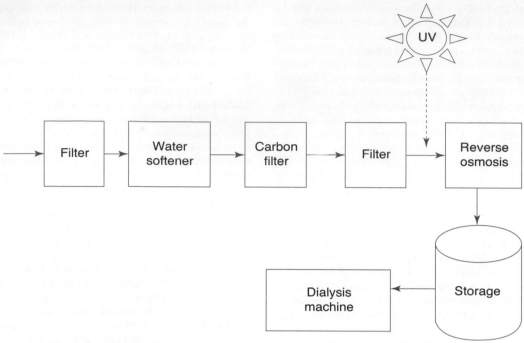

▲ **Figure 50–2.** Water treatment system.

by special filters prior to RO to protect the RO system. In addition, microfilters can be added to enhance the removal of microbial contaminants. Standard quality dialysis fluid is not free from bacteria and endotoxins.

Recently, a trend toward using ultrapure water, especially with use of high-flux dialyzers, has occurred. The term ultrapure water in dialysis refers to pyrogen-free water.

Cappelli G et al: Water treatment for hemodialysis: a 2005 update. Contrib Nephrol 2005;149:42.

Chelamcharla M et al: Dialyzer membranes as determinants of the adequacy of dialysis. Semin Nephrol 2005;25:81.

Huang Z et al: Determinants of small solute clearance in hemodialysis. Semin Dial 2005;18:30.

Ward RA: Ultrapure dialysate. Semin Dial 2004;17:489.

C. Access

In patients with a GFR less than 30 mL/minute, forearm and arm veins that are suitable for use for a permanent hemodialysis access should not be used for venipuncture, the placement of intravenous catheters, or the placement of subclavian catheters or peripherally inserted central catheter (PICC) lines. Discussions regarding the choice of dialysis modality should begin once the patient's estimated GFR is less than 30 mL/minute. Once the patient chooses hemodialysis as

the preferred dialysis modality, a permanent dialysis access should be placed in a timely manner to ensure that this access is functional at the time that the patient initiates chronic hemodialysis therapy. In general, an arteriovenous (AV) fistula should be placed at least 6 months prior to the anticipated start of chronic hemodialysis treatment. This will allow adequate time for any needed revisions to be corrected, eg, arterial stenosis or collateral veins, and still allow adequate time for AV fistula maturation. An AV graft should be placed at least 3–6 weeks prior to the anticipated start of hemodialysis. In addition to a history and physical examination, appropriate preoperative assessment of the patient should include an evaluation of the brachial and radial arteries and peripheral veins of the patient using Doppler ultrasound. In select cases, an evaluation of the central veins should be performed, especially if the patient has had prior internal jugular or subclavian lines.

1. Type of dialysis access

A. ARTERIOVENOUS FISTULAS—The AV fistula is the preferred type of chronic hemodialysis vascular access due to a higher primary and secondary patency rate compared to AV grafts. The preferred order of placement for an AV fistula is a wrist (radial-cephalic) primary AV fistula, any other forearm primary AV fistula, an elbow (brachial-cephalic) primary AV fistula, and a transposed brachial basilic vein fistula. This order of placement helps to maximize the number of fistulas that an individual patient can receive. The initial fistulas should be placed in the nondominant arm.

B. Arteriovenous grafts—An AV graft should be placed only if an AV fistula cannot be placed due to either small veins or marked obesity of the arm that will render cannulation of an AV fistula difficult due to the depth of the access below the skin.

C. Catheters and ports—Uncuffed catheters should be used only in hospitalized patients and only for less than 1 week. A permanent tunneled cuffed catheter or port should be placed as soon as clinically feasible. These tunneled catheters should be placed in the internal jugular vein on the side opposite to an existing or planned AV fistula or graft in order to reduce the risk of central vein stenosis on the side of the permanent access. The position of the tip of the catheter should be verified radiologically. Most uncuffed catheters should have the tip in the superior vena cava. Most cuffed tunneled catheters or ports should have the tip within the right atrium.

Catheters have a high rate of infection, and infection control measures are important to help reduce the rate of infectious complications. Catheters should be examined by trained personnel prior to each dialysis session to assess for possible infection. The catheter dressing should be changed at each dialysis session. The catheter should not be used for any purpose other than dialysis, except in emergencies when no other blood access is available. The use of an antibiotic lock solution may decrease the rate of catheter infections. Catheter lock solutions that can be used include cefazolin (5 mg/mL) with heparin (5000 units/mL) or edetate disodium (EDTA, 30 mg/mL).

2. Monitoring for access dysfunction—Surveillance for access dysfunction on a regular basis may help to improve access patency rates. All permanent accesses should be examined on a regular basis to detect possible stenoses. A high-pitched bruit or an area with a decreased thrill may be suggestive of an area of stenosis and should be evaluated by a fistulogram or other radiologic technique. There are also surveillance techniques that can be used to assess for access dysfunction. Persistent abnormalities in either the physical examination or in the surveillance techniques should result in referral of the patient for a fistulogram or other radiologic procedure.

A. Arteriovenous fistulas—Several techniques can be used to assess for access dysfunction in AV fistulas. In order of preference, these include direct flow measurements, recirculation using a non-urea-based method, and duplex Doppler analysis.

B. Arteriovenous grafts—Techniques that can be used to assess for access dysfunction in AV grafts, in order of

preference, include measurement of intraaccess flow, directly measured static venous pressures, or duplex ultrasound.

3. Correction of access complications

A. Arteriovenous fistulas—A patient should have an evaluation of an AV fistula in the presence of inadequate blood flow, hemodynamically significant venous stenosis, aneurysm formation, or ischemia in the access arm. A stenosis is considered to be hemodynamically significant if it is greater than 50% and is accompanied by abnormal physical findings, persistent abnormal surveillance tests, has had a previous thrombosis, or has resulted in an otherwise unexplained decrease in the measured dose of hemodialysis. Hemodynamically significant stenosis should be corrected by either surgical revision or percutaneous transluminal angioplasty. Thrombosis of an AV fistula should be performed as early as possible after the thrombus is detected in order to increase the chances of a successful declotting.

B. Arteriovenous grafts—A patient should have revision of an AV graft in the presence of either graft degeneration or pseudoaneurysm formation. If a graft has a 50% or greater stenosis in either the venous outflow tract or the arterial inflow tract, and the stenosis is accompanied by abnormal physical findings, decreased access flow, measured static pressure, or the presence of a past thrombosis, then the stenosis should be treated with either surgical revision or percutaneous transluminal angioplasty. Thrombosis of an AV graft should be done in an expeditious manner to increase the chances of a successful declotting. Thrombus can be treated by surgical thrombectomy, mechanical thrombolysis, or pharmacomechanical thrombolysis. An infected AV graft will need treatment with intravenous antibiotics and it will need to be resected if the infection is extensive.

C. Catheters and ports—A catheter or port is considered to be dysfunctional if it is unable to deliver a blood flow rate of at least 300 mL/minute with a prepump arterial pressure of −250 mm Hg. A dysfunctional catheter can be corrected with thrombolytics, endoluminal brush, or if the catheter is incorrectly positioned or of an inadequate length, by catheter replacement. Thrombolytics can be provided using an intraluminal lytic intradialytic lock, an intracatheter thrombolytic infusion, or an interdialytic lock.

The extent of the infection determines how an infected catheter or port should be treated. A catheter exit site infection, in the absence of a tunnel infection, is usually treated with topical antibiotics. All other catheter infections are treated with parenteral antibiotics. The antibiotics used should cover the suspected organisms, which are usually *Staphylococcus* or *Streptococcus*. Definitive antibiotic therapy should be chosen based on the organisms isolated by blood culture. The catheter should be removed if the patient does not have an improvement in clinical status in the first 36–48 hours after the initiation of parenteral antibiotic therapy or if the patient is clinically unstable. Catheter salvage can be attempted if the patient is clinical stable. Under these circumstances, the patient should be treated with parenteral antibiotics for 3 weeks and follow-up blood cultures should be obtained 1 week after the completion of a course of antibiotics. Port infections should be treated according to the manufacturer's recommendations.

Maya ID et al: Vascular access stenosis: comparison of arteriovenous grafts and fistulas. Am J Kidney Dis 2004;44:859.

D. Assessing the Adequacy of Hemodialysis

Providing a dose of dialysis above a certain minimal level can reduce patient mortality and morbidity. The delivered dose of dialysis should be measured monthly by obtaining a predialysis and postdialysis blood sample for blood urea nitrogen (BUN). It is critical that the post-BUN sample be obtained using a standardized method since recirculation can significantly alter the value of the postdialysis BUN. Both the stop flow or slow flow techniques are acceptable methods for obtaining the postdialysis BUN sample. These samples are then used to calculate the dose of dialysis, expressed as Kt/V, where K is the dialyzer clearance for urea, t is the number of minutes of the treatment, and V is the volume of distribution of urea in the body, approximately equal to total body water.

1. Minimum dose of hemodialysis—Results from multiple clinical trials and observational studies suggest that the minimum dose for three times per week hemodialysis is a Kt/V of at least 1.2. To achieve this delivered dose of dialysis, the prescribed Kt/V should be at least 1.3. For patients receiving hemodialysis on a schedule other than three times per week, the minimum standardized dose of dialysis should be an sKt/V of at least 2.0. This level of sKt/V is equivalent to a single pool Kt/V of 1.2 for patients receiving hemodialysis three times per week.

2. Preservation of residual renal function—Several studies in the peritoneal dialysis population suggest that residual kidney function is a more important predictor of outcome than peritoneal clearance. Although there are few data on this subject in hemodialysis patients, it is reasonable to assume that preservation of residual kidney function is also beneficial in these patients. Thus, efforts should be taken to preserve residual kidney function in chronic hemodialysis patients, including the avoidance of nephrotoxins, such as contrast dye, nonsteroidal anti-inflammatory drugs (NSAIDs), and aminoglycosides, and the use of an angiotensin-converting enzyme (ACE) inhibitor or angiotensin receptor blockers (when not contraindicated).

Daugirdas JT et al: Factors that affect postdialysis rebound in serum urea concentration, including the rate of dialysis: results from the HEMO Study. J Am Soc Nephrol 2004;15:194.

E. Alternative Hemodialysis Therapies

Alternative schedules for hemodialysis were first developed in the 1960s. Many of the hemodialysis treatments of that era were performed at home, including nocturnal hemodialysis. These home treatments became less popular after Medicare began to cover the costs of performing hemodialysis treatments in an outpatient setting in 1973. In the past 10 years, there has been a renewed interest in both performing hemodialysis at home and performing hemodialysis more than three times per week on a routine basis.

1. In-center hemodialysis six times per week—Most studies of patients receiving dialysis six times per week (either in-center or at home) have involved small numbers of patients and none includes randomized trials. In general, patients receiving in-center hemodialysis six times per week for less than 4 hours per session report an improvement in quality of life and in control of blood pressure. There does not appear to be an improvement in serum albumin levels, phosphorus levels, or body composition. Some centers have also performed overnight hemodialysis (6–8 hours) three times per week in the dialysis center.

2. Home hemodialysis—Home hemodialysis currently accounts for less than 1% of all hemodialysis treatments in the United States. It is more common in other countries such as New Zealand. Home dialysis can be performed during the day or evening 3–6 days per week or overnight for three to six nights per week. Patients receiving home hemodialysis three times per week in the United States have a lower mortality rate and fewer hospitalizations compared to patients receiving in-center hemodialysis; however, it is unclear if these results are due to selection bias, the modality itself, or some combination of the two. Nocturnal home hemodialysis six times per week is performed in small numbers of patients throughout the developed world. Small studies suggest that patients receiving home nocturnal hemodialysis six nights per week have improved blood pressure control, normal phosphorus levels without the use of phosphate binders, and improved levels of physical activity and quality of life.

Lindsay RM et al: Is more frequent hemodialysis beneficial and what is the evidence? Curr Opin Nephrol Hypertens 2004;13:631.

Pierratos A: Daily nocturnal home hemodialysis. Kidney Int 2004;65:1975.

▶ Complications

A. Hypotension

Hypotension is the most common complication of dialysis. It occurs in up to 30% of hemodialysis treatments. The differential diagnosis is broad. It is often related to an imbalance between fluid removal with dialysis treatment and fluid replacement by the extravascular compartment.

During dialysis, fluid is rapidly removed from the intravascular space. The maintenance of blood pressure despite fluid removal is due to a fluid shift from the extravascular space back into the vascular system. A large weight gain between dialysis treatments is a major risk factor for hypotension. This factor is especially important in patients with diabetic neuropathy, low cardiac ejection fraction, and diastolic dysfunction. A low dialysate sodium concentration, elevated dialysate temperature, excessive fluid removal, or intake of antihypertensive medications prior to treatment can also cause hypotension during dialysis. Patients are advised to limit their food intake prior to or during the dialysis treatment to avoid splanchnic vasodilation and hypotension. If dialysis access is provided by a catheter, bacteremia and early sepsis syndrome need to be considered and empiric antibiotic coverage initiated. Arrhythmias, pericardiac tamponade, sepsis, hemolysis, dialyzer reactions, bleeding, and air embolus are other possible causes of hypotension. Hypotension can result in cardiac ischemia and loss of access secondary to access thrombosis.

If a patient becomes hypotensive during hemodialysis, the ultrafiltration is stopped and the blood flow is decreased. If the patient remains hypotensive, normal saline and occasionally albumin can be infused. To prevent hypotension, intradialytic weight gain has to be limited by minimizing the fluid intake and avoiding salt intake. If the patient is anemic this needs to be corrected. Starting the dialysis with a higher sodium concentration and gradually decreasing the sodium concentration during dialysis (sodium modeling) have been reported to improve hemodynamic stability. However, sodium modeling has been linked to increased intradialytic weight gain and thirst. Increasing the dialysate calcium also improves hemodynamic stability. Lowering the dialysate temperature is also beneficial if it is acceptable to the patient. Recently, midodrine has been used to improve peripheral vasoconstriction in patients who are either not responsive to the above measures or who have autonomic dysfunction. Midodrine is a selective α_1-agonist that is given 1 hour before the initiation of dialysis. The dose can be repeated 1 hour into dialysis. Its use is contraindicated in patients with heart disease, urinary retention, and thyrotoxicosis.

B. Muscle Cramps

Muscle cramps are believed to be related to shifts in fluids and electrolytes. It is an early sign of ultrafiltration down to the patient's dry weight. Quinine is often used off-label for the treatment of leg cramps. Vitamin E intake might also be beneficial for this condition. Infusion of a hypertonic glucose solution (50 mL of 50% dextrose) can provide acute relief.

C. Nausea and Vomiting

Nausea and vomiting are common symptoms, especially during the first hour of dialysis. It is usually associated with hypotension and responds to the treatment of hypotension. It can also be an early symptom of the dysequilibrium syndrome, dialyzer reaction, cardiac or intestinal ischemia, or hypercalcemia. The differential diagnosis is broad and includes reflux disease, gastroparesis, peptic ulcer disease, and gastroenteritis. The treatment is symptomatic.

Bellucci A: Shortness of breath and abdominal pain within minutes of starting hemodialysis. Semin Dial 2004;17:417.

Brouns R, De Deyn PP: Neurological complications in renal failure: a review. Clin Neurol Neurosurg 2004;107:1.

Daugirdas JT: Pathophysiology of dialysis hypotension: an update. Am J Kidney Dis 2004;38(Suppl 4):S11.

Donauer J: Hemodialysis-induced hypotension: impact of technologic advances. Semin Dial 2004;17:333.

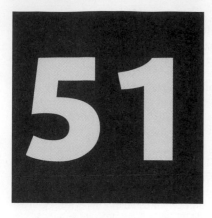

Peritoneal Dialysis

Brenda B. Hoffman, MD

▶ General Considerations

Peritoneal dialysis (PD) is an established form of renal replacement therapy that is used around the world. The concept of continuous ambulatory peritoneal dialysis (CAPD) was first described in 1976. During the 1980s there was rapid growth in the utilization of CAPD in the United States with the development of chronic indwelling PD catheters and the introduction of PD solution in sterile, disposable plastic bags. In the 1990s there was a rapid increase in the number of patients on automated peritoneal dialysis (APD) with the increased interest in dialysis adequacy and the development of simplified, automated cycler machines. In more recent years, however, the growth of PD has decreased in the United States. United States Renal Data System (USRDS) data from 1998 to 2002 indicate that the prevalent PD population decreased by 3.5% per year, with only 8% of prevalent dialysis patients being treated with PD in 2002. In contrast to the experience in the United States, the prevalent number of patients with end-stage renal disease receiving PD has exceeded 60% in other countries, such as in Mexico and Hong Kong. The cause for these differences is likely multifactorial and is related to access to PD, physician expertise, patient mix, and reimbursement.

The selection of dialysis modality is influenced by a number of considerations such as availability and convenience, medical factors, and socioeconomic and dialysis center factors. In general, the one absolute contraindication to chronic PD is an unsuitable peritoneum due to the presence of extensive adhesions, fibrosis, or malignancy. Other relative contraindications do exist (Table 51–1). PD continues to be the preferred dialysis modality for infants and young children, patients with severe hemodynamic instability on hemodialysis, and patients with difficult vascular access. Studies investigating differences in patient mortality between PD and hemodialysis (HD) have been conflicting. Most reports have shown no significant difference in survival between PD and nondiabetic HD patients. Survival by dialysis modality among diabetic patients may vary with age. Some series have found lower survival for older diabetic patients on PD compared to HD. Variable results in these mortality studies have been affected by differences in patient comorbidities, inclusion of prevalent versus incident patients, and the types of analytical methods utilized. Real differences in mortality between PD and HD can be assessed only in prospective, randomly controlled trials that will be very difficult and therefore unlikely to be performed. Technique survival is shorter in PD compared to HD due to peritonitis, peritoneal membrane failure, and patient burnout.

▶ Clinical Findings

PD involves the transport of solutes and water across the peritoneal membrane, which separates the blood in the peritoneal capillaries and the dialysis solution in the peritoneal space. The dialysis solution in the peritoneal space typically contains sodium, chloride, calcium, and lactate and is made hyperosmolar by the addition of various amounts of glucose. The peritoneal membrane as a dialyzer has a surface area that typically ranges from 1 m^2 to 2 m^2 in adults. It is a complex membrane composed of the capillary endothelium and associated basement membrane, the intersitium, the mesothelium, and a stagnant fluid film that overlies the peritoneal membrane. The transport of water and solutes across this membrane best fits a model that describes the presence of three different sized pores in the peritoneal membrane. Large pores that are few in number and thought to represent clefts between endothelial cells allow the transport of macromolecules such as proteins. Numerous small pores are responsible for the transport of small solutes such as urea, creatinine, and cations and anions, while ultrasmall, transcellular pores or aquaporins allow the movement of water only.

In PD, solutes are transported by the processes of diffusion and ultrafiltration. During the course of a PD dwell, smaller solutes such as creatinine, urea, and potassium diffuse down a concentration gradient from the peritoneal capillary blood

Table 51-1. Contraindications to performance of peritoneal dialysis.

Absolute contraindication
Extensive abdominal adhesions or documented loss of peritoneal function

Relative contraindications
Abdominal hernias

Presence of colostomy, ileostomy, nephrostomy, or ileal conduit

Recurrent chronic backache with preexisting disc disease

Severe psychological and social problems

Severe diverticular disease of the colon

Severe neurologic disease, movement disorder, or severe arthritis preventing self care (caregivers can be trained to perform the peritoneal dialysis)

Severe chronic obstructive pulmonary disease

Malnutrition

into the peritoneal dialysis solution. With increasing dwell time, the ratio of dialysate to serum levels approaches 1 (Figure 51–1). Thus, for small solutes such as urea, the removal is maximal at the start of the dwell, when the concentration in the dialysis solution is zero, and gradually decreases during the course of the dwell. Diffusion becomes more restricted as molecular weight increases (ie, urea diffuses faster than creatinine). Glucose, lactate, and calcium will diffuse in the opposite direction, from dialysate into the blood.

Ultrafiltration occurs as a result of an osmotic pressure gradient between the dialysis solution and the peritoneal capillary blood. The dialysis solution is made hypertonic usually by the addition of high concentrations of glucose. Ultrafiltration is maximal at the beginning of a dwell when the osmotic pressure gradient is highest. The osmotic pressure gradient will decrease over time due to the dilution of the glucose by ultrafiltrate and by the diffusion of glucose from the peritoneal cavity into the bloodstream (Figure 51–2). Fluid removal is maximized by using more hypertonic dialysis solutions or by doing more frequent exchanges. During ultrafiltration solutes present in body fluids will be swept along by solvent drag, contributing to overall solute clearance. Water and solutes are also constantly being absorbed from the peritoneal cavity into the lymphatic system and this will counteract both solute and fluid removal.

Not all patients' peritoneal membranes transport solute at the same rate. In clinical practice, a patient's peritoneal membrane transport characteristics can be determined by measuring the creatinine equilibration curve and the glucose absorption curve during a standardized peritoneal equilibration test (PET). Conventionally, the PET involves a 2-L, 2.5% dextrose dwell with dialysate samples taken at 1, 2, and 4 hours and a plasma sample at 2 hours. Net fluid removal is also measured along with the ratio of dialysate glucose at 4 hours to dialysate glucose at time zero. Patients are classified principally into one of four transport categories: high, high-average, low-average, and low (Figure 51–3).

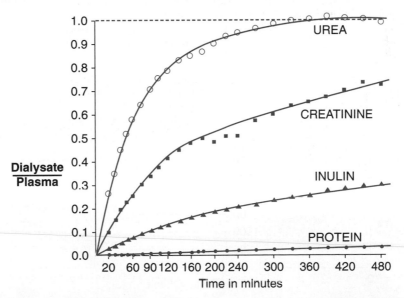

▲ **Figure 51-1.** Dialysate-to-plasma ratio over the period of a dwell using 1.5 g/dL dextrose, 2 L volume. (Reproduced with permission from Popovich RP et al: Continuous ambulatory peritoneal dialysis. Ann Intern Med 1978;88:453.)

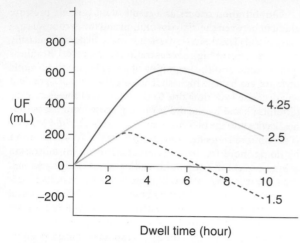

▲ **Figure 51–2.** Ultrafiltration with 1.5, 2.5, and 4.25 g/dL dextrose dialysis solution. (Reproduced with permission from Twardowski ZJ et al: Osmotic agents and ultrafiltration in peritoneal dialysis. Nephron 1986;42:93.)

High transporters will have the fastest equilibration of creatinine, but ultrafiltration will not be as great due to rapid absorption of glucose and dissipation of the osmotic gradient. High transporters also tend to have higher dialysate protein losses. In contrast, low transporters will have less complete equilibration of creatinine, but will have good net ultrafiltration due to the slower absorption of glucose into the bloodstream. Thus, high transporters tend to do better on regimens that have frequent, short duration dwells, such as APD, whereas low transporters tend to do better on regimens with longer duration dwells, such as CAPD. Average transporters are generally able to do well on a variety of PD regimens.

▶ Complications

A. Peritonitis and Catheter-Related Infections

Peritonitis remains a leading complication of PD. It contributes to technique failure, hospitalization, and patient mortality. Peritonitis is thought to occur most often by touch contamination, but may also occur in the setting of a catheter exit site or tunnel infection, by transmural migration of bacteria through the intestinal wall, or rarely by the hematogenous or transvaginal route. Patients with peritonitis usually present with cloudy peritoneal fluid and abdominal pain. When a patient presents with these complaints the abdomen should be drained and the effluent sent for cell count with differential, Gram stain, and culture. At least two of the following three conditions should be present to make the diagnosis of peritonitis: symptoms and signs of peritoneal inflammation, an effluent white blood cell count of more than $100/mm^3$ with at least 50% polymorphonuclear neutrophil cells, and a positive culture from the dialysate. Using appropriate culture techniques an organism can be isolated from the peritoneal fluid in over 80% of cases. Infections due to gram-positive cocci (*Staphylococcus epidermidis* and *Staphylococcus aureus*) tend to be most common (60–70% episodes) compared to infections with gram-negative bacteria (15–25%) or fungi (2–3%). Infection with mycobacteria can also occur but is rare. Peritonitis with multiple organisms or anaerobes should raise the concern of intrabdominal pathology and lead to abdominal computed tomography (CT) scan and surgical evaluation.

Patients who present with signs and symptoms of peritonitis should always be treated empirically with antibiotics. Various antibiotics can be used to treat peritonitis, but empiric therapy must cover both gram-positive and gram-negative organisms. Guidelines outlining empiric antibiotic regimens are published and have changed over the years in

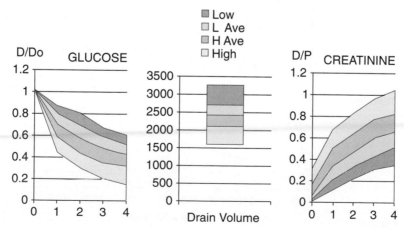

▲ **Figure 51–3.** Peritoneal equilibrium test. (Reproduced with permission from Twardowski ZJ et al: Peritoneal equilibration test. Peritoneal Dial Bull 1987;7:138.)

response to concern over the development of vancomycin-resistant organisms and appreciation of the importance of preservation of residual renal function. Gram-positive organisms may be covered by vancomycin or a cephalosporin, and gram-negative organisms by a third-generation cephalosporin or aminoglycoside. Numerous combinations are possible, but the choice of antibiotics should take into account the patient's infection history and the center's history of resistant organisms. Antibiotics are usually administered by the intraperitoneal route and can be given by intermittent (once daily) or continuous (in each exchange) dosing (Table 51–2). Most patients will show considerable clinical improvement within 48 hours of starting antibiotic therapy. Final antibiotic therapy should be guided by culture results and sensitivities. Treatment should be continued for a total of 2 weeks, while more severe infections due to S aureus, pseudomonas, or multiple gram-negative organisms should be treated for 3 weeks. If there is no clinical improvement after 48 hours, cell counts and cultures should be repeated. Refractory peritonitis is defined as failure to respond to appropriate antibiotics within 5 days and should be managed by catheter removal. Other indications for catheter removal are fungal peritonitis, relapsing peritonitis, peritonitis in the setting of severe exit site or tunnel infection, and infection due to multiple enteric organisms in the setting of a surgical abdomen. During peritonitis the permeability of the peritoneal membrane increases due to inflammation, and patients often will need a more concentrated dialysis solution in order to maintain fluid removal. Protein losses will also increase during peritonitis. Peritonitis is also often associated with increased fibrin clot production that can occlude the dialysis catheter. Heparin can be added to each bag of dialysis solution (500–1000 units/L) to decrease fibrin clot production.

Catheter-related infections can occur at the exit site or in the subcutaneous tunnel. An exit-site infection is defined by the presence of purulent drainage at the catheter–epidermal interface that may or may not be accompanied by erythema, tenderness, or crust formation. A tunnel infection may present as erythema, edema, or tenderness of the subcutaneous tunnel, but may be clinically occult. Exit-site and tunnel infections may be caused by a variety of microorganisms, with S aureus and Pseudomonas aeruginosa being responsible for the majority. A gram stain and culture of exit-site drainage should be performed. Empiric therapy may be initiated immediately and should always cover S aureus. Oral antibiotic therapy is as effective as intraperitoneal therapy. In some cases, intensified local care or a local antibiotic cream may be sufficient. A patient with an exit-site infection that progresses to peritonitis or who presents with an exit site infection in conjunction with peritonitis will usually require catheter removal. Patients should be taught to perform routine exitsite care in order to prevent catheter infections. Daily cleansing with antibacterial soap and water is recommended by most centers. The daily application of mupirocin or gentamicin cream to the exit site has been shown to be effective in reducing catheter infections and related peritonitis.

B. Mechanical Complications

The increased intrabdominal pressure that occurs during PD can be associated with a variety of mechanical complications. Hernias are quite common and can be inguinal, incisional (pericatheter or other), umbilical, or ventral. Risk factors for hernia formation include large dwell volumes, recent abdominal surgery, and polycystic kidney disease. Hernias usually present as painless swelling but can be associated with intestinal strangulation. The performance of a CT scan with

Table 51–2. Intraperitoneal antibiotic dosing for treatment of peritonitis.[1]

	Intermittent (per Exchange, Once Daily)	Continuous (mg/L, All Exchanges)
Cefazolin	15 mg/kg	LD 500, MD 125
Ceftazidime/cephalothin	1000–1500 mg	LD 500, MD 125
Ampicillin/oxacillin/nafcillin	No data	MD 125
Vancomycin	15–30 mg/kg every 5–7 days	LD 1000, MD 25
Gentamicin/netilmicin/tobramycin	0.6 mg/kg	LD 8, MD 4
Amikacin	2.0 mg/kg	LD 25, MD 12
Aztreonam	No data	LD 1000, MD 250

[1]Dosing of drugs in patients with residual renal function (>100 mL/day urine output) should be increased by 25%. LD, loading dose; MD, maintenance dose.

the instillation of intraperitoneal contrast can aid in the diagnosis of a hernia. Treatment usually involves surgical repair with temporary cessation of PD and conversion to hemodialysis. In some situations PD can be resumed postoperatively with low volume exchanges and with the patient supine [as in nocturnal intermittent peritoneal dialysis (NIPD)] in order to maintain low intraabdominal pressure and facilitate healing. Leaks may also occur at the catheter site or through other defects into the abdominal wall. The diagnosis of abdominal wall leaks may sometimes be difficult. Patients may present with decreased ultrafiltration and weight gain due to fluid accumulation in the tissues. Patients with leaks may also present with scrotal or labial edema, which may be difficult to distinguish from fluid migration through a patent processus vaginalis. Abdominal CT with intraperitoneal contrast will assist in making the proper diagnosis in this situation. Leaks can sometimes heal with conversion to NIPD or hemodialysis, but they often will require surgical repair. Hydrothorax formation due to the passage of dialysate through defects in the hemidiaphragm is a rare complication of PD. Thoracentesis will yield a transudative fluid with a very high glucose concentration. Diagnosis can also be made by radionuclide scanning after technetium-labeled albumin is added to the peritoneal fluid and allowed to dwell for several hours. Definitive treatment will usually involve surgical repair of the diaphragmatic defect.

C. Encapsulating Peritoneal Sclerosis

Encapsulating peritoneal sclerosis (EPS) is a rare but serious condition characterized by extensive intraperitoneal fibrosis and encasement of bowel loops. This entity should not be confused with the more benign and subclinical peritoneal fibrosis that can occur in most patients on PD. EPS is typically associated with a progressive loss of ultrafiltration and poor solute transport. Patients may present with bloody effluent, malnutrition, abdominal pain, nausea, and bowel obstruction. The diagnosis is usually based on clinical suspicion and can be confirmed on CT by the presence of peritoneal thickening and calcification along with encapsulation and cocooning of bowel loops. It can also be confirmed by peritoneal biopsy. The cause of EPS is unknown but may be related to prior episodes of severe peritonitis, a reaction to foreign substances such as plasticizers or disinfectants, and an extended duration of peritoneal dialysis. No uniformly successful therapy for EPS exists at this time and mortality remains quite high (>50%). Described treatment strategies have included cessation of PD, bowel rest, and total parenteral nutrition. Surgery may be beneficial but can be technically difficult. Immunosuppression with corticosteroids and azathioprine has been reported in several small series to be beneficial.

D. Ultrafiltration Failure

Fluid balance management is one of the primary functions of renal replacement therapy. PD is an excellent modality for fluid removal due to the continuous, more physiologic nature of this modality. However, there remains an unacceptably high incidence of hypertension and cardiovascular disease in the PD population. Patients are trained to adjust their ultrafiltration by choosing the correct concentration of dextrose in their dialysis solution regimen depending on their dietary intake and volume status. Ultrafiltration failure can be defined as the failure of PD fluid removal to match the volume balance needs of the patient. Patients presenting with the clinical syndrome of volume overload need to be carefully evaluated prior to being labeled with ultrafiltration failure. It is important to consider the numerous factors that can alter fluid balance. Reversible causes such as dietary indiscretion, loss of residual renal function, noncompliance with dialysis, mechanical problems such as leaks or catheter malfunction, and inappropriate dialysis prescription need to be initially ruled out. Inappropriate tailoring of a PD prescription to a patient's transport type (eg, using long dwell times with low glucose concentrations in a high transporter) should not be attributed to technique failure. After these reversible causes of impaired fluid removal have been ruled out, the next diagnostic step is to evaluate the ultrafiltration and transport functions of the peritoneal membrane in parallel (Figure 51–4). This can be accomplished by performing a modification of the standard PET using a 4.25% dextrose solution. A net ultrafiltration volume of less than 400 mL with a 4-hour dwell is considered abnormal. A net ultrafiltration volume greater than 400 mL rules out alterations in peritoneal membrane function and the patient should be reevaluated clinically focusing on dietary indiscretion, noncompliance, inappropriate prescription, or loss of residual renal function.

If the net ultrafiltration volume is less than 400 mL, then small solute transport characteristics should be measured. Patients with a low drain volume and high transport characteristics represent the largest group of patients with ultrafiltration failure. Patients falling into this profile include those with inherently high transport (approximately 10% of patients starting PD) and recent peritonitis and those who have developed high transport during long-term PD. In general it is easy to maintain solute clearance goals in these patients despite a tendency toward clinical volume overload. The combination of low ultrafiltration volume and low transport tends to be rare. This usually represents disruption of the peritoneal membrane or inadequate distribution of the peritoneal fluid such as seen with severe adhesions or encapsulating peritoneal sclerosis. These patients will have inadequate solute clearance and fluid overload and will be difficult to maintain on PD if they have no residual renal function. Patients with low ultrafiltration volume and low average or high average transport may have mechanical problems, high peritoneal/lymphatic absorption rates, or aquaporin deficiency.

General therapeutic strategies to prevent fluid overload include routine monitoring of desired weight, residual renal function, daily ultrafiltration volumes, and PET results.

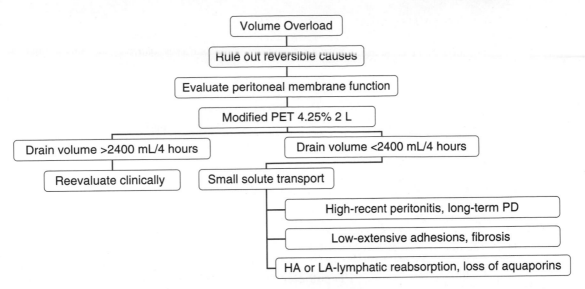

▲ **Figure 51–4.** Evaluation of volume overload in peritoneal dialysis patients.

Dietary counseling concerning salt and fluid intake should be ongoing. Protection of residual renal function should be a priority and high-dose loop diuretics may be used in patients with residual renal function to enhance fluid removal.

Hyperglycemia must be controlled in diabetic patients to allow maintenance of an osmotic gradient and adequate ul-trafiltration. Preservation of peritoneal membrane function by prevention of peritonitis, the timely removal of peritoneal catheters when necessary, and the use of more biocompatible dialysis solutions should also be a priority. Specific therapeutic interventions in patients with poor ultrafiltration and high transport include converting to APD if the patient is undergoing CAPD. With continuous cycling peritoneal dialysis (CCPD) the long daytime dwell may still result in fluid absorption in very high transporters, in which case a manual exchange can be performed in the middle of the day. Another option is to use the polyglucose solution icodextrin in the long dwell cycle. Icodextrin is poorly absorbed and has been shown to be superior to glucose-based solutions in maintaining net ultrafiltration during long dwells. Patients with poor ultrafiltration and low solute transport will be difficult to maintain on PD if they have no residual renal function and transfer to hemodialysis is usually necessary. Therapeutic options for patients with poor ultrafiltration and low or high average transport include the use of icodextrin in long dwells and shorter dwell times for glucose-based exchanges. There are no pharmacologic agents currently available to decrease lymphatic absorption.

E. Metabolic Complications

PD can be associated with a number of metabolic abnormalities. Glucose absorption will vary depending on a patient's transport characteristics, but can amount to 100–150 g/day. This, in addition to the hyperinsulinemia that ensues, can lead to weight gain and possibly also increased atherosclerosis. Glucose absorption is likely responsible for the lipid abnormalities that are commonly seen in PD patients. PD patients typically have high total and low-density lipoprotein (LDL) cholesterol, high triglycerides, and low high-density lipoprotein (HDL) cholesterol. This glucose loading may also result in hyperglycemia requiring the initiation or intensification of diabetes therapy. Protein malnutrition is common in PD patients and is partially due to protein loss across the peritoneum, which can be substantial (>10 g/day) in patients with high peritoneal transport or with peritonitis. PD patients may also have a suppressed appetite due to absorption of glucose during dialysis and a feeling of abdominal fullness. A protein intake of at least 1.2 g/kg is recommended for PD patients.

▶ Treatment

A. Forms of Peritoneal Dialysis

PD is a form of dialysis in which a dialysis solution is instilled in the peritoneal cavity, periodically drained, and exchanged with fresh solution through a single, indwelling peritoneal catheter (Figure 51–5). During each exchange there are inflow, dwell, and outflow periods. In chronic PD these exchanges are repeated according to a fixed schedule in a continuous, daily fashion such as in CAPD or APD. Exchanges may also be done in a more noncontinuous fashion over a fixed period of time such as in intermittent peritoneal dialysis (IPD) performed for acute renal failure.

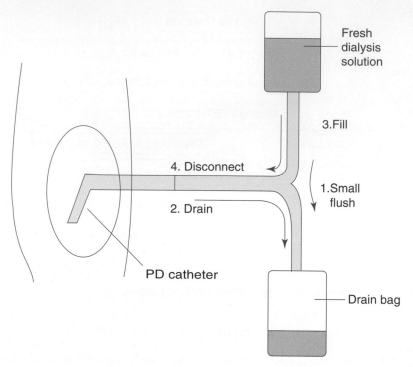

Fresh dialysis solution

3.Fill

4. Disconnect

1.Small flush

2. Drain

PD catheter

Drain bag

▲ **Figure 51–5.** Diagram of a continuous ambulatory peritoneal dialysis exchange. The patient connects the peritoneal dialysis catheter to a Y-set tubing system. A small volume of fresh dialysis solution is flushed directly into the drain bag and then the abdomen is allowed to drain. This washes away any bacteria introduced into the system during the connection of the catheter. Fresh dialysis solution is then instilled and the patient disconnects the catheter from the tubing. The fluid is allowed to dwell for several hours and then the entire cycle is repeated.

1. Continuous ambulatory peritoneal dialysis—In CAPD dialysis solution is constantly present in the abdomen, typically being exchanged four to fives times per day, 7 days per week. The dialysis fluid is exchanged manually by the patient using the force of gravity to drain and fill the abdomen. Actual dialysis prescriptions will vary depending on the individual patient, but typical exchange volumes are usually in the range of 2–3 L with three or four shorter dwell periods occurring during the day and one longer dwell period overnight during sleep.

2. Automated peritoneal dialysis—In APD a cycler machine automatically exchanges fluid into and out of the abdomen for the patient. The cycler draws dialysis solution from larger bags (usually 5 L), which it warms to the desired temperature. An alarm in the cycler is set off when various monitored parameters are disrupted. APD is traditionally divided into CCPD and NIPD. A standard CCPD prescription usually has three or four shorter nighttime dwell periods of 1.5–3.0 L. The patient usually spends between 8 and 10 hours a night on the cycler, disconnects from the cycler in the morning after a final fill is delivered, and then is free to go about daily activities. In CCPD therefore the longer dwell

period occurs over the daytime. In certain situations patients may also complete one or two manual exchanges during the day in order to increase solute clearance or fluid removal. In NIPD the patient drains fully at the end of the night and the abdomen remains "dry" all day. NIPD is usually reserved for patients with significant residual renal function, as solute clearance is usually lower than in CCPD due to the absence of the long daytime dwell period. NIPD may also be employed for patients with mechanical complications such as hernias in order to avoid the increased abdominal pressure that occurs with a full abdomen during ambulation or upright posture. Tidal peritoneal dialysis (TPD) is a form of automated PD in which a constant reserve volume of dialysis solution remains in the peritoneal cavity at all times while smaller tidal volumes of solution are repeatedly instilled into the abdomen by the cycler. TPD has the advantage of eliminating the nondialytic period required for filling and draining dialysis solution, but there is little evidence to suggest that TPD provides greater clearance than CCPD.

3. Intermittent peritoneal dialysis—IPD is a form of PD that is usually performed in a hospital or in a dialysis center. It is usually reserved for patients with acute renal failure or end-stage renal failure and sometimes for patients immediately after catheter placement who are uremic and need more urgent dialysis. The duration of treatment, number of exchanges, dwell times, and total volume of exchange fluid will depend on the individual patient. IPD is usually performed for the patient by healthcare personnel, using an automated cycler or by manual exchange.

B. Apparatus for Peritoneal Dialysis

1. Dialysis solutions—PD solution is manufactured in clear flexible plastic bags in volumes of 1.5–5 L. The electrolyte concentrations in PD solutions commonly have lactate as a buffer and dextrose as the osmotic agent (Table 51–3). Dialysis solutions containing 1.5%, 2.5%, and 4.25% dextrose are routinely marketed in the United States. The true anhydrous dextrose or glucose concentrations in these solutions are 1.36%, 2.27%, and 3.86%, respectively, and this is how the solutions are typically labeled outside of the United States. Glucose is safe, effective, easily metabolized, and inexpensive. However, it is not an ideal osmotic agent because it is rapidly absorbed and can cause metabolic problems such as hyperglycemia, hyperinsulinemia, hyperlipidemia, and obesity. The pH of the dialysis solution must also be kept relatively low to prevent the carmalization of glucose during sterilization. This unphysiologic pH, in addition to nonenzymatic glycation of proteins induced by the glucose, may contribute to long-term pathologic changes in the peritoneal membrane. There has been interest in developing dialysis solutions with alternative osmotic agents that may be more effective than glucose with fewer metabolic and long-term detrimental effects on peritoneal membrane function. A dialysis solution containing the polyglucose molecule icodextrin is now commercially available. Icodextrin is poorly absorbed into the peritoneal bloodstream and therefore its osmotic effect is more sustained than glucose. It can be used during long dwells in patients who have high transport and ultrafiltration failure and it may also be less damaging long term to the peritoneal membrane. Amino acids can also function as osmotic agents and amino acid-containing dialysis solutions are available.

The potential benefit of these solutions is that the absorbed amino acids would replace the obligatory amino acids lost during dialysis and serve as a protein caloric source. However, long-term improvement in nutritional status has not been conclusively demonstrated with these solutions. Lactate has a negative impact on the biologic function of resident cells in the peritoneum and therefore a more biocompatible bicarbonate buffered PD solution using a two-chamber bag system has also been developed.

2. Peritoneal catheters—The PD catheter must permit consistent bidirectional flow of dialysate. Most catheters are flexible silicone or polyurethane tubes with multiple ports in the intraperitoneal segment positioned in the pelvis. The transperitoneal portion of the catheter is implanted within the abdominal wall using one or two cuffs. With the commonly used double-cuffed catheter, the deep cuff is secured within the rectus muscle and the superficial cuff is placed subcutaneously approximately 2 cm from the catheter exit site. Many types of catheters are available for chronic PD, but the double cuff straight Tenckhoff catheter still remains one of the more commonly used. The benefit of one catheter design over another has not been conclusively demonstrated and the catheter used by a PD program primarily depends upon the experience of the clinician inserting the catheters. PD catheters are usually inserted surgically with or without laparoscopy/peritoneoscopy. Catheters may also be placed at the bedside using a trocar and guidewire, although this technique is generally reserved for the placement of temporary, acute PD catheters. PD catheters should be placed in the paramedian or lateral abdominal location with a downwardly directed tunnel to help prevent exit-site infection. PD catheters may also be placed with a presternal exit site. This location is often more desirable in obese patients, patients with ostomies, and children in diapers. The Moncrief–Popovich technique, in which the entire extraperitoneal portion of the catheter is left in a subcutaneous pocket for weeks to months and then later externalized, is thought by some to promote better healing and cuff incorporation. Newly placed catheters are usually flushed with heparinized saline and secured with

Table 51–3. Peritoneal dialysis solutions.

	1.5% Dextrose	2.5% Dextrose	4.25% Dextrose
Dextrose, H_2O	15 g/L	25 g/L	42.5 g/L
Sodium	132 mEq/L	132 mEq/L	132 mEq/L
Calcium	2.5–3.5 mEq/L	2.5–3.5 mEq/L	2.5–3.5 mEq/L
Magnesium	0.5–1.5 mEq/L	0.5–1.5 mEq/L	0.5–1.5 mEq/L
Chloride	95–102 mEq/L	95–102 mEq/L	95–102 mEq/L
Lactate	35–40 mEq/L	35–40 mEq/L	35–40 mEq/L
pH	5.5	5.5	5.5

Table 52–2. Choice of dialytic technique in acute renal failure.[1]

Primary Therapeutic Goal	Clinical Condition	Renal Replacement Therapy
Solute removal	Stable, catabolic	Hemodialysis
	Unstable, catabolic	CAVHD, CVVH, CVVHD, SCUF + HD
	Unstable, noncatabolic	CAVH, CVVH, SCUF + HD, CEPD
Fluid removal	Stable	IIUF
	Unstable	IIUF, SCUF
Solute and fluid removal	Stable	Hemodialysis
	Unstable	CAVHD, CVVH, CVVHD, CAVH + HD, IIUF + HD
Blood detoxification	Unstable	CVVH, CVVHD, CAVH, ?TPE

[1]Optimal modality of renal replacement therapy in acute renal failure according to the clinical status of the patient. IIUF, intermittent isolated ultrafiltration; CEPD, continuous equilibrium peritoneal dialysis; TPE, therapeutic plasma exchange; CAVHD, continuous arteriovenous hemodialysis; CVVH, continuous venovenous hemofiltration; CVVHD, continuous venovenous hemodialysis; SCUF, slow continuous ultrafiltration; HD, hemodialysis; CAVH, continuous arteriovenous hemofiltration.

Reproduced with permission from Golper TA: Continuous renal replacement therapy in acute renal failure. UpToDate 2005;online 13.1.

6. Anticoagulation—Because of the extended contact of patient blood with the foreign extracorporeal circuit and the procoagulant state associated with severe illness and sepsis, continuous anticoagulation is needed to prolong circuit life and deliver the prescribed dose in CRRT. Anticoagulant strategies are continuously evolving because of the difficult balance between the desire to prolong filter life and increased bleeding risk. Both systemic and regional anticoagulation strategies are commonly used, and some centers will also try anticoagulant-free CRRT in patients who are at extraordinarily high risk of bleeding.

A. SYSTEMIC ANTICOAGULATION— Systemic anticoagulants have the advantage of being relatively easy to administer, especially in comparison with citrate anticoagulation. The most commonly used agents are heparins and direct thrombin inhibitors such as argatroban and hirudins.

Unfractionated heparin remains the systemic anticoagulant most often used in the delivery of CRRT. It is usually delivered as a loading dose of ~10–20 U/kg, followed by a maintenance infusion of 3–20 U/kg/hour. Priming of the extracorporeal circuit with heparin is necessary as its negative charge can cause adsorption to the circuit's plastic tubing. It is mainly metabolized by the liver, with the kidney as a minor contributor to overall clearance in those patients with intact kidney function. However, neither dialysis nor hemofiltration clears heparin efficiently, and as such, the half-life of heparin is increased to roughly 40–120 minutes in patients on CRRT. Careful monitoring of clotting times is necessary, with target activated clotting times (ACT) ranging from 140 seconds to 180 seconds or activated partial thromboplastin times of 55–100 seconds. The major complication from unfractionated heparin use is hemorrhage, which occurs in roughly 25–30% of patients in whom heparin is used as the CRRT anticoagulant. Patients with minor bleeding should have their anticoagulation stopped, while patients with serious bleeding may benefit from administration of protamine. Occasionally, heparin-induced thrombocytopenia (HIT) can occur, the first sign of which may be repeated filter clotting. If HIT is diagnosed, another mode of anticoagulation must be used.

Low-molecular-weight (LMW) heparin has been compared to unfractionated heparin in several studies, and has been shown to be of equal efficacy at best, although it does increase the cost. In addition, because monitoring of LMW heparin is more difficult (requiring measurements of factor Xa activity, which are not commonly done at most hospitals) and because it has a much longer half-life than unfractionated heparin (making hemorrhage more problematic), LMW heparin is infrequently used as a mode of systemic anticoagulation in CRRT.

Argatroban works via reversibly binding the active site of thrombin. It is metabolized by the liver, is excreted in the bile, and has a half-life of roughly 40–50 minutes. The usual administration of argatroban requires a constant infusion of 2 μg/kg/minute, with dosing monitored with target activated partial thromboplastin time (aPTT) of roughly twice normal. Because argatroban is not generally cleared by hemofiltration or dialysis, it does not require dose adjustment in the CRRT setting. Because of its relative ease of use, argatroban has become the systemic anticoagulant of choice in patients requiring CRRT with HIT.

Hirudins are also direct thrombin inhibitors, and bind irreversibly to thrombin. Because there is no antidote to hirudin and because monitoring its levels requires performance of the ecorin clotting time (not readily available in most centers), hirudins are rarely used in CRRT.

B. REGIONAL ANTICOAGULATION—Regional citrate anticoagulation has become increasingly popular as centers have become more familiar with its use. Its effect is based on the ability of citrate to chelate calcium (and other divalent cations), which is required at multiple levels of both the intrinsic and extrinsic coagulation cascades. In conceptual terms (Figure 52–3), a citrate-containing solution (most commonly trisodium citrate or acid citrate dextrose-A) is infused just as blood leaves the patient to enter the extracorporeal circuit. The citrate rapidly binds calcium, causing ionized calcium levels to fall and effectively eliminating blood clotting. To prevent hypocalcemia, a calcium infusion is required, which can be administered through a stopcock at the venous return site or through another central venous access. In most protocols, the citrate infusion rate starts at a fixed fraction of blood flow and the calcium infusion starts as a fixed fraction of citrate flow. Prefilter (ie, circuit) and postfilter (ie, patient) ionized calcium levels are drawn periodically to monitor the efficacy of anticoagulation, with target levels being 0.25–0.35 mmol/L and 1.1–1.3 mmol/L, respectively. The rates of the two infusions are then adjusted accordingly to meet those target ranges.

Regional citrate anticoagulation has several advantages over systemic anticoagulation. First, assuming ionized calcium levels in the patient should be normal, there is little to no bleeding risk above the patient's baseline risk. Second, citrate anticoagulation is associated with the longest filter life when compared with other anticoagulant strategies. Lastly, because citrate is metabolized to three bicarbonate molecules in the liver, the citrate can also act as a therapeutic agent in patients with acidosis, obviating or lessening the need for anionic base replacement in the replacement fluids or dialysate.

Conversely, citrate anticoagulation is associated with several complications. If the care team is not mindful that citrate is converted to bicarbonate and can represent a significant base load, severe metabolic alkalosis can occur. To decrease the risk of alkalosis, some centers have begun using high chloride dialysate. However, if nonstandard dialysates are being used, a dedicated sterile pharmacy must be available at all times. In addition, citrate anticoagulation can cause electrolyte abnormalities including hypernatremia (especially if 4% trisodium citrate is used) and hypocalcemia. Lastly, patients who cannot convert citrate to bicarbonate (ie, cirrhotic patients) can develop citrate intoxication, which manifests as an increasing anion gap and is defined as a plasma total calcium/ionized calcium greater than four. This can be treated by attempting to increase the circuit clearance of citrate by decreasing the blood flow rate, by increasing the dialysate flow rate, and/or by decreasing the citrate infusion rate.

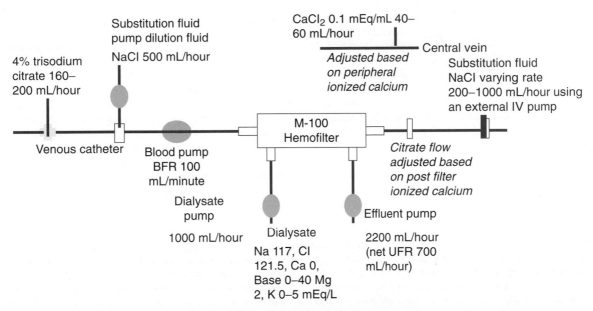

▲ **Figure 52–3.** Continuous renal replacement therapy circuit using regional citrate anticoagulation with the Gambro PRISM machine and M-100 filter. BFR, blood flow rate; UFR, ultrafiltration rate. (Reproduced with permission from Mehta RL: Continuous renal replacement therapy in the critically ill patient. Kidney Int 2005;67:781.)

Thus, although there are many advantages to citrate anticoagulation, it does place a significant burden on the nursing and medical staff to ensure proper monitoring. Nevertheless, it is becoming increasingly popular as a mode of continuous anticoagulation, with much longer circuit lives as compared to heparin.

C. OTHER ANTICOAGULATION STRATEGIES—Prostanoids such as prostacyclin (PGI_2) and its analog epoprostenol have also been used for anticoagulation in CRRT. They function via breakdown of arachidonic acid, thereby strongly blocking cyclooxygenase activity and platelet activation. There is little increased risk of bleeding with this agent, but because both of these compounds are potent arterial vasodilators, symptomatic hypotension can occur. The half-life is quite short (measured in minutes), so hypotensive episodes can be treated easily by stopping the infusion. Though effective, prostanoids are not commonly used because there are no reliable tests to assess their activity and because they are extremely expensive.

7. Fluid management—Fluid management is an integral component of the management of critically ill patients. In the presence of a failing kidney, fluid removal with diuretics is often challenging enough, but when coupled with shock and multiorgan failure, may require dialytic intervention. Over the past decade the general trend has been to use aggressive fluid resuscitation for patients in this setting, with most surgeons and intensivists willing to accept edema as a necessary evil to maintain blood pressure. However, fluid overload itself may be an important independent factor contributing to an adverse outcome, with patient survival plummeting in several series of ICU patients if fluid overload is >10–20% of baseline. This can be explained by recognizing that the fluid excess causes not only superficial edema but also myocardial and gut edema, with resultant vital organ dysfunction and local ischemia. Thus, the goal of fluid management in this setting should be the removal of excess fluid as necessary without compromising cardiac output and hemodynamic stability, all while allowing for the often significant volume of nutritive and pharmacologic support needed for care of the critically ill patient.

Setting targets for fluid removal or replacement is a crucial element of fluid management in CRRT. In non-ICU patients, overall volume assessment based on physical examination, daily weights, and measured intakes and outputs is usually sufficient to appropriately guide therapy. However, in ICU patients, this task is far more treacherous, particularly if large volumes of fluid have been used for resuscitation in short periods of time. Records of weights are often erroneous given the inherent inaccuracy of weighing immobile patients connected to more than one apparatus, and estimates of fluid losses can be unreliable in patients with large insensible losses (eg, patients with burns or on ventilators). The assessment of circulatory capacitance is helped by measurement of central filling pressures, cardiac output, and systemic vascular resistance, but even these measures are prone to measurement error. Thus, it is fairly common to encounter patients who are clearly whole-body volume overloaded but who have an inscrutable intravascular volume status. In this situation, although fluid removal is ultimately required, it may be initially necessary to maintain an adequate intravascular volume by a combination of altering the composition of fluids infused (colloids and blood products) and influencing the systemic resistance. Attempts to manage fluid balance without taking these factors into account may lead to drastic overestimation or underestimation of the patient's needs, resulting in either worsening volume overload or hypotension from intravascular volume depletion.

8. Acid–base and electrolyte management—Derangement of acid–base and electrolyte homeostasis is a common feature of critically ill patients requiring renal replacement therapy. Ultrafiltration further disturbs blood chemistry as there is ongoing loss of bicarbonate and other electrolytes across the filter. The degree of electrolyte loss can essentially be expressed as the total ultrafiltrate/dialysate effluent rate times the plasma concentration of the individual electrolytes. For example, if the ultrafiltration rate is 2 L/hour and the plasma bicarbonate concentration is 25 mEq/L, the patient will be losing 50 mEq of bicarbonate into the waste ultrafiltrate every hour. Thus, management of acid–base and electrolyte balance in CRRT requires ongoing replacement of iatrogenic bicarbonate and electrolyte losses, in addition to the correction of the patient's intrinsic metabolic abnormalities.

Regulation of acid–base status is generally accomplished by adding either lactate or bicarbonate into the dialysate or replacement fluid. The choice of agent for base replacement has been a topic of some controversy, as both have significant advantages and disadvantages. Lactate, which is converted on an equimolar basis to bicarbonate in the liver, has traditionally been used as the base equivalent of choice because it is relatively inexpensive and has a long shelf life. However, its effectiveness is quite dependent on the patient's hepatic function; in patients with liver dysfunction or in patients who require large amounts of base to maintain their blood pH at physiologic levels, the administered lactate may overwhelm the liver's conversion capacity and cause significant hyperlactatemia. Bicarbonate, on the other hand, is physiologic and does not rely on patient's organ function for its buffering action. However, bicarbonate solutions have a short shelf life, and can microprecipitate with calcium if mixed in the same bag. Nevertheless, clinical practice is shifting toward bicarbonate usage, as several studies have suggested that lactate can cause increased catabolism and worsened hemodynamics compared to bicarbonate. Other base replacement agents include citrate and acetate; acetate is not commonly used as it has been associated with cardiovascular instability, particularly in patients with left ventricular dysfunction.

Control of electrolyte levels in CRRT is usually accomplished by either infusing replacement fluids containing appropriate concentrations of electrolytes and/or by diffusive exchange with the proper dialysate. It would seem that electrolyte control in this manner would be similar to intermittent dialysis. However, it is important to recognize that CRRT techniques, while utilizing the same forces for solute and fluid removal, are distinct from intermittent techniques in that time is no longer a limiting factor for blood purification. As such, total solute clearance in CRRT is equal to or greater than IHD over time, and correction of laboratory abnormalities can occur gradually with minimal periods of disequilibrium. Furthermore, because the replacement fluid infusion rate *and* composition can be altered individually, solute balance can be altered while fluid balance can be kept either even, negative, or positive as needed. This degree of control over fluid, solute, and acid–base balance is what makes continuous techniques so versatile and valuable in the ICU setting.

C. Complications

From a procedural standpoint, CRRT is generally well tolerated by patients, especially given the dire state in which most patients treated with CRRT are in. Complications pertaining to the apparatus can arise in almost any part of the circuit, ranging from vascular access failure, circuit clotting, and loss of filter efficiency to mundane problems such as line disconnection. These issues are difficult to predict and may result in significant down-time of therapy.

More serious are acid–base and electrolyte problems, which not only can result in loss of treatment time while the cause is evaluated but can also quickly lead to life-threatening metabolic abnormalities. Because CRRT allows individualization of therapy, changes in acid–base status and electrolyte levels should be highly predictable to the prescribing nephrologists. When unexpected abnormalities arise, it is imperative to distinguish between problems related to the patient's underlying condition, problems resulting from the therapy, and problems caused by true iatrogenic error (Table 52–3). Abnormalities attributable to the patient's condition can be anticipated if there is an understanding of the underlying pathophysiology; unexpected changes should prompt reconsideration of the clinical syndrome if treatment-related and iatrogenic causes of the abnormality are thought to be unlikely. Other anomalies can be ascribed to unintended effects of proper treatment. For example, a patient on citrate anticoagulation who receives multiple citrated blood products can develop overshoot alkalemia from supratherapeutic conversion of citrate to bicarbonate. Lastly, iatrogenic complications do occur, and can result from errors in prescription, formulation, delivery, or interference. Of these, errors in formulation and delivery can have profound and sudden consequences, especially if they involve solutions containing potassium and/or calcium. For example, if a calcium infusion used during

Table 52–3. Nature of acid–base and electrolyte problems with continuous renal replacement therapy.

Type of problem	
Due to patient's condition	Severe metabolic acidosis
	Respiratory acidosis
	Alkalemia
	Hyponatremia or hypernatremia
	Hyperglycemia
	Hyperphosphatemia

Contributed by therapy	Acid–base imbalance
	    Increased base loss
	    Overshoot alkalosis
	    CO_2 retention

	Hyponatremia and hypernatremia
	Hyperglycemia
	Hypophosphatemia

	Citrate accumulation
	    Hypocalcemia
	    Citrate gap
	    Alkalemia

	Hypothermia

Iatrogenic	Inappropriate prescription
	    Inadequate replacement of base
	    No adjustment for dextrose absorption

	Errors in formulation
	    Pharmacy errors
	    Bedside mixing
	    Precipitation of calcium in dialysate bicarbonate

	Errors in delivery
	    Calcium solution used as dialysate
	    Low citrate flow rate

	Interference
	    Change in orders
	    Excess bircarbonate given exogenously
	    Fluid imbalance

Reproduced with permission from Mehta RL: Acid-base and electrolyte management in continuous renal replacement therapy. Blood Purif 2002;20:262.

citrate anticoagulation is mistakenly hung as dialysate, significant hypercalcemia can occur. Alternatively, miscalculation of fluid intake and output can lead to improper administration or removal of volume, which can result in severe overhydration or dehydration. Lastly, problems of interference with the proper therapy can occur if there are misunderstandings between members of the care team as to the treatment plan.

Although complications occur with any procedure or treatment, many of the adverse events associated with administration of CRRT can be prevented or at least mitigated by the institution of safety protocols (eg, cross-checking of solution content or creation of simple flow sheets to aid fluid management). Furthermore, adoption of a multidisciplinary approach in the decision-making process by including members of the medical, nursing, nutrition, and pharmacy staff can help in preventing miscommunication.

D. Recent Technical Innovations

1. High volume hemofiltration—Conventional hemofiltration is able to remove pathologic immune mediators such as inflammatory cytokines, but its ability to do so to any clinically appreciable degree is controversial. Despite the appearance of these mediators in the ultrafiltrate, changes in plasma levels are inconsequential and outcomes are unchanged. However, there is mounting evidence that high-volume hemofiltration (ie, >45 mL/kg/minute ultrafiltration rate) may improve intermediate endpoints, lending credence to the notion that increased plasma water purification may lead to improved outcomes.

2. Hybrid therapies

A. EXTENDED INTERMITTENT TECHNIQUES—Extended intermittent techniques such as slow low-efficiency dialysis (SLED) have incrementally higher dialysis and blood flow rates as compared to continuous techniques but are run typically for 12 hours or less per day. Blood flow rates are classically set at 200 mL/minute and dialysate flow rates at 100 mL/minute. By using a lower blood flow rate, SLED may be less of a hemodynamic stress on the patient. Likewise, by lowering the dialysate flow rate, solute clearance is less efficient per unit time than in IHD, yielding a more gradual change in body solute concentrations. Because the therapy is intended to run for only part of the day or night, procedures and imaging studies can be coordinated to coincide with scheduled downtime. Furthermore, SLED does not require the intensive monitoring that is necessary in CRRT. Preliminary studies have suggested that overall solute clearance and hemodynamic tolerability in SLED may be on a par with CRRT, although large comparative studies have not yet been published. Moreover, SLED does not afford the same high level of hour-to-hour control of fluids, electrolytes, and acid–base parameters possible with CRRT.

B. COUPLED ADSORPTION—As previously described, high levels of proinflammatory cytokines are thought to contribute to poor patient outcomes in sepsis. Research is ongoing in the use of sorbent cartridges that presumably remove these cytokines from the circulation. Strategies for removal include the addition of a sorbent cartridge either in series or in parallel with the hemofilter or in parallel with a plasma filter that has much larger pores than the standard hemofilter. Although these technologies may be beneficial in terms of intermediate endpoints as shown in animals and in small human trials, no large human studies have yet validated their usage. Nevertheless, the concept is intriguing and will warrant much future research.

C. MOLECULAR ADSORBENT RECIRCULATING SYSTEM—Blood purification by traditional dialysis in patients with ESRD is ineffective because many of the toxins produced in liver disease are bound to albumin and are therefore not cleared through the dialysis membrane. In the molecular adsorbent recirculating system (MARS), patient blood is passed through a high-flux dialysis membrane against dialysate enriched in albumin. Although albumin cannot pass through the membrane, albumin-bound toxins can cross the dialysis membrane down their concentration gradients onto "clean" albumin. In small studies this system has been shown to improve recovery from severe hepatic encephalopathy.

D. RENAL TUBULE ASSIST DEVICE—The renal tubule assist device (RAD) was developed based on the premise that while conventional dialysis and CRRT can mimic the kidney's solute and fluid clearance capabilities, they are unable to replace the kidney's endocrinologic activity. The device consists of a conventional hemofiltration system attached in series to a bioreactor cartridge containing approximately 10^9 human proximal tubule cells. Blood is passed through the hemofiltration circuit and then into the assist device, where theoretically the resident proximal tubular cells perform further metabolic functions on the blood before it is returned to the patient. Small human trials have been promising.

Davenport A: Anticoagulation for continuous renal replacement therapy. Contrib Nephrol 2004;144:228.

Gillespie RS et al: Effect of fluid overload and dose of replacement fluid on survival in hemofiltration. Pediatr Nephrol 2004;19:1394.

Humes HD et al: Initial clinical results of the bioartificial kidney containing human cells in ICU patients with acute renal failure. Kidney Int 2004;66:1578.

Mehta RL: Continuous renal replacement therapy in the critically ill patient. Kidney Int 2005;67:781.

Renal Transplantation

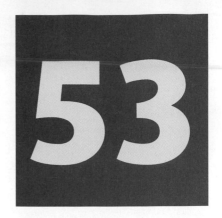

53

Phuong-Thu Pham, MD, Julie Yabu, MD,
Phuong-Chi Pham, MD, &
Alan H. Wilkinson, MD, FRCP

▶ General Considerations

A. Recipient Evaluation

Currently, kidney transplantation is the treatment of choice for patients with end-stage renal disease (ESRD) as it improves both patient survival and quality of life when compared to dialysis. It must be noted, however, that although the risk of death in the first year after transplantation is less than 5%, not all patients qualify for the surgery due to their unacceptably high risk for complications. The transplant evaluation process requires a comprehensive assessment of each patient's medical, surgical, and psychosocial history. A systematic approach should be used in the evaluation of potential renal transplant candidates.

1. The initial evaluation process—Prior to the formal evaluation process, all potential transplant candidates are encouraged to attend a "patient education" session. At the meeting, patients are informed about the medical and surgical risks and benefits of renal transplantation, the necessity for frequent outpatient visits in the early postoperative period, the potential adverse effects of immunosuppression, and the importance of compliance with immunosuppressive therapy. The potential advantages and disadvantages of deceased versus living donor renal transplantation are discussed with the patients and, when possible, with their family members, significant others, and/or friends. Other issues that are addressed include the prolonged waiting time for a deceased donor transplant due to the critical shortage of donor organs and the adverse effects of waiting time on patient and graft survival. In addition, patients are forewarned that various medical and psychosocial conditions may preclude a patient from being a transplant candidate. Absolute and relative contraindications to kidney transplantation are outlined in Table 53–1.

2. General assessment—The routine assessment of a renal transplant candidate includes a detailed history and a thorough physical examination. In particular, it is important to determine the cause of the original kidney disease as it can help in predicting the transplant course and outcome and the risk for disease recurrence. When available, the kidney biopsy report should be reviewed. Patients with ESRD secondary to congenital or genitourinary abnormalities should undergo a voiding cystourethrogram (VCUG) and appropriate urologic evaluation, preferably by the kidney transplant surgeon. Documentation of the patient's residual urine volume from the native kidneys is invaluable in the assessment of graft function in the posttransplant period. A history of familial or hereditary renal disease must be obtained if living related kidney donation is an option. The patients's surgical history should be elicited with special emphasis on previous abdominal operations. A complete physical examination should include a careful assessment for the presence of carotid and peripheral vascular disease. Patients should preferably have a body mass index below 30–35 as obesity is associated with a higher incidence of postoperative complications. In addition to a thorough history and physical examination, patients should also undergo a number of routine laboratory testings and imaging studies as outlined in Table 53–2. Specific risk factors need to be addressed during the transplant evaluation process.

3. Evaluation of risk factors by specific organ system disease

A. Cardiovascular disease and peripheral vascular disease—Cardiovascular disease (CVD) is the leading cause of death after renal transplantation. Deaths with a functioning graft occurring within 30 days after transplantation are due to ischemic heart disease in nearly 50% of cases. A detailed cardiovascular history not only predicts the operative risk but also helps in postoperative cardiac management to improve short-term and long-term cardiac outcomes. Although the determinants of CVD risk in ESRD patients have not been well defined, all patients with CKD should be considered increased cardiac risk candidates. Major conventional risk factors include diabetes

Table 53–1. Contraindications for renal transplantation.

Absolute contraindications
Active malignancy

Active infection

Severe irreversible extrarenal disease

Life expectancy <2 years

Liver cirrhosis (unless combined liver and kidney transplant)

Poorly controlled psychiatric illnesses

Active substance abuse

Relative contraindications
Active peptic ulcer disease[1]

Medical noncompliance

Active hepatitis B virus infection[2]

Morbid obesity

Special considerations
ABO incompatibility[3]

Positive T cell crossmatch[3]

[1]Should be treated prior to transplantation.
[2]Liver biopsy and pretransplant antiviral therapy recommended. Obtain hepatology consult.
[3]Pretransplant desensitization protocols may allow successful transplantation across these barriers.

Table 53–2. Assessment of renal transplant candidate

Laboratory evaluation
Serologies: HIV, hepatitis B and C, CMV, EBV, HSV, RPR

Liver function tests, calcium, phosphate, prothrombin time, partial thromboplastin time

Urinalysis, urine culture

PSA in men >50 years of age[1]

Other evaluation
EKG

Chest x-ray

Colonoscopy if >50 years of age

Abdominal ultrasound in diabetics to evaluate for gallstones

Native renal ultrasound to assess for acquired cystic disease or masses

Pap smear (for women)

Mammogram for women >40 years of age

Cardiac evaluation (see text)

Urologic evaluation if history of bladder/voiding dysfunction, recurrent urinary tract infections (see text)

Immunologic studies
Blood group and HLA typing

HLA antibodies

Crossmatching

CMV, cytomegalovirus; EBV, Epstein–Barr virus; HSV, herpes simplex virus; RPR, rapid plasmin reagin; PSA, prostate-specific antigen; EKG, electrocardiogram.
[1]High-risk patients should be screened at an earlier age (African-Americans, those with two or more first-degree relatives with prostate cancer).

mellitus, hypertension, dyslipidemia, obesity, a history of angina pectoris, congestive heart failure, previous cardiac events, older age, smoking, and family history. Other suggested risk factors include preexisting left ventricular hypertrophy, dialysis for a prolonged period, coronary artery vascular calcification, abnormal electrocardiogram, and hyperhomocysteinemia. Exercise tolerance should be assessed along with cardiac-related symptoms as many patients on dialysis lead sedentary lifestyles and are symptom free. Noninvasive cardiac screening such as nuclear stress test or dobutamine stress echocardiogram is probably adequate for low-risk candidates. However, for those with multiple risk factors, particularly diabetes mellitus and/or previous cardiac events, coronary angiography is warranted. If necessary, coronary angioplasty/stenting or coronary bypass surgery and cardiac rehabilitation should be performed prior to transplantation. In general, high-risk candidates should undergo a formal evaluation by cardiology.

Patients with a history of transient ischemic attacks or cerebrovascular accidents should undergo carotid Doppler studies. When carotid bruits are detected on physical examination in an asymptomatic patient, further diagnostic imaging should be performed at the discretion of the clinician. Evidence of significant stenosis requires vascular surgery consultation. If necessary, carotid endarterectomy should be performed prior to transplantation and patients should be symptom free for at least 6 months prior to transplantation. For those with milder carotid disease, a neurologic consultation and optimal medical management may be sufficient.

Peripheral vascular disease is present in a significant number of renal transplant recipients and is associated with increased morbidity and mortality. Vascular imaging with either a Doppler ultrasound or a noncontrast abdominal/pelvis CT scan is indicated in patients with a history of claudication and/or signs of diminished peripheral arterial pulses (particularly in diabetics) on physical examination. An angiogram should be considered if noninvasive studies suggest the presence of large-vessel disease. Significant aortoiliac disease requires evaluation by the surgical transplant team and may preclude transplantation.

B. MALIGNANCY—Transplant recipients are at greater risk of developing both *de novo* and recurrent malignancy due to the use of immunosuppressants. As the incidence of malignancy increases with the intensity and duration of immunosuppression, a history of immunosuppressive therapy for the native kidneys represents an added risk for posttransplant malignancy. For patients with a history of malignancy, consultation with an oncologist is advisable.

Table 53–3. Malignancy and renal transplantation[1]

Most tumors: wait time of >2 years
No waiting time if cured at the time of transplantation
Incidental renal cell carcinoma
In situ carcinoma
Noninvasive bladder carcinoma
Basal cell skin cancer
Squamous cell carcinoma[2,3]

Waiting time >2 years[3]
Melanoma
Wilms tumor
Renal cell carcinoma
Breast carcinoma
Lymphoma
Colorectal carcinoma
Invasive cervical carcinoma, uterine carcinoma

[1]Certain cancers may recur despite a tumor-free waiting period.
[2]Surveillance.
[3]Oncology evaluation or consultation with the Israel Penn International Transplant Tumor registry at www.ipittr.uc.edu may be invaluable.

Table 53–3 provides general guidelines for minimum tumor-free waiting periods for common malignancies.

C. INFECTIONS—All patients should be assessed for common latent or active infections and questioned for a history of infectious exposures. Active infections including diabetic foot ulcers and osteomyelitis must be fully treated prior to transplantation. A prior history of tuberculosis or untreated tuberculosis exposure requires appropriate posttransplant prophylactic therapy. Patients with an established history of systemic coccidioidomycosis or histoplasmosis or those from an endemic area should undergo appropriate antibody testing. In addition, these patients should be informed of possible disease reactivation with immunosuppressive therapy and indefinite posttransplant azole prophylactic therapy.

A history of immunization should also be obtained to ensure adequate immunizations for common infections prior to transplantation (eg, hepatitis B, pneumovax, and other standard immunizations appropriate for age). An immunization update is mandatory for those who have undergone surgical splenectomy. Infections with the human immunodeficiency virus (HIV) was once considered a contraindication to transplantation due to early reports of serious infectious complications and death following HIV infection transmitted from a transplanted organ or inadvertent transplantation of HIV-infected patients. However, with the advent of effective highly active antiretroviral therapy (HAART) regimens, there have been changing views regarding transplantation in HIV-positive patients. Currently, a number of transplant centers would consider transplantation in stable HIV patients, defined as those with an undetectable HIV viral load, CD4 lymphocyte count >300/mm^3, and absence of opportunistic infections in the previous year. Specific recommendations may vary from center to center and a formal consultation with an infectious disease specialist is recommended.

D. SPECIFIC GASTROINTESTINAL DISEASE EVALUATION—There has been no consensus on whether all asymptomatic renal transplant candidates should be screened for cholelithiasis. Screening is warranted, however, in diabetics and patients with a history of cholecystitis. Pretransplant cholecystectomy is recommended for these patients if there is evidence of cholelithiasis due to the increased risk of life-threatening cholecystitis after transplantation.

E. UROLOGIC EVALUATION—All renal transplant candidates on dialysis should be imaged with a renal ultrasound, computed tomography (CT), or magnetic resonance imaging (MRI) to evaluate for acquired cystic kidney disease and associated renal cell carcinoma if no imaging study has been performed within the previous 3 years. Urinalysis and urine cultures should be performed in all patients with significant residual urine volume. Transplant candidates with a history of recurrent urinary tract infections, voiding symptoms, or ESRD secondary to congenital or genitourinary abnormalities should undergo a VCUG. Persistent hematuria or sterile pyuria may warrant endoscopic evaluation and/or retrograde pyelography. Urodynamic studies may be helpful in patients with a history of lower urinary tract dysfunction and/or urinary incontinence. Patients with bladder dysfunction secondary to neurogenic bladder or chronic infections can often be managed without urinary diversion. In continent patients with lower urinary tract dysfunction, intermittent self-catheterization is a safe and effective alternative to urinary diversion. However, a formal urologic evaluation and patient education during the initial transplant evaluation process are mandatory. Augmentation cystoplasty or urinary diversion procedures may be necessary in patients in whom simple reimplantation into a dysfunctional bladder is not an option. Male transplant candidates with sufficient urine volume and symptoms of outflow tract obstruction due to benign prostatic hypertrophy should undergo prostate resection before transplantation, whereas in anuric patients, the procedure should be postponed until after a successful renal transplant.

F. SPECIAL UROLOGIC CONSIDERATIONS: PRETRANSPLANT NATIVE NEPHRECTOMY—For most patients with autosomal dominant polycystic kidney disease (ADPKD) pretransplant nephrectomy is not routinely recommended. However, unilateral or bilateral pretransplant nephrectomy(ies) may be necessary for those with massively enlarged kidneys, recurrent infection, bleeding, and/or intractable pain. Table 53–4 lists the special indications for pretransplant native nephrectomy. Generally, a minimum of 6 weeks after nephrectomy is recommended prior to transplantation. For

Table 53–4. Indications for pretransplant native nephrectomy.

Absolute indications
Chronic renal parenchymal infection
Recurrent infected stones
Reflux or obstructive megaureter complicated by infection or stone formation
Polycystic kidney disease[1]
Heavy proteinuria
Relative indications
Intractable hypertension[2]
Acquired renal cystic disease[3]

[1]Indicated for massively enlarged kidneys, recurrently infected or bleeding, intractable pain.
[2]Should be individualized.
[3]When there is suspicion for adenocarcinoma.

transplant candidates who undergo preemptive transplantation from a living donor, simultaneous native nephrectomy and transplantation may be performed.

4. Evaluation of risk factors related to specific patient's characteristics

A. ADVANCED AGE—There is no arbitrary age limit for transplantation. The United Network for Organ Sharing organ procurement and transplant network (UNOS OPTN) database reveals that the number of kidney transplants performed in patients >65 years old has more than tripled over the past 10 years. Similar to the younger population, transplantation in the older age group of 60–74 years has been shown to improve survival compared to their wait-listed counterparts. Graft loss from rejection is lower in older compared to younger recipients presumably due to the decreased immune responsiveness in the aged population. It must be noted, however, that older transplant recipients are at increased risk for infectious complications, malignancy related to immunosuppression, and deaths in the early posttransplant period, most often as a consequence of cardiovascular disease. Screening for covert cardiovascular disease and occult malignancy in older potential recipients is, therefore, crucial and mandatory.

B. OBESITY—Obesity is considered a contraindication to transplantation by some centers as it is associated with increased risk of posttransplant complications including delayed graft function, surgical wound infection, and death, particularly from cardiovascular disease. Although there has been no consensus on an acceptable upper limit body mass index (BMI), weight reduction to a BMI of 30–35 kg/m² or less prior to transplantation is recommended. Morbidly obese candidates may benefit from surgery referral for gastric bypass surgery or gastric banding procedure. Data on patient and

graft survival in obese versus nonobese transplant recipients are variable and contradictory. Determination of transplant candidacy in obese patients should, therefore, be assessed on an individual basis rather than reliance on an absolute BMI index. Obese candidates with comorbid conditions such as known coronary artery disease and advanced age are at particularly high risk and may fare better receiving dialysis.

B. Donor Evaluation

This section focuses primarily on the evaluation of the living donor candidate.

1. Evaluation of the living donor—Over the past decade, the number of living donors has steadily increased whereas the number of deceased donor kidneys has remained relatively unchanged. The increased rates of living donation are in part due to excellent patient and graft survival rates achieved with living donor transplant, the advent of laparoscopic donor nephrectomy, and improved patient and public awareness and education. Living donor transplantation offers survival advantages over deceased donor transplantation and permits the prospective recipient to undergo preemptive or elective transplantation at the time of optimal medical health. General guidelines for evaluating a potential donor candidate are described.

A. GENERAL ASSESSMENT—Similar to the evaluation process of the potential recipient, living donor evaluation requires a complete history, physical examination, and psychosocial assessment. A formal psychiatric evaluation by the transplant center is recommended to evaluate for any significant psychiatric problem and any possibility of coercion. The presence of either of these would preclude donation. The mandatory preliminary evaluation of a potential living donor includes determination of ABO blood group compatibility, HLA typing, and cross-matching against the potential recipient. In cases in which more than one donor is available, selection of the best donor depends on the degree of HLA matching and donor age. In addition, biologically related donors are generally preferred over unrelated donors. A suggested routine evaluation and optional testing are listed in Table 53–5.

B. MEDICAL ASSESSMENT OF THE POTENTIAL DONOR—There are significant variations among transplant centers regarding the medical evaluation of living donors, but the universal goals are to ensure that the potential donor (1) is sufficiently healthy to undergo the operation, (2) has normal kidney function with minimal future risk of kidney disease, and (3) represents no risk to the recipient in terms of infection or transmission of malignancy. Absolute and relative contraindications to living kidney donation are listed in Table 53–6.

Measurement of creatinine clearance based on a 24-hour urine collection is generally adequate, although some centers prefer iothalamate or diethylenetriaminepentaacetic acid (DTPA) clearance for a more accurate estimation of the glomerular filtration rate (GFR). A minimum GFR of 80 mL/minute/1.73 m²

Table 53–5. Living donor evaluation

Laboratory tests

Blood group, HLA typing, crossmatch

Urinalysis and urine culture

24-hour urine collection for protein and creatinine clearance or GFR determination by nuclear medicine test

Complete blood count, prothrombin time, partial thromboplastin time, comprehensive metabolic panel including liver function tests, albumin, calcium, phosphorus

Viral serologies: HIV, hepatitis B and C, EBV, CMV, HSV, RPR

Men: PSA level if >50 years of age

Other tests

Electrocardiogram

Chest x-ray

Pap smear (for women)

Mammogram for women >40 years of age

Renal imaging: spiral CT, CT angiogram, or MR angiogram

Further testing depending on age/history/abnormal laboratory findings/family history screening

Colonoscopy

Cardiac screening: echocardiogram, nuclear medicine stress test

Twenty-four hour ambulatory blood pressure monitoring

Renal biopsy

Cystoscopy

PPD skin test

Screening for hypercoagulability

Glucose tolerance test with family history of diabetes mellitus or risk factors for development of diabetes

GFR, glomerular filtration rate; EBV, Epstein–Barr virus; CMV, cytomegalovirus; HSV, herpes simplex virus; RPR, rapid plasmin reagin; PSA, prostate-specific antigen; CT, computed tomography; MR, magnetic resonance; PPD, purified protein derivative.

Table 53–6. Contraindications for living kidney donation[1]

Absolute contraindications

Evidence of renal disease (GFR <80 mL/minute, microalbuminuria or overt proteinuria)

Significant renal or urologic abnormalities

Transmissible infectious disease (HIV infection, hepatitis B, hepatitis C)

Active malignancy

Chronic illness that places patient at significant risk of undergoing surgery

Poorly controlled psychiatric illness or active substance use

Cognitive deficit

Current pregnancy

Hypertension (clinically significant)

Diabetes mellitus

Recurrent nephrolithiasis or bilateral stones

History of thrombotic disorders with risk factors for future events or inherited hypercoagulable states[2]

Relative contraindications

Age <18 or >65 years

Borderline or mild hypertension

Borderline urinary abnormalities in the absence of renal function impairment

Single prior episode of nephrolithiasis without evidence of secondary risk

Obesity

Young donor with risk factors for future development of diabetes mellitus

Jehovah's Witness

[1]Criteria may differ among transplant centers.
GFR, glomerular filtration rate.
[2]For example, the presence of lupus anticoagulant or anticardiolipin antibody, Factor V Leiden, or prothrombin gene mutation (FII-20210).

is required by most centers, considering that unilateral nephrectomy reduces overall renal function by about 20% at long-term follow-up. Renal imaging studies are mandatory to assess the anatomic features of the kidneys, to delineate renal vessels to select one kidney for donation, to determine the most appropriate nephrectomy technique, and to exclude potential donors with incidental masses or fibromuscular dysplasia.

The medical evaluation should specifically probe for possible hereditary renal disease, diabetes, and hypertension. The most commonly encountered hereditary renal disease is ADPKD. For potential donors over the age of 30 years, it is safe to proceed with donor nephrectomy if ultrasound or CT imaging reveals no evidence of cysts. For potential donors between the age of 20 and 30 years, genetic studies such as linkage analysis or direct deoxyribonucleic acid (DNA) sequencing can reliably exclude the presence of ADPKD. These tests, however, are not routinely available. Potential donors

with a family history of Alport's syndrome should be screened for hematuria and hypertension and should undergo special hearing and ocular testing. Alport's syndrome is predominantly transmitted as X-linked and less commonly as autosomal recessive or autosomal dominant. The absence of hematuria in an adult male 20 years of age or older essentially excludes the presence of the genetic defect. Adult female siblings with normal urinalysis have a low risk of being carriers and can safely donate. However, female relatives with persistent hematuria are most likely carriers of the mutation and donation is not advisable. Although genetic testing is possible it is not readily available and generally is not performed.

All potential donors should have a fasting plasma glucose to detect diabetes mellitus or undiagnosed impaired glucose tolerance. The presence of diabetes mellitus would preclude living donation. All individuals with impaired fasting glucose and those with risk factors for developing type 2 diabetes mellitus should undergo a 2 hour oral glucose tolerance test (OGTT). The latter includes first-degree relatives of patients with type 2 diabetes mellitus, obesity, gestational diabetes mellitus, and dyslipidemia. If the OGTT test is normal (<140 mg/dL) and no other risk factors are present, it is reasonable to proceed with the donation process. Individuals with impaired glucose tolerance are at risk for the development of diabetes mellitus and risk factor modifications including exercise and weight reduction or avoidance of excessive weight gain should be emphasized. Potential donors with impaired glucose tolerance should be assessed on an individual basis. Those with mild or borderline impaired glucose tolerance and additional risk factors and those with blood sugar levels in the high range should probably not donate since the higher the blood sugar within the range of impaired glucose tolerance (140–199 mg/dL) or impaired fasting glucose (100–125 mg/dL), the greater the tendency for tolerance to deteriorate.

C. RISKS OF DONATION—Donor nephrectomy is either performed via open nephrectomy or, increasingly more popular, laparoscopic nephrectomy. Acute mortality rates related to open nephrectomy are estimated at 0.03–0.04%. The incidence of postoperative complications including wound infection, pneumonia, ileus, deep vein thrombosis, or pulmonary embolism is approximately 3%. The incidence of testicular pain, paresthesia of L1, and the need for reoperation or conversion from laparoscopic to open donor nephrectomy ranges from 0% to 3% and may vary among centers. The incidence of complications is slightly higher for laparoscopic compared to open nephrectomy. However, with the refinement in surgical techniques and the increasing expertise of the surgeons performing the procedures, comparable postoperative complication rates between the two surgical operations have been reported. The potential advantages of laparoscopic versus open nephrectomy include less donor pain and shorter donor recovery time.

The risk of future development of chronic kidney disease and progression to ESRD in the remaining single kidney has always been a major concern for prospective donors. At long-term follow-up, unilateral nephrectomy reduces renal function by approximately 20%. Similar to the nondonating population, an additional 5 mL/minute loss in GFR per decade occurred after donating. Although data on the effects of nephrectomy on the progression and complications of ESRD are lacking, the UNOS database revealed that of the 48,000 living kidney donors whose donations occurred between 1987 and 2001, 20 (or 0.04%) donors were listed for transplantation. It should also be noted that the baseline lifetime risk of developing ESRD in the general population is about 2–3% for whites and about 7% for African-Americans. Annual medical evaluation of renal function, proteinuria, fasting blood sugar, and blood pressure measurements is warranted after donation.

2. Evaluation of the deceased donor—Whereas the number of patients on the transplant waiting list has steadily increased, the number of deceased donor kidneys has remained far below the growing need, leading to longer waiting times and increased wait-list deaths. One approach to increasing the pool of deceased donor organ supply has been to expand the previously defined criteria for acceptable donor kidneys, such as advanced donor age (>60 years of age), donor comorbid conditions, such as hypertension or diabetes, donor preprocured high serum creatinine level, pediatric donors (<5 years of age), donors after cardiac death (DACD), and donor kidneys with prolonged cold preservation time. Dual kidney transplantation into one recipient from an otherwise nonacceptable donor has also been performed by some centers. More recently, UNOS set forth a new expanded criteria donor (ECD) kidney policy defining donors that meet these criteria. These kidneys are defined by donor characteristics that are associated with a 70% greater risk of kidney graft failure when compared to a reference group of normotensive donors aged of 10–39 years whose cause of death was not a cerebrovascular accident (CVA) and whose terminal serum creatinine was <1.5 mg/dL. The donor factors associated with this increased relative rate of graft failure include age 60 years or older or age 50–59 years with at least one comorbid factor. The latter may include CVA as a cause of death, hypertension, and/or terminal serum creatinine greater than 1.5 mg/dL (Table 53–7). Despite inferior outcomes compared to standard criteria donor kidneys, ECD kidney transplantation offers survival advantages over "wait-listed" continued dialysis. Compared to the younger age group, older recipients (>65 years) had a significant proportional increase in longevity, and compared to patients with nondiabetic nephropathy, more patients with ESRD due to diabetic nephropathy died while awaiting kidney transplantation (4.3% versus 10.8%, respectively, $p < 0.001$). Acknowledging the potential benefits and risks of ECD kidney transplantation compared to maintenance dialysis has led many centers to liberalize the criteria for accepting deceased donor kidneys.

Table 53–8 lists the absolute and relative contraindications to deceased donor donation. However, it should be noted that the acceptance criteria for deceased donor kidneys may be institution specific.

Davis CL: Evaluation of the living kidney donor: current perspectives. Am J Kidney Dis 2004;43:508.

Jordan SC et al: Evaluation of intravenous immunoglobulin as an agent to lower allosensitization and improve transplantation in highly sensitized adult patients with end-stage renal disease: Report of the NIH IG02 Trial. J Am Soc Nephrol 2004;15:3256.

Kendrick E et al: Medical and surgical aspects of kidney donation. In: *Handbook of Kidney Transplantation*, ed 4. Danovitch GM (editor). Lippincott, Williams & Wilkins, 2005.

Siddiqi N et al: Evaluation and preparation of renal transplant candidates. In: *Handbook of Kidney Transplantation*, ed 4. Danovitch GM (editor). Lippincott, Williams & Wilkins, 2005.

Steiner RW, Danovitch GM: The medical evaluation and risk estimation of end-stage renal disease for living kidney donors. In: *Educating, Evaluating, and Selecting Living Kidney Donors*, ed 1. Steiner RW (editor). Kluver Academic Publishers, 2004.

Table 53–7. UNOS definition of expanded criteria kidney donor.

Donor condition	Donor age categories	
	50–59 years	≥60 years
CVA + HTN + creatinine >1.5 mg/dL	X	X
CVA + HTN	X	X
CVA + creatinine >1.5 mg/dL	X	X
HTN + creatinine >1.5 mg/dL	X	X
CVA		X
HTN		X
Creatinine >1.5 mg/dL		X
None of the above		X

UNOS, United Network for Organ Sharing; X, expanded criteria donor; CVA, cerebrovascular accident was cause of death; HTN, history of hypertension at any time.

Complications

Complications following renal transplantation vary over time and can be arbitrarily categorized into those occurring early (the first 1–6 months) or late (after 6 months). We concentrate more on the early complications, describe a basic approach to evaluating renal allograft dysfunction in the immediate and early postoperative period, and discuss the urologic and infectious complications commonly encountered in the first 1–6 months following renal transplantation.

Table 53–8. Contraindications to cadaveric kidney donation.

Transmission of infectious disease
Untreated bacterial sepsis
Acute hepatitis
HIV infection
Hepatitis B surface antigen (HBSAg) positive
High-risk behavior (eg, recent intravenous drug abuse)
Potential metastatic malignancy
History of chronic kidney disease
Age >70 years[1]
Estimated creatinine clearance less than 60 mL/minute[2]
Significant proteinuria
Severe hypertension
Prolonged warm ischemia time (>30–45 minutes)
Prolonged cold ischemia time
Oliguric acute renal failure

[1]Not considered as absolute contraindication by some centers.
[2]Some centers consider double kidney transplantation.

A. Renal Allograft Complications

1. Delayed graft function and primary nonfunction—The term delayed graft function (DGF) has been used to describe marginally functioning grafts that recover function only after several days to weeks. In contrast, the term primary nonfunction is best applied to kidneys that never function where allograft nephrectomy is usually indicated.

The incidence of DGF may range from 10% to 50% in some centers and can often be anticipated based on both recipient and donor factors (Table 53–9). Unless these patients have adequate residual urine output from the native kidneys, most will require temporary dialysis support for volume, hyperkalemia, and/or uremia. The differential diagnoses of DGF are shown in Table 53–10. A systematic approach to the evaluation of DGF may be categorized as prerenal (or preglomerular type), intrinsic, and postrenal. Although uncommon in the early postoperative period, vascular causes of DGF must be excluded.

A. PRERENAL CAUSES OF DELAYED GRAFT FUNCTION—Intravascular volume depletion and nephrotoxic drugs are the more common causes of prerenal dysfunction. Severe intravascular volume depletion is usually suggested by a careful review of the patient's preoperative history and intraoperative report. Knowing the dialysis dry weight and preoperative weight of patients may be invaluable in the assessment of their volume status in the immediate postoperative period. Both calcineurin inhibitors (CNI)—cyclosporine and to a lesser extent tacrolimus—have been shown to cause a dose-related reversible afferent arteriolar vasoconstriction and a "preglomerular type" allograft dysfunction that manifest clinically as delayed recovery of allograft function. Intraoperative direct injection of the calcium channel blocker verapamil into the renal artery may reduce capillary spasm

Table 53–9. Risk factors for delayed graft function due to acute tubular necrosis in cadaveric renal transplantation

Donor factors	Recipient factors
Premorbid factors	Premorbid factors
Age (<10 or >50 years)	African-American (compared to whites)
Donor hypertension	Peripheral vascular disease
Donor macrovascular or microvascular disease Cause of death (cerebrovascular versus traumatic)	Presensitization (PRA >50) Reallograft transplantation
Preoperative donor characteristics	Perioperative and postoperative factors
Brain death stress	Recipient volume contraction
Hypotension, shock	Early high-dose calcineurin inhibitors ± early use of OKT3
Prolonged use of vasopressors	
Preprocurement ATN	
Non-heart-beating donor	
Nephrotoxic agents	
Organ procurement surgery	
Hypotension prior to cross-clamping of aorta	
Traction on renal vasculatures	
Cold storage flushing solutions	
Kidney preservation	
Prolonged warm ischemia time (± contraindication to donation)	
Prolonged cold ischemia time	
Cold storage versus machine perfusion	
Intraoperative factors	
Intraoperative hemodynamic instability	
Prolonged rewarm time (anastomotic time)	

PRA, plasma renin activity; ATN, acute tubular necrosis. Adapted with permission from Pham PT et al: Diagnosis and therapy of graft dysfunction. In: *Chronic Kidney Diseases: Dialysis and Transplantation,* ed 2. Sayegh MH et al (editors). W.B. Saunders, 2005.

Table 53–10. Differential diagnoses of delayed graft function.

Prerenal (or preglomerular type) Volume contraction Nephrotoxic drugs (see text)
Vascular complications Arterial or venous thrombosis Renal artery stenosis
Intrinsic renal Acute tubular necrosis Accelerated acute or acute rejection Thrombotic microangiopathy Recurrence of primary glomerular disease (particularly FSGS)
Postrenal Catheter obstruction Perinephric fluid collection (lymphocele, urine leak, hematoma) Ureteral obstruction   Intrinsic (blood clots, poor reimplantation, ureteral slough)   Extrinsic (ureteral kinking)   Neurogenic bladder   Benign prostatic hypertrophy

FSGS, focal segmental glomerulosclerosis. Adapted with permission from Pham PT et al: Diagnosis and therapy of graft dysfunction. In: *Chronic Kidney Diseases: Dialysis and Transplantation,* ed 2. Sayegh MH et al (editors). W.B. Saunders, 2005.

up to 40%. Other commonly used drugs that may potentially precipitate acute "preglomerular type" allograft dysfunction include angiotensin-converting enzyme inhibitors (ACEI), amphotericin B, nonsteroidal anti-inflammatory drugs (NSAIDs), and contrast dye.

B. Intrinsic renal causes of delayed graft function—Intrinsic renal causes of DGF typically include acute tubular necrosis, acute rejection, thrombotic microangiopathy, and recurrence of glomerular diseases affecting the native kidneys.

(1) Acute tubular necrosis—Posttransplant acute tubular necrosis (ATN) is the most common cause of DGF. The two terms are often used interchangeably although not all cases of DGF are caused by ATN. The incidence of ATN varies widely among centers and has been reported to occur in 20–25% of patients (range 6–50%). The difference in the incidence reported may, in part, be due to the more liberal use of organs from marginal donors by some centers but not by others and/or the difference in the criteria used to define DGF. Unless an allograft biopsy is performed, posttransplant ATN should be a diagnosis of exclusion. In the absence of superimposed hyperacute or acute rejection, ATN typically resolves over several days and, on occasion, up to several weeks (4–6 weeks),

and improve renal blood flow. Most centers have advocated the use of nondihydropyridine calcium channel blockers (ie, diltiazem) to counteract the vasoconstrictive effect of and to allow a reduction in the dose of the calcineurin inhibitors. Their use may permit the cyclosporine dose to be reduced by particularly in recipients of older donor kidneys. Recovery from ATN is usually heralded by a steady increase in urine output associated with a decrease in the interdialytic rise in serum creatinine and eventually in dialysis independence. Prolonged DGF should prompt a diagnostic allograft biopsy to exclude covert acute rejection or other intrinsic causes of allograft dysfunction. The administration of sirolimus in *de novo* renal transplant recipients may prolong DGF duration without adversely affecting 1-year graft survival.

(2) Acute rejection—While hyperacute or accelerated acute rejection due to presensitization may occur immediately following transplantation or after a delay of several days, classic cell-mediated acute rejection is typically seen after the first posttransplant week. Accumulating evidence suggests that there is an interactive effect between ATN and acute rejection. Ischemia reperfusion injury causes upregulation of multiple cytokines and growth factors within the allograft including interleukin-1 (IL-1), IL-2, IL-6, tumor necrosis factor (TNF), interferon-α (IFN-α), and transforming growth factor (TGF)-β. The proinflammatory cytokine response may in turn trigger acute allograft rejection through upregulation of various costimulatory and adhesion molecules as well as through increased expression of MHC class I and class II antigens. It is therefore prudent to perform a diagnostic allograft biopsy with prolonged ATN.

(3) Thrombotic microangiopathy—Thrombotic microangiopathy (TMA) is a well-recognized complication following renal allograft transplantation. It may develop as early as 4 days postoperatively and as late as 6 years posttransplantation. In most cases, calcineurin inhibitors (cyclosporine or tacrolimus) are believed to play a role in the development of this disorder.

Posttransplant TMA may be evident clinically by the typical laboratory findings of intravascular coagulation (such as thrombocytopenia, elevated lactate dehydrogenase levels, and peripheral schistocytes) or it may be covert with inconsistent laboratory findings. In renal allograft recipients, renal dysfunction is the most common manifestation. Thrombocytopenia and microangiopathic hemolysis are often mild or absent. Indeed, the diagnosis of posttransplant TMA is often made on graft biopsies performed to determine the cause of DGF or to rule out acute rejection. Although there have been no controlled trials comparing the different treatment modalities of this condition, dose reduction or discontinuation of the offending agent appears to be pivotal to management. Adjunctive plasmapheresis with fresh frozen plasma (FFP) replacement may offer survival advantages. In transplant recipients with cyclosporine-associated TMA, successful use of tacrolimus immunosuppression has been reported. However, recurrence of TMA in renal transplant recipients treated sequentially with cyclosporine and tacrolimus has been described and clinicians must remain vigilant for signs and symptoms of recurrence of TMA in patients who are switched from cyclosporine to tacrolimus or vice versa. There have been anecdotal reports of the successful use of sirolimus and/or mycophenolate mofetil (MMF) in transplant recipients with calcineurin inhibitor-associated TMA. However, recently, sirolimus has also been reported to cause TMA in renal allograft recipients. Although infrequent, the use of the monoclonal antibody muromonab-CD3 OKT3 has also been associated with the development of posttransplant TMA.

Other potential causative factors of posttransplant-associated TMA include the presence of lupus anticoagulant and/or anticardiolipin antibody, cytomegalovirus infection, and, less frequently, systemic viral infection with parvovirus B19 or influenza A virus. An increased incidence of TMA has also been described in a subset of renal allograft recipients with concurrent hepatitis C virus infection and anticardiolipin antibody positivity.

(4) Recurrence of glomerular disease of the native kidneys—The incidence of recurrent renal disease after renal transplantation and the risk of graft loss from disease recurrence is shown in Table 53–11.

C. POSTRENAL CAUSES OF DELAYED GRAFT FUNCTION—Postrenal DGF is generally due to obstruction and may occur anywhere from the intrarenal collecting system to the level of the bladder-catheter drainage system. The latter is generally due to blood clots and can often be managed by flushing the catheter with saline solution. Nursing care orders should

Table 53–11. Rates of recurrent renal disease after transplantation and risk of graft loss from disease recurrence.[1]

	Recurrence rates %[2]	Graft loss from disease recurrence %[2]
FSGS	30-50	50
IgA nephropathy	30-60	10-30
MPGN I	15-50	30-35
MPGN II	80-100	10-20
Membranous GN	3-30	30
HUS	10-40	10-40
Anti-GBM disease	10	<5
SLE	3-10	<5

[1]Only selected renal diseases are listed. For a more extensive list of estimated rates of recurrence of primary and secondary glomerulopathies, see Sadlier D, O'Meara YM. Recurrent and De Novo renal disease in kidney transplantation. In: *Chronic Kidney Disease: Dialysis and Transplantation*, 2nd ed. Sayegh MH, Pereira BJG, Blake P (eds). WB Saunders, 2005.
[2]Rates reported vary widely among studies of rapamycin.
FSGS, focal segmental glomerulosclerosis; MPGN, membranoproliferative glomerulonephritis; GN, glomerulonephropathy; HUS, hemolytic uremic syndrome; SLE, systemic lupus erythematosus.

routinely include irrigation of the Foley catheter as needed for clots or no urine flow. In patients with persistent gross hematuria, continuous bladder irrigation may be helpful. However, potential serious complications such as bleeding from vascular anastomoses or graft thrombosis should be excluded. Obstructive uropathy due to perinephric fluid collections or extrinsic compression and ureteral obstruction are discussed further under surgical and urologic complications.

D. Vascular complications and renal artery stenosis—Arterial or venous thrombosis generally occurs within the first 2–3 postoperative days but may occur as late as 2 months posttransplant. In most series reported, the incidence of arterial/venous thrombosis ranges from 0.5% to as high as 8% with arterial thrombosis accounting for one-third and us thrombosis for two-thirds of cases. Thrombosis occurring early after transplantation is most often due to surgical complications while late-onset thrombosis is generally due to acute rejection. In patients with initially good allograft function, thrombosis is generally heralded by the acute onset of oliguria or anuria associated with a deterioration of allograft function. Clinically, the patient may present with graft swelling or tenderness and/or gross hematuria. In patients with good residual urine output from the native kidneys but with DGF and an absence of overt signs and symptoms, the diagnosis rests on clinical suspicion and prompt imaging studies. Confirmed arterial or venous thrombosis typically necessitates allograft nephrectomy. Suggested predisposing factors for vascular thrombosis include arteriosclerotic involvement of the donor or recipient vessels, intimal injury of the graft vessels, kidneys with multiple arteries, a younger recipient and/or younger donor age, a history of recurrent thrombosis, the presence of antiphospholipid antibodies (anticardiolipin antibody and/or lupus anticoagulant antibody), and thrombocytosis.

There has been no consensus on the optimal management of recipients with an abnormal hypercoagulability profile such as an abnormal activated protein C resistance ratio associated with factor V Leiden mutation (and to a lesser extent with factor II mutation, prothrombin II 20210 A), antiphospholipid antibody positivity, protein C or protein S deficiency, or antithrombin III deficiency. However, unless contraindicated, perioperative and/or postoperative prophylactic anticoagulation should be considered, particularly in patients with a prior history of recurrent thrombotic events. At our institution, patients with identifiable risk factors are observed intraoperatively for adequacy of hemostasis. If satisfactory, these patients are given a small bolus dose of intravenous heparin (usually 1000 U). Postoperatively, a heparin infusion is continued at 100–300 U/hour. Complete blood counts are checked every 6 hours for the first 24 hours and then daily thereafter. If no bleeding complications are observed, oral warfarin is begun after 48 hours and heparin is continued until a therapeutic INR level is achieved (INR 2.0–2.5). The duration of anticoagulation has not been well defined but lifelong anticoagulation should be considered in high-risk candidates. Transplant of pediatric en bloc kidneys into adult recipients with a history of thrombosis should probably be avoided.

E. Transplant renal artery stenosis—Although transplant renal artery stenosis may occur as early as the first week, it is usually a late complication. Clinically, patients may present with new onset or accelerated hypertension, acute deterioration of graft function, severe hypotension associated with the use of ACEI, recurrent pulmonary edema or refractory edema in the absence of heavy proteinuria, and/or erythrocytosis. The latter, when associated with hypertension and impaired graft function, should raise the suspicion of renal artery stenosis (RAS) (ie, a triad of erythrocytosis, hypertension, and elevated serum creatinine). The presence of a bruit over the allograft is neither sensitive nor specific for the diagnosis of graft renovascular disease. However, a change in the intensity of the bruit or the detection of new bruits warrants an evaluation. Although noninvasive, a radionuclide scan with and without captopril is neither sufficiently sensitive nor specific for detecting transplant RAS (a sensitivity and specificity of 75% and 67%, respectively). Color Doppler ultrasound is highly sensitive and serves well as an initial noninvasive assessment of the transplant vessels. It should be noted, however, that color Doppler ultrasound is limited by its relatively low specificity. CO_2 angiography avoids nephrotoxic contrast agents but its use is not without limitations. Overestimation of the degree of stenosis, bowel gas artifact, and/or patient intolerance have been reported with the use of a CO_2 angiogram. Although gadolinium-enhanced MR angiography has previously been suggested to be an alternative non-nephrotoxic method in identifying transplant renal artery stenosis, its use should be avoided in those with allograft dysfuction due to the well-described association between gadolinium and the development of nephrogenic fibrosing dermopathy (NFD) and systemic fibrosis (NSF). Although invasive, renal angiography remains the gold standard for establishing the diagnosis of RAS.

2. Allograft rejection—Allograft rejection can be classified as hyperacute, accelerated acute, acute, and chronic.

A. Hyperacute rejection—Hyperacute rejection can occur immediately following vascular anastomosis, which can be recognized intraoperatively by the surgeon, or it may occur within minutes to hours after graft revascularization. Grossly, the kidney allograft may appear flaccid or cyanotic and hard, and graft rupture may occur within minutes after revascularization. Hyperacute rejection is mediated by preformed, cytotoxic immunoglobulin G (IgG) anti-HLA class I antibodies that are produced in response to previous exposure to alloantigens through multiple pregnancies, blood transfusions, and/or prior transplants. These antibodies bind to the graft vascular endothelium and activate complement leading to severe vascular injury including thrombosis and obliteration of the graft vasculature. Hyperacute rejection almost uniformly leads to graft loss, and prevention with meticulous cross-match is the mainstay of management. Hyperacute rejection can also occur as a result of ABO blood group incompatibility due to preformed anti-ABO blood group antibodies. With the current pretransplant cytotoxic cross-match as well as ABO-matching policy, hyperacute rejection has become almost nonexistent.

Recently "pretransplant preconditioning" with plasmapheresis and cytomegalovirus hyperimmune globulin (CMVIg) with or without rituximab (a humanized CD20 monoclonal antibody) has allowed renal transplantation to be carried out across a positive cross-match and/or ABO blood group incompatibility without the development of hyperacute rejection. These, however, are currently performed only at experienced transplant centers and a discussion is beyond the scope of this chapter.

B. Accelerated acute rejection (within 24 hours to 7 days)—Accelerated acute rejection occurs after the first 24 hours to 7 days after transplantation and may be mediated by both humoral and cellular mechanisms. Accelerated acute rejection probably represents a delayed amnestic response to prior sensitization. It may be seen after donor-specific transfusions in recipients of living-related donor transplant due to a primed T cell response. Treatment of accelerated acute rejection generally requires aggressive treatment with antibody therapy (OKT3 or antithymocyte antibody), intravenous immunoglobulin (IVIG) with or without adjunctive plasmapheresis. Despite aggressive treatment, accelerated acute rejection commonly results in early graft loss. The T cell flow cytometry cross-match (FCXM) may be useful in the pretransplant evaluation of sensitized or reallograft transplant candidates whose antibody levels may have declined but who can mount a rapid amnestic response upon rechallenge. Transplant across a positive T cell FXCM is associated with a higher rate of early acute rejection episodes. Hyperacute rejection, however, has not been reported as long as the pretransplant cytotoxic cross-match is negative. More recently, various desensitization protocols have been developed to allow successful transplantation in sensitized recipients.

C. Acute rejection—Historically, approximately 30–50% of renal allograft recipients have an episode of acute rejection within the first 6 months after transplantation. With the introduction of mycophenolate mofetil (MMF) and anti-IL-2 receptor antibody (anti-IL-2R) daclizumab and basiliximab into clinical practice, acute rejection rates of 15–30% or less have now been routinely achieved by most transplant programs. In the era of cyclosporine and other potent immunosuppressive agents in general, the classic constitutional symptoms of acute rejection including fevers, chills, myalgias, arthralgias, graft swelling, and/or tenderness are often absent. Patients are usually nonoliguric and a rise

in serum creatinine may be the only sign of acute rejection. Elevated blood pressure or worsening hypertension may be variably present. Noninvasive imaging studies such as renal Doppler ultrasound or renal radioisotope flow scan is neither sufficiently sensitive nor specific in the diagnosis of acute rejection. Although invasive, allograft biopsy remains the most accurate means of differentiating acute rejection from other causes of acute deterioration of allograft function.

3. Treatment of acute rejection—Because the treatment of acute rejection is a specialized area overseen by the kidney transplant team, the reader is referred to specialty reviews and textbooks for this information.

B. Surgical and Urologic Complications

1. Perinephric fluid collections—Symptomatic perinephric fluid collections in the early postoperative period can be due to lymphoceles, hematoma, urinoma, or abscesses. Lymphoceles are collections of lymph caused by leakage from severed lymphatics. They typically develop within weeks after transplantation. Most lymphoceles are small and asymptomatic. Generally, the larger the lymphocele, the more likely it is to produce symptoms and require treatment, although very small but strategically placed lymphoceles can result in ureteral obstruction. Lymphoceles may also compress the iliac vein leading to ipsilateral leg swelling or deep vein thrombosis or occasionally produce urinary incontinence due to bladder compression.

Lymphoceles are usually detected by ultrasound either as an incidental finding or during an evaluation of allograft dysfunction. They appear as a roundish, sonolucent, septated mass. Hydronephrosis may be present with a lymphocele adjacent to or compressing the ureter. Generally, the clinical presentation and ultrasound appearance can distinguish a lymphocele from other types of perinephric fluid collections, such as a hematoma or urine leak. Needle aspiration reveals a clear fluid with a creatinine concentration similar to that of serum in the case of a lymphocele, while that of a urine leak would have a much higher concentration.

No therapy is necessary for the common, small, asymptomatic lymphocele. Percutaneous aspiration should be performed if a ureteral leak, obstruction, or infection is suspected. The most common indication for treatment is ureteral obstruction. If the cause of the obstruction is simple compression resulting from the mass effect of the lymphocele, percutaneous drainage alone usually suffices. The ureter is often narrowed and may need to be reimplanted because of its involvement in the inflammatory reaction in the wall of the lymphocele. Repeated percutaneous aspirations are not advised because they seldom lead to dissolution of the lymphocele and often result in infection. Infected or obstructing lymphoceles can be drained externally. Sclerosing agents such as povidone-iodine, tetracycline, or fibrin-glue can be instilled into the cavity with variable results. Lymphoceles can also be marsupialized into the peritoneal cavity, where the fluid is reabsorbed.

An obstructed hematoma is best managed by surgical evacuation. Urinoma or evidence of a urine leak should be treated without delay. A small leak can be managed expectantly with insertion of a Foley catheter to reduce intravesical pressure. This maneuver may occasionally reduce or stop the leak altogether. Persistent allograft dysfunction, particularly in a symptomatic patient, often necessitates early surgical exploration and repair. Infected perinephric fluid collections should be treated by external drainage or open surgery in conjunction with systemic antibiotics.

2. Ureteral obstruction—Ureteral obstruction occurs in 2–10% of renal transplants and is usually manifested by painless impairment of graft function due to the lack of innervation of the engrafted kidney. Hydronephrosis may be minimal or absent in early obstruction, whereas low-grade dilation of the collecting system secondary to edema at the ureterovesical anastomosis may be seen early posttransplantation and does not necessarily indicate obstruction. A full bladder may also cause mild calyceal dilation due to ureteral reflux and repeat ultrasound with an empty bladder should be performed. Persistent or increasing hydronephrosis on repeat ultrasound examinations is highly suggestive of obstruction. A renal scan with furosemide washout may help support the diagnosis, but it does not provide clear anatomic detail. Although invasive, the placement of a percutaneous nephrostomy tube with an antegrade nephrostogram is the most effective way to visualize the collecting system and can be both diagnostic and therapeutic.

Blood clots, a technically poor reimplantation, and ureteral slough are common causes of early acute obstruction after transplantation. Ureteral fibrosis secondary to either ischemia or rejection can cause an intrinsic obstruction. The distal ureter close to the ureterovesical junction is particularly vulnerable to ischemic damage due to its remote location from the renal artery and hence its compromised blood supply. Ureteral fibrosis associated with polyoma BK virus is a newly recognized cause of ureteral obstruction in the setting of renal transplantation. Ureteral kinking, lymphocele, pelvic hematoma or abscess, and malignancy are potential causes of extrinsic obstruction. Calculi are uncommon causes of transplant ureteral obstruction.

Definitive treatment of ureteral obstruction due to ureteral strictures consists of either endourologic techniques or open surgery. Intrinsic ureteral scars can be treated effectively by endourologic techniques in an antegrade or retrograde approach. A stent is left indwelling to bypass the ureteral obstruction and can be removed cystoscopically after 2–6 weeks. Routine ureteral stent placement at the time of transplantation may be associated with a lower incidence of early postoperative obstruction. Extrinsic strictures or strictures that are longer than 2 cm are less likely to be amenable to percutaneous techniques and are more likely to require surgical treatment, as do strictures that fail endourologic incision. Obstructing calculi can be managed by endourologic techniques or by extracorporeal shock wave lithotripsy.

C. Infectious Complications

Despite the routine use of prophylactic therapy against common bacterial, viral, and opportunistic pathogens in the perioperative and postoperative period, infection remains an important cause of morbidity and mortality after organ transplantation. The time to occurrence of different infections in immunocompromised transplant recipients follows a "timetable" pattern.

In the first month after transplantation, infections are most frequently caused by bacterial microorganisms. Similar to those following any major surgical procedure, the sources of infection after solid organ transplantation include surgical wounds, surgical drainage catheters, an indwelling Foley catheter, bacteremia from vascular access devices, aspiration pneumonia, and urinary tract infections (UTIs). Potential sources of infection specific to renal transplant recipients include perinephric fluid collections due to lymphoceles, wound hematomas or urine leaks, indwelling urinary stents, and anatomic or functional genitourinary tract abnormalities such as ureteral stricture or vesicoureteric reflux and neurogenic bladder. Although bacterial pathogens may vary from center to center, UTIs in renal transplant recipients are commonly caused by *Enterococcus* spp., Enterobacteriaceae, and *Pseudomonas aeruginosa*. Preventive and prophylactic measures to reduce UTIs include early Foley catheter removal and antibiotic prophylaxis. The use of trimethoprim-sulfamethoxazole or ciprofloxacin prophylaxis effectively reduces the frequency of UTIs to less than 10% and essentially eliminates urosepsis unless urine flow is obstructed. Although strict aseptic surgical techniques and the perioperative use of the first generation cephalosporins reduce the incidence of wound infections, nonmodifiable risk factors include the presence of diabetes mellitus and obesity at the time of transplant. Weight reduction prior to transplantation should therefore be encouraged.

After the first posttransplant month, infections with immunomodulating viruses including cytomegalovirus (CMV), herpes simplex virus (HSV), varicella zoster virus (VZV), Epstein–Barr virus (EBV), hepatitis B virus (HBV), and hepatitis C virus (HCV) may occur either due to the overall state of immunosuppression, exogenous infection, or reactivation of latent disease. Repeated courses of antibiotics and corticosteroid therapy increase the risk of fungal infections whereas infections with immunomodulating viruses may render the patients more susceptible to opportunistic infections. Causative opportunistic agents include *Pneumocystis jiroveci*, *Aspergillus spp.*, *Listeria monocytogenes*, *Nocardia species*, and *Toxoplasma gondii*. Trimethoprim prophylaxis eliminates *P jiroveci* pneumonia (PCP) and reduces the incidence of *L monocytogenes* meningitis, *Nocardia* spp. infection, and *T gondii*. Beyond 6 months following transplantation, the risk of infection in patients with good allograft function is similar to that of the general population, with community-acquired respiratory viruses constituting their major infective

Table 53–12. Suggested prophylactic therapy for recipients of renal transplants.

	Comments
Trimethoprim-sulfamethoxazole (TMP/SMX)	Its routine use reduces or eliminates the incidence of PCP, *Listeria monocytogenes, Norcardia asteroides,* and *Toxoplasma gondii* In renal transplant recipients, TMP/SMX reduces the incidences of UTI from 30–80% to less than 5–10%
Monthly intravenous or aerosolized pentamidine >dapsone[1] > atovaquone[2]	Replaces TMP/SMX for patients with sulfa allergies
Nystatin 100,000 U/mL, 4 mL qpc and qhs	For fungal prophylaxis
Acyclovir, valganciclovir, ganciclovir	For CMV prophylaxis see Table 53–12

PCP, *Pneumocystis carinii*; UTI, urinary tract infection; CMV, cytomegalovirus.
[1]Check for glucose-6-phosphate dehydrogenase deficiency prior to initiation of therapy.
[2]In order of efficacy.

agents. These patients are usually maintained on a relatively low level of immunosuppression. In contrast, patients who experience multiple episodes of rejection requiring repeated exposure to heavy immunosuppression are the most likely candidates for chronic viral infections and superinfection with opportunistic organisms. Causative opportunistic pathogens include *P jiroveci, L monocytogenes, N asteroides,* and *Crytococcus neoformans.* Geographically, restricted mycoses include coccidioidomycosis, histoplasmosis, blastomycosis, and paracoccidioidomycosis. In high-risk candidates, lifelong prophylactic therapy has been advocated. Suggested prophylactic therapy in renal transplant recipients in shown in Table 53–12.

1. Cytomegalovirus—CMV infection occurs primarily after the first month posttransplantation and continues to be a significant cause of morbidity the first 6 months after organ transplantation. CMV infection may occur in the setting of primary infection in a seronegative recipient *(donor seropositive, recipient seronegative),* reactivation of endogenous latent virus *(donor seropositive or seronegative, recipient seropositive),* or superinfection with a new virus in a seropositive recipient *(donor seropositive, recipient seropositive).* Primary CMV infection often results in more severe disease than reactivation or superinfection. The clinical manifestations of CMV infection span the spectrum of asymptomatic seroconversion, mononucleosis-like

syndrome, or flu-like illness with fever and leukopenia, and/or thrombocytopenia to widespread tissue invasive disease. The latter may result in clinical hepatitis, esophagitis, gastroenteritis, colitis, pneumonia, and allograft dysfunction. Donor and recipient seropositive status and the use of blood products from CMV seropositive donors are well-established risk factors for CMV infection. Other factors associated with an increased risk of CMV infection include the use of antilymphocyte antibodies, prolonged or repeated courses of antilymphocyte preparations, episodes of allograft rejection, comorbid illnesses, and neutropenia. Management of CMV infection consists of preventive (prophylactic and/or preemptive therapy) and therapeutic measures. Prophylactic therapy involves antiviral therapy beginning in the immediate postoperative period whereas preemptive therapy involves treatment of those who are found to seroconvert during surveillance studies. Treatment of established CMV disease consists of 2–3 weeks of intravenous ganciclovir followed by a 2- to 4-month course of oral ganciclovir or valganciclovir. In patients slow to respond to therapy the addition of CMV hyperimmune globulin can be of therapeutic benefit. Although oral valganciclovir provides good bioavailability, its use in the treatment of CMV disease has not been well studied. A suggested CMV prophylaxis protocol is shown in Table 53–13.

2. *Candida* fungal infections—*Candida* spp. are the most common fungal pathogens encountered in the immunocompromised transplant recipients, with *C albicans* and *C tropicalis* accounting for 90% of the infections followed by *C glabrata.* Diabetes mellitus, high-dose corticosteroids, and broad spectrum antibacterial therapy predispose patients to mucocutaneous candidal infections such as oral candidiasis, intertriginous candidal infections, candidal esophagitis, candidal vaginitis, and candidal UTIs. Superficial infections involving the mouth or intertriginous areas can be treated with nystatin and topical chlortrimazole whereas candidal UTIs require amphotericin B bladder washing or systemic antifungal therapy with fluconazole, amphotericin B (preferably in the lipid preparation), or caspofungin for fluconazole-resistant species. Whenever possible, foreign objects such as a bladder catheter, surgical drains (such as a percutaneous nephrostomy tube), and urinary stents should be removed.

3. Polyomavirus infection—The polyomaviruses are non-enveloped double-stranded DNA viruses. BK and JC viruses are the two strains associated with disease in humans and are named after the initials of the patients in whom they were first isolated. Over the past decade BK virus-associated nephropathy has emerged as an important cause of allograft failure following renal transplantation, whereas the pathogenic role of JC virus in allograft nephropathy remains to be defined.

Table 53–13. Cytomegalovirus (CMV) prophylaxis protocol.[1]

For CMV (−) recipients of a CMV (−) organ
Acyclovir 400 mg daily (or valganciclovir 450 mg daily) × 3 months
CMV DNA every 2 weeks × 3 months

For CMV (−) recipients of a CMV (+) organ
During antibody treatment DHPG[2] 2.5 mg/kg intravenously every day
Following antibody treatment valganciclovir 900 mg orally every day × 6 months
If no antibody treatment: valganciclovir 900 mg every day for 6 months
CMV DNA every 2 weeks × 3 months

For CMV (+) recipients of a CMV (−) organ
During antibody treatment DHPG 2.5 mg/kg intravenously every day
Following antibody treatment valganciclovir 900 mg orally every day × 6 months
If no antibody treatment: acyclovir 400 mg daily (or valganciclovir 450 mg daily) × 3 months
CMV DNA every 2 weeks × 3 months

For CMV (+) recipients of a CMV (+) organ
During antibody treatment DHPG 2.5 mg/kg intravenously every day
Following antibody treatment valganciclovir 900 mg orally every day × 6 months
If no antibody treatment: acyclovir 400 mg daily (or valganciclovir 450 mg daily)[3] × 3 months
CMV DNA every 2 weeks × 3 months

[1]If CMV status is unknown, give 9-(1,3-dihydroxy-2-propoxymethyl) guanine (DHPG) intravenously until the CMV status is determined.
[2]Dose adjustment for renal function is necessary.
[3]Although low-dose valganciclovir 450 mg daily has been shown to be effective, recent guidelines from the Canadian Society of Transplantation Consensus Workshop on CMV management recommend dosing valganciclovir 900 mg daily for CMV (+) recipients of a CMV (+) organ (kidney, liver, pancreas, heart). Am J Transplant 2005: 218.

BK virus is a ubiquitous human virus with a peak incidence of primary infection in children 2–5 years of age and a seroprevalence rate of greater than 60–90% among the adult population worldwide. Following primary infection, the BK virus preferentially establishes latency within the genitourinary tract and frequently reactivates in the setting of immunosuppression. In renal transplant recipients, the BK virus has been shown to be associated with a range of clinical syndromes including asymptomatic viuria with or without viremia, ureteral stenosis and obstruction, interstitial nephritis, and BK allograft nephropathy. In most series it has been reported that 30–40% of renal transplant recipients develop BK viuria, 10–20% develop BK viremia, and 2–5% develop BK nephropathy (BKN).

BK nephropathy most commonly presents with an asymptomatic rise in serum creatinine between 2 and 60 months (median 9 months). The diagnosis of BKN is made by allograft biopsy showing BK virus inclusions in renal tubular and glomerular epithelial cells. Variable degrees of interstitial inflammation, degenerative changes in tubules, and focal tubulitis can be seen and may mimic acute tubular necrosis (ATN) or acute rejection. In the absence of classic histologic findings, distinguishing between BKN, acute rejection, and the concomitant presence of both processes can be a diagnostic challenge. Additional ancillary studies such as immunohistochemistry, *in situ* hybridization, or electron microscopy are required to confirm the diagnosis. Urine cytology for decoy cells or quantitative determinations of viuria and of viral load in blood have been proposed as surrogate markers for the diagnosis of BKN. In the late stage of BKN, few characteristic intranuclear inclusions are seen and the histopathologic changes are indistinguishable from those of chronic allograft nephropathy including interstitial fibrosis and scarring.

There has been no well-defined protocol for the treatment of BKN. The current mainstay of treatment includes a reduction or discontinuation of antimetabolites in conjunction with a judicious reduction in calcineurin inhibitor therapy or other components of the immunosuppressive regimen. The level of reduction in immunosuppression, however, has not been clearly defined. Switching from tacrolimus to cyclosporine or to sirolimus has resulted in resolution of BKN and viremia/viuria in anecdotal case reports. Adjunctive antiviral therapy with cidofovir or leflunomide has been used with variable response rates. Low-dose cidifovir (0.25–0.33 mg/kg intravenously biweekly) may be of therapeutic benefit in refractory cases. Despite various treatment strategies, up to 30–50% of patients with established BKN experienced a progressive decline in renal function and graft loss. Early diagnosis and intervention may improve the prognosis. Intensive monitoring of urine and serum for BK by polymerase chain reaction (PCR) during the first year posttransplantation and preemptive withdrawal of immunosuppression have been shown to be associated with resolution of viremia and an absence of BK nephropathy without acute rejection or graft loss. More recently, an independent panel of experts have suggested that all renal transplant recipients should be screened for BKV replication in the urine (1) every 3 months during the first 2 years posttransplant, (2) when allograft dysfunction is noted, and (3) when an allograft biopsy is performed. A positive screening result should be confirmed in <4 weeks and assessed by quantitative assays (eg, BKV DNA or RNA load in plasma or urine). A definitive diagnosis of BKN requires an allograft biopsy. In the absence of active viral replication, patients with graft loss due to BKN can safely undergo retransplantation. Active surveillance for BK virus reactivation after transplantation is recommended.

Crew RJ et al: De novo thrombotic microangiopathy following treatment with sirolimus: report of 2 cases. Nephrol Dial Transpl 2005;20:203.

Fishman JA, Ramos E: Infection in renal transplant recipients. In: *Chronic Kidney Disease, Dialysis, and Transplantation*, ed 2. Perira BJG et al (editors). Elsevier Saunders, 2005.

Kubak BM et al: Infections in kidney transplantation. In: *Handbook of Kidney Transplantation*, ed 4. Danovitch GM (editor). Lippincott, Williams & Wilkins, 2005.

Pham PT et al: Diagnosis and therapy of graft dysfunction. In: *Chronic Kidney Disease: Dialysis and Transplantation*, ed 2. Sayegh MH et al (editors). W.B. Saunders, 2005.

Pham PT et al: Management of the transplant recipient in the early postoperative period. In: *Oxford Textbook of Clinical Nephrology*, ed 3. Davison AM et al (editors). Oxford University Press, 2005.

Singer J et al: The transplant operation and its surgical complications. In: *Handbook of Kidney Transplantation*, ed 4. Danovitch GM (editor). Lippincott, Williams & Wilkins, 2005.

Stallone G et al: Addition of sirolimus to cyclosporine delays the recovery of delayed graft function but does not affect 1-year graft function. J Am Soc Nephrol 2004;15(1):228.

Warren DS et al: Successful renal transplantation across simultaneous ABO incompatible and positive crossmatch barriers. Am J Transplant 2004;4:561.

Wali RK et al: BK virus-associated nephropathy in renal allograft recipients: rescue therapy by sirolimus-based immunosuppression. Transplantation 2004;74:1069.

Williams JW et al: Leflunomide for polyoma type BK nephropathy. N Engl J Med 2005;352:1157.

▶ Treatment

In this section the mechanisms of action of various immunosuppressive agents, the basic principles of immunosuppressive protocols, the use of immunosuppressive agents in the treatment of acute rejection, and the potential adverse effects of immunosuppressive medications and important drug–drug interaction are discussed.

A. The Three-Signal Model of Alloimmune Responses

T cell activation requires three signals (Figure 53–1). The first signal (*signal 1*) is initiated by the binding of the alloantigen on the surface of antigen-presenting cells (APCs) to the T cell receptor (TCR)–CD3 complex. *Signal 2* is a non-antigen-specific costimulatory signal provided by the engagement of CD80 and CD86 on the surface of APCs with CD28 on T cells. These dual signals activate the intracellular pathways that trigger T cells to activate IL-2 and other growth-promoting cytokine genes. IL-2 will in turn engage its receptor and activate the mammalian target of rapamycin (mTOR) pathway to provide *signal 3*, and lead to cell proliferation. If a T cell receptor is triggered without the accompanying costimulatory *signal 2*, the T cell is driven into an anergic state in which it is both inactivated and refractory to later

activation when all necessary activation elements are present. These observations have led to the concept of induction of graft tolerance or adaptation through agents that target the costimulatory pathways.

Immunosuppressive agents that target *signal 1* include the monoclonal antibody OKT3 and polyclonal antibodies such as antithymocyte globulins directed against the CD3 molecule and a variety of T cell markers. The calcineurin inhibitors cyclosporine and tacrolimus inhibit intracellular *signal 1* transduction. There are currently no clinically approved agents that target *signal 2*, although LEA29Y, which binds CD80 and CD86 with high affinity and inhibits the costimulatory pathway, is a new promising agent that is currently in phase II clinical trials. Agents that target *signal 3* include baxiliximab and daclizumab, which are humanized monoclonal antibodies targeted against the IL-2 receptor, and sirolimus, which blocks *signal 3* by preventing cytokine receptors from activating the cell cycle. Lymphocyte proliferation, which requires the synthesis of purine and pyrimidine nucleotides, is inhibited by the antimetabolites azathioprine and MMF. The sites of actions of other immunosuppressive agents that are under clinical development are shown in Figure 53–1.

B. Immunosuppressive Drugs in the Three-Signal Model

1. Anti-CD3 monoclonal antibodies—The monoclonal antibody muromonab-CD3, also known as OKT3, is a murine IgG_2 monoclonal antibody targeting the ε-chain of the CD3 receptor complex. The subsequent deactivation of the CD3 complex causes the T cell receptor to undergo endocytosis. The latter process renders the T cells ineffectual and within an hour of OKT3 administration the T cells disappear from the circulation as a result of opsonization and subsequent removal from the circulation by mononuclear cells in the liver and spleen. After the first dose, OKT3 can cause an initial transient T cell activation and release of several cytokines including IL-2, TNF, IFN-γ, and IL-6 that are responsible for the "first dose cytokine release syndrome." Clinically, patients may develop fevers, chills, rigors, headaches, pulmonary edema, and, less commonly, aseptic meningitis, acute respiratory distress syndrome (ARDS), and encephalopathy. To alleviate the severity of the cytokine release syndrome patients should be kept euvolemic and premedicated with intravenous methylprednisolone, diphenhydramine hydrochloride, and acetaminophen. Repeated use of OKT3 can result in loss of efficacy due to the potential development of high titers of neutralizing human antimurine antibodies.

2. Polyclonal antithymocyte globulin: antithymocyte γ-globulin and thymoglobulin—Polyclonal antithymocyte globulin (ATG) is obtained by immunizing animals with human lymphoid cells. Antithymocyte γ-globulin (ATGAM) is produced by immunization of horses with human lymphoid material whereas thymoglobulin is made by immunizing rabbits with human lymphoid tissue. The immune

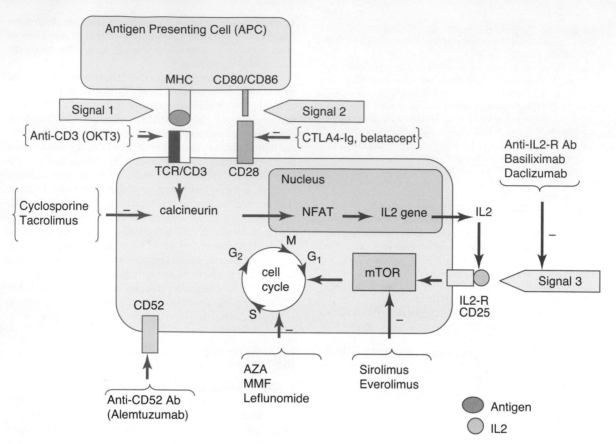

▲ **Figure 53–1.** The three-signal model of the alloimmune responses. Alemtuzumab binds to CD52 on T and B cells, causing cell lysis and profound and prolonged lymphocyte depletion. Leflunomide (Arava) inhibits *de novo* pyrimidine synthesis. APC, antigen-presenting cell; MHC, major histocompatibility complex; TCR/CD3, T cell receptor/CD3 complex; NFAT, nuclear factor of activated T cells; IL-2R; IL-2 receptor; Ab, antibody; AZA, azathioprine; MMF, mycophenolate mofetil; mTOR, mammalian target of rapamycin.

sera are harvested and processed to obtain purified globulin. The resultant product contains antibodies targeting against a number of T cell surface markers including CD3, CD4, and CD8. Similar to OKT3, the polyclonal antibodies are xenogeneic proteins and can induce a number of side effects including fevers, chills, and arthralgia. ATG, however, does not cause the severe first-dose reactions seen with OKT3. Other severe adverse reactions such as serum-sickness syndrome and anaphylaxis are rarely seen. Nevertheless, patients receiving ATG should also be premedicated as with OKT3.

3. The calcineurin inhibitors: cyclosporine and tacrolimus—Cyclosporine is a highly hydrophobic cyclic endecapeptide isolated from *Tolypocladium inflatum* Gams, whereas tacrolimus is a macrocyclic lactone isolated from actinomycetes. Despite their distinct chemical structures, cyclosporine and tacrolimus share a common mechanism

of action. The adverse effects of cyclosporine include nephrotoxicity, hypertension, hyperlipidemia, gingival hyperplasia, posttransplant diabetes mellitus (PTDM), neurotoxicity, hirsutism, and, less commonly, thrombotic microangiopathy. Commonly encountered laboratory abnormalities include hyperkalemia, hypomagnesemia, and hyperuricemia. The adverse effects of tacrolimus are similar to those of cyclosporine but with a lower incidence of hypertension, hyperlipidemia, hirsutism, gingival hyperplasia, and hyperuricemia, and a higher incidence of PTDM, neurotoxicity, gastrointestinal disturbances, and alopecia. Recently, monitoring of cyclosporine levels 2 hours after administration (C_2, compared to the trough level, C_0) may better reflect drug exposure thereby avoiding overexposure or underexposure to the drug. The former may alleviate nephrotoxicity whereas the latter may prevent acute rejection episodes. Trough drug level monitoring is required for tacrolimus.

4. Target of rapamycin inhibitors: sirolimus and everolimus—Sirolimus (rapamycin) is a macrocyclic lactone isolated from *Streptomyces hygroscopicus*. It was discovered in 1975 in the region of Rapa Nui, Easter Island. Sirolimus was first shown to inhibit the growth of yeast and fungi and was subsequently explored as an antitumor and immunosuppressive agent. Everolimus is an analog of sirolimus with a shorter half-life but with similar immunosuppressive mechanism and side effect profile. Although sirolimus is structurally related to tacrolimus and both engage the same FKBP-12, sirolimus has a mechanism of action that is distinct from that of tacrolimus. Commonly encountered adverse effects of sirolimus and everolimus include hyperlipidemia, particularly hypertriglyceridemia, increased CNI nephrotoxicity, mouth ulcers, thrombocytopenia, and impaired wound healing. Other reported side effects include proteinuria, peripheral edema, delayed recovery from ATN or delayed graft function, reduced testosterone concentration, and pulmonary toxicity.

5. Humanized anti-CD25 monoclonal antibodies: basiliximab and daclizumab—Basiliximab (Simulect) is a genetically engineered murine—human *chimeric* monoclonal antibody consisting of a variable region of murine origin and a human constant region. Daclizumab (Zenapax) is a *humanized* monoclonal antibody consisting of a murine hypervariable antibody-binding site and a human IgG$_1$ framework (Figure 53–2). Both agents target the α chain of the IL-2 receptor (CD25 or Tac) thereby blocking *signal 3*. Unlike OKT3 or ATG that target all T cells, the anti-IL-2 receptor inhibitors bind only to activated T cells that have up-regulated the α chain of the IL-2 receptor, hence complementing the effect of the CNIs. In contrast to OKT3 and the ATGs, basiliximab and daclizumab have a prolonged serum half-life and lack immunogenicity, presumably due to the "more humanized" nature of the constructs. Clinical trials leading to their approval for use in renal transplantation revealed minimal toxicity.

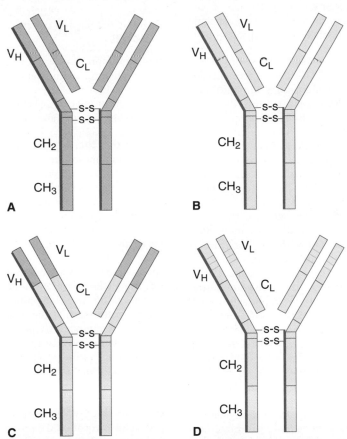

▲ **Figure 53–2.** Chimeric versus humanized monoclonal antibodies (mAbs)(basiliximab versus daclizumab). **A:** The structures of the fully xenogeneic mouse mAb. **B:** Human mAb. **C:** Basiliximab, a mouse–human chimeric mAb. **D:** Daclizumab, a humanized mAb. Chimeric mAbs consist of human constant regions (CH) and mouse heavy and light chain variable (V$_H$, V$_L$) regions. In contrast, humanized mAbs consist of human IgG$_1$ frameworks and only the complementary determining regions (shown as red stripes) are of mouse origin.

6. Antimetabolite agents: azathioprine and mycophenolic acid

A. AZATHIOPRINE (IMURAN)—The immunosuppressive mechanism of action of azathioprine (AZA) is related to its inhibition of gene replication and consequent T cell activation. It is a purine analog that is incorporated into cellular deoxyribonucleic acid (DNA) where it inhibits purine nucleotide synthesis and interferes with the synthesis and metabolism of ribonucleic acid (RNA). AZA was the first immunosuppressive agent introduced into clinical transplantation and was widely used with steroids as maintenance immunosuppression until the introduction of cyclosporine in the early 1980s. With the dramatic improvement in graft survival seen with cyclosporine, AZA became the second-line immunosuppressive agent and later became an adjunctive agent in a triple regimen that consisted of cyclosporine, prednisone, and AZA. With the advent of the newer inhibitor of nucleoside synthesis MMF, AZA has largely been replaced by MMF as adjunctive immunosuppressive therapy. The use of AZA has been associated with bone marrow toxicity, leukopenia, macrocytosis, and, less commonly, hepatotoxicity.

B. MYCOPHENOLATE MOFETIL—MMF is a semisynthetic derivative of mycophenolic acid (MPA), a fermentation product of the fungus penicillium. After oral administration, MMF is rapidly and completely converted to MPA, which is a reversible inhibitor of the rate-limiting enzyme inosine monophosphate dehydrogenase (IMPDH) required in the *de novo* synthesis of purines. In contrast to other cell types that can use the *salvage* pathway for the production of guanosine nucleotides from guanine, lymphocytes are primarily dependent on *de novo* purine biosynthesis. Hence, depletion of guanosine nucleotides by MPA has relative selective antiproliferative effects on B and T lymphocytes. Three large multicenter studies have shown that MMF was more effective than AZA in the prevention of acute rejection episodes in recipients of deceased donor renal transplants when used in combination with cyclosporine and prednisone. Consequently, it was approved by the Food and Drug Administration (FDA) in 1995 for use in rejection prophylaxis in renal transplantation. The most common adverse effects of MMF are related to the gastrointestinal tract and include diarrhea, nausea, vomiting, flatulence, and dyspepsia. Dose reduction or transient discontinuation of the drug or dividing the dose into three or four times a day often results in symptomatic relief. The enteric-coated formulation of MPA (Myfortic), developed to improve gastrointestinal tolerability, has not been shown to be significantly better than the original formulation, although there tends to be fewer gastrointestinal side effects. Leukopenia and anemia are common hematologic adverse effects of MPA that often resolve with dose reduction or transient drug discontinuation.

7. Corticosteroids

Steroids have been used in the prevention and treatment of episodes of acute rejection since the early 1960s. The immunosuppressive effect of steroids is due to specific immunologic processes as well as to nonspecific immunosuppressant and anti-inflammatory responses. Steroids inhibit the expression of several cytokine gene including IL-1, IL-2, IL-3, IL-6, TNF, and IFN. As a result, essentially all stages of T cell activation are inhibited. Nonspecific immunosuppressive effects of steroids may include redistribution of lymphocytes from the vascular compartment back to lymphoid tissues, inhibition of monocyte migration to inflammatory sites, and inhibition of the synthesis and action of chemoattractants and vasodilators. Well-established adverse effects of steroids include growth impairment, weight gain, Cushing's facies, avascular necrosis, osteoporosis, impaired wound healing, cataracts, hyperlipidemia, and posttransplant glucose intolerance or diabetes mellitus.

C. Drug–Drug Interactions

Important drug–drug interactions are shown in Table 53–14.

D. Basic Principles of Immunosuppressive Protocols

Immunosuppression for transplantation can be classified into induction, maintenance therapy, and treatment of acute rejection. The use of immunosuppressive agents in the treatment of acute rejection is discussed under postoperative complications and management.

1. Induction therapy—Induction therapy is referred to the intense immunosuppression in the first day or weeks after transplantation. Both polyclonal and monoclonal antibodies have been used for induction therapy since the 1970s after it was demonstrated that antilymphocyte globulin (ALG) reduced the episodes of acute rejection in renal transplant recipients. Their beneficial effect is derived from depleting the recipients of CD3-positive cells at the time of transplantation. Although OKT3 and thymoglobulin were initially approved for use as antirejection therapy, these agents have increasingly been used as induction agents under different contexts such as rejection prophylaxis in high-immunologic-risk recipients (such as those with high panel reactive antibodies or retransplant recipients), DGF, and, more recently, in corticosteroid avoidance or withdrawal protocols and in CNI-sparing regimens. The use of lymphocyte-depleting antibodies, however, is not without severe adverse effects. ATGAM, thymoglobulin, and OKT3 use has been associated with an increased incidence of posttransplant lymphoproliferative disease, CMV infections, and other infectious complications. Adequate CMV prophylaxis should be an integral part of the antibody treatment protocol.

Induction therapy with the anti-IL-2R monoclonal antibodies daclizumab and basiliximab, the "so-called nondepleting antibodies," became popular in the early 2000s when phase III clinical trials revealed that patients receiving these agents had significantly lower acute rejection rates compared to those

Table 53–14. Drug–drug interactions.[1]

Drugs that decrease the CNI level by induction of P450 activity

Antituberculous drug	Rifampin > rifabutin
Anticonvulsants	Barbiturates > phenytoin > carbamazepine
Antidepressant herbal preparation	*Hypericum perforatum* (St.John's wort)
Others (less well established/case reports)	Nafcillin, intravenous trimethoprim, imipenem, cephalosporins, terbinafine

Drugs that increase the CNI level by inhibition of P450 or by competition for its pathways

Calcium channel blockers[2]	Verapamil, diltiazem > amlodipine, nicardipine
Antifungal agents	Ketoconazole, fluconazole, itraconazole
Antibiotics	Erythromycin > other macrolide antibiotics[3]
Antiretroviral agents (protease inhibitors)	clarithromycin, josamycin, ponsinomycin
Others (less well established)	Ritonavir (used alone or in combination; ritonavir/lopinavir "kaletra")
	Amiodarone, carvedilol, allopurinol, bromocriptine, chloroquine

Important drugs/food that increase the absorption of CNIs

Metoclopramide

Grapefruit juice

Drugs that may potentiate CNI toxicity

Amphotericin, aminoglycosides,

NSAIDs

Sirolimus

Lipid-lowering agents

The statins[4] or HMG-CoA reductase inhibitors + CNI (particularly cyclosporine) have a much greater risk of myopathy/rhabdomyolysis

[1]This table provides only a general guideline. Physicians should see drug packet inserts for full drug–drug interactions. CNI, calcineurin inhibitor; NSAIDs, nonsteroidal anti-inflammatory drugs; HMG-CoA, 3-hydroxy-3-methylglutaryl coenzyme A.

[2]Nifedipine, isradipine, and felodipine have minimal effects on CNI levels.

[3]Azithromycin does not increase CNI levels.

[4]The lowest dose should be introduced; any increase in dose requires close monitoring. Cases of acute renal failure have been seen with lovastatin.

who did not receive induction therapy. Studies comparing the effectiveness and safety of basiliximab versus thymoglobulin induction therapy in low-immunologic-risk patients showed similar acute rejection rates and overall outcome. However, a higher incidence of side effects was seen in patients receiving thymoglobulin. In contrast, studies involving high-immunologic-risk patients [defined as retransplants, plasma renin activity (PRA) >20%, those with expected delayed graft function, six antigen mismatch, and African-American recipients] demonstrated a significantly lower incidence of acute rejection and graft loss in patients receiving thymoglobulin.

Although the choice of induction therapy with depleting (ATGAM, thymoglobulin, OKT3) versus nondepleting (basiliximab, daclizumab) antibodies is largely center dependent, in general, the lymphocyte-depleting antibodies are being used in high-immunologic-risk patients due to their greater efficacy, whereas the nondepleting antibodies are used in low-to moderate-risk candidates due to their more favorable side-effect profile. Thymoglobulin has essentially displaced ATGAM and OKT3 because of its greater efficacy and lack of severe first-dose reaction, respectively.

2. Maintenance immunosuppression—The CNIs cyclosporine and tacrolimus have been the mainstay of maintenance immunosuppression for the past one and a half to two decades. A traditional or "conventional" immunosuppressive protocol generally consists of a CNI (cyclosporine or tacrolimus), an antimetabolite (AZA or MMF), and prednisone, with or without induction therapy. With the introduction of sirolimus and the availability of newer agents used for induction therapy, CNI-sparing or steroid-withdrawal protocols are being increasingly used by a number of transplant centers. Although the choice of immunosuppressive therapy varies widely among centers, the ultimate goal of the transplant physician is to select a regimen that will optimize graft and patient survival while minimizing adverse effects. Reducing acute rejection rates, minimizing nephrotoxicity, lowering the incidence of dyslipidemia, post-transplant diabetes mellitus, and hypertension, and minimizing cosmetic side effects are among the important factors to consider when selecting an immunosuppressive regimen.

A. Tacrolimus versus cyclosporine—In general, tacrolimus is the preferred agent in adolescents and young women because of its lack of significant cosmetic changes and in higher immunologic risk recipients because of its somewhat greater immunosuppressive potency compared to cyclosporine. Several comparative studies have demonstrated that compared to cyclosporine, tacrolimus-based immunosuppression is associated with a lower incidence of acute rejection episodes, although this has not consistently been shown to translate into improving graft survival rates. Independent investigators have also suggested that steroid withdrawal may be safer for tacrolimus- than for cyclosporine-treated patients.

Compared to cyclosporine, tacrolimus has been shown to have a more favorable effect on hypertension and the lipid profile and is often preferred over cyclosporine in recipient

Table 53–15. Immunosuppressive protocols.

Conventional immunosuppressive protocol
Antibody induction at the discretion of the clinician

CNI-based: Cyclosporine or tacrolimus

+ Prednisone

+ Adjunctive agent: MMF or azathioprine

Current commonly used standard immunosuppressive protocols
IL-2R antibody induction[1]

CNI-based: Cyclosporine or tacrolimus

+ Prednisone

+ Adjunctive agent: MMF or sirolimus

Steroid-withdrawal protocols[2]
IL-2R antibody induction + corticosteroids (rapid taper followed by withdrawal at the discretion of the transplant physician)

CNI + MMF (or sirolimus) maintenance therapy

CNI-withdrawal protocols[3]
Induction therapy

Sirolimus + prednisone + cyclosporine (discontinued at 3 months posttransplant)

Sirolimus + prednisone maintenance therapy

CNI, calcineurin inhibitor; MMF, mycophenolate mofetil; IL-2R, interleukin 2R.
[1]Routinely used by most transplant programs in low- to moderate-risk renal transplant recipients.
[2]Used in low-risk renal transplant recipients [first transplant, non-sensitized or low plasma renin activity (PRA) candidates, non-African-Americans].
[3]Preliminary results revealed increased acute rejection rates at 12 months. Further studies are needed.

with difficult to control hypertension or severe dyslipidemia; however, recent studies have shown that conversion from cyclosporine trough level monitoring (C_0) to 2 hour cyclosporine peak level monitoring (C_2) in stable renal transplant recipients results in improvement in hypertension and hyperlipidemia control. In recipients who are at increased risk for posttransplant impaired glucose tolerance or posttransplant diabetes mellitus, cyclosporine may be the preferred agent. These recipients may include African-Americans, Hispanics, and recipients who are older, obese, and/or have a strong family history of type 2 diabetes mellitus. Recent studies demonstrated that the incidence of diabetes mellitus might be reduced when lower trough tacrolimus levels are used.

B. Sirolimus—In low-immunologic-risk recipients, sirolimus has increasingly been used in CNI-sparing or steroid-withdrawal protocols. Complete cyclosporine withdrawal in a regimen consisting of cyclosporine, sirolimus, and a corticosteroid has been shown to increase the risk of late acute rejection, particularly among high-risk transplant recipients. Clinically significant adverse effects of sirolimus when used in combination therapy with a CNI may include an increase in CNI nephrotoxicity and worsening dyslipidemia, particularly hypertriglyceridemia. Drug level monitoring, particularly in the early posttransplant period, is mandatory. In patients with gastrointestinal intolerance to MMF, sirolimus has been used as an adjunctive agent in combination therapy with a CNI. Although sirolimus may theoretically be the drug of choice in recipients with a history of malignancy or who develop malignancy posttransplant due to its antiproliferative or "antitumor" effect, further studies are needed.

C. Azathioprine versus mycophenolate mofetil—Three phase III clinical trials have shown that MMF is more effective than AZA in the prevention of acute rejection in recipients of deceased donor kidney transplant when used in combination therapy with cyclosporine and prednisone. Hence AZA has largely been replaced by MMF as an adjunctive immunosuppressive therapy.

Table 53–15 lists some of the commonly used immunosuppressive regimens. However, it should be noted that the choice of an immunosuppressive regimen should best be individualized.

Cianco G et al: A randomized long-term trial of tacrolimus and sirolimus versus tacrolimus and mycophenolate mofetil versus cyclosporine (Neoral) and sirolimus in renal transplantation. I. Drug interactions and rejection at one year. Transplantation 2004;77:244.

Cianco G et al: A randomized long-term trial of tacrolimus and sirolimus versus tacrolimus and mycophenolate mofetil versus cyclosporine (Neoral) and sirolimus in renal transplantation. II. Survival, function and protocol compliance at 1 year. Transplantation 2004;78(2):252.

Cianco G et al: The use of Campath-1H as induction therapy in renal transplant: preliminary results. Transplantation 2004;78(3):426.

Cittero F et al: Results of a three-year prospective study of C2 monitoring in long-term renal transplant recipients receiving cyclosporine microemulsion. Transplantation 2005;79(7):802.

Danovitch GM: Immunosuppressive medications and protocols for kidney transplantation. In: *Handbook of Kidney Transplantation*, ed 4. Danovitch GM (editor). Lippincott, Williams & Wilkins, 2005.

First R, Fitzsimmons WE: Modified release tacrolimus. Yonsei Med J 2004;45(6):1127.

Halloran PF: Immunosuppressive drugs for kidney transplantation. N Engl J Med 2004;351:2715.

Pham PT et al: Sirolimus-associated pulmonary toxicity. Transplantation 2004;77:1215.

Vicenti F, Rostaing L: Rationale and design of the DIRECT Study; a comparative assessment of the hyperglycemic effects of tacrolimus and cyclosporine following renal transplantation. Contemp Clin Trials 2005;26:17.

Webster AC et al: Interleukin 2 receptor antagonist for renal transplant recipients: a meta-analysis of randomized trials. Transplantation 2004;77:166.

Diabetic Nephropathy

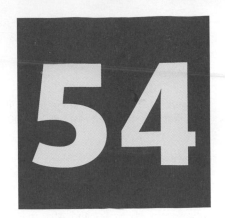

Yalemzewd Woredekal, MD, & Eli A. Friedman, MD

ESSENTIALS OF DIAGNOSIS

► Afflicts 35–40% of type 1 and type 2 diabetics with an increasing incidence associated with type 2 diabetes mellitus.

► An initial period of glomerular hyperfiltration.

► Progressively increasing proteinuria.

► A gradual decline in the glomerular filtration rate (GFR).

► Results in renal failure.

▶ General Considerations

Diabetic nephropathy is a serious public health concern because it has become the leading cause of end-stage renal disease (ESRD) in most developed countries and is associated with increased cardiovascular mortality. Tracking both the incidence and prevalence of ESRD attributed to diabetes underscores its annual growth rate over the past decade in excess of 9%. According to the 2004 report of the U.S. Renal Data System (USRDS), in 2002, of 419,263 patients in the United States receiving either dialytic therapy or a kidney transplant, 149,614 had diabetes, a prevalence rate of 35.6%. The incidence rate was 44.5% in 2002, with 42,665 of 149,614 new (incident) cases of ESRD attributed to diabetes (Figure 54–1). This increase is mainly attributed to an increase in the occurrence of diabetes, especially type 2 diabetes; the extended life span of diabetic patients due to improved management of comorbid conditions; and the acceptance of patients for replacement therapy who in the past were excluded.

Diabetic nephropathy is characterized by an initial period of glomerular hyperfiltration associated with progressively increasing proteinuria, followed by a gradual decline in the GFR, eventually resulting in renal failure. Diabetic nephropathy afflicts 35–40% of type 1 and type 2 diabetic patients. While the natural history of diabetic nephropathy is well studied in type 1 diabetic patients, recent studies have shown a similar course of diabetic nephropathy in type 2 diabetic patients as well. In the past 2 decades, much has been learned about the possible pathogenesis of diabetic nephropathy leading to the development and use of specific therapies that have been effective in slowing progression to renal failure.

A cumulative incidence of diabetic nephropathy has been documented after 20–25 years of diabetes in both type 1 and type 2 individuals. Recent studies demonstrated that present treatment strategies substantially reduce the progression and incidence of diabetic nephropathy in type 1 diabetes. For example, a study from Sweden showed a substantial decline in albuminuria after 25 years of diabetes from 30% in patients in whom diabetes developed from 1961 to 1965 to 8.5% in those with onset from 1966 to 1970 and 13% in those diagnosed from 1971 to 1975. Similarly, the Steno Diabetes Center reported that in the same cohorts, the cumulative incidence of diabetic nephropathy after 20 years fell from 31.3% to 13.7%. Improved glycemic control, better control of blood pressure, and reduced prevalence of smoking were associated with the lower incidence of nephropathy.

In contrast to the decreasing incidence of diabetic nephropathy in type 1 diabetes, the incidence of diabetic nephropathy associated with type 2 diabetes mellitus has been increasing over the past 50 years, so that in the United States about 44% of all patients beginning ESRD replacement therapy have diabetes compared to 25–50% in Europe and about 25% in Australia. The incidence of diabetic nephropathy is about 1–2% per year in patients with type 1 diabetes.

Among young nonwhite patients with type 2 diabetes, such as Pima Indians, Japanese, and African-Americans, the incidence of nephropathy is similar to that of type 1 diabetes. However, the incidence of diabetic nephropathy is much lower in elderly white type 2 diabetic patients than in nonwhite patients.

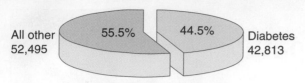

▲ **Figure 54–1.** New end-stage renal disease patients with diabetes, reported at 44.5% in 2003.

Several large population-based studies found substantial racial and ethnic differences in the incidence rate of ESRD attributed to type 2 diabetes. The highest incidence of ESRD secondary to diabetes has been reported in Native Americans followed by Hispanics and African-Americans. In Pima Indians the cumulative incidence of ESRD after the onset of clinically detectable proteinuria is 40% at 10 years and 61% at 15 years. By contrast, ESRD developed in only 11% of white patients after 10 years of proteinuria and in 17% after 15 years. These ethnic and racial differences in the incidence of diabetic nephropathy reflect a complex and still poorly understood interplay between genetic and environmental factors.

Among patients starting renal replacement therapy, the incidence of diabetic nephropathy doubled from the years 1991 to 2001. Fortunately, the rate of increase is slowing down, probably because of adoption in clinical practice of several measures that contribute to the early diagnosis and delay of diabetic nephropathy, thereby slowing the progression to clinically noted renal disease. However, implementation of effective preemptive therapy in diabetic patients falls far below desirable goals.

Nordwall M et al: Declining incidence of severe retinopathy and persisting decrease of nephropathy in an unselected population of type I diabetes—the Linkoping Diabetes Complication Study. Diabetologia 2004;47:1266.

Rossing K et al: Progression of nephropathy in type 2 diabetic patients. Kidney Int 2004;66:1596.

US Renal Data System: USRDS 2004 Annual Data Report: Bethesda, MD, National Institutes of Health, National Institute of Diabetes and Digestive and Kidney Diseases, 2004.

▶ **Pathogenesis**

The key to the development of diabetic nephropathy is hyperglycemia, which is postulated to mediate its effects in several different ways. First, glucose in high concentrations may be directly toxic to cells, altering cell growth and gene and protein expression, thus increasing extracellular matrix (ECM) and growth factor production. Second, hyperglycemia may induce its adverse effect indirectly through the formation of metabolic end products such as oxidative and glycation products. *In vitro*, transforming growth factor (TGF)-β modulates ECM production in glomerular mesangial and epithelial cells. In addition, TGF-β inhibits the synthesis of collagenases and stimulates production of metalloproteinase inhibitors, an effect that could lead to reduced degradation of ECM and hence ECM accumulation. High glucose concentrations also increase TGF-β mRNA expression in renal cells, stimulating TGF-β mRNA expression and bioactivity, cellular hypertrophy, and collagen transcription in proximal tubules, providing *in vitro* evidence for a role of TGF-β in the development of diabetic nephropathy.

Three of several pathways by which hyperglycemia may induce diabetic nephropathy are actively being explored.

A. Advanced Glycation End-Products

In health, reducing sugars such as glucose react nonenzymatically and reversibly with free amino groups in proteins to form small amounts of stable Amadori products (eg, hemoglobin A_{1c}) through Schiff base adducts. In normal aging, spontaneous further irreversible modification of proteins by glucose results in the formation of advanced glycation endproducts (AGEs), a heterogeneous family of biologically and chemically reactive compounds with cross-linking properties. This process of protein modification is amplified by the high ambient glucose concentration present in diabetes. In cultured glomerular endothelial and mesangial cells *in vitro*, glycated albumin and AGE-rich proteins have been shown to enhance the expression of type IV collagen and TGF-β1 and increase protein kinase C (PKC) activity. When performed under physiological glucose conditions, *in vitro* studies provide evidence that early glycation products may contribute to the pathogenesis of diabetic glomerulopathy independently of glucose.

Aminoguanidine, a hydrazine-like compound, reacts with early glycation products inhibiting further AGE formation. Aminoguanidine retards the development of nephropathy and other complications of diabetes in long-term experimental rats.

Other AGE inhibitors and AGE cross-link breakers are able to ameliorate diabetic nephropathy in experimental animals.

B. Aldose Reductase Pathway

The enzyme aldose reductase (AR) converts a variety of toxic aldehyde derivatives from lipid peroxidation to inactive alcohol.

AR is the rate-limiting enzyme in the polyol pathway, and facilitates the reduction of glucose to sorbitol. Sorbitol dehydrogenase converts sorbitol to fructose using nicotinamide adenine dinucleotide (NAD). In hyperglycemia, when the pathway of glucose to glucose-6-phosphate is saturated, excess glucose enters the polyol pathway and aldose reductase is activated, resulted in an accumulation of sorbitol. In *in vitro* experiments in mesangial cells, increased expression of glucose transporter 1 leads to increased AR expression and activity along with sorbitol accumulation and increased

PKC-α protein levels, promoting stimulation of matrix protein synthesis. Numerous experimental and clinical studies with different AR inhibitors (ARI) implicate the diabetes-induced increased flux of glucose through the polyol pathway in the development of diabetic retinopathy and neuropathy; however, only a few studies have investigated the influence of ARI in diabetic nephropathy.

C. Diacylglycerol-Protein Kinase C Activation

PKC is a family of serine-threonine kinases, consisting of at least 10 structurally related isoforms that regulate a variety of cell functions including proliferation, gene expression, cell differentiation, cell migration, and apoptosis. *In vitro* studies have shown that PKC is activated in vascular tissues and glomerular mesangial cells exposed to high glucose concentration. Activated PKC increases production of cytokines and ECM and vasoconstrictor endothelin-1. These changes contribute to basement membrane thickening, vascular occlusion, and increased permeability. Several PKC inhibitors used in experimental diabetes yielded promising results.

Ruboxistaurin (LY333531) mesylate, a bisindolymaleimide, shows a high degree of specificity within the protein kinase gene family for inhibiting PKC-β isoforms. In experimental rodent models of diabetes, ruboxistaurin normalized glomerular hyperfiltration, decreased urinary albumin excretion, and reduced glomerular TGF-β1 and ECM protein production, despite continued hypertension and hyperglycemia.

Kouroedov A et al: Selective inhibition of protein kinase C beta2 prevents acute effects of high glucose on vascular cell adhesion molecule-1 expression in human endothelial cells. Circulation 2004;110(1):91.

Nobe K et al: Novel diacylglycerol kinase inhibitor selectively suppressed an U46619-induced enhancement of mouse portal vein contraction under high glucose condition. Br J Pharmacol 2004;143(1):166.

Tsugawa T et al: Alteration of urinary sorbitol excretion in WBN-kob diabetic rats—treatment with an aldose reductase inhibitor. J Endocrinol 2004;181:429.

► Clinical Findings

A. Symptoms and Signs

In health, daily urinary excretion of albumin is less than 25 mg. Diabetic nephropathy follows a characteristic course starting with microalbuminuria defined as albuminuria ranging from 30–299 mg/24 hours or 20–199 μg/minute to overt proteinuria defined as albuminuria ≥300 mg/24 hours or ≥200 μg/minute and worsening azotemia. There are several clinical similarities between diabetic nephropathy in patients with type 1 diabetes and in patients with type 2 diabetes; however, the clinical course differs in some respects between these two groups. In patients with type 1 diabetes in whom nephropathy develops the clinical course is relatively well defined. Nephropathy usually becomes clinically evident

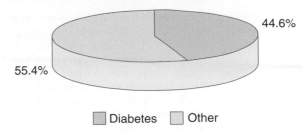

44.6%

55.4%

☐ Diabetes ☐ Other

▲ **Figure 54–2.** Schematic presentation of the progression of diabetic nephropathy. Diabetes and incidence of other end-stage renal diseases, 1998–2002.

after 15–25 years of diabetes and almost always progresses to ESRD.

However, because of the frequently insidious onset of type 2 diabetes, the advanced age of many patients, and the common presence of coexisting vascular disease and hypertension, early renal involvement is frequently missed. In elderly patients with type 2 diabetes, it is not always clear whether renal failure is due solely to or even caused by diabetes. However, in young patients with type 2 diabetes, recent studies have shown a course similar to that in type 1 diabetes. Thus, the clinical course of diabetic nephropathy is best defined in type 1 diabetes and proceeds through several stages (Figure 8–2).

B. Laboratory Findings

1. Stage 1: glomerular hyperfiltration and renomegally—At the onset of type 1 diabetes, the GFR is above normal up to 140% in the majority of individuals. No single pathogenesis fully explains both the nephromegaly and glomerular hyperfiltration characteristic of type 1 diabetes; a correlation between renal enlargement and glomerular hyperfiltration has been inferred from the correction of both perturbations after the establishment of euglycemia. Intensive insulin therapy normalizes hyperglycemia and corrects glomerular hyperfiltration; the GFR begins to decline within 8 days of initiation of insulin therapy and falls further during 3 months of insulin treatment. A substantial subset of individuals (~25–40%) with type 1 diabetes achieving usual levels of plasma glucose under insulin therapy continues to manifest a persistently elevated GFR; it is within this subgroup of hyperfiltering diabetic patients that the initial reductions in the GFR are first noted, with progression to clinical nephropathy.

Glomerular hyperfiltration has also been reported in patients with a recent diagnosis of type 2 diabetes mellitus and is positively correlated with the development of proteinuria.

2. Stage 2: early glomerular lesion—Expansion of the glomerular mesangial matrix and thickening of the glomerular basement membrane (GBM) are subtle morphologic changes noted 2–5 years after the onset of type 1 diabetes and persists for many years. During this stage of morphologic change, transient and recurrent microalbuminuria may be the only clinical evidence of renal involvement. A supplemental perspective of the early glomerular changes in type 2 diabetes is provided by the study of kidneys from nondiabetic donors transplanted into diabetic recipients. In biopsies of these recipient kidneys, the same sequence of changes—mesangial matrix expansion and GBM thickening within 3–5 years after transplant—was observed. Reversal of these sequential changes in type 1 diabetes has been noted after 10 years of euglycemia afforded by a functioning pancreas transplant. Stages 1 and 2 of diabetic nephropathy are usually clinically silent since the estimation of the GFR and renal biopsy are not performed routinely. However, early mesangial and basement membrane abnormalities are often seen on renal biopsy in stages 1 and 2, if this is performed.

3. Stage 3: microalbuminuric stage—In the early 1980s, studies in type 1 diabetic patients linked the presence of increased amounts of albumin in the urine, measured by immunoassay, to the subsequent development of overt diabetic nephropathy 10–14 years later.

Microalbuminuria is defined as increased urinary albumin excretion (UAE) (30–300 mg/24 hours or 20–200 μg/minute) not detected by standard bedside tests (dipstick) commonly employed to detect proteinuria. Several methods for quantifying low concentrations of urinary albumin are available, including radioimmunoassay, enzyme-linked immunoassay, and nephelometric immunoassay; a semiquantitative dipstick test has also been introduced (Micro-Bumintest, Miles Laboratories, Elkhart, IN).

A timed urine collection, either 24 hours or overnight, is the reference standard for assessment of microalbuminuria. Because of high intraindividual variability, transient elevations of proteinuria in the microalbuminuric range occur frequently, and clinical assessment should therefore be based on at least three measurements taken over 3–6 months. Persistent microalbuminuria is confirmed when at least two out of three consecutive, timed urine collections are in the range of 20–200 μg/minute.

Several factors can confound the assessment of microalbuminuria, including urinary tract infection, heavy exercise, high dietary protein intake, congestive heart failure, and acute febrile illness. For accurate evaluation, testing should be postponed if these factors are present.

There is accumulating evidence suggesting that the risk of developing diabetic nephropathy and cardiovascular disease starts when UAE values are still within the normoalbuminuric range. After 10 years of follow-up, the risk of diabetic nephropathy was 29 times greater in patients with type 2 diabetes with UAE values >10 μg/minute. The same was true for patients with type 1 diabetes. This favors the concept that the risk associated with UAE is a continuum, as is the case with blood pressure levels.

Although microalbuminuria has been considered a risk factor for macroalbuminuria, not all patients progress to this stage and some may regress to normoalbuminuria. In earlier studies ~80% of type 1 diabetic patients with microalbuminuria progressed to proteinuria over a period of 5–15 years. In recent studies, only 30–45% of microalbuminuric patients progressed to proteinuria over 10 years. This change might be the consequence of more intensive glycemic and blood pressure control strategies.

Without specific intervention, as detailed below, once microalbuminuria becomes constant, a progressive decline in renal functional reserve marking a downhill course toward clinical renal failure is usual. Typically, albumin excretion increases by about 25 μg/minute/year, while the GFR remains normal or elevated. The GFR begins to decline, at a variable although individually constant rate, once the amount of microalbuminuria exceeds 70 μg/minute. Blood pressure is higher in type 1 diabetic patients with microalbuminuria than in normoalbuminuric patients, although not necessarily higher than 140/90 mm Hg. The combination of microalbuminuria and high blood pressure leads to near-term (5–15 years) deterioration to clinical nephropathy.

4. Stage 4: clinical nephropathy—Following a variable interval, usually after several years of microalbuminuria, the GFR declines below normal for age and gender and proteinuria is detectable by dipstick. Proteinuria, defined as albumin excretion greater than 300 mg/day, is the universal hallmark noted in diabetic nephropathy. Once overt nephropathy develops, blood pressure is usually elevated, and there is a progressive decline in the GFR that can be assessed as an absolute decline in milliliters/minute per year.

In most patients with overt nephropathy and type 1 diabetes, the decrease in the GFR approaches linearity and is of the order of 11 mL/minute per year. In a prospective study, 227 white type 2 diabetic patients with nephropathy for 6.5 years (range 3–17 years) had a decline in the GFR of 5.2 mL/minute/year. In multivariate regression analysis, higher baseline albuminuria, systolic blood pressure, hemoglobin A_{1c} (HbA_{1c}), heavy smoking, and the presence of diabetic retinopathy were significantly associated with an increased rate of decline in the GFR. In the subset of diabetic patients who manifest nephropathy in both type 1 and type 2 diabetes, proteinuria is duration related, increasing in time to a florid nephrotic syndrome (proteinuria of more than 3.5 g/day coupled with hypoalbuminemia and hyperlipidemia). Anasarca develops in diabetic nephrotic patients at a higher serum albumin concentration than in nondiabetic patients, an observation probably explained by the fact that glycation of albumin leads to enhanced transcapillary permeability compared to normal albumin. Nearly 100% of diabetic patients who have reached the azotemic phase of diabetic nephropathy have coincident retinopathy when examined by fluorescein angiography; the absence of diabetic retinopathy in advanced renal disease is reason to doubt the diagnosis of diabetic nephropathy.

It should be kept in mind that because diabetic patients are at equal risk for unrelated renal disease, the quest for a renal diagnosis should be pursued, including renal biopsy, whenever the course does not fit the usual pattern of diabetic nephropathy, most often signaled by the absence of diabetic retinopathy and albuminuria, a rapid increase in serum creatinine, and the presence of active urinary sediment.

5. Stage 5: end-stage renal disease—As noted above, after 20–30 years of type 1 diabetes, about 30–40% of patients manifest irreversibly failed kidneys. Prospective studies of populations with a high prevalence of type 2 diabetes such as blacks, Hispanics, and Native American tribes indicate that the interval between diagnosis of type 2 diabetes and onset of ESRD ranges from 5 years to 25 years. But because the diagnosis of type 2 diabetes may be delayed until a clinical complication or comorbidity is apparent, the timetable is imprecise. As the GFR decreases the uremic symptoms and signs become apparent and renal replacement therapy is needed.

C. Imaging Studies

The central pathologic change in the diabetic kidney is overproduction and impaired degradation of ECM components that lead to their accumulation in the basement membranes and mesangial region of the glomerulus.

Light microscopy findings show an increase in the solid spaces of the tuft, most frequently observed as coarse branching of solid material. An extensive accumulation of matrix is also seen as a nodule and the lesion is known as Kimmelstiel–Wilson nodules. Hyalin deposits may be seen in Bowman's capsule ("capsular drop") and in the expanded mesangium. Diffuse global glomerular sclerosis, tubular atrophy, and interstitial fibrosis are late manifestations of the disease.

Immunofluorescence microscopy may show deposition of immunoglobulin G and albumin along the GBM in a linear pattern.

Electron microscopy shows thickening of the GBM in a very early stage of diabetic nephropathy, concomitant with the increase of mesangial matrix. In advanced disease, the mesangial regions occupy a large proportion of the tuft, with prominent matrix.

The severity of diabetic glomerulopathy has been gauged in some studies by the thickness of the basement membrane and mesangium and matrix expressed as a fraction of appropriate spaces (eg, volume fraction of mesangium/glomerulus, matrix/mesangium, or matrix/glomerulus).

D. Special Tests

Screening for diabetic nephropathy in type 1 diabetic patients is recommended 5 years after diagnosis; for type 2 diabetic patients screening should be started when diabetes is diagnosed since at least 7% of newly diagnosed patients have microalbuminuria. Furthermore, in type 1 diabetic patients with poor glycemic control, high blood pressure, and poor

lipid regulation, the prevalence of microalbuminuria before 5 years may be as high as to 18%. It follows that in type 1 diabetes, screening for microalbuminuria is reasonable 1 year after diabetes is diagnosed. If microalbuminuria is absent, screening should be repeated annually in both type 1 and type 2 diabetic patients.

The first step in the screening and diagnosis of diabetic nephropathy is to measure albumin in a spot urine sample, collected either as the first urine in the morning or at random. Results of albumin measurements in spot urine collection may be expressed as a urinary albumin concentration (mg/L) or as a urinary albumin-to-creatinine ratio (mg/g or mg/mmol). The upper limit of 17 mg/L in a random urine specimen has a sensitivity of 100% and a specificity of 80% for the diagnosis of microalbuminuria using a 24-hour timed urine collection as the reference standard. All positive tests should be confirmed in two out of three samples collected over a 3- to 6-month period due to the known day-to-day variability in urinary albumin excretion.

Screening should not be performed in the presence of conditions that increase UAE such as urinary tract infection, hematuria, acute febrile illness, vigorous exercise, and heart failure. Although measurement of UAE is the cornerstone for diagnosing diabetic nephropathy, some patients with either type 1 or type 2 diabetes may have a decreased GFR with a normal UAE. In patients with type 1 diabetes, this finding is more frequent in women with long-standing diabetes, hypertension, and/or retinopathy. Therefore, the GFR and UAE should be routinely estimated for proper screening of diabetic nephropathy.

American Diabetes Association: Nephropathy in diabetes (Position Statement). Diabetes Care 2004;27(Suppl 1):S79.

MacIsaac RJ et al: Nonalbuminuric renal insufficiency in type 2 diabetes. Diabetes Care 2004;27:195.

Rossing K et al: Progression of nephropathy in type 2 diabetic patients. Kidney Int 2004;66:1596.

▶ Treatment

A. Early Treatment of Risk Factors

Early treatment of risk factors for diabetic nephropathy will slow and/or prevent its progression. These risk factors include hyperglycemia, hypertension, smoking, and dyslipidemia. These are also risk factors for cardiovascular disease that should be vigorously treated.

1. Intensive glycemic control—The importance of strict glycemic control in preventing diabetic nephropathy has been confirmed by large clinical trials in both type 1 and type 2 diabetes. In the Diabetes Control and Complications Trial (DCCT), intensive treatment of diabetes reduced the incidence of microalbuminuria by 39%. Furthermore, patients randomized to strict glycemic control had a long-lasting reduction of 40% in the risk for development of microalbuminuria and hypertension 7–8 years after the end of the DCCT. Similarly, the UK Prospective Diabetes Study (UKPDS) of type 2 diabetes reported a 30% reduction in the risk of developing microalbuminuria in the intensively treated group as compared to the conventionally treated group.

The effect of strict glycemic control on the progression from microalbuminuria to macroalbuminuria and on the rate of renal function decline in macroalbuminuric patients is still controversial.

In the DCCT study, intensified glycemic control did not decrease the rate of progression to macroalbuminuria in patients with type 1 diabetes who were microalbuminuric at the beginning of the study. In another prospective study of 115 patients with diabetes and renal impairment, 50 with type 1 diabetes and 65 with type 2 diabetes, no relationship between HbA_{1c} and fall in creatinine clearance was seen over a 7-year period. However, in two-combined analysis of the large Steno study better glycemic control was associated with a fall in the urinary albumin excretion rate and a decreased decline in the GFR. Similarly, in 18 patients with type 1 diabetes and diabetic nephropathy prospectively followed for 21 months, a direct relationship was noted between fall in the GFR and HbA_{1c}, with the greatest fall in the GFR occurring in those with the highest HbA_{1c}.

There are fewer details on the natural history of treated type 2 diabetes, although one study based in Japan randomized 110 patients with type 2 diabetes and 55 patients with retinopathy and microalbuminuria to receive either multiple injection therapy or conventional insulin therapy over a 6-year period. The cumulative percentage of progression of nephropathy in the multiple insulin therapy group was 11.5% as compared to 32.0% in the conventional insulin therapy group.

To date, no large trial of intensive therapy has been reported in overt nephropathy in either type 1 or type 2 diabetes. This lack of evidence of efficacy might be due to the complexity of delivering tight glycemic control and the increased risk of hypoglycemia in patients with impaired renal function. Therefore, intensive treatment of diabetes aiming at a HbA_{1c} <7% (The American Diabetes Association standard) should be pursued as early as possible to prevent the development of microalbuminuria.

2. Intensive blood pressure control—Multiple studies on the effect of pharmacologic induction of normotension in type 1 and type 2 diabetic patients with persistent microalbuminuria indicate that urinary albumin excretion may be reduced while clinically evident nephropathy is postponed and perhaps prevented. Hypertension is common in diabetic patients, even when renal involvement is not present. About 40% of type 1 and 70% of type 2 diabetic patients with normoalbuminuria have blood pressure levels <140/90 mm Hg.

In both type 1 and type 2 diabetic patients with overt diabetic nephropathy, blood pressure reduction, whether with angiotensin-converting enzyme (ACE) inhibitors or non-ACE inhibitors, reduces albuminuria, delays progression of nephropathy, postpones renal insufficiency, and improves survival. As a key example in UKPDS, a reduction in systolic blood pressure from 154 mm Hg to 144 mm Hg reduced the risk for the development of microalbuminuria by 29%.

Although retardation of the decline in the GFR has been shown with other antihypertensive medications, blockade of the renin–angiotensin system (RAS) with ACE inhibitors or angiotensin receptor blockers (ARBs) is thought to confer an additional "renoprotective" benefit on preserving renal function.

The sixth report of the Joint National Committee on Prevention, Detection, Evaluation, and Treatment of High Blood Pressure first published the recommendation that the target level of blood pressure in diabetes be reduced to at or below 130/85 mm Hg. Similarly, the American Diabetes Association adapted the recommendation in 1999. Continuing this theme, a consensus report of the National Kidney Foundation (NKF) advises that the blood pressure goal should be less than 130/80 mm Hg for nonproteinuric patients and 125/70 mm Hg for those with proteinuria. To achieve this degree of blood pressure reduction usually necessitates more than one antihypertensive drug plus a willing patient. The ideal drug combination is far from clear. Few data compare combination drugs with single agents. One study examined the added antihypertensive effect of 12.5 mg of hydrochlorothiazide (HCTZ) in patients with diabetic nephropathy and GFR values within normal ranges. These patients were initially treated with an ACE inhibitor (cilazapril) or an α-blocker (doxazosin). A mean decline of 15 mm Hg in systolic blood pressure (SBP) and 8 mm Hg in diastolic blood pressure (DBP) was obtained. Addition of HCTZ induced a further decline in SBP of 8 mm Hg and in DBP of 5 mm Hg. The combination also gained a greater reduction in the urinary albumin excretion rate.

ACE inhibitors are the drugs of choice for the treatment of hypertension and for retarding the decline in renal function in diabetic patients. Evidence that ACE inhibitors are indeed renoprotective against deterioration of renal failure was afforded by a study that demonstrated a significant decline in primary endpoints (doubling of serum creatinine and the development of ESRD) in the cohort treated with captopril. Seven years later, the EUCLID study, which was done in 18 European centers, randomized type 1 diabetic patients with normoalbuminuria or microalbuminuria to treatment with an ACE inhibitor (lisinopril) or a placebo. After 24 months, there was a significant difference favoring the lisinopril cohort both in terms of mean UAE and in the ratio of transition from normoalbuminuria to microalbuminuria. Similar benefits of ACE inhibitors have also been seen in patients with type 2 diabetes. The MICRO-HOPE study involved 1140 patients with type 2 diabetes and microalbuminuria randomized to ramipril 10 mg/day or a placebo. The blood pressure of all patients was to be kept at normal (target) values permitting the addition of other medications. The study aim was to determine whether ACE inhibition has organ protective effects independent of its antihypertensive action. Sustaining this thesis, at 4.5 years ramipril-treated patients had a combined primary outcome risk reduction of 25%, with myocardial infarction being decreased by 22%, stroke by 33%, cardiovascular death by 37%, and total mortality by 24%. There was a slower rise in UAE in ramipril-treated patients while fewer patients on ramipril progressed from microalbuminuria to macroalbuminuria.

ARBs are antihypertensive agents that inhibit the renin–angiotensin system by selectively blocking the AT_1 subtype of A_{11} receptors. A renoprotective effect of ARBs was proven by the results of three large international prospective controlled studies published in one issue of the *New England Journal of Medicine*. These three studies enrolled type 2 diabetic patients with microalbuminuria or overt proteinuria and renal impairment. The renoprotective effect of irbesartan and losartan was established as these agents not only reduced albuminuria but also, over period of 2–4 years, significantly retarded the decline in the GFR and decreased the proportion of patients progressing to end-stage renal failure.

These three studies, in addition to the MICRO-HOPE and EUCLID studies, provide a strong rationale for the use of ACE inhibitors and/or ARBs in diabetic patients with nephropathy. The present standard of care for proteinuric diabetic patients is based on the inclusion of ACE inhibitors or ARBs. Recently, several studies have indicated benefits from dual blockade of the renin–angiotensin system by ACE inhibitors plus ARBs as noted by a greater reduction in albuminuria and blood pressure in combination-treated diabetic patients compared to the maximal dose of an ACE inhibitor alone.

3. Dietary protein restriction—In health and in diabetes, dietary protein intake modulates renal hemodynamics. Several reports suggest that in type 1 diabetes, ingestion of a high protein diet increases the risk of nephropathy. It is also known that protein restriction is effective in alleviating the symptoms of uremia and may delay the need for dialysis. Beyond symptomatic relief, a reduced protein intake is advocated to slow or/and prevent a decline in renal function. The proposed mechanism for halting progression is the reduction in hyperfiltration that occurs in the remaining nephrons after renal injury is established. A benefit from dietary protein restriction was noted in a small prospective randomized controlled study of 35 patients with type 1 diabetes and clinical nephropathy. The low-protein diet contained 0.6 mg/kg/day and patients were followed for a mean period of 35 months. A 4-fold decrease in the rate of fall of the GFR was found in the low-protein diet group compared to controls after 3 months. The mean urinary protein excretion fell by 24% in the study group but rose by 22% in the control group. At the end of the study, the reduction in proteinuria in the study population was only 6%, whereas the controls had a 24% increase. Adding to the case for dietary protein restriction, it was found that albumin excretion rates decreased when patients with microalbuminuria were fed a predominantly vegetarian diet in the absence of significant change in either blood glucose control or arterial blood pressure. Although a clear benefit of dietary restriction has not been shown in a large randomized prospective trial, based on these small positive clinical studies a protein intake of <0.8 g/kg is a reasonable regimen for patients with macroalbuminuria with further restriction as the GFR falls.

4. Lipid-lowering drugs—Hyperlipidemia is a risk factor for the development of vascular disease including nephropathy in both rat models of diabetes and human type 1 and type 2 diabetes. The effect of lipid reduction by antihyperlipidemic agents on the progression of diabetic nephropathy has not been established. Although large prospective trials of the effect of treatment of dyslipidemia on the progression of diabetic nephropathy have not been reported, some evidence indicates that lipid reduction by antihyperlipidemic agents preserves the GFR and decreases proteinuria in diabetic patients.

A recent randomized, double-blind placebo-controlled study compared simvastatin and diet versus placebo and diet on albuminuria in 39 patients with type 1 diabetes and nephropathy. Although not attaining significance, the rise in albuminuria was slower in the simvastatin-treated cohort compared to placebo over 2 years. A meta-analysis on lipid-lowering therapy on progression of renal disease assessed 13 prospective controlled trials, seven of which were exclusively in diabetic patients. Lipid lowering was associated with a lower rate of decline in renal function compared to controls ($p = 0.008$) inducing beneficial effects equivalent to ACE inhibition in the preservation of renal function. The discerned effect on the GFR did not correlate with either the type of lipid-lowering agent or the etiology of renal disease. As for other components of renoprotection, large prospective clinical trials with longer follow-up are needed to validate the value of lipid-lowering agents.

However, as cardiovascular disease is the number one cause of death in diabetic patients with nephropathy, optimizing lipid control is now a standard of care.

5. Cessation of cigarette smoking—Convincingly, a linkage between cigarette smoking and progression of diabetic nephropathy has been established. The effect of cigarette smoking on diabetic renal and retinal complications in 359 type 1 diabetic patients was assessed. The prevalence of an increased rate of albumin excretion was 2.8 times higher in smokers than in those who do not smoke. Even after correction for glycohemoglobin level and duration of diabetes, smoking was a significant factor in their logistic regression model for albuminuria. Significant improvement in urinary albumin excretion was noted when subjects ceased smoking. Similar findings were reported in patients with type 2 diabetes and nephropathy. As is true for preventing pulmonary and cardiovascular disease, reducing or quitting smoking should be part of all regimes for renoprotection in diabetic patients.

B. Uremia Therapy

Although normalizing blood pressure, optimizing glycemic control, and adhering to a low-protein diet may retard the development and progression of diabetic nephropathy, many diabetic patients still progress to ESRD. Continuing empathetic interactions as renal function deteriorates builds confidence and minimizes panic, despair, and frantic behavior as the need for ESRD therapy becomes pressing. Patients with diabetic nephropathy should be referred to a nephrologist early in the course of their disease in order to optimize their pre-ESRD care. Reports from both Europe and the United States found that a high proportion of patients with diabetic nephropathy are referred to a nephrologist late in the course of their disease, resulting in suboptimal treatment.

Management of diabetic patients with progressive renal insufficiency is a challenge because of comorbid conditions that accompany the nephropathy. These preexisting comorbid conditions (cardiovascular disease, retinopathy, cerebrovascular and peripheral vascular disease) play a major role in the decreased survival of diabetic patients on renal replacement therapy. In practice, a team of collaborating specialists optimize the pre-ESRD diabetic care. This team should include a nephrologist, diabetologist, nutritionist, cardiologist, ophthalmologist, podiatrist, and other specialists when necessary. Pre-ESRD management of diabetic patients with advanced renal failure includes sustaining a hemoglobin level above 11 g/dL by administering erythropoietin and supplemental iron, minimizing metabolic bone disease due to secondary hyperparathyroidism by use of phosphate binders, along with use of synthetic vitamin D and/or calcimimetics. Potential familial kidney donors should be interviewed and tissue typed; when hemodialysis appears to be likely, preserving forearm cutaneous veins by avoiding venous punctures and intravenous catheters and maintaining good nutritional status are essential.

C. Renal Replacement Therapy

Diabetic patients with ESRD have options for renal replacement therapy similar to nondiabetic patients. For diabetic ESRD patients those options include hemodialysis, peritoneal dialysis, kidney transplant alone, and a combined pancreas and kidney transplant, which is unique to diabetic patients. Before a patient is assigned a specific modality of renal replacement therapy, it is important that patients and their families be properly informed about the advantages and disadvantages of each treatment option.

Selecting the treatment that is best for a particular patient is made by considering the patient's age, level of education, severity of comorbid conditions, social and family support, and geographic location. Once the decision for a preferred option is made, preparation for renal replacement therapy should be started. For instance, an arteriovenous fistula should be established in patients who will be undergoing hemodialysis, and a peritoneal catheter should be inserted in those who will be treated with peritoneal dialysis. As a general guide, renal replacement therapy is initiated when the GFR of a diabetic patient falls to 10–15 mL/minute.

D. Maintenance Hemodialysis

As reported in the USRDS 2004 registry, 75% of all diabetic patients with ESRD are treated with hemodialysis (center or home), 7.4% with peritoneal dialysis [continuous ambulatory peritoneal dialysis (CAPD) or continuous cyclic peritoneal dialysis (CCPD)], and 17% receive a functioning kidney transplant. Hemodialysis treatment for diabetic patients is similar to that for nondiabetic patients. An ideal hemodialysis regimen consists of three weekly dialysis sessions, each lasting 3.5–4.5 hours, as determined by individual blood chemistry and clinical response during which extracorporeal blood flow is maintained at 300–500 mL/minute.

The survival and rehabilitation of diabetic patients on maintenance hemodialysis are distinctly inferior to those of nondiabetic patients, mainly because of preexisting severe vascular disease. Peripheral vascular calcification in middle-sized arteries plus atherosclerosis of small vessels may pose a challenge for the vascular surgeon attempting to construct a vascular access in a diabetic patient. Although the preferred vascular access is an arteriovenous fistula, preexisting vascular disease limits its utility in diabetic patient, who have a primary fistula failure rate of 30–40%. A less desirable, but necessary alternative vascular access can be constructed using a polytetrafluoroethylene graft, which has a half-life in excess of 1 year.

The proportion of arteriovenous fistulas compared to grafts can be increased in diabetic patients by careful preoperative investigation to select an adequate location for initial placement to the fistula. Large-diameter arteries and veins, frequently requiring use of the elbow region, are employed, thereby avoiding an initial polytetrafluoroethylene graft. Continuous surveillance by a nephrologist and the dialysis staff concerning early elective access revision and avoidance of thrombosis improves the viability of the primary fistulas. Complications of vascular access are the leading cause of hospitalization in diabetic patients with ESRD undergoing hemodialysis.

Glycemic control in diabetic patients undergoing dialysis is difficult. Insulin dosage is more complex because of unrecognized gastroparesis, which disconnects absorption of ingested food from timed insulin administration and because of reduced renal insulin catabolism, which results in the prolonged action of exogenous insulin. This combination causes erratic glucose regulation complicated by frequent hypoglycemic episodes, a potentially serious complication. Glycemic control should remain a priority in the dialyzed diabetic patient as it may retard further complications of microvascular disease. Survival during the long-term management of ESRD in diabetes has been linked to the quality of glycemic control achieved.

Although the survival of diabetic patients on dialysis has been improving over the past decade, morbidity and mortality remain significantly higher than in those without diabetes. This grim reality is mostly attributed to the progression of comorbid conditions. Cardiovascular disease, infections, and withdrawal from dialysis are the leading cause of mortality in patients with diabetes and ESRD.

E. Peritoneal Dialysis

Peritoneal dialysis is a satisfactory alternative mode of dialytic therapy available for diabetic ESRD patients. In the United States, peritoneal dialysis is applied to only 7% of all diabetic patients on renal replacement therapy. As is true for hemodialysis, preparation of the patient for CAPD, the most frequently utilized form of peritoneal dialysis, necessitates education, repetitive explanation, and facilitating surgery to insert an intraperitoneal permanent catheter. CAPD can be mastered as a home regimen in about 4 weeks. An alternative to manual cycling of the dialysate is the use of a mechanical cycling device in a CCPD regimen, which can be performed during sleep.

CAPD offers some advantages over hemodialysis, such as freedom from a machine, performance at home, reduced cardiovascular stress, better preservation of renal function, avoidance of heparin, and less dietary restrictions. However, the disadvantages of peritoneal dialysis include the risk of peritonitis, the high rate of technical failure, and less adequate dialysis when residual renal function is low.

Some nephrologists consider peritoneal dialysis as the preferred choice of treatment for diabetic ESRD patients. Indeed, the CAPD or CCPD may be life sustaining when vascular access sites for hemodialysis have been exhausted, or in those with severe congestive heart failure, angina, or severe dialysis-related hypotension. Peritoneal dialysis involves less vascular stress because of its relatively slow ultrafiltration rate coupled with less rapid solute removal.

During the course of both CAPD and CCPD, there is a constant risk of peritonitis as well as a gradual decrease in peritoneal surface area, which may ultimately prove to be insufficient for adequate dialysis. Diabetic patients on CAPD experience twice as many hospitalization days as nondiabetic patients: peritonitis accounts for 30–50% of these hospital days.

Of the two major options in dialytic therapy for ESRD in diabetes, the USRDS consistently reports superior survival in those treated by hemodialysis, except in those under age 45 years, compared to peritoneal dialysis. However, there are few studies reporting equivalent patient survival for peritoneal dialysis versus hemodialysis in the first 2 years of treatment. The two leading causes of death in diabetic CAPD patients are cardiovascular events and infection.

F. Kidney Transplantation

In the 1970s and early 1980s many transplant programs excluded diabetic ESRD patients from consideration for renal transplantation. However, in centers that performed transplants during this period, the survival of diabetic patients receiving transplants exceeded that of diabetic patients remaining on dialysis. Today, the improved management of diabetic and uremic complications established kidney transplantation as the preferred form of treatment for diabetic ESRD patients.

Although the survival of diabetic ESRD patients after renal transplantation is continuously improving, over a 5-year period it is 10–20% below that of patients with other causes of renal disease. A further decrease in survival of diabetic renal transplant recipients after 5 or more years is the consequence of coronary, cerebral, and other macrovascular diseases. The most recent analysis of patient survival in diabetic kidney transplant recipients indicated 93.7% 1-year and 85.5% 3-year survival for recipients of grafts from deceased donors and 95.4% 1-year and 91.3% 3-year survival for those receiving living donor transplants. The annual death rates of transplant recipients are approximately one-third those of diabetic patients remaining on dialysis. In fairness, it must be noted that a strong selection bias extracts the fittest patients for kidney transplants leaving a residual pool of dialysis patients with extensive life-threatening comorbidities.

To respond to the real risk of cardiac events in diabetic renal transplant recipients and to assess the extent of cardiovascular disease present prior to transplantation, at least annual reassessment with noninvasive studies in asymptomatic high-risk patients should be performed.

G. Pancreas Transplantation

Over the past decade, highly successful results have been reported in type 1 diabetic patients for pancreatic transplants inserted concurrently with a renal allograft. Although combined pancreas and kidney transplants do not result in an increase in immediate perioperative mortality, perioperative morbidity is markedly increased over that of a kidney transplant alone. Almost 13,000 pancreas transplants were reported to the international Pancreas Transplant Registry from 1966 through September 1999, with 75% of them performed in the United States. The majority of pancreas transplants in the United States have been combined kidney–pancreas transplants (SPK). One year patient survival has improved from 90% for 1987–1988 cases to 95% for 1995–1996 cases. In addition, pancreas graft survival has improved from 74% to 85% at 1 year for the same time period; kidney graft survival improved from 83% to 91%. Solitary pancreas transplants, either pancreas alone (PTA) or pancreas after kidney transplant (PAK), constitute only a small proportion of the total pancreas transplants in the United States. Graft survival of PTA or PAK is worse compared to SPK. Early reports have surprisingly found a substantial survival benefit for pancreas plus kidney transplants in type 2 diabetic ESRD patients.

Chuahirun T et al: Cigarette smoking exacerbation and its cessation ameliorates renal injury in type 2 diabetes. Am J Kidney Dis 2004;327:57.

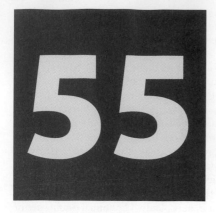

Pregnancy & Renal Disease

Priya Anantharaman, MD,

Rebecca J. Schmidt, DO, &

Jean L. Holley, MD

PREGNANCY-INDUCED ANATOMIC AND PHYSIOLOGIC CHANGES

1. Anatomic Changes in Pregnancy

Kidney size increases by approximately 1 cm during pregnancy. The urinary collecting system (renal calyces, pelvis, and ureters) dilates. Hormonal and mechanical forces are thought to account for ureteral dilation as early as 6 weeks gestation. In the later stages of pregnancy, mechanical compression of the ureter against the pelvic brim may lead to hydroureter and hydronephrosis. Hydronephrosis occurs on the right in 90% of cases due to dextrorotation of the uterus by the sigmoid colon.

In rare instances this becomes a clinically significant cause of obstructive uropathy. The dilated collecting systems can hold up to 300 mL of urine and hence serve as a reservoir for bacteria. The dilated urinary tract also allows for urinary stasis and increases the risk of pyelonephritis in pregnant women with asymptomatic bacteriuria.

2. Physiologic Changes in Pregnancy

Renal physiologic changes are characterized by marked vasodilation, which leads to increases in glomerular filtration rate (GFR) and renal plasma flow (RPF). These changes occur early in the first trimester and peak increases in GFR and RPF to 50% above baseline are seen by the end of the first trimester. The filtration fraction (GFR/RPF) falls significantly, indicating a greater rise in effective RPF. Creatinine production is unchanged in pregnancy but creatinine clearance is increased, resulting in lower levels of serum creatinine; the normal creatinine value during pregnancy is <0.8 mg/dL (see Table 55–1).

Increased urinary excretion of protein, amino acids, uric acid, glucose, and calcium occurs as a result of the elevated GFR. Hence, proteinuria in pregnancy is considered abnormal when it exceeds 300 mg/day compared with an upper limit of normal of 150 mg/day in the nonpregnant population. Uric acid clearance also increases in pregnancy and serum uric acid levels in pregnant women usually do not exceed 4.5 mg/dL by the third trimester.

3. Electrolytes & Acid Base Changes

Pregnancy is associated with significant changes in water metabolism. Serum osmolality falls by 5–10 mOsmol/kg as a result of several forces. The serum osmostat is reset as suggested by normal responses to water loading and water deprivation despite a lower serum osmolality. There is a decrease in the osmotic thresholds for thirst and arginine vasopressin (AVP) release. Enhanced catabolism of AVP by release of placental vasopressinases leads to transient diabetes insipidus and in some women is severe enough to warrant treatment. Total body water increases by 6–8 L, most of which is extracellular. Plasma volume increases throughout pregnancy by 1.1–1.6 L, resulting in a plasma volume of 4.7–5.2 L, 30–50% above that in nonpregnant women. This is accompanied by the retention of 900–1000 mEq of sodium, which contributes to the mild edema seen in some pregnant women. Red blood cell mass increases 20–30% above baseline by the end of pregnancy. The proportionally greater increase in intravascular volume relative to red cell mass results in the dilutional or physiologic anemia of pregnancy.

Serum sodium falls by 5 mEq/L due to resetting of the osmostat (Table 55–1). Hyponatremia during pregnancy parallels the increased release of human chorionic gonadotropin (hCG), which appears to mediate these changes via the release of relaxin. Serum potassium levels are normal despite increased serum aldosterone, perhaps due to the potassium-sparing effects of elevated progesterone levels in pregnancy. Elevated progesterone levels stimulate hyperventilation and cause mild respiratory alkalosis, resulting in a slight increase in arterial pH and a fall in plasma bicarbonate concentrations by about 4 mEq/L. Total serum calcium levels fall in pregnancy but ionized calcium remains normal.

Table 55–1. Normal laboratory values in pregnancy.

Blood urea nitrogen (BUN), mg/dL	7–10
Creatinine, mg/dL	0.3–0.6
Creatinine clearance, mL/minute	150–200
Uric acid, mg/dL	3.2–4
Sodium, mEq/L	130–135
24-hour urine protein, mg	<300
Arterial pH	7.4–7.45
Pco_2, mm Hg	27–32
HCO_3, mEq/L	18–21

Accelerated renal and placental production of calcitriol leads to increased gastrointestinal absorption of calcium and absorptive hypercalciuria with urine calcium as high as 300 mg/day. Serum parathyroid hormone (PTH) concentrations are lower than normal, partly in response to higher serum levels of calcitriol.

4. Hemodynamic Changes in Pregnancy

Profound changes in cardiovascular physiology and systemic hemodynamics are required to accommodate the increased metabolic demand of normal pregnancy. Pregnancy is accompanied by a rise in cardiac output and fall in mean arterial blood pressure and systemic vascular resistance (Figure 55–1). Cardiac output increases by 30–50% (1.8 L/minute) above prepregnancy values. Increased preload

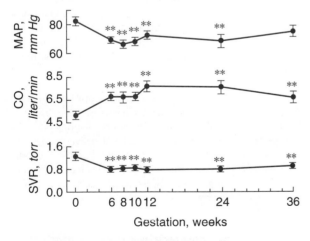

▲ **Figure 55–1.** Systemic hemodynamic changes throughout early human pregnancy. Mean arterial pressure (MAP) and cardiac output (CO) increase significantly in early gestation in association with a fall in systemic vascular resistance (SVR). (Modified with permission from Chapman AB et al: Temporal relationships between hormonal and hemodynamic changes in early human pregnancy. Kidney Int 1998;54:2056.)

(due to increased blood volume), decreased afterload (due to decreased systemic vascular resistance), and the increase in maternal heart rate account for the rise in cardiac output. Cardiac output in pregnant women is affected significantly by changes in posture that compromise preload by compression of the inferior vena cava by a gravid uterus.

The fall in systemic vascular resistance (SVR) is manifested by a fall in blood pressure, which begins by the end of the first trimester. Blood pressure falls to 10 mm Hg below baseline by the second trimester, declining to a mean of 105/60 mm Hg. In the third trimester, the diastolic blood pressure gradually increases to nonpregnant values by term. Mechanisms underlying the fall in SVR and subsequent vasodilation include decreased vasopressor responsiveness to angiotensin II and norepinephrine, enhanced production of the vasodilatory factors prostacyclin and nitric oxide, and decreased aortic stiffness.

The renin–angiotensin–aldosterone system (RAS) is highly activated in normal human pregnancies. Plasma renin activity (PRA) increases 4-fold in the first trimester and continues to rise until approximately 20 weeks gestation. The increase in PRA stimulates increased secretion of aldosterone. The activation of the RAS is thought to be secondary, in response to vasodilation and a decrease in blood pressure.

EFFECT OF KIDNEY DISEASE ON PREGNANCY

Table 55–2 summarizes the two issues involved in chronic kidney disease/end-stage renal disease (ESRD) and pregnancy: the effects of kidney disease on pregnancy (course, complications, and outcome) and the effects of pregnancy on kidney disease.

1. Infertility

▶ General Considerations

Pregnancy is not common in women on dialysis. Fertility rates in patients with ESRD are extremely low and are difficult to quantify accurately. Chronic kidney disease (CKD) is also associated with infertility.

Table 55–2. Relationship between pregnancy and kidney disease.

Effects of pregnancy on kidney disease	Effects of kidney disease on pregnancy
Worsening proteinuria	Infertility
Loss of kidney function	Preterm delivery
Hypertension and preeclampsia	IUGR
	Decreased fetal survival
	Preeclampsia

IUGR, intrauterine growth retardation.

▶ Clinical Findings

The reproductive hormonal milieu in patients with ESRD remains an enigma. Elevated levels of follicle-stimulating hormone (FSH) and luteinizing hormone (LH) and low levels of free testosterone are common in men with ESRD.

Women with ESRD are usually amenorrheic or have irregular menstrual cycles. The frequency of menstruation in women of childbearing age with ESRD is variable, between 10% and 42%. Anovulatory cycles commonly occur even among menstruating women with ESRD. In contrast to women with ESRD, premenopausal women with normal kidney function have both tonic and cyclic components of gonadotropin secretion. The tonic component is regulated through basal gonadotropin secretion; the cyclic component is regulated through the midcycle surge of LH and its effects on the hypothalamus. The ovarian dysfunction in women on dialysis is characterized by the absence of cyclic gonadotropin release, presumably hypothalamic in origin. Menopause tends to occur earlier among women on dialysis.

Prolactin levels are elevated in both men and women on dialysis due to increased production and reduced renal clearance. Strikingly high numbers of women on hemodialysis (70–90%) and most peritoneal dialysis patients have hyperprolactinemia. Because of all of these factors, successful conception in dialysis patients is rare. Pregnancy is more common in kidney transplant recipients and in women with chronic kidney disease.

Holley JL: The hypothalamic-pituitary axis in men and women with chronic kidney disease. Adv Renal Replac Ther 2004;11:337. [PMID: 15492969]

2. Fetal Outcomes
▶ General Considerations

The difficulties of conception notwithstanding, successful pregnancies in dialysis-dependent patients are rare: of 115 pregnancies reported by the European Dialysis and Transplant Association, 23% carried to term. Fetal outcomes have improved over time: the percentage of pregnancies with surviving infants reported from the United States was 21% prior to 1990 and 52% from 1990 to 1991. The U.S. registry of pregnancy in dialysis patients reported that 42% of pregnancies resulted in a surviving infant, 7.5% in neonatal death, 6% in still birth, 32% in spontaneous abortion, and 10.5% in therapeutic abortion. Only 12% of the therapeutic abortions were performed due to pregnancy complications. Women who started dialysis during their pregnancy, conceived close to the point of requiring dialysis, or experienced a rapid decline in kidney function during their pregnancy have fairly good infant survival (73.6%) compared to that in women who conceived after starting dialysis (40% infant survival).

▶ Complications
A. Prematurity

Prematurity and low-birth-weight babies are, unfortunately, the norm. Most deliveries in women who conceive on dialysis are premature (mean gestational age 32.4 weeks) and 36% of these infants weighed less than 1500 g at birth. Long-term medical and developmental problems are also common in these children and are due to prematurity and low birth weights rather than the azotemic intrauterine environment.

B. Polyhydramnios

Polyhydramnios, which can precipitate preterm labor and postpartum infant complications, is an important fetal complication in pregnancies in women with CKD. It is thought to be the result of increased fetal diuresis in response to high maternal blood urea nitrogen levels. The resulting fetal azotemia resolves rapidly after delivery but can lead to volume depletion and electrolyte imbalance from the ensuing osmotic diuresis.

▶ Treatment

Obstetric management of these infants involves preventing preterm labor and appropriate fetal surveillance and timing of delivery. Strategies to prevent preterm labor include cautious use of magnesium or indomethacin in women with polyhydramnios. Magnesium levels must be closely monitored to avoid toxicity and consequent respiratory distress. Indomethacin can result in the loss of residual renal function and hyperkalemia, necessitating the initiation of dialysis or an increase in dialysis dose. Mid trimester losses may be prevented by monitoring dialysis patients for cervical shortening or cervical incompetence.

The timing of delivery is controversial. In most dialysis patients, preterm labor or an obstetric complication necessitates early delivery. Some obstetricians prefer delivery at 34–36 weeks if fetal lung maturity can be demonstrated. In transplant recipients and those with CKD, delivery is delayed until the onset of labor as long as maternal and fetal conditions remain optimal. A multidisciplinary team of health care providers including nephrologists, obstetricians, perinatologists, and dialysis providers is needed to ensure optimal care for the pregnant woman with CKD or ESRD.

EFFECTS OF PREGNANCY ON KIDNEY DISEASE

▶ General Considerations

Pregnancy may influence the course of kidney disease. Importantly, women with CKD do not have the normal pregnancy-associated increase in GFR. Overall, the pregnancy outcome is usually favorable in women with mild CKD, serum creatinine less than 1.4 mg/dL, and normal blood pressure early in pregnancy. Several case series suggest that women who conceive with a serum creatinine greater than 1.4 mg/dL experience a more rapid deterioration in kidney function than their nonpregnant counterparts with similar degrees of kidney function. In a study of 82 pregnancies in 67 women with a serum creatinine level of 1.4 mg/dL or greater at conception or in their first trimester, 20% of women had a decline in kidney function during pregnancy and 23% had a decline by the first 6 weeks postpartum. At 6 months postpartum, 8% of women recovered kidney function to their baseline values and an additional 10% had deterioration in kidney function. Women with a baseline creatinine exceeding 2.0 mg/dL experienced the greatest decrease in kidney function: 10% of this group had a rapid loss of kidney function and progressed to ESRD within 1 year of delivery. Women with pregnancy-associated deterioration in kidney function account for approximately 20% of women requiring dialysis in pregnancy. Obstetric complications include a high rate of preterm delivery (59%) and fetal growth retardation (37%). The infant survival rate was 93%.

Complications

Proteinuria usually increases in pregnant women with CKD. Hypertension occurs or is exacerbated in most women with underlying kidney disease and usually requires antihypertensive medications. The Registry of Pregnancy in Dialysis Patients reported that 79% of pregnant patients with ESRD were hypertensive and 48% experienced a blood pressure greater than 170/110 mm Hg during their pregnancy. In women with moderate to severe CKD, the frequency of hypertension rose from 28% at baseline to 48% in the third trimester. Maternal mortality, although rare, has certainly been reported.

Kidney disease that develops during pregnancy is usually due to new onset glomerulonephritis, lupus nephritis, interstitial nephritis, or acute renal failure. The evaluation of kidney disease during pregnancy includes the measurement of kidney function, serologic testing, and ultrasonography. Renal biopsy is rarely employed and is reserved for unexplained deterioration in renal function or severe nephritic syndrome. There is no role for a renal biopsy in pregnancy beyond 32 weeks.

1. Diabetic Nephropathy & Pregnancy
General Considerations & Complications

Pregnancy in women with diabetes mellitus is relatively common. The presence of diabetic nephropathy (urine albumin excretion >300 mg/day) at conception is a significant risk factor for perinatal morbidity and mortality. Preeclampsia superimposed upon diabetic nephropathy enhances the risk for preterm delivery and intrauterine growth retardation.

Among women with gestational diabetes, the prevalence of preeclampsia is 10–20%. The frequency of preeclampsia is higher with increasing severity of diabetes and in those

with proteinuria at conception. Preterm delivery may be as high as 30% in women with preeclampsia. Diabetic women with microalbuminuria (urine albumin excretion of 30–300 mg/day) are also likely to develop preeclampsia, a risk similar to that of women with diabetic nephropathy. Preeclampsia also substantially increases the prevalence of their preterm delivery.

Early reports suggested pregnancy had little effect on the long-term progression of diabetic nephropathy, but recent reports contradict this. The progression of kidney disease is accelerated in 45% of pregnant women with diabetic nephropathy. A significant elevation in maternal blood pressure and proteinuria with nephrotic syndrome develops in most (71%) of these pregnancies. Infant birth weight correlates with gestational age and maternal kidney function: 71% of infants are appropriate for gestational age, 16% are small for gestational age, and 13% are large for gestational age. A prepregnancy history of tight glycemic control, a urine albumin excretion of less than 500 mg/day, and angiotensin-converting enzyme inhibitor (ACEI) therapy have been linked to a prolonged protective effect on maternal kidney function and more favorable pregnancy outcomes.

2. Pregnancy & Antiphospholipid Antibody Syndrome
General Considerations

Systemic lupus erythematosus (SLE) is a disease often seen in women of childbearing age. Signs of active SLE early in pregnancy herald a hazardous course. As with other nephropathies, the presence of hypertension and elevated creatinine level increases the risk of complications. Antiphospholipid syndrome (APS) can be primary or secondary. Secondary APS is associated with SLE, other collagen vascular diseases, and malignancy. APS is associated with arterial and/or venous thrombosis and recurrent fetal loss, particularly in the second trimester, and is usually accompanied by mild to moderate thrombocytopenia and elevated titers of antiphospholipid antibodies (aPLs). aPLs, either anticardiolipin antibodies of the IgG or IgM serotype or the lupus anticoagulant, link the seemingly disparate syndromes of recurrent pregnancy loss with spontaneous thrombosis and suggest that the placenta and systemic blood vessels may in some way be targets of autoantibodies with similar phospholipid specificity. Preliminary classification criteria for APS are described in Table 55–3. This classification of pregnancy loss recognizes that a preterm live birth accompanied by severe preeclampsia or severe placental insufficiency is comparable to fetal loss late in pregnancy.

Prevention

Preconception counseling and close maternal–fetal monitoring are recommended during all pregnancies of aPL-positive women. Recommendations for pharmacologic treatment are

Table 55–3. Preliminary classification criteria for APS.[1]

Clinical criteria
Vascular thrombosis

1. One or more clinical episodes of arterial, venous, or small-vessel thrombosis in any tissue or organ.

2. Thrombosis confirmed by imaging or Doppler studies or histopathology, with the exception of superficial venous thrombosis.

3. For histopathologic confirmation, thrombosis should be present without significant evidence of inflammation in the vessel wall.

Pregnancy morbidity

1. One or more unexplained deaths of a morphologically normal fetus at or beyond the tenth week of gestation, with normal fetal morphology documented by ultrasound or by direct examination of the fetus.

2. Or one or more premature births of a morphologically normal neonate at or before week 34 of gestation because of severe preeclampsia or severe placental insufficiency.

3. Or three or more unexplained consecutive spontaneous abortions before the tenth week of gestation, with maternal anatomic or hormonal abnormalities and paternal and maternal chromosomal causes excluded.

Laboratory criteria

1. Anticardiolipin antibody of IgG and/or IgM isotype in blood, present in medium or high titer, on at least two occasions at least 6 weeks apart, measured by standard enzyme-linked immunosorbent assay for β_2-glycoprotein I-dependent anticardiolipin antibodies.

2. Or lupus anticoagulant present in plasma, on two or more occasions at least 6 weeks apart, detected according to the guidelines of the International Society on Thrombosis and Hemostasis.

[1]Definite antiphospholipid syndrome (APS) is considered to be present if at least one of the clinical and one of the laboratory criteria are met.

Modified with permission from Derksen RHWM et al: Management of the obstetric antiphospholipid syndrome. Arthritis Rheum 2004;50(4):1028.

controversial and specific to a woman's clinical and obstetric history. Combination aspirin and heparin therapy has been recommended. Warfarin is contraindicated during pregnancy (Table 55–4) but can be used in the postpartum period. Both heparin and warfarin are safe for nursing mothers. Primary aPL syndrome and aPL syndrome with SLE are treated similarly.

▶ Complications

Maternal complications include arterial and venous thrombosis, thrombotic microangiopathy, and increased risk of preeclampsia (18–50%). An association between severe preeclampsia and aPL has been reported. The presence of lupus anticoagulant is a strong predictor of a pregnancy-associated thrombotic event; anticardiolipin antibody was less

predictive. A past thrombotic event posed a strong risk and a past history of intrauterine growth retardation (IUGR) or fetal death predicted IUGR in the current pregnancy. Survival rates of neonates born to aPL-positive women are 62–84%. High rates of prematurity (37–43%), fetal distress (50%), and IUGR (30%) have been reported.

Derksen RHWM et al: Management of the obstetric antiphospholipid syndrome. Arthritis Rheum 2004;50:1028. [PMID: 15077285]

MANAGEMENT OF WOMEN WITH CHRONIC KIDNEY DISEASE BEFORE & DURING PREGNANCY

▶ Prevention

Preconception counseling is important in patients with CKD, after kidney transplantation, and while on dialysis. ACEIs and angiotensin receptor blockers (ARBs) are contraindicated in pregnancy (Table 55–4). ACEIs and ARBs disrupt fetal vascular perfusion and renal function and are associated with oligohydramnios, severe fetal renal dysfunction, fetal growth retardation, pulmonary hypoplasia, limb contractures, and calvarial hypoplasia mediated via the suppression of the fetal renin–angiotensin system. Studies have shown no adverse effects from exposure to ACEIs/ARBs in the first trimester of pregnancy. Thus, inadvertent exposure to ACEIs/ARBs in the first trimester may not warrant termination of pregnancy. Also, women with CKD who are on ACEIs/ARBs need not be advised to terminate the medication prior to planned conception as long as there is some assurance that pregnancy can be diagnosed promptly and ACEIs/ARBs stopped at that time.

Alwan S et al: Angiotensin II receptor antagonist treatment during pregnancy. Birth Defects Res A Clin Mol Teratol 2005;73:123. [PMID: 15669052]

1. Dialysis & Pregnancy

▶ General Considerations

Diagnosing pregnancy can be difficult in dialysis patients. Results of urine pregnancy tests are not reliable, even if patients are not anuric. hCG levels may be mildly elevated even in nonpregnant patients on dialysis, hence, pregnancy may need to be confirmed by ultrasound.

There is no evidence to suggest that fetal or maternal outcomes are influenced by dialysis modality. The usual methods of selecting a dialysis modality can be employed if dialysis is started during pregnancy. Peritoneal dialysis has the theoretical advantage of gradual ultrafiltration and solute clearance, but peritoneal dialysis may be relatively contraindicated in patients with gestational diabetes due to the possibility of dialysate-induced hyperglycemia.

Table 55–4.   Medications in pregnancy.

Medication	Safety issues	Comments
Common medications in CKD/ESRD		
1. Erythropoietin	Safe to use	Limited data.
2. Iron	Safe to use	Low dose intravenous iron recommended
3. Vitamin D	Widely used	Limited data
4. Heparin	Safe to use	Minimize dose of heparin
5. Coumadin	Not safe	Teratogenic
Common medications in kidney transplantation		
1. Prednisone	Safe to use	Fetal adrenal insufficiency
2. Cyclosporine	Safe to use	IUGR
3. Tacrolimus	Not safe to use	Severe IUGR, renal failure, and hyperkalemia
4. Mycophenolate mofetil	Not safe to use	Teratogenic in animals
5. Azathioprine	Widely used	Fetal neutropenia, teratogenic in high doses
6. Polyclonal antibodies and OKT3	Not safe to use	Very limited data
Common medications in hypertension		
1. ACE inhibitors, ARBs	Not safe to use	Fetal oligohydramnios pulmonary hypoplasia, skeletal deformities
2. Diuretics	Not safe to use	Maternal volume depletion; fetal thrombocytopenia, hemolytic anemia, jaundice
3. β-Blockers	Not safe to use	Fetal bradycardia, hypoglycemia, respiratory distress
4. Labetalol	Widely used	Limited data
5. α-Methyldopa	Safe to use	Limited long-term follow-up shows no developmental problem in children
6. Clonidine	Not safe to use	Limited data
7. Calcium channel blockers	Safe to use	Potentiates the hypotensive effect of magnesium; limit use to refractory hypertension
8. Hydralazine	Safe to use	Given intravenously for acute, severe hypertension

CKD, chronic kidney disease; ESRD, end-stage renal disease; IUGR, intrauterine growth retardation; ACE, angiotensin-converting enzyme; ARBs, angiotensin receptor blockers.

▶ Treatment

A. Dialysis Prescription

The dialysis dose is an important consideration in pregnant patients because intensive dialysis results in a prolonged period of gestation, improved infant survival, and fewer maternal complications. A cumulative weekly dialysis dose exceeding 20 hours per week is recommended. The Registry for Pregnancy in Dialysis Patients reported improved pregnancy outcome in patients who conceived before dialysis therapy was initiated, suggesting that residual renal function and increased clearance of uremic toxins contribute to better outcomes. These women had lower rates of premature birth, low birth weight, and perinatal mortality than those who conceived after starting dialysis. They also had a lower incidence of polyhydramnios and a reduced risk for intradialytic hypotension.

Intensive hemodialysis may be achieved by daily dialysis or nocturnal hemodialysis. Appropriate modifications include a high potassium, low calcium, and low bicarbonate dialysis bath. Daily dialysis treatments (5–6 days/week) will also allow gentle ultrafiltration and avoid rapid hemodynamic changes during the treatment. Patients with hypertension may require intensive ultrafiltration, which may contribute to intradialytic hypotension. Because of the expected increase in plasma volume with pregnancy, vigilant attention must be paid to the changing dry weight of the pregnant dialysis patient. Patients on peritoneal dialysis who cannot tolerate large volume exchanges may need more frequent exchanges. A combination of daytime continuous ambulatory peritoneal dialysis (CAPD) and nighttime continuous cycling peritoneal dialysis (CCPD) may be necessary to achieve dialysis adequacy. Heparin can be used safely for anticoagulation during hemodialysis as it does not cross the placenta and hence is not teratogenic (Table 55–4).

B. Anemia

The anemia of kidney disease is likely to worsen in hemodialysis patients during gestation. Hemoglobin below 8 g/dL poses a significant risk to the fetus. Erythropoietin is safe during pregnancy; there are no reports of teratogenicity. Erythropoietin requirements increase by 50–100% during pregnancy in patients on hemodialysis. Iron deficiency is also common in pregnancy and supplemental oral iron is often prescribed. Intravenous iron can cause acute iron toxicity in the fetus, hence small doses are recommended if there is a poor response to oral agents.

C. Nutrition

Protein intake must be increased to meet the needs of pregnancy. Achieving adequate protein intake may be particularly difficult in patients on peritoneal dialysis. Potassium intake will also need to be increased, especially if dialysis is performed 5–6 days per week. Water-soluble vitamins such as folic acid should be dosed to meet increased demand and loss during dialysis.

Holley JL, Reddy SS: Pregnancy in dialysis patients: a review of outcomes, complications, and management. Semin Dial 2003;16:384. [PMID: 12969392]

Shemin D: Dialysis in pregnant women with chronic kidney disease. Semin Dial 2003;16:379. [PMID: 12969390]

2. Pregnancy after Kidney Transplantation
▶ General Considerations

Fertility is usually restored following kidney transplantation. The incidence of pregnancy can be as high as 12% in transplant recipients of childbearing age; 90% of these pregnancies succeed once they pass the first trimester if the preconception creatinine is ≤1.5 mg/dL.

Women with good allograft function usually experience a physiologic increase in GFR during pregnancy. Short-term effects of glomerular hyperfiltration may manifest as proteinuria, but urinary protein excretion usually returns to baseline values by 3 months postpartum. However, proteinuria in the first trimester of pregnancy indicates underlying kidney disease that may worsen during pregnancy, especially in the setting of uncontrolled hypertension. From an immunologic standpoint, the risk of acute rejection during pregnancy is no different than that expected for nonpregnant controls. Acute rejection rates of 3–9% have been reported.

▶ Clinical Findings

A. Blood Pressure in Pregnant Transplanted Women

In pregnant kidney transplant recipients, blood pressure tends to increase after 20 weeks gestation, making it difficult to distinguish between accelerated hypertension and preeclampsia. Calcineurin inhibitors promote hyperuricemia, making elevated uric acid levels a poor marker of preeclampsia in women taking cyclosporine or tacrolimus. Hypertension and preeclampsia have been reported in 25–40% of pregnancies and the incidence of preeclampsia is four times greater in kidney transplant recipients than in the general population. If hypertension is present at conception, a 5-fold greater risk of worsening hypertension or superimposed preeclampsia exists.

B. Effects of Pregnancy on Allograft Function

The effects of pregnancy on graft function are controversial. Some case–control studies suggest that pregnancy has no adverse effect on allograft function. One controlled study reported poor graft survival: 69% at 10-year follow-up compared to 100% in the control group. The National Transplantation Pregnancy Registry (NTPR) reports a rejection rate of 11% and a 7.5% rate of graft loss at 2 years in patients treated with cyclosporine. Most studies suggest that the two criteria most strongly affecting long-term kidney function are serum creatinine at the time of conception and the interval between transplant and conception. Patients with a serum creatinine of less than 1.5 mg/dL did not have any adverse renal outcome.

▶ Complications

Infectious complications pose a significant problem for pregnant renal transplant recipients. Bacterial infections occur with increased incidence; 40% of patients have urinary tract infections. Pregnant transplant patients should therefore have monthly urine cultures. Opportunistic infections may also pose risks to the fetus. Reactivation of cytomegalovirus (CMV) in pregnancy may cause infection in the fetus. Up to 10% of infants with congenital CMV infection have microcephaly, mental retardation, or perinatal death; 5–15% may have late manifestations such as deafness and learning disabilities. The efficacy of treatment to prevent CMV disease in the fetus has not been established and treatment is reserved for serious maternal infections.

Herpes simplex infection during pregnancy is problematic only when the infection occurs close to the onset of labor. Acyclovir can be safely used in this situation. Toxoplasmosis in the mother may result in neonatal infection in 25–65% of cases and should be treated with sulfadiazine and pyrimethamine or spiromicin, even if the mother is not seriously ill. Hepatitis B can be transmitted vertically to the fetus and 80% of infants born to hepatitis B carriers become carriers themselves. Hepatitis B immune globulin and vaccination are effective in preventing 95% of infections in the neonate. Hepatitis C is a relatively common problem in dialysis patients and in those with kidney transplants. Vertical transmission is thought to be low, but there are no good approaches to prevention.

▶ Treatment

The effects of immunosuppressive drugs on infants of pregnant kidney transplant recipients have not been studied long-term and it is not known whether the risk for childhood cancer or infertility is increased (Table 55–4). Prednisone crosses the placenta in the form of prednisolone and may cause adrenal insufficiency or thymic hypoplasia in infants. These side effects appear minimal when the dose of prednisone is less than 15 mg/day. Azathioprine has been associated with small-for-gestational age babies and myelosuppression in the fetus. Calcineurin inhibitors have not been linked to congenital abnormalities but have been associated with increased risk of small-for-gestational age and very-low-birth weight infants. Tacrolimus, in particular, has been associated with neonatal anuria and hyperkalemia (Table 55–4). There are no data on the use of mycophenolate mofetil in pregnancy. The effects of polyclonal antibodies on the fetus are also unknown. Pregnancy in women with kidney disease requires a multidisciplinary team approach involving nephrologic, obstetric, and pediatric health care providers to maximize the likelihood of good maternal and fetal outcomes.

Armenti VT et al: Report from the National Transplantation Pregnancy Registry (NTPR): outcomes of pregnancy after transplantation. Clin Transpl 2003;123. [PMID: 15387104]

Stratta P et al: Pregnancy in kidney transplantation: satisfactory outcomes and harsh realities. J Nephrol 2003;16:792. [PMID: 14736006]

ACUTE RENAL FAILURE IN PREGNANCY

 ESSENTIALS OF DIAGNOSIS

▶ Rising blood urea nitrogen (BUN) and creatinine levels.

▶ Elements of history that suggest a specific cause.

▶ Will need a complete blood count (CBC) and platelet count and liver function tests.

▶ Urine analysis, especially urine protein.

▶ General Considerations

Acute renal failure in pregnancy is uncommon but can be severe, requiring dialysis. Any of the causes of acute renal failure occurring in the nonpregnant population may also occur during pregnancy, but there are some specific causes of acute renal failure during pregnancy that must be considered. Determining the type of acute renal failure in a pregnant woman will depend on the history, especially the timing of the acute renal failure in terms of the pregnancy (eg, in the first, second, or third trimester or postpartum), the presence or absence of preeclampsia, findings on urine analysis (especially proteinuria, white blood cells, red blood cells), and associated laboratory abnormalities, especially anemia, platelet count, liver transaminases and bilirubin, and tests of coagulation (prothrombin time and partial thromboplastin time).

Because plasma volume is increased in normal pregnancy, normal BUN and creatinine levels are lower in pregnancy than in the nonpregnant state (Table 55–1). Thus, during pregnancy, a creatinine >0.8 mg/dL and a BUN >14 mg/dL are abnormal and consistent with kidney disease (either acute or chronic).

1. Prerenal or Hemodynamic Causes of Acute Renal Failure in Pregnancy

 ESSENTIALS OF DIAGNOSIS

▶ Rising BUN and creatinine.

▶ History, physical examination, and laboratory data consistent with volume depletion, sepsis, or hemorrhage.

▶ General Considerations

Hyperemesis gravidarum and hemorrhage may cause acute renal failure in pregnancy as a result of volume depletion. Sepsis-induced acute renal failure in pregnancy is most often associated with abortion, especially in the developing world and in areas where therapeutic abortion is illegal. Most cases of prerenal acute renal failure in pregnancy occur early in the pregnancy. As in the nonpregnant state, prerenal causes of acute renal failure in pregnancy may progress to acute tubular necrosis (ATN). Prerenal acute renal failure must be distinguished from postrenal (obstruction) and intrinsic acute renal failure.

▶ Clinical Findings

A. Symptoms and Signs

The history and physical examination will suggest volume depletion and/or hemodynamic compromise. Abruptio placentae may precede hemorrhage and is also associated with cortical necrosis.

B. Laboratory Findings

Evidence of intact kidney tubular function (low urine sodium, low urine fractional excretion of sodium and fractional excretion of urea) may often accompany prerenal acute renal failure. An elevated BUN:creatinine ratio may also be seen.

▶ Treatment & Prognosis

Treatment of prerenal acute renal failure in pregnancy is to correct the underlying cause, ie, replete lost volume or blood and treat sepsis. With timely and appropriate treatment, progressive acute renal failure (ATN) may be avoided with an excellent chance of complete recovery of kidney function.

> Finkielman JD et al: The clinical course of patients with septic abortion admitted to an intensive care unit. Inten Care Med 2004;30:1097. [PMID: 15007546]

2. Postrenal Acute Renal Failure in Pregnancy

 ESSENTIALS OF DIAGNOSIS

▶ Rising BUN and creatinine in a pregnant woman.
▶ Obstruction of the urinary tract.

▶ General Considerations

Moderate dilation of the urinary collecting system is usual during pregnancy. This "functional" hydronephrosis is commonly more prominent on the right side, usually with preservation of normal kidney function. In rare cases, acute renal failure can occur if the degree of obstruction is great. In such cases, kidney function often normalizes if the woman is placed in the lateral recumbent position (relieving uterine pressure on the ureters), thereby confirming the diagnosis. In some cases, urologic intervention or delivery is needed to relieve the obstruction and resolve the acute renal failure.

3. Intrinsic Acute Renal Failure in Pregnancy

 ESSENTIALS OF DIAGNOSIS

▶ Rising BUN and creatinine.
▶ Exclusion of prerenal and postrenal causes of acute renal failure.

▶ General Considerations

Although most cases of pyelonephritis during pregnancy do not result in acute renal failure, acute pyelonephritis can cause acute renal failure during pregnancy. As in the nonpregnant population, ATN, acute interstitial nephritis, and acute glomerulonephritis may also cause acute renal failure in a pregnant woman. In such cases, the history, physical examination, and urine analysis will usually lead to these diagnoses. However, there are some specific causes of acute renal failure that are seen only during pregnancy or are associated primarily with pregnancy. These include the acute renal failure seen with preeclampsia/eclampsia, acute fatty liver of pregnancy (AFLP), thrombotic microangiopathies [hemolytic uremic syndrome (HUS), thrombotic thrombocytopenic purpura (TTP), and HELLP syndrome (hemolysis with a microangiopathic blood smear, elevated liver enzymes, and a low platelet count)], and cortical necrosis.

4. Preeclampsia/Eclampsia-Associated Acute Renal Failure

 ESSENTIALS OF DIAGNOSIS

▶ Typically develops late in the third trimester.
▶ Preeclampsia does not occur before 20 weeks of gestation.
▶ Preeclampsia = hypertension, edema, and proteinuria.

▶ General Considerations

Kidney function is usually normal or near normal in women with preeclampsia unless hemodynamic instability develops with excessive bleeding or disseminated intravascular coagulation (DIC) occurs. Mild degrees of kidney dysfunction may be seen with preeclampsia, likely because of reduced glomerular permeability. Delivery of the fetus usually results in resolution of the preeclampsia in 24–48 hours. Severe preeclampsia may also present with thrombotic microangiopathic acute renal failure (see below and the section on eclampsia/preeclampsia).

5. Thrombotic Microangiopathies

 ESSENTIALS OF DIAGNOSIS

▶ Thrombocytopenia.
▶ Microangiopathic anemia.
▶ Normal prothrombin time.
▶ Abnormal kidney function.
▶ Usually occurs late in pregnancy or early postpartum.

▶ General Considerations

It can be difficult to make a specific diagnosis when acute renal failure associated with thrombocytopenia and microangiopathic hemolytic anemia occurs late in pregnancy. In addition to TTP and HUS, severe preeclampsia and HELLP (hemolysis with a microangiopathic blood smear, elevated liver enzymes, and a low platelet count) can cause acute renal failure as a result of thrombotic microangiopathy. Although TTP and HUS are considered distinct entities, because their clinical presentations are often indistinguishable, they are best considered as part of a spectrum of disease. Differentiating severe preeclampsia or HELLP from TTP-HUS is important for both therapeutic and prognostic reasons. The most useful distinguishing features are the timing of the onset of acute renal failure and the blood pressure and urine protein during the pregnancy.

▶ Clinical Findings

A. Symptoms and Signs

Severe preeclampsia is more common than TTP-HUS and usually presents with proteinuria, hypertension, and edema late in pregnancy. TTP-HUS often occurs postpartum without an antecendent history of pregnancy-associated hypertension or proteinuria. When TTP-HUS occurs antepartum, it often presents early in the second or even during the first trimester. Importantly, unlike TTP-HUS, acute renal failure with preeclampsia and HELLP usually resolves with delivery.

B. Laboratory Findings

Thrombocytopenia and microangiopathic anemia are the cardinal findings. Elevated liver enzymes may occur with TTP-HUS, but if they are extremely high, it should suggest HELLP (Figure 55–2). Patients with TTP generally have very low levels of plasma ADAMTS13 while HELLP is associated with only mildly to moderately low ADAMTS13 levels.

▶ Differential Diagnosis

In addition to severe preeclampsia and HELLP, acute renal failure occurring late in pregnancy may also be associated with AFLP, disseminated intravascular coagulation with sepsis, hemorrhage, or obstetric catastrophe (eg, abruptio placentae). The differential diagnosis may also include severe ATN and cortical necrosis. In most cases, the clinical history and laboratory findings will narrow the diagnostic possibilities.

▶ Treatment

The optimal treatment of TTP-HUS in pregnancy is the same as in the nonpregnant population. Plasma infusion with or without plasma exchange is the mainstay of treatment and has significantly improved mortality. Renal replacement therapy may be required depending on the clinical circumstances. The treatment of HELLP is more controversial, although delivery is clearly indicated. Some of the abnormal laboratory results may transiently worsen after delivery, but usually normalize within postpartum week one.

▶ Prognosis

Before the use of plasma exchange, the mortality of pregnancy-associated TTP-HUS approached 90%. Today, with appropriate treatment, mortality has improved, although a significant proportion of women may be left with CKD or, less often, ESRD requiring dialysis.

George JN: The association of pregnancy with thrombotic thrombocytopenic purpura-hemolytic uremic syndrome. Curr Opin Hematol 2003;10:339. [PMID: 12913787]

Lattuada A et al: Mild to moderate reduction of a von Willebrand factor cleaving protease (ADAMTS13) in pregnant women with HELLP microangiopathic syndrome. Haematologica 2003;88:1029. [PMID: 12969811]

Vesely SK et al: Pregnancy outcomes after recovery from thrombotic thrombocytopenic purpura-hemolytic uremic syndrome. Transfusion 2004;44:1149. [PMID: 15265118]

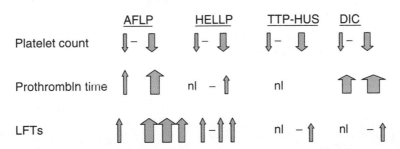

▲ **Figure 55–2.** Laboratory values in acute renal failure due to thrombotic microangiopathy and disseminated intravascular coagulation. AFLP, acute fatty liver of pregnancy; HELLP, hemolysis with elevated liver enzymes and low platelets; TTP-HUS, thrombotic thrombocytopenic purpura–hemolytic uremic syndrome; DIC, disseminated intravascular coagulation; LFTs, liver function tests.

6. Acute Fatty Liver of Pregnancy

▶ Jaundice and liver dysfunction.

▶ Occurs at the end of pregnancy or in early puerperium.

▶ Usually simultaneous coagulation disorders.

▶ Liver biopsy is diagnostic.

▶ General Considerations

AFLP is characterized by microvesicular fatty infiltration of hepatocytes without necrosis or inflammation. This disorder is unique to human pregnancy and is relatively uncommon, occurring in one in 7000–16,000 deliveries. It usually occurs late in pregnancy, close to term. Some patients may present after delivery.

▶ Pathogenesis

As with Reye's syndrome, microvesicular fatty infiltration is seen histologically with AFLP. Affected women may have an inherited enzyme deficiency in β-oxidation of fatty acids that predisposes them to AFLP. The accumulation of long-chain 3-hydroxyacyl metabolites produced by the fetus or the placenta is toxic to the maternal liver and may be the cause of the disease.

▶ Clinical Findings

A. Symptoms and Signs

Women with AFLP often present with nausea and vomiting, abdominal pain, lethargy, jaundice, headache, bleeding, or altered mental status due to hepatic encephalopathy. However, in some patients incidentally elevated liver test results lead to the diagnosis.

B. Laboratory Findings

See Figure 55–2. Abnormal liver function tests occur with modest to severe elevations of aminotransferase. The platelet count is normal unless progression to DIC has occurred. In such cases, antithrombin III levels will be low. In severe cases of AFLP, elevations of ammonia may occur as well as profound hypoglycemia. Acute renal failure occurs in up to 60% of cases.

C. Imaging Studies

Imaging studies are primarily used to exclude hepatic infarct or hematoma. Fat may be seen on ultrasound or computed tomography (CT) of the liver but is rarely diagnostic.

D. Special Tests

Liver biopsy is diagnostic and shows pericentral pallor with lobular disarray and vacuolization of the centrizonal hepatocytes. Special stains should be done to identify the microvesicular fat. Because of the coagulopathy accompanying AFLP, liver biopsy caries a high risk of bleeding and is reserved for cases in which the diagnosis is in doubt and/or treatment is being delayed.

▶ Differential Diagnosis

Acute renal failure associated with severe preeclampsia, HELLP, and thrombotic microangiopathies comprises the diagnostic possibilities (Figure 55–2). Hepatic infarction or hematoma and other causes of acute liver failure should be excluded.

▶ Treatment

Treatment is delivery after stabilization. Supportive therapy is usually required and may include monitoring in an intensive care unit. Glucose infusion and reversal of the associated coagulopathy are usually required.

▶ Prognosis

Today most women recover without sequelae, but a mortality rate of 10% has been reported. AFLP can recur in subsequent pregnancies. One out of four infants born to women with AFLP will have an inherited disorder of long-chain 3-hydroxyacyl CoA dehydrogenase deficiency (LCHAD). When stressed, such infants are at risk of fatal nonketotic hypoglycemia. Additionally, some forms of LCHAD deficiency are associated with neonatal dilated cardiomyopathy or progressive neuromyopathy.

7. Cortical Necrosis

▶ Seen with complications of pregnancy, eg, abruptio placentae, placenta previa, amniotic fluid embolism, prolonged intrauterine death.

▶ Usually associated with severe renal ischemia and/or DIC.

▶ Abrupt onset of oliguria or anuria.

▶ Often a triad of anuria, gross hematuria, and flank pain.

▶ General Considerations

Bilateral cortical necrosis is an unusual cause of acute renal failure, but when seen it often occurs in the obstetric setting. It usually follows a complication of pregnancy and is associated with DIC and/or severely impaired renal blood flow. Cortical necrosis is usually diagnosed clinically and confirmed radiologically by finding hypoechoic or hypodense areas of renal cortex on ultrasound or CT scan. Renal calcification on plain film may be seen 1–2 months after the event. There is no specific treatment for cortical necrosis and many women require chronic dialysis; 20–40% may have some recovery of kidney function and be left with CKD. Most women with acute renal failure from cortical necrosis will remain dialysis dependent.

PREECLAMPSIA & ECLAMPSIA

 ESSENTIALS OF DIAGNOSIS

▶ A systolic blood pressure exceeding 140 mm Hg or a diastolic blood pressure exceeding 90 mm Hg.

▶ Proteinuria that may be in the nephrotic range.

▶ Eclampsia = grand mal seizure activity in a pregnant woman with preeclampsia.

▶ General Considerations

Preeclampsia is defined as the development of new onset hypertension and proteinuria in a pregnant woman after 20 weeks gestation. A significant increase in blood pressure in a previously normotensive woman during pregnancy should raise suspicion for the diagnosis. Proteinuria in excess of 300 mg in a 24-hour period is abnormal during pregnancy and should raise the possibility of preeclampsia.

Preeclampsia occurs in 3–14% of pregnancies. Most cases are mild and very few occur in pregnant women less than 34 weeks gestation. For unclear reasons, primigravid women less than 20 years of age are at highest risk for developing preeclampsia. Many factors are recognized as risks for preeclampsia, including higher blood pressure at the start of pregnancy, large maternal body size, preexisting hypertension, antiphospholipid syndrome, advanced maternal age (exceeding 35–40 years), preexisting diabetes, multiple pregnancies, and vascular or rheumatologic disease. A family history of preeclampsia raises the risk 2- to 5-fold and recent studies suggest that a paternal genetic factor might also contribute to defective placentation and the subsequent evolution of preeclampsia.

Eclampsia is recognized by the new onset of grand mal seizures in a pregnant woman with preeclampsia. Eclampsia develops in 2% and 0.5% of severe and mild preeclamptic women, respectively, and is more common in nonwhite nulliparous women of low socioeconomic status. Eclamptic seizures are typically short lived and do not result in

neurologic deficit. The cause of eclamptic seizures is not known.

▶ Pathogenesis

Abnormal placentation, placental ischemia, and endothelial dysfunction play supportive and integrated roles in the pathogenesis of preeclampsia. Abnormal trophoblastic invasion of the endothelium and maternal spiral arteries and the impaired trophoblast differentiation that follows preclude formation of the low resistance highly capacitant uteroplacental circulation. Placental ischemia is thought to elaborate circulating factors that culminate in maternal endothelial dysfunction, extreme renal vasoconstriction, and the clinical correlates of hypertension, arteriole thrombosis, and multiorgan failure. Genetic predisposition may pose a risk as well and both maternal and paternal contributions may be operative.

Chaiworapongsa T et al: Evidence supporting a role for blockade of the vascular endothelial growth factor system in the pathophysiology of preeclampsia. Young Investigator Award. Am J Obstet Gynecol 2004;190.1541. [PMID: 15284729]

Solomon CG, Seely EW: Preeclampsia—searching for the cause. N Engl J Med 2004;12:350. [PMID: 14764924]

Wang X et al: A proinflammatory cytokine response is present in the fetal placental vasculature in placental insufficiency. Am J Obstet Gynecol 2003;189:1445. [PMID: 14634584]

▶ Prevention

Several agents have been studied to prevent preeclampsia but none has definitively been shown to reduce the risk. These include aspirin, calcium, fish oil, and vitamins C and E, the latter two for their purported antioxidant effect. A preventive role for the selective serotonin-2 receptor antagonist ketaserin has been suggested, but further study of its potential to mitigate endothelial cell vasoconstriction via serotonin blockade is needed.

Only aspirin has been confirmed to be safe, but its efficacy in preventing preeclampsia remains unclear. Aspirin may modestly reduce the risk in moderate to high-risk pregnant women but is not recommended for use in low-risk pregnancies. In addition, aspirin has not been shown to be of benefit when pregnancy-induced hypertension has developed. Aspirin also does not prevent progression of preeclampsia to HELLP. The risk of bleeding diathesis in the latter increases the risks associated with aspirin.

Coomarasamy A et al: Aspirin for prevention of preeclampsia in women with historical risk factors: a systematic review. Obstet Gynecol 2003;101:1319. [PMID: 12798543]

Duley L et al: Antiplatelet agents for preventing pre-eclampsia and its complications. Cochrane Database Syst Rev 2004;1: CD004659. [PMID: 14974074]

▶ Clinical Findings

A. Symptoms and Signs

Symptoms and signs include the gradual development of hypertension, proteinuria, and edema, which all typically manifest in the late third trimester. Preeclampsia rarely presents before 20 weeks gestation, but symptoms can begin as early as 24 weeks (the late second trimester) or as late as immediately before delivery or even early postpartum. Primigravidas with hypertension, edema, and proteinuria most likely have preeclampsia and can be definitively diagnosed by the presence of two or more criteria. A rise in blood pressure from baseline, even to a level considered within normal range, constitutes risk and should be considered a clue to preeclampsia. While blood pressure increases usually occur in the second trimester, hypertension per se does not usually manifest until late in the third trimester. The diagnosis is confirmed by finding increased blood pressure on two occasions at least 6 hours, but no more than 7 days, apart. Edema is typical of normotensive pregnancy but may be abrupt and severe in preeclampsia and occurs in the face of decreased intravascular volume. Neurologic manifestations of preeclampsia include headache, blurred vision, scotoma, and cortical blindness. The latter is rare and signifies severe preeclampsia.

All signs and symptoms of preeclampsia generally resolve within 2–6 weeks after delivery.

B. Laboratory Findings

Urinary dipstick-positive proteinuria is an important clue, although not all preeclamptic women present with proteinuria. The 24-hour urine measurement for total protein remains the gold standard for quantifying proteinuria. However, a random or spot urine protein-to-creatinine ratio from nontimed specimens can be helpful in identifying significant proteinuria. Routine urinalysis (dipstick for protein) alone is not sensitive enough to rule out significant proteinuria. Proteinuria in preeclampsia typically evolves gradually and may reach a nephrotic range; hence, its absence should not be cause for excluding preeclampsia from the differential diagnosis of hypertension in pregnancy.

In addition to proteinuria, preeclamptic women may have thrombocytopenia (secondary to increased platelet turnover), hyperuricemia, hypocalcemia, and microangiopathic hemolytic anemia. The presence of hemolysis may not be obvious if the hemoconcentration is significant enough to mask anemia. Hemolysis in the presence of elevated liver enzymes suggests the evolution of the HELLP syndrome. Hemoconcentration, proteinuria, and hyperuricemia suggest preeclampsia, and although liver enzymes may be elevated in mild or moderate preeclampsia, severe elevations (greater than 2-fold), in conjunction with proteinuria >5 g/24 hours, increased creatinine, and thrombocytopenia suggest severe preeclampsia. Elevated lactate dehydrogenase

and a smear indicative of hemolysis support the diagnosis of HELLP.

C. Imaging Studies

Imaging of the uterine artery by Doppler flow can be used to assess risk. Reductions in flow within uterine and/or umbilical arteries suggest risk for impending preeclampsia. Diastolic notching of the arcuate vessels of the uterus and high resistive indices have been used as predictive tests. However, neither has adequate positive predictive value to warrant their routine use even in high-risk patients.

D. Special Tests

Urinary placental growth factor (PlGF) may be useful in predicting the future development of preeclampsia. PlGF appears to rise normally in women destined to have preeclampsia but nadirs at a level lower than in women without preeclampsia. Placental peptide measurements may be employed in the future to assess for preeclamptic risk, although studies of their potential use are currently experimental.

Conde-Agudelo A et al: World Health Organization systematic review of screening tests for pre-eclampsia. Obstet Gynecol 2004;104:1367. [PMID: 15572504]

Levine RJ et al: Urinary placental growth factor and risk of preeclampsia. JAMA 2005;293:77. [PMID: 15632339]

Papageorghiou AT et al: The role of the uterine artery Doppler in predicting adverse pregnancy outcome. Best Pract Res Clin Obstet Gynecol 2004;18:383. [PMID: 15183134]

▶ Differential Diagnosis

Preeclampsia is a clinical diagnosis. The differential diagnosis includes chronic hypertension, gestational hypertension, new onset essential hypertension, and acute exacerbation of underlying kidney disease. Other diseases that can present with various combinations of hypertension, coagulopathy, and liver and renal dysfunction include primary liver disease, TTP-HUS, pancreatitis, diseases characterized by thrombocytopenia such as lupus, or even gestational thrombocytopenia.

The presence of liver enzyme abnormalities, hemoconcentration, and perhaps hemolysis is not typical in chronic hypertension and should prompt suspicion for preeclampsia. Further, chronic hypertension will not resolve postpartum as can be expected with preeclampsia.

Gestational hypertension may present with mild proteinuria late in the third trimester. However, both the increase in blood pressure and the elevated urinary protein excretion resolve shortly after delivery and typically without complications. Gestational hypertension that occurs earlier in gestation is more likely to evolve into preeclampsia and should be treated as such. Similarly, gestational hypertension with symptoms of severe preeclampsia, headache, growth restriction, or features suggestive of HELLP should be treated as preeclampsia.

New onset hypertension may be difficult to distinguish from preeclampsia, particularly in young, nulliparous women. The development of hypertension in a pregnant woman prior to 20 weeks gestation favors a diagnosis of new onset essential hypertension. The normal physiologic fall in blood pressure that occurs in the early stages of pregnancy may mask the presence of underlying but as yet undiagnosed hypertension.

▶ Complications

Eclampsia is the major complication of untreated or unsuccessfully treated preeclampsia. Eclampsia occurs in 0.5% of mild and 2% of severe preeclampsia. Eclamptic seizures are indistinguishable from tonic–clonic seizures of other etiologies and are treated differently (see the section on treatment). In the 15–20% of preeclamptic women who do not have proteinuria, seizures may help retrospectively distinguish preeclampsia from chronic or new onset hypertension.

The timing of eclampsia is variable with approximately 50% of cases occurring prior to term, one-third at term, 25% postpartum, and less than 10% at 31 weeks. The pathogenesis of eclampsia is unclear, although cerebral hemorrhage and edema are thought to play a central role.

HELLP is likely a form of severe preeclampsia, but its classification in this regard remains controversial. HELLP develops in 10–20% of women with preeclampsia/eclampsia. Importantly, HELLP is an indication for delivery to avoid hepatic complications, such as rupture, infarct, and hemorrhage. Signs and symptoms include abdominal pain, commonly occurring in the right upper quadrant or epigastrium, nausea, vomiting, and elevated blood pressure. Proteinuria less commonly accompanies symptoms, occurring in 15–20% of cases.

The diagnostic criteria for HELLP include signs of microangiopathic hemolytic anemia (peripheral blood smear with schistocytes, hyperbilirubinemia or elevated lactate dehydrogenase, and decreased haptoglobin), thrombocytopenia, and elevated liver enzymes (Figure 55–2). The latter can be increased in preeclampsia, but in the presence of the other laboratory abnormalities noted above, HELLP should be considered. Delivery is indicated for women with HELLP who are past 34 weeks gestation and who exhibit signs and symptoms of multiorgan failure, DIC, renal failure, abruptio placentae, liver failure, or hemorrhage.

Sibai BM: Diagnosis, controversies and management of the syndrome of hemolysis, elevated liver enzymes, and low platelet count. Obstet Gynecol 2004;103:981. [PMID: 15121574]

▶ Treatment

A. Preeclampsia

Expectant treatment of preeclampsia includes close fetal and maternal monitoring and treatment of moderate to severe hypertension. Medical intervention is considered appropriate when the systolic blood pressure reaches 170 mm Hg or the diastolic blood pressure reaches 104 mm Hg with an ultimate target of 140–150 mm Hg systolic and 90–105 mm Hg diastolic. α-Methyldopa is the antihypertensive medication of choice because it has a long history of use in pregnancy without complications (Figure 55–2). Diuretics and β-blockers are generally avoided, but calcium channel blockers and, acutely, hydralazine and labetalol may be used (Figure 55–2). Severe preeclampsia is an indication for delivery and should prompt consideration of magnesium sulfate therapy, the drug of choice for primary prevention of eclampsia in women with severe preeclampsia. Gestational hypertension, when severe, should be treated as preeclampsia.

B. Eclampsia

This obstetric emergency poses significant risk of death or neurologic sequelae. In addition to general stabilization measures, intravenous magnesium sulfate is the drug of choice for treating eclamptic seizures. Calcium gluconate may be needed if symptoms of hypocalcemia evolve. Anticonvulsant agents such as phenytoin may be used, but in general are less effective than magnesium sulfate in preventing recurrent seizures. Moderate to severe hypertension (systolic pressure greater than 160 mm Hg and diastolic pressure greater than 105 mm Hg) should be treated with labetalol or hydralazine. No benefit of treating mild hypertension has been shown.

C. HELLP

As with eclampsia, management of HELLP syndrome includes maternal and fetal stabilization, therapy for hypertension to a target of less than 160/105 mm Hg, consideration of magnesium sulfate, and timely delivery for women after 34 weeks gestation. Corticosteroids are administered for pregnancies less than 34 weeks to optimize fetal lung maturation.

Sibai BM: Magnesium sulfate prophylaxis in preeclampsia: lessons learned from recent trials. Am J Obstet Gynecol 2004;190:1520. [PMID: 15284724]

▶ Prognosis

A. Preeclampsia

Multiparous women with a history of preeclampsia have a 3-fold increased risk of recurrent preeclampsia in subsequent pregnancies. Mild preeclampsia occurring near term in primagravid women is associated with a good outcome, rapid fall in blood pressure, and a 5–7% recurrence rate. Both severe preeclampsia and preeclampsia occurring early in pregnancy are associated with an increased risk of recurrence as well as an increased risk of developing chronic hypertension.

Women with a history of preeclampsia are at increased risk for cardiovascular disease and as many as 78% develop chronic hypertension. Risk of stroke is increased 3-fold in women with a history of preeclampsia.

B. HELLP

There is currently no therapy known to prevent recurrent HELLP. Prognosis for mothers with HELLP is generally good with only 1% maternal mortality. There is a 2–19% risk of recurrence and a 20% risk of preeclampsia in subsequent pregnancies.

C. Eclampsia

One-third of eclampsia is not preventable. Those with the earliest symptoms of preeclampsia are at highest risk of recurrence and/or a bad outcome. Maternal death occurs at a rate of 0–13.9% and is highest in women with early onset of eclampsia (eg, prior to 28 weeks). Complications of eclampsia occur in a large number of women (70%).

Chames MC et al: Subsequent pregnancy outcome in women with a history of HELLP syndrome at 28 weeks of gestation. Am J Obstet Gynecol 2003;188:1504. [PMID: 12824985]

Aging & Renal Disease

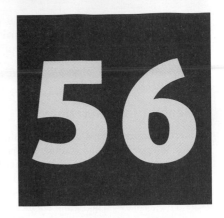

Nada B. Dimkovic, MD, &
Dimitrios G. Oreopoulos, MD

As the elderly population continues to grow, the diagnosis and treatment of renal diseases become challenges for the everyday nephrology practice. Although elderly patients are prone to the same diseases of the kidney as younger patients, the diagnostic criteria are not so clearly defined. Anatomic and functional age-induced changes often overlap pathologic processes. The resulting reduced renal function decreases the individual's capacity to respond to a variety of stresses and has important clinical implications for diagnosis and treatment. Comorbid conditions, the absence of classic symptoms, "symptomless" conditions in those with impaired consciousness, and the poor correlation between clinical presentation and the etiology of disease make the diagnosis of renal diseases in the elderly even more difficult. Finally, several pathologic conditions of the kidneys might occur simultaneously in the elderly.

ACUTE RENAL FAILURE

▶ General Considerations

Acute renal failure (ARF) is more frequent in elderly patients than in younger patients and it is often due to multiple causes. Predisposing factors are age-related changes in renal structure and function. The incidence of ARF is estimated to involve 6–10% of all admissions of the elderly to an acute medical service.

▶ Pathogenesis

The most frequent causes of ARF are nephrotoxic drugs, sepsis, and hypoperfusion. Radiocontrast-induced ARF and postoperative ARF are still very frequent (occurring in about 17% and 25% of cases, respectively).

▶ Clinical Findings

About 50% of the patients with ARF have a prerenal etiology and the majority of them have only mild renal impairment. Oliguria is not a prominent finding in ARF in the elderly and

cases of nonoliguric ARF may go unrecognized. This may result in overdosing patients with renally excreted medications (digitalis, gentamicin). Hypophosphatemia and hypokalemia, when present, most probably reflect the severity of the underlying disease or malnutrition.

▶ Treatment

The treatment of patients with ARF requires careful monitoring of fluid and electrolyte balance. It is very important to prevent malnutrition since hypercatabolism is a frequent finding in elderly patients with ARF; nutritional support should be implemented during the early phase since such patients may lose about 0.5 kg of body mass per day. On the other hand, fluid restriction will delay recovery from ARF and lead to a deterioration in central nervous system function. In patients with advanced renal failure standard dialytic techniques including slow continuous methods should be applied.

▶ Prognosis

The prognosis differs depending on the underlying disease since age itself does not have a significant impact on the prognosis of patients with ARF. The aged kidney retains the capacity to recover from acute ischemic or toxic injury over several weeks. However, care should be taken to avoid nephrotoxins, radiocontrast agents, and volume depletion. The overall mortality rates correlate with the severity of clinical disease ranging between 40% and 60%. Aortic aneurysm repair had very high mortality (as high as 100% in some series) but recent introduction of endovascular repair has decreased this substantially. Other causes of acute renal failure such as hepatic failure, shock, and renovascular disease also have high mortality. Patients with intrinsic renal failure had a higher than expected mortality rate possibly because of delays in diagnosis. A higher mortality rate was also seen in obstructive uropathy in the elderly, which is caused by malignant diseases more often than in younger patients. The prognosis is negatively influenced by malnutrition and high urea and creatinine levels. Of those patients who survive to discharge, about 60% have complete recovery of renal function and the remaining have some degree of renal impairment not requiring dialysis.

GLOMERULAR DISEASES

▷ General Considerations

Glomerular diseases have a similar or slightly higher incidence in the elderly than in younger adults. The disease spectrum is similar to that in younger populations with the main presenting features being proteinuria and hematuria.

Renal biopsy, as a diagnostic marker, remains the gold standard for diagnosis, with no significant increase in complication rates as compared to younger patients. Still, some age-related differences exist with regard to difficulties in distinguishing lesions of chronic ischemia from previous proliferative glomerulonephritis (GN) and focal sclerosing GN. Elderly patients who undergo renal biopsy have a greater incidence of nephrotic syndrome or acute renal failure than younger patients: Idiopathic GN is the most common underlying diagnosis followed by secondary GN and unclassified GN.

1. NEPHROTIC SYNDROME

▷ General Considerations

Nephrotic syndrome is the most common reason for renal biopsy in the elderly. The underlying reasons include membranous nephropathy (an almost three times higher incidence than in the overall population), minimal change disease (MCD), amyloidosis, and multiple myeloma. Focal segmental glomerulosclerosis and immunoglobulin A (IgA) nephropathy are less common than in younger patients.

2. MEMBRANOUS NEPHROPATHY

▷ General Considerations

Out of all cases of membranous nephropathy in the elderly, about 80% are idiopathic and 20% are secondary to solid organ tumors and drugs.

▷ Clinical Findings

A full clinical examination, chest x-ray, CT scan of the abdomen, and stool examination should be performed as screening tests. Apart from nephrotic proteinuria, which is a usual finding, elderly patients have hypertension, hematuria, and renal impairment at the time of biopsy more frequently than younger patients.

▷ Treatment

Treatment with prednisone and chlorambucil has a favorable effect, but remission rates were lower, the time to remission was longer, and the severity of side effects was higher. The recommended dose of chlorambucil is 0.1 mg/kg/day for 3–6 months with or without low-dose corticosteroids.

3. MINIMAL CHANGE NEPHROPATHY

▷ General Considerations

The typical presentation of minimal change nephropathy (MCN) in elderly patients is nephritic syndrome. Again, microscopic hematuria, hypertension, and renal impairment are more frequent at the time of presentation than in younger patients.

▷ Complications

Complications resulting from hypoalbuminemia, hyperlipidemia, and hypercoagulability include thrombotic events, infections, and progressive cardiovascular disease.

▷ Treatment

Treatment with a standard immunosuppressive regimen can be used, but for a longer duration than in younger patients. Corticosteroid-resistant patients may benefit from chlorambucil, cyclophosphamide, or cyclosporine A, but with a risk of bone marrow depression.

4. FOCAL SEGMENTAL GLOMERULOSCLEROSIS

▷ General Considerations

This is not the usual form of glomerulonephritis in the elderly.

▷ Clinical Findings

Heavy proteinuria is a typical presentation of disease, which is often associated with some degree of renal impairment.

▷ Treatment

A trial of corticosteroids for 3 months (or even an additional 3 months if there is no response) should be considered. Angiotensin-converting enzyme inhibitors (ACEIs) and angiotensin II receptor blockers (ARBs) have an antiproteinuric effect and should be used either before trial of steroids or simultaneously with steroids.

5. PROLIFERATIVE GLOMERULONEPHRITIS

▷ General Considerations

Immune complex deposition, antineutrophylic cytoplasmic antibody (ANCA), and antiglomerular basement membrane (anti-GBM) antibodies may cause proliferative GN with the clinical findings and course of disease similar to those found in younger patients. Elderly patients tend to present with much higher serum creatinine levels and a higher incidence of hypertension and refractory renal impairment. Standard immunosuppressive therapy in elderly patients appears to be as effective as in younger patients in terms of short-term prognosis, but there is a higher risk of complications with immunosuppression.

▶ Clinical Findings

Crescentic GN can be associated with immune deposits (as seen in severe IgA nephropathy or lupus nephritis) or with pauci-immune disease without immune deposits (Wegener's granulomatosis, anti-GBM disease, and polyarteritis nodosa). The clinical presentation includes nausea, anorexia, malaise, edema, arthralgia, and myalgia. Symptoms of pyrexia, rash, and hemoptysis suggest a diagnosis of vasculitis. Renal manifestations include hematuria (microscopic or macroscopic), hypertension, and oliguria. Serum ANCA levels, anti-GBM levels, antinuclear factor, complement, immunoglobulin levels, and renal biopsy help distinguishing the different syndromes.

▶ Treatment

A standard immunosuppressive regimen with steroids and cyclophosphamide is indicated.

6. Systemic Disorders Causing Glomerular Diseases

▶ General Considerations

As in the overall population, glomerular diseases are associated with diabetes, myeloma, systemic lupus erythematosus, and systemic bacterial infections and no specific findings for elderly patients have been described compared to younger patients.

▶ Clinical Findings

Acute poststreptococcal glomerulonephritis (APSGN) originates more often from pyodermal than from throat infection. Therefore antideoxyribonuclease B is a more specific test than antistreptolysin O titer in elderly patients with APSGN. Oliguria is a more frequent finding most probably because of underlying age-related renal changes. The outcome of disease is similar to that in younger patients and most patients recover renal function.

RENOVASCULAR DISEASE

1. Ischemic Nephropathy

▶ General Considerations

Ischemic nephropathy (or insufficient renal perfusion) includes two entities: Renal macrovascular disease or renal artery stenosis (RAS) and microvascular diseases, which affect intrarenal arteries.

The prevalence of RAS is difficult to estimate, but according to some data age is a significant multivariate predictor

for RAS (>50%). The prevalence of significant RAS is ~50% in hypertensive patients >55 years of age who have coexistent coronary artery disease (CAD) or peripheral vascular disease (PVD). The risk factors include age, hypertension, diabetes, and evidence of vascular disease elsewhere in the body.

▶ Clinical Findings

A. Symptoms and Signs

Disease should be suspected in patients who have flash pulmonary edema, unresponsive hypertension, and generalized vascular disease, in those who develop ARF after mild hypotension or with use of ACEIs or ARBs, and in cases of renal impairment of unknown etiology.

B. Imaging Studies

Diagnostic procedures include duplex ultrasonography, captopril renal scintigraphy, and magnetic resonance (MR) and computed tomographic (CT) angiography using the gold standard of intra-arterial angiography.

▶ Complications

The disease is often undetected and if left untreated stenosis will progress over a few years.

▶ Treatment

Therapy includes angioplasty, angioplasty with stenting, and surgery. The initial success of angioplasty is high (90–95%), but restenosis occurs in up to 25% of patients. Stents inserted into the renal arteries have improved long-term results. Surgical procedures include aortorenal bypass, transaortic renal endarterectomy, hepatorenal or gastroduodenal renal bypass (for right-side stenosis), splenorenal bypass (for left-side stenosis), extraanatomic revascularization, and autotransplantation. Even though results with surgery are very good, the treatment is not always recommended due to the progressive decline in renal function even after successful revascularization.

Microvascular disease of the kidney has not been extensively studied and it is suggested to be a cause of many cases of end-stage renal disease (ESRD) of "unknown etiology."

2. Atheroembolic Disease

▶ General Considerations

Atheroembolic disease may be a consequence of myocardial infarction, atrial fibrillation, subacute bacterial endocarditis, extensive surgery, and angiography. Although uncommon, it may cause both acute and chronic renal failure.

▶ Clinical Findings

Clinical finding may be absent or include severe flank pain and tenderness, hematuria, pyrexia, renal failure, and hypertension. In case of cholesterol embolism, patients may experience a sudden increase in serum creatinine, signs of peripheral embolism in the limbs, confusional state, gut ischemia, and peripheral eosinophilia after arterial catheterization or systemic heparinization. Small emboli are difficult to diagnose; major emboli are defined by pyelography, renal scan, and aortography. Cholesterol embolism is confirmed by renal biopsy (intravascular cholesterol crystals) and skin or muscle biopsy.

▶ Treatment

Therapy includes thrombolytic agents given intraarterially. The final renal function depends on the collateral renal blood flow.

SYSTEMIC DISEASES & KIDNEYS IN THE ELDERLY

1. DIABETIC NEPHROPATHY
▶ General Considerations

Type 2 diabetes is more common in the elderly and diabetic nephropathy is a frequent finding at the time of diagnosis. Therefore, the National Kidney Foundation recommends that patients aged 70 years or older with non-insulin-dependent diabetes mellitus should test their urine for microalbuminuria (albumin excretion of 30–300 mg/24 hours in at least two urine samples within 6–12 weeks). Apart from glycemic control, progression of nephropathy is influenced by two independent risk factors: hypertension and diabetic dyslipidemia.

▶ Treatment

Strict glycemic control, reduction of blood pressure to less than 130/80 mm Hg, and introduction of ACEIs and/or angiotensin II receptor blockers (independently of blood pressure) are advised if microalbuminuria or proteinuria is present. The antihypertensive protocol recommended by the National Kidney Foundation Hypertension and Diabetes Working Group suggests a combination of ACEIs and diuretics as initial therapy. If the resting pulse rate exceeds 84/minute or in case of coexisting cardiac disease, β-blockers may be introduced in combination with ACEIs and/or angiotensin II receptor blockers. Special attention should be paid to subclinical RAS in elderly patients with close monitoring of serum creatinine. A self-limited decline in renal function of up to 30% within the first 4 months is acceptable if the baseline serum creatinine is less than 250 μmol/L. Even in that case, there is continued benefit after 3 years of therapy. Although dyslipidemia has been considered a risk factor for disease progression, there are no clear data indicating that lipid-lowering agents reduce the rate of progression.

2. MULTIPLE MYELOMA
▶ General Considerations

Multiple myeloma is more frequent in older than in younger people. Renal failure is a consequence of myeloma

glomerulopathy, tubular toxic effects of light chains, cast formation and intratubular obstruction, hypercalcemia, hyperuricemia, and cryoglobulinemia. Contributing factors are dehydration and nephrotoxic drugs.

▶ Treatment

Management usually involves chemotherapy with renal support. Hyperuricemia and hypercalcemia secondary to chemotherapy should be avoided by adequate hydration and the use of allopurinol.

▶ Prognosis

The prognosis depends on a variety of paraproteins, the stage of myeloma, and the type of chemotherapy. Biopsy may help predict prognosis; light chain deposits have the best prognosis. A good survival of myeloma patients on dialysis has been reported. Peritoneal dialysis has been recommended as the treatment of choice due to a better clearance of immunoglobulins, a reduction in the tubular toxic effect of the light chains, and a reduced incidence of hyperviscosity syndrome.

OBSTRUCTIVE NEPHROPATHY

The most common cause of urinary obstruction in old age is benign prostatic hypertrophy; age does not have a major effect on the prevalence or clinical presentation of nephrolithiasis and renal tumors. The increased intrapelvic pressure caused by a urinary obstruction is being transmitted back through the tubular lumina and induces atrophy of the renal parenchyma. After prostatectomy, renal plasma flow increases slightly, but glomerular filtration does not change in most of the cases.

URINARY TRACT INFECTIONS & PYELONEPHRITIS

1. URINARY TRACT INFECTIONS IN THE ELDERLY
▶ General Considerations

Predisposing factors for urinary tract infections in the elderly include structural and functional abnormalities of the urinary tract, comorbidity, invasive instrumentation/operations, and bacterial virulence. The most common causes of obstruction are benign prostatic hypertrophy, carcinoma, changes of the bladder neck, malformations, nephrolithiasis and ureterolithiasis, and uterine prolapse and descensus of the vagina in females. The most important functional impairments are due to diabetes, stroke, Parkinson's disease, motor neuron disease, and spinal injury.

▶ Prevention

An important factor for urinary tract infection in the elderly is the use of indwelling catheters. If a catheter is left *in situ* for longer periods of time, there is a risk of developing polymicrobial bacteriuria or chronic pyelonephritis. Therefore, removal of the catheter is recommended at the earliest time. Older patients are more susceptible to the consequences of instrumentation and surgical operations involving genitourinary tract.

▶ Clinical Findings

Bacterial virulence factors affect the ability of an organism to attach to human uroepithelial cells and are related to the severity of infection. These factors include fimbria, which increase the attachment of the organism to cells (P and S fimbriae), toxins secreted by the organisms (α-hemolysin, cytotoxic necrotizing factor-1, enterobactin), and proteins that allow the organism to alter complement activation. These virulence factors are modulated by genes triggered by signals such as temperature, pH, and the oxygen level of the tissues.

▶ Treatment

A short-term course of antibiotic therapy for those manifesting significant bacteriuria for the first time is indicated regardless of symptoms. Although therapy does not protect against renal damage, it is helpful in mitigating distressing symptoms.

Cotrimaxazole or amoxicillin is recommended for uncomplicated urinary tract infections. Penicillin and aminoglycoside or quinolone therapy are the therapies of choice for catheter-associated infections.

Acute pyelonephritis is treated with intravenous antibiotics with ampicillin and an aminoglycoside or a third-generation cephalosporin or a quinolone. At the same time, an evaluation for reversible causes should be done (obstruction, nephrolithiasis, cysts, neoplasia).

2. BACTERIURIA IN THE ELDERLY
▶ General Considerations

The risk of bacteriuria increases with age. Older, sicker, and less mobile patients are more susceptible to urinary infection and this reflects a general condition rather than a causal relationship.

▶ Clinical Findings

Significant bacteriuria occurs in up to 20% of the population aged 65 years and over. The incidence of bacteriuria increases more in intermittently catheterized hospitalized patients (about 50%) than in noncatheterized ones (about 43%). The commonest microorganisms seen in urine culture in uncomplicated infections are *Escherichia coli*, *Klebsiella* spp., *Staphylococcus saprophyticus*, *Enterococcus* spp., and *Proteus* spp. *Pseudomonas* and *Candida* spp. are more frequent in catheterized patients. No long-term sequelae of bacteriuria are seen in the elderly. The relationship among bacteriuria, lower urinary tract infection, and upper urinary tract infection in the elderly is not clear.

Asymptomatic bacteriuria is defined as ≥100,000 colony-forming units/mL urine on two or more consecutive occasions without any clinical symptoms. The prevalence of asymptomatic bacteriuria increases with age and functional debility. It is estimated at 9.3% in women aged 65 years or more, increasing to 20–50% in women over 80 years. Of men over 80 years 6–20% may have asymptomatic bacteriuria. Screening for bacteriuria is not recommended unless patients have some indicators of infection (incontinence, frequency, dysuria). In the elderly, a leukocyte count above 10 cells/mm^3 in the urinary sediment does not correlate with infection and therefore it should not be used as a valid diagnostic marker.

▶ Treatment

Treatment for 2 weeks is recommended only in those with previous frequent urinary tract infections, in patients who have a structural defect in their urinary tract, and in those with a history of renal transplantation and prior to a urologic procedure. Urine bacteriology should be rechecked 4 weeks after the discontinuation of treatment.

3. PYELONEPHRITIS
▶ General Considerations

Autopsy data revealed that the prevalence of pyelonephritis in the elderly ranges from 20% to 28%. Infections with fastidious organisms are more frequent (*Lactobacilli*, *Ureaplasma urealyticum*, *Gardnerella vaginalis*, *Staphylococcus saphrophyticus*, *Corynebacterium* spp., and certain strains of *Streptococcus* spp.) than in younger people. An important feature of chronic pyelonephritis is that older patients have an asymptomatic course of disease; it is clinically diagnosed in only about 20% of those patients detected at autopsy. In addition, many cases are diagnosed accidentally during admission into a hospital for other reasons or even at advanced stages including uremia. Postinfectious inflammatory mechanisms may induce prolonged damage in the renal interstitium after the disappearance of bacteria from the tissue.

OTHER CAUSES OF RENAL DISEASE

1. ALLERGIC INTERSTITIAL NEPHRITIS
▶ General Considerations

The elderly are very often subject to polypharmacy and medications are a common cause of renal disease. The most frequent drugs causing allergic interstitial nephritis are antibiotics (penicillin and sulfonamides), analgesics, anti-inflammatory drugs, anticoagulants, diuretics, anticonvulsants, allopurinol, metals (lithium), and immunosuppressive drugs (azathioprine).

▶ Clinical Findings

Nonsteroidal anti-inflammatory drugs (NSAIDs) induce renal failure by interference with prostaglandin release and by inducing acute or chronic allergic interstitial nephritis usually without classic symptoms of allergy or eosinophilia.

▶ Treatment

Withdrawal of the drug is usually sufficient treatment and steroid therapy is rarely required.

2. RADIOCONTRAST NEPHROTOXICITY

▶ General Considerations

Age itself is not a risk factor for the nephrotoxic effect of radiocontrast materials. However, predisposing factors for radiocontrast nephrotoxicity are more frequent in the elderly and include subclinical renal disease, diabetes, congestive heart failure, and dehydration. The volume of contrast used and the use of nonionic contrast of high osmolality are two additional factors that may stress nephrotoxicity.

▶ Prevention

Nephrotoxicity may be prevented by proper hydration with saline or hypotonic saline for a minimum of 12 hours and oral N-acetylcysteine (600 mg orally twice daily on the day before and on the day of administration of the contrast agent).

▶ Clinical Findings

Radiocontrast agents cause vacuolization of the cells in the proximal tubule possibly by intense local vasoconstriction, which may damage the kidneys of high-risk elderly patients.

The use of carbon dioxide as a contrast and fenoldopan (a dopamine agonist) at the time of the procedure decreases the prevalence of nephrotoxicity. There are no clear data indicating that the use of mannitol, furosemide, or renal vasodilator agents during the procedure may improve the outcome.

3. RENAL PAPILLARY NECROSIS

▶ General Considerations

Renal papillary necrosis is ischemic necrosis of the papillae and the medullary pyramid. It is most commonly a complication of the severe form of chronic pyelonephritis, unilateral renal artery stenosis, and prolonged consumption of analgesics, especially phenacetin.

▶ Clinical Findings

The patient usually has hematuria, renal colic, and often a high fever.

▶ Treatment

In the majority of cases relief of the obstruction caused by necrotic papilla leads to improved renal function. The disease has a rapid course toward uremia and, if untreated, death.

CHRONIC RENAL FAILURE & RENAL REPLACEMENT THERAPY

▶ General Considerations

The number of elderly patients who need renal replacement therapy (RRT) for ESRD grows steadily coincident with the overall aging of the population and with the increasing frequency with which elderly patients are accepted for such treatment. The most rapid growth among all new ESRD patients is in those who are 65–74 years of age. Individual countries show a marked variation in their trends in the use of RRT, possibly reflecting the variability in the accessibility to health care worldwide.

Elderly patients are less likely than younger patients to have ESRD secondary to GN (except in Japan where the number of elderly patients with GN is increasing) but are more likely to have renal failure due to type 2 diabetes and/or hypertension and to renal vascular disease. Such patients have many comorbid conditions that make therapy considerably more difficult and require multidisciplinary work and special knowledge of geriatric medicine.

Experience with elderly patients with renal diseases and uremia is still limited. For ethical reasons, there are very few comparative studies and no randomized, prospective studies have been conducted. In addition, these studies are based on populations that differ considerably in both medical and social characteristics.

▶ Treatment

A. Predialysis Management and Initiation of Dialysis

In elderly patients, chronic renal failure is characterized by an absence of classic symptoms, the nonspecific nature of the presenting symptoms, the presence of comorbid conditions, and by interference with the interpretation of findings by the aging process. Therefore these patients require regular screening for comorbid conditions, screening for cancer [prostate-specific antigen (PSA), Pap smear, mammography, renal ultrasound or CT, X-ray], review of medications with an emphasis on over-the-counter drugs, the possibility of drug interactions, dosing, adequate vaccination, examination of feet, especially in diabetics, and, if necessary, psychiatric and social intervention.

The elderly show a poor correlation between serum creatinine and glomerular filtration rate and therefore it is preferable to monitor creatinine clearance measured or calculated from serum creatinine. Salt intake should be limited to 4–5 g/L/day and regular clinical monitoring of fluid overload and/or dehydration is advisable. Severe constipation, which is frequent in the elderly, may exacerbate hyperkalemia. In the predialysis phase [chronic kidney disease (CKD) stages 3–4], the use of recombinant human erythropoietin (rh-EPO) may improve the quality of life (QOL) and prevent left ventricular hypertrophy. Strict dietary protein restriction is often unnecessary (acceptable ingestion: 60–70 g protein/day). Also, to avoid acidosis, special attention should be paid to serum bicarbonate levels.

Late referral to a nephrology unit is significantly related to early death. On some occasions, it is not that the elderly are not referred early, but that the nephrologist may have delayed initiation of dialysis due to misleading serum creatinine levels. Therefore, the National Kidney Foundation Disease Outcomes Quality Initiative (NKF-DOQI) guidelines suggest that regular estimations of weekly creatinine clearance to avoid late initiation of dialysis should be performed. An early referral may provide better salt and water balance and better control of anemia, leading to a decrease in overall morbidity and mortality. Initiation of dialysis should be recommended before uremic symptoms become overt and particularly before there is evidence of malnutrition. A low serum albumin level, a dietary protein intake <0.7 g/kg/day, weight loss, and a decrease in muscle mass indicate the need for dialysis.

B. Chronic Hemodialysis

In most countries hospital hemodialysis, which is the principal form of RRT in the elderly, offers many advantages. Dialysis is performed by nurses, the treatment time is shorter, it allows for socialization with staff and other patients, and there is continuous follow-up by the medical team.

Crucial to successful hemodialysis is the presence of a functional vascular access. Proper planning for such an access requires comprehensive evaluation with respect to earlier placement of vascular catheters, the presence of a cardiac pacemaker on a prosthetic cardiac valve, the presence of enlarged axillary lymph nodes, and past radiation therapy. Diabetes and hypertension, the most frequent causes of ESRD in the elderly, are associated with abnormal blood vessels. A good forearm Brescia–Cimino arteriovenous fistula is the ideal form of vascular access whatever the patient's age. However, there is a higher primary failure rate and shorter survival with this form of access in the elderly. Among the various vascular substitutes, the homologous saphenous vein graft proved to be superior to other synthetic grafts. In some elderly patients, particularly those with diabetes, synthetic grafts can be very useful. Vascular-access thrombosis associated with rh-EPO therapy was more common in elderly patients for both native arteriovenous fistulas and grafts. In cases of late referral, "trial dialysis," and a failed arteriovenous fistula, both cuffed and noncuffed catheters may provide suitable vascular access.

Hemodialysis is more likely to precipitate cardiovascular instability in the elderly. Some investigators reported more frequent episodes of hypotension during dialysis and/or postdialysis, which may be a risk factor for falls. In elderly patients who have autonomic dysfunction and a low cardiac reserve, hypotension during hemodialysis may be a consequence of rapid ultrafiltration. Also, the incidence of arrhythmias increases progressively with age and in such patients arrhythmias could be a risk factor for cardiac death. While on hemodialysis, elderly patients may develop gastrointestinal bleeding due to gastritis, duodenal ulceration, and angiodysplasia.

Although it is rarely used, home dialysis is a highly successful therapeutic option. Individuals on home hemodialysis have few dialysis-related complications.

C. Chronic Peritoneal Dialysis

Chronic peritoneal dialysis (CPD) offers many advantages including good control of hypertension, independence from hospitals, simplicity of access, better cardiovascular stability (less hypotension and fewer arrhythmias), and slow solute removal. A family member may perform such dialysis and the patient does not need to go to the hospital three times a week. On the other hand, patients are at higher risk of complications such as malnutrition, which is more frequent in the elderly than in younger peritoneal dialysis (PD) patients and which is highly correlated with mortality. In addition, low initial albumin levels correlate with mortality among elderly patients on continuous ambulatory peritoneal dialysis (CAPD) and cachexia is a frequent cause of death.

Elderly patients with uremia have an increased risk of infection because they suffer from immunodeficiency, malnutrition, and high rates of bowel disease, which may explain the higher rates of peritonitis among the elderly on PD. Bedridden patients tend to have an even higher rate of peritonitis. Catheter-related complications are infrequent among elderly patients on PD, probably because they are less active than younger patients. The higher incidence of hernias (incisional, inguinal) in elderly PD patients has been attributed to weakness of the abdominal wall.

Hospitalization rates are higher among elderly than among younger patients, especially among those of African descent and diabetics. The duration of stay varies between 5.5 and 23.1 in-hospital days.

PD is not used extensively among the elderly because they are unable to perform dialysis by themselves; about 61.2% of very old patients (above 80 years) need help with dialysis exchanges, exit-site care, and medication. Many patients older than 65 years suffer from comorbid conditions such as depression, dementia, impaired vision, and decreased physical and mental activity, all of which significantly impair self-performance of PD. However, given a network of medical, nursing, and social support, the elderly can perform PD (especially automated PD) successfully at home.

D. Renal Transplantation

Renal transplantation may be successful in the elderly; perioperative survival is comparable to that among younger recipients. However, in Europe, only 2% of patients older than 65 years and less than 0.3% of patients older than 75 years receive renal transplants, except in Norway, where transplantation is the primary mode of therapy for patients 60–65 years old. Lower transplantation rates among the elderly may be explained not only by selection bias but also by a shortage of organ donation; older patients tend to have fewer living donors and younger persons are less willing to donate a kidney to an older relative than to a younger one. The shortage of kidneys could be improved in older recipients by using kidneys from older cadaveric donors. Kidneys from elderly donors may be suitable for elderly recipients who have lower muscle mass and less metabolic demands coupled with decreased immunologic reactivity, thus allowing the use of less aggressive immunosuppressive regimens without increasing rejection rates. However, special attention should be paid to age and size matching between donor and recipient and to cold ischemia time, which should be as short as possible. No differences in kidney survival were found in a comparison of elderly patients previously treated by hemodialysis or CAPD. Over the past 10 years the improvement in overall patient and graft survival rates may be related to increased experience with the use of newer immunosuppressive regimes [United States Renal Data System (USRDS), Canadian Organ Replacement Register (CORR)] in the elderly.

E. Social Issues

With the growing number of elderly patients requiring dialysis, an increasing number need assisted care.

1. Home-care nursing—Trained home-care nurses may provide the elderly with comfortable and safe home dialysis without reliance on family members. Also, the low rate of infection and hospitalization and the avoidance of transportation in this high-risk population achieve significant savings. The rates of peritonitis and exit-site infection are not significantly different between those who had assisted dialysis by a home-care nurse and those on self-dialysis. The home-care nurse may assist in the treatment of episodes of peritonitis and other complications, thereby contributing to a lower total hospitalization rate.

2. Rehabilitation and chronic care dialysis units—Rehabilitation and chronic care dialysis units (RCDUs) may provide dialysis, physiotherapy, a rehabilitation program, and occupational therapy for those patients who cannot return home or who cannot be placed in a nursing home. Such units achieve significant reduction in costs compared to hospital treatment and this cost reduction is not accompanied by any deterioration in the elderly person's QOL.

3. Dialysis in the nursing home—An increasing number of the elderly will live in a nursing home in the future. A substantial number of nursing homes still refuse to introduce dialysis into everyday care because they believe that the ESRD elderly population is difficult to care for, because they lack knowledge about dialysis and renal diet and lack adequate storage space for machines and supplies, and because there is poor communication with the renal team.

Although hemodialysis is the mode most used in nursing homes, published data are limited and, until now, there have been no control trials. Nursing home residents on hemodialysis spend about 15 hours in the dialysis unit per week; this coupled with transportation time takes time away from rehabilitation and social activities. The need for transportation may be overcome by building the dialysis center within or adjacent to a skilled nursing facility.

PD in nursing homes offers many advantages and allows flexibility in schedules for patients and for staff. In this regard, automated PD (APD) or nightly PD frees the patients' daytime for nursing home activities, increases socialization, and results in better rehabilitation, which improves their QOL. Patients on PD in nursing homes and day care centers have a lower survival rate than the general CAPD population. This is probably a reflection of patient selection because patients in nursing homes are significantly older and have many comorbid conditions. It seems that rates of peritonitis do not differ significantly from those in the overall noninstitutionalized elderly.

F. Ethical Issues

Dialysis in the elderly is a life-extending treatment, and, for many, these are lives of quality. However, some older individuals elect to cease dialysis because of QOL issues. For this reason, health care professionals should be completely honest when educating patients and their families regarding the burdens associated with living on dialysis. They cannot make this decision for others but should share their knowledge and experience and advise patients without projecting their own prejudices. With respect to the decision-making process, the first published guidelines that appeared in 1993 were personal and did not reflect the opinion of the majority. A set of consensus guidelines, published by the NKF in 1996, allowed all patients to explore their own options. Finally, the American Society of Nephrology and the Renal Physicians Association published evidence-based guidelines in 2000. All of these publications emphasize that they are just guidelines and not rules; they also emphasize the difficulties of the decision-making process arising from the heterogeneous nature of both providers and the patient population. None of the guidelines recommend mandatory standards for the determination of the patient's candidacy for dialysis.

Sometimes neither the medical team nor the patient or family members find it easy to reach a decision. In that case, the patient should be offered a period of trial dialysis, say for of 30–90 days. All guidelines recommend that dialysis not be offered to patients with a known serious terminal illness or patients who have serious mental impairment as a result of stroke, Alzheimer's disease, or neurologic dysfunction. Also, patients on dialysis who develop a terminal illness or become demented should be offered the option of discontinuing dialysis. Patients choosing to withdraw from dialysis should know that they will receive ongoing active, caring treatment to minimize suffering and prevent pain.

Withdrawal from dialysis is more frequent among elderly patients, particularly among those living in a nursing home. However, this high discontinuation rate among elderly patients is not due to dialysis per se but rather to associated social and medical circumstances.

Cassidy MJD, Sims RJA: Dialysis in the elderly. New possibilities, new problems. Minerva Urolog Nephrol 2004;56:305.

Fehrman-Ekhom I, Skeppholm L: Renal function in the elderly (>70 years old) measured by means of iohexol clearance, serum creatinine, serum urea and estimated clearance. Scand J Urol Nephrol 2004;38:73.

Vistoli F et al: Kidney transplantation from donors aged more than 65 years. Transplant Proc 2004;36:481.

Yamagata K et al: Age distribution and yearly changes in the incidence of ESRD in Japan. Am J Kidney Dis 2004;43(3):433.

Interventional Nephrology: Endovascular Procedures

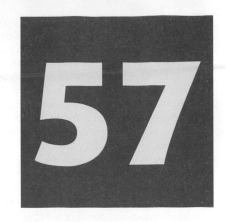

Theodore F. Saad, MD

ISSUES IN INTERVASCULAR PROCEDURES

Over the past decade, there has been a resurgence of interest by nephrologists in the management of hemodialysis vascular access. The early days of dialysis were marked by advances in vascular access conceived and developed by visionary nephrologists, including the Scribner shunt and the Brescia-Cimino arteriovenous (AV) fistula. Without these means of obtaining reliable repeated blood access, the delivery of chronic hemodialysis would not have been possible. Some nephrologists have maintained this primary role in the creation and maintenance of vascular access, particularly in Europe. One successful example reported the construction of a series of 748 consecutive native AV fistulas, with 2 year assisted access survival rates in diabetics and non-diabetics ranging from 75% to 96%. During the 1970s and 1980s, at least in the United States, interest and involvement in vascular access largely faded. This may have been due to exciting progress in what were perceived to be more scientifically rewarding areas of study, as opposed to the relatively mundane "plumbing" problems of vascular access. Certainly neither technical proficiency nor rigorous academic attention to vascular access was emphasized in most nephrology training centers in the United States during that time. In many programs and practices management of vascular access was left exclusively to the surgeons. At the same time, particularly in the United States, there was increased promotion and utilization of synthetic polytetrafluoroethylene (PTFE) grafts in favor of native AV fistulas. This shift may have been driven by marketing and reimbursement practices, poor long-term venous access catheters available for use as "bridges" to native fistulae, and increasing emphasis on short, high efficiency dialysis treatments. The result for the United States nephrology community was a large hemodialysis patient population with a high prevalence of PTFE grafts, a low usage of AV fistulas, and perhaps incidentally, the highest dialysis patient mortality of all industrialized nations. In 1999, 49% of hemodialysis patients in the

United States were dialyzing with AV grafts, 28% with native fistulas, and 23% with venous catheters.

During this period of a rapidly growing hemodialysis patient population, increasing PTFE graft utilization, and decreased involvement of nephrologists in the management of vascular access problems, there was a predictable crisis in the access-related medical care of these patients. Management of access dysfunction and thrombosis was largely "reactive" and primarily utilized open surgical techniques. The role of venous stenosis in contributing to AV graft thrombosis and failure was underappreciated. In the late 1980s, interventional radiologists began to recognize these problems and applied their tools and techniques to treating access dysfunction. A method for declotting AV hemodialysis grafts using pharmacomechanical thrombolysis and angioplasty was reported in 1991. Numerous other reports and variations on this method followed, with increasing acceptance of percutaneous interventions in the management of hemodialysis access dysfunction. Largely, however, nephrologists remained on the periphery, as vascular access continued to be the province of the vascular surgeon and more recently interventional radiologists. This collaboration of expert subspecialties might have been all that was needed to provide timely, high-quality hemodialysis access care. Undeniably, in some settings, this was the case. However, while access dysfunction was of critical and immediate importance to the patient, dialysis unit, and nephrologist, for many programs this could not be the first priority for the surgeons or radiologists, creating a service void and an opportunity for improvement in care.

The central role of vascular access in the care of patients on hemodialysis cannot be overemphasized. Comprehensive medical care of the hemodialysis patient includes management of uremia, hypertension, sodium and water balance, anemia, mineral metabolism, metabolic bone disease, and nutritional status. This care cannot be properly delivered unless there is reliable, efficient blood access for dialysis. Leaving this critical aspect of care entirely in the hands of others puts the patient and the nephrologist at a significant disadvantage. Under ideal circumstances, when the skills and priorities of the multispecialty access team come together, patient care may be very well served. Conversely, if the appropriate surgical or interventional services cannot be delivered in a timely fashion, the patient may suffer in terms of delayed dialysis, temporary venous hemodialysis access, unnecessary hospitalization, or other avoidable morbidity. This also may result in a significantly greater financial burden to the health care system.

In the early 1990s, this problem was recognized and confronted by Dr. Gerald Beathard in Austin, Texas. He acquired the necessary training, adapted the reported interventional radiology techniques, and developed a nephrology-run service for percutaneous management of vascular access. He then liberally shared this expertise, training many nephrologists from various practices and backgrounds, this author included. It is a remarkable fact that all interventional nephrologists practicing in the United States can trace their roots directly back to Dr. Beathard. As these nephrologists brought these techniques to their practices, the field of "interventional nephrology" was effectively born. When nephrologists began to perform these access-related percutaneous interventions, the first priorities were to master the techniques, establish suitable facilities in which to work, and then deal with the multitude of day-to-day access failures, largely centered on the PTFE graft. While this led to an immediate and dramatic improvement in care, it was very evident that the poor performance of PTFE grafts compared to native AV fistulas was contributing to an excessively high rate of access failure and hence a large volume of percutaneous interventions. This was good business, but very bad medicine. This realization led to the next phase in the evolution of interventional nephrology, which was to take on comprehensive vascular access management for the patient on hemodialysis. To improve vascular access outcomes, it would be folly to address only the technical aspects of percutaneous interventions. To achieve optimal vascular access, the following aspects of care take on equal or greater importance.

- Preservation of peripheral veins for native AV fistulas.
- Avoidance of peripherally inserted central venous catheters and subclavian catheters.
- Judicious use of internal jugular vein tunneled hemodialysis catheters for temporary hemodialysis access.
- Early referral to a surgeon for construction of a native AV fistula.
- Education and selection of surgical colleagues willing and able to master the techniques for the creation of a native AV fistula.
- Preoperative imaging of veins and arteries, including ultrasound vein mapping and venography.
- Evaluation and treatment of a poorly functioning or immature AV fistula.

- Conversion from a failing PTFE graft to a "secondary" native AV fistula.
- Maintenance of a complete and accurate clinical database with regular quality analysis including rates of usage of AV fistulas and catheters success rates of technical procedures, complications, and patient satisfaction.

Another essential principle must be recognized in order to provide optimal hemodialysis access care: For each scenario of access dysfunction, there is a "best solution." There has been a tendency for vascular access solutions to follow "the path of least resistance" or, worse yet, "the path of greatest reimbursement," both of which may be very different from the optimal pathway. From the perspective of the interventionist, there is the temptation to view all problems as best solved using percutaneous means. However, there are clearly situations in which surgical solutions are preferable and should be employed. This of course works both ways. It would be equally poor care to perform frequent, repeated percutaneous thrombectomies and angioplasties on a failing PTFE graft as it would be to attempt an open surgical declot of a fistula that thrombosed due to central venous stenosis. Knowing the anatomy and history of each patient is the critical element that allows these judgments to be made correctly. In this regard, keeping a detailed clinical database is essential. This allows the operator to fully assess the vascular access problem at hand, make the most appropriate management decision based upon the history and known anatomic factors, and perform the necessary procedure with the lowest risk and best possibility of a successful outcome.

When a patient presents with access dysfunction, a timely solution is required. This may represent an urgent problem such as a thrombosed AV fistula that requires immediate intervention to salvage the access and provide dialysis. Although arguably not a true "medical emergency," restoration of fistula or graft function is of paramount importance to the care of the patient on hemodialysis, with potentially grave implications for both short-term and long-term morbidity and mortality. Other access problems may be less immediate, such as prolonged bleeding from needle puncture sites related to venous outflow stenosis; this may not prevent dialysis, but puts the patient at risk, may lead to access thrombosis, and should be dealt with before it becomes an urgent problem. Other access problems may be relatively elective in nature, such as the evaluation of limb swelling associated with central venous stenosis or a slowly enlarging pseudoaneurysm. In all cases, the goal of an interventional program should be to address each problem in an appropriate timely fashion, minimizing disruption of the dialysis schedule of patients. Nephrologists are in an ideal position to provide these services when equipped with the necessary skills, allowing for seamless delivery of care and management of dialysis-related problems as required before, during, and after an interventional procedure. Alternatively, there are many practices in which excellent care and service are provided by interventional radiologists or vascular surgeons. The title of the individual responsible for vascular access interventions is not as important as his or her knowledge, skill, availability, and willingness to work with surgeons, nephrologists, and the dialysis staff as part of a multidisciplinary access management team.

The American Society of Diagnostic and Interventional Nephrology (ASDIN) was founded in 2000 to promote the proper application of procedures in the practice of nephrology. These include diagnostic ultrasound imaging and peritoneal dialysis catheter placement in addition to the full complement of percutaneous interventions required for management of hemodialysis vascular access. A central goal of this society was to develop standards for training, certification, and accreditation relative to these diagnostic and interventional disciplines. These were published in 2003 and remain the only standards specific to these procedures. Previously there were no specific standards and there was tremendous variation in the training and credentialing requirements of health care facilities. It is expected that with increasing awareness and acceptance of these criteria in the United States and elsewhere, interventional training will become more uniform and rigorous, ultimately improving the quality of care offered as well as patient outcome. Over the past several years, interventional nephrology training programs have become established at some U.S. academic centers. As these centers develop, they should be expected to advance the standard for training, quality, and clinical research related to vascular access.

CORE ENDOVASCULAR PROCEDURES

The core procedures of interventional nephrology include the placement and management of venous hemodialysis catheters, diagnostic imaging of AV accesses and native veins, percutaneous angioplasty, and percutaneous thrombectomy of occluded AV access. Other related procedures include the placement of venous stents, the ligation or embolization of native fistula accessory branches, and the implantation of subcutaneous venous hemodialysis access ports.

▶ Venous Hemodialysis Catheters

Venous catheters are the least desirable method of hemodialysis access. In a sense, every placement of a venous catheter represents a failure to prepare a native fistula in advance of initiating dialysis as well as a failure to detect a dysfunctional AV access and to intervene preemptively either to maintain its function or to create a new alternative access. Nevertheless, venous catheters are an unavoidable necessity for many patients who do not have functional AV access. For most interventional nephrologists, insertion of tunneled dialysis catheters is the first and most basic procedure acquired, building on the common skill of temporary hemodialysis catheter placement. Nevertheless, the risks of this procedure should not be understated, with the potential for severe

injury to major central vessels from large-bore catheters and dilators. The use of real-time ultrasound guidance is widely considered to be essential for safe and efficient venipuncture based on higher procedural success rates and fewer complications compared to the use of landmarks only. The low posterior approach to the right internal jugular vein is ideal; this keeps the catheter low on the neck, with minimal patient discomfort and a good cosmetic result, and creates a smooth bend of the catheter that avoids kinking. Fluoroscopy is also recommended for proper catheter tip positioning, although there is limited evidence to support this requirement. There is general agreement that the performance of chronic dialysis catheters is optimized when the catheter tips are placed in the right atrium, and Disease Outcomes Quality Initiative (DOQI) guidelines support this approach. Nevertheless, this remains controversial, and achieving the desired tip position is difficult, even with fluoroscopy and careful attention to anatomic landmarks. In any case, to achieve the best possible outcomes, the operator must adhere to a meticulous sterile surgical technique, utilize ultrasound guidance for venipuncture, and pay careful attention to tip positioning using fluoroscopic and/or landmark guidance. Figure 57–1A shows a poorly placed left internal jugular vein tunneled dialysis catheter, with a high vein puncture from the anterior approach, a tight bend with the catheter kinked, and its split tips extending only into the superior vena cava. This catheter did not function for dialysis. Figure 57–1B shows the catheter replaced with a new Ash-Split catheter (Medcomp, Harleysville, PA), using the right internal jugular vein puncture from a low posterior approach with a smooth bend in the neck. In Figure 57–1C, the new catheter tips are shown extending into the high right atrium, yielding excellent catheter function as required for delivery of hemodialysis.

Over the past several years, two totally implantable venous hemodialysis access devices have been developed: the LifeSite hemodialysis valve (Vasca Inc., Tewksbury, MA) (Figure 57–2), and the Dialock Access System (Biolink Inc., Norwell, MA). In the United States, only the LifeSite device became available. The LifeSite system consisted of two independently implanted subcutaneous valves, each connected to a single-lumen catheter placed into the right atrium. These were accessed using 14-gauge needles through a "buttonhole" tract. Disinfection with isopropyl alcohol before and after each dialysis needle access was essential to reduce serious device infections. The LifeSite system provided improved device survival and lower rates of infection than conventional tunneled dialysis catheters. Interventional nephrologists have been instrumental in the LifeSite clinical trials and the application of the LifeSite device in practice. However, considerably greater time, skill, risk, and expense were associated with the implantation of these devices, factors that had to be weighed when considering the use of these devices versus the use of a conventional venous catheter. There is also a significant "learning curve" for both the implanting physician and the dialysis nursing staff, requiring a number of patients to be

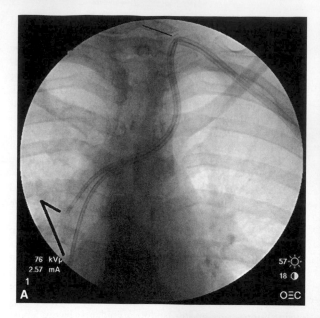

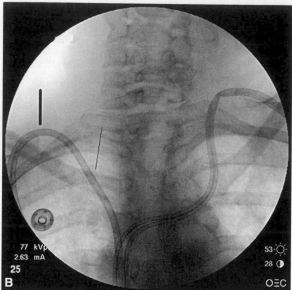

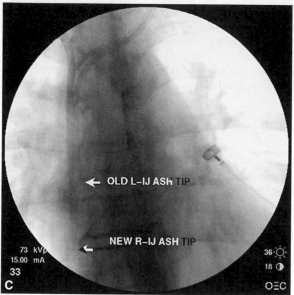

▲ **Figure 57–1.** *A:* Poorly placed left internal jugular vein tunneled cuffed hemodialysis catheter using a high-anterior approach. The bend is sharply kinked in the neck (fine line) and the tips are in the superior vena cava (bold lines). Blood flow was insufficient to support hemodialysis. *B:* The same patient with a properly placed right internal jugular catheter using a low-posterior approach (fine line), with a smooth bend in the neck (bold line), prior to removal of a faulty catheter. *C:* The same patient showing the new right internal jugular vein catheter tips extending into the right atrium. (Courtesy of TF Saad.)

maintained in a program with the LifeSite device in order to achieve consistent successful results.

Because the product did not gain wide acceptance in most nephrology communities, the manufacturing company, Vasca Inc., eventually decided to withdraw LifeSite from the market in 2005.

▶ Arteriovenous Access Dysfunction

Stenosis associated with AV grafts due to neointimal hyperplasia typically occurs at or near the venous anastomosis. This may be triggered by turbulent blood flow, the shear force on the vessel wall, and material compliance mismatch

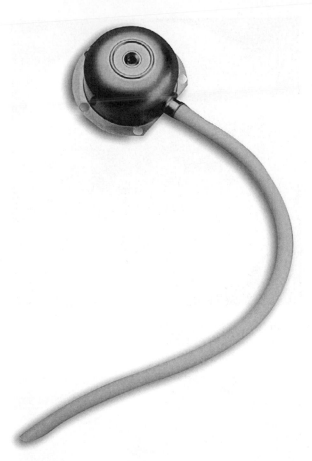

▲ **Figure 57–2.** LifeSite hemodialysis valve and cannula system available as a totally implanted long-term temporary or chronic venous hemodialysis access. Two separate valves and cannulas are utilized for blood draw and return with 14-gauge needles inserted via a buttonhole tract into each valve.

between the synthetic graft and vein. Proliferation of smooth muscle cells, endothelial cells, and fibroblasts leads to stenosis, as seen in Figure 57–3. The pathophysiology of stenosis affecting native AV fistulas is not as well studied or understood and may involve different factors in the absence of a surgically constructed venous anastomosis or synthetic material. Trauma to the vein during surgical manipulation or from intravenous catheters may be a contributing factor. Stenosis may also affect other sites in the AV access system, whether native fistula or synthetic graft. These include the arterial anastomosis (Figure 57–4), the fistula or draining peripheral vein (Figures 57–5 and 57–6), the central veins (Figure 57–7), or in the case of synthetic grafts, the body of the graft itself. Left untreated, progressive stenosis will lead to a reduction in access blood flow, ineffective hemodialysis, and ultimately access thrombosis.

Numerous studies have evaluated the role of screening and preemptive intervention for stenosis associated with synthetic AV hemodialysis grafts in maintaining function and preventing thrombosis. These studies are based on the premise that graft dysfunction and thrombosis are commonly associated with stenosis of the venous outflow, typically at the venous anastomosis. Outflow obstruction will result in diminished AV access flow, with a large pressure gradient across the stenosis, causing pressures within the access to rise toward arterial pressure. The utility of a good history and physical examination of the access should not be underestimated in detecting stenosis. Prolonged needle site bleeding, or an excessively pulsatile quality of the access, without a prominent "thrill" may indicate outflow stenosis or poor flow that may predispose the patient to thrombosis. Early studies suggested that elevated pressures measured through the venous dialysis needle during hemodialysis were predictive of PTFE graft thrombosis, and that preemptive angioplasty of these lesions was effective in reducing the rate of graft thrombosis. This relatively crude technique may be enhanced by a reduction of dialysis circuit flows, by more sophisticated analysis of dynamic venous pressure screening, or by measurement of static pressures within the graft in the absence of dialysis circuit flow. A number of studies have shown that the periodic measurement of access flow rates is useful in detecting graft stenosis, with intervention for low or reduced flow leading to reduced graft thrombosis. However, this remains somewhat controversial, and it is not clear that preemptive intervention results in longer overall access survival.

It should be noted that there are no comparable published studies evaluating screening and intervention for native AV fistulas despite the fact that this is the preferred form of hemodialysis access. As the nephrology community in the United States successfully transitions to a patient population dominated by native fistulas rather than synthetic grafts, questions concerning surveillance and intervention for failing PTFE grafts will become less relevant.

▶ Percutaneous Transluminal Angioplasty

Angioplasty of a vascular stenosis is an essential tool in the management of hemodialysis access dysfunction. The principles and techniques of percutaneous angioplasty are well established, and these must be mastered by the interventional nephrologist, radiologist, or surgeon performing the procedure. There is considerable controversy as to whether angioplasty is an "effective therapy." While it is almost always possible to dilate a stenosis and achieve an anatomically improved appearance, it is not clear that this will result in a sustained resolution of stenosis or improved long-term access patency. Elastic recoil may occur immediately following an apparently successful angioplasty. The angioplasty procedure itself is injurious to the vessel and may promote rapid restenosis. There are clearly lesions that will respond more favorably to surgical correction with

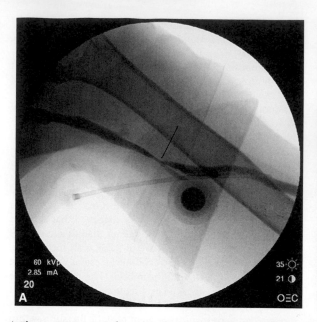
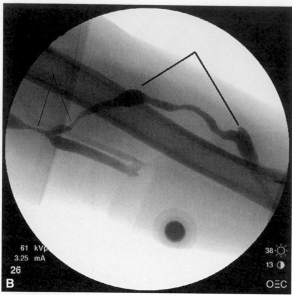

▲ **Figure 57–3.** ***A:*** Left upper arm polytetrafluoroethylene graft with severe stenosis at the venous anastomosis to the proximal brachial vein. ***B:*** Left upper arm polytetrafluoroethylene graft with graft pseudoaneurysms (bold lines) and stenosis at the venous anastomosis to the proximal brachial vein (fine lines). (Courtesy of TF Saad.)

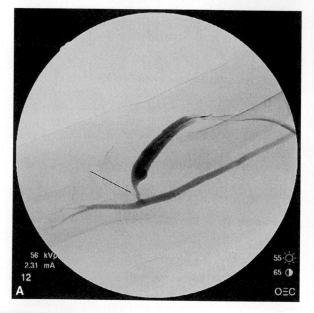
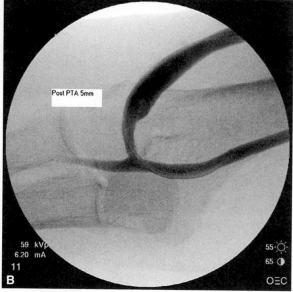

▲ **Figure 57–4.** ***A:*** Right upper arm cephalic vein arteriovenous fistula with poor flow due to severe stenosis at the arterial anastomosis and contiguous portion of the cephalic vein. ***B:*** Arterial anastomosis following 5-mm balloon angioplasty with improved fistula flow and performance. (Courtesy of TF Saad.)

improved duration of patency compared to percutaneous treatment.

It should be noted that some venous stenoses, especially those related to native AV fistulas, are quite resistant to expansion but may be successfully dilated using specialized cutting balloons or ultrahigh-pressure angioplasty. Conventional angioplasty balloons are rated with "burst pressures" of 12–15 atm and are typically operated at pressures up to 50% greater than this rating. Even this pressure may not be sufficient to dilate certain resistant lesions, which may require the

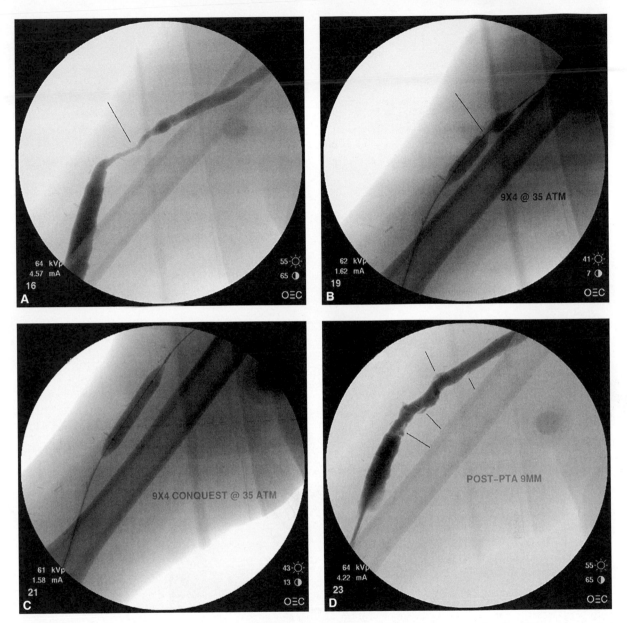

▲ **Figure 57–5. A:** Right upper arm brachial artery to transposed cephalic vein arteriovenous fistula with severe stenosis in the mid cephalic vein near the surgical "swing point." On examination there was prominent fistula pulsation and poor thrill. **B:** Ultrahigh pressure 9-mm angioplasty using a Conquest balloon (Bard Peripheral Vascular Inc., Tempe, AZ) at 35 atm, with persistent severe balloon waist. **C:** Balloon waist effaced after sustained angioplasty at >35 atmospheres. **D:** Postangioplasty image shows resolution of stenosis, associated with an improved palpable thrill on examination. Note the ragged appearance of the fistula lumen at the angioplasty site. (Courtesy of TF Saad.)

use of ultrahigh-pressure balloons, such as the Conquest balloon (Bard Peripheral Vascular Inc., Tempe, AZ), with burst pressure ratings of 30 atm. Figure 57–5A shows a right upper arm cephalic vein fistula referred for evaluation of excessive dialysis needle-site bleeding. On physical examination the fistula was firm and markedly pulsatile, with a poor palpable

thrill. Severe stenosis was demonstrated in the mid portion of the upper-arm cephalic vein, correlating with the history and physical findings. The lesion was extremely resistant to angioplasty (Figure 57–5B), ultimately responding with sustained inflation at ultrahigh pressure, >35 atm (Figure 57–5C). Postangioplasty there was improved flow, with restoration of

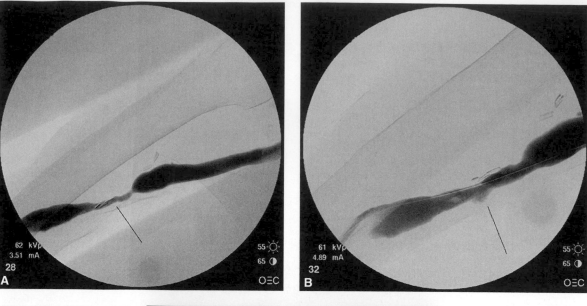

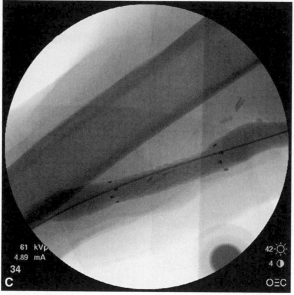

▲ **Figure 57–6.** **A:** Right upper arm basilic vein fistula with severe stenosis at the junction of the basilic to brachial vein, rapidly recurrent following angioplasty 1 and 2 months previously. **B:** Postangioplasty using an ultrahigh pressure Conquest (Bard Peripheral Vascular Inc., Tempe, AZ) balloon at >35 atm. Early postangioplasty recoil and mild extravasation (fine line) with persistent poor flow and prominently pulsatile examination. **C:** Following placement of a 10 mm × 40 mm Fluency tracheobronchial stent graft (Bard Peripheral Vascular Inc., Tempe, AZ) with elimination of stenosis and restoration of good flow and thrill. There was subsequent excellent fistula function without need for reintervention at 10 months follow-up. (Courtesy of TF Saad.)

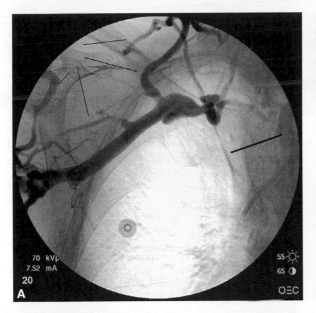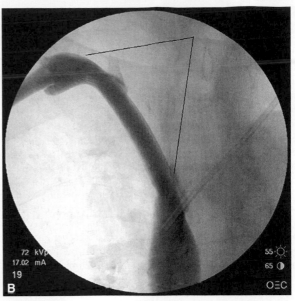

▲ **Figure 57–7.** **A:** Cancer patient receiving hemodialysis via a right upper extremity polytetrafluoroethylene graft presented with severe right arm swelling. There was a history of multiple previous subclavian vein catheters. Right subclavian stenosis and near occlusion of right brachiocephalic vein (bold line) were associated with venous hypertension evidenced by numerous dilated collateral veins (fine lines). Note the left-sided infusion catheter tip in the superior vena cava. **B:** Following angioplasty to 12 mm and placement of a right subclavian and brachiocephalic vein 14 mm × 40 mm Wallstent biliary endoprosthesis (Boston Scientific, Natick, MA). Margins of the stent do not have radiopaque markers (fine lines). (Courtesy of TF Saad.)

a palpable thrill; a fistulogram demonstrated improved stenosis along with a ragged vessel lumen likely representing an intimal tear and disruption (Figure 57–5D). This indicates that the angioplasty procedure itself is injurious to the vessel and may incite local factors leading to further neointimal hyperplasia, contributing to eventual restenosis.

Percutaneous Thrombectomy

Prior to the 1990s, management of AV access thrombosis was almost exclusively surgical. Diagnosis of associated venous stenosis was limited, and there was very little preventive intervention. Since the first publications of percutaneous methods for declotting AV grafts, many devices and techniques for declotting hemodialysis access have been reported. For the most part, no one method or device has been shown to have any advantage over others in terms of procedural success, complications, or duration of access patency. The principal determinant of outcome is the correction of underlying stenoses or other conditions responsible for the thrombosis. The most notable progress has been made in the management of native AV fistula thrombosis. Until very recently, salvage of a thrombosed native fistula was not considered possible. Several studies have now shown that results of percutaneous native fistula

thrombectomy can be excellent, ranging from 76% to 94%. Most of these studies, and our own technique of thrombus aspiration, involve a combination of pharmacologic thrombolysis and/or mechanical clot removal or maceration, with no proven difference in efficacy or safety between different methods. Long-term secondary fistula patency after successful declotting is also quite favorable, with 50–86% remaining patent at 24 months. It should be emphasized that to achieve this secondary or "assisted" patency and to avoid repeated thrombosis, other percutaneous interventions may be required. In the United States, as we continue to improve our utilization of native fistulas, and in other countries in which this has already been achieved, there clearly will be more emphasis on the application of percutaneous interventional techniques for the maintenance of native fistula function. Furthermore, as we attempt to create functional fistulas in more patients with poor quality veins, it is likely that the rate of native fistula dysfunction and thrombosis will be higher in these "marginal" fistulas than in those previously reported.

Venous Stents

The role of endovascular stents in the management of stenosis associated with AV hemodialysis access is poorly defined and rather controversial. This remains in sharp contradistinction to coronary and renal artery stenosis, where primary stent placement is widely accepted to be the appropriate standard for most lesions. No such clear data exist to demonstrate improved outcomes of stents versus simple angioplasty in hemodialysis vascular access applications. In general, a stent should not be placed at a site where a definitive surgical revision would be technically feasible, given the opportunity for prolonged access function following surgical revision. Stent placement should be considered only after the failure of conventional angioplasty, due to either immediate recoil, rupture, or repeated rapid restenosis, or in the management of complete vessel occlusions.

There are a variety of self-expanding metallic stents suitable for this purpose, although only the stainless-steel Wallstent endoprosthesis (Boston Scientific, Natick, MA) has been approved in the United States for a central venous indication. Other stents have biliary, tracheobronchial, or arterial indications, but are commonly utilized in the venous system "off-label." These are primarily nitinol (nickel-titanium alloy) stents, which have improved radial force, flexibility, and other material property advantages compared to stainless-steel stents. A recent uncontrolled, retrospective study utilized the nitinol SMART Stent (Cordis/Johnson & Johnson, Warren, NJ) for treatment of central or peripheral vein stenosis and demonstrated a primary patency of 14.9 and 8.9 months, respectively. This study also suggested that the SMART Stent conferred longer periods of intervention-free access patency than angioplasty alone. Clearly further study will be needed to determine the appropriate indications for venous stents. It is possible that drug-eluting stents used for treatment of AV hemodialysis access stenosis may result in less rapid or severe restenosis, by inhibiting local proliferative responses. One of the challenges for the interventional nephrology community is to take the lead on such studies and advance the clinical scientific basis for vascular access care.

Potential sites for stent placement include the peripheral draining veins related to a native fistula (Figure 57–6) or synthetic graft, central veins (Figures 57–7 and 57–8), graft venous anastomosis, or intragraft for the treatment of stenosis. Covered stent grafts may be particularly useful for the treatment of graft or fistula pseudoaneurysms in situations in which open surgical repair is not practical. Figure 57–9A shows a left upper arm PTFE graft segment with multiple large pseudoaneurysms resulting from difficult needle cannulation and poor closure of needle puncture sites. An 8 mm × 80 mm Fluency tracheobronchial stent graft (Bard Peripheral Vascular Inc., Tempe, AZ) was placed with complete exclusion of the pseudoaneurysms (Figure 57–9B).

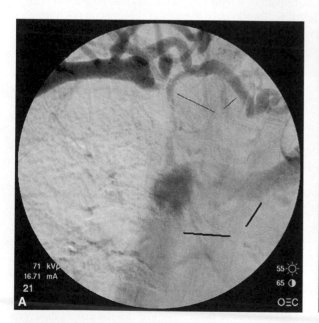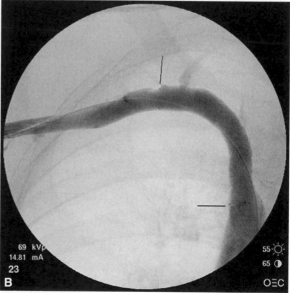

▲ **Figure 57–8.** ***A:*** Patient with a right upper arm graft for hemodialysis with severe right upper extremity edema. There was right subclavian and brachiocephalic vein occlusion with extensive venous collateral engorgement (fine lines). Note the delayed filling of the left innominate vein and superior vena cava (bold lines) via collaterals. ***B:*** Following angioplasty to 12 mm and placement of a right subclavian and brachiocephalic vein 14 mm × 60 mm SMART Stent (Cordis/Johnson & Johnson, Warren, NJ) with dramatic resolution of collateral venous flow. Note the radiopaque markers at the stent margins (fine lines). (Courtesy of TF Saad.)

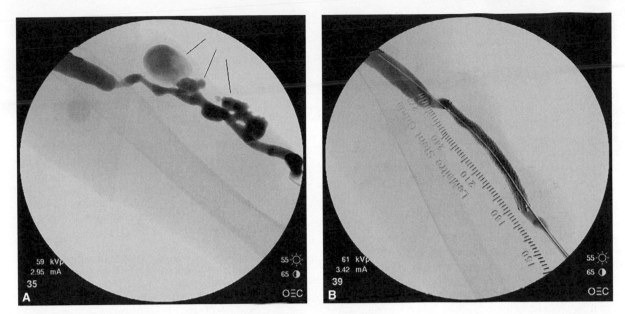

▲ **Figure 57–9.** **A:** Left upper arm polytetrafluoroethylene graft segment with multiple large pseudoaneurysms (fine lines) resulting from difficult needle cannulation and poor closure of needle puncture sites. **B:** An 8 mm × 80 mm Fluency tracheobronchial stent graft (Bard Peripheral Vascular Inc., Tempe, AZ) was placed with complete exclusion of the pseudoaneurysms. (Courtesy of TF Saad.)

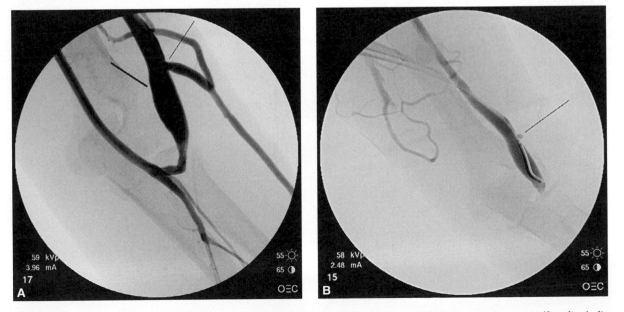

▲ **Figure 57–10.** **A:** Left upper arm brachial artery-to-cephalic vein fistula with a single large accessory vein (fine line) diverting flow from the cephalic vein (bold line). **B:** Ligation of the accessory vein was performed with elimination of flow in this vessel on repeat fistulogram. Note the small stump at the origin of the ligated branch (fine line). (Courtesy of TF Saad.)

▶ Fistula Accessory Branch Ligation

To be usable for hemodialysis access, a native fistula must have sufficient flow through an accessible vein or veins. In selected cases, accessory veins may divert flow from the dominant fistula vein into branches that are not suitable for needle access. This may leave insufficient flow through the dominant vein for dialysis, especially when there is relatively poor blood delivery due to small or diseased peripheral arteries, low blood pressure, or poor cardiac output. In these circumstances, in addition to correcting any flow-limiting stenosis, ligation or embolization of accessory veins may result in improved fistula performance. This can be done using minimally invasive techniques, with immediate confirmation of successful branch occlusion. Figure 57–10A shows an upper-arm brachial artery-to-cephalic vein fistula with a single accessory vein diverting flow from the preferred vessel; this fistula was not functioning well for hemodialysis due to inadequate maturation of the vessel and ongoing difficulty with needle access. Ligation of the accessory vein was performed, with elimination of flow into this vessel on repeat fistulogram (Figure 57–10B). When selecting accessory veins for occlusion, great care must be taken not to sacrifice veins that might eventually be suitable for needle cannulation or useful for a surgical revision. Furthermore, collateral veins that are providing outflow due to occlusion or stenosis of the dominant vein should never be sacrificed. In these cases, the outflow stenosis should be corrected before any vein branches are considered expendable.

THE FUTURE OF INTERVENTIONAL NEPHROLOGY

Interventional nephrology is an exciting and rapidly evolving field. It is extremely important to address and resolve the critical vascular access problems that arise in patients on hemodialysis. Our ability to provide timely, efficient, high-quality, and cost-effective service is central to the care of these patients and to the operation of our dialysis units and practices. Our role as nephrologists also provides multiple opportunities for improvements in vascular access, including early vein preservation, the creation of AV access in advance of the need for dialysis, the minimization of venous catheter use, monitoring and screening for access dysfunction, and planning for the creation of secondary native fistulas in anticipation of impending access failure. Working closely with surgeons, radiologists, nurses, and dialysis technicians, our challenge is to continue to improve the quality of access care that is provided to patients on dialysis. Improved hemodialysis access care and enhanced outcomes will result in higher native fistula rates, lower patient morbidity and mortality, reduced requirements for inpatient care, and reduced costs to the health care system.

Asif A et al: Venous mapping using venography and the risk of radiocontrast-induced nephropathy. Semin Dialysis 2005;18:239.

Beasley C et al: Fistula first: an update for providers. Nephrol News Issues 2004;18:88.

Churchill DN, Moist LM: Is percutaneous transluminal angioplasty an effective intervention for arteriovenous graft stenosis? Semin Dialysis 2005;18:190.

Clark TWI: Nitinol stents in hemodialysis access: J Vasc Interv

Clark TWI, Rajan DK: Treating intractable venous stenosis: present and future therapy. Semin Dialysis 2004;17:4.

Saad TF, Vesely TM: Venous access for patients with chronic kidney disease: J Vasc Interv Radiol 2004;15:1041.

Trerotola SO et al: Hemodialysis-related venous stenosis: treatment with ultrahigh-pressure angioplasty balloons. Radiology 2004;231:259.

Vogel PM, Parise C: SMART stent for salvage of hemodialysis access grafts. J Vasc Interv Radiol 2004;15:1051.

White JJ et al: Treatment of hemodialysis AV graft stenosis: stents resurgent. Kidney Int 2005;67:772.

Interventional Nephrology: Peritoneal Dialysis Catheter Procedures

58

Stephen R. Ash, MD, FACP

▶ General Considerations

In addition to being a continuous daily home therapy, peritoneal dialysis (PD) offers a number of advantages for end-stage renal disease (ESRD) patients. Nevertheless, PD remains an underutilized form of renal replacement therapy. Recent data demonstrate that over 50% of ESRD patients in the United States prefer and request PD as the modality of choice for renal replacement therapy. However, only 12% of ESRD patients are initiated on this form of therapy. A variety of factors including timely insertion of PD access are likely responsible for the dramatic underutilization of PD. Recent attention has focused on increasing the use of this important modality of renal replacement therapy. To this end, interventional nephrologists have taken the initiative in performing PD access-related procedures, including catheter insertion, catheter removal, and repositioning of a migrated catheter. The safety and success of PD access-related procedures by nephrologists have been well documented.

This chapter provides a review of PD catheter types, catheter placement procedures, and management of some catheter-related complications. It emphasizes the importance, feasibility, and advantages of PD access procedures by nephrologists.

▶ Chronic Peritoneal Catheters

A. Types

Chronic PD catheters are designed to be used for many months or years. They are constructed of soft materials ssuch as silicone rubber or polyurethane. The intraperitoneal portion usually contains 1-mm side holes, although one version has linear grooves or slots rather than side holes. All chronic PD catheters have one or two extraperitoneal Dacron cuffs that promote a local inflammatory response. This produces a fibrous plug that fixes the catheter in position, preventing fluid leaks and bacterial migration around the catheter. Chronic PD catheters are the most successful of all transcutaneous access devices, with longevity measured in years rather than days to months. Peritoneal access failure, however, is still a source of frustration for all continuous ambulatory peritoneal dialysis (CAPD) programs, and it is the reason why about 25% of patients drop out. Increasing the success of a CAPD program requires optimal use of peritoneal catheters. Currently, the method of catheter placement has more effect on outcome than catheter choice.

As shown in Figure 58–1, at first there appears to be a bewildering variety of chronic PDs. However, each portion of the catheter has only a few basic design options.

There are four designs of the intraperitoneal portion:

1. Straight Tenckhoff, with an 8-cm portion containing 1-mm side holes.

2. Curled Tenckhoff, with a coiled 16-cm portion containing 1-mm side holes.

3. Straight Tenckhoff, with perpendicular discs (Toronto-Western, rarely used).

4. T-fluted catheter (Ash Advantage) a T-shaped catheter with grooved limbs positioned against the parietal peritoneum.

There are three basic shapes of the subcutaneous portion between the muscle wall and the skin exit site:

1. Straight or gently curved.

2. A 150° bend or arc (Swan Neck).

3. A 90° bend, with another 90° bend at the peritoneal surface (Cruz "Pail Handle" catheter).

There are three positions and designs for Dacron cuffs:

1. A single cuff around the catheter, usually placed in the rectus muscle but sometimes on the outer surface of the rectus.

2. Dual cuffs around the catheter, one in the rectus muscle and the other in the subcutaneous tissue.

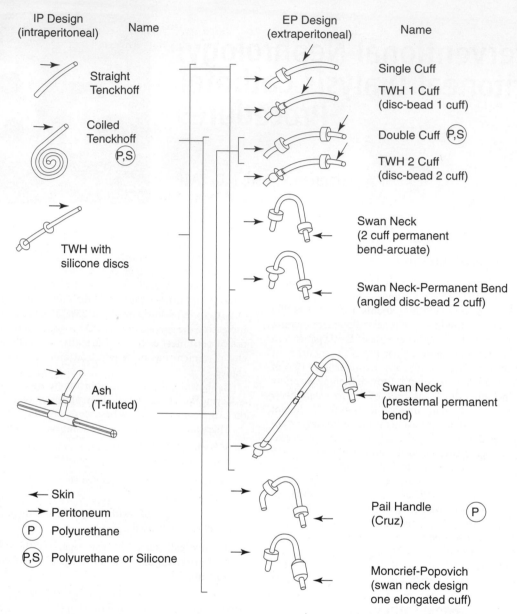

IP Design (intraperitoneal) Name

- Straight Tenckhoff
- Coiled Tenckhoff (P,S)
- TWH with silicone discs
- Ash (T-fluted)

← Skin
→ Peritoneum
(P) Polyurethane
(P,S) Polyurethane or Silicone

EP Design (extraperitoneal) Name

- Single Cuff
- TWH 1 Cuff (disc-bead 1 cuff)
- Double Cuff (P,S)
- TWH 2 Cuff (disc-bead 2 cuff)
- Swan Neck (2 cuff permanent bend-arcuate)
- Swan Neck-Permanent Bend (angled disc-bead 2 cuff)
- Swan Neck (presternal permanent bend)
- Pail Handle (Cruz) (P)
- Moncrief-Popovich (swan neck design one elongated cuff)

▲ **Figure 58–1.** Currently available peritoneal catheters; combinations of intraperitoneal and extraperitoneal designs.

3. A disc-ball deep cuff with the parietal peritoneum sewn between the Dacron disc and silicone ball (Toronto–Western and Missouri catheters).

There are three internal diameters, each having an outer diameter of approximately 5 mm (Figure 58–2).

1. 2.6 mm, the standard Tenckhoff catheter size.
2. 3.1 mm, the Cruz catheter.
3. 3.5 mm, the Flexneck catheter.

There are two materials of construction:

1. Silicone rubber (nearly all catheters).
2. Polyurethane (Cruz catheter).

The various intraperitoneal designs are all created to diminish outflow obstruction. The shape of the curled Tenckhoff catheter and the discs of the Toronto-Western catheter hold visceral peritoneal surfaces away from the side holes of the catheter. The grooves of the Advantage catheter distribute

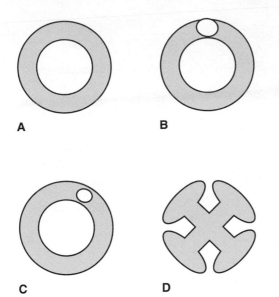

▲ **Figure 58–2.** Comparison of cross-sectional dimensions of the intraperitoneal portion of several peritoneal catheters: **A:** Flexneck Tenckhoff catheter (silicone). **B:** Cruz Tenckhoff catheter (polyurethane). **C:** Standard Tenckhoff catheter (silicone). **D:** One intraperitoneal limb of the T-fluted catheter (Ash Advantage, silicone).

flow over the surface of the limbs that contact the parietal peritoneum, providing a much larger surface area for drainage than the side holes provide. An irritated omentum attaches firmly to the side holes of a catheter but only weakly to the grooves on a catheter (as demonstrated by the Blake surgical drain, with grooves on the catheter surface).

The subcutaneous catheter shapes all provide a lateral or downward direction of the exit site, which minimizes the risk of exit infection. An upward-directed exit site collects debris and fluid, increasing the risk of exit-site infection.

The optimal location for the standard deep cuff is within the rectus muscle. The subcutaneous cuff provides additional protection from bacterial contamination of the subcutaneous tunnel. The disc-ball deep cuff provides security of position of the catheter, since with the peritoneum sewn between the Dacron disc and intraperitoneal ball the catheter is fixed in position and cannot migrate outward. Similarly, the T shape of the Advantage catheter places the intraperitoneal limbs against the parietal peritoneum, preventing outward migration of the catheter.

The larger internal diameter of the Cruz and Flexneck catheters provides lower hydraulic resistance and more rapid dialysate flow during the early phase of outflow. In the latter part of outflow, the resistance to flow is determined mostly by the spaces formed by peritoneal surfaces as they approach the catheter, rather than the inside of the catheter. The Advantage catheter provides much larger entry ports for drainage of peritoneal fluid; limited clinical studies have demonstrated faster drainage of the peritoneum in the early and late phases of outflow and a decrease in residual peritoneal volume at the end of outflow.

The material from which peritoneal catheters are constructed has not affected the incidence of complications. There is no decrease in the incidence of peritonitis or omental attachment leading to outflow failure with polyurethane catheters, although they do have a weaker bond to the Dacron cuff, and loosening of this bond can create pericatheter leaks.

B. Proper Location of Components

There is general agreement on the proper location of the components of chronic PD catheters (Figure 58–3):

1. The intraperitoneal portion should be between the parietal and visceral peritoneum and directed toward the pelvis to the right or left of the bladder.

2. The deep cuff should be within the medial or lateral border of the rectus sheath.

3. The subcutaneous cuff should be approximately 2 cm from the skin exit site.

Placing the deep cuff within the abdominal musculature promotes tissue ingrowth and therefore avoids pericatheter hernias, leaks, catheter extrusion, and exit-site erosion. At the parietal peritoneal surface, the squamous epithelium reflects along the surface of the catheter to reach the deep cuff. If the deep cuff is outside the muscle wall, the peritoneal extension creates a potential hernia. At the skin surface, the stratified squamous epithelium follows the surface of the catheter until it reaches the superficial cuff. If the exit site is longer than 2 cm, the squamous epithelium disappears and granulation tissue is left, leading to an exit site with continued "weeping" of serous fluid; the potential for exit site infection is therefore increased.

Some peritoneal catheters have components that provide greater fixation of the deep cuff within the musculature. When the Missouri and Toronto-Western catheters are placed, the parietal peritoneum is closed between the ball (inside the peritoneum) and disc (outside the peritoneum). When the T-fluted (Ash Advantage) catheter is placed, the wings open in position adjacent to the parietal peritoneum and perpendicular to the penetrating tube. With these catheters, outward migration of the catheter is impossible.

When placing peritoneal catheters it is best to choose a deep cuff location that is free of major blood vessels (Figure 58–4).

C. Methods of Implantation

PD catheter insertion can be accomplished by any one of three techniques: the dissective or surgical, the blind or modified Seldinger, and the peritoneoscopic. The dissective

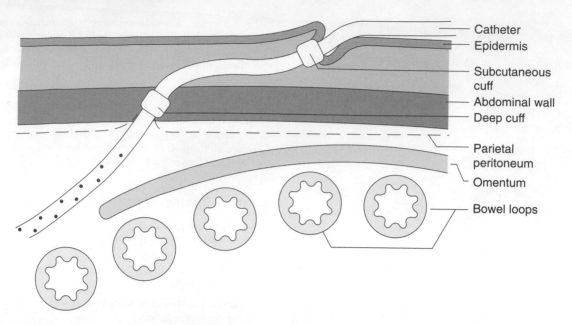

Catheter
Epidermis
Subcutaneous cuff
Abdominal wall
Deep cuff
Parietal peritoneum
Omentum
Bowel loops

▲ **Figure 58–3.** Proper relationship of peritoneal cuffs to the abdominal musculature, parietal and visceral peritoneum, and skin exit site for the straight Tenckhoff catheter.

technique utilized by most surgeons places the catheter by minilaparotomy, usually under general anesthesia. In the blind or modified Seldinger technique a needle is inserted into the abdomen, a guide wire is placed, a tract is dilated, and the catheter is inserted through a split sheath, all without visualization of the peritoneal cavity. Peritoneoscopic insertion uses a small (2.2-mm-diameter) optical peritoneoscope (Y-TEC Scope) for direct inspection of the peritoneal cavity and identification of a suitable site for the intraperitoneal portion of the catheter.

There are advantages and disadvantages of each technique of catheter placement, and the overall success of the catheters is as dependent upon the skill and experience of the physician performing the procedure as the method of placement. Each procedure has unique advantages and problems.

Dissective techniques securely place the deep cuff within the abdominal musculature. The techniques can be performed without any specialized equipment except for a stylet to straighten the catheter. Some types of catheters require surgical placement, such as the disc-and-ball Missouri or Toronto-Western catheters. The incision in the abdominal musculature requires surrounding tissues to first heal the wound and then grow into the deep cuff before the deep cuff is secure. Pericatheter leaks are frequent if the catheter is used immediately after placement. The dissective approach provides no visualization of adhesions and free spaces within the peritoneum. The catheter tip is advanced by "feel" and may be advanced to press against loops of bowel, or near adhesions, leading to early outflow failure of the catheter.

Blind placement procedures are convenient, can be performed anywhere in a hospital, and have the advantage of being low in cost. The needle, guidewire, dilators, and sheath are often packed in a kit with the peritoneal catheter. Bowel perforation is an occasional complication, usually not recognized until the catheter has been completely placed and is flushed. No visualization of the peritoneal space is provided to avoid impingement of the catheter tip on adhesions or visceral surfaces. The deep cuff is usually left just outside of the abdominal musculature, not within the rectus sheath.

Peritoneoscopic placement allows the best visualization of the peritoneal space. This avoids placing the catheter under bowel loops, under omentum, or against adhesions. The Quill expands to allow the deep cuff to advance into the musculature. The Y-TEC procedure can be performed in any room in the hospital. Specialized equipment must be purchased, however, and the physician must have some training in peritoneoscopic techniques. Of the three techniques, only the latter allows for direct visualization of the intraperitoneal structures. The use of this technique, most commonly employed by nephrologists, is rapidly expanding. Peritoneoscopic placement varies from laparoscopic techniques by using a much smaller scope and puncture size, only one peritoneal puncture site, a device to advance the cuff into the musculature, air in the peritoneum rather than CO_2, and local rather than general anesthesia.

The preference of one technique over another must take into account the incidence of complications (pericatheter leakage, exit site and tunnel infection), the long-term

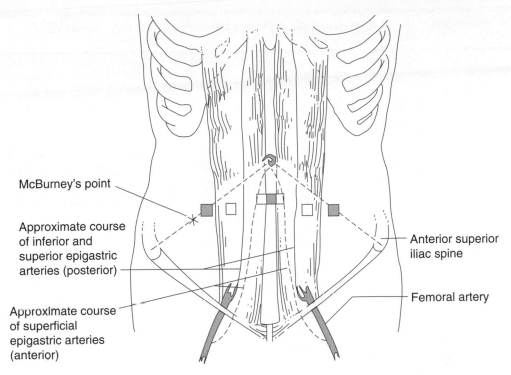

▲ **Figure 58–4.** Major blood vessels and landmarks of the anterior abdominal wall. Open squares represent the preferred and safest points for the location of the deep cuff of a chronic peritoneal catheter within the medial or lateral border of the rectus muscle. Solid squares indicate the external landmarks used during blind insertion of a needle or cannula at the start of peritoneoscopic or blind catheter placement: One-half of the distance between the anterior superior iliac spine for the lateral border of the rectus and 2 cm below the umbilicus for the medial border of the rectus.

McBurney's point

Approximate course of inferior and superior epigastric arteries (posterior)

Approximate course of superficial epigastric arteries (anterior)

Anterior superior iliac spine

Femoral artery

catheter survival associated with each technique, the costs, ease, and timely insertion of the catheter, and factors contributing to risk of mortality (general anesthesia). To this end, peritoneoscopic placement of PD catheters by nephrologists has been rigorously compared to the surgical and the blind technique (Table 58–1). Both randomized and nonrandomized studies have documented the superiority of the peritoneoscopic technique in terms of a lower incidence of catheter complications (infection, outflow failure, pericatheter leak) and increased catheter survival. The avoidance of various complications by peritoneoscopic placement may relate to the decreased tissue dissection required with this technique. Extensive dissection (incising/splitting the rectus sheath/muscle as well as incising the parietal peritoneum) in the surgical technique may lead to loose attachment of the catheter to the abdominal wall, thereby increasing the incidence of pericatheter leaks, subsequent tunnel infection and peritonitis, and catheter loss.

Peritoneoscopic insertion of a PD catheter by a nephrologist can be safely performed in a procedure room, an interventional laboratory, or an intensive care unit using standard precautions for infection control. Conversely, the dissective

surgical technique requires a surgeon, operating room facilities and staff, and anesthesia services. In addition, a second admission and surgical procedure for catheter exteriorization may be required for catheters that are buried on placement. The surgical approach introduces delays and restrictions inherent in the system and increases costs. At our center, the average time between the initial contact with the interventional nephrology team and PD catheter insertion was markedly shortened to 6.4 ± 0.9 days (mean $\pm$ SE), in contrast to the prior 34.3 ± 1.6 day (mean $\pm$ SE) delay when catheters were placed by the surgeon. Since tissue dissection is minimal with the peritoneoscopic technique, the postoperative course is brief and the catheter can be used immediately for some schedule of PD (such as with overnight exchanges with the patient at rest, dry during the day). A 2- to 3-week postoperative period for complete wound healing is recommended before implementing CAPD.

Mortality risk from general anesthesia varies with the American Society of Anesthesia (ASA) physical status categories. These range from class I to V. Class I includes patients with no physiologic or psychologic stress (minimal risk) and class V describes patients with severe systemic

Table 58–1. Comparison of the blind, dissective, and peritoneoscopic technique utilizing a double-cuff Tenckhoff catheter.

Investigator (year)[1]	Number of patients	Mean follow-up (months)	Infectious complications	Outflow failure	Subcutaneous leaks
Blind or Seldinger technique					
Bierman (1985)	222	24.0	0.12	0.36	0.03
Valenti (1985)	30	13.7	n/a	n/a	0.26
Zappacosta (1991)	101	36.0	0.15	0.07	0.03
Nebel (1991)	49	9.6	0.05	0.30	0.02
Swartz (1990)	134	12.3	0.75	0.11	0.22
Scalamonga (1994)	110	20.0	0.10	0.02	n/a
Ozener (2001)	133	17	0.20	0.09	0.07
Average		18.9	0.23	0.16	0.11
Peritoneoscopic/laparoscopic technique					
Khanna (1981)	132	13.3	0.19	0.07	0.07
Rottenbourg (1981)	48	12.0	n/a	n/a	0.30
Odor (1985)	150	6.1	0.10	0.33	0.00
Twardowski (1985)	83	18.0	0.50	0.11	n/a
Swartz (1990)	79	12.1	0.88	0.14	0.10
Piraino (1991)	228	36.0	1.00	0.04	0.06
Shyr (1994)	43	18	0.46	0.07	0.00
Rugiu (1996)	134	27.0	0.50	0.20	0.08
Gadallah (1999)	72	24	0.13	0.08	0.11
Ozener (2001)	82	21.2	0.27	0.16	0.05
Average		17.6	0.45	0.13	0.09
Dissective or surgical technique					
Ash (1983)	61	10.0	0.02	0.04	0.05
Handt (1984)	98	27.0	0.15	0.00	0.00
Cruz (1989)	150	12.0	0.01	0.01	0.01
Adamson (1992)	100	10.0	0.01	0.04	0.09
Swartz (1993)					
Chadha (1994)	70	24	0.04	0.07	n/a
Scott (1994)	30	12.0	0.10	0.1	0.00
Copley (1996)	135	8.7	0.21	0.07	0.04
Gahallah (1999)	76	24	0.02	0.07	0.01
Average		18.4	0.07	0.04	0.01

[1]Bierman M et al: Perit Dial Bull 1985;5:229. Valenti G et al: Perit Dial Bull 1985;5:39. Zappacosta AR et al: ASAIO Trans 1991;37:13. Nebel M et al: Adv Perit Dial 1991;7:208. Swartz R et al: Perit Dial Int 1990;10:231. Scalamogna A et al: Perit Dial Int 1994;14:S81 (Abstr). Ozener C et al: Nephrol Dial Transplant 2001;16:1893. Khanna R et al: Perit Dial Bull 1981;1:24. Rottembourg J et al: Perit Dial Bull 1981;1:123. Odor A et al: Perit Dial Bull 1985;5:226. Twardowski ZJ et al: Perit Dial Bull 1885;5:219. Shyr YM: Perit Dial Int 1994;14:401. Piraino B et al: Perit Dial Int 1991;11:64. Rugiu C et al: Perit Dial Int 1996;16:S54 (Abstr). Gadallah MF et al: Am J Kidney Dis 1999;33:118. Ash SR et al: Perit Dial Bull 1983;3:8. Handt AD, Ash SR: Perspect Perit Dial 1984;2:30. Cruz C et al: Perit Dial Int 1989;9:S1 (Abstr). Adamson AS et al: Nephrol Dial Transplant 1992;7:855. Swartz DA et al: Perit Dial Int 1993;S31 (Abstr).Chadha I et al: Perit Dial Int 1994;14:S89 (Abstr). Scott PD et al: Perit Dial Int 1994;14:289. Copley JB et al: Perit Dial Int 1996;16:S330.

disturbances. For class II patients (mild-to-moderate systemic disturbances, such as essential hypertension, diabetes, or anemia) mortality is estimated at 3/1000. The mortality rate increases with moderate-to-severe disturbances reaching 1.8% for class III and 7.8% for class IV patients. ESRD patients usually have multiple complex and advanced medical problems. Therefore, avoiding general anesthesia and its inherent risk is a major advantage. Utilizing local anesthesia for PD catheter placement avoids the risks of general anesthesia. Among methods of placement, the peritoneoscopic method (performed by nephrologists, generally) has the lowest incidence of infectious complications over the life of the catheters. This may relate to the decreased amount of tissue trauma and smaller incision size of the peritoneoscopic placement versus dissective placement and better assurance that the cuff is placed within the muscle versus blind placement. Outflow failure and leaks are comparable between peritoneoscopic placement and surgical dissection, but are higher with blind placement. This relates to the lack of peritoneal visualization during positioning of the catheter with blind techniques and to the positioning of the cuff outside the rectus sheath rather than within the rectus muscle (in general).

There are also differences in the use of catheters according to the method of placement. Peritoneoscopically placed catheters may be used for PD treatments immediately to support the patient without the need for hemodialysis in almost any schedule that does not include full volume of the peritoneum during times of activity. This includes night-time cycler therapy or overnight exchanges, but excludes full-volume CAPD. Some surgically placed catheters may also be used immediately, but this involves modifying the technique. One approach is to angle the catheter course through the rectus muscle, separating the site of penetration of the anterior and posterior rectus sheaths and maintaining the cuff position in the middle of the rectus muscle.

In summary, with optimal training in PD catheter insertion, a nephrologist can perform PD catheter placement safely and successfully. The American Society of Diagnostic and Interventional Nephrology (ASDIN) has established accreditation guidelines for training centers and certification guidelines for individual physicians to obtain the necessary skills in PD catheter placement. Although two nephrologists would be ideal, a PD access placement program can be successfully initiated by a single trained nephrologist. When peritoneal catheter insertion is performed by nephrologists, a variety of advantages can occur for the patient, some related to the procedure of peritoneoscopy and some related to the timeliness and continuity of care (Table 58–2). However, the success of the procedure is tantamount to patient benefit. The placement of PD catheters should be performed by the physician with the best outcomes, using whatever technique is most successful in their hands.

Effects of Design on Catheter Success

Randomized, prospectively controlled studies have generally shown little effect of catheter design on the success of peritoneal catheters, although one study demonstrated a longer 3-year survival of coiled versus straight Tenckhoff catheters.

Table 58–2. Potential procedural advantages of peritoneal dialysis catheter insertion by an interventional nephrologist.

Interventional nephrologist	Surgeon
Timely initiation of therapy	Unnecessary delays often present
Operating room not required	Operating room time and scheduling required
Anesthesia services not required	Anesthesia services required
Local anesthesia used	General anesthesia used (usually)
Less dissection	More dissection
Rectus sheath/muscle and peritoneum intact	Rectus sheath and peritoneum incised
Direct intraperitoneal visualization	No intraperitoneal visualization
Decreased incidence of complications	Higher incidence of complications
Longer catheter survival	Shorter catheter survival
Complete understanding of the renal disease	Minimal understanding of renal disease
Cost effective	Higher cost
Continuity of care	Lack of continuity of care
May help to counteract peritoneal dialysis underutilization	No evidence to counteract peritoneal dialysis underutilization
Effective communication	Increased number of middle men and decreased communication

Data from Asif A et al: Semin Dial 2003;16:266. Ash SR: Semin Nephrol 2002;22:221. Ash SR: Nephrol News Issues 1993;7:33. Ash SR: Adv Perit Dial 1998;14:75. Ash SR et al: Perit Dial Bull 1983;3:8–12. Ash SR: Semin Dial 1992;5:199. Gadallah MF et al. Adv Perit Dial 2001;17:122. Gadallah MF et al: Am J Kidney Dis 2000;35:301.

If properly placed, dual-cuff Tenckhoff catheters have a lower incidence of exit-site infection and longer lifespan than single-cuff catheters, although properly placed single-cuff catheters can work as well. Curled Tenckhoff catheters have a lower incidence of outflow failure than straight catheters. Swan neck catheters have a lower incidence of exit-site infection than those with straight subcutaneous segments. Nonrandomized studies of specific catheters have indicated various advantages, including the fact that catheters with the best fixation of the deep cuff (such as the Missouri and Advantage catheters) have a very low incidence of exit-site infection.

Some silicone Tenckhoff catheters, such as the Flexneck, have a larger internal diameter and thinner walls (Figure 58–2). These catheters are more pliable and create less tension between deep and superficial cuffs during normal patient activities. This may result in a lower incidence of pericatheter leaks and hernias and fewer exit-site and tunnel erosions, although any real advantages are as yet unproven. A problem with Flexneck catheters is that they are prone to crimping in the subcutaneous tunnel if they are angled sharply. If physicians follow a template to create the subcutaneous tunnel with a gentle downward curve, crimps in the subcutaneous tract are eliminated. Flexneck catheters, such as the Cruz catheter, have a higher rate of inflow and initial outflow than catheters with standard, smaller internal diameters. Rapidity of flow at the end of outflow for the Cruz catheter is partly due to the 90° angle of the catheter at the parietal surface, which positions the coiled portion next to the parietal peritoneal surface. Catheters constructed from polyurethane (such as the Cruz) have excellent strength and biocompatibility. The glue bonding of the Dacron cuffs to the catheters, however, often fails within 1–2 years of use, resulting in pericatheter leaks and sometimes infections.

The Advantage catheter contains a straight portion that is adjacent to the parietal peritoneum, ensuring a stable position without extrusion of the deep cuff or exit site erosion (similar to the disc-ball catheters and the older Lifecath catheter). Advantage catheters placed in patients beginning PD and those with previous Tenckhoff failures demonstrate a 1-year survival of 90%, higher than the 50–80% survival of Tenckhoff catheters in numerous studies (Figure 58–5). During follow-up of 42 patients with Advantage catheters in place for up to 4 years, only one patient developed a pericatheter leak (resolved by delaying CAPD), and no patient developed a pericatheter hernia or late exit infection. The outflow rate of PD fluid is on average equal to the best functioning Tenckhoff catheters (including the large internal diameter Flexneck catheters). The total outflow volume is more consistent with the Advantage catheter. In CAPD exchanges with the same glucose concentration and dwell time the Advantage catheter has a standard deviation of 2% versus 10% for Tenckhoff catheters. The more consistent peritoneal outflow is probably due to more complete drainage of the peritoneum, with a diminished residual volume, but this has also not been proven. Diminished residual volume is important, since if residual volume is decreased by 300–500 mL, the inflow volume can be increased by the same amount, thus increasing the peritoneal clearance by 10–20% without increasing patient discomfort by overfilling the abdomen.

Advantage peritoneal catheters may diminish the risk of outflow failure, but do not eliminate this risk. The mechanism of outflow failure is different from that in Tenckhoff catheters. The omentum does not directly attach to the intraperitoneal portion of the catheter, but rather surrounds the long, slotted catheter intraperitoneal limbs and traps them against the parietal peritoneum. Infusion of iodine dye during fluoroscopy demonstrates that the dye does not pass freely in many directions out of the grooves of the

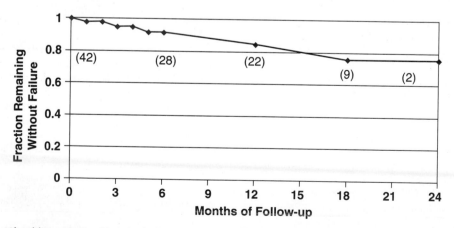

▲ **Figure 58–5.** Lifetable analysis of survival of the Advantage peritoneal dialysis catheter placed in patients with previous Tenckhoff catheter failures and in patients new to peritoneal dialysis.

catheter, but rather stays near the catheter and exits from the ends of the intraperitoneal limbs. Laparoscopic removal of adhesions from around the catheter can often result in a perfectly functioning PD catheter. The negative features of the Advantage catheter include the fact that it is somewhat more complicated to insert, either during dissection or by peritoneoscopy. A special slotted "Key Tube" and guide are needed to hold the ends of the catheter together so that it can be inserted through the Quill guide or through a peritoneal opening. The catheter opens automatically when the tube and guide are retracted. Another problem with this catheter is that if the peritoneal fluid contains a considerable amount of blood or fibrin the small openings between the fluted limbs and the central T portion can block off. This usually resolves with some in/out flushes by a 20-mL syringe with saline, but sometimes tissue plasminogen activator infusion is necessary.

All PD catheters can serve as a nidus for infection, requiring removal in cases of persistent peritonitis. None of the new designs or materials has changed this. Peritoneal catheters with a long-term and effective antibacterial surface are still an elusive goal, but several new approaches to sterilization of biofilm are now being evaluated. Another challenge is to limit the growth of adventitial tissue around and onto catheters, such as in fibrous sheathing of central venous catheters and omental attachment to peritoneal catheters. Of course, these materials would have to be applied to the intravascular or intraperitoneal surfaces of the catheters and not in the subcutaneous space or on the cuffs.

New Placement Techniques

Several recent publications have described the use of laparoscopic techniques for the placement of peritoneal catheters. These techniques use the same 5- to 10-mm-diameter trocars generally used for laparoscopic surgery. These are much larger than the 2.2-mm peritoneoscope used in the Y-TEC system, and usually require general anesthesia and automated inflation equipment. The catheter is inserted through a large cannula into the abdomen, and it is difficult to ensure that the deep cuff is placed within the musculature until after the cannula is removed. In spite of the excellent visualization of the peritoneum with laparoscopic placement techniques, several studies have shown that catheters placed in this manner have a high frequency of pericatheter leak due to the large hole made in the musculature. As opposed to catheters placed with specially designed equipment, those placed by the laparoscopic technique have no advantage in terms of longevity over those placed by dissection. However, laparoscopy does provide knowledge of intraperitoneal anatomy that may be helpful in the placement of PD catheters in patients with previous surgeries and multiple adhesions. In fact, the visibility of the peritoneum is considerably greater than with the small peritoneoscope. Additionally, adhesion lysis is possible as is repositioning of the catheters using laparoscopy. In difficult cases laparoscopy, versus dissective placement, may be the preferable technique.

Burying the Peritoneal Dialysis Catheter

Traditional surgical implantation of Tenckhoff catheters involves immediate exteriorization of the external segment through the skin, so that the catheter can be used for supportive PD or for intermittent infusions during the "break-in" period. To prevent blockage and to confirm function, the catheter is flushed weekly with saline or dialysate; each exchange carries the same risk of peritonitis as in CAPD therapy. The catheter must also be bandaged and the skin exit site must be kept clean in the weeks after placement to avoid bacterial contamination of the exit site. The patient must therefore be trained in some techniques of catheter care. It has always been difficult to decide when to place a PD catheter in a patient with chronic renal insufficiency. If the catheter is placed too early, the patient may spend weeks to months caring for a catheter that is not used for dialysis. If the catheter is placed after the patient becomes uremic, it is often used for PD therapy without a "break-in" period.

A placement technique has been devised in which the entire peritoneal catheter can be buried under the skin some weeks to months before it needs to be used. The catheter burying technique was first described for placement of a modified Tenckhoff catheter with a 2.5-cm-long superficial cuff, but the technique has been adopted for standard dual-cuff Tenckhoff catheters. In the original technique the external portion of the catheter was brought through a 2- to 3-cm skin exit site (much larger than the usual 0.5 cm incision). The catheter was then tied off with silk suture and coiled and placed into a "pouch" created under the skin. The skin exit site was then closed. Weeks to months later, the original skin exit site was opened and the free end of the catheter was brought through the original skin large exit site.

The goal of burying the PD catheter was to allow ingrowth of tissue into the cuffs of the catheter without the chance of bacterial colonization and to allow a transcutaneous exit site to be created after the tissue had fully grown into the deep and subcutaneous cuffs. Burying the catheter effectively eliminated early pericatheter leaks and decreased the incidence of peritonitis. In 66 months of follow-up, patients with a buried Tenckhoff catheter had 0.017–0.37 infections per year versus 1.3–1.9 infections per year in control patients. In a study of 26 buried Tenckhoff catheters, the incidence of infection during PD was 0.8 infections per year and the incidence of catheter-related peritonitis was only 0.036 per patient-year. A retrospective study confirmed a significantly lower rate of catheter infection and peritonitis in patients who had buried catheters and a significantly longer catheter life, although the procedure was not effective when used for single-cuff catheters.

The incidence of exit-site infections is not generally decreased in patients with catheters that are buried and exteriorized, which may be explained by the increase in trauma near the exit site that occurs during burying and exteriorizing the catheter. A large exit site is created when the catheter is buried and a similarly large site is recreated when the catheter is exteriorized. Creating a "pouch" under the skin requires a considerable amount of dissection and trauma near the exit site. The size of the pocket limits the length of the catheter that can be coiled and buried under the skin, which limits the external length of the catheter after exteriorization. The exit site must be opened widely to remove the catheter, because the coil rests in a position distant from the skin exit site. Subcutaneous adhesions to the silk suture around the catheter further restrict removal. Increased trauma near the exit site during placement and exteriorization of the catheter may have caused an increased incidence of early exit infection with this technique. In a study of "embedded" catheters in 26 adult patients (with a mean subcutaneous residence of 79.5 days) two patients developed local seromas and 12 developed subcutaneous hematomas (five of which were revised surgically). There were a number of flow problems at catheter "activation": Nine patients developed fibrin thrombi (two requiring operative clearance) and four patients had omental catheter obstruction (four requiring omentectomy). When burying the Tenckhoff catheter using standard techniques there were a total of 27 complications in 26 catheter placements, with 13 of these complications requiring corrective surgery.

When catheters are placed by the Y-TEC procedure the Quill and cannula of the system can be reassembled and used to bury the external portions of dual-cuff Tenckhoff and Advantage catheters. The catheter exit site is made slightly larger than the standard exit site. The Quill and cannula are inserted through this exit site to create a long, straight tunnel for the external end of the catheter. The catheter is blocked with an internal plug rather than an external silk suture. We have used this technique to bury and then remove over 40 Tenckhoff and Advantage catheters. There have been only a few early complications—insignificant hematoma (3%), seroma (0%), exit infection (3%), or outflow failure (0%)—and all catheters have functioned after exteriorization. Nephrologists can bury and exteriorize PD catheters with greater ease and less trauma than with surgical procedures and possibly obtain improved results.

In planning for hemodialysis of patients with ESRD, it is common practice to place fistulas or grafts several months before the need for initiation of dialysis, so that they can "mature" before use. PD catheters also "mature" after placement, with fibrous tissue ingrowth into the cuffs and the development of a fibrous tunnel. The fully ingrown catheter is more resistant to infection of the cuffs and the surface of the catheter. The technique of burying PD catheters after placement allows this maturation to occur before use of the catheter, much as with fistulas and grafts. It also allows the time of catheter insertion to be separated from the time of catheter use and avoids the patient having to learn how to care for the catheter site or observe the catheter site for potential complications. At the time of initiation of dialysis, the patient and physician can focus attention on the proper performance of the technique and patient response rather than on the function of the catheter. The patient can be trained in full-volume CAPD techniques rather than in "break-in" or cycler techniques used for immediately exteriorized catheters.

A curious aspect of the burying technique is that it seems contrary to "the rules" of catheter break-in. In immediately exteriorized catheters, it is necessary to infuse and drain the dialysate or saline (with or without heparin) at least weekly to prevent outflow failure or obstruction of the catheter. However, with the completely buried catheter, there is no infusion of any fluid for periods of up to 1 year. This may be possible because in the exteriorized catheter, stress and strain on the catheter and its compliance allow some fluid to enter and exit the side holes during patient movement. The buried catheter has less motion and with a secure blockage there is very little fluid inflow/outflow through the holes during normal activity. Furthermore, the infusion of saline or dialysate during break-in techniques adds a bioincompatible fluid to the abdomen at a time before the catheter is "biolized" or protein/lipid coated. The catheter becomes biolized in the absence of dialysate or saline in the peritoneum. When PD is begun, the catheter is already biolized and less likely to develop omental attachment, even in patients with an active omentum.

▶ Catheter Removal

In general, a physician who places a device is responsible for following the success of the device and removing it when complications require removal or when it is no longer needed. Removal of a PD catheter can be safely performed by nephrologists without significant discomfort under local anesthesia, although Toronto=Western catheters require more dissection and the patient may require conscious sedation. The procedure should be done only with a sterile technique, good lighting, antiseptic skin preparation (including the catheter near the skin), and draping typical of a procedure done in a surgical suite or outpatient surgery room (a drape to cover the primary incision, deliberately excluding the exit site, since the exit site and catheter, even when treated with antiseptic, cannot be considered clean). Here too, an operating room is not needed as the procedure can be performed in a procedure room using standard precautions for infection control.

Removal of Missouri or Toronto–Western type catheters is a little more complicated, since the Dacron disc rests next to the peritoneum and develops fibrous adhesions to the peritoneum and the posterior rectus sheath. These catheters are generally placed by surgeons and should be removed by the surgeons who placed them.

▶ Complications of Catheter Insertion

A variety of issues surround the procedure for PD catheter insertion. These include migration of a catheter, placement of a catheter in a patient with prior abdominal surgery, and bowel perforation following insertion of a PD catheter.

A. Visceral Perforation

Bowel perforation is the most feared complication of peritoneoscopic insertion of a PD catheter and is the most important factor preventing nephrologists from performing this procedure. Although the risk of bowel perforation following insertion of a PD catheter is minimal, nephrologists performing this procedure should be well versed in diagnosing this complication promptly and managing the patient effectively.

The true incidence of bowel perforation with the peritoneoscopic technique is unknown. A recent study evaluating 750 PD catheter insertions performed by nephrologists utilizing the peritoneoscopic technique found the incidence of this complication to be 0.8%. However, numerous other studies do not report a single episode of bowel perforation. In contrast, the incidence of visceral perforation using the dissective technique has been reported to range from 1% to 1.4%. Whereas some investigators suggest that this complication should be treated with surgical intervention, successful conservative management of bowel perforation using bowel rest and intravenous antibiotics has also been reported.

Introduction of a trocar (diameter 2.2 mm) into the abdominal cavity is likely responsible for bowel injury when a PD catheter is inserted using the peritoneoscopic technique. Bowel injuries due to the introduction of insufflation needles, trocars, rigid catheters, and colonoscopic examinations have been reported. The majority of these perforations are usually small and seal spontaneously. These "miniperforations" close within 24–48 hours, most likely secondary to omental adherence. The majority of small perforations are self-sealing and do not require surgical intervention.

In summary, the peritoneoscopic technique of PD catheter insertion allows the nephrologist to make the diagnosis of bowel perforation immediately and implement therapeutic measures promptly. Nephrologists can successfully manage these patients conservatively with close monitoring of vital signs, serial abdominal examination, bowel rest, and broad spectrum intravenous antibiotics. With this approach patients who do not need surgical intervention can be identified and unnecessary laparotomy can be avoided. Clinical deterioration and signs of peritoneal irritation should prompt a surgical consult.

B. Migration and Repositioning

PD catheter migration to the upper abdomen is not uncommon (15–35%) and usually leads to outflow problems and catheter failure. The condition is suspected by encountering flow problems and is confirmed by plain abdominal X-ray. A variety of techniques have been used to combat migration with long-term success rates of 27–48%.

C. Previous Abdominal Surgery

A history of previous abdominal surgery could result in significant intraperitoneal adhesions and has been identified as a relative contraindication to PD. Nevertheless, catheter insertion can be successfully accomplished in this population; a history of abdominal surgery does not necessarily increase the risk of bowel perforation. The common notion that "patients with previous abdominal surgery are not the best candidates for peritoneal dialysis" should be discouraged. Since the peritoneoscopic technique identifies intraperitoneal adhesions, assesses their extent, and determines a suitable site for catheter placement, patients with a history of prior abdominal surgery should not be routinely denied this modality (Figure 58–5). PD catheter insertion can be successfully performed in this population with a high rate of success (>95%).

D. Underutilization

PD is an underutilized form of renal replacement therapy. Only 12% of patients with ESRD utilize this form of dialysis in the United States. A variety of factors have been deemed responsible. Of these, modality choice presentation followed by swift catheter insertion is of critical importance. Unnecessary delays in catheter insertion may leave patients who choose PD with a modality that they did not desire. At least two separate studies have documented a positive impact of PD access surgery by nephrologists on underutilization of PD.

▶ Conclusions

PD access-related procedures can be safely and successfully performed by nephrologists with excellent catheter outcome data. There are a variety of advantages, including the timely initiation of therapy, when the catheter insertion is performed by a nephrologist. However, nephrologists must obtain optimal training and develop the necessary skills to perform these procedures. ASDIN is actively engaged in promoting the performance of PD access-related procedures by nephrologists and developing training centers at academic medical centers. At every dialysis center, selected nephrologists should consider expanding their role to perform PD access-related procedures in order to provide timely delivery of this aspect of ESRD care.

Poisonings & Intoxications

James F. Winchester, MD, &
Donald A. Feinfeld, MD

Because of modern medical approaches mortality from poisoning is low. However, severe poisoning in certain groups of patients is associated with a high mortality: poisons with toxic metabolites (eg, methanol, ethylene glycol, and acetaminophen), poisons inducing metabolic changes (eg, salicylates), and poisons that produce deep coma (eg, phenobarbital). This chapter will discuss the role of forced diuresis and modern dialysis techniques used to treat poisoning, and will give the clinician guidance in the appropriate use of these treatments applied to drug or chemical intoxication. We will use real case reports to illustrate these points.

The cumulative American Association of Poison Control Center (AAPCC) database now contains 33.8 million human poison exposures. During 2003, 2,395,582 human exposures were reported by 64 participating poison centers, reflecting an increase of 0.7% compared to the 2002 AAPCC report, and an increase of 10.5% over the exposures reported in 2000. Although the majority of cases were managed at home, in 2003, 525,710 cases required treatment in a health care setting and 1106 patients died; 134,619 patients were treated with single dose activated charcoal, 7875 were treated by alkalinization, 1509 received hemodialysis, and 27 received hemoperfusion.

MULTIPLE DOSE ACTIVATED CHARCOAL

One method of removing toxins from the body is the administration of multiple doses of activated charcoal. Charcoal given acutely decreases the absorption of toxins from the gastrointestinal tract, but has also been recommended in repeated doses in the hope of trapping toxic substances from the enterohepatic recirculation. However, although there is some experimental evidence that this mode of therapy can decrease the half-life of many xenobiotics, there are only a few toxic substances for which multidose charcoal administration has been shown to be effective. According to the American Academy of Clinical Toxicology, these include carbamazepine, dapsone, phenobarbital, quinine,

and theophylline. One recent study in volunteers suggests that repeated doses of superactivated charcoal may have some detoxification benefit up to 3 hours after acetaminophen ingestion. However, two other volunteer studies conclude that multidose activated charcoal may not be effective more than 1 hour after acetaminophen overdose. Multidose activated charcoal has also been reported to reduce death and serious arrhythmias in yellow oleander poisoning (Table 59–1).

FORCED DIURESIS & URINARY ALKALINIZATION

Many substances are eliminated by the kidneys if they are filtered and not reabsorbed or if they are actively secreted by the tubules into the urine. Filtration occurs freely for smaller molecules (<5000 Da) that are not highly bound to plasma proteins such as albumin. Phenobarbital is such a substance. For such substances to be excreted effectively, they must remain largely in the tubular fluid as they traverse the nephron.

If a substance is cleared by filtration and kidney function is good, it is important to maintain that level of function in order to continue elimination of that substance. It is therefore crucial to support the patient's extracellular fluid volume by giving appropriate intravenous saline, ie, to maintain a good diuresis. However, the concept of overhydrating a patient to

Table 59–1. Substances for which multidose activated charcoal is indicated.

Carbamazepine
Dapsone
Phenobarbital
Quinine
Theophylline
Acetaminophen (up to 1 hour after ingestion)
Yellow oleander

"force" a diuresis has not been shown to be of benefit in poisoning and risks overloading the left ventricle. Repletion and maintenance of extracellular volume are always indicated, especially in salicylate poisoning, where there is usually a loss of about 2 L in the adult. The patient should be monitored for signs of volume overload or depletion.

The natural ability of the kidneys to clear the blood of many substances is also enhanced by the kidneys' secretion of substances into the urine. The tubules take up many xenobiotics that circulate in plasma, even if they are bound to proteins, and move them into the lumen to be excreted. There are separate transport pathways for anions (such as penicillin) and cations (such as gentamicin).

Renal excretion of a particular xenobiotic can be increased if there is a form of the substance that is less readily reabsorbed back into the blood from the tubular lumen. Many drugs and toxins are weak acids or bases that diffuse back into tubular cells in their neutral form but are poorly absorbed as anions or cations. For this reason, if the pH of the urine can be maintained such that the nonreabsorbable ionized form is favored, there will be greater net excretion of that substance (Table 59–2). In general, anionic substances (such as salicylate) are best excreted at a higher urine pH (above 7), whereas cationic drugs (such as phencyclidine) are best excreted at a low urine pH (below 5.5). This phenomenon is called "diffusion trapping." It is seen in the case of urinary ammonium, which is the main route of renal hydrogen ion excretion. Ammonia freely diffuses from the tubular lumen into the cells and the blood. However, in the relatively acid urine pH, most of the ammonia takes up hydrogen ions, and the resultant ammonium ion is trapped in the tubular lumen to be readily excreted.

However, the clearance of many drugs and chemicals is not substantially increased by this maneuver. Not all ionizable substances have their excretion enhanced by manipulation of urine pH. This is usually because their volume of distribution V_d is high (Table 59–3). Substances that remain exclusively (or nearly so) in total body water will have a lower V_d than those with a high affinity for lipid or protein and that appear to dissolve in a much greater quantity of water than their plasma levels indicate (digoxin is a good example).

Table 59–3. Volume of distribution and protein binding of selected drugs in a 70-kg person.

Drug	Volume of distribution		Protein binding (%)
	L/kg	L	
Acetylsalicylic acid	0.1–0.2	7–14	50–90
Amitriptyline	15	1050	95
Digoxin	6.8	476	2
Phenobarbital	50	49	51

Adjusting the urine pH is effective only if the V_d is low and if an altered urine pH has actually been shown to be effective in enhancing removal of the toxin.

In the case of xenobiotics that are weak bases, such as phencyclidine, no advantage has been shown in acidifying the urine to enhance the drug's excretion. Acidifying the blood in an attempt to accomplish this leads to metabolic acidosis, which can worsen the patient's condition. On the other hand, renal excretion of a number of weak acids is markedly enhanced by urinary alkalinization (Table 59–4). Of these, the most important is salicylate, whose excretion can be quadrupled if the urinary pH is 7.5 or above. It is unclear, however, why this is so, since the pK_a for salicylic acid is 3.0. At a urine pH of 6.0, 99.9% of the salicylate should already be ionized and therefore not reabsorbed. Mechanisms other than diffusion trapping may explain the enhanced salicylate excretion at higher urine pH.

In the past, the Done nomogram has been used to estimate the toxicokinetics of salicylate in moderate to severe overdoses. Some clinicians use this nomogram to calculate the endogenous clearance of salicylate. Unfortunately, the Done calculations were established in children and assume first-order kinetic clearance of salicylate from the body, in which the excretion of a drug is proportional to the concentration of that drug in body fluids. In fact, in severe salicylate poisoning, several elimination pathways for the drug become saturated, and the clearance becomes zero order, ie, there is a constant rate of drug removal per time, independent of concentration.

Table 59–2. Dissociation constants pK_a for various drugs.

Acids		Bases	
Drug	pK_a	Drug	pK_a
Acetylsalicylic acid	3.49	Amphetamine	9.9
Amobarbital	7.7	Phencyclidine	8.5
Barbital	7.91		

Table 59–4. Substances for which urinary alkalinization improves excretion.

Salicylate
Mecoprop
2,4-Dichlorophenoxyacetic acid (2,4-D)
Methotrexate
Phenobarbital (but not as effective as multidose activated charcoal)
Chlorpropamide (usually responds to supportive treatment)
Diflunisal (not of clinical usefulness)

The renal excretion of two herbicides, 2,4-dichlorophenoxyacetic acid (2,4-D) and mecoprop, is also increased at a higher urine pH. Alkalinizing the urine may also help to eliminate overdoses of methotrexate. The excretion of phenobarbital and chlorpropamide is also augmented by urinary alkalinization, but this is rarely useful since the former is better eliminated by multidose activated charcoal and the latter usually responds to supportive care with glucose infusion (Table 59–2).

DIALYSIS TECHNIQUES USED IN POISONING

Many substances can be removed by hemodialysis and hemoperfusion.

▶ Principles of Dialysis in Relationship to Drug Removal

These principles have been discussed elsewhere in this book. Factors governing drug removal are solute (or drug) size, its lipid–water partition coefficient (or lipid solubility), the degree to which it is protein bound, its volume of distribution, and the presence of a concentration gradient promoting constant removal of the drug or chemical moiety. The physical factors governing drug removal by the dialyzer are blood flow rate through the dialyzer, dialysate flow rate, dialyzer surface area, and the characteristics of the specific membrane.

For drugs (usually about 300 Da) that are diffusible across semipermeable membranes solute removal rates (clearance) increase with increasing blood flow rate. For solutes greater than 300 Da, the rate of diffusion across the membrane is less, the concentration gradients across the membrane remain high, and increasing flow rates have a decreased effect on drug clearance rates. For larger drugs, the removal rate can be increased by increasing the surface area or by choosing a high permeability membrane. The latter is the preferred method.

▶ Clearance

Clearance of drugs and chemicals follows the same principle as that used to calculate solute clearance by the kidney. Clearance is given by the following formula:

$$Clearance = Q_b[(A - V)/A]$$

where A is arterial or inlet concentration and V is venous or outlet concentration of the drug going through the dialyzer and Q_b is the blood flow rate through the dialyzer. The ratio $A - V/A$ is the drug extraction ratio (ER) across the dialyzer.

▶ Hemodialysis

The procedure for hemodialysis in poisoning is identical to that used in a Stage V chronic kidney disease (CKD) patient with one or two exceptions.

In a drug intoxicated hypotensive patient who requires pressor agents to maintain an adequate blood pressure, if pressors are administered through the dialysis blood lines they should be placed distal to the drug-removing device since they are readily removed through the hemodialysis membrane or sorbent. Pressor requirements may need to be increased during the procedure even if pressors are administered in a completely separate line for the same reason.

If dialysate regeneration systems using a sorbent system (the REDY system) are used in the treatment of patients who have been poisoned, there is the theoretical risk of sorbent saturation, and drug removal rates may decrease over time.

▶ Sorbent Hemoperfusion

Hemoperfusion was quite popular for the treatment of poisoning in the 1970s and 1980s. Currently in the United States activated charcoal hemoperfusion devices, but not resin hemoperfusion devices, are available for clinical use.

Certain resins have been shown to be most effective for removal of lipid-soluble drugs, with drug clearance rates from blood often exceeding those achieved by charcoal hemoperfusion; these are available in Europe. A partial list of the available hemoperfusion devices is given in Table 59–5. Hemoperfusion relies on the physical process of adsorption. For many drugs clearance was better than with hemodialysis. The hemoperfusion circuit for treatment of drug intoxication can but need not be combined with dialysis in certain situations (particularly when there is a serious acidosis shown to be corrected by bicarbonate dialysate). The manufacturers Instructions for Use should be followed since some devices come "dry" and others need to be flushed with saline, and heparinization protocols differ. The most efficient drug removal is achieved with blood flow rates of approximately 300 mL/minute. Even in the hypotensive patient lower blood flow rates achieve significant drug removal.

Removal of lipid-soluble drugs, such as glutethimide and methaqualone, was far more efficient with XAD-4 resin hemoperfusion than with activated charcoal. Modern dialyzers with high permeability may be of greater efficiency than those used in the 1970s and 1980s, and a reappraisal of dialysis versus charcoal hemoperfusion in poisoning may be called for (see Case 3 below). However, the spectrum of drugs taken in overdose situations in the twenty-first century is quite different from that used in the late twentieth century, and studies to reexamine drugs that are obsolete may never be done.

Table 59–5. Available hemoperfusion devices.

Manufacturer	Device	Sorbent type
Clark	Biocompatible system	Charcoal
Gambro	Adsorba	Charcoal
Braun	Haemoresin	XAD-4 resin

Complications of Hemoperfusion

The principal side effect of hemoperfusion with charcoal or resin preparations is platelet depletion of about 30% or greater, which may or may not give rise to clinical bleeding problems. Reductions in serum calcium and serum glucose and transient decreases in white blood cell counts, usually mild, may be seen. A mild reduction of 1–2°F in body temperature is expected, due to no rewarming in the extracorporeal circuit, and frequent body temperatures should be taken in deeply comatose patients. The decreases in platelet concentration usually return to normal within 24–48 hours following a single hemoperfusion.

Criteria for Hemodialysis in Poisoning

The prime consideration in the decision to employ extracorporeal techniques to remove poisons is based on the clinical features of poisoning, particularly if the patient's condition deteriorates progressively despite intensive supportive therapy.

Suggested clinical criteria are outlined in Table 59–6. These criteria should be used along with the plasma concentrations of common drugs (Table 59–7), above which hemodialysis or hemoperfusion should be considered. Table 59–8 lists the reported dialyzable drugs; many of these reports are single case reports, since it has been difficult to undertake controlled studies. In addition, it cannot be overstated that a large number of these reports are anecdotal, but critical review of drug removal rates indicates that those drugs not enclosed in parentheses are most efficiently removed. For further information see Aronoff et al (1999).

Hemoperfusion & Hemodialysis with Chelating Agents

In patients on dialysis, aluminum and iron intoxication can be treated with deferoxamine in conjunction with dialysis (continuous ambulatory peritoneal dialysis or hemodialysis) or hemoperfusion for removal of the deferoxamine–aluminum or deferoxamine–iron complex. Clinical improvement in the osteomalacia component of renal osteodystrophy is seen after aluminum is removed. Encephalopathy, iron overload, and anemia also improve.

Heavy metals and their salts are not removed efficiently by dialysis or hemoperfusion alone. During hemodialysis, metal removal may be enhanced with chelating agents, such as N-acetylcysteine or cysteine. On the other hand, removal of mercury and thallium by hemoperfusion appears modest at best.

IMMUNOPHARMACOLOGY IN POISONING

Digoxin antibodies, specifically the Fab fragments, neutralize digoxin and reduce any toxicity. Recrudescence of digoxin poisoning has been reported 24–48 hours after administration of Fab antibodies in renal failure patients. In a kinetic analysis of elderly and renally impaired patients with digoxin and digitoxin poisoning, it was suggested that the dose of Fab antibodies should be the same as for young patients or those with normal renal function. In digoxin poisoning the elimination halftime of digoxin in anephric patients can be substantially reduced with the addition of hemoperfusion.

CASE REPORTS

Case 1: Methanol Intoxication

A 32-year-old male with no significant past history drank a bottle of windshield washer fluid as he was being arrested in an attempt to avoid going straight to jail. He was promptly brought to the emergency department where he was evaluated. His only symptom at the time was nausea without vomiting. He denied chest pain, dyspnea, headache, diaphoresis, and visual disturbances. His blood pressure (BP) was 146/86 mm Hg, temperature (T) 98.7°C, pulse (P) 106 and regular, and respiration (R) 14 rpm. Examination of the head, eyes (including fundi), neck, lungs, heart, chest, abdomen, nervous system, and extremities was entirely normal.

Table 59–7. Plasma concentrations of common poisons above which hemodialysis (HD) or hemoperfusion (HP) should be considered.[1]

Drug	Serum concentration		Method of choice
	μg/mL	mmol/L	
Salicylates	800	5000	HD
Theophylline	400	2200	HP>HD
Paraquat	0.1	0.5	HP>HD
Methanol	50		HD

[1]Suggested concentrations only: in mixed intoxications clinical condition may not reflect drug concentrations.

Table 59–6. Clinical considerations for hemodialysis or hemoperfusion in poisoning.

1. Progressive deterioration despite intensive care
2. Severe intoxication with hypoventilation, hypothermia, and hypotension
3. Predisposition to complications of coma (eg, chronic obstructive pulmonary disease)
4. Impaired normal drug excretory function due to hepatic, cardiac, or renal insufficiency
5. Poisoning with agents with metabolic and/or delayed effects, eg, methanol, ethylene glycol
6. Intoxication with a drug or poison that can be extracted at a rate exceeding endogenous elimination

Table 59–8. Drugs and chemicals removed with hemodialysis and hemoperfusion (not well removed).

Antimicrobials/anticancer
Acyclovir
(Amantadine)
Amikacin
Amoxicillin
(Amphotericin)
Ampicillin
(Azathioprine)
(Azithromycin)
Azlocillin
Aztreonam
Bacitracin
Bredinin
Busulphan
Capreomycin
Carbenicillin
Cefaclor
Cefadroxil
Cefamandole
Cefazolin
Cefixime
Cefmenoxime
Cefmetazole
(Cefonicid)
(Cefoperazone)
Ceforamide
(Cefotaxime)
Cefotetan
Cefotiam
Cefoxitin
Cefpirome
Cefroxadine
Cefsulodin
Ceftazidime
(Ceftriaxone)
Cefuroxime
Cephacetrile
Cephalexin
Cephalothin
(Cephapirin)
Cephradine
(Chloramphenicol)
(Chloroquine)
Cilastatin
Ciprofloxacin
(Clarithromycin)
Clavulinic acid
(Clindamycin)
(Cloxacillin)
Colistin
Cyclophosphamide
(Cycloserine)
Dibekacin
(Dicloxacillin)
Didanosine
(Doxycycline)
(Enoxacin)

(Erythromycin)
Ethambutol
(Floxacillin)
(Fluconazole)
5-Fluorocytosine
5-Fluorouracil
Fluroxacin
Foscarnet
Fosfomycin
Ganciclovir
Gentamicin
Imipenem
Isoniazid
(Itraconazole)
Kanamycin
(Ketoconazole)
Mecillinam
(Methicillin)
(Methotrexate)
Metronidazole
(Mezlocillin)
(Miconazole)
(Minocycline)
Moxalactam
(Nafcillin)
Neomycin
Netilmicin
Nitrofurantoin
(Norfloxacin)
Ofloxacin
Ornidazole
PAS (*p*-aminosalicylate)
Penicillin
(Pentamidine)
Piperacillin
(Praziquantel)
Pyrizinamide
(Quinine)
(Ribavirin)
(Rifampin)
Sisomicin
Streptomycin
Sulfisoxazole
Sulfonamides
Temocillin
Tetracycline
Ticarcillin
Tinidazole
Tobramycin
Trimethoprim
(Vancomycin)
Vidarabine
Zidovudine

Barbiturates
Amobarbital
Aprobarbital

Barbital
Butabarbital
Cyclobarbital
Pentobarbital
Phenobarbital
Quinalbital
(Secobarbital)

Nonbarbiturate hypnotics, sedatives, tranquilizers, anti-convulsants, muscle relaxants
Carbamazepine
Atenolol
Baclofen
Betaxolol
(Bretylium)
(Calcium channel blockers)
Captopril
Carbromal
Chloral hydrate
(Chlordiazepoxide)
Clonidine
(Diazepam)
(Diazoxide)
(Diphenylhydantoin)
(Diphenylhydramine)
Ethchlorvynol
Ethiamate
Ethosuximide
Gallamine
Glutethimide
(Heroin)
Meprobamate
(Methaqualone)
Methsuximide
Methyprylon
Paraldehyde
Primidone
Valproic acid

Cardiovascular agents
Acebutolol
N-Acetylprocainamide
(Amiodarone)
Amrinone
(Digoxin)
Enalapril
(Encainide)
(Flecainide)
Fosinopril
(Lidocaine)
Lisinopril
Methyldopa
Metoprolol
Nadolol
(Ouabain)
(Pindolol)

Practolol
Procainamide
Propranolol
Quinapril
(Quinidine)
Ramipril
Sotatol
(Timolol)
Tocainide

Alcohols
2-Butoxyethanol
Ethanol
Ethylene glycol
Isopropanol
Methanol

Analgesics, antirheumatics
Acetaminophen
Acetophenetidin
Acetylsalicylic acid
Colchicine
Methylsalicylate
(D-Propoxyphene)
Salicylic acid

Antidepressants
(Amitriptyline)
Amphetamines
(Imipramine)
Isocarboxazid
Moclobemide
Monoamine oxidase inhibitors
(Pargylline)
(Phenelzine)
Tranylcypromine
(Tricyclics)

Solvents, gases
Acetone
Camphor
Carbon monoxide
(Carbon tetrachloride)
(Eucalyptus oil)
Thiols
Toluene
Trichloroethylene

Plants, animals, herbicides, insecticides
Alkyl phosphate
Amanitin
Demeton sulfoxide
Dimethoate
Diquat
Glufosinate
Methylmercury complex
Oleander toxin

Table 59–8. *Continued*

Plants, animals, herbicides, insecticides	Aniline	Thiocyanate	Lithium
(Organophosphates)	Borates	Ranitidine	(Magnesium)
Paraquat	Boric acid		(Mercury)[1]
Snake bite	(Chlorpropamide)	**Metals, inorganics**	Phosphate
Sodium chlorate	Chromic acid	(Aluminum)[1]	Potassium
Star fruit toxin	(Cimetidine)	Arsenic[1]	(Potassium dichromate)[1]
Potassium chlorate	Dinitro-{it}O{end}-cresol	Barium	Sodium
	Folic acid	Bromide	Strontium
Miscellaneous	Mannitol	(Copper)[1]	(Thallium)[1]
Acipimox	Methylprednisolone	Formate	(Tin)
Allopurinol	4-Methylpyrazole	Iodine	(Zinc)
Aminophylline	Sodium citrate	(Iron)[1]	
	Theophylline	(Lead)[1]	

[1]Removed with a chelating agent.

Laboratory data showed serum osmolality 390 mOsm/kg, Na 138 mEq/L, K 6.3 mEq/L, Cl 99 mEq/L, CO_2 23 mEq/L, blood urea nitrogen (BUN) 11 mg/dL, creatinine 0.8 mg/dL, and glucose 96 mg/dL. Urinalysis was normal; the methanol level was 227 mg/dL.

The patient was begun promptly on intravenous ethanol and subsequently given fomepizole. The following day he had pH 7.376, Pco_2 44.2, Po_2 86.9, and HCO_3 25.3. His ethanol level was 159.9 mg/dL. Hemodialysis was performed and the methanol level fell to 59 mg/dL. By the following day it had rebounded to 90 mg/dL and a second hemodialysis was performed on day 3, with the methanol level falling to 28 mg/dL. At no time during the hospitalization was the patient significantly acidotic, and his ophthalmologic examination remained normal. He was discharged asymptomatic to jail on the fifth hospital day. This case illustrates that prompt inhibition of alcohol dehydrogenase can entirely prevent both the life-threatening acidosis and the ocular complications. The use of fomepizole eliminates the need for continual monitoring of the patient's ethanol level, which was formerly necessary when ethanol was the only available alcohol dehydrogenase blocker; however, giving fomepizole does not obviate the use of hemodialysis. The course of hospitalization can be considerably shortened by dialyzing out the methanol, even if a second procedure is necessary. Furthermore, if acidosis has set in, dialysis quickly corrects it. In cases of severe methanol intoxication, as in this case, dialysis may avoid the need to give a second dose of fomepizole.

▶ Case 2: Ethylene Glycol Poisoning

A previously healthy 28-year-old man was hospitalized 3 hours after drinking 280 mL of antifreeze containing 95% ethylene glycol. He was tremulous and agitated but not obviously intoxicated. His BP was 137/88 mm Hg, T 98.8°F, P 88 bpm, and R 24 rpm. His head, eyes, neck, lungs, heart, abdomen, neurologic system, and extremities were all normal.

Laboratory data showed serum osmolality 362 mOsm/kg, Na 146, K 4.5, Cl 110, and CO_2 11. BUN was 10 mg/dL and creatinine 1.1 mg/dL. Arterial pH was 7.17, Pco_2 26, and Po_2 105. The serum ethylene glycol level was 303 mg/dL. The urine had no protein, glucose, or cells, but contained numerous envelope- and needle-shaped crystals. The patient was loaded with saline and ethanol and was subsequently hemodialyzed. At no time did the patient show any decrease in renal function. Timed collections of blood and urine for ethylene glycol were performed before and after hemodialysis. Endogenous renal clearance of ethylene glycol was 27.5 mL/minute, while hemodialysis clearance of ethylene glycol was 136.6 mL/minute. By 30 hours after ingestion the patient's ethylene glycol level was zero. The patient was discharged after 72 hours with no target organ damage from the ingestion. This case illustrates that prompt administration of an alcohol dehydrogenase blocker (ethanol or fomepizole) can prevent injury to the kidneys, heart, and brain; hemodialysis clearance of ethylene glycol is about five times greater than the endogenous clearance of the toxin; and because it is so much more efficient, hemodialysis is an important means of rapidly reducing the amount of ethylene glycol and its metabolites in the body and can substantially shorten the hospital stay.

▶ Case 3: Aluminum Intoxication

A 75-year-old female was admitted from another hospital 8 days following irrigation of the bladder with a 1% alum solution (aluminum potassium sulfate) for intractable hemorrhagic cystitis. Her mental status had been impaired from postirrigation day 3 and a serum Al drawn on day 3 was reported 5 days later to be 423 µg/L. Six hours after a 500 mg infusion of deferoxamine she was dialyzed for 4 hours using a 2 M^2 high-flux dialyzer for 4 hours. Because of past reports that charcoal hemoperfusion was superior to hemodialysis, she was treated on day 2 with a 4 hour hemoperfusion 6 hours after the same dose of deferoxamine. Total (chelated and nonchelated) Al extraction by the devices was calculated.

Although starting at a lower extraction ratio than hemo-perfusion (20% versus 38%), hemodialysis had an average extraction ratio of 24% versus an average of 16% because of saturation of the hemoperfusion device (extraction was only 5% at 2 and 4 hours). In addition, the patient had no changes in platelets during hemodialysis, but profound thrombo-cytopenia after hemoperfusion. The patient was subse-quently treated with chelation and hemodialysis alone. This illustrates the need to reappraise older literature in light of improvements in dialysis.

Case 4: Salicylate Poisoning

A 22-year-old college student was found wandering in the residence hall. She was examined at the student health center where she was found to be irritable, confused, tachypneic, and mildly hypotensive. Her roommate called the student health center to report that the patient had just broken up with her boyfriend, and that she had found some pills lying on the bathroom floor and an empty aspirin container. This prompted transfer of the patient to a tertiary care center where she was found to be acidemic (pH 7.24) and hypoka-lemic, with a salicylate concentration of 75 mg/dL. Shortly after admission it was noticed that she was somnolent. This prompted admission to the medical intensive care unit where hemodialysis was performed via a femoral vein catheter. Within 2 hours her acidosis had improved (pH 7.34) and the salicylate concentration was 35 mg/dL and by 4 hours her pH was 7.4 and the salicylate concentration was 20 mg/dL. Dialysis was discontinued. This case illustrates that central nervous system (CNS) changes in the presence of acidemia reflect CNS trapping of salicylate and an urgency to correct the pH with bicarbonate dialysate and that salicylate is an ideally dialyzable drug (although protein binding is high, the bond is weak and the molecule traverses dialysis membranes easily).

Aronoff G et al (Eds): *Drug Prescribing in Renal Failure.* American College of Physicians, 1999.

Hörl WH et al: *Replacement of Renal Function by Dialysis,* ed 5. Kluwer Academic Publishers, 2004.

Proudfoot AT et al: Position paper on urine alkalinization. J Toxicol Clin Toxicol 2004;42:1.

Watson WA et al: 2003 annual report of the American Association of Poison Control Centers Toxic Exposure Surveillance System. Am J Emerg Med 2004;22:335.

Index

Page numbers with "t" and "f" indicate table and figure.

Abdominal X-ray, 147
Acetaminophen, 26t
Acetate, 50
Acetazolamide, 13, 44, 112, 137
Acetohydroxamic acid (AHA), 348
Acetylcysteine, 198
Achlorhydria, 65
Acid–base disorders
    degree of elevation of the plasma [HCO₃ –], 42–43
    and normal mechanism, 46
    $PaCO_2$ in, 42
    treatment, 54
Acid–base homeostasis, 460
Acid–base management, in renal insufficiency, 196–197
Acidemia, 184
Acinetobacter baumanii, 329
Acquired cystic kidney disease
    clinical findings, 420
    differential diagnosis, 420
    essentials of diagnosis, 420
    general considerations, 420
    treatment, 420
Acquired reflux nephropathy, 337
    pathogenesis, 337–340
    symptoms and signs, 341
Acquired renal scarring, 339
Acral or circumoral paresthesias, 55
α-actinin-4, 223
Acute alcoholic cirrhosis, 105
Acute bacterial prostatitis
    clinical findings, 336
    differential diagnosis, 336
    essentials of diagnosis, 335
    general considerations, 335
    treatment, 336
Acute coronary syndromes, in CKD, 167
Acute glomerulonephritis, 94
Acute interstitial nephritis (AIN), 94, 125t
    clinical features of, 124–125
Acute kidney failure, 226
Acute kidney injury (AKI), 297
    clinical findings, 94
    complications, 94–96
    essentials of diagnosis, 89
    general considerations, 89
    pathogenesis, 90–93
    prevention, 93–94
    prognosis, 98
    treatment, 96–98
Acute lymphoblastic leukemia, 70
Acute lymphocytic leukemia, 117
Acute nephrocalcinosis, 117
Acute-on-chronic respiratory acidosis, 58–59
Acute pancreatitis, 67, 83

Acute phosphate nephropathy, 325
Acute poststreptococcal glomerulonephritis (APSGN). *See*
    Poststreptococcal glomerulonephritis, acute (APSGN)
Acute prostatitis, 313
Acute pyelonephritis, 320–321, 337
    clinical findings, 332
    differential diagnosis, 332
    essentials of diagnosis, 332
    general considerations, 332
    prognosis, 333–335
    treatment, 332–333
Acute renal and respiratory failure, 257t
Acute renal failure (ARF), 117, 285, 321t
    due to NSAIDs, 138
    in elderly, 507–508
    from therapeutic agents
        ACE inhibitors, 132–134
        acyclovir, 127–129
        adefovir, 130
        aminoglycosides, 125–127
        amphotericin B, 132
        ARBs, 132–134
        carboplatin, 134–135
        cidofovir, 130
        cisplatin, 134–135
        classification of drugs based on pathophysiologic categories, 125t
        essentials in diagnosis, 124
        foscarnet, 129–130
        general considerations, 124–125
        hydroxyethylstarch, 131–132
        indinavir, 130–131
        intravenous immunoglobulin (IVIG), 131–132
        lithium, 136–137
        NSAIDs, 137
        tenofovir, 130
        vancomycin, 127
    toxicity of acyclovir, 127
Acute respiratory acidosis, 58
Acute rhabdomyolysis, 5
Acute tubular cell injury, 91
Acute tubular necrosis (ATN), 2t, 4, 9, 28, 91–92, 93, 96, 103, 120, 124, 125t
    ATIN from, 316
Acute tubulointerstitial disease (ATID), 124
Acute tubulointerstitial nephritis (ATIN), 2t, 313–318
    from acute tubular necrosis (ATN), 316–317
    algorithm for the diagnosis and treatment, 318f
    drugs causing, 315t
Acute uncomplicated cystitis
    clinical findings, 330–331
    differential diagnosis, 331
    essentials of diagnosis, 330
    general considerations, 330
    treatment, 331–332
Acute uncomplicated pyelonephritis, 333t

Acute uremia, 98
Acyclovir, 127–129, 315t
Acyclovir-induced ARF, 129
Acyclovir-induced nephropathy, 129
Acyclovir-resistant mucocutaneous herpes simplex
    infections, 129
ADAMTS 13, 288–289, 291–292
Addison's disease, 8
Adefovir, 130
Adenoma sebaceum, 414
Adenosine-induced renal vasoconstriction, 115
Adenosine monophosphate (AMP), 70
Adenosine triphosphate (ATP), 70
    production, 50
Adrenal cancer, 37
β_2-adrenergic agonists, 33f, 79, 387
β_3-adrenergic receptors, 110
African-Americans
    cardiovascular and related complications, 376
    chronic kidney disease, 376–377
    congestive heart failure (CHF), 376
    dietary salt intake, 375
    end-stage renal disease (ESRD) in, 295, 374
    and ESRD, 149
    hypertension, 374–378
    stroke, 376
    study of treatment with ramipril, 206
    therapeutic lifestyle changes, 377, 377t–378t
AL amyloidosis, 282
Albumin, 6, 20, 107, 159, 182, 185, 211, 258, 287
    257, 286
    for nephrotic syndrome, 21
Albuminuria, 358
Albuterol, 41
Alclofenac, 315t
Alcoholic hepatitis, 107
Alcoholic ketoacidosis, 49
Alcoholic myopathy, 77, 109
Aldosterone, 79
    antagonists, 227
    blockers, 13, 15
    functions of, 366
    hypertension, 369
Aldosterone-producing adenoma, 367
Alemtuzumab, 273
Alendronate, 63, 70
Alkalemia, 32
Alkalinization
    of K salts, 38
    of the urine, 112
Allantoin, 122
Allergic interstitial nephritis, 511–512
Allopurinol, 93, 122, 125, 315t, 419
Alport's syndrome, 225, 258
    clinical findings, 423
    complications, 424
    differential diagnosis, 423–424
    essentials of diagnosis, 422
    general considerations, 422
    pathogenesis, 422–423

prognosis, 424
    treatment, 424
Aluminum hydroxide, 122
Aluminum intoxication, management of, 180
Aluminum levels, plasma, 176
Alveolar CO_2 concentration, 54
Alveolar ventilation, 46, 55
Ambulatory blood pressure monitoring
    (ABPM), 354, 397
American diet, 79
Amikacin, 126
Amiloride, 15, 19, 38, 45, 368, 370
Aminoaciduria, 50, 74
Aminoglycoside-induced nephrotoxicity, 126
Aminoglycosides, 37, 92, 104, 107, 125–126, 333
    dosing guidelines, 127t
Aminoglycoside toxicity, 150
Aminolevulinate dehydrase (ALAD), 325
5-aminosalicylates, 125
Amitriptyline, 26t
Amlodipine, 206
Ammonium acid urate stones, 349
Ammonium chloride, 44
Amorphous debris, 116
Amoxicillin, 263, 315t
Amphetamine derivatives, 110–111
Amphotericin, 92
Amphotericin B, 37, 83, 132, 334
Ampicillin, 315t
Amyloid fibril, 281
Amyloidosis, 174–175, 232
    classification and nomenclature for the, 282t
    clinical findings, 282–283
    differential diagnosis, 283
    essentials of diagnosis, 281
    general considerations, 281
    pathogenesis, 281–282
    primary, 282
    prognosis, 284
    symptoms and signs, 282–283
    treatment, 283–284
Analgesia, 56
Analgesic abuse nephropathy (AAN)
    clinical findings, 323
    essentials of diagnosis, 322
    general considerations, 322–323
    pathogenesis, 323
    treatment, 323
Anemia, 65, 96, 167, 498
    of CKD
        pathogenesis, 155
        prognosis, 159
        treatment, 156–159
    in Goodpasture's syndrome, 255
    normocytic normochromic, 263
    prevention and treatment, 166
    shunt nephritis, 264
    treatment, 208
Angiography, 165
Angiomyolipomata, 414–415

Angiotensin-converting enzyme (ACE) inhibitors, 13, 15, 17, 38, 52, 90, 102, 107, 124, 132–134, 143, 152, 166, 188, 192, 198, 207–208, 234, 245, 293, 301, 325, 344, 355, 361, 364–365, 367, 376, 386, 429

Angiotensin II antagonists, 77, 102, 107

Angiotensin receptor blockers (ARBs), 38, 90, 132–134, 143, 152, 166, 188, 204, 207, 234, 245, 325, 355, 386, 429

Animal models, of renal disease, 202

Anion gap, 313
    diagnosis, 52–53
    high, 48–49
    normal, 49–52
    serum, 47–48

Anorexia, 82, 151, 159, 182
    correction of, 198–199

Antacid abuse, 75

Antacids, 85

Antegrade pyelography, 5

Antegrade ureteropyelograms, 147

Antiarrhythmic agents, 34

Antibiotic prophylaxis, 107, 344

Antibiotics, 262–263, 290, 333, 336, 447

Anti-C5 monoclonal antibody, 240

Anticoagulation strategies, 460–461

Anticoagulants, 290

Antidepressants, 26t

Antidiuretic hormone (ADH), 22, 79

Anti-GBM disease, 256

Anti-GBM ELISA assays, 258

Antihypertensive agents, 227, 293

Antihypertensive therapy, 391

Anti-immunoglobulin (Ig) G renal deposits, 260

Antimineralocorticoid receptor antagonist treatment, 15

Antineutrophil cytoplasmic antibodies (ANCA), 215, 260, 277
    associated glomerulonephritis, 269
    MPO, 269
    SVV, 267
    testing, 267, 269
    vasculitis, 270, 274

Antineutrophilic cytoplasmic antibody (ANCA)-associated systemic vasculitis, 255, 257

Antinuclear antibody (ANA), 212

Antiphospholipid syndrome, 290
    clinical findings, 294–295
    essentials of diagnosis, 294
    general considerations, 294
    treatment, 295

Antiplatelet agents, 290

Antiplatelet and anticoagulant therapy, 253

Antipsychotics, 26t

Antipyretics, 56

Antistreptolysin O (ASO) titers, 215, 260

Anxiety, 55, 67

Anxiety-related hyperventilation, 56

Aortic coarctations
    clinical findings, 372
    differential diagnosis, 372
    essentials of diagnosis, 372
    general considerations, 372

    prognosis, 373
    treatment, 372

Aortoplasty, 372

Apathy, 42

Apnea, 86

Apoptosis, 91

Apparent mineralocorticoid excess (AME)
    clinical findings, 369
    essentials of diagnosis, 369
    general considerations, 369
    prognosis, 369–370
    symptoms and signs, 369
    treatment, 369

"Apparent mineralocorticoid excess" (AME) syndrome, 37

Aquaporin-2 channel, 136

Aristolochic acid nephropathy
    clinical findings, 325
    essentials of diagnosis, 324
    general considerations, 325
    treatment, 325

Arm cuff systolic BP values, 380–381

Arrhythmias, 371

Arterial blood flow, effective, 90

Arterial portion, of body fluids, 7

Arteriography, 362–363

Arteriosclerosis, in CKD, 162

Arteriovenous (AV) fistulas, 162

Artifactual and hyperphosphatemia, 70

ART, 300

Ascites formation, overflow theory of, 18

Ascorbic acid, 327

Asphyxiating thoracic dystrophy, 413

Aspirin, 56, 166, 267, 295, 315t

Atelectasis, 20

Atenolol, 393

Atheroembolic disease, 93

Atheroembolic renal disease, 252, 313

Atheroembolism, 116

Atherosclerosis (ASO), 72, 360

Atherosclerotic renal artery stenosis, 362, 365

AT II receptor blockers (ARB), 361, 364–365, 367

Atrial natriuretic peptide, 114

Autoimmune anticardiolipin antibodies, 294

Autoregulation process, 401

Autosomal dominant hypophosphatemic rickets (ADHR), 75–76

Autosomal dominant polycystic kidney disease
    clinical findings, 406–408
    differential diagnosis, 408
    distinguishing features of, 409t
    essentials of diagnosis, 405
    general considerations, 405
    treatment, 408–411

Autosomal recessive polycystic kidney disease
    clinical findings, 412–413
    differential diagnosis, 413
    essentials of diagnosis, 411
    general considerations, 411–412
    treatment, 413

Azapropazone, 315t

Azathioprine, 271–274, 278–279, 315t

Azotemia, 9, 94, 117, 119, 130, 132, 260, 263
Azotemic pseudodiabetes, 152
Aztreonam, 315t

Babinsky sign, 151
Back sprain, 111
Bacterial cholangitis, 413
Bacterial infections, in FSGS, 226
Bacterial peritonitis, 107
Bacterial virulence, 338
Bacteriuria, 332
Balkan nephropathy, 327–328
Bardet–Biedl syndrome, 413
Bartter syndrome, 37, 43, 45, 80
Basolateral bicarbonate, 46
B cell dyscrasia, 282
B cell lymphoma, 287
B cell neoplasia, 285
B cell surface antigen CD20, 308
Beckwith–Wiedemann syndrome, 419
Bence Jones (myeloma) cast nephropathy, 281, 285
    clinical findings, 287
    differential diagnosis, 287
    essentials of diagnosis, 286
    general considerations, 286–287
    pathogenesis, 287
    treatment, 287
Bence Jones protein, 287
Benign prostatic hypertrophy, 1, 93
Benzathine penicillin, 261
Berlin Questionnaire, 373
Berylliosis, 62
Bethanidineb, 315t
Bicarbonate concentration, plasma, in normal
        individual, 46
Bicarbonate solutions, 460
Bicarbonate wasting, 50
Bilateral adrenal hyperplasia, 37
Bilirubin analysis, of urine, 3t
Bismuth salts, 315t
Bisphosphonates, 64, 65t, 70
BK polyoma virus infection, 320
BK virus nephropathy, 320
Bladder cancer, 6
Bladder catheter, 334
Bladder dynamics, abnormal, 339
Bladder outlet obstruction, 146
β-blockers, 13, 40, 355, 367, 371, 376, 381, 387
α/β-blockers, 409, 413
Blood cells analysis, of urine, 3t
Blood chemistry, in nephrolithiasis, 346
Blood pressure control, in CKD, 152
Blood pressure elevation, in scleroderma renal
        crisis, 293
Blood urea nitrogen (BUN), 3t
    ATIN, 313
    in CKD, 152
    due to AKI, 89

impact of aminoglycoside-induced nephrotoxicity
        manifestations, 126
    as indication of ECF, 9
    metabolic acidosis, 49
    monitoring in CIN patients, 116
    in nephrotic syndrome, 212
    post NSAID therapy, 143
    in rhabdomyolysis, 111
Blurred vision, 57
Body fluid distribution, 8t
Body water excess, 27
Bolus intravenous therapy, 127
Bone anabolism, 71f
Bone breakdown and formation, 61
Bone disease, 53
Bone manifestations, in chronic kidney disease (CKD), 151
Bone marrow aspirates, 282
Bone resorption, 61
    and hyperphosphatemia, 70
Bone turnover, 61
Bowman's space, 256
BP in preeclampsia, 390
Bradycardia, 86
Brisk water diuresis, 27
Bronchial alveolar lavage, 269
Bronchoscopy, 269
B-type natriuretic peptides, 7, 11–13
Bulimia, 43
Bumetanide, 14, 125
BUN to serum creatinine ratio, in prerenal azotemia, 90
Burkitt's lymphoma, 70, 117
Burned patients and hypernatremia, 28
Burning on urination, 6

C5-9, 235
Cachexia, 1
Cadmium-induced CIN, 325
Calcidiol, 66
Calcific uremic arteriolopathy (CUA), 174
Calcimimetic agents, 64, 179
Calcimimetics, 73
Calcineurin inhibitor, 227
Calcineurin inhibitor induced nephropathy
    clinical findings, 324
    essentials of diagnosis, 324
    general considerations, 324
    treatment, 324
Calcineurin inhibitors, 200, 226–227, 295
Calciphylaxis, 72
Calcitonin, 65t, 79
Calcitriol, 60–63, 67–68, 178
Calcium, 181
    intake in CKD, 193
Calcium acetate, 73, 177
Calcium carbonate, 177, 197
Calcium channel blockers (CCBs), 166, 293, 355, 365, 367, 387–388,
        396, 413
Calcium gluconate, 41

Calcium intake, in metabolic alkalosis, 43
Calcium monohydrogen phosphate (brushite), 351
Calcium oxalate, 93, 131, 345
Calcium phosphate, 131
Calcium phosphate stones, 345
Calcium salts, 73
Calcium-sensing receptor, 62
Calcium stones, treatment for, 349–352
Ca^{2+}/Mg^{2+} sensing receptor (CaSR), 80
Campylobacter enteritis, 246
Candesartan, 206
Candida spp., 329, 334
Captopril, 206, 315t, 393
Captopril scintigraphy/renography, 362
Captopril-stimulated plasma renin activity test, 364
Carbamazepine, 315t
Carbamazepine–oxycarbazepine, 26t
Carbenicillin, 315t
Carbenoxolone, 369
Carbonic anhydrase (CA) inhibitors, 44
Carbon monoxide poisoning, 109
Carbonyl compounds, 185
Carboplatin, 134–135
Cardiac arrhythmias, 34, 42–43, 45, 160
Cardiac pacing devices, 34
Cardiac troponins, 164
Cardiovascular manifestations, in chronic kidney disease (CKD), 151
    clinical findings, 163–165
    essentials of diagnosis, 160
    general considerations, 160
    pathogenesis, 161–163
    prevention and treatment, 165–168
    prognosis, 168–169
Carnitine, 191
Carnitine deficiency, 191
Carnitine palmityltransferase deficiency, 109
Caroli's disease, 412
Castelman's disease, 284
Catecholamine-producing tumors, 370
Catecholamines, 371
Catheter-associated UTI (CAUTI), 334
Catheter placements, 334
Catheter-related infections, 447
Cationic proteins, 47
C5b-9, 229–230
C3 convertase (C3bBb) activity, 249
CD4 and CD8 T lymphocytes, 326
CD2AP, 223
Cefaclor, 315t
Cefamandole, 315t
Cefazolin, 315t
Cefepime, 333
Cefotaxime, 315t
Cefoxitin, 315t
Ceftazidime, 333
Celecoxib, 139
Cellular necrosis, 114
Cellulitis, 219
C3eNef, 260
Central brain stem herniation syndrome, 86

Central pontine myelinolysis (CPM), 23
Cephalexin, 263, 315t
Cephalosporins, 93, 125, 314, 333
Cephalothin, 315t
Cerebral edema, 22, 27–28, 54
Cerebral salt wasting, 25
Cerebral vasospasm, 56
Cervical cancer, 93
Cervical malignancy, 1
Chest radiographs, 13, 256
Chinese herb nephropathy. *See* Aristolochic acid nephropathy
Chlamydia, 185, 326
Chlorambucil, 237
Chloride-depletion metabolic alkalosis (CDA), 44
Chloride shunt, 51
Chlorothiazide, 17
Chlorpromazine, 295
Chlorpropamide, 26t, 315t
Chlorthalidone, 315t
Cholangitis, 412
Cholecalciferol, 61
Cholestasis, 101–102
Chronic hypercalciuria, 68
Chronic hypokalemia, 327
Chronic interstitial nephritis (CIN), 130
    heavy metal induced, 325–326
    immune mediated, 326–327
    medication-related, 322–325
    metabolic, 327
    others, 327–328
    primary/idiopathic, 320
    secondary, 320–322
Chronic kidney disease (CKD), 2, 17, 69, 72, 74, 113, 138, 297, 325. *See also* Cardiovascular manifestations, in chronic kidney disease (CKD); Nutritional issues, in chronic kidney disease (CKD)
    African-Americans, 376–377
    annual screening guidelines for, 203t
    bone manifestations, 151
    cardiovascular manifestations, 151
    classification and management recommendations, 150t
    clinical findings, 150–152, 203–204
    complications, 204
    definition, 149
    effects of angiotensin II levels, 202
    endocrine and metabolic manifestations, 152
    essentials of diagnosis, 201
    gastrointestinal manifestations, 151
    general considerations, 201
    glomerular hemodynamic factors, 201
    hematologic manifestations, 151
    and hypertension, 357–358
    neurologic manifestations, 151
    pathogenesis, 149–150, 201–202
    prevention, 150, 202–203
    prognosis, 154, 209
    and proteinuria, 202
    screening of individuals, 150
    skin manifestations, 150–151
    treatment, 152–154, 204–208

Chronic obstructive pulmonary disease (COPD), 58
Chronic peritoneal dialysis (CPD), 513
Chronic pyelonephritis, 321–322
Chronic renal failure (CRF), in SCD
  clinical findings, 434
  differential diagnosis, 434
  essentials of diagnosis, 433
  general considerations, 433
  pathogenesis, 433–434
  prevention, 434
  treatment, 434–435
Chronic respiratory acidosis, 58
Chronic tubulointerstitial nephritis (CTIN), 320–321, 321f
  causes of, 322t
  clinical features of, 321t
Chronic tubulointerstitial nephropathy (CTIN), 136
Churg–Strauss syndrome, 266–267
Chvostek sign, 42, 67, 80, 119
Cidofovir, 130
Cigarette smoking and Goodpasture's syndrome, 255
Cimetidine, 1, 44, 125, 315t
Cinacalcet, 67, 73, 159
Ciprofloxacin, 125, 315t, 336
Cirrhosis, 11, 23, 26. *See also* Hepatic cirrhosis
  hemodynamic changes in, 99–100
  NSAID therapy, 142, 144
Cirrhotic ascites, 19
Cisplatin, 37, 83, 91t, 134–135
Cisplatin-induced CIN, 325
Citrate, 345
  anticoagulation, 460
  clearance, 82
Cl⁻ deficit, treatment for, 44
Clofibrate, 26t, 315t
Clonidine, 387
Clotting inhibitors, 211
Cloxacillin, 315t
Clozapine, 315t
C3 nephritic factor, 249, 250t, 251
Coagulation profile, of renal patients, 5
Cocaine, 110–111
Cocidioidomycosis, 62
Cockroft–Gault formula, 1–2, 3t
Cofactor deficiency, 159
COL4A3, COL4A4, and *COL4A5* genes, 422
COL4A3 and *COL4A4* genes, 425
Colistin, 315t
Collagen-vascular disorders, 291–292
Collecting duct diuretics, 13
Collecting duct proton secretion, 46, 51
  collection methods, 53
Colloid solutions, 103
Colon resection, 351
Coma, 62, 76, 80, 151
Compensatory processes, to arterial underfilling, 7, 12
Complicated UTI, 333
Compound papillae, 338, 338f
Computed tomography (CT), 4, 152, 165, 283, 322, 333, 372, 408
Computed tomography scan with contrast enhancement, 4t
Computed tomography scan without contrast, 4t

Congenital chloridorrhea, 44
Congenital hemihypertrophy, 419
Congenital reflux nephropathy, 337, 343
  pathogenesis, 339–340
  symptoms and signs, 341
Congestive heart failure (CHF), 1, 2t, 9, 23, 27, 33, 89, 109, 133, 160
  African-Americans, 376
  differential diagnosis, 13
  essentials of diagnosis, 11
  imaging studies, 13
  laboratory findings, 12–13
  NSAID therapy, 142, 144
  symptoms and signs, 12
  treatment, 13–15
Conjunctivitis, 267
Conn syndrome, 37
Continuous ambulatory peritoneal dialysis (CAPD), 175
Continuous arteriovenous hemodialysis (CAVHD), 97
Continuous positive airway pressure (CPAP), during sleep, 373
Continuous renal replacement therapy (CRRT), 96–97
  complications, 453
  general considerations, 453
  treatment
    clinical considerations, 456–461
    modalities, 453–456
    technical innovations, 462
Continuous venovenous hemodiafiltration (CVVHDF), 97
Continuous venovenous hemodialysis (CVVHD), 97
Continuous venovenous hemofiltration (CVVH), 97
Contrast-induced nephropathy (CIN)
  clinical findings, 115–116
  differential diagnosis, 116
  essentials of diagnosis, 113
  general considerations, 113
  hyperosmolarity, 114
  mechanism of, 114f
  pathogenesis, 114
  prevention, 114–115
  prognosis, 116
  strategies for, 115t
  treatment, 116
Contrast nephropathy, 150
Converting enzyme inhibitors, 13
CO_2 production, role in the development of respiratory acidosis, 59
Core endovascular procedures
  arteriovenous access dysfunction, 520–521
  fistula accessory branch ligation, 528
  percutaneous thrombectomy, 525
  percutaneous transluminal angioplasty, 521–525
  venous catheters, 519–520
  venous stents, 525–526
Cornea (band keratopathy), 72
Coronary artery disease and hypertension, 356–357
Coronary artery disease (CAD), 356–357, 360
Coronary heart disease, 35
Cortical scarring, 431
Corticosteroids, 117, 219, 226, 235–236, 245, 254, 271, 278, 307, 311
Corynebacterium urealyticum, 329
Costochondral swelling or bending, 74
Cotrimoxazole, 315t

C1q deposition, 231
C1q nephropathy, 225
Craniotabes, 74
C-reactive protein (CRP), 185, 373
Creatine kinase (CK), 109
    muscle type (CKMM), 110
    myocardial bound (CKMB) isoform, 111
Creatinine clearance, 99, 452
Creatinine level
    ATIN, 313
    in CIN, 115
    determination, 1–2, 3t
    factors affecting, 3t
    in nephrotic syndrome, 212
    post NSAID therapy, 143
    and use of aldosterone blockers, 15
Crescentic glomerulonephritis, 233, 263
CREST (calcinosis, Raynaud's phenomenon, esophagitis,
        sclerodactyly, telangiectasias) syndrome, 293
Crow–Fukase syndrome, 284
Crush injuries, 70
Cryglobulins, 260
Cryoablation, 418
Cryocoagulation, 418
Cryoglobulinemia, 247, 302–303
    gender differences, 304
    Hepatitis C virus-related, 303–305
Cryoglobulinemic glomerulonephritis, 305
Cryoglobulinemic MPGN, 252
Cryoglobulinemic vasculitis, 268
Cryoglobulin-related MPGN, 215
Cryoglobulins, 260, 302–303, 304t, 305, 307
Cryosupernatant (cryoprecipitate-poor plasma) infusion, 292
Crystal-induced ARF, 124
Crystalloid administration, 10
Crystalluria, 131
Crystal nephropathy, 125
C trachomatis, 336
Cuprophane, 182
Cushing syndrome, 31, 37, 369, 384
Cyanotic congenital heart disease, 223
Cyclic AMP (cAMP), 136
Cyclooxygenase (COX)-2 inhibitors, 138–139, 139t
Cyclophilin inhibitors, 291
Cyclophosphamide, 26t, 227, 237, 267, 270–271, 278–279, 307, 327
Cyclosporin, 83, 92, 267
Cyclosporine, 40, 110, 226, 237–238, 245, 278, 315t, 324
CYP11B1 gene, 368
CYP17 gene, 368
Cystatin C, 94
Cyst decompression, 410
Cyst hemorrhages, 406, 410
Cystic diseases, of kidney, 405–421
Cystine stone, treatment for, 348–349
Cystinuria, 345
Cystitis. See Acute uncomplicated cystitis
Cystoscopy, 147, 467
Cytochrome P450-3A4 hepatic metabolism, 132
Cytokine release engender progressive tubulointerstitial
        fibrosis, 230

Cytokines, 101
Cytomegalovirus (CMV) infections, 129
Cytopenia, 412
Cytoplasmic carbonic anhydrase II, 46
Cytotoxic T cells, 125
Cytotoxic therapy, 70

Dantrolene, 110
Darbepoetin-alfa (AraNESP), 158
Deep tendon reflexes (DTR), 83
Deep venous thrombosis, 212, 218
Delirium, 57, 80
Delta HCO$_3$, 53
Dementia, 67
Dent's disease, 345
Deoxycorticosterone (DOC), 37
11-deoxycortisol, 368
Depression, 67
Desmopressin acetate (dDAVP), 26t, 30–31
Dextrose (D$_5$W), 27
D–form, of IIUS, 288
DFO treatment, 180
Diabetes, 72
    and hypertension, 356
Diabetes insipidus, 28–30
Diabetes mellitus, 11, 83, 182
Diabetic ketoacidosis, 38, 49, 54, 70, 73, 75–76, 83
    Δanion gap to ΔHCO$_3$ ratio, 53
Diabetic myonecrosis, 109
Diabetic nephropathy, 153, 205, 232
    clinical findings, 485–487
    essentials of diagnosis, 483
    general considerations, 483–484
    pathogenesis, 484–485
    treatment
        early treatment of risk factors, 487–489
        kidney transplantation, 491
        maintenance hemodialysis, 490–491
        pancreas transplantation, 491
        peritoneal dialysis, 491
        renal replacement therapy, 490
        uremia therapy, 489–490
Dialysate calcium, 73
Dialysis, 31, 41, 121, 126, 130, 151, 429
Diarrhea, 25, 35, 49, 82
Diarrheal illnesses, 82
Diazepam, 315t
Diclofenac, 315t
Didronel (disodium etidronate), 70
Dietary hyperoxaluria, 351
Dietary magnesium, 79
Dietary NaCl, 10
Dietary nutrient intake, in CKD. See Energy intake, in CKD
Dietary phosphorus intake, in CKD, 193
Dietary protein intake
    in CKD, 187–188
    in MN, 234
Dietary recommendations, for renal osteodystrophy, 177

Differential renal vein renin determinations, 364
Diffuse renal abnormalities, 343f
Diflunisal, 315t
DiGeorge's syndrome, 66
Digitalis glycosides, 13
Digoxin, 34–35
1,25-dihydroxycholecalciferol, 75, 181, 184
1,25-dihydroxyvitamin D_3, 76, 326
    synthesis, 119
1,25-dihydroxyvitamin D (calcitriol) deficiency, 66
Diltiazem, 358
Diphenhydramine, 132
2,3-diphosphoglycerate, 76
Dipstick examination, 3–4, 3t, 93, 313
    for hematuria, 5–6
    in nephrotic syndrome, 212
Distal convoluted tubule (DCT) diuretics, 13
    action of, 15
    life of, 17
    magnesium reabsorption in, 80
Distal renal tubular acidosis, 51–52, 146, 321t, 351
Distal tubular acidosis (RTA type 1), 38
Distal tubule dysfunction, 37
Distal urinary acidification, 146
Distended bladder, 146
Diuretic resistance
    algorithm for the treatment of, 16f
    clinical findings, 15–17
    essentials of diagnosis, 15
    general considerations, 15
    laboratory findings, 17
    symptoms and signs, 15–17
    treatment, 17–18
Diuretics, 12–13, 33, 35, 93, 114, 325, 356, 388, 390, 413. *See also*
        Loop diuretics; Thiazide diuretics
    bioavailability of, 14
    as a cause of renal magnesium wasting, 82
    and cirrhotic patients with refractory ascites, 101
    combination therapy, 17, 17t
    complications of, 15t
    effect on ECF, 136
    for heart failure, 13
    for hepatic cirrhosis, 20
    and hepatorenal syndrome, 106–108
    hypermagnesemia, 87
    for nephrotic syndrome, 21
    physiological classification of, 14t
Diverticulitis, 332
Dizziness, 55–56
Docosahexaenoic acid (DHA), 245
Dopamine, 104, 114
Doxazosin, 371
Doxercalciferol, 178
D-penicillamine, 229, 232, 315t, 349
Drug-induced AIN. *See* Acute interstitial nephritis (AIN)
Drug-induced glomerulonephritis, 125
Dryness, of the mucous membranes, impact, 8
Duplex Doppler ultrasound, 147, 152, 363
Dysarthria, 76, 151
Dyskalemia, 32

Dyslipemia, 208
Dysmorphic kidneys, 337
Dysplasia, 340
Dyspnea, 55
Dyspneic patients, 12
Dysuria, 6

EBV renal scarring, 320
ECG abnormalities, 41, 34f
Echocardiogram, 13
Echogenicity and renal disease, 4
Eclampsia, 383, 503–506
Ectopic corticotropin production, 369
Ectopic corticotropin-secreting tumors, 369
Ectopy, 35
Eculizumab, 240
Edema, 367
    APSGN, 260
    in diuretic-induced renal impairment, 106–107
    in FSGS, 224
    HUS, 288
    loop diuretic treatment for, 14
    MN, 231
    in nephritic syndrome, 215
    from nephrotic syndrome, 13
    in nephrotic syndrome, 211, 213
Edematous disorders
    compensatory processes, 7
    general considerations, 11
Effective arterial blood volume (EABV), 7
Ehlers–Danlos syndrome, 419
Eicosanoids, 140
Eicosapentaenoic acid (EPA), 245
Electrocardiogram (ECG), 34, 118–119
Electrolyte abnormalities and hypovolemia, 9
Electrolyte disturbances, associated with symptomatic magnesium
        depletion, 80
Electrolyte homeostasis, 460
Electron beam computerized tomography (EBCT), 165
Emphysematous pyelonephritis, 335
Encapsulating peritoneal sclerosis (EPS), 448
Encoded glycoproteins (E1 and E2), 302
Endemic (Balkan) nephropathy (EN), 327–328
Endocarditis-associated glomerulonephritis
    clinical findings, 262
    essentials in diagnosis, 262
    general considerations, 262
    immunoglobulin deposition in, 262
    pathogenesis, 262
    prognosis, 263
    treatment, 263
Endocrine and metabolic manifestations, in chronic kidney disease
        (CKD), 152
Endocrine disorders, of uremia, 184
Endocrine hypertension, 366
Endocrinopathy, 284
Endothelin-1, 100
Endothelin receptor antagonists, 105, 114

Endotoxins, 101
End-stage kidney disease (ESKD), 73, 271
End-stage renal disease (ESRD), 149, 160, 201, 233, 271, 284, 286,
    296, 297, 360, 412, 423, 463
    calcification, 163
    cause of, 248
    estimated risk in reflux nephropathy, 343–344
    soft-tissue and vascular calcification in, 174
Energy intake, in CKD, 189, 190t
Enteric hyperoxaluria, 351
Enterobacter spp., 329
Enterococcus fecalis, 263
Enterococcus spp., 329, 332
Env, 298
Enzyme-linked immunosorbent assay (ELISA), 256, 270
Eosinophils, 93
Eosinophiluria, 316
Ephedra compounds, 111
Epidermal growth factor receptor (EGFR), 72
Epimembranous glomerulonephritis, 229
Epinephrine, 32
Epithelial neoplasms, 415
Epithelial sodium channel (ENaC), 47f, 52
Epithelioid angiomyolipomata, 415
Eplerenone, 19
Epoetin-alfa, 158
Epogen, 158
Eprex, 159
Epstein–Barr virus (EBV), 320, 326
Erythema of the oropharyngeal mucosa, 267
Erythrocyte sedimentation rate (ESR), 212
Erythromycin, 110, 315t
Erythropoietin (rHuEPO), cloned, 156
Erythropoietin therapy, for anemia of CKD, 158
    resistance to, 159
Escherichia coli, 226, 320, 322, 332, 335, 338, 406
    UTIs with, 329
Escherichia coli 0157:H7, 288–289
Esophageal and/or gastric varices, 412
Estradiol, 56
Estrogen–progesterone treatment, on breast cancer, 64
Etanercept, 274
Ethacrynic acid, 315t
Ethambutol, 315t
Ethanol, 75
Ethylenediamine tetraacetic acid (EDTA), 325
Ethylene glycol, 93, 327
Ethylene glycol (antifreeze), 49
Ethylene glycol intoxication, treatment, 49
Euvolemia, 23
Euvolemic hypernatremia, 31
Euvolemic hyponatremia, 26–27
Excretory urography, 420
Exercise-induced muscle injury, 111
Extracellular fluid (ECF) volume expansion, as treatment for CIN,
    115
Extracellular fluid volume (ECF), disorders of, 7
    in children and treatment, 10t
    clinical features, 9
    contraction with high levels of renin and aldosterone, 38

and dietary NaCl intake, 8
and diminished turgor, 8
edematous disorders, 11
hypovolemia, 8–11
impact of changes in pulse rate and arterial pressure, 9
impact of serum magnesium concentrations, 79
impact on kidney, 9
K translocation, 32
oral rehydration solutions (ORS), 11t
prerenal azotemia, 9
routes of losses, 8
salt intake impacts, 33
secondary hyperaldosteronism and, 37
and signs of diuretic resistance, 15
symptoms of, 8
Extracorporeal albumin dialysis, 105
Extracorporeal shock wave lithotripsy (ESWL), 148, 345
Extramembranous nephropathy, 229
Exudative-proliferative glomerulonephritis, 307

Fabrazyme, 429
Fabry disease
    clinical findings, 427–428
    differential diagnosis, 428
    essentials of diagnosis, 426
    general considerations, 426–427
    pathogenesis, 427
    treatment, 428–429
Facial angiofibromas, 413
Factor H deficiency, 288
Factor H replacement, 289
"False-positive" antibody test, 285
Familial hematuria, 422
Familial hypocalciuric hypercalcemia, 62
Familial hypocalciuric hypercalcemia (FHH), 63
Fanconi's syndrome, 50, 75, 126, 130, 321t
Females, creatinine clearance in, 2
Fenclofenac, 315t
Fenofibrate, 315t
Fenoldopam, 114
Fenoprofen, 315t
Fever, 28, 56, 59, 65, 93–95, 104, 111, 116, 124–125, 131–132,
    136, 138, 215, 226, 239, 252, 261, 264, 289, 291, 304,
    316–317, 320, 326, 330, 332, 334–335, 349, 406–407, 410,
    412, 415, 420, 431, 473, 475, 478, 512
FGF23, 76
Fibric acid derivatives, 110
Fibrillary glomerulonephritis, 307
Fibrillogenesis, 307
Fibrin, 289
Fibrinolytics, 290
Fibroblast growth factor (FGF)23, 70
Fibromuscular disease, 362
Fibromuscular disease (FMD), 360
Fibromuscular dysplasia, 361
Fibromyalgia, 111
Fibronectin accumulation, 124–125
Fibrosis, 125

Fish oils, 245
Flaccid paralysis, 33–34
Flaccid skeletal muscle paralysis, 86
Fludrocortisone, 10
Fluid management, 460
Fluoroquinolones, 333, 410
Fluoxetine, 26t
Fluphenazine, 26t
Flurbiprofen, 139t
Foam cells, 322
Focal glomerulosclerosis (FGS), 300
Focal necrotizing glomerulonephritis, 257
Focal renal abnormalities, 342f
Focal segmental glomerulosclerosis (FSGS), 217, 232, 252, 342
    blood chemistries, 225
    clinical findings, 224–225
    clinical presentation, 222
    collapsing, 225
    complications, 226
    differential diagnosis, 225–226
    epidemiology, 222
    essentials of diagnosis, 222
    genetic mutations associated with, 224t
    with HIV infection, 225
    pathogenesis
        primary, 223
        secondary, 223
    pathologic findings, 222–223
    prognosis, 227
    secondary causes, 224t
    treatment, 226–227
Folate metabolite tetrahydrofolic acid, 191
Folic acid, 181, 191, 200
Fomepizole, 93
Foscarnet, 37, 92, 129–130, 315t
Foscarnet-induced renal failure, 129
Fractional excretion of HCO$_3$ (FEHCO$_3$), 51
Fractional excretion of magnesium (FE$_{Mg}$), 81
Frank potassium cardiotoxicity, 112
Frank symptomatic cryoglobulinemia, 303
Free-oxygen radicals, 339
Fresh frozen plasma (FFP), 292
Fuchsin orange G-stain (AFOG), 255
Fulminant hepatitis, 70
Fungal diseases, 62
Funguria, 334
Furosemide, 95
Furosemide, 13–14, 18–19, 21, 65t, 94, 96, 125, 135, 220, 315t
    combination with albumin, 21

Gadodiamide, 67
Gadolinium, 5
Gadolinium MRA, 363
Gadoversetamide, 67
Gag, 298
Gallium nitrate, 65t
Gardnerella vaginalis, 329
Gas gangrene, 110

Gastrocystoplasty, 44
Gastrointestinal bicarbonate wasting, 49
Gastrointestinal bleeding, 101, 104
Gastrointestinal losses, in hypernatremia, 28
Gastrointestinal manifestations, in chronic kidney disease (CKD), 151
Generalized edema, 11
Genetic autosomal recessive disorder. See 11β-hydroxylase deficiency
Gentamicin, 126, 315t
Gestational diabetes insipidus, 30
Gestational hypertension, 383
Giant cell arteritis, 265
GI dyspepsia, 143
Gitelman's syndrome, 37, 43
Glitazones, 198
Glomerular basement membrane (GBM), 229, 307
Glomerular diseases, 1–2t, 313. See also Immunoglobulin A nephropathy (IgAN)
    drug-induced, 125
    in elderly, 508–509
Glomerular filtration rate (GFR), 1, 83, 92f, 354
    and acute kidney injury (AKI), 89
    and aristolochic acid, 325
    in calculation of load of HCO$_3$, 50
    and CKD, 149
    effect of intratubular hyperosmolality, 114
    effects of angiotensin II, 91
    intratubular crystal formation and, 119
    lithium-induced nephropathy, 324
    malnutrition and, 182, 183f
    in metabolic acidosis, 48
    in metabolic alkalosis, 43
    in MN, 230
    MPGN, 250
    NSAID therapy, 142, 142f
    observed in MIDD, 284
    subclinical decrements in CIN patients, 116
Glomerular hematuria, 251
Glomerular proteinuria, 6
Glomeruli with focal segmental sclerosis, 233
Glomerulonephritis, 6, 93–94, 104, 124, 214, 242, 276
Glomerulopathy, 202
Glomerulopathy, in SCD
    clinical findings, 434
    differential diagnosis, 434
    essentials of diagnosis, 433
    general considerations, 433
    pathogenesis, 433–434
    prevention, 434
    treatment, 434–435
Glomerulosclerosis, 149, 212, 233
Glomerulosclerosis, nodular, 286
Glucagon, 79
Glucocorticoid deficiency, 26
Glucocorticoids, 37, 65t, 327
Glucocorticoid therapy, 64
Glucose, 23
Glucose content analysis, of urine, 3t
Glucose-6-phosphate dehydrogenase deficiency, 122

Glucosuria, 130
Glycemic control, in CKD, 208
Glyceraldehyde-3-phosphate dehydrogenase (GAPDH), 260
Glycine, 23
β_2-glycoprotein I, 294
Glycosaminoglycans, 345
Glycosuria, 50, 112
Glycyrrhetinic acid, 37
Glycyrrhiza glabra, 369
Gold, 229
Gold salts, 315t
Goodpasture's syndrome, 93, 214–216, 268
  clinical findings, 255–257
  differential diagnosis, 257
  essentials of diagnosis, 255
  general considerations, 255
  prognosis, 258
  protocol for treatment of acute, 257t
  symptoms and signs, 255–256
  treatment, 257–258
Gordon's syndrome, 52
GPIIb-IIIa antagonists, 167
G protein (Rheb), 414
Granular casts, 126
Granulomatous diseases, 62–63, 64
Griseofulvin, 315t
GTP-binding proteins, 235
Guillain–Barré syndrome, 58
Gynecomastia, 19

HAART therapy, 300–301
Haloperidol, 26t
Hansel's stain, 313
HBV DNA, 308
HCl therapy, 44
HCO$_3$ blood concentration, prior to metabolic acidosis, 52
HCO$_3$ - impairment, 42, 46
  for acute respiratory acidosis, 58
  for chronic respiratory acidosis, 58
  due to excretion of bicarbonate, 50
  in response to respiratory alkalosis, 55
HCO$_3$ transportation, 46, 47f
Headache, 57
Heart failure, in CKD, 162
  prevention and treatment, 167–168
  symptoms and signs, 163
Heavy chain deposition (HCDD), 284
HELLP syndrome, 389, 392
Hematologic manifestations, in chronic kidney disease (CKD), 151
Hematuria, 1, 3, 104, 112, 218, 222, 231, 245, 259–260, 276, 313, 346, 406
  in elderly individuals, 6
  family history, 6
  in females, 5
  gross, 5
  microscopic, 5
Hematuria in SCD
  clinical findings, 430–431

differential diagnosis, 431
essentials of diagnosis, 430
general considerations, 430
pathogenesis, 430
treatment, 431–432
Heme pigments, 112
Hemodiafiltration (HDF), 456
Hemodialysis, 44, 63, 97, 513
  alternative therapy, 442
  assessment of adequacy, 442
  complications, 442–443
  general considerations, 437
  and increased losses of nutrients, 182
  treatment
    access, 440–442
    apparatus, 437–440
    indications for starting chronic dialysis therapy, 437
Hemodialysis dialysate, 96
Hemofiltration, 115, 457
Hemoglobin, 111
Hemoglobin A$_{1C}$ (HbA$_{1C}$), 203
Hemoglobinopathies, 159
Hemoglobinuria, 5
Hemolysis, 77
Hemolytic anemia, 292
Hemolytic uremic syndrome (HUS), 93, 328
  clinical findings, 288–289
  differential diagnosis, 289–290
  essentials of diagnosis, 288
  general considerations, 288
  treatment, 290–291
Hemophilia, 131
Hemoptysis, 255
Henle, loop of, 79, 82, 87, 114, 137, 140, 340
Henoch–Schönlein purpura (HSP), 93, 251–252
  clinical findings, 246–247
  differential diagnosis, 247
  essentials of diagnosis, 246
  general considerations, 246
  pathogenesis, 246
  prognosis, 247–248
  treatment, 247
Hepacivirus, 302
Heparin, 235
Hepatan, 125
Hepatic cirrhosis, 13, 33
  essentials of diagnosis, 18
  general considerations, 18
  treatment, 18–20
Hepatic disease, 82
Hepatic dysfunction, 100–101
Hepatic fibrosis, 11
Hepatitis B and C, 229
Hepatitis B-associated MN, 232
Hepatitis B core antigen (HBcAg), 232, 311
Hepatitis B e antigen (HBeAg), 308
Hepatitis B surface antigen (HbsAg), 232, 308–309
Hepatitis B virus, 130
Hepatitis B virus-associated PAN, 267
Hepatitis B virus-associated renal diseases

Hepatitis B virus-associated renal diseases (*Cont.*)
  clinical findings, 309–311
  essentials of diagnosis, 308
  general considerations, 308
  pathogenesis, 308–309
  pathology, 310f
  treatment, 311–312
Hepatitis B virus virology, 308
Hepatitis C-associated cryoglobulinemia, 253–254
Hepatitis C MPGN, 254
Hepatitis C virus-associated renal diseases
  clinical findings, 303–307
  essentials of diagnosis, 302
  general considerations, 302
  pathogenesis, 303
  treatment, 307–308
Hepatitis C virus (HCV) coinfection, 131
Hepatitis C virus-related cryoglobulinemia, 303–305
Hepatitis C virus virology, 302
Hepatorenal syndrome, 18
  clinical findings, 102–103
  defined, 99
  diagnostic criteria for, 100t
  differential diagnosis, 103–104
  essentials of dignosis, 99
  general considerations, 99
  pathogenesis, 99–102
  prevention, 106–107
  prognosis, 107–108
  treatment, 104–106
  type 1, 99
  type 2, 99
  urinary sodium excretion in, 99
Hepatosplenomegaly, 304, 413
Heroin, 223
High anion gap metabolic acidosis, 48–49
High-density lipoprotein (HDL), 152
High turnover renal bone disease, 170–172
Histamine 2-receptor blocker, 44
Histoplasmosis, 62
HIV-associated nephropathy (HIVAN)
  clinical findings, 300
  essentials of diagnosis, 296
  general considerations, 296–298
  pathogenesis, 298–300
  treatment, 300–301
HIV transgene, 298
HLA B8DR3, 254
HLA-DR2, 230
HLA-DR3, 230
HLA DR7 and DR1, 255
Hodgkin's disease, 62
Hollenhorst plaque, 116
Home BP measurements, 354
Homocysteine, 191
24-hour urine collection, 3t
  assessment of urinary magnesium excretion, 81
  determination, 2
  in diagnosing excessive intake of sodium chloride intake, 17
  for FSGS, 224–225
  lithium-induced nephropathy, 324

  measurement of sodium urinary excretion, 396
  measure of proteinuria, 204
  potassium excretion, 36
  proteinuria, 6
  stone analysis, 346–347
Human immunodeficiency virus (HIV) infection, 26
"Hungry bone" syndrome, 66
Hydralazine, 295, 389
Hydraulic conductivity, 11
Hydrochloric acid (arginine, lysine), 50
Hydrochlorothiazide, 13, 17, 315t, 388
Hydronephrosis, 93, 147
β-hydroxybutyrate, 48–49
Hydroxychloroquine, 295
25-hydroxycholecalciferol, 184
Hydroxyethylstarch, 131–132
11β-hydroxylase deficiency
  clinical findings, 368
  essentials of diagnosis, 368
  general considerations, 368
  treatment, 369
1-hydroxylase gene, 66
3-hydroxy-3-methylglutaryl coenzyme A (HMGCoA) reductase
    inhibitors, 92, 110, 166, 199, 227, 234
11 β-hydroxysteroid dehydrogenase type 2, 37
25- hydroxyvitamin D (calcidiol), 61–63, 68, 75, 213
Hyperaldosteronism, 15, 31, 33, 37, 395–396
Hypercalcemia, 34, 43, 83, 111, 175, 287, 326, 327
  clinical findings, 61–63
  differential diagnosis, 63
  essentials of diagnosis, 60
  pathogenesis, 60–61
  prognosis, 64
  treatment, 63–64
Hypercalcemia of malignancy, 62
Hypercalciuria, 51, 63, 327, 419
Hypercalciuria-related nephrolithiasis, 326
Hypercapnia, 57, 59
Hyperchloremic metabolic acidosis, 48, 146
Hypercholesterolemia, 185, 212
Hypercoaguable state, in nephrotic syndrome, 219
Hyperdynamic circulation, 100
Hyperfiltration, 433–435
Hyperglycemia, 449
Hyperhomocysteinemia, 161, 200
Hyperkalemia, 19, 39, 93, 94–95, 111, 118–119, 121, 133, 139, 144,
    152, 261, 370, 400
  chronic, 40
  diagnosis and complications, 39–40
  due to reduced renal K excretion, 40
  essentials of diagnosis, 39
  treatment, 40–41
Hyperkalemia (Type 4) RTA, 321t
Hyperkalemic cardiotoxicity, 112
Hyperkalemic distal renal tubular acidosis, 52–53
  causes, 52t
Hyperlipidemia, 150, 213, 231
Hypermagnesemia, 152
  causes, 86t
  clinical findings, 85–87
  essentials of diagnosis, 85

general considerations, 85
life-threatening, 87
prevention, 87
symptoms and signs, 86t
treatment, 85–87, 86t
Hypermineralocorticoidism, 37
Hypernatremia
approach to, 29f
differential diagnosis
with an increased extracellular volume, 30–31
with low extracellular volume, 28
with a normal extracellular volume, 28
essentials of diagnosis, 28
general considerations, 28
symptoms and signs, 28
treatment, 31
Hyperosmolality, 28
Hyperoxaluria, 327
Hyperparathyroidism, 60, 159, 180
Hyperphosphatemia, 67, 93, 96, 119, 122,
129, 152
causes, 70t
clinical findings, 72
development of secondary hyperparathyroidism and renal
osteodystrophy, 72
essentials of diagnosis, 69
pathogenesis, 69–71
role of kidneys in, 69–70
treatment, 72–73
Hyperprolactinemia, 152
Hypersensitivity angiitis, 125t
Hypersensitivity vasculitis, 247
Hypertension, 34, 133. *See also* Primary
aldosteronism
in ADPKD patients, 406
APSGN, 260
cardiovascular and related complications, 376
chronic kidney disease (CKD) and, 357–358
in CKD, 203
congestive heart failure and, 356
coronary artery disease and, 356–357
diabetes and, 356
in FSGS, 224
in high-risk populations
African-Americans, 374–378
elderly, 379–382
pregnancy, 382–393
HUS, 288
kidney function tests for, 354
lead nephropathy, 325
in metabolic alkalosis, 42
in MIDD, 285
in obstructive uropathy, 146
patients with scleroderma, 293
and physical inactivity, 375
prevention and treatment, 166
primary
clinical evaluation, 353–355
complications, 355
essentials of diagnosis, 353
general considerations, 353

prevention, 353
treatment, 355–358
public health interventions, 353
reflux nephropathy, 342
secondary, 359–373
steroid-induced side effects, 220
stroke and, 357
treatment of, 205
xanthogranulomatous pyelonephritis, 322
Hypertensive emergencies and urgencies
cardiovascular emergencies, 402t
catecholamine-excess states, 402t–403t
clinical findings, 401
complications, 403
differential diagnosis, 401
essentials of diagnosis, 401
general considerations, 401
neurologic emergencies, 402t
pathogenesis, 401
pregnancy-related conditions, 403t
prognosis, 403
renal emergencies, 402t
signs/symptoms and other findings, 402t–403t
treatment, 403
Hyperthyroidism, 13, 350
Hyperthyroid periodic paralysis, 36
Hypertriglyceridemia, 190, 212
Hypertrophy, 111
Hyperuricemia, 93, 119, 153, 327, 419
Hyperuricosuria, 50, 327
with calcium oxalate stones, 350–351
Hyperventilation, 53, 56, 59
in respiratory alkalosis, 55
Hypervitaminosis D, 63
Hypervolemic hypernatremia, 31
Hypervolemic hyponatremia, 23
treatment, 27
Hypoalbuminemia, 11, 44, 60, 111, 186, 213, 218, 231
Hypoaldosteronism, 40
Hypocalcemia, 34–35, 93, 112, 119, 122, 129, 152, 212
associated renal failure, 68
cardiac abnormalities, 67
causes of, 67
of chronic hypoparathyroidism, 68
clinical findings, 67
diagnosis of, 67
differential diagnosis, 67–68
essentials of diagnosis, 64
neuropsychiatric manifestations, 67
pathogenesis, 64–67
phosphate-induced, 72
symptomatic, 68
and tetany, 72
treatment, 68
pharmacologic therapy for, associated with
cancer, 65t
Hypocapnia, 55
Hypocitraturia, 350–351, 419
Hypocomplementemia, 232, 252
Hypogammaglobulinemia, 218, 285
Hypokalemia, 15, 33–34, 42, 51, 83, 129, 351, 361, 366–367

Hypokalemia (*Cont.*)
  diagnosis and complications, 35–38
  essentials of diagnosis, 35
  extrarenal losses, 36t
  rapid expansion of cell mass, 36t
  renal losses, 36, 36t
  transcellular shift, 36t
  treatment, 38–39
Hypokalemic alkalosis, 9, 369
Hypokalemic metabolic alkalosis, 9
Hypomagnesemia, 15, 45, 66–68, 75, 83, 129
  among alcoholics, 83
  causes, 82t
  clinical findings, 80–81
  clinical manifestations of, 80t
  due to sequestration of magnesium into the bone
      compartment, 81
  effect on parathyroid hormone (PTH), 81
  essentials of diagnosis, 80
  etiology & differential diagnosis, 81–83
  inherited disorders of magnesium handling associated
      with, 84t
  prevention, 85
  treatment, 83–85
Hyponatremia, 15, 96, 139, 144, 152, 153
  clinical findings, 22–23
  differential diagnosis
    with excess extracellular volume, 26
    with extracellular volume depletion, 24–25
    with a low plasma osmolality and elevated urine
        osmolality, 24
    with low plasma osmolality and low urine
        osmolality, 24
    with normal extracellular volume, 25–26
    with a normal or high plasma osmolality, 23–24
  drugs associated with, 26t
  essentials of diagnosis, 22
  general considerations, 22
  laboratory findings, 23
  pathogenesis, 22
  primary cause of, 22
  symptoms and signs, 22–23
  in terms of water movement, 22, 24
  treatment
    euvolemic hyponatremia, 26–27
    hypervolemic hyponatremia, 27
    hypovolemic hyponatremia, 27
Hypoosmolality, 23–24
Hypoparathyroidism, 64–66, 70
Hypophosphatemia, 129–130
  associated with a cardiomyopathy, 77
  on cardiovascular system, 77
  causes of, 74t
  on central nervous system, 76
  clinical findings, 76–78
  consequences of severe, 77t
  definition, 73
  essentials of diagnosis, 73
  on hematopoietic system, 77
  and milk, 78

on musculoskeletal system, 77
  pathogenesis, 74–76
  and phosphate deficiency, 77
  renal effects, 77–78, 77t
  risk factors, 74t
  signs and symptoms of, 76
  skeletal defects, 77
  symptomatic, 78
  treatment, 78
Hypophysectomy, 31
Hyporeflexia, 34
Hyporeninemic hypoaldosteronism, 40
  treatment, 41
Hypotension, 1, 2t, 442–443
Hypothyroidism, 13, 26
Hypotonic fluid loss, in hypernatremia, 28
Hypoventilation, 42
  elimination of CO_2, 57
Hypovolemia
  complications, 9–10
  differential diagnosis, 9
  essentials of diagnosis, 8
  general considerations, 8
  imaging studies, 9
  laboratory findings, 9
  prognosis, 10–11
  special tests, 9
  symptoms and signs, 8–9
  treatment, 10
Hypovolemic hypernatremia, 31
Hypovolemic hyponatremia, 27
Hypoxia, 42, 56–57, 109
Hysteroscopy, 23

Ibuprofen, 315t
Idiopathic acute interstitial nephritis, 317
Idiopathic cyclic edema, 11
Idiopathic hypercalciuria (IH), 349–350
Idiopathic hypocomplementemic interstitial
        nephritis, 327
Idiopathic MN, 229
Idiopathic monoclonal gammopathy, 303
Idiopathic polyarteritis nodosa, 267
Ifosfamide, 26t
IgA ANCA, 246
IgA nephropathy, 6
IgG and IgM rheumatoid factor (RF), 302
Image-guided percutaneous radiofrequency ablation, 418
Imipenem-cilastin, 333
Immobilization, 63
Immunofluorescence microscopy, 231
Immunofluorescence staining, 225
Immunoglobulin A nephropathy (IgAN), 190, 214, 225, 252
  clinical findings, 243
  differential diagnosis, 245
  diseases associated with, 243t
  essentials of diagnosis, 242
  general considerations, 242

pathogenesis, 242–243
prognosis, 246
symptoms and signs, 243
treatment, 245
Immunoglobulin G (IgG), 131, 229, 257, 314
Immunologic glomerulonephritis, 93
Immunosuppressive therapy, for MN, 235–240
Immunotactoid glomerulopathy, 307
Indapamide, 315t
Indinavir, 130–131, 315t
Indinavir-induced urolithiasis, 131
Indomethacin, 138, 315t
Infective endocarditis (IE), 262
Inflammation, 182
in CKD patients, 184–185, 184t
Infliximab, 267
Insterstitial fluid volume, significance, 11
Insulin-like growth factor 1 (IGF-1), 98
Interferons, 315t
Interferon-α therapy, 117, 253
Interleukin-2, 315t
Interleukin-1 (IL-1), 159, 182
Interleukin (IL) 4, 217
Interleukin-6 (IL-6), 182, 279
Interleukins (IL), 62
Intermediate-density lipoproteins (IDL), 190
Interstitial edema, 13
Interstitial fibrosis, 56, 254, 338
Interstitial nephritis, 51, 93
Intervascular procedures, issues with, 517–519
Interventional nephrology, prospects, 528
Intestinal malabsorption, 75
Intracellular buffering, 46
Intracranial aneurysms (ICAs), 407, 411
Intracranial arterial dolichoectasia, 407
Intradialytic parenteral nutrition (IDPN), 198
Intrarenal acute kidney injury, 91–93
Intrarenal reflux, 337–338
Intratubular hyperosmolality, 114
Intravascular volume depletion, 1
Intravenous cyclophosphamide, 272
Intravenous γ-globulin (IVIg), 220
Intravenous hydration therapy, 121
Intravenous immunoglobulin (IVIG), 131–132, 267, 290
Intravenous pyelography, 4t
Intravenous pyelography (IVP), 147, 322, 363
Intravenous quinolones, 336
Intravenous tocolytic therapy, 38
Intravenous urography (IVU), 341–342
Intrinsic acute kidney injury, 91t
Ionized hypocalcemia, 130
Iron deficiency and erythropoietin, 159
Iron supplementation, for anemia of CKD, 157–158
Ischemic heart disease (IHD), 160
in CKD, 163
prevention and treatment, 166–167
Isoniazid, 315t
Isoosmolar contrast media, 115
Isosorbide dinitrate, 389
Isotonic saline, 39

Jejunoileal bypass procedures, 327
Jugular vein, 12
Jugular venous pressure, 9
Juxtamedullary nephrons, 222

Kaliuresis, 37
Kawasaki's disease, 265–267
Kerley-B lines, 13
Ketanserin, 389
Ketoacidosis, 45, 48–49, 54
Ketoacids, 49
Ketones, 53
Ketones analysis, of urine, 3t
Ketonuria, 75
Ketoprofen, 315t
Kidney biopsy, 152, 243
amyloidosis, 282
for the management of ANCA glomerulonephritis, 269
Kidney function tests, for hypertension, 354
Kidneys. See also Chronic kidney disease (CKD)
crystal nephropathy, 125
damages in TLS, 121
drug toxicity of, 124
enlargement of, 322
impact of antiphospholipid syndrome, 294
and myoglobin, 112
in obstructive uropathy, 146
and patients with IgAN, 242–243
and renal disease, 4
role in hyperphosphatemia, 69–70
role in magnesium homeostasis, 79
role in regulating acid–base balance, 46
role in regulating of HCO_3, 46
systemic diseases affecting, 104t
Kidney stones, 321t, 347
Kidney transplantation, 254, 351, 491
Klebsiella pneumoniae, 329, 332, 335
Klebsiella spp., 329, 406
Klotho gene, 72
K-sparing diuretic, 19
Kyphoscoliosis, 58
Kyphosis, 74

Labetalol, 371, 387, 393
Laboratory abnormalities, in nephrotic syndrome, 212
B-lactam antibiotics, 314
Lactic acidosis, 45, 48–49, 53, 54
Lamivudine, 311f, 312
Lanthanum carbonate, 73, 177
Laparoscopy, 23
Large vessel vasculitis, 265
Laxatives, 85
L-carnitine, 191
LC deposit disease (LCDD), 284–285
Lead-induced CIN, 325–326
Lead nephropathy, 325

Left ventricular end diastolic pressure (LVEDP), 12
Left ventricular hypertrophy, 162, 376
   prevention and treatment, 165–166
   symptoms and signs, 163
Legionella, 110
Leiomyomatosis, 423
Leukemia (blast crisis), 76
Leukocyte exterase analysis, of urine, 3t
Leukocytoclastic vasculitis, 302
Leukocytopenia, 413
Leukocytosis, 111, 332, 336
Leukotrienes, 100
Levofl oxacin, 336
Licorice-flavored chewing tobacco, 369
Liddle syndrome, 37
   clinical findings, 370
   essentials of diagnosis, 370
   treatment, 370
Life-style modifications, 356t
Life-threatening pulmonary hemorrhage, 255
Light chain deposition disease, 232
Lincomycin, 315t
Lipid-lowering agents, 227
Lipid peroxidation, 235
Lipid profiles, 212
Lipid therapy, 199–200
Lisinopril, 206
Lithium, 63, 136–137
Lithium-induced renal disease
   clinical findings, 323–324
   essentials of diagnosis, 323
   general considerations, 323
   treatment, 324
Lithium nephrotoxicity, 324f
Livedo reticularis, 93
Liver, systemic diseases affecting, 104
Liver cirrhosis, 99
Liver diseases, complicated by renal diseases, 103t
Liver dysfunction, 100
Liver pathology, 407–408
Liver transplantation, 20, 106
Loop diuretics, 13, 33, 35, 96
   action of, 15
   bioavailability of, 14
   ceiling doses of, 14t
   and chronic kidney disease, 17
   complications associated with high doses, 18
   continuous infusion of, 18t
   effects of, 37
      lithium reabsorption process, 137
   hypermagnesemia, 87
   and hypokalemia, 35
   initiation of diuresis, 27
   and metabolic alkalosis, 43
   myeloma cast nephropathy, 287
   for nephrotic syndrome, 21
   TLS, 121
   treatment of edema, 13
Losartan, 395
Low-molecular-weight heparin (LMWH), 167

Low-salt diet, 13, 31, 153
Low turnover renal bone disease, 172–173
Lupus anticoagulants, 294
Lupus erythematosus, 182
Lupus nephritis (LN), 214, 245, 268, 307
   clinical findings, 276–277
   clotting diathesis, 277
   complications, 277–278
   differential diagnosis, 277
   essentials of diagnosis, 276
   general considerations, 276
   Heymann nephritis animal model, 276
   prognosis, 280
   serologic testing, 277
   treatment, 278–279

Macroglossia, 282
Macroscopic hematuria, due to IgAN, 245
Magnesium, food sources of, 79
Magnesium balance disorders
   general considerations, 79–80. *See also* Hypermagnesemia;
      Hypomagnesemia
Magnesium carbonate, 178
Magnesium-containing antacids, 73
Magnesium intake
   in CKD, 192
   daily, 79
Magnesium oxide, oral, 45
Magnesium retention test, 81
Magnetic resonance angiography (MRA), 363
   with gadolinium contrast, 5
Magnetic resonance imaging (MRI), 5, 322, 372
Magnetic resonance urography (MRU), 147
Mag-Tab SR, 84
Malabsorption syndromes, 66
Males, creatinine clearance in, 2
Malignant hyperthermia, 110
Malnutrition, 159
   in CKD, 181–182
      causes, 182–185
      inflammation complex and clinical outcome, 185–187
   in nephrotic syndrome, 213
Malnutrition– inflammation complex syndrome (MICS), 186
B2M amyloid fi brils, 174
Mannitol, 13, 23, 37, 94, 114
Matrix GLA protein, 72
McArdle's syndrome, 109, 112
Mean arterial pressure (MAP), 379
Meckel–Gruber syndrome, 413
Medium-sized vessel vasculitides, 265–266
Medullary cystic disease
   clinical findings, 419
   essentials of diagnosis, 418
   general considerations, 418–419
   treatment, 419
Medullary sponge disease
   clinical findings, 419–420
   differential diagnosis, 420

essentials of diagnosis, 419
general considerations, 419
treatment, 420
Mefenamic acid, 315t
Megalin, 126, 229–230
Meloxicam, 315t
Melphalan-prednisone therapy, 283
Membrane cofactor protein (MCP), 249
Membranoproliferative glomerulonephritis, 286, 307
Membranoproliferative glomerulonephritis (MPGN), 211, 306f
    in adult patients, 251, 253–254
    associated with HCV infection, 302
    clinical findings, 250–252
    complications, 252
    differential diagnosis, 252
    essentials of diagnosis, 249
    etiology, 250t
    general considerations, 249
    pathogenesis, 249–250
    pathology in, 251–252
    in pediatric patients, 252–253
    prevention, 250
    prognosis, 254
    recurrence posttransplantation, 254
    symptoms and signs, 250–251
    treatment, 252–254
    type I and II, 232
Membranous lupus nephritis, 278t
Membranous nephropathy (MN), 252
    animal model experiments, 229
    clinical findings, 231–232
    complications, 233–234
    differential diagnosis, 232–233
    Ehrenreich and Churg "staging" of glomerular
        morphology in, 232t
    essentials of diagnosis, 229
    general considerations, 229
    pathogenesis, 229–231
    prognosis, 240
    relapse subsequent to a complete remission (CR), 234
    risk of progression, 233t
    secondary, 230t
    treatment, 234–240
Mental obtundation, 62
Mental retardation, 67
Meropenem, 333
Mesalamine, 125
Mesalazine (5-ASA), 315t
Mesangial contraction, 100
Mesenteric vasculitis, 304
Metabolic acidosis, 33, 38, 78, 95, 139, 144, 370
    adverse effects, 53 54
    anion gaps, 47–52
    causes, 45–46, 48t, 50t
    clinical findings, 53–54
    differential diagnosis of, 47–48
    due to salicylate intoxication, 49
    essentials of diagnosis, 45
    gastrointestinal causes, 49–50
    general considerations, 45–46

intravenous sodium bicarbonate for, 96
    in oliguric acute renal failure, 48
    pathogenesis, 46–53
    in patients with AKI, 95–96
    renal causes, 50–52
    respiratory compensation, 46–47
    treatment, 54
Metabolic alkalosis, 32, 34
    chloride-depletion (CDA), 44
    classification by pathogenesis, 43t
    degree of elevation of the plasma [HCO$_3$ –], 42–43
    differential diagnosis, 43–44
    essentials of diagnosis, 42
    general considerations, 42
    laboratory findings, 43
    potassium depletion impacts, 45
    prognosis, 45
    symptoms and signs, 42–43
    transient states of, 44
    treatment, 44–45
Metabolic encephalopathy, 76
Metabolic myopathies, 109
Metamphetamine (MDMA or Ecstacy), 26t
Metanephric mesenchyme, 340
Metastatic carcinoma, 93
Methanol intoxication, treatment, 49
Methanol (wood alcohol), 49
Methenamine silver, 309
Methicillin, 315t
Methionine, 191
Methotrexate (MTX), 125, 267, 273
Methoxyflurane, 327
Methyldopa, 387, 393
α-Methyldopa, 315t
3,4-methylenedioxymethamphetamine (MDMA), 110
α-methylnorepinephrine, 387
Metolazone, 17
Metoprolol, 393
Mezlocillin, 315t
Microalbuminuria, 3t, 205–206
Microangiopathic hemolytic anemia, 288–289, 293
β$_2$-microglobulin, 326
Microscopic hematuria, 5
Microscopic polyangiitis (MPA), 266, 267t
Microvascular thrombosis, 294
Midodrine, 105, 443
Milk-alkali syndrome, 43, 45, 63
Mineralocorticoid, synthetic, 10
Mineralocorticoid deficiency, 25
Mineralocorticoid hypertension, 366t
Mineralocorticoid receptor blockers, 367
Mineralocorticoids, 37, 43, 45
Minimal change disease (MCD), 232
    children with, 219
    clinical findings, 218–219
    complications, 219
    differential diagnosis, 219
    essentials of diagnosis, 217
    general considerations, 217
    pathogenesis, 217

Minimal change disease (*Cont.*)
  prognosis, 220–221
  selected secondary causes of, 219t
  symptoms and signs, 218
  treatment, 219–220
Minimal change nephrotic syndrome (MCNS), 222
Minocycline, 315t
Mithramycin, 65t
Mitomycin-C, 291
Modification of Diet in Renal Disease (MDRD) Study formula, 1–2
Molecular absorbent recirculating system (MARS), 105, 462
Monoclonal gammopathy of uncertain significance (MGUS), 281–282
Monoclonal immunoglobulin deposition disease (MIDD)
  clinical findings, 285–286
  differential diagnosis, 286
  essentials of diagnosis, 284
  general considerations, 284
  myeloma cast nephropathy, 286
  pathogenesis, 284–285
  prognosis, 286
  treatment, 286
Monoclonal LCs, 282
Monoclonal rheumatoid factors (mRF), 302
MPA, 266–267
Mucocutaneous candidiasis, 65
Mucocutaneous lymph node syndrome, 266
Multiple dose activated charcoal, 540
Multiple endocrine neoplasia (MEN), 371
Multiple endocrine neoplasia syndromes (type 1 or 2), 61
Multiple myeloma (MM), 62, 281, 303
Muscle contraction disorders. *See* Rhabdomyolysis
Muscle cramps, 34
Muscle fibrosis, 112
Muscle twitching, 80
Muscle wasting, 53
Muscle weakness, 34
Mycelex, 271
Mycobacterium tuberculosis, 269, 329
Mycophenolate mofetil (MMF), 220, 227, 238, 245, 253, 278, 278t, 317
Mycoplasma hominis, 329
Myeloma cast nephropathy, 285
Myeloma kidney, 286–287
Myocardial fibrosis, 162
Myocardial infarction (MI), 161
Myoclonic movements, 151
Myocyte depolarization, 35
Myocytes, 32
Myoglobin, 109, 111
Myoglobinuria, 5, 93, 111

N-Acetylcysteine, 94
N- acetylcysteine (NAC), 114
Na channel blockers, 14, 38
Nafcillin, 315t
NaHCO$_3$ therapy, 38
Na-hippurate, 38

Na-β-hydroxybutyrate, 38
Na-K-ATPase pumps, 32–33, 36
Na-penicillin, 38
Naproxen, 315t
Narcotics, 26t
Nasogastric suction, 35, 38
Native valve endocarditis, 263
Natriuresis, 7, 13
Nausea, 124, 129, 151, 332, 443
Nef gene, 299
Neoplastic renal disease, 322
Nephrectomy, 344, 413
Nephrin, 223
Nephritic syndrome
  acute, 260
  clinical findings, 214–215
  complications, 215
  differential diagnosis, 215
  essentials of diagnosis, 214
  general considerations, 214
  pathogenesis, 214
  prevention, 214
  prognosis, 215–216
  treatment, 215
Nephritis-associated plasmin receptor (NAPlr), 260
Nephritis (HSPN), 246
Nephrocalcinosis, 51, 64, 68, 121, 369
Nephrocalcinosis, acute, 119
Nephrogenic diabetes insipidous, 29–31, 30t, 34, 43, 126, 129–130, 321t
Nephrolithiasis, 5, 64, 68, 93, 131, 322, 406, 410
  clinical findings, 346–347
  complications, 348
  differential diagnosis, 348
  essentials of diagnosis, 345
  general considerations, 345
  pathogenesis, 345–346
  prevention, 346
  prognosis, 352
  treatment, 348–352
Nephronophthisis
  clinical findings, 419
  essentials of diagnosis, 418
  general considerations, 418
  treatment, 419
Nephropathia epidemica, 317
Nephrotic edema, 20
Nephrotic syndrome (NS), 13, 23, 26, 66, 231, 252, 263
  clinical findings, 211–212
  complications, 212–213
  differential diagnosis, 212
  essentials of diagnosis, 20, 211
  general considerations, 20, 211
  NSAID therapy, 142
  pathogenesis, 20, 211
  prevention, 211
  prognosis, 214
  treatment, 21, 213–214
Nephrotoxins, 92
Net acid excretion, 46

Netilmicin, 126
Neurofibromatosis type 1, 371
Neurogenic diabetes insipidus, 30t
Neuroleptic malignant syndrome, 111
Neurologic manifestations, in chronic kidney disease (CKD), 151
Neuromuscular irritability, 42, 80
Neutraphos tablets, 78
N gonorrhea, 336
Nicotine, 26t
Nicotinic acid, 110
Nifedipine, 261, 393
Nitric oxide, 101, 114
Nitrite analysis, of urine, 3t
Nitrofurantoin, 315t
Nitrogen appearance (nPNA), 185
Nitroprusside, 261, 389
Nocturia, 12, 203
Noncaseating granulomas, 326
Nondiabetic CKD, 206–207
Nondihydropyridine CCBs, 358
Nondihydropyridine (DHP)-CCBs, 356
Non-Hodgkin's lymphomas, 62, 117, 304–305
Nonimmunosuppressive therapy, for MN, 234–235
Nonoliguric renal insuffi ciency, 126
Nonpharmacologic treatment, for CKD
    physical activities, 204
    role of dietary protein restriction, 204–205
Nonsteroidal antiinflammatory drugs (NSAIDs), 13, 21, 26t, 31, 40,
        91, 104, 124–125, 137, 229, 235, 287, 293, 325
    in cirrhosis, 102
    classes of, 139t
    clinical findings, 143–144
    complications, 144
    differential diagnosis, 144
    efficacy and toxicity, 139
    epidemiology, 138
        antiinflammatory drug-associated acute renal failure, 138–139
    gastrointestinal (GI) complications, 138
    induced-ATIN, 314–316
    pathogenesis, 139–143
    prognosis, 144
    renal syndromes associated with, 139t
        risk factors, 140–143, 142t
    treatment for toxicity, 144
Nonstructural (from NS2 to NS5) proteins, 302
Nonsuppurative lymphadenopathy, 267
Nontraumatic rhabdomyolysis, 70
Norepinephrine, 32, 77, 104
Norfloxacin, 315t
Normomagnesemic magnesium depletion, 81
Nosocomial UTIs, 333
Nphs1 promoter, 299
Nuclear renal scan, 342
Nuclear scintigraphy, 164–165
Numbness, 76
Nutrition, in acute kidney injury, 98
Nutritional issues, in chronic kidney disease (CKD)
    clinical findings, 187–189
    complications, 189–197
    essentials of diagnosis, 181
    general considerations, 181
    pathogenesis, 181–187
    protein–energy malnutrition in, 181–182
    treatment, 197–200
Nutritional management, of renal transplant patients, 199–200

Obesity-related glomerulopathy, 225
Obstructive nephropathy, 2t, 510
Obstructive uropathy, 152
    clinical findings, 146–147
    complications, 148
    differential diagnosis, 147–148
    essentials of diagnosis, 146
    etiologies, 147t
    general considerations, 146
    during pregnancy, 147–148
    prevention, 146
    and stones, 147
    symptoms and signs, 146
    treatment, 148
    urinary tract dilation as obstruction, 148
    in women, 147
Obtundation, 76
Octreotide, 105
Ocular defects, 423
Oliguria, 89, 96, 99, 113, 115, 256, 389
Omega-3 fatty acids, 190, 245
Omeprazole, 44, 315t
Oncogenic osteomalacia, 76
"Onion skin" appearance, 289
Oral calcitriol therapy, 178
Oral phosphates and hyperphosphatemia, 69
Oral potassium salts, 38t
Oral rehydration solutions (ORS), 10, 11t
Oral sodium phosphate solutions (OSPS), 325
Organic K salts, 38
Organic renal disease, 103–104
Organomegaly, 284
Ornipressin, 104
Orthopnea, 12
Orthostatic hypotension, 382
Orthostatic proteinuria, 6
Osler maneuver, 397
Osler's nodes, 263
Osmolal gap, 52
Osmotic diuresis, 114
Osmotic nephrosis, 131
Osteitis fibrosa cystica, 72
Osteoblasts, 61
Osteoclasts, 61
Osteocytes, 61
Osteodystrophy, 413
Osteogenesis, 72
Osteomalacia, 74
Osteopontin, 72, 345
Osteoporosis, 69–70
Osteoprotegerin, 72
Overdiuresis, 104

Overt diabetic nephropathy, 206
Overt edema, 12
Oxacillin, 315t
Oxalate, 327
Oxidant-mediated endothelial injury, 294
Oxidants, 185
Oxidative stress, 181
Oxygen administration methods, 57
Oxytocin, 26t

P aeruginosa, 333, 335
Pamidronate, 63, 65t, 70
P-ANCA immunofl uorescent pattern, 269
Pancreatitis, 182
Papillary collecting duct ectasia, 412
Papillary necrosis, 321t
Papilledema, 284
Paracellin-1 (claudin-16), 80
Paracentesis, 20, 101
Paracentesis, aggressive, 104
Paradoxic aciduria, 43
Paralytic ileus, 34
Paraproteinemias, 252
Parasympathetic blockade, 86
Parathyroidectomy, 66–68, 179–180
Parathyroid hormone (PTH), 60, 170, 350
    absence of, effects, 61
    dysregulation of, 61
    effect of hypomagnesemia, 81
    and hypocalcemia, 67–68
    intact, 62
Paresthesias, 34, 76
Parkinsonian syndrome, 67
Paroxysmal nocturnal dyspnea, 12
Patient compliance and BP control, 397
Patient-related contraindications, for renal biopsy, 5
Pauci-immune crescentic glomerulonephritis, 215, 268
Pauci-immune small vessel vasculitis, 247
PCO$_2$ concentration, in respiratory alkalosis, 55
Pedal edema, 12
Pediatric chronic HBV, 309
Pegylation, 307
Penicillin clindamycin, 263
Penicillin G, 315t
Penicillins, 15, 93, 125, 314
Pentamidine, 83, 92
Pentoxifylline, 105
P-450 enzymes, 66
Percutaneous coronary angiography, 165
Percutaneous drainage, 335
Percutaneous nephrostomy, 147
Percutaneous renal artery intervention, 365
    for fibromuscular dysplasia, 365
Percutaneous renal biopsy, 5
Pericarditis, 160
Periodic acid–Schiff stain, 309
Peripheral arterial vasodilation theory, 18
Peripheral blood eosinophilia, 116

Peripheral edema, 20, 203
Peripheral neuropathy, 284, 304
Peripheral vascular disease (PVD), 160
    in CKD, 163
        prevention and treatment, 168
    investigation of, 165
Peritoneal catheters, 451–452
Peritoneal dialysis catheter procedures
    catheter removal, 538
    chronic peritoneal catheters, 529–538
    complications with catheter insertion, 538–539
    general considerations, 529
Peritoneal dialysis (PD), 97, 182
    clinical findings, 444–446
    complications, 446–449
    general considerations, 444
    prognosis, 452
    treatment, 449–452
Peritoneal equilibration test (PET), 445
Peritoneal protein, 182
Peritonitis, 182, 219
Phagocytosis, 339
pH analysis, of urine, 3t
pH balance
    in acid–base disorders, 54
    in respiratory acidosis, 57
    in respiratory alkalosis, 54–55
Phenazopyridine, 5
Phenindione, 315t
Phenobarbital, 315t
Phenothiazine, 5, 315t
Phenoxybenzamine, 371
Phenylbutazone, 138, 315t
Phenylpropanolamine, 315t
Phenytoin, 21, 315t
Pheochromocytomas, 371, 384
    clinical findings, 371
    complications, 371
    differential diagnosis, 371
    essentials of diagnosis, 370
    general considerations, 370–371
    prognosis, 371–372
    treatment, 371
PHEX gene, 76
Phlebotomy, 39
Phosphate-binding agents, 177–178
Phosphate depletion, 83
Phosphate repletion, 65t
Phosphatonins, 76
Phosphaturia, 50, 75
Phosphorus (Pi) concentrations, serum inorganic, 69
    balance of, 70
    dietary, 73
    ethanol effects on, 75
    in hypophosphatemia, 74
    impact of acute, 72
    skeletal defects with Pi depletion, 77
    therapy, 76, 78
    transcellular shift of, 70
Photocoagulation, 418

Pi deficiency syndrome, 77
Pigeon chest, 74
Pigment nephropathy, 111–112
Pigmenturia, 112
Piperacillin, 315t
Piroxicam, 315t
Pitting edema, 12
PKD gene, 405
Placental growth factor (PlGF), 390
Plasma cell dyscrasia, 281
Plasma infusion, 290
Plasma osmolality, 22–23, 23f, 24
Plasmapheresis, 215, 227, 253, 267, 271, 290, 307
Plasma renin activity (PRA), 37, 367
Platelet-derived growth factor (PDGF), 259
Platelet dysfunction, treatment of, 153
Platelet inhibitors, 292
Platins, 134
Platinum excretion, 134
P mirabilis, 335
Pneumococcal pneumonia, 110
Pneumocystis carinii, 269
Pneumocystis prophylaxis, 271
Pneumonia, 219
Podocin, 223
Podocyte architecture, 224f
Podocytes, 299
POEMS, 284, 286
Poisoning, treatment of
    case examples
        aluminum Intoxication, 545–546
        ethylene glycol poisoning, 545
        methanol intoxication, 543–545
        salicylate poisoning, 546
    dialysis techniques, 542–543
    forced diuresis & urinary alkalinization, 540–542
    immunopharmacology, 543
    multiple dose activated charcoal, 540
Pol, 298
Polyarteritis nodosa (PAN), 93, 247, 265–267, 309
Polyarteritis nodosum, 214
Polycystic kidney disease (PKD), 152, 408
Polycystic liver disease (PLD), 406–407, 411
Polycythemia, 146
Polydipsia, 29
Polyethylene glycol (PEG), 307
Polyglandular autoimmune syndrome type I, 65
Polymorphous erythematosus rash, 267
Polymyalgia rheumatica, 265
Polymyxin acid, 315t
Polysulfone hemodialyzers, 182
Polyuria, 29, 129, 135, 313, 412–413
Portal hypertension, 99–100
Portosystemic shunting, 20, 413
Postcoital prophylaxis, 332
Postobstructive diuresis, 148
Postoperative hyponatremia, 26
Postparacentesis circulatory dysfunction, 107
Postprandial insulin release, 32
Postrenal acute kidney injury, 93

Postrenal disease, 1
Poststreptococcal glomerulonephritis, acute (APSGN)
    clinical findings, 260
    clinical manifestations in children, 260
    complications, 261
    differential diagnosis, 261
    essentials of diagnosis, 259
    general considerations, 259–260
    prognosis, 261
    treatment, 261
Potassium balance disorder. See also Hyperkalemia; Hypokalemia
    clinical findings, 33–35
    clinical manifestations of an abnormal plasma [K], 34
    depletion impacts, 44–45
    effects on cardiac conduction, 35
    electrocardiographic tracings with hypokalemia and hyperkalemia, 34f
    general considerations, 32
    impact of acute K shifts, 35
    pathogenesis, 32–33
Potassium bicarbonate ($KHCO_3$), 38
Potassium chloride (KCl), 38
Potassium deficiency, 109
Potassium intake, in CKD, 192
Potassium physiology
    absorption in the small intestine, 32
    changes, 121
    homeostatic mechanisms, 32
    impact of acid–base abnormalities, 32
    individual intakes, 32
    load in cortical collecting duct (CCD), 32–33, 33f
    role in cell functions, 32
    transcellular balance, 32
Potassium replacement salts, 38
Potassium-rich foods, 38
Potter's phenotype, 412
Prazosin, 371
Prednisone, 220, 278t, 301, 317
Preeclampsia, 383, 389–392, 503–506
    risk factors, 390t
Pregnancy
    acute fatty liver of, 502
    acute renal failure in, 498–502
    after kidney transplantation, 498–499
    anatomic changes in, 492
    antiphospholipid syndrome (APS) and, 495–496
    changes in water metabolism, 492–493
    cortical necrosis, 502–503
    diabetic nephropathy and, 495
    dialysis and, 496–498
    eclampsia, 503–506
    effects of kidney disease, 493
        fetal outcomes, 494
        infertility, 493–494
    effects on kidney disease, 494–495
    hemodynamic changes in, 493
    management of chronic kidney disease during, 496–497
    physiologic changes in, 492
    preeclampsia, 503–506
    thrombotic microangiopathies, 500–501

Renal tubular acidosis (RTA type 2), 38
Renal tubular defects, 75
Renal tubular epithelial (RTE) cells, 116, 144
Renal tubule assist device (RAD), 462
Renal ultrasonography, 4, 4t
Renal ultrasound, 120
Renal vasoconstriction, 101
Renal vein thrombosis, 212
Renal volume losses, in hypovolemia, 23
Renal water excretion, 7
Renin–aldosterone axis abnormality, 52
Renin–angiotensin–aldosterone system (RAAS), 134t, 143, 146, 260, 360–361
Renin–angiotensin system (RAS), 301
Renovascular diseases, in elderly, 509–510
Renovascular hypertension, 384
    animal model studies, 360–361
    clinical clues, 360
    clinical findings, 361–364
    epidemiology, 360
    essentials of diagnosis, 359
    etiology, 360, 360t
    general considerations, 360
    MAG3 uptake, 362
    pathogenesis, 360–361
    plasma renin activity (PRA), 362
    renal functions in, 362
    stages of experimental, 361
    target organ damage (TOD) from, 361
    treatment, 364
Respiratory acid–base disorders, 54
Respiratory acidosis, 32
Respiratory acidosis
    clinical findings, 57–58
    clinical manifestations, 57t
    complications, 59
    CO_2 production, role in the development of, 59
    differential diagnosis, 58–59
    essentials of diagnosis, 57
    general considerations, 57
    pathogenesis, 57
    prevention, 57
    prognosis, 59
    treatment, 59
Respiratory alkalosis, 49, 67
    causes of, 56t
    clinical findings, 55
    clinical manifestations, 55t
    complications, 56
    differential diagnosis, 55–56
    essentials of diagnosis, 54
    general considerations, 55
    pathogenesis, 55
    prevention, 55
    prognosis, 56
    treatment, 56
Respiratory depression, 86
Respiratory tract infection, upper, 6
Restlessness, 57
Retin-A, 63

Retinal hamartomas, 414
Retinal hemangioblastomas, 418
Retrograde pyelography, 5
Retrograde ureterograms, 147
Retroperitoneal bleeding, 406
Retroperitoneal fibrosis, 93, 148
Retroperitoneal lymphoma, 93
Rev, 298
Reverse epidemiology, of cardiovascular risk factors, 186
Rhabdomyolysis, 34, 66–67, 93, 234, 430
    causes, 110–111, 110t
    clinical findings, 111
    differential diagnosis, 111–112
    elevation of blood urea nitrogen (BUN), 111
    elevations of muscle enzymes, 111
    essentials of diagnosis, 109
    general considerations, 109
    pathogenesis, 109–111
    prevention, 111
    prognosis, 112
    treatment, 112
Rhythm disturbances, in CKD, 151
Ribavirin, 215, 307–308
Rickets, 74–75
Rifampicin, 315t
Rifampin, 5, 125
Rifampin-induced ATIN, 314
Ringer's lactate, 10
Rituximab, 117, 239–240, 292, 308
Rofecoxib, 139

Sagittal sinus thrombosis, 218
Salicylate intoxication, impact, 49
Salmonella, 289
Salt-losing nephropathy, 25
Salt-wasting disorders, of the kidney, 8, 8t
    clinical features, 9
Sarcoidosis, 64, 175, 326
S aureus, 447
Schizophrenia, 24
Scleroderma, 292
Scleroderma renal crisis, 290
    clinical findings, 293
    essentials of diagnosis, 292
    general considerations, 292–293
    treatment, 293
Sclerotic bone lesions, 284
Secondary hyperaldosteronism, 37
Secondary polydipsia, 28
Seizures, 115, 392
Selective serotonin reuptake inhibitor (SSRI), 25, 26t
Self-measurement of BP (SMBP), 397
Sensipar. See Cinacalcet
Sensorineural hearing loss (SNHL), 423
Sensory abnormalities, in CKD, 151
Sepsis, 91, 336
    renal vasoconstriction in, 91
Serotonin$_2$ receptor blockers, 389

Serratia species, 264
Serum amyloid P (SAP), 283
Serum chloride, measurement of, 47
Serum creatinine, 67. *See* Creatinine level
Serum protein electrophoresis (SPEP), 212
Serum rheumatoid factor titers, 260
Sevelamer, 73
Sevelamer hydrochloride, 177
Sex steroids, 79
Shiga-like toxin bacteria, 288
Shigella, 289
Shohl's solution (sodium citrate), 54
Shunt nephritis, 307
   clinical findings, 264
   essentials of diagnosis, 264
   general considerations, 264
   pathogenesis, 264
   treatment, 264
Sickle cell anemia, 223
Sickle cell disease, 159
Sickle cell nephropathy, 430–435
Simple papillae, 338, 338f
Single nephron glomerular filtration rate (SNGFR), 201
Sinusoidal portal hypertension, 105
Sjögren's syndrome-associated CIN, 326
Sjögren syndrome, 51, 351
Skimmed milk, 78
Skin manifestations, in chronic kidney disease (CKD), 150–151
Skin turgor, 8
Sleep apnea
   clinical findings, 373
   essentials of diagnosis, 373
   general considerations, 373
   pathogenesis, 373
   prognosis, 373
   treatment, 373
Slow continuous ultrafiltration (SCUF), 97, 456
Slow-Mag containing magnesium chloride, 84
Smad6, 72
Small bowel bypass surgery, 82
Small vessel vasculitides, 267–268
Small vessel vasculitis (SVV), 265
Sodium, fractional excretion, 4, 7, 14, 17
Sodium bicarbonate, 93, 115, 153
Sodium chloride
   excretion, as treatment of heart failure, 13
   renal retention and intake, 17, 20
Sodium concentration, serum, 31
   diabetes insipidus, 29
   hypovolemia, 23
Sodium concentration, serum, significance, 9
Sodium intake
   and CKD, 192
   and congestive heart failure, 13
Sodium loss, in hypernatremia, 28
Sodium nitroprusside, 403
Sodium polystyrene sulfate, 121
Sodium-restricted diet, for FSGS, 227
Sodium salicylate, 138
Sodium supplementation, 132

Spiral computed tomography, 147
Spiral (helical) computed tomography scanning, 363
Spironolactone, 13, 18–19, 45, 368, 399
Splanchnic arteriovenous shunts, 18
Splanchnic circulation, 100
Splanchnic nerve blockade, 410
Splenectomy, 292, 413
Splenic lymphomas, 305
Spontaneous bacterial peritonitis, 20, 101
Staphylococcal endocarditis, 263
Staphylococcus aureus, 322, 329, 446
Staphylococcus epidermidis, 446
Staphylococcus saprophyticus, 329
Starling's law, 11
Statin monotherapy, 112
Statins, 110, 198, 234–235
Stem cell transplants, 283
Stenosis, 361
Stone analysis, 346
Stool potassium excretion, 41
Streptococcal cationic exotoxin B, 260
Streptococcal glomerulonephritis, 245
Streptococcal infection, 260
Streptococci of M types 47, 49, 55, and 57, 259
Streptococcus aureus, 262–264
Streptococcus bovis endocarditis, 262
Streptococcus epidermidis, 264
Streptococcus pneumoniae, 213, 226
Streptococcus viridans, 262
Streptococcus zooepidemicus, 259, 261
Streptokinase, 315t
Struvite stone, treatment for, 348
Subependymal giant cell astrocytomas, 414
Subependymal nodules, 414
Sulfasalazine, 315t
Sulfinpyrazone, 315t
Sulfonamides, 93, 125, 315t
Sulfosalicylic acid (SSA), 287
Sulfosalicylic acid test (SSA), 6
Sulfuric acid (cysteine, methionine), 50
Sulindac, 315t
Superimposed preeclampsia, 383
Supine position, renal perfusion in, 12
Sustained low-efficiency dialysis (SLED), 97
Symptomatic acute hypernatremia, 31
Symptomatic chronic hypernatremia, 31
Symptomatic hyponatremia, 27
Synchronized intermittent mechanical ventilation (SIMV), 56
Syndrome of inappropriate antidiuretic hormone (SIADH), 24–26
   essential diagnostic criteria, 25t
Systemic anticoagulation, 458
Systemic diseases, in elderly, 510
Systemic infections, 70
Systemic leukocytoclastic vasculitis, 246–247
Systemic lupus erythematosis (SLE), 51, 229, 247, 276, 289, 292, 327, 385
Systemic lupus erythematosis (SLE) nephritis, 252
Systemic streptococcal infections, 110
Systemic vasculitis, 302
Systolic Hypertension in the Elderly Program (SHEP), 379

Tachyarrhythmias, 80
Tachycardia, 103
Tachyphylaxis, 63
Tacrolimus, 40, 227, 238, 245, 324
Tacrolimus nephrotoxicity, 92
Takayasu's arteritis, 265
Tamm–Horsfall proteins, 112, 287
Tamoxifen, 117
Tat, 298
Tatasuke syndrome, 284
T cell effector responses, 293
Technetium-99m diethylenetriaminepentaacetic acid (DTPA), 362
Technetium- 99m dimercaptosuccinic acid (^{99m}Tc-DMSA), 342
Teicoplanin, 315t
Tenofovir, 130
Terazosin, 371
Terlipressin, 104–105
Tetany, 67, 72
Tetracycline, 315t
Thalassemia, 159
Thalidomide, 283
Theophylline, 115
Therapeutic Lifestyle Changes (TLC) diet, 190, 191t
Thiazide diuretics, 17, 31, 33, 35, 37, 41, 125, 153, 356, 367, 370
    as an effect of autosomal recessive genetic disorders, 37
    as a cause of renal magnesium wasting, 82
    effect on ECF, 136
    and renal calcium reabsorption, 63
Thick ascending limb (TAL), 79
Thin basement membrane nephropathy (TBMN), 425
Thioradazine, 26t
Third spacing of fluids, 1
Thirst mechanism, in hypernatremia, 28, 31
Thrombocytopenia, 288, 293, 295, 317, 413
Thrombocytosis, 39, 284
Thromboembolic phenomena, 218
Thrombosis, 212
    in FSGS, 226
Thrombotic microangiopathies (TMAs), 252, 288
    etiologies, 289t
Thrombotic microangiopathy, 125t, 277, 293
Thrombotic thrombocytopenic purpura (TTP), 328
    classic pentad of, 292
    clinical findings, 292
    essentials of diagnosis, 291
    general considerations, 291–292
    lactate dehydrogenase (LDH) levels, 292
    neurologic symptoms, 292
    renal signs and symptoms, 292
    treatment, 292
Thromboxane A_2 (TXA$_2$), 140
Thyroid-stimulating hormone (TSH), 152
Thyrotoxicosis, 36
Ticlopidine, 291
Titratable acid (TA) formation, 46
Tobramycin, 126
Tolmetin, 315t
Torsemide, 14
Total parenteral nutrition (TPN), 82
Toxicity, of aminoglycosides, 125–126

Trace elements
    defined, 193
    requirements in CKD, 193–195
Transcellular shift and hyperphosphatemia, 70
Transferrin, 211
Transforming growth factor (TGF)-β, 202
Transient bicarbonaturia, 43
Transjugular Intrahepatic Portosystemic Stent Shunt (TIPS), 18, 105, 108
Transrectal ultrasound (TRUS), 336
Transtubular potassium gradient (TTKG), 36, 143
Transurethral resection of the prostate, 23
Tremor, 80, 151
Tremors, 57
Triamterene, 38, 45, 125, 315t
Trichrome stain, 309
Triglyceride levels, in CKD, 190
Trimethoprim, 1, 334
Trimethoprim-sulfamethoxazole (TMP/SMX), 131, 273, 331–332, 334, 410
Tris (hydroxymethyl) aminomethane (THAM), 54
Troponins, 164
Trousseau sign, 42, 67, 80
TRPC6, 223
TSC genes, 413–414
Tube feeding, 198
Tuberculosis, 62, 175
Tuberous sclerosis complex
    clinical findings, 414–416
    differential diagnosis, 416
    essentials of diagnosis, 413
    features of, 414t
    general considerations, 413–414
    renal manifestations of, 415t
    treatment, 416
Tubular atrophy, 254
Tubular dysfunction, in SCD
    clinical findings, 433
    essentials of diagnosis, 432
    general considerations, 432
    pathogenesis, 432
    treatment, 433
Tubular obstruction, 125t
Tubulointerstitial diseases, 1, 2t. *See* Acute interstitial nephritis (AIN)
    clinical findings, 315–317
    differential diagnosis, 317
    general considerations, 313
    pathogenesis, 314–315
    treatment, 317
Tubulointerstitial fibrosis, 233
Tubulointerstitial inflammation, 301
Tubulointerstitial lesions, 150
Tubulointerstitial nephritis with uveitis syndrome
    clinical findings, 326
    differential diagnosis, 326–327
    essentials of diagnosis, 326
    general considerations, 326
    pathogenesis, 326

prognosis, 327
treatment, 327
Tumoral calcinosis, 70
Tumor growth factor (TGF)-α, 72
Tumor lysis syndrome, 70, 72, 94, 327
  acute renal failure (ARF) associated with, 117, 119
  associated with hyperkalemia, 118–119, 121
  azotemia with, 119
  characteristic laboratory abnormalities, 118t
  clinical consequence of, 117
  clinical findings, 118–120
  differential diagnosis, 120–121
  disturbances of calcium and phosphorus, 119
  electrolyte disturbances, 121
  essentials of diagnosis, 117
  general considerations, 117
  hyperuricemia associated with, 119
  hypocalcemia and hyperphosphatemia, 119, 122
  prevention, 118
  prognosis, 122–123
  risk factors associated with, 117
  treatment, 121–122
Tumor necrosis factor (TNF), 62, 159
Tumor necrosis factor (TNF)-α, 182, 223, 235, 259
Type IV renal tubular acidosis, 52–53, 53t

UDP-N-acetyl-α-D-galactosamine: polypeptide N-
    acetylgalactosaminyltransferase 3 (GALNT3) gene, 70
Ultrafiltration, 18
Ultrasonography, 326
Urate oxidase, 122
Ureaplasma urealyticum, 329
Uremia, 9, 115, 182, 261
Uremic fetor, 151
Uremic pericarditis, 151
Uremic syndrome, clinical and laboratory manifestations
    of the, 150t
Uremic toxins, 182, 184
Ureteric bud-metanephric mesenchyme interaction,
    abnormal, 339–340
Ureteric obstruction, 148
Urethral catheterization, 336
Uric acid, 111
  in TLS, 119–120
Uric acid stone, treatment for, 349
Urinalysis
  acute bacterial prostatitis, 335–336
  acyclovir toxicity, 129
  APSGN, 260
  in CIN patients, 116
  evaluation of patients with ARF due to TLS, 119–120
  for FSGS, 224–225
  IgAN, 242
  indices, 4
  interpretation, 3t–4t
  microscopic examination, 4
  for nephritic syndrome, 214–215
  nephronophthisis and medullary cystic disease, 419

nephropathia epidemica, 317
  in nephrotic syndrome, 212
  and patterns of findings, 4
  stone analysis, 346
Urinary alkalinization, 93
Urinary bicarbonate wasting, 50, 130
Urinary retention, 146
Urinary stasis, 146
Urinary tract infections (UTIs), 5, 329–336
  catheter-associated, 334
  in diabetics, 335
  in elderly, 510–511
  in men, 333–334
  during pregnancy, 334–335
  risk factors for, 330t
Urine alkalinization, 122
Urine concentration defect, 406
Urine crystallization, 122
Urine osmolality, 25
Urine protein electrophoresis (UPEP), 212
Urine urea nitrogen (UUN), 188
Urine uric acid/creatinine ratio, utility of, 120
Urolithiasis, 131
Urosepsis, 332
Uveitis, 326

Valdecoxib, 139
Valproate sodium, 315t
Valsartan treatment, 206
Valvular heart disease, 160, 162
Valvular heart diseases, 407
Vancomycin, 127, 263, 315t
  dose determination in adults, 128t–129t
Vancomycin-induced nephrotoxicity, 127
Vanillylmandelic acid (VMA), 371
Variceal bleeding, 412
Vascular calcification, 165
Vascular disease, 1, 2t, 233
  in CKD, 162–163
Vascular endothelial growth factor (VEGF), 217, 390
Vascular manifestations, in ADPKD, 407
Vascular mineralization, 72
Vasculitides, 2t
  clinical findings, 269–270
  complications, 270–272
  differential diagnosis, 270
  essentials in diagnosis, 265
  general considerations, 265–268
  names and definitions of, 266t
  pathogenesis, 268
  prognosis, 274–275
  risk of relapse, 275
  treatment, 272–274
Vasculitis, 252
Vasoconstrictive effects, of norepinephrine, 101
Vasoconstrictors, 100
Vasopressin analogues, 7, 22, 26t, 29–30, 104–105
Vasopressors, 91–92

VDRL test, 294
Venipuncture, 39
Ventilation–perfusion (V/Q) matching, impaired, 54, 57–59
Ventricular arrhythmias, 115, 293
Ventricular hypertrophy, 366
Verapamil, 358, 395
Very low-density lipoprotein (VLDL), 152, 190
Vesicoureteral reflux (VUR), 5, 225, 321, 337, 339
VHL gene, 417
Vif, 298, 299
Vincristine, 26t
Vincristine–adramycin–dexamethasone (VAD) regimen, 286
Visceral amyloid deposits (VAD), 283
Vitamin A, 196
Vitamin B$_6$, 181, 191
Vitamin B$_{12}$ deficiency, 65
Vitamin C, 181
Vitamin D, 60–61, 79
    analogs, 159
    binding protein, 211, 213
    deficiency, 66, 74, 184, 212
    refractory rickets, 74–75
    sterols, 178–179
Vitamin E, 196, 227, 443
Vitamin K, 196
Vitamin requirements, in CKD, 195–196
Voiding cystourethrography, 152
Vomiting, 23, 25, 35, 38, 42–43, 124, 129, 151, 332, 443
Von Hippel–Lindau disease
    classification, 417t
    clinical findings, 417–418
    differential diagnosis, 418
    essentials of diagnosis, 416
    general considerations, 416–417
    treatment, 418
Von Willebrand cleaving factor (vWF), 289, 291
Voriconazole, 132
Vpr, 298–299
Vpu, 298–299
V$_2$-receptor antagonists, 27

Waldenström macroglobulinemia, 287, 303
Warfarin, 315t

Warfarin therapy, 295
Water deficit, estimation of, 31
Water deprivation test, 29
    interpretation, 30t
Water diuresis, 7
Water-hammer effect, 339
Water intake
    for maintenance of ECF volume, 10
    myeloma cast nephropathy, 286
    requirements in CKD, 192
Water loss, in hypernatremia, 28–29
Water movement and hyponatremia, 22–24
Water replacement therapy, 31
Water-soluble vitamins, 182
Wegener's granulomatosis, 93, 214–216, 266–268, 270
Western blotting, 256
Western diets, 8
White-coat effect, 395
White-coat hypertension, 354, 384
White coat syndrome, 380
Wilms tumor suppressor (WT1), 223
WNK1, 370
WNK4, 370
Wolff–Parkinson–White (WPW) syndrome, 414
Woodchucks, 309
Wright's stain, 316

Xanthine oxidase, 122
Xanthogranulomatous pyelonephritis, 322
X-linked form of the disease (XLAS), 422–424
X-Linked hypophosphatemic (XLH) rickets, 75–76

Zaroxylin®, 17
Zinc, 181
Zoledronate, 65t
Zolendronic acid, 63
Zollinger–Ellison syndrome, 44
Zymogen precursor (SPE B), 260